AMYOTROPHIC LATERAL SCLEROSIS

Edited by **Martin H. Maurer**

Amyotrophic Lateral Sclerosis
Edited by Martin H. Maurer

Published by InTech

Janeza Trdine 9, 51000 Rijeka, Croatia

Publishing Process Manager Adriana Pecar

Technical Editor Teodora Smiljanic

Cover Designer InTech Design Team

Additional hard copies can be obtained from orders@intechopen.com

Amyotrophic Lateral Sclerosis, Edited by Martin H. Maurer
p. cm.
978-953-307-806-9

For EU product safety concerns:
IN TECH d.o.o., Prolaz Marije Krucifikse Kozulić 3, 51000 Rijeka, Croatia,
info@intechopen.com or visit our website at intechopen.com.

Meet the editor

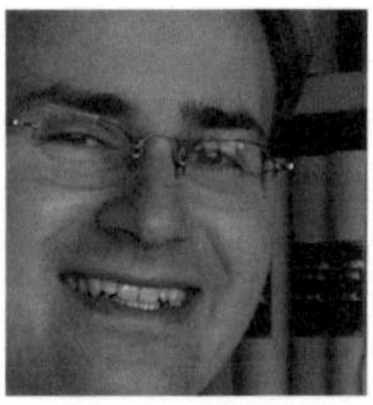

Martin H. Maurer graduated from medical school at the University of Heidelberg, Germany, and McGill University, Montréal, Canada, in 1999 – receiving his MD in 1999. As a post-doctoral fellow in 2003 at the Johns Hopkins University, Baltimore, Md., USA, he concentrated on neurological diseases and was appointed Assistant Professor of Physiology in 2005 and Associate Professor of Physiology in 2007 at the University of Heidelberg. From 2007-08, he was a research group leader in the biotech industry. In 2009-10, he did clinical work in pediatrics, and since 2011 in child and adolescent psychiatry at the Mariaberg Hospital, Germany. His main research interests include neural stem cell differentiation, growth factors in the brain (EPO, VEGF, G-CSF), and neuropsychopharmacology.

Contents

Preface

"It is right it should be so;
Man was made for joy and woe;
And when this we rightly know,
Thro' the world we safely go."
(William Blake, Auguries of Innocence, c. 1803)

When Amyotrophic Lateral Sclerosis first was described and defined as a disease entity in the middle of the 19th century, very little was know about its pathophysiology, nor any form of treatment. The early reports collected signs and symptoms and noted the disease progression. Subsequently, interest arose in the cause of the disease, and with the emergence of molecular techniques, a broad field of pathophysiological hypotheses emerged.

In this book, the reader will find a compilation of state-of-the-art reviews about the etiology, epidemiology, and pathophysiology of ALS, the molecular basis of disease progression and clinical manifestations, the genetics familial of ALS, as well as novel diagnostic criteria in the field of electrophysiology. An overview over all relevant pharmacological trials in ALS patients is included. Moreover, current advances and future trends in ALS research are presented.

The chapters assembled in Part 1, Pathophysiology and Methodology in ALS Research, introduce the current concept of disease pathophysiology and present the techniques currently used ALS research, including data mining, gene expression profiling, and animal models.

In Chapter 1, "Amyotrophic Lateral Sclerosis: An Introduction to Treatment and Trials" by Martin H. Maurer, the author introduces the spectrum of disorders and diseases subsumed by "motor neuron disease". By defining the diagnostic criteria of the disease, the author summarizes the pathophysiological basis of ALS, which has become the foundation for translational research, known as the "from bench to bedside" principle. But for ALS, this approach did not work, and the author describes the reasons and the current recommendations for ALS trials. He then provides an inventory of nearly all clinical trials conducted in ALS patients with pharmacological intervention, including compounds currently under investigation.

Johnathan Cooper-Knock, Joanna J. Bury, Laura Ferraiuolo, Emily F. Goodall, Pamela J. Shaw, and Janine Kirby contribute to chapter 2, "Gene Expression Profiling and it's Application in Amyotrophic Lateral Sclerosis", in which they introduce principles and methods of gene expression profiling. Then the authors review sources and results from in vitro and in vivo models of ALS, as well as from human samples.

Chapter 3, "Dynamic meta-analysis as a therapeutic prediction tool for Amyotrophic Lateral Sclerosis" by Cassie S. Mitchell and Robert H. Lee introduces a novel method for literature data mining which is called dynamic meta-analysis. The authors provide a step-by-step flow chart and demonstrate the method in a feasibility study in the G93A SOD1 mouse model. Their findings indicate that dynamic meta-analysis can be used to predict treatment outcomes in a high-throughput manner.

In Chapter 4, François Berthod and François Gros-Louis describe in their chapter "In vivo and in vitro models to study Amyotrophic Lateral Sclerosis" experimental models for ALS research, including invertebrate models such as C. elegans and drosophila, as well as vertebrate models such as mouse, rat, zebrafish, dog, and pig. Additionally, they provide information about in vitro models including organotypic slice cultures, spinal cord cell cultures, motor neuron cultures, stem cell cultures and oocyte cultures.

Chapter 5, "Advantages and pitfalls in experimental models of ALS" by Marina Boido, Elisa Buschini, Antonio Piras, Giada Spigolon, Valeria Valsecchi, Letizia Mazzini and Alessandro Vercelli provides an in-depth review of the animals models for ALS which are currently available. The authors describe the animal model and the underlying genetic mutation for superoxide dismutase 1 (SOD1), TAR DNA-binding protein-43 (TDP-43), and rare mutations, such as alsin, vescicle-associated membrane protein B (VAPB), vascular endothelial growth factor (VEGF), and cytoskeletal protein mutations such as dynactin, neurofilaments, peripherin, and tau. Moreover, spontaneous mutation models, i.e. the Wobbler (Wbl), neuromuscular degeneration (NMD), progressive motor neuronopathy (PMN), Wasted (Wst), Legs at odd angles (LOA), Cramping 1 (CRA) mice are included. Additionally, a section on in vitro models is added. The authors reflect paradigmatically also on the problems of animal models with regard to translational research: Does the animal model "mimic" the motor disabilities in ALS patients? Or, is the underlying gene mutation similar to the human disease? The provocative chapter makes the reader thinking about our research models.

In chapter 6, "Electrophysiological abnormalities in SOD1 transgenic models in Amyotrophic Lateral Sclerosis: the commons and differences" by Sherif M. Elbasiouny, Katharina A. Quinlan, Tahra M. Eissa, and Charles J. Heckman, the authors provide a review chapter on the electrophysiological abnormalities in the most common mouse model for ALS, the SOD1-G93A transgenic mouse, and compare the results of the in vivo studies to other animal models of ALS.

The authors discuss both changes in the motor neuron anatomical properties and changes in the motor neuron electrical properties, including (1) input resistance, with the influence factors tissue preparation and extracellular calcium concentration, (2) action potential and afterhyperpolarization, (3) persistent inward currents, (4) motoneuron gain and firing activity, and (5) motoneuron excitability.

In chapter 7, "Molecular and electrical abnormalities in the mouse model of Amyotrophic Lateral Sclerosis", Katharina A. Quinlan, Sherif M. Elbasiouny and C.J. Heckman review altered electrophysiological properties of ALS motor neurons and the underlying molecular events. The authors first introduce ALS animal models, then provide a timeline of deficits and emphasize the role of calcium in disease pathology. Subsequent parts of the chapter discuss transport processes, mitochondrial deficiency and energy balance, as well as protein degradation and endoplasmic reticulum stress for disease progression. Then the authors point out non-cell autonomous deficits based on the interplay of astrocytes and glutamate excitotoxicity.

Part 2, "Signalling Pathways and Molecular Pathophysiology" summarizes the main findings and hypotheses with regard to mitochondrial dysfunction and the role of Cu/Zn-superoxide dismutase, as well as the influence of reactive nitrogen species, protein aggregates, and the kynurenine pathway as paradigmatic examples of disease biochemistry.

Chapter 8, "Role of mitochondrial dysfunction in motor neuron degeneration in ALS" by Luz Diana Santa-Cruz, Uri Nimrod Ramírez-Jarquín and Ricardo Tapia contains the role of mitochondrial dysfunction in ALS. In the first part, the authors summarize the mechanisms of motor neuron death in ALS with regard to its pathophysiology involved, including excitotoxicity, axonal transport deficits, oxidative stress, and inflammation. In the second part, the authors concentrate on mitochondrial deficits in ALS with regard to the basic mechanisms.

In Chapter 9, Alexander Panov, Nury Steuerwald, Valentin Vavilin, and Svetlana Dambinova introduce the "Role of Neuronal Mitochondrial Metabolic Phenotype in Pathogenesis of ALS" as a general overview on the characteristics of mitochondria in the central nervous system with regard to their role in energy metabolism of the brain. Then, the authors discuss the formation of reactive oxygen species and the failure of their detoxification by mitochondria in the pathogenesis of ALS. They distinguish between functional differences between mitochondria isolated from the brain and the spinal cord.

Chapter 10, "Mutant Cu/Zn-superoxide dismutase induced mitochondrial dysfunction in amyotrophic lateral sclerosis" by Jari Koistinaho and Gundars Goldsteins reviews SOD1 biochemistry in the pathogenesis of ALS. The authors discuss the disease mechanisms of SOD1 translocation to mitochondria and SOD1 activity in the mitochondrial intermembrane space as well as mechanisms for mutant SOD1 toxicity in mitochondria.

Chapter 11, "Folding and Aggregation of Cu,Zn-Superoxide Dismutase" by Helen R. Broom, Heather A. Primmer, Jessica A.O. Rumfeldt, Peter Stathopulous, Kenrick. A.

Vassall, Young-Mi Hwang, and Elizabeth M. Meiering reviews the biochemical mechanisms of SOD1 toxicity. The authors introduce factors which influence protein folding, stability and aggregation. Then they review structure and function of Cu, Zn-Superoxide Dismutase (SOD1), and reveal biochemical mechanisms of folding, unfolding and misfolding, as well as aggregation of SOD1 with regard to the pathogenesis of ALS

In Chapter 12, "Oxidative modifications of Cu, Zn-superoxide dismutase (SOD1)-the relevance to amyotrophic lateral sclerosis (ALS)" by Seiichi Nagano, the author reviews the biochemistry of SOD1 toxicity with regard to the copper-mediated oxidative toxicity. Moreover, conformational changes of the SOD1 molecule and oxidative stress by cysteine oxidation are explained for both familial and sporadic forms of ALS.

In Chapter 13, "Reactive Nitrogen Species in Motor Neuron Apoptosis", Maria Clara Franco and Alvaro G. Estévez review the role of reactive nitrogen species in the pathogenesis of ALS. They describe the reaction pathways leading to toxic by- and end-products, such as peroxynitrite, and nitrotyrosine, and the biochemical pathways involving reactive nitrogen species, which lead to motor neuron disease. In ALS, namely apoptosis and SOD1 toxicity contribute to the fatal events in disease development.

In Chapter 14, Yoshiaki Furukawa contributes a review chapter on "Protein aggregates in pathological inclusions of amyotrophic lateral sclerosis" where he summarizes the current knowledge about the pathological inclusions of superoxide dismutase 1 (SOD1), TAR DNA-binding protein-43 (TDP-43), and the Fused in Sarcoma (FUS) protein. He discusses the relevant inclusion bodies for ALS patients, animal models, and in vitro models, respectively. Moreover, biochemical mechanisms of SOD1 aggregation, such as post-translational modifications such as disulfide reduction, are reviewed.

In Chapter 15, "Involvement of the kynurenine pathway in amyotrophic lateral sclerosis", Guillemin Gilles introduces the kynurenine pathway as a major route for the catabolism of the amino acid tryptophan, which is also involved in the synthesis of the neurotransmitter serotonin (5-hydroxy tryptamin), or melatonin. The author proposes that the kynurenine pathway is involved in the pathogenesis of ALS by linking several pathophysiological models, such as glutamate excitotoxicity, oxidative stress, non-cell-autonomous mechanism and apoptosis. Moreover, the role of quinolinic acid (QUIN) as neurotoxic substance discussed. The second part of the chapter contains a discussion on the neuropharmacology in ALS research with regard to compounds influencing the kynurenine pathway.

Part 3 of the book, "Cellular Pathophysiology, the Immune System and Stem Cell Strategies" collects novel findings based on cellular approaches.

Chapter 16, "The astrocytic contribution in ALS: inflammation and excitotoxicity" by Kim Staats and Ludo van den Bosch provides a deeper insight into the role of astrocytes in ALS. The author's review the role of astrocytes in the two pathogenetic processes - inflammation and excitotoxicity - which have great implications in disease pathophysiology and progression in ALS.

In Chapter 17, John D. Lee, Jia Y. Lee, Stephen M. Taylor, Peter G. Noakes, and Trent M. Woodruff review in their chapter “Innate immunity in ALS” the contribution of the innate immune system to disease progression in ALS. The authors define the role of the complement system and review the role of toll-like receptors (TLRs) and the receptor for advanced glycosylation end products (RAGEs) in the pathophysiology of ALS. In the last part of their chapter, the authors provide a clinical outlook by modulating neuroinflammation. The inhibition of the complement 5a receptor, or other factors in the cascade, may be a future topic for discussion.

In Chapter 18, "TNF-alpha role in ALS: new hypotheses for future therapeutic approaches", Cristina Cereda, Stella Gagliardi, Emanuela Cova, L. Diamanti, and Mauro Ceroni describe the role of TNF-alpha in signal transduction processes which are related to ALS pathophysiology. They discuss the somewhat controversial role of the cytokine with regard to its interaction with the SOD1 gene.

In Chapter 19, “Stem Cell Application for Amyotrophic Lateral Sclerosis: Growth Factor Delivery and Cell Therapy” by Masatoshi Suzuki, Chak Foon Tso, and Michael G. Meyer, the authors introduce an overview over growth factors and gene therapy in ALS. They review strategies and sites of growth factor delivery in the disease and discuss the rationale for cell replacement strategies, such as motor neuron replacement, or astrocyte replacement, as well as the rationale for the neuroprotection strategy by growth factor delivery, including a immunomodulatory effect. They review data on translational research, where genetically engineered stem cells have been used for growth factor delivery, for example, using GDNF.

Chapter 20, "Glial Cells as Therapeutic Targets for ALS" by Amanda M. Haidet-Phillips and Nicholas J. Maragakis, the authors introduce the role of glial cells in disease formation and progression in ALS. They review the contributions of the different types of non-neural cells in the central nervous system, mainly those of astrocytes and microglia to the pathogenesis of ALS and discuss the still undefined role of oligodendrocytes. In the second part of their chapter, the authors review disease models of ALS involving glial cells. In the third part, they discuss therapeutic strategies for targeting glial cells, either by cell therapy, genetic reprogramming, or gene targeting.

Part 4 id dedicated to “Human Genetics in ALS”. In this part of the book, the reader will find an overview of the results of recent genetic studies in ALS research, compiling all information of genes which are involved in ALS pathophysiology.

In Chapter 21, "Genetics of amyotrophic lateral sclerosis" by Max Koppers, Michael van Es, Leonard H. van den Berg, Jan H. Veldink, and R. Jeroen Pasterkamp, the authors review the genetics of both sporadic and familial ALS. In the first part of their chapter, the authors provide an insight into the current knowledge of gene mutations involved in the pathogenesis of familial ALS. Then, they provide an overview over mutation involved in sporadic ALS. In the second part of their chapter, the authors focus paradigmatically on two genomic regions associated with sporadic ALS, namely, chromosomal regions 9p21.2 and 19p13.11. They discuss the evidence for the association within these regions as well as the function of the genes found in these regions.

Chapter 22, "Genetics of Familial Amyotrophic Lateral Sclerosis" by Emily F. Goodall, Joanna J. Bury, Johnathan Cooper-Knock, Pamela J. Shaw and Janine Kirby contains all important information on genes involved in the disease. Although only 5 percent of all ALS cases are caused by inheritable mutations in the ALS genes and with the majority of familial cases being clinically and pathologically indistinguishable from the sporadic cases, the genetics of familial ALS is necessary to approach the disease. Its results can be used to generate genetic models of ALS, to investigate the mechanisms of motor neuron degeneration, to identify therapeutic targets, and to screen for candidate therapeutic agents. In the second part of their chapter, the authors provide insight into advances in the sequencing technology, which allow sequencing large genomes and finding novel genetic mutations. These techniques may help finding novel genes involved in familial ALS.

Chapter 23, "A major genetic factor at chromosome 9p implicated in Amyotrophic Lateral Sclerosis (ALS) and Frontotemporal Lobar Degeneration (FTLD)" by Ilse Gijselinck, Kristel Sleegers, Christine van Broeckhoven, and Marc Cruts reviews the latest findings on genetic studies focussing on chromosome 9p21. On this chromosome, common genetic features of ALS and fronto-temporal lobar degeneration (FTLD) have been localized.

In Part 5, "Clinical Research in ALS", contains reviews and collections of original data obtained from ALS patients. It summarizes clinical recommendations such as for rehabilitation and palliative care, nutrition, and respiratory function. Moreover, results of electrophysiological studies are presented which aimed at finding parameters for disease progression and prognosis. In the final section of this part, the main issues in patient communication, ortheses and human-computer interactions, as well as insights in neuropsychology and neuropsychiatry of ALS patients are discussed.

The Latin word "pallium" describes a special cloak. Thus, palliative care means that the patient is sheltered by the means provided by the caregivers. In Chapter 24, "Multidisciplinary rehabilitation in Amyotrophic Lateral Sclerosis", Louisa Ng and Fary Khan review aspects of clinical rehabilitation in ALS, where rehabilitation means, that the patient is enabled to take part in daily life activities at the best of remaining competences. In the first part of their chapter, they define the setting for a prosperous rehabilitation and describe the needs of a care-giving surrounding of the patients, including family, specialized health care professionals, and the social environment, including friends and spiritual guidance. In the second part of their review, the authors address all questions of practical issues during the day and the night. They discuss the points of respiratory dysfunction, communication, swallowing and nutrition, exercise, mobility and activities of daily living, incontinence and sexuality, pain, fatigue and sleep disorders, cognition and behavioural impairment, pseudobulbar affect, and psychosocial issues. Of note, they provide a subsection on end-of-life issues, where ethical issues come to an immediate focus.

In Chapter 25, "Assessment and management of respiratory dysfunction in patients with Amyotrophic Lateral Sclerosis" by Daniele Lo Coco, Paolo Volanti, Domenico De Cicco, Antonio Spanevello, Gianluca Battaglia, Santino Marchese, Alfonsa Claudia Taiello, Rossella Spataro and Vincenzo La Bella, the authors provide a review on one of the most threatening problems in the disease progression of ALS, respiratory dysfunction. Respiratory dysfunction is not only part of the disabling course of the disease, but also contributes to the cause of death. The authors discuss the evaluation of pulmonary function. In the following sections, non-invasive mechanical ventilation, invasive mechanical mentilation, and physiotherapy are reviewed in the light of prevention of deterioration and symptomatic therapy.

Chapter 26, "Nutritional care in Amyotrophic lateral sclerosis: an alternative for the maximization of the nutritional state" by Luciano Bruno de Carvalho-Silva discusses the current management of nutritional care in ALS patients based on physiological parameters such as body composition and functional measurements. He also provides practical clinical recommendations for the preparation of suitable food both in clinical and everyday aspects.

In Chapter 27, "The electrodiagnostic methods macro-EMG and MUNE to assess disease severity and monitor patients with Amyotrophic Lateral Sclerosis: overview and own experience", Ferdinando Sartucci, Tommaso Bocci, Lucia Briscese, Chiara Pecori, Chiara Rossi, and Fabio Giannini present own original data from electrophysiological studies in ALS patients. The report that Motor Unit Number Estimation (MUNE) techniques can be a useful tool to assess and evaluate pharmacological interventions, such as treatment with riluzole.

The first part of Chapter 28, "Protection of motor neurons in pre-symptomatic individuals carrying SOD1 mutations: Results of motor unit number estimation (MUNE) electrophysiology" by Arun Aggarwal, provides a review of mechanisms and patterns of motor neuron loss involved in ALS disease progression with regard to the genetic components of familial ALS. In the second part, the author contributes own original data of an electrophysiological study in unsymptomatic individuals who carry specific SOD1 mutations. The chapter ends with a number of case studies.

The chapter shows nicely which heavy burden genetic testing can impose on carriers of genetic mutations, and it should also make us think about our narrow definition of a "healthy" person and a patient.

Chapter 29, "Communication Impairment in ALS patients -- Assessment and Treatment" by Paolo Bongioanni reviews the impaired communication of ALS patients resulting from speech and language deficits, as well as non-verbal communication impairments by paralysis which deteriorate writing and gesture. The authors discusses the methods and techniques for assessing the severity of motor deficits with a focus on dysphonia and dysarthria.

In the second part of his chapter, the author reviews rehabilitation approaches, including gaze-controlled high-tech communication aids and brain-computer interface-based devices. He points out that, besides the improvement in assisted care, the dignity of the patients has to stand in the center of our help strategies.

Chapter 30, "Human Computer Interactions for Amyotrophic Lateral Sclerosis Patients" by Ali Bülent Uşaklı describes novel applications and developments for human computer interactions (HCIs). With deteriorating muscle function, communication and autonomy is impaired. Therefore, devices have been developed for daily life activities. The author summarizes recent advances in the field of controlling these devices by electrical brain activity, eye movement and haemoglobin levels in the blood.

In Chapter 31, "Overview of cognitive function in ALS, with special attention to the temporal lobe: Semantic fluency and rating the approachability of faces" by Heike Schmolck, Paul E. Schulz, and Michele K. York, the authors introduce a field of research which came into the focus of interest only recently: cognitive function is impaired in ALS, which led to the hypothesis of a continuum of ALS and certain types of dementia.

In the first part of the chapter, the authors provide original data on a study which showed an unusual response pattern when ALS patients were asked to judge unfamiliar faces in a social context, suggesting amygdala dysfunction. In the second part of their chapter, original data on phonemic and semantic verbal fluency showed impaired temporal lobe function, contributing to the novel understanding of the disease also with lesions outside the motor system.

Although a considerable amount of research, both pre-clinical and clinical, has been conducted during recent years, Amyotrophic Lateral Sclerosis (ALS) remains one of the mysterious diseases of the 21st century. Great efforts have been made to develop pathophysiological models and to clarify the underlying pathology, and with novel instruments in genetics and transgenic techniques, the aim for finding a durable cure comes into scope. On the other hand, most pharmacological trials failed to show a benefit for ALS patients, but major improvements in clinical care could be achieved. *Amyotrophic Lateral Sclerosis* documents the relevant findings and provides the current knowledge for the research community.

Martin H. Maurer
University of Heidelberg
Germany

Part 1

Pathophysiology and Methodology

1

Amyotrophic Lateral Sclerosis: An Introduction to Treatment and Trials

Martin H. Maurer
Dept. of Physiology and Pathophysiology, University of Heidelberg
Germany

1. Introduction

There are several synonyms for Amyotrophic Lateral Sclerosis (ALS) which include Motor Neuron Disease (MND), Charcot's disease, and Lou Gehrig's disease. The latter is named after the American baseball professional Lou Gehrig, who died of ALS in the 1940s (Miller, 2011).
The symptoms of motor neuron disease (MND) have first been described by several neurologists by the mid-19th century. The French neurologist Charcot defined the nosological entity "amyotrophic lateral sclerosis" (ALS) some years later (historic aspects of ALS are reviewed in (Eisen, 2007; Mitsumoto et al., 2006; Oliveira & Pereira, 2009; Rowland, 2001; Wijesekera & Leigh, 2009)).
In the present understanding, MND comprehends a spectrum of different neurodegenerative syndromes which show a common neuropathology, i. e. the progressive degeneration of motor neurons.
These syndromes include the "classical" ALS, progressive bulbar palsy (PBP), progressive muscular atrophy (PMA), primary lateral sclerosis (PLS), flail arm syndrome (Vulpian-Bernhardt syndrome), flail leg syndrome, and ALS with multi-system involvement (e.g., Fronto-Temporal Dementia, FTD) (**Fig. 1**) (reviewed in Lillo & Hodges, 2009; Silani et al., 2011).

2. Diagnostic criteria

2.1 Clinical features

The diagnosis of ALS is based on a catalogue of criteria specified by the World Federation of Neurology (www.wfneurology.org). These criteria are known as the "El Escorial" criteria, named after the Spanish historic site El Escorial. The original criteria of 1994 (Brooks, 1994; Mitsumoto, 1997) have been revised in 1998 (Brooks et al., 2000; Ross et al., 1998), which are known as the "Airlie House" criteria, named after the conference site at Warrenton, VA, U.S.A. In 2006, a consensus conference at Awaji-shima defined criteria of electromyographic and nerve conduction measurements for the diagnosis of ALS (de Carvalho et al., 2008).
The clinical features comprehend the presence of (i) lower motorneuron (LMN) signs such as the loss of muscle strength, muscular atrophy, fasciculations, hyporeflexia, hypotonicity or flaccidity, or muscle cramps, in at least two limbs; (ii) upper motorneuron (UMN) signs such as extensor plantar responses, spasticity, or pathologic hyperreflexia, in at least one region (bulbar, cervical, or lumbosacral), and (iii) the progression of the disease defined as increasing symptomatic impairment by history in the same region or new regions (Ferguson & Elman, 2007).

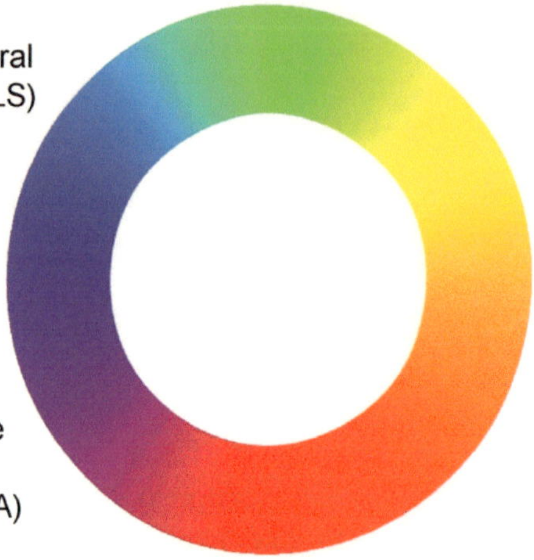

Fig. 1. Spectrum of motor neuron disease (MND). Currently, the understanding of MND comprehends a variety of neurodegenerative syndromes with progressive degeneration of motor neurons.

Neuropathological findings defining the MND spectrum are, on the cellular level, the progressive degeneration of upper and/or lower motor neurons, respectively, and on the molecular level, the presence of intraneuronal inclusion bodies which are immunopositive for ubiquitin-(Ub) and the 43 kB TAR DNA-binding protein (TDP-43) (reviewed in Colombrita et al., 2011; Geser et al., 2010), named Bunina, or Hirano, inclusion bodies (Rowland, 2009).

Moreover, sensory signs (except those attributable to aging), neurogenic sphincter abnormalities, other progredient diseases of the central nervous system (CNS) or peripheral nervous system (PNS) must be absent. Additionally, ALS-like syndromes must be ruled out. These include myelopathy, structural lesions of the spinal cord, multifocal motor neuropathy, hyperthyroidism, hyperparathyroidism, hematologic malignancy associated with monoclonal gammopathy, lead poisoning, a history of radiation to the CNS, and hexosaminidase A deficiency in patients younger than 30 years of age.

The revised criteria defined a certain probability level for the diagnostic criteria (Brooks et al., 2000), which have been questioned by the later electrophysiological consensus (de Carvalho et al., 2008; Sathasivam, 2010).

At present, a consensus conference has defined morphological markers by MRI, which may lead to a biomarker for ALS diagnosis (Kiernan et al., 2011; Turner et al.).

2.2 Neuropsychiatry of ALS

Only in recent years, psychiatric and behavioural symptoms of ALS patients came into the focus of interest. It has become clear that psychiatric symptoms are not only secondary phenomena of a disabilitating disease, but are also inherent and specific in ALS. On the other hand, the etiopathological connections remain unknown.

With regard to the diagnoses and prevalence of these in ALS patients, there are only few data available, which are summarized in **Table 1**.

Psychiatric Diagnosis	Prevalence (percentages, rounded) and reference
Depression	30(Atassi et al., 2011; Lillo et al., 2011); 15 (Ferentinos et al., 2011); 10 (Kurt et al., 2007)
Dementia	10 (Lillo et al., 2011)
Stereotypical behavior	20 (Lillo et al., 2011)
Reduction in motivation	80 (Lillo et al., 2011)
Apathy	40 (Lillo et al., 2011)
Cognitive impairment	50 (Woolley & Jonathan, 2008)
Sleep disturbances	Unknown (Hetta & Jansson, 1997)
Fatigue	Unknown
Psychosis	Unknown

Table 1. Common psychiatric symptoms and diagnoses reported in ALS patients.

In the following paragraphs, I will shortly describe the major psychiatric abnormalities in ALS patients and current findings.

2.2.1 Dementia

In the concept of a "continuum" of TDP-43 proteinopathies (Geser et al., 2009), ALS is classified together with fronto-temporal dementia (Giordana et al., 2011; Lillo & Hodges, 2009; Nakano, 2000; Woolley & Jonathan, 2008; Yoshida, 2004; Zago et al., 2011). This has also been shown on the morphological level (Tsujimoto et al., 2011).
Another pathophysiological pathway discussed in the pathogenesis of FTD is the progranulin pathway (Sleegers et al., 2010).
Cognitive impairment and frontal lobe dysfunction is seen in about 40-60% of ALS patients (Abrahams et al., 1996; Evdokimidis et al., 2002; Witgert et al., 2009).

2.2.2 Sleep

In the current understanding, it is difficult to distinguish whether psychiatric abnormalities in ALS patients are integral part of the CNS disease, or if they are a secondary phenomenon. For example, sleep disturbances are a common problem in ALS patients, but besides anxiety, they may also result from reduced mobility, muscle cramps, or swallowing problems (Hetta & Jansson, 1997).

2.2.3 Fatigue

Fatigue is also a common problem in ALS patients, which does not describe physical exhaustion, but a pathological state of mind (Jackson & Bryan, 1998; Lou, 2008).

2.2.4 Depression and anxiety

The patients know about the devastating nature of ALS with only a short survival time remaining at the point of time at diagnosis, with a deteriorating quality of life, and without a pharmacological treatment option towards "healing". Therefore, a high prevalence of depression and anxiety in ALS patients would be expected. On the other hand, prevalence rates for depression in ALS patients range from 0-44% in the literature, whereas structured interviewing according to DSM-IV criteria reveals rates of 9-11% (Averill et al., 2007; Ferentinos et al., 2011; Kurt et al., 2007). Prevalence rates for anxiety in ALS have been reported with 0-30% (Kurt et al., 2007). Interestingly, the rate of depression and anxiety is not as high as expected (Huey et al., 2010; McLeod & Clarke, 2007; Norris et al., 2010), which means that the quality of life addressed by an individual is not dependent on the remaining lifetime.

2.2.5 Psychosis

The association of schizophrenia with ALS has been reported (Enns et al., 1993; Howland, 1990; Yase et al., 1972), but the pathophysiological interrelation remains unknown. There have been reports on a familial association (Burnstein, 1981).

3. Measuring the disease

The use of ALS assessment techniques such as rating scales is to monitor disease progression , to make outcome parameters in clinical trials comparable; and to predict efficacy of therapeutic strategies (Cudkowicz et al., 2004).

Typical ALS assessment techniques comprehend (i) global scales which are based on clinical observation, (ii) measuring of the muscular strength, (iii) electrophysiological testing, and (iv) the assessment of the quality of life.

3.1 Clinical assessment scales

Global scales subsume (i) scores based on subjective or historic data, such as the ALS functional rating scale (ALSFRS) (Cedarbaum & Stambler, 1997; The ALS CNTF treatment study (ACTS) phase I-II Study Group, 1996), and the ALS severity scale (ALSSS) (Hillel et al., 1989), (ii) scores based on clinical tests such as the Norris scale (Norris et al., 1974), or the Appel scale (Appel et al., 1987), and (iii) scales used both for ALS and other diseases such as the Schwab and England global rating scale (Schwab & England, 1969), or the modified Ashworth spasticity scale (Bohannon & Smith, 1987).

3.2 Muscular function testing

Measuring of the muscular strength includes quantitative tests, maximum voluntary isometric contraction, handheld dynamometry, Jamar grip strength, manual muscle testing. Moreover, the spirometric measurement of the forced vital capacity and maximum voluntary ventilation can also be included in muscle tests.

3.3 Electrophysiological measurements

Electrophysiological testing includes compound muscle action potentials (CMAPs) and motor unit number estimate (MUNE) (Shefner et al., 2011) or the motor unit number index (MUNIX) (Nandedkar et al., 2010; Neuwirth et al., 2011).

A consensus conference has defined electrophysiological criteria for the diagnosis of ALS (de Carvalho et al., 2008).

3.4 Assessment of the quality of life

The quality of life is assessed by questionnaires such as the Short form - 36 (SF-36), Short form - 12 (SF-12), ALSQ-40, or the Sickness Impact Profile (reviewed in Epton et al., 2009; McGuire et al., 1997; Williams et al., 2008).

4. The pathophysiological rationale for therapeutic interventions

4.1 Pathophysiology of motor neuron degeneration in ALS

Pathophysiological mechanisms involved in ALS include (reviewed in Mitsumoto et al., 2006; Wijesekera & Leigh, 2009):

- genetic factors (reviewed in Pasinelli & Brown, 2006; Robberecht, 2002; Ticozzi et al., 2011),
- excitotoxicity (reviewed in Bogaert et al., 2011; Foran & Trotti, 2009),
- oxidative stress (reviewed in Kaur & Ling, 2008; Orrell et al., 2008),
- mitochondrial and SOD1 dysfunction (reviewed in Benatar, 2007; Shi et al., 2010; Valentine et al., 2005),
- impaired axonal transport (reviewed in Costa et al., 2010),
- apoptosis and cell death (reviewed in Sathasivam et al., 2001),
- neurofilament and protein aggregation such as TDP-43 proteinopathies (reviewed in Geser et al., 2010; Worrall et al., 2000),
- neuro-inflammation (reviewed in Graber & Dhib-Jalbut, 2009; Holmoy, 2008; Lipton et al., 2007; Weydt & Moller, 2005), and
- the lack or dysfunction of neurotrophic factors (reviewed in Maurer et al., 2008; Siciliano et al., 2010; Traynor et al., 2006).

These pathophysiological mechanisms all end in motor neuron degeneration as the final pathway in disease progression (reviewed in Bruijn et al., 2004; Carlesi et al., 2011; Thatte & Dahanukar, 1997).

To address the genetic influence in ALS, two databases have been established. The ALSoD database (alsod.iop.kcl.ac.uk) contains detailed information about genes involved in ALS pathophysiology, and the ALSGene database lists genetic association studies (www.alsgene.org) (Lill et al., 2011).

4.2 Pathophysiological considerations in the planning of ALS treatment strategies

Most pre-clinical trials in ALS research started with the pathophysiological model of the disease. In counteracting the pathophysiology of the disease, motor neuron survival and stabilization of motor neuron function is increased (reviewed in Bedlack et al., 2007; Carlesi et al., 2011; Fornai et al., 2011; Ilieva et al., 2009; Pradat et al., 2010; Silani et al., 2011).

Current strategies for treatment concepts reach for counteracting the individual pathophysiological actors. They including the following groups of agents:

- Anti-excitotoxicitory drugs. Excitotoxicity is mainly modulated by the release of glutamate and contributes to an acute toxicity. Typical molecules involved are the NMDA and AMPA receptors and the glial glutamate transporter Excitatory amino-acid transporters type-2 (EAAT2), which is regulating most of the extracellular glutamate concentration.

- Anti-aggregation drugs. Cellular aggregates of proteins, such as the Bunina bodies, occur in the neuronal somata of ALS patients. The prevention of these cellular aggregates may also increase the survival of motor neurons. The subcellular component involved in the degradation of aggregates is the endoplasmic reticulum (ER). Defects in ER function may contribute to the formation of the protein aggregates, as well as the inhibition of the proteasome.
- Suppliers of cellular energy. In ALS, mitochondrial dysfunction contributes to the cellular energy loss. Thus the prevention of neuronal energy depletion may increase and prolong neuronal survival.
- Anti-oxidants. The generation of reactive oxygen species (ROS), such as H_2O_2, can produce major damage to the neuron. Thus specialized cellular systems exist in the cell to prevent oxidative damage. One of these systems include [Cu,Zn]-superoxide dismutase-1 (SOD1), of which mutations in humans can induce ALS.
- SOD1 reduction techniques. The clearance of the mutated and dysfunctional SOD1 protein may also positively influence motor neuron survival.
- Inducers of intraaxonal transport. Molecules that signal damage in the bouton terminal are transported to the neuronal soma. In ALS, this transport is retricted, thus the damage information reaches the peri-nuclear area only delayed.
- Drugs supporting nerve-muscle transmission. Defects in the transmission at the neuromuscular junction may contribute to disease progress.
- Stabilizers of the neuro-vascular unit. The loss of proteins at the tight junctions may disrupt the neuro-vascular unit. Thus molecules stabilizing the tight junctions may ameliorate the supply of neurons with substrates.
- Anti-inflammatory compounds. Neuroinflammation plays a role in the chronic detrimental processes occurring in the immediate microenvironment of the neuron.
- Neuroprotectants. Since neurodegeneration is the general mechanism in ALS progression, neuroprotective drugs may prevent or slow down neuronal break-down.
- Anti-apoptotic compounds. Cell death is the ultimate reason in the apoptotic cascade. Thus compounds preventing cell death may contribute to increased survival of motor neurons.
- Growth factors. Growth factors such as G-CSF, VEGF, GDNF and others can both stimulate the growth of novel neurons (neurogenesis) and the repair of damaged neurons (neuroregeneration).
- Various techniques whereby muscles can be strengthened even in an environment where motor neurons are degenerating, thus maintaining motor function.
- Gene therapy. In these approaches, the expression of endogenous proteins, such as growth factors, are used to increase
- Stem cell therapies. The transplantation of various sources, such as bone-marrow derived stem cells (BMSC), mesenchymal stem cells (MSC), or neuronal stem cells (NSC), may support the microenvironment and thus the survival of motor neurons, or supply new motor neurons by replacing apoptotic cells.

5. Clinical trials in ALS

5.1 Programmed failure in clinical trials for ALS?

In the typical process of drug development, preclinical data such as biochemical assays, cellular assays, and rodent models for the disease, lead to positive results with regard to predefined outcome parameters, for example, the increase in muscle strength, or survival time. For all of the drugs listed in the next section, promising preclinical data have been provided and published (for review, see (Ludolph & Sperfeld, 2005)). But why did the majority of the clinical trials fail, when preclinical data have been so promising?

Three major points came to my notice, when reviewing the literature: First, the animal models (mouse, rat, drosophila etc.) may either not sufficiently reflect the human pathology, or the animal pathology does not reflect human conditions (discussed in Green, 2002; Kiernan et al., 2011; Scott et al., 2008). Second, "ALS" is a clinical but not a pathophysiological entity. Thus, the inter-personal variability between patients is too big, and the inclusion criteria are too broad. Third, the design of the clinical trials may be insufficient (Aggarwal & Cudkowicz, 2008; Fornai et al., 2011; Kiernan et al., 2011; Maragakis, 2009), including:

- the number of subjects is too small,
- the time for follow-up is too short,
- the power of the study is calculated too low,
- the inclusion criteria are too broad,
- the outcome measures are not well-defined and comparable, or insufficient.

In future clinical trials, these issues should be discussed and included into the design of clinical ALS trials (Borasio, 1997).

5.2 Consensus guidelines for ALS trials

Therefore, a round table has been established to agree on minimal criteria for a "good" clinical trial (Miller et al., 1999). Of note, there have been substantial efforts also in other diseases such as stroke research to agree on clinical and pre-clinical guidelines for research, such as the "Stroke Therapy Academic Industry Roundtable (STAIR)" (STAIR - Stroke Treatment Academic Industry Roundtable, 2006).

In the following paragraphs, I will shortly summarize the consensus guidelines for ALS trial. The prerequisite for any ALS trial should be a substantial diagnosis according to the criteria defined by the World Federation of Neurology (see above). Moreover, the inclusion criteria should be handled strictly, including that both sporadic and familial ALS can be entered into the trial. The age of the patients should be limited between 18 and 85 years of age. Symptoms should show a disease progression within the first six months after onset, but not more than five years. Additionally, also exclusion criteria have been defined, for example, the patients should not show sensory abnormalities, dementia, other neurological diseases, they should not suffer from any uncompensated medical illness, substance abuse, or psychiatric illness. Of note, the patients should not be taking any other investigational drug.

The endpoints of the trial must be defined in advance, for example, survival time, muscle strength, or ventilator dependence are common endpoints. All trials should include a control group.

The quality of life should be assessed in every efficacy trial. The statistical analysis must be sound and planned with sufficient power. Any co-medication must be carefully re-considered.

Since there has been an early release of information about the efficacy in clinical ALS trials, which had to be revoked after thorough analysis, any information with regard to the efficacy of an investigational drug should only be released when peer-reviewed publication is at least imminent (with the exception of scientific meetings). The investigator is responsible for any conflict of interest.

The design of ALS trials should comprehend three phases (Brooks, 1997). In phase I, toxicity and pharmacokinetics is tested. In phase II (pilot, exploratory, or screening trials) information is gathered about dose finding, preliminary efficacy, and further safety observations. In phase III, definitive efficacy and safety is evaluated. Phase I trials should incorporate a placebo control group and the follow-up should be at least six months. Phase II trials may use placebo controls, historic controls, or a crossover design. If the prospective therapeutic value aims at improvement of signs and symptoms, such as increased muscle strength or ameliorated function, the follow-up should be at least six months, whereas trials aiming at stabilization or slowing of deterioration should observe the patients' condition for at least 12 months (Bedlack, 2010). All phase III trials should be placebo-controlled. The endpoints should include at least the survival time, assessment of strength measured by maximum voluntary isometric contraction, pulmonary function, and functional performance by the ALS rating scale. Of course, an independent data and safety monitoring board should be established.

Of note, since survival times are rather short, many patients feel desperate and take unapproved medication out of the reach of a clinical trial. By establishing these consensus guidelines, this potentially dangerous drug use may be reduced (Ross, 2009).

5.3 Overview over drug candidates in clinical ALS trials

In the following "inventory" of clinical trials in ALS, I will give an overview over drug candidates used in ALS trials. I have included all interventional clinical trials registered at Clinicaltrials.gov (http://clinicaltrials.gov/). Information on these trials can be obtained by accessing the website http://ClinicalTrials.gov/show/NCTxxx, where xxx stands for the registration number shown below.

Since there have been various clinical trials in the era before Clinicaltrials.gov required registration, and before a consensus conference established criteria for ALS trials (Miller et al., 1999), I have included some information on earlier trials. On the other hand, I excluded case reports, trials with nutritional supplements, and non-pharmacological therapeutic procedures such as plasma exchange, whole-body irridation, hyperbaric oxygenation, balneotherapy, cervico-dorsal electroshock therapy, adrenal cortex injection or stem cell injection, even when the stem cells are used as vehicles and vectors for the expression of biologicals.

Of note, this inventory is neither comprehensive, nor does it contain all available references due to space restriction. It is mainly based on a selective literature search in the PubMed database, and summarizes recent reviews in the field (Carlesi et al., 2011; Miller et al., 2005; Siciliano et al., 2010; Zinman & Cudkowicz, 2011; Zoccolella et al., 2009).

5.3.1 N-acetylcysteine

The anti-oxidant N-acetylcysteine did not show efficacy in a phase II clinical trial (Louwerse et al., 1995).

5.3.2 AEOL-10150

AEOL-10150 is a metalloporphyrin scavenging reactive oxygen species (ROS) (Orrell, 2006). It has been tested for safety and tolerability in three phase I trials, but further development has been halted.

5.3.3 Amantadine (1-adamantylamine, 1-aminoadamantane)

Amantadine shows a weak NMDA receptor antagonism and anti-cholinergic effects. In a cross-over study with guanidine, no benefits for ALS patients have been described (Munsat et al., 1981).

5.3.4 Anakinra

Anakinra is a recombinant antibody directed against the interleukin-1 receptor (IL-1R). IL-1 is involved in sustaining the neuroinflammatory process. Treatment with anakinra in the G93A-SOD1 transgenic mouse model of ALS extended the lifespan of the animals and decreased neuroinflammation (Meissner et al., 2010). Thus blocking of the IL-1R may be a potential target in decreasing the speed of ALS progression (van der Meer & Simon, 2010). Currently, a phase II study (NCT01277315), designed as a riluzole add-on study, investigates the safety and tolerability of anakinra in ALS.

5.3.5 Antioxidants

In a systematic review, no evidence for a benefit of anti-oxidant treatment with regard to survival, neither alone, nor in combination, has been described (Orrell et al., 2008). The antioxidants administered in ALS patients included vitamin E, acetylcysteine, L-methionine, and selenium.

5.3.6 Arimoclomol (BRX-220)

The small molecule arimoclomol is a co-inducer of heat-shock proteins (Phukan, 2010), namely of HSP70 (Brown, 2007). Thus it may be used to increase endogenous cellular protein repair and to prevent misfolding, or aggregation, of proteins by activating molecular chaperones (Kalmar & Greensmith, 2009).

Arimoclomol was tested in two phase II studies to evaluate safety and efficacy in ALS patients (NCT00561366) and to find a dose range and to determine pharmacokinetic parameters (NCT00244244) (Cudkowicz et al., 2008; Lanka et al., 2009).

Currently, arimoclomol is tested in a phase II/III trial in patients with SOD1-positive fALS (NCT00706147).

5.3.7 Arundic acid (ONO-2506)

Arundic acid is an enantiomeric, three carbon atom homolog of valproic acid, with anti-inflammatory and anti-glutamatergic effects (de Paulis, 2003).

It was tested in two phase II studies, designed as riluzole add-on, in clinical ALS trials for long-term safety (NCT00694941) and safety and efficacy (NCT00403104). The original evaluation of the trials did not show statistically significant differences between groups, but the subgroup analysis showed a possible positive effect for patients in early stages, namely within 14 months after onset of symptoms. On the other hand, patients with longer disease onset showed negative outcome (Thomas Meyer, 2005).

5.3.8 AVP-923 (Zenvia)

AVP-923 is a combinational formulation containing dextromethorphan hydrobromide, which is an NMDA antagonist and sigma-1 receptor agonist, and quinidine sulphate, which inhibits the cytochrome P450 2D6 (CYP2D6) enzyme. Dextromethorphan hydrobromide shows a high first pass metabolism in the liver, where it is metabolized by CYP2D6. Thus the addition of quinidine sulphate increases the bioavailability of dextromethorphan hydrobromide (Olney & Rosen, 2010).

AVP-923 was tested in two phase III trials in ALS patients with pseudobulbar affect (PBA), which is characterized by emotional dysregulation, such as uncontrollable outbursts of laughing or crying that are inappropriate to the emotions being experienced (Garnock-Jones, 2011; Olney & Rosen, 2010). The study showed that AVP-923 ameliorates symptoms of PBA in ALS patients and improved quality of life and quality of relationships (Brooks et al., 2004).

5.3.9 Azathioprine

The immunosuppressant azathioprine in combination with prednisolone did not show a benefit in ALS patients (Werdelin et al., 1990).

5.3.10 Brain-derived neurotrophic factor (BDNF)

The neuroprotective growth factor BDNF has been evaluated in a phase I/II clinical trial which reported a trend for prolonged survival after subcutaneous infusion (The BDNF Study Group & Bradley, 1995), a result which could not be reproduced in the subsequent phase III clinical trial (The BDNF Study Group (Phase III), 1999). The intrathecal administration was safe and well-tolerated (Ochs et al., 2000).

5.3.11 Branched-chain amino acids (BCAA)

The branched-chain amino acids comprehend leucine, isoleucine, and valine.

In clinical trials, branched chain amino acids did not show a beneficial effect in ALS patients (Tandan et al., 1996).

5.3.12 Bromocriptine

The dopamine agonist bromocriptine did not show a benefit in ALS patients (Szulc-Kuberska et al., 1990).

5.3.13 Buspirone

The anxiolytic agent buspirone did not show a benefit in ALS patients (The ALS Association, 2010).

5.3.14 Ceftriaxone

Ceftriaxone is a ß-lactam antibiotic which also shows anti-oxidant and anti-excitotoxity effects (Traynor et al., 2006).

Currently, ceftriaxone is evaluated in a phase III clinical trial in patients with ALS (NCT00349622).

5.3.15 Celecoxib

Celecoxib is an inhibitor of cyclooxygenase-2 (COX-2), an enzyme which promotes inflammation by releasing of inflammatory substances, such as prostaglandin E(2) (PGE2).

The rationale of celecoxib treatment is the reduction of PGE2 in the cerebrospinal fluid (CSF), thus preventing neuroinflammation and neuronal loss.
In a phase II clinical trial (NCT00355576), celecoxib did not show a beneficial effect on the decline in muscle strength, motor unit number estimates, vital capacity, ALS Functional Rating Scale-Revised, and overall survival (Cudkowicz et al., 2006). Moreover, PGE2 levels in the CSF were not elevated at baseline and did not decline during treatment (Cudkowicz et al., 2006). In this trial, celecoxib was combined with creatinine and/or minocycline (Gordon et al., 2008).

5.3.16 Ciclosporine A

The immunosuppressant cyclosporine A did not show a benefit in ALS patients (Appel et al., 1988).

5.3.17 Ciliary neurotrophic factor (CNTF)

CNTF is a neurotrophic factor with neuroprotective properties.
It has been tested in two clinical trials finding no effect on disease progression (ALS CNTF Treatment Study Group, 1996; Miller et al., 1996), but an increased trend of adverse effects (Miller et al., 1996).

5.3.18 Cistanche total glycosides (CTGs)

The glycosidic extract of the plant *Cistanche spp.* has a long tradition in its medicinally use in Traditional Chinese Medicine (TCM). It has been described as a neuroprotective agent in a mouse model of Parkinson's Disease (PD) (Li et al., 2008). Currently, Cistanche Total Glycosides are investigated in a phase II trial (NCT00753571). Of note, the CTGs are the only agents in registered ALS trials without a defined chemical composition, which may impose problems in future comparability to other medications and effectiveness of different preparations.

5.3.19 CK-2017357

With regard to the loss of skeletal muscle strength, the substituted urea derivative CK-2017357 is claimed to activate the muscle protein troponin in fast skeletal muscle fibres. A proposed mode-of-action is sensitizing the sarcomere to calcium, thus the neuro-muscular transmission is amplified, thus muscle power increases and the time to musclular fatigue is delayed (von Haehling et al., 2010).
A phase IIa study (NCT01089010) was completed in 2010 and showed a trend towards short-term improvements in grip-strength and respiration parameters.

5.3.20 Coenzyme Q10

Coenzyme Q10 has been proposed to inhibit neurodegeneration. In a phase II clinical trial, it was well tolerated and safe (Ferrante et al., 2005), but showed no efficacy in a phase II futility trial (NCT00243932) (Kaufmann et al., 2009; Levy et al., 2006).

5.3.21 Creatine

Creatine acts as anti-oxidant and is a mitochondrial co-factor.
It has been evaluated in several phase II clinical trials (NCT00070993, NCT00005674, NCT00005766) which reported no beneficial effect in ALS patients (Groeneveld et al., 2003; Shefner et al., 2004), as well as a phase III clinical trial (NCT00069186) (Rosenfeld et al., 2008).

Creatine supplementation temporarily increased maximal isometric power in ALS patients (Mazzini et al., 2001).
In a phase I dose-escalation trial, creatine concentrations in the brain increased after oral administration (Atassi et al., 2010).
Currently, creatine is evaluated in a phase II clinical trial (NCT01257581) in combination with tamoxifen in ALS patients.

5.3.22 Cyclophosphamide

The immunosuppressant cyclophosphamide showed only a temporary amelioration of symptoms in ALS patients without a long-term benefit (Gourie-Devi et al., 1997).

5.3.23 Dexpramipexole (R-(+) pramipexole; RPPX; KNS-760704)

Dexpramipexole is a synthetic amino-benzothiazole and the (+)-enantiomer of pramipexole which has dopaminergic activity and is a mitochondrial neuroprotectant by scavenging reactive oxygen and nitrogen species (RONS) (Cheah & Kiernan, 2010; Gribkoff & Bozik, 2008).
In earlier studies, RPPX reduced oxidative stress in sporadic ALS patients (Pattee et al., 2003). RPPX has been found to be safe and tolerable (Bozik et al., 2010; Wang et al., 2008), but did not change ALSFRS-R (NCT00140218, NCT00600873, NCT00596115, NCT00647296) (Wang et al., 2008). In the open-label extension protocol, RPPX caused a non-significant reduction in the slope of decline in the ALSFRS-R score (NCT00931944) (Wang et al., 2008).
RPPX is currently evaluated in a phase III study (NCT01281189) in ALS patients.

5.3.24 3,4-Diaminopyridine (DAP)

The potassium channel blocker DAP did not show a benefit in ALS patients (Aisen et al., 1996; Aisen et al., 1995). Currently, the drug is re-evaluated after a phase I safety study (Bertorini et al., 2011).

5.3.25 Dronabinol

Dronabinol is a synthetic Δ9-tetrahydrocannabinol (Delta-9-THC, Δ9-THC, THC).
It has been tested in a phase II study (NCT00812851) in ALS patients suffering from muscular cramps, where no subjective improvement of cramp intensity has been seen (Weber et al., 2010).

5.3.26 Edaravone (MCI-186; NSC 2629)

Edavarone is an anti-oxidant free radical scavenger (Takahashi, 2009).
It has been tested in several phase II/III clinical trials (NCT00330681, NCT00415519, NCT00424463) for safety and efficacy. A phase II study found a possible delay in the progression of functional motor symptoms in ALS patients (Yoshino & Kimura, 2006).

5.3.27 Erythropoietin (EPO)

EPO is a hematopoietic growth factor with neuroprotective properties (Maurer et al., 2008).
Moreover, EPO exhibited anti-inflammatory and anti-apoptotic effects.
It has been evaluated in a phase II trial, finding no effects on survival and functional outcome (Lauria et al., 2009).

5.3.28 Escitalopram

Escitalopram is a selective serotonin reuptake inhibitor (SSRI) and used clinically as an antidepressant.

It has been tested in a phase III clinical trial (NCT00965497) for the improvement of depressive symptoms and the quality of life in ALS patients.

5.3.29 Gabapentin

Gabapentin is an anti-convulsant with anti-glutamatergic effects, which have been proposed to slow down neuronal pathology (Welty et al., 1995).

It has been tested in a phase II trial finding a smaller slope in arm strength decrase (Miller et al., 1996), but a subsequent phase III trial has not shown beneficial effects of (Miller et al., 2001). No effects on neuronal integrity have been found in an MR spectroscopy study (Kalra et al., 2003).

5.3.30 Gangliosides

Gangliosides are derivatives of sialylated glycosphingolipids containing one to five sialic acids at various anomeric linkage sites to the core glycan. They modulate the effect of nerve growth factor and activate protein kinase (DeFelice & Ellenberg, 1984; Rapport, 1990).

Gangliosides have been tested in several clinical trials without benefit for ALS patients (Bradley et al., 1984; Harrington et al., 1984; Lacomblez et al., 1989).

5.3.31 Glatiramer acetate

Glatiramer acetate is a random polymer composed of four amino acids that are found in myelin basic protein (MBP). It has been proposed that it inhibits neuroinflammation, stimulates anti-glutamatergic growth factor effects.

In a phase II clinical trial (NCT00326625), glatiramer acetate has not shown any beneficial effect in ALS patients (Meininger et al., 2009).

5.3.32 Granulocyte colony stimulating Factor (G-CSF; AX200)

G-CSF is a hematopoietic growth and maturation factor with neuroprotective and neuroregenerative effects (reviewed in Maurer et al., 2008).

G-CSF has been evaluated in a phase II study (NCT00298597) in ALS patients, finding no differences with regard to functional outcome between study groups, but slowing the progression of white matter tract destruction (Duning et al., 2011). In a second phase II trial (NCT00397423), the authors reported preliminary data on 13 patients with slower disease progression (Zhang et al., 2009). Another clinical trial did not report statistically significant differences between study and control group (Nefussy et al.), but a trend towards slowing down disease progression.

5.3.33 Growth hormone (GH, Somatropin)

Human growth hormone (hGH) stimulates the production and release of insulin-like growth factor I (IGF-1) which induces cell proliferation and differentiation (Rosenbloom, 2009).

GH has evaluated in a phase II trial (NCT00635960) with no effects on disease progression (Sacca et al., 2011).

5.3.34 GSK1223249

GSK1223249 is a humanised monoclonal antibody which counteracts the inhibition of neurite outgrowth by Nogo-A. Currently, GSK1223249 is evaluated in a phase I study (NCT00875446) for safety in ALS patients.

5.3.35 Guanidine

In a clinical trial, guanidine caused severe side effects such as acute paralysis (Norris et al., 1974; Norris et al., 1974). In a cross-over study with amantadine, no benefits for ALS patients have been described (Munsat et al., 1981).

5.3.36 Indinavir

The antiviral drug indinavir did not show a benefit in ALS patients (Scelsa et al., 2005).

5.3.37 Insulin-like growth factor-1 (IGF-1)

IGF-1 is a growth factor stimulated by the human growth hormone (hGH). It induces cell proliferation and differentiation (Rosenbloom, 2009).

Whereas a first trial of IGF-1 in ALS patients reported a slower disease progression of functional impairment and a higher quality of life score (Lai et al., 1997), a subsequent study did not find beneficial effects after 9 months of treatment (Borasio et al., 1998). A phase III clinical trial (NCT00035815) found no beneficial effects after 2 years of treatment in ALS patients (Sorenson et al., 2008).

5.3.38 Interferon

The immunomodulators interferon-alpha (Dalakas et al., 1986; Mora et al., 1986) and interferon-beta (Beghi et al., 2000; Bouche et al., 1986) did not show a benefit in ALS patients.

5.3.39 ISIS 333611 (ISIS-SOD1$_{Rx}$)

ISIS 333611 is an antisense oligonucleotide inhibitor of Cu/Zn superoxide dismutase (SOD1) (Smith et al., 2006). Currently, a phase I (NCT01041222) investigates the safety, tolerability, and activity familial ALS caused by SOD1 gene mutations.

5.3.40 Isoprinosine

The antiviral drug isoprinosine did not show a benefit in ALS patients (Fareed & Tyler, 1971; Percy et al., 1971).

5.3.41 Lamotrigine

Lamotrigine is an anti-epileptic drug with anti-excitotocicity effects. It has been tested in two clinical trials (Eisen et al., 1993; Ryberg et al., 2003) showing no effects on disease progression.

5.3.42 Lecithin

The term lecithin describes a group compounds consisting of phosphoric acid, choline, fatty acids, glycerol, glycolipids, triglycerides, and phospholipids. Typical members comprehend phosphatidylcholine, phosphatidylethanolamine, and phosphatidylinositol.

In a clinical trial, lecithin did not show a benefit in ALS patients (Kelemen et al., 1982).

5.3.43 Leuprorelin (Leuprolide)

Leuprorelin is a is a nonapeptide and a GnRH analog.
It has been tested in a phase II study in combination with testosterone (NCT00004771), the results are awaited.

5.3.44 Levamisole

Levamisole is a synthetic imidazothiazole derivative with anti-helmintic and immunomodulatory effects. In a clinical trial, no beneficial effects have been seen for ALS patients (Olarte & Shafer, 1985).

5.3.45 Lithium

Lithium has been described as inductor of autophagy and anti-oxidant. Clinically, it is used as mood stabilizer.
In a phase II study (EudraCT), lithium did not show efficacy with regard to survival and keeping of patient autonomy (Chio et al.).
In another phase II study, lithium was reported to delay disease progression (Fornai et al., 2008), but in a follow-up, riluzole add-on phase II study (NCT00818389), lithium has been proven to be safe and well tolerated in ALS patients, but did not slow disease progression (Aggarwal et al.). Due to these findings, two other studies of lithium are currently not recruiting patients (NCT00925847, NCT00790582).

5.3.46 Memantine

Memantine non-competitive antagonist at the NMDA and AMPA glutamate receptors with low affinity.
In two phase II/III clinical trials (NCT01020331, NCT00409721), memantine was safe and tolerated, but no efficacy has been found in ALS patients (de Carvalho et al., 2010).

5.3.47 Methylcobalamin (E0302, mecobalamin)

Methylcobalamin is an analog of vitamin B12, which reduces the concentration of homocystein, an excitatory amino acid which showed toxic effects on motor neurons by inducing apoptosis.
ALS patients treated with high doses of methylcobalamin (MeCbl) showed an increase in compound muscle action potential amplitudes (CMAPs) after 4 weeks of treatment (Kaji et al., 1998). It increased the decline in ALS patients with regard to becoming respirator-bound (Izumi & Kaji, 2007).
Methylcobalamin is currently evaluated in two phase III studies (NCT00445172, NCT00444613) in ALS patients

5.3.48 Minocycline

Minocycline has been described as anti-apoptotic and anti-inflammatory.
In a phase III study (NCT00047723), minocycline showed harmful effects of minocycline in ALS patients (Gordon et al., 2007).

5.3.49 Modafinil

Modafinil is a psychostimulant clinically used for the treatment of narcolepsy and other sleep disorders.

It is currently evaluated in a phase IV study (NCT00614926) for the treatment of fatigue in ALS patients.

5.3.50 Naloxone

The μ opioid receptor antagonist naloxone did not show a benefit in ALS patients (Silani et al., 1983).

5.3.51 Neostigmine

The cholinesterase inhibitor did not show a benefit in ALS patients (Aquilonius et al., 1986).

5.3.52 Nimodipine

The calcium channel antagonist nimodipine showed no beneficial effect in a clinical trail in ALS patients (Miller et al., 1996).

5.3.53 NP001

NP001 is a small molecule regulator of macrophage activation, which aims at restoring the neuroprotective state of macrophages, reducing inflammation, and normalizing the neuronal microenvironment.
NP001 has been tested in a phase I trial (NCT01091142) for safety and tolerability. It is currently evaluated in a subsequent phase II clinical trial (NCT01281631).

5.3.54 Olanzapine

Olanzapine is an atypic neuroleptic drug used in psychiatry for the treatment of schizophrenia and other psychoses. One of its effects is also weight gain. In ALS patients, an involuntary weight loss of more than 10 percent of the original body weight correlates with an increased mortality. Thus treatment with olanzapine might increase the body weight, or, at least, keep it constant.
Currently, olanzapine is evaluated in a phase II/III study (NCT00876772) in ALS patients.

5.3.55 Olesoxime (TRO19622)

Olesoxime is a neuroprotective agent with a cholesterol-like structure which is thought to act at the mitochondrial membrane (Bordet et al., 2010; Martin, 2010).
Currently, olesoxime is evaluated in a phase II/III trial (NCT00868166) as add-on to riluzole and a phase II/III safety extension study (NCT01285583).

5.3.56 Penicillamine

The metal ion chelating agent penicillamine did not show a benefit in ALS patients (Conradi et al., 1982).

5.3.57 Pentoxifylline

Pentoxifylline is an anti-apoptotic drug. It has been tested in a riluzole add-on phase II clinical trial, which did not show efficacy, but increased mortality (Meininger et al., 2006).

5.3.58 Phthalazine

The inhibitor of cyclic adenosine monophosphate (cAMP) phosphodiesterase and cyclic guanine monophosphate (cGMP) phosphodiesterase phthalazinol did not show a benefit in ALS patients (Engel & Brooks, 1980).

5.3.59 Physostigmine

The acetylcholine esterase inhibitor physostigmine did not show a benefit in ALS patients (Norris et al., 1993).

5.3.60 Pioglitazone

Pioglitazone activates the nuclear receptor peroxisome proliferator-activated receptor gamma (PPAR-γ) (Gillies & Dunn, 2000; Kiaei, 2008). It has been used as anti-diabetic drug in diabetes type 2.

In phase II clinical trial (NCT00690118), pioglitazone was found to be save and well-tolerated, but showed no effect on ALS disease progression (Ludolph et al., 2010).

In a riluzole add-on phase II study (NCT00919555), pioglitazone is currently evaluated in combination with tretinoin.

5.3.61 Prednisolone

The immunosuppressant prednisolone in combination with azathioprine did not show a benefit in ALS patients (Werdelin et al., 1990).

5.3.62 Pyrimethamine

The anti-malaria drug pyrimethamine was found to reduce SOD1 levels in vitro and in vivo in rodents as well as in humans (Lange, 2008).

Pyrimethamine is currently evaluated in a phase I/II trial (NCT01083667) for tolerability, safety, and efficacy in familial ALS.

5.3.63 Rasagiline

Rasagiline is a monoamine oxidase type B inhibitor with neuroprotective effects.

Rasagiline is currently evaluated in a phase II clinical trial (NCT01232738).

5.3.64 Riluzole

Riluzole is an anti-glutamatergic drug (Cheah et al., 2010; R.G. Miller et al., 2007).

In two clinical trials, riluzole showed a moderate increase of about two months in survival after 21 and 18 months of treatment, respectively (Bensimon et al., 1994; Lacomblez et al., 1996). An open-label phase IV study (NCT00542412) found a longer survival in riluzole-treated patients of 92 days in median.

In subsequent population-based trials, older patients and patients with bulbar-onset had the biggest beneficial effect of riluzole, but the effects were transient and lost after longer periods of observation (Traynor et al., 2003; Zoccolella et al., 2007).

5.3.65 SB-509

SB-509 is an engeineered zinc finger protein which up-regulates the transcription of the pro-angiogenic vascular entothelial growth factor A (VEGF-A) (Liu et al., 2001), which is also neuroprotective and neuroregenerative (Maurer et al., 2008)

SB-509 is currently evaluated in a phase II clinical trial (NCT00748501).

5.3.66 Selegiline

The anti-depressant drug selegiline is an inhibitor of monoamino oxidase B.
It has been tested in several clinical trials without benefit for ALS patients (Jossan et al., 1994; Lange et al., 1998; Mazzini et al., 1994).

5.3.67 Snake venom

Modified snake venom as neurotoxin did not show a benefit in ALS patients (Rivera et al., 1980).

5.3.68 Sodium phenylbutyrate

Sodium phenylbutyrate acts as a histone deacetylase inhibitor, therefore it improves transcription and stimulates post-transcriptional pathways.
In a phase II study (NCT00107770), sodium phenylbutyrate was safe and well tolerated (Cudkowicz et al., 2009).

5.3.69 Sodium valproate

Valproic acid (VPA) is a histone deacetylase inhibitor that showed antioxidative and antiapoptotic properties and reduced glutamate toxicity. It is used as antiepileptic drug.
In a phase II clinical trial (NCT00136110), VPA has been found safe but not effective with regard to survival and disease progression (Piepers et al., 2009).

5.3.70 Talampanel (GYKI 53405)

Talampanel is a derivated benzodiazepine which is a non-competitive antagonist at the AMPA glutamate receptor.
It has been evaluated in a phase II trial (NCT00982150) which showed safety and tolerability (Pascuzzi et al., 2010), whereas a subsequent phase II study (NCT00696332) did not show efficacy in ALS patients (reviewed in Carlesi et al., 2011).

5.3.71 Tamoxifen

The selective estrogen receptor modulator tamoxifen is an inhibitor of protein kinase C, which is a mediator in neuroinflammation.
It has been evaluated in a phase II study (NCT00214110) in ALS patients (Brooks et al., 2005) and was recommended for a phase III trial (mentioned in Traynor et al., 2006).
Currently, tamoxifen is evaluated in a phase II clinical trial (NCT01257581) in combination with creatine in ALS patients.

5.3.72 Tauroursodeoxycholic acid (TUDCA)

In preclinical data, tauroursodeoxycholic acid (TUDCA) has been found to be neuroprotective, antioxidative, and antiapoptotic in rat models of neurodegenerative diseases such as stroke (Rodrigues et al., 2002) and Huntington's disease (Keene et al., 2002).
TUDCA is currently evaluated in a phase II study (NCT00877604) for safety and efficacy.

5.3.73 TCH346

TCH 346 showed neuroprotective effects by binding glyceraldehydes-3-phosphate dehydrogenase (GAPDH) (Mück-Seler & Pivac, 2000).
It has been evaluated in three phase II studies (NCT00230074, NCT00072709, NCT00036413), where it showed no beneficial effects in ALS (R. Miller et al., 2007).

5.3.74 Testosterone

The sexual hormone testosterone has been tested in a phase II study in combination with leuprolide (NCT00004771), the results are awaited.

5.3.75 Tetrahydroaminoacridine (Tacrine, THA)

The reversible inhibitor of cholinesterase THA did not show a benefit in ALS patients (Askmark et al., 1990).

5.3.76 Thalidomide

Thalidomide is a small molecule which has been used as a sedative drug in the 1950s-1960s. Due to its teratogenic and neuropathic adverse effects, its use was discontinued until the 1990s, when thalidomide was introduced in oncology for its anti-angiogenic effects.

With regard to clinical trials in ALS, thalidomide was tested in a phase II clinical trial (NCT00140452) (Stommel et al., 2009), with no improvement in the ALS Functional Rating Scale (ALSFRS) and pulmonary function testing (PFT) curves after nine months of thalidomide treatment. Moreover, thalidomide showed severe side effects, and did not affect anti-inflammatory cytokine levels.

A second phase II clinical trial (NCT00231140) was terminated after severe adverse effects (Thomas Meyer, 2005).

5.3.77 L-Threonine

The hydroxylated essential amino acid L-threonine did not show a benefit in ALS patients (Blin et al., 1992; Tandan et al., 1996).

5.3.78 Thyreotropin releasing hormone (TRH, Protirelin)

TRH has been tested in a larger number of clinical trials, but none of them showed a benefit in ALS patients (Brooke et al., 1986; Brooks et al., 1987; Caroscio et al., 1986; Congia et al., 1991; Hawley et al., 1987; Imoto et al., 1984; Klimek et al., 1989; Klimek et al., 1988; Miller & Warnick, 1989; Mitsumoto et al., 1986; Munsat et al., 1992; Patrignani et al., 1992; Serratrice et al., 1985; Stober et al., 1985; Thielen et al., 1987; Yamane et al., 1986).

5.3.79 Tilorone

The antiviral drug tilorone did not show a benefit in ALS patients (Olson et al., 1978).

5.3.80 Tocopherol (Vitamin E)

The anti-oxidant tocopherol has been evaluated in two phase II clinical trials, where tocopherol has been as add-on medication to riluzole in ALS patients. Both studies reported safe and well-tolerated drug administration, but no beneficial effect for ALS patients (Desnuelle et al., 2001; Graf et al., 2005). In a retrospective case-control study, high dosage of tocopherol decreased the risk of developing ALS (Veldink et al., 2007).

5.3.81 Topiramate

Topiramate is an anti-convulsant with anti-glutamatergic effects. It has been tested in a clinical trial without benefit for ALS patients, but with an increased rate of life-threatening side effects (Cudkowicz et al., 2003).

5.3.82 Transfer factor

The antiviral agent transfer factor did not show a benefit in ALS patients (Jonas et al., 1979; Olarte et al., 1979).

5.3.83 Tretinoin (all-*trans* retinoic acid)

Tretinoin is the all-trans form of retinoic acid. It has various effects in the nervous system, including neuroprotection and neuroregeneration (for review, see (Lee et al., 2009)).
In a riluzole add-on phase II study (NCT00919555), tretinoin is currently evaluated in combination with pioglitazone.

5.3.84 Trypan blue and trypan red

The antimicrobial agents trypan blue and trypan red did not show a beneficial effect in ALS patients (Montanari & Pessina, 1955; Schwob & Bonduelle, 1952).

5.3.85 Vascular endothelial growth factor (VEGF, sNN0029)

VEGF is a neuroprotectice and angiogenic growth factor (Maurer et al., 2008). It is currently tested in a phase I/II clinical trial (NCT00800501) for safety and tolerability. Of note, VEGF must be administered into the CSF.

5.3.86 Verapamil

The calcium channel antagonist verapamil showed no beneficial effect in a clinical trail in ALS patients (Miller et al., 1996).

5.3.87 Xaliproden (SR57746)

The 5HT1R agonist xaliproden is neurotrophic and neuroprotective. It has been evaluated in phase II/III trials, which showed modest effects on vital capacity, but not on survival of ALS patients (Lacomblez et al., 2004; Meininger et al., 2004).

5.3.88 YAM80

There is no drug information available for YAM80 searching literature and chemical databases. YAM80 is evaluated in a phase II study (NCT00886977) for safety and efficacy in ALS patients.

5.3.89 Zidovudine

The antiviral drug zidovudine did not show a benefit in ALS patients (Westarp et al., 1993).

5.3.90 Preclinical agents

The following agents have shown promising results in preclinical assessment, but no clinical trials have been conducted:
Azathioprine, glycine, the tripeptide zVAD-fmk, AM-1241, celastrol, dantrolene, nordihydroguaiaretic acid, RO-28-2653, L-arginine, 5-hydroxytryptophan, N-acetylated alpha-linked acidic dipeptidase, mechano-growth factor (MGF), hepatocyte growth factor (HGF), glial-derived neurotrophic factor (GDNF), promethazine and other anti-histaminergic drugs, calcium disodium EDTA, toluloxy propane, ammonium tetramolybdate (for details, see (Mitsumoto, 2009; Zoccolella et al., 2007)), and cannabis (Carter et al., 2010).

5.3.91 "Alternative" therapeutic approaches

Since most clinical trials in ALS did not show a benefit for ALS patients, a number of "alternative" or off-label cures have been propagated. Besides severe ethical issues, these treatments are of experimental nature, but not in the sense of a registered trial.
Some ALS patients who are desperately looking for a relief, tend to participate in these treatments, although they have to pay large amounts of money by themselves, and no proven, or replicable outcome has been reported in a peer-reviewed journal.
To evaluate some of these treatments, the ALSUntangled group (www.alsuntangled.com), which is based on social networking of patients, clinicians, and scientists (Bedlack & Hardiman, 2009), reports sporadically on these treatments (see homepage for open and completed investigations).

6. Outlook

ALS remains a mysterious disease with a limited life expectancy and a deteriorating condition, although efforts in basic and clinical research brought some light in the understanding of pathophysiological aspects of MND.
With dozens of failed neuropharmacological trials in ALS, the current concept of the design of clinical trials in ALS patients must be reevaluated, as well as the pre-clinical models.
Future research may concentrate on the definition of ALS, maybe by the use of biomarkers, and on translational aspects, that is, how to transfer pre-clinical results into successful clinical treatment.

7. Abbreviations

ALS, amyotrophic lateral sclerosis
ALSFRS, ALS functional rating scale
ALSSS, ALS severity scale
CNS, central nervous system
FTD, Fronto-Temporal Dementia
LMN, lower motor neuron
MND, motor neuron disease
PBP, progressive bulbar palsy
PLS, primary lateral sclerosis
PMA, progressive muscular atrophy
ROS, Reactive oxygen species
SOD1, [Zn, Cu] Superoxide dismutase type 1
UMN, upper motor neuron

8. Acknowledgments

The author has been supported by grants of the European Union within the Framework Program 7, the Germany Ministry of Research and Education (BMBF) within the National Genome Research Network NGFN-2, the German Research Foundation DFG, the intramural program of the Medical Faculty of the University of Heidelberg, the Steuben-Schurz Society, and the Estate of Friedrich Fischer.

9. References

Abrahams, S., Goldstein, L.H., Kew, J.J., Brooks, D.J., Lloyd, C.M., Frith, C.D. & Leigh, P.N. (1996). Frontal lobe dysfunction in amyotrophic lateral sclerosis. A PET study. *Brain*, Vol. 119, No. Pt 6, pp. 2105-2120.

Aggarwal, S. & Cudkowicz, M. (2008). ALS drug development: reflections from the past and a way forward. *Neurotherapeutics*, Vol. 5, No. 4, pp. 516-527.

Aggarwal, S.P., Zinman, L., Simpson, E., McKinley, J., Jackson, K.E., Pinto, H., Kaufman, P., Conwit, R.A., Schoenfeld, D., Shefner, J. & Cudkowicz, M. (2010). Safety and efficacy of lithium in combination with riluzole for treatment of amyotrophic lateral sclerosis: a randomised, double-blind, placebo-controlled trial. *Lancet Neurol*, Vol. 9, No. 5, pp. 481-488.

Aisen, M.L., Sevilla, D., Edelstein, L. & Blass, J. (1996). A double-blind placebo-controlled study of 3,4-diaminopyridine in amytrophic lateral sclerosis patients on a rehabilitation unit. *J Neurol Sci*, Vol. 138, No. 1-2, pp. 93-96.

Aisen, M.L., Sevilla, D., Gibson, G., Kutt, H., Blau, A., Edelstein, L., Hatch, J. & Blass, J. (1995). 3,4-diaminopyridine as a treatment for amyotrophic lateral sclerosis. *J Neurol Sci*, Vol. 129, No. 1, pp. 21-24.

ALS CNTF Treatment Study Group. (1996). A double-blind placebo-controlled clinical trial of subcutaneous recombinant human ciliary neurotrophic factor (rHCNTF) in amyotrophic lateral sclerosis. . *Neurology*, Vol. 46, No. 5, pp. 1244-1249.

Appel, S.H., Stewart, S.S., Appel, V., Harati, Y., Mietlowski, W., Weiss, W. & Belendiuk, G.W. (1988). A double-blind study of the effectiveness of cyclosporine in amyotrophic lateral sclerosis. *Arch Neurol*, Vol. 45, No. 4, pp. 381-386.

Appel, V., Stewart, S.S., Smith, G. & Appel, S.H. (1987). A rating scale for amyotrophic lateral sclerosis: description and preliminary experience. *Ann Neurol*, Vol. 22, No. 3, pp. 328-333.

Aquilonius, S.M., Askmark, H., Eckernas, S.A., Gillberg, P.G., Hilton-Brown, P., Rydin, E. & Stalberg, E. (1986). Cholinesterase inhibitors lack therapeutic effect in amyotrophic lateral sclerosis. A controlled study of physostigmine versus neostigmine. *Acta Neurol Scand*, Vol. 73, No. 6, pp. 628-632.

Askmark, H., Aquilonius, S.M., Gillberg, P.G., Hartvig, P., Hilton-Brown, P., Lindstrom, B., Nilsson, D., Stalberg, E. & Winkler, T. (1990). Functional and pharmacokinetic studies of tetrahydroaminoacridine in patients with amyotrophic lateral sclerosis. *Acta Neurol Scand*, Vol. 82, No. 4, pp. 253-258.

Atassi, N., Cook, A., Pineda, C.M., Yerramilli-Rao, P., Pulley, D. & Cudkowicz, M. (2011). Depression in amyotrophic lateral sclerosis. *Amyotroph Lateral Scler*, Vol. 12, No. 2, pp. 109-112.

Atassi, N., Ratai, E.M., Greenblatt, D.J., Pulley, D., Zhao, Y., Bombardier, J., Wallace, S., Eckenrode, J., Cudkowicz, M. & Dibernardo, A. (2010). A phase I, pharmacokinetic, dosage escalation study of creatine monohydrate in subjects with amyotrophic lateral sclerosis. *Amyotroph Lateral Scler*, Vol. 11, No. 6, pp. 508-513.

Averill, A.J., Kasarskis, E.J. & Segerstrom, S.C. (2007). Psychological health in patients with amyotrophic lateral sclerosis. *Amyotroph Lateral Scler*, Vol. 8, No. 4, pp. 243-254.

Bedlack, R. & Hardiman, O. (2009). ALSUntangled (ALSU): a scientific approach to off-label treatment options for people with ALS using tweets and twitters. *Amyotroph Lateral Scler*, Vol. 10, No. 3, pp. 129-130.

Bedlack, R.S. (2010). Amyotrophic lateral sclerosis: current practice and future treatments. *Curr Opin Neurol*, Vol. 23, No. 5, pp. 524-529.

Bedlack, R.S., Traynor, B.J. & Cudkowicz, M.E. (2007). Emerging disease-modifying therapies for the treatment of motor neuron disease/amyotropic lateral sclerosis. *Expert Opin Emerg Drugs*, Vol. 12, No. 2, pp. 229-252.

Beghi, E., Chio, A., Inghilleri, M., Mazzini, L., Micheli, A., Mora, G., Poloni, M., Riva, R., Serlenga, L., Testa, D. & Tonali, P. (2000). A randomized controlled trial of recombinant interferon beta-1a in ALS. Italian Amyotrophic Lateral Sclerosis Study Group. *Neurology*, Vol. 54, No. 2, pp. 469-474.

Benatar, M. (2007). Lost in translation: treatment trials in the SOD1 mouse and in human ALS. *Neurobiol Dis*, Vol. 26, No. 1, pp. 1-13.

Bensimon, G., Lacomblez, L. & Meininger, V. (1994). A controlled trial of riluzole in amyotrophic lateral sclerosis. ALS/Riluzole Study Group. *N Engl J Med*, Vol. 330, No. 9, pp. 585-591.

Bertorini, T.E., Rashed, H., Zeno, M., Tolley, E.A., Igarashi, M. & Li, Y.D. (2011). Effects of 3-4 diaminopyridine (DAP) in motor neuron diseases. *J Clin Neuromuscul Dis*, Vol. 12, No. 3, pp. 129-137.

Blin, O., Pouget, J., Aubrespy, G., Guelton, C., Crevat, A. & Serratrice, G. (1992). A double-blind placebo-controlled trial of L-threonine in amyotrophic lateral sclerosis. *J Neurol*, Vol. 239, No. 2, pp. 79-81.

Bogaert, E., d'Ydewalle, C. & Van Den Bosch, L. (2011). Amyotrophic lateral sclerosis and excitotoxicity: from pathological mechanism to therapeutic target. *CNS Neurol Disord Drug Targets*, Vol. 9, No. 3, pp. 297-304.

Bohannon, R.W. & Smith, M.B. (1987). Interrater reliability of a modified Ashworth scale of muscle spasticity. *Phys Ther*, Vol. 67, No. 2, pp. 206-207.

Borasio, G.D. (1997). Amyotrophic lateral sclerosis: lessons in trial design from recent trials. *J Neurol Sci*, Vol. 152 Suppl 1, No. 1, pp. S23-28.

Borasio, G.D., Robberecht, W., Leigh, P.N., Emile, J., Guiloff, R.J., Jerusalem, F., Silani, V., Vos, P.E., Wokke, J.H. & Dobbins, T. (1998). A placebo-controlled trial of insulin-like growth factor-I in amyotrophic lateral sclerosis. European ALS/IGF-I Study Group. *Neurology*, Vol. 51, No. 2, pp. 583-586.

Bordet, T., Berna, P., Abitbol, J.-L. & Pruss, R.M. (2010). Olesoxime (TRO19622): A Novel Mitochondrial-Targeted Neuroprotective Compound. *Pharmaceuticals*, Vol. 3, No. 2, pp. 345-368.

Bouche, P., Hanin, B. & Castaigne, P. (1986). Effects of intrathecal interferon therapy in amyotrophic lateral sclerosis. *Neurology*, Vol. 36, No. 5, pp. 735-736.

Bozik, M.E., Mather, J.L., Kramer, W.G., Gribkoff, V.K. & Ingersoll, E.W. (2010). Safety, Tolerability, and Pharmacokinetics of KNS-760704 (Dexpramipexole) in Healthy Adult Subjects. *J Clin Pharmacol*.

Bradley, W.G., Hedlund, W., Cooper, C., Desousa, G.J., Gabbai, A., Mora, J.S., Munsat, T.L. & Scheife, R. (1984). A double-blind controlled trial of bovine brain gangliosides in amyotrophic lateral sclerosis. *Neurology*, Vol. 34, No. 8, pp. 1079-1082.

Brooke, M.H., Florence, J.M., Heller, S.L., Kaiser, K.K., Phillips, D., Gruber, A., Babcock, D. & Miller, J.P. (1986). Controlled trial of thyrotropin releasing hormone in amyotrophic lateral sclerosis. *Neurology*, Vol. 36, No. 2, pp. 146-151.

Brooks, B., Sanjak, M., Roelke, K. & al., e. (2005). Phase 2B randomized dose ranging clinical trial of tamoxifen, a selective estrogen receptor modulator [SERM], in ALS:

sensitivity analyses of discordance between survival and functional outcomes with long-term follow-up. *Amyotroph Lateral Scler Other Motor Neuron Disord*, Vol. 6, No. Suppl 1, pp. 118.

Brooks, B.R. (1994). El Escorial World Federation of Neurology criteria for the diagnosis of amyotrophic lateral sclerosis. Subcommittee on Motor Neuron Diseases/Amyotrophic Lateral Sclerosis of the World Federation of Neurology Research Group on Neuromuscular Diseases and the El Escorial "Clinical limits of amyotrophic lateral sclerosis" workshop contributors. *J Neurol Sci*, Vol. 124 Suppl, pp. 96-107.

Brooks, B.R. (1997). Clinical evaluation of ALS drugs. *Neurology*, Vol. 48, No. Suppl 4, pp. S23-S27.

Brooks, B.R., Miller, R.G., Swash, M. & Munsat, T.L. (2000). El Escorial revisited: revised criteria for the diagnosis of amyotrophic lateral sclerosis. *Amyotroph Lateral Scler Other Motor Neuron Disord*, Vol. 1, No. 5, pp. 293-299.

Brooks, B.R., Sufit, R.L., Montgomery, G.K., Beaulieu, D.A. & Erickson, L.M. (1987). Intravenous thyrotropin-releasing hormone in patients with amyotrophic lateral sclerosis. Dose-response and randomized concurrent placebo-controlled pilot studies. *Neurol Clin*, Vol. 5, No. 1, pp. 143-158.

Brooks, B.R., Thisted, R.A., Appel, S.H., Bradley, W.G., Olney, R.K., Berg, J.E., Pope, L.E. & Smith, R.A. (2004). Treatment of pseudobulbar affect in ALS with dextromethorphan/quinidine: a randomized trial. *Neurology*, Vol. 63, No. 8, pp. 1364-1370.

Brown, I.R. (2007). Heat shock proteins and protection of the nervous system. *Ann N Y Acad Sci*, Vol. 1113, pp. 147-158.

Bruijn, L.I., Miller, T.M. & Cleveland, D.W. (2004). Unraveling the mechanisms involved in motor neuron degeneration in ALS. *Annu Rev Neurosci*, Vol. 27, pp. 723-749.

Burnstein, M.H. (1981). Familial amyotrophic lateral sclerosis, dementia, and psychosis. *Psychosomatics*, Vol. 22, No. 2, pp. 151-157.

Carlesi, C., Pasquali, L., Piazza, S., Lo Gerfo, A., Caldarazzo Ienco, E., Alessi, R., Fornai, F. & Siciliano, G. (2011). Strategies for clinical approach to neurodegeneration in amyotrophic lateral sclerosis. *Arch Ital Biol*, Vol. 149, No. 1, pp. 151-167.

Caroscio, J.T., Cohen, J.A., Zawodniak, J., Takai, V., Shapiro, A., Blaustein, S., Mulvihill, M.N., Loucas, S.P., Gudesblatt, M., Rube, D. & et al. (1986). A double-blind, placebo-controlled trial of TRH in amyotrophic lateral sclerosis. *Neurology*, Vol. 36, No. 2, pp. 141-145.

Carter, G.T., Abood, M.E., Aggarwal, S.K. & Weiss, M.D. (2010). Cannabis and amyotrophic lateral sclerosis: hypothetical and practical applications, and a call for clinical trials. *Am J Hosp Palliat Care*, Vol. 27, No. 5, pp. 347-356.

Cedarbaum, J.M. & Stambler, N. (1997). Performance of the Amyotrophic Lateral Sclerosis Functional Rating Scale (ALSFRS) in multicenter clinical trials. *J Neurol Sci*, Vol. 152 Suppl 1, pp. S1-9.

Cheah, B.C. & Kiernan, M.C. (2010). Dexpramipexole, the R(+) enantiomer of pramipexole, for the potential treatment of amyotrophic lateral sclerosis. *IDrugs*, Vol. 13, No. 12, pp. 911-920.

Cheah, B.C., Vucic, S., Krishnan, A.V. & Kiernan, M.C. (2010). Riluzole, neuroprotection and amyotrophic lateral sclerosis. *Curr Med Chem*, Vol. 17, No. 18, pp. 1942-1199.

Chio, A., Borghero, G., Calvo, A., Capasso, M., Caponnetto, C., Corbo, M., Giannini, F., Logroscino, G., Mandrioli, J., Marcello, N., Mazzini, L., Moglia, C., Monsurro, M.R., Mora, G., Patti, F., Perini, M., Pietrini, V., Pisano, F., Pupillo, E., Sabatelli, M., Salvi, F., Silani, V., Simone, I.L., Soraru, G., Tola, M.R., Volanti, P. & Beghi, E. (2010). Lithium carbonate in amyotrophic lateral sclerosis: lack of efficacy in a dose-finding trial. *Neurology*, Vol. 75, No. 7, pp. 619-625.

Colombrita, C., Onesto, E., Tiloca, C., Ticozzi, N., Silani, V. & Ratti, A. (2011). RNA-binding proteins and RNA metabolism: a new scenario in the pathogenesis of Amyotrophic lateral sclerosis. *Arch Ital Biol*, Vol. 149, No. 1, pp. 83-99.

Congia, S., Tronci, S., Ledda, M., Porcella, A. & Coppola, G. (1991). Low doses of TRH in amyotrophic lateral sclerosis and in other neurological diseases. *Ital J Neurol Sci*, Vol. 12, No. 2, pp. 193-198.

Conradi, S., Ronnevi, L.O., Nise, G. & Vesterberg, O. (1982). Long-time penicillamine-treatment in amyotrophic lateral sclerosis with parallel determination of lead in blood, plasma and urine. *Acta Neurol Scand*, Vol. 65, No. 3, pp. 203-211.

Costa, J., Gomes, C. & de Carvalho, M. (2010). Diagnosis, pathogenesis and therapeutic targets in amyotrophic lateral sclerosis. *CNS Neurol Disord Drug Targets*, Vol. 9, No. 6, pp. 764-778.

Cudkowicz, M., Qureshi, M. & Shefner, J. (2004). Measures and markers in amyotrophic lateral sclerosis. *NeuroRx*, Vol. 1, No. 2, pp. 273-283.

Cudkowicz, M.E., Andres, P.L., Macdonald, S.A., Bedlack, R.S., Choudry, R., Brown, R.H., Jr., Zhang, H., Schoenfeld, D.A., Shefner, J., Matson, S., Matson, W.R. & Ferrante, R.J. (2009). Phase 2 study of sodium phenylbutyrate in ALS. *Amyotroph Lateral Scler*, Vol. 10, No. 2, pp. 99-106.

Cudkowicz, M.E., Shefner, J.M., Schoenfeld, D.A., Brown, R.H., Jr., Johnson, H., Qureshi, M., Jacobs, M., Rothstein, J.D., Appel, S.H., Pascuzzi, R.M., Heiman-Patterson, T.D., Donofrio, P.D., David, W.S., Russell, J.A., Tandan, R., Pioro, E.P., Felice, K.J., Rosenfeld, J., Mandler, R.N., Sachs, G.M., Bradley, W.G., Raynor, E.M., Baquis, G.D., Belsh, J.M., Novella, S., Goldstein, J. & Hulihan, J. (2003). A randomized, placebo-controlled trial of topiramate in amyotrophic lateral sclerosis. *Neurology*, Vol. 61, No. 4, pp. 456-464.

Cudkowicz, M.E., Shefner, J.M., Schoenfeld, D.A., Zhang, H., Andreasson, K.I., Rothstein, J.D. & Drachman, D.B. (2006). Trial of celecoxib in amyotrophic lateral sclerosis. *Ann Neurol*, Vol. 60, No. 1, pp. 22-31.

Cudkowicz, M.E., Shefner, J.M., Simpson, E., Grasso, D., Yu, H., Zhang, H., Shui, A., Schoenfeld, D., Brown, R.H., Wieland, S. & Barber, J.R. (2008). Arimoclomol at dosages up to 300 mg/day is well tolerated and safe in amyotrophic lateral sclerosis. *Muscle Nerve*, Vol. 38, No. 1, pp. 837-844.

Dalakas, M.C., Aksamit, A.J., Madden, D.L. & Sever, J.L. (1986). Administration of recombinant human leukocyte alpha 2-interferon in patients with amyotrophic lateral sclerosis. *Arch Neurol*, Vol. 43, No. 9, pp. 933-935.

de Carvalho, M., Dengler, R., Eisen, A., England, J.D., Kaji, R., Kimura, J., Mills, K., Mitsumoto, H., Nodera, H., Shefner, J. & Swash, M. (2008). Electrodiagnostic criteria for diagnosis of ALS. *Clin Neurophysiol*, Vol. 119, No. 3, pp. 497-503.

de Carvalho, M., Pinto, S., Costa, J., Evangelista, T., Ohana, B. & Pinto, A. (2010). A randomized, placebo-controlled trial of memantine for functional disability in amyotrophic lateral sclerosis. *Amyotroph Lateral Scler*, Vol. 11, No. 5, pp. 456-460.

de Paulis, T. (2003). ONO-2506. Ono. *Curr Opin Investig Drugs*, Vol. 4, No. 7, pp. 863-867.

DeFelice, S.L. & Ellenberg, M. (1984). Gangliosides--clinical overview. *Adv Exp Med Biol*, Vol. 174, pp. 625-628.

Desnuelle, C., Dib, M., Garrel, C. & Favier, A. (2001). A double-blind, placebo-controlled randomized clinical trial of alpha-tocopherol (vitamin E) in the treatment of amyotrophic lateral sclerosis. ALS riluzole-tocopherol Study Group. *Amyotroph Lateral Scler Other Motor Neuron Disord*, Vol. 2, No. 1, pp. 9-18.

Duning, T., Schiffbauer, H., Warnecke, T., Mohammadi, S., Floel, A., Kolpatzik, K., Kugel, H., Schneider, A., Knecht, S., Deppe, M. & Schabitz, W.R. (2011). G-CSF prevents the progression of structural disintegration of white matter tracts in amyotrophic lateral sclerosis: a pilot trial. *PLoS One*, Vol. 6, No. 3, pp. e17770.

Eisen, A., Stewart, H., Schulzer, M. & Cameron, D. (1993). Anti-glutamate therapy in amyotrophic lateral sclerosis: a trial using lamotrigine. *Can J Neurol Sci*, Vol. 20, No. 4, pp. 297-301.

Eisen, A.A. (2007). Historical aspects of motor neuron diseases, In: *Handbook of Clinical Neurology Motor Neuron Disorders and Related Diseases*, Eisen, A.A. & Shaw, P.J. (Eds.), pp. 1-11, Elsevier B.V., Amsterdam.

Engel, W.K. & Brooks, B.R. (1980). Phthalazinol, thrombocytopenia, and amyotrophic lateral sclerosis. *Arch Neurol*, Vol. 37, No. 5, pp. 320.

Enns, M.W., Barakat, S.M. & Brown, J.H. (1993). Amyotrophic lateral sclerosis presenting with psychosis. *Psychosomatics*, Vol. 34, No. 5, pp. 453-455.

Epton, J., Harris, R. & Jenkinson, C. (2009). Quality of life in amyotrophic lateral sclerosis/motor neuron disease: a structured review. *Amyotroph Lateral Scler*, Vol. 10, No. 1, pp. 15-26.

Evdokimidis, I., Constantinidis, T.S., Gourtzelidis, P., Smyrnis, N., Zalonis, I., Zis, P.V., Andreadou, E. & Papageorgiou, C. (2002). Frontal lobe dysfunction in amyotrophic lateral sclerosis. *J Neurol Sci*, Vol. 195, No. 1, pp. 25-33.

Fareed, G.C. & Tyler, H.R. (1971). The use of isoprinosine in patients with amyotrophic lateral sclerosis. *Neurology*, Vol. 21, No. 9, pp. 937-940.

Ferentinos, P., Paparrigopoulos, T., Rentzos, M., Zouvelou, V., Alexakis, T. & Evdokimidis, I. (2011). Prevalence of major depression in ALS: Comparison of a semi-structured interview and four self-report measures. *Amyotroph Lateral Scler*, Vol. 12, No. 4, pp. 297-302.

Ferguson, T.A. & Elman, L.B. (2007). Clinical presentation and diagnosis of Amyotrophic Lateral Sclerosis. *NeuroRehabilitation*, Vol. 22, pp. 409-416.

Ferrante, K.L., Shefner, J., Zhang, H., Betensky, R., O'Brien, M., Yu, H., Fantasia, M., Taft, J., Beal, M.F., Traynor, B., Newhall, K., Donofrio, P., Caress, J., Ashburn, C., Freiberg, B., O'Neill, C., Paladenech, C., Walker, T., Pestronk, A., Abrams, B., Florence, J., Renna, R., Schierbecker, J., Malkus, B. & Cudkowicz, M. (2005). Tolerance of high-dose (3,000 mg/day) coenzyme Q10 in ALS. *Neurology*, Vol. 65, No. 1, pp. 1834-1836.

Foran, E. & Trotti, D. (2009). Glutamate transporters and the excitotoxic path to motor neuron degeneration in amyotrophic lateral sclerosis. *Antioxid Redox Signal*, Vol. 11, No. 7, pp. 1587-1602.

Fornai, F., Longone, P., Cafaro, L., Kastsiuchenka, O., Ferrucci, M., Manca, M.L., Lazzeri, G., Spalloni, A., Bellio, N., Lenzi, P., Modugno, N., Siciliano, G., Isidoro, C., Murri, L.,

Ruggieri, S. & Paparelli, A. (2008). Lithium delays progression of amyotrophic lateral sclerosis. *Proc Natl Acad Sci U S A*, Vol. 105, No. 6, pp. 2052-2057.

Fornai, F., Meininger, V. & Silani, V. (2011). Future therapeutical strategies dictated by pre-clinical evidence in ALS. *Arch Ital Biol*, Vol. 149, No. 1, pp. 169-174.

Garnock-Jones, K.P. (2011). Dextromethorphan/Quinidine: in pseudobulbar affect. *CNS Drugs*, Vol. 25, No. 5, pp. 435-445.

Geser, F., Lee, V.M. & Trojanowski, J.Q. (2010). Amyotrophic lateral sclerosis and frontotemporal lobar degeneration: a spectrum of TDP-43 proteinopathies. *Neuropathology*, Vol. 30, No. 2, pp. 103-112.

Geser, F., Martinez-Lage, M., Robinson, J., Uryu, K., Neumann, M., Brandmeir, N.J., Xie, S.X., Kwong, L.K., Elman, L., McCluskey, L., Clark, C.M., Malunda, J., Miller, B.L., Zimmerman, E.A., Qian, J., Van Deerlin, V., Grossman, M., Lee, V.M. & Trojanowski, J.Q. (2009). Clinical and pathological continuum of multisystem TDP-43 proteinopathies. *Arch Neurol*, Vol. 66, No. 2, pp. 180-189.

Gillies, P.S. & Dunn, C.J. (2000). Pioglitazone. *Drugs*, Vol. 60, No. 2, pp. 333-343; discussion 344-335.

Giordana, M.T., Ferrero, P., Grifoni, S., Pellerino, A., Naldi, A. & Montuschi, A. (2011). Dementia and cognitive impairment in amyotrophic lateral sclerosis: a review. *Neurol Sci*, Vol. 32, No. 1, pp. 9-16.

Gordon, P.H., Cheung, Y.K., Levin, B., Andrews, H., Doorish, C., Macarthur, R.B., Montes, J., Bednarz, K., Florence, J., Rowin, J., Boylan, K., Mozaffar, T., Tandan, R., Mitsumoto, H., Kelvin, E.A., Chapin, J., Bedlack, R., Rivner, M., McCluskey, L.F., Pestronk, A., Graves, M., Sorenson, E.J., Barohn, R.J., Belsh, J.M., Lou, J.S., Levine, T., Saperstein, D., Miller, R.G. & Scelsa, S.N. (2008). A novel, efficient, randomized selection trial comparing combinations of drug therapy for ALS. *Amyotroph Lateral Scler*, Vol. 9, No. 4, pp. 212-222.

Gordon, P.H., Moore, D.H., Miller, R.G., Florence, J.M., Verheijde, J.L., Doorish, C., Hilton, J.F., Spitalny, G.M., MacArthur, R.B., Mitsumoto, H., Neville, H.E., Boylan, K., Mozaffar, T., Belsh, J.M., Ravits, J., Bedlack, R.S., Graves, M.C., McCluskey, L.F., Barohn, R.J. & Tandan, R. (2007). Efficacy of minocycline in patients with amyotrophic lateral sclerosis: a phase III randomised trial. *Lancet Neurol*, Vol. 6, No. 12, pp. 1045-1053.

Gourie-Devi, M., Nalini, A. & Subbakrishna, D.K. (1997). Temporary amelioration of symptoms with intravenous cyclophosphamide in amyotrophic lateral sclerosis. *J Neurol Sci*, Vol. 150, No. 2, pp. 167-172.

Graber, J.J. & Dhib-Jalbut, S. (2009). Protective autoimmunity in the nervous system. *Pharmacol Ther*, Vol. 121, No. 2, pp. 147-159.

Graf, M., Ecker, D., Horowski, R., Kramer, B., Riederer, P., Gerlach, M., Hager, C., Ludolph, A.C., Becker, G., Osterhage, J., Jost, W.H., Schrank, B., Stein, C., Kostopulos, P., Lubik, S., Wekwerth, K., Dengler, R., Troeger, M., Wuerz, A., Hoge, A., Schrader, C., Schimke, N., Krampfl, K., Petri, S., Zierz, S., Eger, K., Neudecker, S., Traufeller, K., Sievert, M., Neundorfer, B. & Hecht, M. (2005). High dose vitamin E therapy in amyotrophic lateral sclerosis as add-on therapy to riluzole: results of a placebo-controlled double-blind study. *J Neural Transm*, Vol. 112, No. 5, pp. 649-660.

Green, A.R. (2002). Why do neuroprotective drugs that are so promising in animals fail in the clinic? An industry perspective. *Clin Exp Pharmacol Physiol*, Vol. 29, No. 11, pp. 1030-1034.

Gribkoff, V.K. & Bozik, M.E. (2008). KNS-760704 [(6R)-4,5,6,7-tetrahydro-N6-propyl-2, 6-benzothiazole-diamine dihydrochloride monohydrate] for the treatment of amyotrophic lateral sclerosis. *CNS Neurosci Ther*, Vol. 14, No. 3, pp. 215-226.

Groeneveld, G.J., Veldink, J.H., van der Tweel, I., Kalmijn, S., Beijer, C., de Visser, M., Wokke, J.H., Franssen, H. & van den Berg, L.H. (2003). A randomized sequential trial of creatine in amyotrophic lateral sclerosis. *Ann Neurol*, Vol. 53, No. 4, pp. 437-445.

Harrington, H., Hallett, M. & Tyler, H.R. (1984). Ganglioside therapy for amyotrophic lateral sclerosis: a double-blind controlled trial. *Neurology*, Vol. 34, No. 8, pp. 1083-1085.

Hawley, R.J., Kratz, R., Goodman, R.R., McCutchen, C.B., Sirdofsky, M. & Hanson, P.A. (1987). Treatment of amyotrophic lateral sclerosis with the TRH analog DN-1417. *Neurology*, Vol. 37, No. 4, pp. 715-717.

Hetta, J. & Jansson, I. (1997). Sleep in patients with amyotrophic lateral sclerosis. *J Neurol*, Vol. 244, No. 4 Suppl 1, pp. S7-9.

Hillel, A.D., Miller, R.M., Yorkston, K., McDonald, E., Norris, F.H. & Konikow, N. (1989). Amyotrophic lateral sclerosis severity scale. *Neuroepidemiology*, Vol. 8, No. 3, pp. 142-150.

Holmoy, T. (2008). T cells in amyotrophic lateral sclerosis. *Eur J Neurol*, Vol. 15, No. 4, pp. 360-366.

Howland, R.H. (1990). Schizophrenia and amyotrophic lateral sclerosis. *Compr Psychiatry*, Vol. 31, No. 4, pp. 327-336.

Huey, E.D., Koppel, J., Armstrong, N., Grafman, J. & Floeter, M.K. (2010). A pilot study of the prevalence of psychiatric disorders in PLS and ALS. *Amyotroph Lateral Scler*, Vol. 11, No. 3, pp. 293-297.

Ilieva, H., Polymenidou, M. & Cleveland, D.W. (2009). Non-cell autonomous toxicity in neurodegenerative disorders: ALS and beyond. *J Cell Biol*, Vol. 187, No. 6, pp. 761-772.

Imoto, K., Saida, K., Iwamura, K., Saida, T. & Nishitani, H. (1984). Amyotrophic lateral sclerosis: a double-blind crossover trial of thyrotropin-releasing hormone. *J Neurol Neurosurg Psychiatry*, Vol. 47, No. 12, pp. 1332-1334.

Izumi, Y. & Kaji, R. (2007). [Clinical trials of ultra-high-dose methylcobalamin in ALS]. *Brain Nerve*, Vol. 59, No. 10, pp. 1141-1147.

Jackson, C.E. & Bryan, W.W. (1998). Amyotrophic lateral sclerosis. *Semin Neurol*, Vol. 18, No. 1, pp. 27-39.

Jonas, S., Wichter, M. & Spitler, L. (1979). Amyotrophic lateral sclerosis: failure of transfer factor therapy. *Ann Neurol*, Vol. 6, No. 1, pp. 84.

Jossan, S.S., Ekblom, J., Gudjonsson, O., Hagbarth, K.E. & Aquilonius, S.M. (1994). Double blind cross over trial with deprenyl in amyotrophic lateral sclerosis. *J Neural Transm Suppl*, Vol. 41, pp. 237-241.

Kaji, R., Kodama, M., Imamura, A., Hashida, T., Kohara, N., Ishizu, M., Inui, K. & Kimura, J. (1998). Effect of ultrahigh-dose methylcobalamin on compound muscle action potentials in amyotrophic lateral sclerosis: a double-blind controlled study. *Muscle Nerve*, Vol. 21, No. 12, pp. 1775-1778.

Kalmar, B. & Greensmith, L. (2009). Activation of the heat shock response in a primary cellular model of motoneuron neurodegeneration-evidence for neuroprotective and neurotoxic effects. *Cell Mol Biol Lett*, Vol. 14, No. 2, pp. 319-335.

Kalra, S., Cashman, N.R., Caramanos, Z., Genge, A. & Arnold, D.L. (2003). Gabapentin therapy for amyotrophic lateral sclerosis: lack of improvement in neuronal integrity shown by MR spectroscopy. *AJNR Am J Neuroradiol*, Vol. 24, No. 3, pp. 476-480.

Kaufmann, P., Thompson, J.L., Levy, G., Buchsbaum, R., Shefner, J., Krivickas, L.S., Katz, J., Rollins, Y., Barohn, R.J., Jackson, C.E., Tiryaki, E., Lomen-Hoerth, C., Armon, C., Tandan, R., Rudnicki, S.A., Rezania, K., Sufit, R., Pestronk, A., Novella, S.P., Heiman-Patterson, T., Kasarskis, E.J., Pioro, E.P., Montes, J., Arbing, R., Vecchio, D., Barsdorf, A., Mitsumoto, H. & Levin, B. (2009). Phase II trial of CoQ10 for ALS finds insufficient evidence to justify phase III. *Ann Neurol*, Vol. 66, No. 2, pp. 235-244.

Kaur, C. & Ling, E.A. (2008). Antioxidants and neuroprotection in the adult and developing central nervous system. *Curr Med Chem*, Vol. 15, No. 29, pp. 3068-3080.

Keene, C.D., Rodrigues, C.M., Eich, T., Chhabra, M.S., Steer, C.J. & Low, W.C. (2002). Tauroursodeoxycholic acid, a bile acid, is neuroprotective in a transgenic animal model of Huntington's disease. *Proc Natl Acad Sci U S A*, Vol. 99, No. 16, pp. 10671-10676.

Kelemen, J., Hedlund, W., Murray-Douglas, P. & Munsat, T.L. (1982). Lecithin is not effective in amyotrophic lateral sclerosis. *Neurology*, Vol. 32, No. 3, pp. 315-316.

Kiaei, M. (2008). Peroxisome Proliferator-Activated Receptor-gamma in Amyotrophic Lateral Sclerosis and Huntington's Disease. *PPAR Res*, Vol. 2008, pp. 418765.

Kiernan, M.C., Vucic, S., Cheah, B.C., Turner, M.R., Eisen, A., Hardiman, O., Burrell, J.R. & Zoing, M.C. (2011). Amyotrophic lateral sclerosis. *Lancet*, Vol. 377, No. 9769, pp. 942-955.

Klimek, A., Stepien, H. & Szulc-Kuberska, J. (1989). [THyroliberin test in patients with amyotrophic lateral sclerosis]. *Pol Tyg Lek*, Vol. 44, No. 43-45, pp. 918-920.

Klimek, A., Szulc-Kuberska, J., Czernielewska-Rutkowska, I. & Gluszcz-Zielinska, A. (1988). [Treatment of amyotrophic lateral sclerosis with TRH]. *Neurol Neurochir Pol*, Vol. 22, No. 3, pp. 206-210.

Kurt, A., Nijboer, F., Matuz, T. & Kubler, A. (2007). Depression and anxiety in individuals with amyotrophic lateral sclerosis: epidemiology and management. *CNS Drugs*, Vol. 21, No. 4, pp. 279-291.

Lacomblez, L., Bensimon, G., Douillet, P., Doppler, V., Salachas, F. & Meininger, V. (2004). Xaliproden in amyotrophic lateral sclerosis: early clinical trials. *Amyotroph Lateral Scler Other Motor Neuron Disord*, Vol. 5, No. 2, pp. 99-106.

Lacomblez, L., Bensimon, G., Leigh, P.N., Guillet, P. & Meininger, V. (1996). Dose-ranging study of riluzole in amyotrophic lateral sclerosis. Amyotrophic Lateral Sclerosis/Riluzole Study Group II. *Lancet*, Vol. 347, No. 9013, pp. 1425-1431.

Lacomblez, L., Bouche, P., Bensimon, G. & Meininger, V. (1989). A double-blind, placebo-controlled trial of high doses of gangliosides in amyotrophic lateral sclerosis. *Neurology*, Vol. 39, No. 12, pp. 1635-1637.

Lai, E.C., Felice, K.J., Festoff, B.W., Gawel, M.J., Gelinas, D.F., Kratz, R., Murphy, M.F., Natter, H.M., Norris, F.H. & Rudnicki, S.A. (1997). Effect of recombinant human insulin-like growth factor-I on progression of ALS. A placebo-controlled study. The North America ALS/IGF-I Study Group. *Neurology*, Vol. 49, No. 6, pp. 1621-1630.

Lange, D. (2008). Pyrimethamine as a therapy for SOD1 associated fALS: early findings. *Amyotrophic Lateral Sclerosis*, No. Suppl. 1, pp. 46.

Lange, D.J., Murphy, P.L., Diamond, B., Appel, V., Lai, E.C., Younger, D.S. & Appel, S.H. (1998). Selegiline is ineffective in a collaborative double-blind, placebo-controlled trial for treatment of amyotrophic lateral sclerosis. *Arch Neurol,* Vol. 55, No. 1, pp. 93-96.

Lanka, V., Wieland, S., Barber, J. & Cudkowicz, M. (2009). Arimoclomol: a potential therapy under development for ALS. *Expert Opin Investig Drugs,* Vol. 18, No. 12, pp. 1907-1918.

Lauria, G., Campanella, A., Filippini, G., Martini, A., Penza, P., Maggi, L., Antozzi, C., Ciano, C., Beretta, P., Caldiroli, D., Ghelma, F., Ferrara, G., Ghezzi, P. & Mantegazza, R. (2009). Erythropoietin in amyotrophic lateral sclerosis: a pilot, randomized, double-blind, placebo-controlled study of safety and tolerability. *Amyotroph Lateral Scler,* Vol. 10, No. 5-6, pp. 410-415.

Lee, H.P., Casadesus, G., Zhu, X., Lee, H.G., Perry, G., Smith, M.A., Gustaw-Rothenberg, K. & Lerner, A. (2009). All-trans retinoic acid as a novel therapeutic strategy for Alzheimer's disease. *Expert Rev Neurother,* Vol. 9, No. 11, pp. 1615-1621.

Levy, G., Kaufmann, P., Buchsbaum, R., Montes, J., Barsdorf, A., Arbing, R., Battista, V., Zhou, X., Mitsumoto, H., Levin, B. & Thompson, J.L. (2006). A two-stage design for a phase II clinical trial of coenzyme Q10 in ALS. *Neurology,* Vol. 66, No. 5, pp. 660-663.

Li, W.W., Yang, R. & Cai, D.F. (2008). [Protective effects of Cistanche total glycosides on dopaminergic neuron in substantia nigra of model mice of Parkinson's disease]. *Zhongguo Zhong Xi Yi Jie He Za Zhi,* Vol. 28, No. 3, pp. 248-251.

Lill, C.M., Abel, O., Bertram, L. & Al-Chalabi, A. (2011). Keeping up with genetic discoveries in amyotrophic lateral sclerosis: The ALSoD and ALSGene databases. *Amyotroph Lateral Scler,* Vol. 12, No. 4, pp. 238-249.

Lillo, P. & Hodges, J.R. (2009). Frontotemporal dementia and motor neurone disease: overlapping clinic-pathological disorders. *J Clin Neurosci,* Vol. 16, No. 9, pp. 1131-1135.

Lillo, P., Mioshi, E., Zoing, M.C., Kiernan, M.C. & Hodges, J.R. (2011). How common are behavioural changes in amyotrophic lateral sclerosis? *Amyotroph Lateral Scler,* Vol. 12, No. 1, pp. 45-51.

Lipton, S.A., Gu, Z. & Nakamura, T. (2007). Inflammatory mediators leading to protein misfolding and uncompetitive/fast off-rate drug therapy for neurodegenerative disorders. *Int Rev Neurobiol,* Vol. 82, pp. 1-27.

Liu, P.Q., Rebar, E.J., Zhang, L., Liu, Q., Jamieson, A.C., Liang, Y., Qi, H., Li, P.X., Chen, B., Mendel, M.C., Zhong, X., Lee, Y.L., Eisenberg, S.P., Spratt, S.K., Case, C.C. & Wolffe, A.P. (2001). Regulation of an endogenous locus using a panel of designed zinc finger proteins targeted to accessible chromatin regions. Activation of vascular endothelial growth factor A. *J Biol Chem,* Vol. 276, No. 14, pp. 11323-11334.

Lou, J.S. (2008). Fatigue in amyotrophic lateral sclerosis. *Phys Med Rehabil Clin N Am,* Vol. 19, No. 3, pp. 533-543, ix.

Louwerse, E.S., Weverling, G.J., Bossuyt, P.M., Meyjes, F.E. & de Jong, J.M. (1995). Randomized, double-blind, controlled trial of acetylcysteine in amyotrophic lateral sclerosis. *Arch Neurol,* Vol. 52, No. 6, pp. 559-564.

Ludolph, A.C., Kassubek, J., Meyer, T. & Group, T.G.A.S. (2010). Phase II study of pioglitazone in ALS. *Abstract Book of the 21st International Symposium on ALS/MND,* pp. 45.

Ludolph, A.C. & Sperfeld, A.D. (2005). Preclinical trials--an update on translational research in ALS. *Neurodegener Dis*, Vol. 2, No. 3-4, pp. 215-219.

Maragakis, N.J. (2009). Rethinking a drug treatment failure on a traditional ALS target. *Exp Neurol*, Vol. 216, No. 2, pp. 254-257.

Martin, L.J. (2010). Olesoxime, a cholesterol-like neuroprotectant for the potential treatment of amyotrophic lateral sclerosis. *IDrugs*, Vol. 13, No. 8, pp. 568-580.

Maurer, M.H., Schabitz, W.R. & Schneider, A. (2008). Old friends in new constellations--the hematopoetic growth factors G-CSF, GM-CSF, and EPO for the treatment of neurological diseases. *Curr Med Chem*, Vol. 15, No. 14, pp. 1407-1411.

Mazzini, L., Balzarini, C., Colombo, R., Mora, G., Pastore, I., De Ambrogio, R. & Caligari, M. (2001). Effects of creatine supplementation on exercise performance and muscular strength in amyotrophic lateral sclerosis: preliminary results. *J Neurol Sci*, Vol. 191, No. 1-2, pp. 139-144.

Mazzini, L., Testa, D., Balzarini, C. & Mora, G. (1994). An open-randomized clinical trial of selegiline in amyotrophic lateral sclerosis. *J Neurol*, Vol. 241, No. 4, pp. 223-227.

McGuire, D., Garrison, L., Armon, C., Barohn, R.J., Bryan, W.W., Miller, R., Parry, G.J., Petajan, J.H. & Ross, M.A. (1997). A brief quality-of-life measure for ALS clinical trials based on a subset of items from the sickness impact profile. The Syntex-Synergen ALS/CNTF Study Group. *J Neurol Sci*, Vol. 152 Suppl 1, No. 1, pp. S18-22.

McLeod, J.E. & Clarke, D.M. (2007). A review of psychosocial aspects of motor neurone disease. *J Neurol Sci*, Vol. 258, No. 1-2, pp. 4-10.

Meininger, V., Asselain, B., Guillet, P., Leigh, P.N., Ludolph, A., Lacomblez, L., Robberecht, W. & Pentoxifylline European Group. (2006). Pentoxifylline in ALS: a double-blind, randomized, multicenter, placebo-controlled trial. *Neurology*, Vol. 66, No. 1, pp. 88-92.

Meininger, V., Bensimon, G., Bradley, W.R., Brooks, B., Douillet, P., Eisen, A.A., Lacomblez, L., Leigh, P.N. & Robberecht, W. (2004). Efficacy and safety of xaliproden in amyotrophic lateral sclerosis: results of two phase III trials. *Amyotroph Lateral Scler Other Motor Neuron Disord*, Vol. 5, No. 2, pp. 107-117.

Meininger, V., Drory, V.E., Leigh, P.N., Ludolph, A., Robberecht, W. & Silani, V. (2009). Glatiramer acetate has no impact on disease progression in ALS at 40 mg/day: a double- blind, randomized, multicentre, placebo-controlled trial. *Amyotroph Lateral Scler*, Vol. 10, No. 5-6, pp. 378-383.

Meissner, F., Molawi, K. & Zychlinsky, A. (2010). Mutant superoxide dismutase 1-induced IL-1beta accelerates ALS pathogenesis. *Proc Natl Acad Sci U S A*, Vol. 107, No. 29, pp. 13046-13050.

Miller, M.C. (2011). Commentary. Did Lou Gehrig have Lou Gehrig's disease? *Harv Ment Health Lett*, Vol. 27, No. 8, pp. 8.

Miller, R., Bradley, W., Cudkowicz, M., Hubble, J., Meininger, V., Mitsumoto, H., Moore, D., Pohlmann, H., Sauer, D., Silani, V., Strong, M., Swash, M. & Vernotica, E. (2007). Phase II/III randomized trial of TCH346 in patients with ALS. *Neurology*, Vol. 69, No. 8, pp. 776-784.

Miller, R.G., Bryan, W.W., Dietz, M.A., Munsat, T.L., Petajan, J.H., Smith, S.A. & Goodpasture, J.C. (1996). Toxicity and tolerability of recombinant human ciliary neurotrophic factor in patients with amyotrophic lateral sclerosis. *Neurology*, Vol. 47, No. 5, pp. 1329-1331.

Miller, R.G., Gelinas, D. & O'Connor, P. (2005). *Amyotrophic lateral sclerosis* Demos Medical Publishing, 1-932603-06-9, New York.

Miller, R.G., Mitchell, J.D., Lyon, M. & Moore, D.H. (2007). Riluzole for amyotrophic lateral sclerosis (ALS)/motor neuron disease (MND). *Cochrane Database Syst Rev*, Vol. 24, No. 1, pp. CD001447.

Miller, R.G., Moore, D., Young, L.A., Armon, C., Barohn, R.J., Bromberg, M.B., Bryan, W.W., Gelinas, D.F., Mendoza, M.C., Neville, H.E., Parry, G.J., Petajan, J.H., Ravits, J.M., Ringel, S.P. & Ross, M.A. (1996). Placebo-controlled trial of gabapentin in patients with amyotrophic lateral sclerosis. WALS Study Group. Western Amyotrophic Lateral Sclerosis Study Group. *Neurology*, Vol. 47, No. 6, pp. 1383-1388.

Miller, R.G., Moore, D.H., 2nd, Gelinas, D.F., Dronsky, V., Mendoza, M., Barohn, R.J., Bryan, W., Ravits, J., Yuen, E., Neville, H., Ringel, S., Bromberg, M., Petajan, J., Amato, A.A., Jackson, C., Johnson, W., Mandler, R., Bosch, P., Smith, B., Graves, M., Ross, M., Sorenson, E.J., Kelkar, P., Parry, G. & Olney, R. (2001). Phase III randomized trial of gabapentin in patients with amyotrophic lateral sclerosis. *Neurology*, Vol. 56, No. 7, pp. 843-848.

Miller, R.G., Munsat, T.L., Swash, M. & Brooks, B.R. (1999). Consensus guidelines for the design and implementation of clinical trials in ALS. World Federation of Neurology committee on Research. *J Neurol Sci*, Vol. 169, No. 1-2, pp. 2-12.

Miller, R.G., Petajan, J.H., Bryan, W.W., Armon, C., Barohn, R.J., Goodpasture, J.C., Hoagland, R.J., Parry, G.J., Ross, M.A. & Stromatt, S.C. (1996). A placebo-controlled trial of recombinant human ciliary neurotrophic (rhCNTF) factor in amyotrophic lateral sclerosis. rhCNTF ALS Study Group. *Ann Neurol*, Vol. 39, No. 2, pp. 256-260.

Miller, R.G., Shepherd, R., Dao, H., Khramstov, A., Mendoza, M., Graves, J. & Smith, S. (1996). Controlled trial of nimodipine in amyotrophic lateral sclerosis. *Neuromuscul Disord*, Vol. 6, No. 2, pp. 101-104.

Miller, R.G., Smith, S.A., Murphy, J.R., Brinkmann, J.R., Graves, J., Mendoza, M., Sands, M.L. & Ringel, S.P. (1996). A clinical trial of verapamil in amyotrophic lateral sclerosis. *Muscle Nerve*, Vol. 19, No. 4, pp. 511-515.

Miller, S.C. & Warnick, J.E. (1989). Protirelin (thyrotropin-releasing hormone) in amyotrophic lateral sclerosis. The role of androgens. . *Arch Neurol*, Vol. 46, No. 3, pp. 330-335.

Mitsumoto, H. (1997). Diagnosis and progression of ALS. *Neurology*, Vol. 48, No. S4, pp. 2S-8S.

Mitsumoto, H. (Eds.). (2009). *Amyotrophic lateral sclerosis. A guide for patients and families.* (3rd), Demos Medical Publishing, New York.

Mitsumoto, H., Przedborski, S. & Gordon, P. (Eds.). (2006). *Amyotrophic Lateral Sclerosis. Current Science and Approaches to Therapy* Taylor & Francis Group, 978-0-8247-2924-0, New York.

Mitsumoto, H., Salgado, E.D., Negroski, D., Hanson, M.R., Salanga, V.D., Wilber, J.F., Wilbourn, A.J., Breuer, A.C. & Leatherman, J. (1986). Amyotrophic lateral sclerosis: effects of acute intravenous and chronic subcutaneous administration of thyrotropin-releasing hormone in controlled trials. *Neurology*, Vol. 36, No. 2, pp. 152-159.

Montanari, M. & Pessina, G. (1955). [Trypan red in therapy of amyotrophic lateral sclerosis and of myelopathic muscular atrophy]. *Rass Int Clin Ter*, Vol. 35, No. 6, pp. 197-206.

Mora, J.S., Munsat, T.L., Kao, K.P., Finison, L.J., Hedlund, W., Bradley, G.A., Scheife, R. & Georgiades, J.A. (1986). Intrathecal administration of natural human interferon alpha in amyotrophic lateral sclerosis. *Neurology*, Vol. 36, No. 8, pp. 1137-1140.

Mück-Seler, D. & Pivac, N. (2000). TCH-346 (Novartis). *IDrugs*, Vol. 3, No. 5, pp. 530-535.

Munsat, T.L., Easterday, C.S., Levy, S., Wolff, S.M. & Hiatt, R. (1981). Amantadine and guanidine are ineffective in ALS. *Neurology*, Vol. 31, No. 8, pp. 1054-1055.

Munsat, T.L., Taft, J., Jackson, I.M., Andres, P.L., Hollander, D., Skerry, L., Ordman, M., Kasdon, D. & Finison, L. (1992). Intrathecal thyrotropin-releasing hormone does not alter the progressive course of ALS: experience with an intrathecal drug delivery system. *Neurology*, Vol. 42, No. 5, pp. 1049-1053.

Nakano, I. (2000). Frontotemporal dementia with motor neuron disease (amyotrophic lateral sclerosis with dementia). *Neuropathology*, Vol. 20, No. 1, pp. 68-75.

Nandedkar, S.D., Barkhaus, P.E. & Stalberg, E.V. (2010). Motor unit number index (MUNIX): principle, method, and findings in healthy subjects and in patients with motor neuron disease. *Muscle Nerve*, Vol. 42, No. 5, pp. 798-807.

Nefussy, B., Artamonov, I., Deutsch, V., Naparstek, E., Nagler, A. & Drory, V.E. (2010). Recombinant human granulocyte-colony stimulating factor administration for treating amyotrophic lateral sclerosis: A pilot study. *Amyotroph Lateral Scler*, Vol. 11, No. 1-2, pp. 187-193.

Neuwirth, C., Nandedkar, S., Stalberg, E., Barkhaus, P.E., Carvalho, M.D., Furtula, J., Dijk, J.P., Baldinger, R., Castro, J., Costa, J., Otto, M., Sandberg, A. & Weber, M. (2011). Motor Unit Number Index (MUNIX): A novel neurophysiological marker for neuromuscular disorders; test-retest reliability in healthy volunteers. *Clin Neurophysiol*, Vol. 2011, pp. 9.

Norris, F.H., Jr., Calanchini, P.R., Fallat, R.J., Panchari, S. & Jewett, B. (1974). The administration of guanidine in amyotrophic lateral sclerosis. *Neurology*, Vol. 24, No. 8, pp. 721-728.

Norris, F.H., Jr., Fallat, R.J. & Calanchini, P.R. (1974). Increased paralysis induced by guanidine in motor neuron disease. *Neurology*, Vol. 24, No. 2, pp. 135-137.

Norris, F.H., Tan, Y., Fallat, R.J. & Elias, L. (1993). Trial of oral physostigmine in amyotrophic lateral sclerosis. *Clin Pharmacol Ther*, Vol. 54, No. 6, pp. 680-682.

Norris, L., Que, G. & Bayat, E. (2010). Psychiatric aspects of amyotrophic lateral sclerosis (ALS). *Curr Psychiatry Rep*, Vol. 12, No. 3, pp. 239-245.

Ochs, G., Penn, R.D., York, M., Giess, R., Beck, M., Tonn, J., Haigh, J., Malta, E., Traub, M., Sendtner, M. & Toyka, K.V. (2000). A phase I/II trial of recombinant methionyl human brain derived neurotrophic factor administered by intrathecal infusion to patients with amyotrophic lateral sclerosis. *Amyotroph Lateral Scler Other Motor Neuron Disord*, Vol. 1, No. 3, pp. 201-206.

Olarte, M.R., Gersten, J.C., Zabriskie, J. & Rowland, L.P. (1979). Transfer factor is ineffective in amyotrophic lateral sclerosis. *Ann Neurol*, Vol. 5, No. 4, pp. 385-388.

Olarte, M.R. & Shafer, S.Q. (1985). Levamisole is ineffective in the treatment of amyotrophic lateral sclerosis. *Neurology*, Vol. 35, No. 7, pp. 1063-1066.

Oliveira, A.S. & Pereira, R.D. (2009). Amyotrophic lateral sclerosis (ALS): three letters that change the people's life. For ever. *Arq Neuropsiquiatr*, Vol. 67, No. 3A, pp. 750-782.

Olney, N. & Rosen, H. (2010). AVP-923, a combination of dextromethorphan hydrobromide and quinidine sulfate for the treatment of pseudobulbar affect and neuropathic pain. *IDrugs*, Vol. 13, No. 4, pp. 254-265.

Olson, W.H., Simons, J.A. & Halaas, G.W. (1978). Therapeutic trial of tilorone in ALS: lack of benefit in a double-blind, placebo-controlled study. *Neurology*, Vol. 28, No. 12, pp. 1293-1295.

Orrell, R.W. (2006). AEOL-10150 (Aeolus). *Curr Opin Investig Drugs*, Vol. 7, No. 1, pp. 70-80.

Orrell, R.W., Lane, R.J. & Ross, M. (2008). A systematic review of antioxidant treatment for amyotrophic lateral sclerosis/motor neuron disease. *Amyotroph Lateral Scler*, Vol. 9, No. 4, pp. 195-211.

Pascuzzi, R.M., Shefner, J., Chappell, A.S., Bjerke, J.S., Tamura, R., Chaudhry, V., Clawson, L., Haas, L. & Rothstein, J.D. (2010). A phase II trial of talampanel in subjects with amyotrophic lateral sclerosis. *Amyotroph Lateral Scler*, Vol. 11, No. 3, pp. 266-271.

Pasinelli, P. & Brown, R.H. (2006). Molecular biology of amyotrophic lateral sclerosis: insights from genetics. *Nat Rev Neurosci*, Vol. 7, No. 9, pp. 710-723.

Patrignani, J., Proano, J. & Morales, M.D. (1992). [Treatment of amyotrophic lateral sclerosis with daily intrathecal TRH. A year's experience. Pilot study II]. *Neurologia*, Vol. 7, No. 1, pp. 4-9.

Pattee, G.L., Post, G.R., Gerber, R.E. & Bennett, J.P., Jr. (2003). Reduction of oxidative stress in amyotrophic lateral sclerosis following pramipexole treatment. *Amyotroph Lateral Scler Other Motor Neuron Disord*, Vol. 4, No. 2, pp. 90-95.

Percy, A.K., Davis, L.E., Johnston, D.M. & Drachman, D.B. (1971). Failure of isoprinosine in amyotropic lateral sclerosis. *N Engl J Med*, Vol. 285, No. 12, pp. 689.

Phukan, J. (2010). Arimoclomol, a coinducer of heat shock proteins for the potential treatment of amyotrophic lateral sclerosis. *IDrugs*, Vol. 13, No. 7, pp. 482-496.

Piepers, S., Veldink, J.H., de Jong, S.W., van der Tweel, I., van der Pol, W.L., Uijtendaal, E.V., Schelhaas, H.J., Scheffer, H., de Visser, M., de Jong, J.M., Wokke, J.H., Groeneveld, G.J. & van den Berg, L.H. (2009). Randomized sequential trial of valproic acid in amyotrophic lateral sclerosis. *Ann Neurol*, Vol. 66, No. 2, pp. 227-234.

Pradat, P.F., Attarian, S., Camdessanche, J.P., Carluer, L., Cintas, P., Corcia, P., Echaniz-Laguna, A., Gonzalez-Bermejo, J., Guy, N., Nicolas, G., Perez, T., Soriani, M.H., Vandenberghe, N. & Verschueren, A. (2010). [Research in amyotrophic lateral sclerosis: what is new in 2009?]. *Rev Neurol (Paris)*, Vol. 166, No. 8-9, pp. 683-698.

Rapport, M.M. (1990). Implications of altered brain ganglioside profiles in amyotrophic lateral sclerosis (ALS). *Acta Neurobiol Exp (Wars)*, Vol. 50, No. 4-5, pp. 505-513.

Rivera, V.M., Grabois, M., Deaton, W., Breitbach, W. & Hines, M. (1980). Modified snake venom in amyotrophic lateral sclerosis. Lack of clinical effectiveness. *Arch Neurol*, Vol. 37, No. 4, pp. 201-203.

Robberecht, W. (2002). Genetics of familial amyotrophic lateral sclerosis and ethical aspects, In: *Motor Neuron Disease*, Kuncl, R.W. (Eds.), pp. 75-93, Saunders, Philadelphia, PA.

Rodrigues, C.M., Spellman, S.R., Sola, S., Grande, A.W., Linehan-Stieers, C., Low, W.C. & Steer, C.J. (2002). Neuroprotection by a bile acid in an acute stroke model in the rat. *J Cereb Blood Flow Metab*, Vol. 22, No. 4, pp. 463-471.

Rosenbloom, A.L. (2009). Mecasermin (recombinant human insulin-like growth factor I). *Adv Ther*, Vol. 26, No. 1, pp. 40-54.

Rosenfeld, J., King, R.M., Jackson, C.E., Bedlack, R.S., Barohn, R.J., Dick, A., Phillips, L.H., Chapin, J., Gelinas, D.F. & Lou, J.S. (2008). Creatine monohydrate in ALS: effects on strength, fatigue, respiratory status and ALSFRS. *Amyotroph Lateral Scler*, Vol. 9, No. 5, pp. 266-272.

Ross, E. (2009). Unapproved drug use: compassionate or cause for concern? *Lancet Neurol*, Vol. 8, No. 2, pp. 136-137.

Ross, M.A., Miller, R.G., Berchert, L., Parry, G., Barohn, R.J., Armon, C., Bryan, W.W., Petajan, J., Stromatt, S., Goodpasture, J. & McGuire, D. (1998). Toward earlier diagnosis of amyotrophic lateral sclerosis: revised criteria. rhCNTF ALS Study Group. *Neurology*, Vol. 50, No. 3, pp. 768-772.

Rowland, L.P. (2001). How amyotrophic lateral sclerosis got its name: the clinical-pathologic genius of Jean-Martin Charcot. *Arch Neurol*, Vol. 58, No. 3, pp. 512-515.

Rowland, L.P. (2009). T.L. Bunina, Asao Hirano, and the post mortem cellular diagnosis of amyotrophic lateral sclerosis. *Amyotroph Lateral Scler*, Vol. 10, No. 2, pp. 74-78.

Ryberg, H., Askmark, H. & Persson, L.I. (2003). A double-blind randomized clinical trial in amyotrophic lateral sclerosis using lamotrigine: effects on CSF glutamate, aspartate, branched-chain amino acid levels and clinical parameters. *Acta Neurol Scand*, Vol. 108, No. 1, pp. 1-8.

Sacca, F., Quarantelli, M., Rinaldi, C., Tucci, T., Piro, R., Perrotta, G., Carotenuto, B., Marsili, A., Palma, V., De Michele, G., Brunetti, A., Brescia Morra, V., Filla, A. & Salvatore, M. (2011). A randomized controlled clinical trial of growth hormone in amyotrophic lateral sclerosis: clinical, neuroimaging, and hormonal results. *J Neurol*, Vol. 2011, pp. [Epub ahead of print].

Sathasivam, S. (2010). Motor neurone disease: clinical features, diagnosis, diagnostic pitfalls and prognostic markers. *Singapore Med J*, Vol. 51, No. 5, pp. 367-372; quiz 373.

Sathasivam, S., Ince, P.G. & Shaw, P.J. (2001). Apoptosis in amyotrophic lateral sclerosis: a review of the evidence. *Neuropathol Appl Neurobiol*, Vol. 27, No. 4, pp. 257-274.

Scelsa, S.N., MacGowan, D.J., Mitsumoto, H., Imperato, T., LeValley, A.J., Liu, M.H., DelBene, M. & Kim, M.Y. (2005). A pilot, double-blind, placebo-controlled trial of indinavir in patients with ALS. *Neurology*, Vol. 64, No. 7, pp. 1298-1300.

Schwob, R.A. & Bonduelle, M. (1952). [Trypan blue and trypan red in the treatment of amyotrophic lateral sclerosis; application to the treatment of multiple sclerosis]. *Sem Hop*, Vol. 28, No. 39, pp. 1637-1642.

Scott, S., Kranz, J.E., Cole, J., Lincecum, J.M., Thompson, K., Kelly, N., Bostrom, A., Theodoss, J., Al-Nakhala, B.M., Vieira, F.G., Ramasubbu, J. & Heywood, J.A. (2008). Design, power, and interpretation of studies in the standard murine model of ALS. *Amyotroph Lateral Scler*, Vol. 9, No. 1, pp. 4-15.

Serratrice, G., Desnuelle, C., Guelton, C., Meyer-Dutour, A., Richard, P., Braguer, D. & Crevat, A. (1985). [Trial of thyrotropin-releasing factor in amyotrophic lateral sclerosis]. *Presse Med*, Vol. 14, No. 8, pp. 487-488.

Shefner, J.M., Cudkowicz, M.E., Schoenfeld, D., Conrad, T., Taft, J., Chilton, M., Urbinelli, L., Qureshi, M., Zhang, H., Pestronk, A., Caress, J., Donofrio, P., Sorenson, E., Bradley, W., Lomen-Hoerth, C., Pioro, E., Rezania, K., Ross, M., Pascuzzi, R., Heiman-Patterson, T., Tandan, R., Mitsumoto, H., Rothstein, J., Smith-Palmer, T., MacDonald, D. & Burke, D. (2004). A clinical trial of creatine in ALS. *Neurology*, Vol. 63, No. 9, pp. 1656-1661.

Shefner, J.M., Watson, M.L., Simionescu, L., Caress, J.B., Burns, T.M., Maragakis, N.J., Benatar, M., David, W.S., Sharma, K.R. & Rutkove, S.B. (2011). Multipoint incremental motor unit number estimation as an outcome measure in ALS. *Neurology*, Vol. 2011, No. [epub ahead of print], pp. 15.

Shi, P., Gal, J., Kwinter, D.M., Liu, X. & Zhu, H. (2010). Mitochondrial dysfunction in amyotrophic lateral sclerosis. *Biochim Biophys Acta*, Vol. 1802, No. 1, pp. 45-51.

Siciliano, G., Carlesi, C., Pasquali, L., Piazza, S., Pietracupa, S., Fornai, F., Ruggieri, S. & Murri, L. (2010). Clinical trials for neuroprotection in ALS. *CNS Neurol Disord Drug Targets*, Vol. 9, No. 3, pp. 305-313.

Silani, V., Meininger, V. & Fornai, F. (2011). Introducing Amyotrophic lateral sclerosis. *Arch Ital Biol*, Vol. 149, No. 1, pp. 1-4.

Silani, V., Messina, S., Poletti, B., Morelli, C., Doretti, A., Ticozzi, N. & Maderna, L. (2011). The diagnosis of Amyotrophic lateral sclerosis in 2010. *Arch Ital Biol*, Vol. 149, No. 1, pp. 5-27.

Silani, V., Perini, M., Fayoumi, Z.M. & Scarlato, G. (1983). Naloxone of no benefit in amyotrophic lateral sclerosis. *Ann Neurol*, Vol. 13, No. 2, pp. 222.

Sleegers, K., Cruts, M. & Van Broeckhoven, C. (2010). Molecular pathways of frontotemporal lobar degeneration. *Annu Rev Neurosci*, Vol. 33, pp. 71-88.

Smith, R.A., Miller, T.M., Yamanaka, K., Monia, B.P., Condon, T.P., Hung, G., Lobsiger, C.S., Ward, C.M., McAlonis-Downes, M., Wei, H., Wancewicz, E.V., Bennett, C.F. & Cleveland, D.W. (2006). Antisense oligonucleotide therapy for neurodegenerative disease. *J Clin Invest*, Vol. 116, No. 8, pp. 2290-2296.

Sorenson, E.J., Windbank, A.J., Mandrekar, J.N., Bamlet, W.R., Appel, S.H., Armon, C., Barkhaus, P.E., Bosch, P., Boylan, K., David, W.S., Feldman, E., Glass, J., Gutmann, L., Katz, J., King, W., Luciano, C.A., McCluskey, L.F., Nash, S., Newman, D.S., Pascuzzi, R.M., Pioro, E., Sams, L.J., Scelsa, S., Simpson, E.P., Subramony, S.H., Tiryaki, E. & Thornton, C.A. (2008). Subcutaneous IGF-1 is not beneficial in 2-year ALS trial. *Neurology*, Vol. 71, No. 22, pp. 1770-1775.

Stober, T., Schimrigk, K., Dietzsch, S. & Thielen, T. (1985). Intrathecal thyrotropin-releasing hormone therapy of amyotrophic lateral sclerosis. *J Neurol*, Vol. 232, No. 1, pp. 13-14.

Stommel, E.W., Cohen, J.A., Fadul, C.E., Cogbill, C.H., Graber, D.J., Kingman, L., Mackenzie, T., Channon Smith, J.Y. & Harris, B.T. (2009). Efficacy of thalidomide for the treatment of amyotrophic lateral sclerosis: a phase II open label clinical trial. *Amyotroph Lateral Scler*, Vol. 10, No. 5-6, pp. 393-404.

Szulc-Kuberska, J., Klimek, A., Stepien, H. & Woszczak, M. (1990). [Clinical trial of the treatment of amyotrophic lateral sclerosis with bromocriptine]. *Neurol Neurochir Pol*, Vol. 24, No. 1-2, pp. 37-41.

Takahashi, R. (2009). Edaravone in ALS. *Exp Neurol*, Vol. 217, No. 2, pp. 235-236.

Tandan, R., Bromberg, M.B., Forshew, D., Fries, T.J., Badger, G.J., Carpenter, J., Krusinski, P.B., Betts, E.F., Arciero, K. & Nau, K. (1996). A controlled trial of amino acid therapy in amyotrophic lateral sclerosis: I. Clinical, functional, and maximum isometric torque data. *Neurology*, Vol. 47, No. 5, pp. 1220-1226.

Thatte, U. & Dahanukar, S. (1997). Apoptosis: clinical relevance and pharmacological manipulation. *Drugs*, Vol. 54, No. 4, pp. 511-532.

The ALS CNTF treatment study (ACTS) phase I-II Study Group. (1996). The Amyotrophic Lateral Sclerosis Functional Rating Scale. Assessment of activities of daily living in patients with amyotrophic lateral sclerosis. . *Arch Neurol*, Vol. 53, No. 2, pp. 141-147.

The BDNF Study Group (Phase III). (1999). A controlled trial of recombinant methionyl human BDNF in ALS. *Neurology*, Vol. 52, No. 7, pp. 1427-1433.

Thielen, T., Stober, T. & Schimrigk, K. (1987). Therapeutic trial of intrathecal thyrotropin-releasing hormone (TRH) and a TRH-analogue in amyotrophic lateral sclerosis (ALS). *Adv Exp Med Biol*, Vol. 209, pp. 305-308.

Ticozzi, N., Tiloca, C., Morelli, C., Colombrita, C., Poletti, B., Doretti, A., Maderna, L., Messina, S., Ratti, A. & Silani, V. (2011). Genetics of familial Amyotrophic lateral sclerosis. *Arch Ital Biol*, Vol. 149, No. 1, pp. 65-82.

Traynor, B.J., Alexander, M., Corr, B., Frost, E. & Hardiman, O. (2003). An outcome study of riluzole in amyotrophic lateral sclerosis--a population-based study in Ireland, 1996-2000. *J Neurol*, Vol. 250, No. 4, pp. 473-479.

Traynor, B.J., Bruijn, L., Conwit, R., Beal, F., O'Neill, G., Fagan, S.C. & Cudkowicz, M.E. (2006). Neuroprotective agents for clinical trials in ALS: a systematic assessment. *Neurology*, Vol. 67, No. 1, pp. 20-27.

Tsujimoto, M., Senda, J., Ishihara, T., Niimi, Y., Kawai, Y., Atsuta, N., Watanabe, H., Tanaka, F., Naganawa, S. & Sobue, G. (2011). Behavioral changes in early ALS correlate with voxel-based morphometry and diffusion tensor imaging. *J Neurol Sci*, Vol. 307, No. 1-2, pp. 34-40.

Turner, M.R., Grosskreutz, J., Kassubek, J., Abrahams, S., Agosta, F., Benatar, M., Filippi, M., Goldstein, L.H., van den Heuvel, M., Kalra, S., Lule, D. & Mohammadi, B. (2011). Towards a neuroimaging biomarker for amyotrophic lateral sclerosis. *Lancet Neurol*, Vol. 10, No. 5, pp. 400-403.

Valentine, J.S., Doucette, P.A. & Zittin Potter, S. (2005). Copper-zinc superoxide dismutase and amyotrophic lateral sclerosis. *Annu Rev Biochem*, Vol. 74, pp. 563-593.

van der Meer, J.W. & Simon, A. (2010). Blocking IL-1beta to slow down progression of ALS? *Proc Natl Acad Sci U S A*, Vol. 107, No. 29, pp. 12741-12742.

Veldink, J.H., Kalmijn, S., Groeneveld, G.J., Wunderink, W., Koster, A., de Vries, J.H., van der Luyt, J., Wokke, J.H. & Van den Berg, L.H. (2007). Intake of polyunsaturated fatty acids and vitamin E reduces the risk of developing amyotrophic lateral sclerosis. *J Neurol Neurosurg Psychiatry*, Vol. 78, No. 4, pp. 367-371.

von Haehling, S., Stepney, R. & Anker, S.D. (2010). Advances in understanding and treating cardiac cachexia: highlights from the 5th Cachexia Conference. *Int J Cardiol*, Vol. 144, No. 3, pp. 347-349.

Wang, H., Larriviere, K.S., Keller, K.E., Ware, K.A., Burns, T.M., Conaway, M.A., Lacomis, D., Pattee, G.L., Phillips, L.H., 2nd, Solenski, N.J., Zivkovic, S.A. & Bennett, J.P., Jr. (2008). R+ pramipexole as a mitochondrially focused neuroprotectant: initial early phase studies in ALS. *Amyotroph Lateral Scler*, Vol. 9, No. 1, pp. 50-58.

Weber, M., Goldman, B. & Truniger, S. (2010). Tetrahydrocannabinol (THC) for cramps in amyotrophic lateral sclerosis: a randomised, double-blind crossover trial. *J Neurol Neurosurg Psychiatry*, Vol. 81, No. 10, pp. 1135-1140.

Welty, D.F., Schielke, G.P. & Rothstein, J.D. (1995). Potential treatment of amyotrophic lateral sclerosis with gabapentin: a hypothesis. *Ann Pharmacother*, Vol. 29, No. 11, pp. 1164-1167.

Werdelin, L., Boysen, G., Jensen, T.S. & Mogensen, P. (1990). Immunosuppressive treatment of patients with amyotrophic lateral sclerosis. *Acta Neurol Scand*, Vol. 82, No. 2, pp. 132-134.

Westarp, M.E., Bartmann, P., Rossler, J., Geiger, E., Westphal, K.P., Schreiber, H., Fuchs, D., Westarp, M.P. & Kornhuber, H.H. (1993). Antiretroviral therapy in sporadic adult amyotrophic lateral sclerosis. *Neuroreport*, Vol. 4, No. 6, pp. 819-822.

Weydt, P. & Moller, T. (2005). Neuroinflammation in the pathogenesis of amyotrophic lateral sclerosis. *Neuroreport*, Vol. 16, No. 6, pp. 527-531.

Wijesekera, L.C. & Leigh, P.N. (2009). Amyotrophic lateral sclerosis. *Orphanet J Rare Dis*, Vol. 4, No. 3, pp. 3.

Williams, M.T., Donnelly, J.P., Holmlund, T. & Battaglia, M. (2008). ALS: Family caregiver needs and quality of life. *Amyotroph Lateral Scler*, Vol. 9, No. 5, pp. 279-286.

Witgert, M., Salamone, A.R., Strutt, A.M., Jawaid, A., Massman, P.J., Bradshaw, M., Mosnik, D., Appel, S.H. & Schulz, P.E. (2009). Frontal-lobe mediated behavioral dysfunction in amyotrophic lateral sclerosis. *Eur J Neurol*, Vol. 17, No. 1, pp. 103-110.

Woolley, S.C. & Jonathan, S.K. (2008). Cognitive and behavioral impairment in amyotrophic lateral sclerosis. *Phys Med Rehabil Clin N Am*, Vol. 19, No. 3, pp. 607-617, xi.

Worrall, B.B., Rowland, L.P., Chin, S.S. & Mastrianni, J.A. (2000). Amyotrophy in prion diseases. *Arch Neurol*, Vol. 57, No. 1, pp. 33-38.

Yamane, K., Osawa, M., Kobayashi, I. & Maruyama, S. (1986). Treatment of amyotrophic lateral sclerosis with thyrotropin-releasing hormone (TRH). *Jpn J Psychiatry Neurol*, Vol. 40, No. 2, pp. 179-187.

Yase, Y., Matsumoto, N., Azuma, K., Nakai, Y. & Shiraki, H. (1972). Amyotrophic lateral sclerosis. Association with schizophrenic symptoms and showing Alzheimer's tangles. *Arch Neurol*, Vol. 27, No. 2, pp. 118-128.

Yoshida, M. (2004). Amyotrophic lateral sclerosis with dementia: the clinicopathological spectrum. *Neuropathology*, Vol. 24, No. 1, pp. 87-102.

Yoshino, H. & Kimura, A. (2006). Investigation of the therapeutic effects of edaravone, a free radical scavenger, on amyotrophic lateral sclerosis (Phase II study). *Amyotroph Lateral Scler*, Vol. 7, No. 4, pp. 241-245.

Zago, S., Poletti, B., Morelli, C., Doretti, A. & Silani, V. (2011). Amyotrophic lateral sclerosis and frontotemporal dementia (ALS-FTD). *Arch Ital Biol*, Vol. 149, No. 1, pp. 39-56.

Zhang, Y., Wang, L., Fu, Y., Song, H., Zhao, H., Deng, M., Zhang, J. & Fan, D. (2009). Preliminary investigation of effect of granulocyte colony stimulating factor on amyotrophic lateral sclerosis. *Amyotroph Lateral Scler*, Vol. 10, No. 5-6, pp. 430-431.

Zinman, L. & Cudkowicz, M. (2011). Emerging targets and treatments in amyotrophic lateral sclerosis. *Lancet Neurol*, Vol. 10, No. 5, pp. 481-490.

Zoccolella, S., Beghi, E., Palagano, G., Fraddosio, A., Guerra, V., Samarelli, V., Lepore, V., Simone, I.L., Lamberti, P., Serlenga, L. & Logroscino, G. (2007). Riluzole and amyotrophic lateral sclerosis survival: a population-based study in southern Italy. *Eur J Neurol*, Vol. 14, No. 3, pp. 262-268.

Zoccolella, S., Santamato, A. & Lamberti, P. (2009). Current and emerging treatments for amyotrophic lateral sclerosis. *Neuropsychiatr Dis Treat*, Vol. 5, pp. 577-595.

2

Insights Arising from Gene Expression Profiling in Amyotrophic Lateral Sclerosis

Johnathan Cooper-Knock, Joanna J. Bury, Laura Ferraiuolo, Emily F. Goodall, Pamela J. Shaw and Janine Kirby
Sheffield Institute for Translational Neuroscience, University of Sheffield, Sheffield, United Kingdom

1. Introduction

Gene expression profiling has been used extensively in multiple fields of research to compare disease and control samples, to investigate mechanisms of disease, to identify subtypes within a heterogeneous clinical phenotype and to establish responses to a specific treatment. In addition, it can also be used to determine the function of a gene, to monitor changes over time, or for discovering cell specific expression or responses.

This chapter will initially explain the principles of gene expression profiling, before discussing the sources of samples, along with their advantages and limitations, and will then summarise the research to date regarding the application of gene expression profiling to amyotrophic lateral sclerosis (ALS).

2. What is gene expression profiling?

The primary application of gene expression profiling is to use a glass slide containing oligonucleotides or cDNA sequences, termed a microarray, to quantify the amount of individual RNA transcripts that are present in a particular cell or tissue. RNA is extracted, fluorescently labelled and then hybridized to the microarray. A linear amplification step can also be performed prior to labelling to ensure sufficient RNA is generated from low yields of RNA extracted from small sample sizes. The quantity of labelled RNA binding to each oligonucleotide or cDNA sequence on the microarray determines the intensity of fluorescence at that location and thus allows quantification of the RNA transcripts in the initial sample (Stoughton 2005).

Comparison of the expression of transcripts between sample groups allows identification of transcripts which are differentially expressed between the groups. The large number of genes simultaneously interrogated by a microarray means that the resulting data are amenable to study the expression of inter-related clusters of genes such as those involved in known functional categories or specific pathways. Changes in expression level of a particular gene do not take into account regulation at the level of translation. However, the functional impact of a differentially expressed gene can be subsequently established by assaying the encoded protein expression or function.

The advent of next generation sequencing, and specifically the sequencing of all RNA molecules in a quantitative manner, has recently become an alternative, though expensive method for measuring levels of gene expression. However, this has the potential to add further knowledge and value to the application of gene expression profiling to disease.

3. Uses of gene expression profiling

Quantification of the transcriptome has been a useful mechanism for both discovering and defining mechanisms of pathogenesis in ALS (Cox et al 2010; Ferraiuolo et al 2007; Kirby et al 2005; Kirby et al 2011). In particular lists of differentially expressed genes can be usefully converted to functional 'themes' by an enrichment analysis (Hosack et al 2003). Various categorisations exist, including the gene ontology (GO) and Kyoto encyclopaedia of genes and genomes (KEGG), which classify genes according to molecular function, biological process, cellular component or a known biological pathway.

A frequent application of gene expression profiling has been the development of putative biomarkers via a supervised classification approach (Booij et al 2011; Nagasaka et al 2005; Scherzer et al 2007). The large number of targets quantified simultaneously by gene expression profiling is essential for biomarker discovery, as it allows an unbiased survey of the most informative RNA transcripts. A reliable biomarker(s) for defining pathogenesis and prognosis in ALS has yet to be established, though gene expression profiling is one of the methodologies currently being used to establish an ALS biomarker(s).

4. Sources of material for studying ALS

In ALS, the vulnerable cells are the motor neurones, located in the motor cortex, brainstem and spinal cord. Since motor neurones cannot be sampled during life, model systems, such as neuronal-like cells in culture and animals carrying mutant transgenes, have been used to study the neurodegenerative process. In addition to sampling post-mortem material from patients, peripheral tissue from living patients (and neurologically normal controls) has been used as a source material for applying gene expression profiling to ALS.

4.1 Cellular models of ALS

Neuronal cell lines, both human (e.g. SH-SY5Y) and rodent (e.g. PC12), have been used as a model to investigate mechanisms of neurodegeneration. However, one of the most widely used cellular models for examining the molecular pathophysiology underpinning the neurodegenerative disease process in ALS is the mouse spinal cord/neuroblastoma cell line NSC-34 (Cashman et al 1992). Immortalized NSC-34 cells recapitulate many of the characteristics of motor neurones whilst maintaining their ability to proliferate in culture; thus providing a continual resource of motor neurone-like cells (Cashman et al 1992; Durham et al 1993). In particular, they have proved a robust model of mutant copper zinc superoxide dismutase-1 (*SOD1*) associated familial ALS (FALS), as they can be transfected with vectors carrying normal or mutant forms of the human *SOD1* gene (Durham et al 1997; Menzies et al 2002a; Menzies et al 2002b). Cellular models of TDP-43-related ALS, caused by mutation of the TAR DNA binding protein gene (*TARDBP*) are being generated (Duan et al 2010; Igaz et al 2009), though sustained over-expression of the wild-type and mutant proteins is proving problematic due to the toxicity of both the wild-type and mutant over-expressed proteins and the tight auto-regulation of TDP-43 (Budini & Buratti 2011).

Gene expression profiling of cell lines transfected with ALS associated genes provides a genetically homogenous cell population uncontaminated by non-neuronal astrocytes and other types of glial cells, which are present in the central nervous system (CNS). Furthermore, environmental conditions can easily be manipulated and tightly controlled *in vitro* so as to reduce the impact of external confounding factors on gene expression. The limitations of this type of model system include the fact that NSC-34 cell lines (or other neuronal cell lines) are continually dividing cells, rather than post-mitotic cells and they are unable to mirror the effects of cellular interactions that occur between the different cell populations *in situ* (Kirby et al 2011).

Primary neuronal and astrocytic cells can be isolated from embryonic mice and short-term cultures generated for microarray analysis. These cells more closely mirror those present in the CNS, though the primary neuronal cultures, as they are post-mitotic cells, have a limited lifespan of 7-10 days. In contrast, cultured primary astrocytes are able to proliferate in culture. Whilst co-cultures or separated co-cultures allow a degree of interaction between the two cell types, these types of mixed cultures have not yet been used for microarray analysis in ALS.

4.2 Animal models of ALS

Transgenic mice expressing mutant forms of ALS-related genes provide a source of RNA for microarray analysis. For investigating the mechanisms of *SOD1*-related neurodegeneration, mice over-expressing the human p.G93A or mouse p.G86R mutant forms of the SOD1 protein ($SOD1^{G93A}$ or $SOD1^{G86R}$) have been used as they develop an age dependent neuromuscular condition; the motor function symptoms and histopathological features have been extensively characterised and resemble those observed in both *SOD1*-related ALS and classical ALS patients (Gurney et al 1994; Ripps et al 1995). In contrast, over-expression of wild-type human SOD1 ($SOD1^{WT}$) does not produce an overt motor phenotype, supporting a toxic gain of function by the mutant SOD1 protein as the mechanism by which the mutant proteins cause cell death. In contrast, mouse models over-expressing either wild-type or mutant TDP-43 show a neurodegenerative phenotype (Igaz et al 2011; Stallings et al 2010).

One of the major advantages of using animal models for microarray analysis is the ability to examine animals at different ages in order to investigate the progression of disease, an approach that is unattainable in human post-mortem tissue. Valuable insights regarding onset of disease can be established in pre-symptomatic and early symptomatic disease stages since these represent time points at which the identification of key novel targets for therapeutic intervention could be best placed to rescue vulnerable neuronal cell populations before the development of irreversible neuronal injury (Ferraiuolo et al 2007). In addition, sampling of specific cell types from the CNS allow gene expression changes to be identified which include the effects of interactions with neighbouring cells.

Backcrossing of the $SOD1^{WT}$ and $SOD1^{G93A}$ mice with C57Bl6 mice has led to the formation of $SOD1^{WT}$ and $SOD1^{G93A}$ mice on a homogeneous background (Ferraiuolo et al 2007). The use of these mice for microarray analysis and the use of non-transgenic littermates as controls have proven effective in reducing inter-individual genetic variability to ensure the generation of consistent and reliable gene expression data.

4.3 Human post-mortem material

Human post-mortem brain and spinal cord specimens derived from clinically and pathologically confirmed cases of ALS can be used in comparisons with age, gender and ethnically matched neurologically normal controls and are a pivotal source of RNA for gene expression profiling in ALS. Brain and spinal cord represent the tissues that are most susceptible to the underlying neurodegenerative disease process. However, there are a number of limitations that should be taken into account when using this tissue. First and foremost, the transcriptional changes that are detected are reflecting the terminal stage of disease, with the majority of vulnerable neuronal cells having already undergone cell death (Sharp et al 2006). Therefore, it can be difficult to distinguish whether the changes detected are due to the survival response in the remaining cells, initiation of a cell death pathway (if the cells are beginning to die), or whether the changes are present in response to a pathogenic trigger (Lederer et al 2007). Secondly, samples, and particularly control material, are difficult to obtain and often in short supply. This restricts the sample sizes that can be used, which has a negative impact upon the statistical power of such studies. Considerable heterogeneity exists between individuals in disease and control groups and gene expression changes may also be influenced by post-mortem interval, variability in brain pH, degree of neuroinflammation and sample type including white versus grey matter or cortical motor neurones versus spinal motor neurones. Furthermore, *ex vivo* RNA degradation, particularly during sample preparation, should also be taken into consideration (Maes et al 2007).

RNA extraction protocols are faster and more straightforward for whole tissue homogenates. However, the inclusion of a heterogeneous mixture of cell populations may in effect blur the distinctive profile emanating from the neuronal cells that are most affected in ALS (Kirby et al 2011). In comparing the gene expression profiles generated from diseased tissue to that of healthy controls there is also the added issue of a shift in the proportion of different cell populations within the sample as neurodegeneration is characterised by the loss of motor neurones and the active proliferation of non-neuronal microglia and macrophages (Dangond et al 2004). Laser capture microdissection (LCM) may be a more expensive and laborious technique but is beneficial in studying a neuronal enriched cell population (Jiang et al 2005). It also is noteworthy that in comparison to primary cultures these cells have had the benefit of being embedded within their natural environment where physiologically relevant cross talk has taken place with neighbouring cells and tissues (Ferraiuolo et al 2007).

4.4 Human peripheral tissue samples

Peripheral tissue such as whole venous blood, cultured skin fibroblasts and muscle biopsy material offer an attractive and readily accessible resource for microarray analysis in ALS. Samples can be collected longitudinally, particularly as the collection of blood is relatively non-invasive and sampling techniques can be standardized across research centres (Highley et al 2011; Saris et al 2009; Shtilbans et al 2011; Tsuang et al 2005).

Blood is classified as a fluid connective tissue composed of plasma (55%), erythrocytes (43%), leukocytes (0.5%) and platelets (1.5%) which continuously permeates and interacts with every other tissue and organ of the mammalian body. It is in a permanent state of renewal and is known to play a pivotal role in physiological homeostasis, cellular immunity and inflammation (Mohr & Liew 2007). Since 80% of the genes routinely expressed within the CNS have also been detectable in circulating blood cells it is anticipated that there are quantifiable changes in the levels of these gene transcripts which have the potential to act as a sentinel of disease (Liew et al 2006). Evidence suggests that the shear abundance of endogenous alpha and beta globin messenger RNA (mRNA), which constitutes up to 70% of

erythrocytic mRNA transcripts, masks the expression of less abundant genes of potential biological significance as a result of their high signal intensity on the microarray (Wright et al 2008). Thus, strategies have been developed and evaluated to remove these transcripts present in the RNA samples from whole blood (Liu et al 2006). Alternatively, fractionation of peripheral blood mononuclear cells (PBMCs) can also be used though the additional processing steps involved in isolating the PBMCs can introduce spurious artifactual alterations in gene expression that are not attributable to the disease (Whitney et al 2003).
Fibroblasts are not known to have any direct involvement in ALS, though they provide a model with the genetic background of the individual and have the added value of being a source for the generation of induced pluripotent stem cells (iPS) or for the direct manipulation into motor neuronal cells (Dimos et al 2008; Son et al 2011). In addition, fibroblasts have been shown to reflect changes in patients with neurodegenerative disease (Aguirre et al 1998; Hoepken et al 2008; Mortiboys et al 2008) and their gene expression profiles distinguish pre-symptomatic individuals from those of controls (Nagasaka et al 2005). In contrast to fibroblasts, skeletal muscle is severely affected by the disease. Whilst muscle biopsies are the most invasive sample to collect, they are a useful source for gene expression profiling, as they provide a window into the mechanisms involved in the neuromuscular degeneration that occur in ALS during life (Dadon-Nachum et al 2011; Dupuis & Loeffler 2009).

5. Results from use of cellular models of ALS

Gene expression profiling of the widely used NSC34 cellular model of *SOD1*-related FALS identified a marked degree of transcriptional repression in the presence of the $SOD1^{G93A}$ mutation (Kirby et al 2005). These repressed genes included a group of antioxidant response (ARE) genes or "programmed cell life" genes that are regulated by the Nrf2 transcription factor (Figure 1). Reduced expression of *Nrf2* and selected downstream targets was seen at both the RNA and protein levels in the cellular model and *NRF2* dysregulation was also demonstrated in isolated motor neurones from *SOD1*-related ALS cases. Subsequent work by Sarlette and colleagues has shown that *NRF2* transcription and translation is also decreased in SALS cases (Sarlette et al 2008). Most recently, it has been demonstrated that activation of *Nrf2* in NSC34 *SOD1*-related ALS cell models, primary motor neurone and astrocyte co-cultures and in the $SOD1^{G93A}$ mouse model all improve neuronal survival (Neymotin et al 2011; Vargas et al 2008a).
Primary astrocyte cultures prepared from mutant SOD1 rodent models have been shown to increase motor neuronal death in co-cultures (Nagai et al 2007; Vargas et al 2006). To investigate this effect, gene expression profiling was performed on RNA isolated from astrocyte cultures generated from $SOD1^{G93A}$ rats (and litter mate controls). Perhaps surprisingly, there were limited differences in the transcriptional profiles of transgenic and non-transgenic astrocytes (Vargas et al 2008b). However, of the two genes most dysregulated, regulator of differentiation (*Rod1*) and decorin (*Dcn*), both showed consistent changes in asymptomatic and early symptomatic rats, implicating components of RNA processing and the extracellular matrix as contributors early in the disease process (Figure 1).
Primary neuronal cultures originating from $SOD1^{G93A}$ mice and subjected to oxidative stress (H_2O_2) or excitotoxicity (NMDA), demonstrated a greater level of cell death, compared to non-transgenic cultures (Boutahar et al 2011). Microarray analysis detected cytoskeletal remodelling and vesicular transport related genes as increased in response to oxidative

stress, whilst genes involved in the ubiquitin-proteasome system and cytokines were increased following excitotoxicity (Figure 1). Several of these pathways have already been implicated as playing a pathogenic role in ALS and add further support to the idea that the proposed disease mechanisms are mutually compatible.

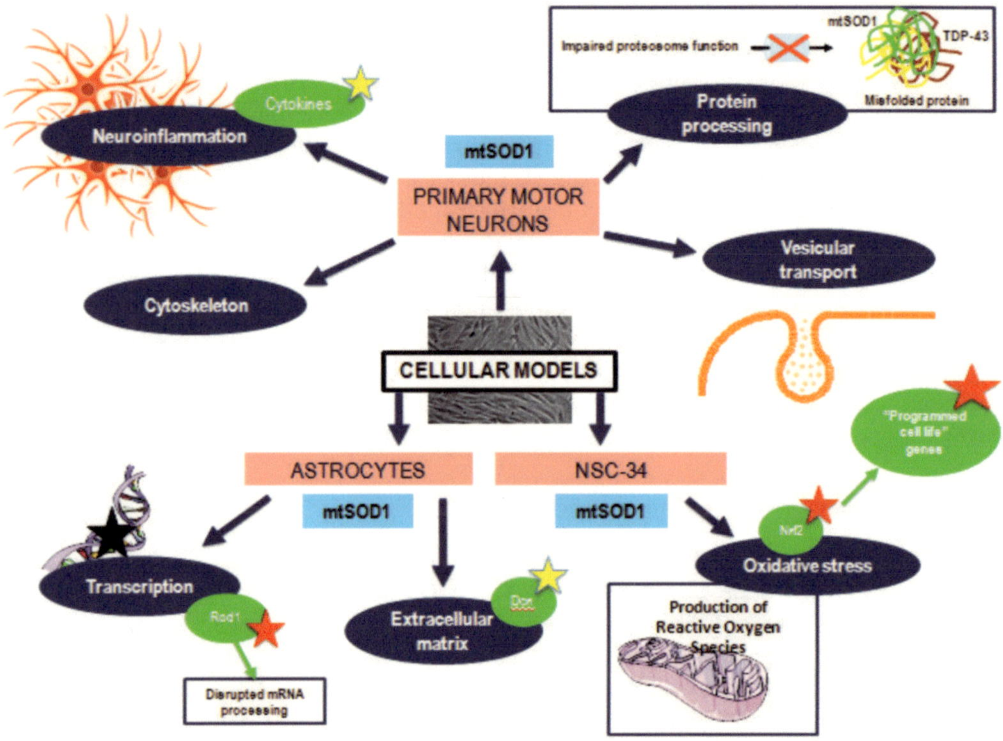

Fig. 1. Summary of prominent pathways arising from GEP of Cellular Models. Important changes in the transcriptome have been highlighted by green labels; yellow stars indicate up-regulation, red stars indicate down-regulation. Blue squares outline functional consequences of changes in the transcriptome. Further details are discussed in the text.

6. Results from use of animal models of ALS

6.1 Gene expression profiling of mixed cell type CNS samples

Microarray analysis of whole spinal cord homogenates from ALS mouse models have been performed by several research groups in order to obtain a global view of changes in the CNS prior to and during disease. Results from $SOD1^{G93A}$ mice have shown that inflammation, apoptosis and adaptive responses to metal ion dysregulation are the main pathways activated in both pre-symptomatic mice and during the disease process (Olsen et al 2001; Yoshihara et al 2002) (Figure 2). Analysis of the $SOD1^{L126delTT}$ transgenic mouse, which results in a truncated SOD1 protein, also showed pre-symptomatic changes related to the reactive gliosis which is occurring in the spinal cord (Fukada et al 2007).

Recently, transgenic mice carrying mutant TDP-43 have also contributed to better understanding the different mechanisms involved in ALS. Transgenic mice induced to express human TDP-43 without the nuclear localization signal (hTDP43-delNLS) developed signs of motor spasticity, neurone loss in forebrain regions and corticospinal tract degeneration (Igaz et al 2011). Microarray analysis of hTDP43-delNLS expression in the cortex of mutant mice, following 2 weeks induction of the mutant protein, detected dramatic changes in gene expression, with the most enriched pathway being chromatin assembly (Figure 2). Interestingly, after only 2 weeks of hTDP43-delNLS induction, markers of inflammation and neuronal loss were unchanged.

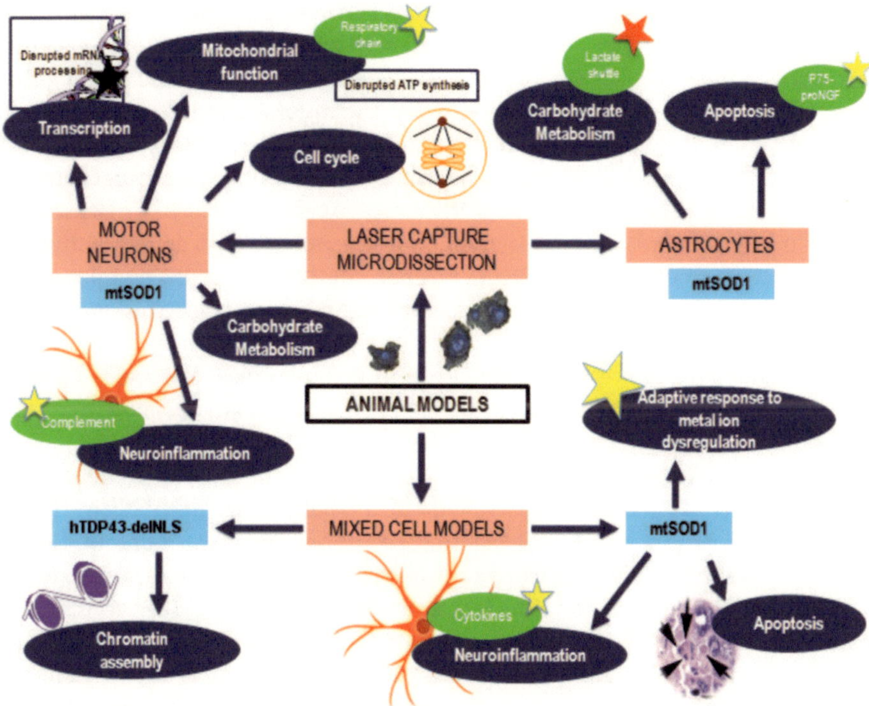

Fig. 2. Summary of prominent pathways arising from GEP of Animal Models. Important changes in the transcriptome have been highlighted by green labels; yellow stars indicate up-regulation, red stars indicate down-regulation. Blue squares outline functional consequences of changes in the transcriptome. Further details are discussed in the text.

Although these studies have greatly contributed to present knowledge on the transcriptional changes occurring in ALS, the analysis of a mixed cell population within the CNS has several disadvantages. This kind of approach does not identify which cell population is responsible for the transcriptional changes observed and only detects those transcripts most highly differentially expressed, with subtle but potential pivotal gene expression changes masked as well as changes in genes differentially expressed in one cell type, but not in others.

6.2 Gene expression profiling of laser capture microdissection isolated cell types

In order to overcome the limitations of using mixed cell population samples, dissection of single cells from complex tissues using LCM has been applied to identify the contribution of different cell types to the degenerative process occurring in ALS.

Several studies have determined the changes in gene expression occurring in motor neurones isolated from the spinal cord of mutant SOD1^{G93A} mice at different stages during the disease; from the pre-symptomatic stage to paralysis (Ferraiuolo et al 2007; Perrin et al 2005). The first report described transcriptional analysis of motor neurones isolated from SOD1^{G93A} mice bred on a mixed background and no differentially expressed genes were detected in the pre-symptomatic mice (Perrin et al 2005). However, in contrast to the whole tissue homogenates, motor neurones did not show activation of apoptotic genes, suggesting that cell death signals derive from other cell types in the spinal cord (Figure 2).
In the second publication, microarray analysis was carried out on SOD1^{G93A} mice bred on a homogeneous background; this enabled important changes in the motor neurones at the pre-symptomatic stage of disease, mainly involved in carbohydrate metabolism and transcription, to be detected (Ferraiuolo et al 2007). The upregulation of transcripts encoding proteins involved in the energy production pathway, i.e. tricarboxylic acid cycle and respiratory chain, suggested that motor neurones were trying to compensate for their increased energy needs in response to ongoing stress. At the late stage of disease, increased expression of transcripts involved in reactivation of the cell cycle (as an alternative pathway of cell death), and complement activation (a mechanism through which motor neurones can attract cells from the immune system), and down-regulation of transcription-related genes were identified (Figure 2).
To complement the gene expression profiling of motor neurones, astrocytes isolated from SOD1^{G93A} mice at the pre-symptomatic stage of disease were isolated and used for microarray analysis (Ferraiuolo et al 2011a). This enabled the cross-talk between the motor neurones and astrocytes at this very early time point to be interrogated. Interestingly, astrocytes displayed a marked impairment of carbohydrate metabolism (Figure 2). Comparing the expression profiles of the two cell types from the same SOD1^{G93A} mice highlighted that the metabolic impairment observed in motor neurones could derive from the lack of provision of substrates, i.e. lactate, from the astrocytes, and led to the conclusion that the lactate shuttle (the mechanism through which motor neurones and astrocytes combine metabolism and signalling through lactate and glutamate), is impaired. In addition, the activation of an important neuronal cell death pathway involving p75 and its ligand pro nerve growth factor (proNGF) was established. Gene expression profiling of SOD1^{G93A} astrocytes demonstrated that these cells expressed high levels of *Ngf,* while the motor neurones over-expressed the p75 receptor. *In vitro* data confirmed the dysregulation of both pathways and preliminary data from human ALS biosamples supported these findings from the murine model.

6.3 Gene expression profiling of peripheral tissue from mouse models

Microarray technology has also been applied to peripheral tissues from the SOD1^{G86R} mouse model (Gonzalez de Aguilar et al 2008). Profiling of the skeletal muscles revealed that the major expression changes happen at onset of disease, when muscles are activating pathways involved in detoxification and regeneration, but also cell death and tissue degradation. These findings revealed that while motor neurones are degenerating, muscles are undergoing major remodelling trying to compensate for muscle damage with new myogenesis. Whilst over-expression of transcripts such as cyclin-dependent kinase inhibitor-1A (*Cdkn1a*) and growth arrest-and DNA damage-inducible gene-45 (*Gadd45*) could be mediating apoptosis of myofibres resulting in muscle atrophy, increased expression B cell translocation gene-1 (*Btg1*), growth differentiation factor-5 (*Gdf5*) and myogenic factor-6 (*Myf6*) are potent activators of new fibre formation.

7. Results from use of human post-mortem material

7.1 Gene expression profiling of mixed cell type CNS samples

Multiple studies have utilised gene expression profiling of post mortem mixed cell samples from ALS patients and controls; these have either focused on using samples from the motor cortex (Lederer et al 2007; Wang et al 2006) or from the spinal cord (Dangond et al 2004; Malaspina et al 2001; Offen et al 2009). The majority used sporadic ALS (SALS) cases, though Dangond et al also sampled two FALS cases, one of which carried an *SOD1* mutation (Dangond et al 2004). Despite the different tissues profiled and the different platforms utilised, the studies showed some consistent results: All of the studies recorded altered gene expression related to inflammation and Malaspina and colleagues detected an increase in glial fibrillary acidic protein (*GFAP*), indicating active astrogliosis (Figure 3). In addition, a number of the studies discovered differential expression related to cytoskeleton function, protein processing and the antioxidant response, in agreement with other lines of research in ALS (Ferraiuolo et al 2011b).

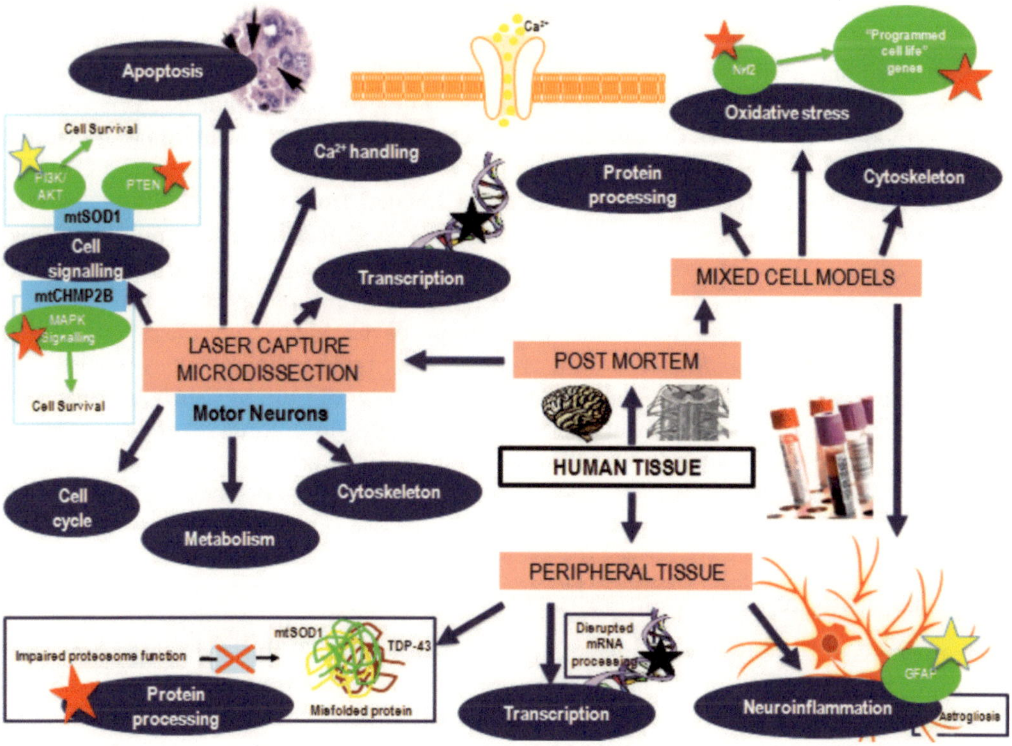

Fig. 3. Summary of prominent pathways arising from GEP of Human Tissue. Important changes in the transcriptome have been highlighted by green labels; yellow stars indicate up-regulation, red stars indicate down-regulation. Blue squares outline functional consequences of changes in the transcriptome. Further details can be found in the text.

7.2 Gene expression profiling of laser capture microdissection isolated cell types

As with the mouse models, in order to determine those genes differentially expressed in the vulnerable cell type, LCM has been used in post-mortem material to isolate the motor neurones from the spinal cord.

Motor neurones isolated from SALS cases and neurologically normal controls were shown to have distinct gene expression profiles compared to those generated from ventral horn homogenates, particularly with respect to those genes down-regulated in motor neurones (Jiang et al 2005). The motor neurones showed differential expression of genes associated with the cytoskeleton and evidence of decreased transcription, whilst cell death-associated genes and those involved in cell signalling were increased (Figure 3). In addition, cell cycle related genes were also reported as dysregulated, supporting the theory that inappropriate activation of the cell cycle in these post-mitotic cells leads to cell death. A follow-up study demonstrated that expression of several of these genes also correlated with pathological markers, such as phosphorylated neurofilament and ubiquitinated protein accumulations as well as motor neurone loss (Jiang et al 2007).

Gene expression profiling of isolated motor neurones has also been performed on ALS cases which carry genetic mutations in the *SOD1* and chromatin modifying protein 2B (*CHMP2B*) genes (Cox et al 2010; Kirby et al 2011). Motor neurones from *SOD1*-related cases of ALS showed increases in genes in the protein kinase B/phosphatidylinositol-3 kinase (AKT/PI3K) cell survival pathway, with concomitant decreases in negative regulators such as phophastase and tensin homologue (*PTEN*) (Kirby et al 2011) (Figure 3). Further work demonstrated that inhibition of PTEN led to increased activation of the AKT/PI3K pathway and increased neuronal survival in cell models including primary motor neurone cultures. Thus, activation of the AKT/PI3K pathway was proposed as a candidate for future therapeutic strategies.

The transcriptional profiles from motor neurones isolated from the *CHMP2B*-related ALS cases were distinct from those in *SOD1*-related cases (Cox et al 2010). These motor neurones showed dysregulation of genes involved in the classical and p38 MAPK signalling pathways, gene changes predicted to reflect reduced autophagy and repression of translation (Figure 3). The functional implication of *CHMP2B* mutations on cellular mechanisms was demonstrated by the presence of large cytoplasmic vacuoles and impairment of autophagy in a cellular model transfected with mutant *CHMP2B*, consistent with the microarray findings (Cox et al 2010). Interestingly, differential expression of genes encoding proteins responsible for calcium handling and cell cycle genes, as well as those genes involved in transcription, signalling and metabolism, was detected in both genetic subtypes.

8. Results from use of human peripheral tissue

Gene expression profiling has been conducted on blood and fibroblasts from ALS patients (Highley et al 2011; Saris et al 2009; Zhang et al 2011). Microarray analysis of SALS and control blood samples was followed by hierarchical clustering of all genes found to be significantly expressed in all samples after normalisation (Saris et al 2009). The method identified five clusters; two of which were able to differentiate between ALS and control samples. These clusters were replicated in a further two cohorts of patients and controls, demonstrating that such an analysis, which takes into account the interdependence of gene expression, is a means of reducing the false negative rate when subsequently detecting differential gene expression. This work also provided evidence that peripheral blood is a valuable medium for studying ALS. In addition, there was a correlation with the CNS tissue studies, as the blood in ALS patients showed a decrease in genes associated with protein processing and RNA post-transcriptional modification, as well as increases in genes associated with inflammation.

A more recent study performed gene expression profiling on peripheral blood mononuclear cells from patients with SALS (Zhang et al 2011). These cells showed an up-regulation of genes associated with immune activation in response to lipopolysaccharide (LPS), which correlated with an elevation of plasma LPS. Unfortunately, no correlation between expression of these genes and disease progression was provided.

Transcriptional profiles of fibroblasts from patients with SALS, FALS and controls have been shown to be informative in distinguishing the different genetic variants from each other, as well as from SALS patients, by their gene expression profiles and specifically the level of alternative splicing (Highley et al 2011). The FALS samples were derived from patients with mutations in *SOD1* and *TARDBP*. Using microarrays which interrogate every exon of every gene, it was demonstrated that there was a significant amount of aberrant splicing in the samples with a *TARDBP* mutation which was replicated to a lesser degree in the SALS samples and virtually absent in the samples with a *SOD1* mutation (Figure 3). In support of this, other work has identified aberrant splicing in cell and animal models with depletion of TDP-43 (Polymenidou et al 2011; Tollervey et al 2011).

9. The future of gene expression profiling in ALS

9.1 RNA sequencing (RNA-seq)

The advent of next generation sequencing has evolved to enable quantitative parallel sequencing of RNA transcripts from isolated cells and tissues. There are a number of advantages of next generation RNA sequencing over the microarray platform which in general extend from the fact that there is no reliance on the pre-designed probes which are present on the microarrays. In contrast, the methodology aims to sequence every base of every transcript of RNA. This leads to a better detection rate of known transcripts and splicing events and the detection of RNA transcripts (both coding and non-coding) which have not previously been described and therefore have no specific probe (Sultan et al 2008). As there is no reliance on probes, the problem of cross hybridisation is avoided. In addition, because each base in each transcript is sequenced, as well as providing information about expression level and alternative splicing, the sequencing also provides information about sequence variability within the RNA (Wang et al 2009). The biggest challenge to RNA sequencing, however, is the analysis of the large amounts of data produced which is substantially more than the read out of even the most comprehensive microarray. Not least among these challenges is the problem of mapping the RNA sequences to the genome, as in contrast to DNA sequencing, the absence of introns can lead to substantial difficulties (Sutherland et al 2011).

9.2 Role of microRNAs in ALS

This chapter has focused on the mRNA that is translated into protein. However, although 90% of eukaryotic genomic DNA is transcribed, only 1-2% actually encodes protein. The vast majority of transcribed material is comprised of non-coding RNA (ncRNA) and there is increasing evidence to support functional roles for at least a subset of these transcripts (Kaikkonen et al 2011). There are broadly two types of ncRNA, infrastructural (including transfer RNA and small nuclear RNA) and regulatory RNA (including microRNA, Piwi-interacting RNA and small interfering RNA). The function of ncRNAs remains largely unknown. However, research into microRNA (miRNA) has led the field in recent years. miRNAs are a class of small, ncRNA molecules predicted to post-transcriptionally regulate at least one third of human genes (Lewis et al 2005). Each miRNA can potentially target hundreds of genes and play key regulatory roles in a diverse range of pathways including development, differentiation and pathological processes such as neurodegeneration (Enciu et al 2011). The study of miRNA in ALS is at a very early stage. However, given the proposed role for TDP-43 in miRNA biogenesis and the recent discovery of a beneficial effect of miRNA-206 in the mutant SOD1 mouse model, this will be an interesting area of investigation for the future (Buratti et al 2010; Williams et al 2009)

9.3 Biomarkers in ALS

There is no diagnostic test for ALS, so diagnosis currently relies upon clinical assessment involving the exclusion of "ALS-mimic" syndromes (such as multifocal motor neuropathy and cervical radiculomyelopathy), causing an average delay of one year from symptom onset to a confirmed diagnosis (Silani et al 2011; Zoccolella et al 2006). In such a rapidly progressive disease this delay is a significant obstacle to potential neuroprotective therapies. ALS is clinically heterogeneous, with multiple subtypes associated with different survival times and symptoms making prognosis challenging. This heterogeneity is also a confounding factor for clinical trials as patient phenotype will impact upon survival data and may influence responses to therapeutic intervention, with some subtypes more responsive to therapy than others (Turner et al 2009). Robust biomarkers would therefore be valuable for the initial diagnosis of disease, the classification of various subtypes, monitoring responses to therapeutic agents and tracking disease progression (Turner et al 2009). Gene expression profiling offers a useful tool for biomarker discovery allowing patient and control biofluids, such as blood and CSF, to be compared on a genome wide scale. These tools have already been employed to improve classification and diagnosis of multiple diseases including neurodegenerative conditions such as Huntington's disease and Parkinson's disease (Borovecki et al 2005; Scherzer et al 2007).

10. Conclusion

In conclusion, microarray analysis has been pivotal in understanding the transcriptional alterations occurring in response to genetic mutations associated with ALS and the sporadic disease (SALS). The cellular model has generated a therapeutic target and transcriptional activation of *Nrf2* is currently being assessed *in-vivo*. Use of spinal cord and peripheral tissues from transgenic mouse models has provided a mechanism to look at the progression of the disease and specifically to identify early changes in the motor neurones and astrocytes. These dysregulated pathways provide future therapeutic targets. In addition, gene expression profiling has allowed crucial insights into the mechanisms affecting different areas of the motor system, with the combination of LCM and microarray technology able to discriminate changes in specific cell types and understand how these affect each other and contribute to disease progression. Finally, the use of human material has begun to allow the distinctions between genetic and sporadic disease to be differentiated as well as providing further candidates for therapeutic approaches. In the future, gene expression profiling of larger, consistently collected patient samples has the potential to generate robust and reliable prognostic and diagnostic biomarkers, which will ultimately be applicable for use in the clinic.

11. Acknowledgments

PJS and JK are funded by the European Community's Health Seventh Framework Programme (FP7/2007-2013) under grant agreement 259867 and by the Motor Neurone Disease Association (MNDA). EFG is also funded by the MNDA.

12. References

Aguirre T, Van Den Bosch L, Goetschalckx K, Tilkin P, Mathijs G, et al. 1998. Increased sensitivity of fibroblasts from amyotrophic lateral sclerosis patients to oxidative stress. *Ann Neurol* 43:452-7

Booij BB, Lindahl T, Wetterberg P, Skaane NV, Saebo S, et al. 2011. A gene expression pattern in blood for the early detection of Alzheimer's disease. *J Alzheimers Dis* 23:109-19

Borovecki F, Lovrecic L, Zhou J, Jeong H, Then F, et al. 2005. Genome-wide expression profiling of human blood reveals biomarkers for Huntington's disease. *Proc Natl Acad Sci U S A* 102:11023-8

Boutahar N, Wierinckx A, Camdessanche JP, Antoine JC, Reynaud E, et al. 2011. Differential effect of oxidative or excitotoxic stress on the transcriptional profile of amyotrophic lateral sclerosis-linked mutant SOD1 cultured neurons. *J Neurosci Res* 89:1439-50

Budini M, Buratti E. 2011. TDP-43 Autoregulation: Implications for Disease. *J Mol Neurosci*

Buratti E, De Conti L, Stuani C, Romano M, Baralle M, Baralle F. 2010. Nuclear factor TDP-43 can affect selected microRNA levels. *FEBS J* 277:2268-81

Cashman NR, Durham HD, Blusztajn JK, Oda K, Tabira T, et al. 1992. Neuroblastoma x spinal cord (NSC) hybrid cell lines resemble developing motor neurons. *Dev Dyn* 194:209-21

Cox LE, Ferraiuolo L, Goodall EF, Heath PR, Higginbottom A, et al. 2010. Mutations in CHMP2B in lower motor neuron predominant amyotrophic lateral sclerosis (ALS). *PLoS ONE* 5:e9872

Dadon-Nachum M, Melamed E, Offen D. 2011. The "dying-back" phenomenon of motor neurons in ALS. *J Mol Neurosci* 43:470-7

Dangond F, Hwang D, Camelo S, Pasinelli P, Frosch MP, et al. 2004. Molecular signature of late-stage human ALS revealed by expression profiling of postmortem spinal cord gray matter. *Physiol Genomics* 16:229-39

Dimos JT, Rodolfa KT, Niakan KK, Weisenthal LM, Mitsumoto H, et al. 2008. Induced pluripotent stem cells generated from patients with ALS can be differentiated into motor neurons. *Science* 321:1218-21

Duan W, Li X, Shi J, Guo Y, Li Z, Li C. 2010. Mutant TAR DNA-binding protein-43 induces oxidative injury in motor neuron-like cell. *Neuroscience* 169:1621-9

Dupuis L, Loeffler JP. 2009. Neuromuscular junction destruction during amyotrophic lateral sclerosis: insights from transgenic models. *Curr Opin Pharmacol* 9:341-6

Durham HD, Dahrouge S, Cashman NR. 1993. Evaluation of the spinal cord neuron X neuroblastoma hybrid cell line NSC-34 as a model for neurotoxicity testing. *Neurotoxicology* 14:387-95

Durham HD, Roy J, Dong L, Figlewicz DA. 1997. Aggregation of mutant Cu/Zn superoxide dismutase proteins in a culture model of ALS. *J Neuropathol Exp Neurol* 56:523-30

Enciu AM, Popescu BO, Gheorghisan-Galateanu A. 2011. MicroRNAs in brain development and degeneration. *Mol Biol Rep* 10.1007/s11033-011-0973-1:(Epub ahead of print)

Ferraiuolo L, Heath PR, Holden H, Kasher P, Kirby J, Shaw PJ. 2007. Microarray analysis of the cellular pathways involved in the adaptation to and progression of motor neuron injury in the SOD1 G93A mouse model of familial ALS. *J Neurosci* 27:9201-19

Ferraiuolo L, Higginbottom A, Heath P, Barber S, Greenald D, et al. 2011a. Dysregulation of astrocyte-motor neuron cross-talk in mutant SOD1 related amyotrophic lateral sclerosis. *Brain* (In Press)

Ferraiuolo L, Kirby J, Grierson AJ, Sendtner M, Shaw PJ. 2011b. Molecular and cellular pathways of motor neuron injury in amyotrophic lateral sclerosis. *Nat Rev Neurology* (In Press)

Fukada Y, Yasui K, Kitayama M, Doi K, Nakano T, et al. 2007. Gene expression analysis of the murine model of amyotrophic lateral sclerosis: studies of the Leu126delTT mutation in SOD1. *Brain Res* 1160:1-10

Gonzalez de Aguilar JL, Niederhauser-Wiederkehr C, Halter B, De Tapia M, Di Scala F, et al. 2008. Gene profiling of skeletal muscle in an amyotrophic lateral sclerosis mouse model. *Physiol Genomics* 32:207-18

Gurney ME, Pu H, Chiu AY, Dal Canto MC, Polchow CY, et al. 1994. Motor neuron degeneration in mice that express a human Cu,Zn superoxide dismutase mutation. *Science* 264:1772-5

Highley JR, Hewamadduma C, Jansweijer JA, Kirby J, Heath PR, et al. 2011. Amyotrophic lateral sclerosis-causing TARDBP (TDP-43) mutations cause widespread dysregulation of mRNA splicing in cell lines from human patients. *PLoS ONE* (Under Review)

Hoepken HH, Gispert S, Azizov M, Klinkenberg M, Ricciardi F, et al. 2008. Parkinson patient fibroblasts show increased alpha-synuclein expression. *Exp Neurol* 212:307-13

Hosack DA, Dennis G, Jr., Sherman BT, Lane HC, Lempicki RA. 2003. Identifying biological themes within lists of genes with EASE. *Genome Biol* 4:R70

Igaz LM, Kwong LK, Chen-Plotkin A, Winton MJ, Unger TL, et al. 2009. Expression of TDP-43 C-terminal Fragments in Vitro Recapitulates Pathological Features of TDP-43 Proteinopathies. *J Biol Chem* 284:8516-24

Igaz LM, Kwong LK, Lee EB, Chen-Plotkin A, Swanson E, et al. 2011. Dysregulation of the ALS-associated gene TDP-43 leads to neuronal death and degeneration in mice. *J Clin Invest* 121:726-38

Jiang YM, Yamamoto M, Kobayashi Y, Yoshihara T, Liang Y, et al. 2005. Gene expression profile of spinal motor neurons in sporadic amyotrophic lateral sclerosis. *Ann Neurol* 57:236-51

Jiang YM, Yamamoto M, Tanaka F, Ishigaki S, Katsuno M, et al. 2007. Gene expressions specifically detected in motor neurons (dynactin 1, early growth response 3, acetyl-CoA transporter, death receptor 5, and cyclin C) differentially correlate to pathologic markers in sporadic amyotrophic lateral sclerosis. *J Neuropathol Exp Neurol* 66:617-27

Kaikkonen MU, Lam MT, Glass CK. 2011. Non-coding RNAs as regulators of gene expression and epigenetics. *Cardiovasc Res* 90:430-40

Kirby J, Halligan E, Baptista MJ, Allen S, Heath PR, et al. 2005. Mutant SOD1 alters the motor neuronal transcriptome: implications for familial ALS. *Brain* 128:1686-706

Kirby J, Ning K, Ferraiuolo L, Heath PR, Ismail A, et al. 2011. Phosphatase and tensin homologue/protein kinase B pathway linked to motor neuron survival in human superoxide dismutase 1-related amyotrophic lateral sclerosis. *Brain* 134:506-17

Lederer CW, Torrisi A, Pantelidou M, Santama N, Cavallaro S. 2007. Pathways and genes differentially expressed in the motor cortex of patients with sporadic amyotrophic lateral sclerosis. *BMC Genomics* 8:26

Lewis BP, Burge CB, Bartel DP. 2005. Conserved seed pairing, often flanked by adenosines, indicates that thousands of human genes are microRNA targets. *Cell* 120:15-20

Liew CC, Ma J, Tang HC, Zheng R, Dempsey AA. 2006. The peripheral blood transcriptome dynamically reflects system wide biology: a potential diagnostic tool. *The Journal of Laboratory and Clinical Medicine* 147:126-32

Liu J, Walter E, Stenger D, Thach D. 2006. Effects of globin mRNA reduction methods on gene expression profiles from whole blood. *J Mol Diagn* 8:551-8

Maes OC, Xu S, Yu B, Chertkow HM, Wang E, Schipper HM. 2007. Transcriptional profiling of Alzheimer blood mononuclear cells by microarray. *Neurobiology of Aging* 28:1795-809

Malaspina A, Kaushik N, de Belleroche J. 2001. Differential expression of 14 genes in amyotrophic lateral sclerosis spinal cord detected using gridded cDNA arrays. *J Neurochem* 77:132-45

Menzies FM, Cookson MR, Taylor RW, Turnbull DM, Chrzanowska-Lightowlers ZM, et al. 2002a. Mitochondrial dysfunction in a cell culture model of familial amyotrophic lateral sclerosis. *Brain* 125:1522-33

Menzies FM, Grierson AJ, Cookson MR, Heath PR, Tomkins J, et al. 2002b. Selective loss of neurofilament expression in Cu/Zn superoxide dismutase (SOD1) linked amyotrophic lateral sclerosis. *J Neurochem* 82:1118-28

Mohr S, Liew CC. 2007. The peripheral-blood transcriptome: new insights into disease and risk assessment. *Trends Mol Med* 13:422-32

Mortiboys H, Thomas KJ, Koopman WJ, Klaffke S, Abou-Sleiman P, et al. 2008. Mitochondrial function and morphology are impaired in parkin-mutant fibroblasts. *Ann Neurol* 64:555-65

Nagai M, Re DB, Nagata T, Chalazonitis A, Jessell TM, et al. 2007. Astrocytes expressing ALS-linked mutated SOD1 release factors selectively toxic to motor neurons. *Nat Neurosci* 10:615-22

Nagasaka Y, Dillner K, Ebise H, Teramoto R, Nakagawa H, et al. 2005. A unique gene expression signature discriminates familial Alzheimer's disease mutation carriers from their wild-type siblings. *Proc Natl Acad Sci U S A* 102:14854-9

Neymotin A, Calingasan NY, Wille E, Naseri N, Petri S, et al. 2011. Neuroprotective effect of Nrf2/ARE activators, CDDO ethylamide and CDDO trifluoroethylamide, in a mouse model of amyotrophic lateral sclerosis. *Free Radic Biol Med* 51:88-96

Offen D, Barhum Y, Melamed E, Embacher N, Schindler C, Ransmayr G. 2009. Spinal cord mRNA profile in patients with ALS: comparison with transgenic mice expressing the human SOD-1 mutant. *J Mol Neurosci* 38:85-93

Olsen MK, Roberds SL, Ellerbrock BR, Fleck TJ, McKinley DK, Gurney ME. 2001. Disease mechanisms revealed by transcription profiling in SOD1-G93A transgenic mouse spinal cord. *Ann Neurol* 50:730-40

Perrin FE, Boisset G, Docquier M, Schaad O, Descombes P, Kato AC. 2005. No widespread induction of cell death genes occurs in pure motoneurons in an amyotrophic lateral sclerosis mouse model. *Hum Mol Genet* 14:3309-20

Polymenidou M, Lagier-Tourenne C, Hutt KR, Huelga SC, Moran J, et al. 2011. Long pre-mRNA depletion and RNA missplicing contribute to neuronal vulnerability from loss of TDP-43. *Nat Neurosci* 14:459-68

Ripps ME, Huntley GW, Hof PR, Morrison JH, Gordon JW. 1995. Transgenic mice expressing an altered murine superoxide dismutase gene provide an animal model of amyotrophic lateral sclerosis. *Proc Natl Acad Sci U S A* 92:689-93

Saris CG, Horvath S, van Vught PW, van Es MA, Blauw HM, et al. 2009. Weighted gene co-expression network analysis of the peripheral blood from Amyotrophic Lateral Sclerosis patients. *BMC Genomics* 10:405

Sarlette A, Krampfl K, Grothe C, Neuhoff N, Dengler R, Petri S. 2008. Nuclear erythroid 2-related factor 2-antioxidative response element signaling pathway in motor cortex and spinal cord in amyotrophic lateral sclerosis. *J Neuropathol Exp Neurol* 67:1055-62

Scherzer CR, Eklund AC, Morse LJ, Liao Z, Locascio JJ, et al. 2007. Molecular markers of early Parkinson's disease based on gene expression in blood. *Proc Natl Acad Sci U S A* 104:955-60

Sharp FR, Lit L, Xu H, Apperson M, Walker W, et al. 2006. Genomics of brain and blood: progress and pitfalls. *Epilepsia* 47:1603-7

Shtilbans A, Choi SG, Fowkes ME, Khitrov G, Shahbazi M, et al. 2011. Differential gene expression in patients with amyotrophic lateral sclerosis. *Amyotroph Lateral Scler* 12:250-6

Silani V, Messina S, Poletti B, Morelli C, Doretti A, et al. 2011. The diagnosis of Amyotrophic lateral sclerosis in 2010. *Arch Ital Biol* 149:5-27

Son EY, Ichida JK, Wainger BJ, Toma JS, Rafuse VF, et al. 2011. Conversion of Mouse and Human Fibroblasts into Functional Spinal Motor Neurons. *Cell Stem Cell* DOI: 10.1016/j.stem.2011.07.014:(Epub ahead of print)

Stallings NR, Puttaparthi K, Luther CM, Burns DK, Elliott JL. 2010. Progressive motor weakness in transgenic mice expressing human TDP-43. *Neurobiol Dis* 40:404-14

Stoughton RB. 2005. Applications of DNA microarrays in biology. *Annu Rev Biochem* 74:53-82

Sultan M, Schulz MH, Richard H, Magen A, Klingenhoff A, et al. 2008. A global view of gene activity and alternative splicing by deep sequencing of the human transcriptome. *Science* 321:956-60

Sutherland GT, Janitz M, Kril JJ. 2011. Understanding the pathogenesis of Alzheimer's disease: will RNA-Seq realize the promise of transcriptomics? *J Neurochem* 116:937-46

Tollervey JR, Curk T, Rogelj B, Briese M, Cereda M, et al. 2011. Characterizing the RNA targets and position-dependent splicing regulation by TDP-43. *Nat Neurosci* 14:452-8

Tsuang MT, Nossova N, Yager T, Tsuang MM, Guo SC, et al. 2005. Assessing the validity of blood-based gene expression profiles for the classification of schizophrenia and bipolar disorder: a preliminary report. *Am J Med Genet B Neuropsychiatr Genet* 133B:1-5

Turner MR, Kiernan MC, Leigh PN, Talbot K. 2009. Biomarkers in amyotrophic lateral sclerosis. *Lancet Neurol* 8:94-109

Vargas MR, Johnson DA, Sirkis DW, Messing A, Johnson JA. 2008a. Nrf2 activation in astrocytes protects against neurodegeneration in mouse models of familial amyotrophic lateral sclerosis. *J Neurosci* 28:13574-81

Vargas MR, Pehar M, Cassina P, Beckman JS, Barbeito L. 2006. Increased glutathione biosynthesis by Nrf2 activation in astrocytes prevents p75NTR-dependent motor neuron apoptosis. *J Neurochem* 97:687-96

Vargas MR, Pehar M, Diaz-Amarilla PJ, Beckman JS, Barbeito L. 2008b. Transcriptional profile of primary astrocytes expressing ALS-linked mutant SOD1. *J Neurosci Res* 86:3515-25

Wang XS, Simmons Z, Liu W, Boyer PJ, Connor JR. 2006. Differential expression of genes in amyotrophic lateral sclerosis revealed by profiling the post mortem cortex. *Amyotroph Lateral Scler* 7:201-10

Wang Z, Gerstein M, Snyder M. 2009. RNA-Seq: a revolutionary tool for transcriptomics. *Nat Rev Genet* 10:57-63

Whitney AR, Diehn M, Popper SJ, Alizadeh AA, Boldrick JC, et al. 2003. Individuality and variation in gene expression patterns in human blood. *Proc Natl Acad Sci U S A* 100:1896-901

Williams AH, Valdez G, Moresi V, Qi X, McAnally J, et al. 2009. MicroRNA-206 delays ALS progression and promotes regeneration of neuromuscular synapses in mice. *Science* 326:1549-54

Wright C, Bergstrom D, Dai H, Marton M, Morris M, et al. 2008. Characterization of globin RNA interference in gene expression profiling of whole-blood samples. *Clinical chemistry* 54:396-405

Yoshihara T, Ishigaki S, Yamamoto M, Liang Y, Niwa J, et al. 2002. Differential expression of inflammation- and apoptosis-related genes in spinal cords of a mutant SOD1 transgenic mouse model of familial amyotrophic lateral sclerosis. *J Neurochem* 80:158-67

Zhang R, Hadlock KG, Do H, Yu S, Honrada R, et al. 2011. Gene expression profiling in peripheral blood mononuclear cells from patients with sporadic amyotrophic lateral sclerosis (sALS). *J Neuroimmunol* 230:114-23

Zoccolella S, Beghi E, Palagano G, Fraddosio A, Samarelli V, et al. 2006. Predictors of delay in the diagnosis and clinical trial entry of amyotrophic lateral sclerosis patients: a population-based study. *J Neurol Sci* 250:45-9

3

Dynamic Meta-Analysis as a Therapeutic Prediction Tool for Amyotrophic Lateral Sclerosis

Cassie S. Mitchell and Robert H. Lee
Georgia Institute of Technology and Emory University, Atlanta, Georgia, United States

1. Introduction

In this chapter, we present a new method, dynamic meta-analysis, which allows the examination of the underlying system dynamics of ALS utilizing the wealth of existing published experimental and/or clinical literature. We perform a small-scale feasibility study of the G93A SOD1 mouse model to show that dynamic meta-analysis can also be utilized to predict treatment outcomes in a high-throughput manner.

1.1 Leveraging the wealth of data

In 2010 alone, 980 articles were specifically published on the fatal neurodegenerative disease Amyotrophic Lateral Sclerosis (ALS), and the cumulative total literature base for this single intractable pathology exceeds 10,300 articles, according to a PubMed search. One might think that with this wealth of information we would have ALS well in hand. Yet, there is no available, life-extending treatment despite the extensive and detailed information obtained by thousands of researchers at the cost of billions of dollars. ALS remains one of the most intractable neurological diseases; there is no apparent quick fix, no smoking gun, and no obvious answers—just mountains of intertwined experimental observations recorded across a host of individual publications. Furthermore, ALS has been remarkably resistant to reductionistic attempts to pinpoint the underlying problem. Potential contributing defects, mutations, and regulatory failures have been cited across a broad range of categories, including axonal transport (Bilsland, Sahai et al.), cellular chemistry (Hayward, Rodriguez et al. 2002), energetics (Shi, Gal et al.), excitotoxicity (Roy, Minotti et al. 1998), free radicals (Bogdanov, Ramos et al. 1998), genetic damage (Nagano, Murakami et al. 2002), inflammation (King, Dickson et al. 2009), necro-apoptosis (Vukosavic, Dubois-Dauphin et al. 1999), proteomics (Wood, Beaujeux et al. 2003), as well as systemic origin (Dobrowolny, Aucello et al. 2008). Yet experimental correction or "treatment" of any individually identified potential contributor has failed to translate into clinically significant and reproducible results (Peviani, Caron et al.).

1.2 Identifying and utilizing the system dynamics of ALS for combination therapy

Based on current evidence, ALS may exhibit system-level abnormalities that emerge from the complexities and interactions of their underlying mechanisms (Mitchell 2009; Rothstein

2009). Like an engineering control loop with many elements that ends up with an unstably high feedback gain, ALS may initiate from the combined effects of many small deviations that, in and of themselves, might be considered normal. To address multiple contributors and their interactions, a distributed intervention like combination therapy is necessary. Combination treatment strategies are typically based on the assumed presence of system-level synergistic interactions, which could amplify the desired treatment effects. Thus, before a combination treatment can even be developed, the system dynamics and potential synergistic interactions must first be revealed. That is, we cannot "treat", for example, a high-loop gain abnormality if we are not aware of its existence and have no means to measure it. A further limitation to combination treatment research is the combinatorial explosion of treatment possibilities (often hundreds to thousands) that must be experimentally explored—a daunting task that is neither financially nor temporally feasible. What is needed is a tool or method that can both identify and utilize ALS pathology dynamics to pre-screen treatment combinations in silico, such that treatment combinations predicted to have the highest efficacies could be experimentally assessed first, and thus greatly speed the time from ALS treatment discovery to potential clinical treatment success.

1.3 Dynamic meta-analysis as a means of experimental and clinical prediction

Here we examine the use of a novel and innovative form of meta-analysis, which we call *dynamic meta-analysis*, as a tool that enables the necessary examination of system-level ALS pathology dynamics as well as the prediction of ALS combination treatment outcomes. Traditional meta-analysis, which aggregates the results of multiple, heavily overlapping clinical/epidemiological studies into a larger virtual study from which relationships across a broader array of conditions can be examined and overall statistical power can be increased, has been successfully used to examine individual clinical treatments (Miller, Mitchell et al. 2007; Pastula, Moore et al. 2010).

Much can and has been honed from using traditonal meta-analysis to examine clinical trials. However, clinical trials lack the advantages of in vitro and in vivo experimental models where we can perform protocols and obtain mechanistic insight that is not possible in human studies alone. To examine the dynamics of ALS in order to develop successful ombination therapies, we really need to examine the individual interactions and regulation of multipe cellular- and system-level interactions, which are either too complex, too inaccessible, or inappropriate for human experimentation. The ALS literature, particularly through superoxide dismutase 1 mouse models (G93A, G85R, etc), identified several such interactions and their regulation. What is needed is a method by which we can integrate the individual studies, each of which study different aspects of ALS (axonal transport, excitotoxicity, apoptosis, etc.), into the quilt that is ALS. This indeed does sound like a task for meta-analysis.

However, traditional meta-analysis is not an option for examining experimental literature. The ALS experimental literature base is simultaneously much larger than any single collection of clinical trials, and much less overlapping than clinical protocols. Dynamic meta-analysis overcomes the constraints of traditional meta-analysis by allowing the implicit inclusion of system interactions and explicit inclusion of time, two key ingredients necessary to examine pathology dynamics and subsequent combination treatments. In short, dynamic meta-analysis provides a manageable means to integrate the experimental data published by thousands of researchers into a unified view from which new ALS treatments and treatment combinations can be explored.

While a major strength of dynamic meta-analysis is that it does provide an approach for aggregating and recapitulating experimental studies, its application is by no means limited to experimental studies. The same method can certainly be used to dynamically examine clinical stuides. The advantages of the implicit inclusion of interactions and explict inclusion of time still apply.

1.4 G93A SOD1 mouse model as a test bed for dynamic meta-analysis

In this chapter we perform a small dynamic meta-analysis feasibility study utilizing the G93A SOD1 ALS mouse model literature to illustrate the potential power of dynamic meta-analysis to reveal key system dynamics, identify treatment strategies, and predict combination treatment outcomes in ALS. This model, developed over 15 years ago, is still the primary experimental model used to investigate ALS mechanisms and treatments.

2. The dynamic meta-analysis method

In this section, we provide the foundation, overview, and detailed processes involved in dynamic meta-analysis. The methods are generalized, such that they could be applied to any experimental or clinical dataset. We use the G93A SOD1 model as our detailed example of the construction, implementation, and analysis required for dynamic meta-analysis in this section. However, we reserve the specific dynamic meta-analysis predictions for the G93A SOD1 mouse model for the 3. Results section.

2.1 Traditional meta-analysis as a foundation

Traditional meta-analysis leverages an a priori model of relationships to generate a system-wide phenomenological model of the system. What makes this approach effective is the statistical weight of all the measured data behind the regressed coefficients. However, its limitations are that it does not explicitly permit the inclusion of time or the implicit examination of metric interactions. The a priori model used in traditional meta-analysis is based on the idea that all systems can be locally approximated algebraically as first order (essentially $\Delta Y = B \cdot \Delta X$ where X and Y are metrics within the system and B is a regression constant of proportionality). The a priori model is typically illustrated in the form of the meta-regression equation:

$$Y = B_1 \cdot X_1 + B_2 \cdot X_2 + B_3 \cdot X_3 + B_4 \cdot X_4 \ldots \quad (1)$$

2.2 Mathematical basis of "dynamic" meta-analysis

The central novel premise behind dynamic meta-analysis is that relationships in biological systems are better conceptualized as a first order differential equation ($dY/dt = B \cdot X$). Such an a priori model utilizing rates of change treats system relationships much like chemical reactions. Clearly, for much of what constitutes a biological system a reaction metaphor is not just a good approximation, it is literally true. Thus, the meta-regression equation for dynamic meta-analysis becomes

$$dY_1/dt = B_1 \cdot X_1 + B_2 \cdot X_2 + B_3 \cdot X_3 + B_4 \cdot X_4 \ldots \quad (2)$$

where X's are various effectors within the system, Y is one (of many) affected metrics and B's are the interaction gain coefficients. With this meta-regression equation, the concept of time is introduced explicitly. Therefore, dynamic meta-analysis can incorporate experimental data from differing time-points and predict effects over time. These traits make dynamic meta-analysis unique, even when compared to advanced meta-analysis methods such as network analysis (Trelle, Reichenbach et al. 2011). While network analysis does use comparative relationships, it does not include interactions or show how relationship ratios change over time. Thus, where traditional or even advanced meta-analysis produces a static set of linear relationships, dynamic meta-analysis produces a set of differential equations. This results in an innovative way to examine pathology dynamics as we can look at how metrics change and interact over time rather than being limited to how they correlate at a single point in time. Currently, the only other available technique capable of implictly including interactions and explicity including time is relational modeling (Mitchell, 2009; Mitchell and Lee, 2008). In fact, dynamic meta-analysis is, itself, one form of relational modeling. However, traditional relational models typically do not provide the desired statistical weight of dynamic meta-analysis since only one primary study is included per interaction.

2.3 Overview of the dynamic meta-analysis process

Dynamic meta-analysis is similar to traditional meta-analysis in that it utilizes literature searches, inclusion/exclusion critieria, and data aggregation techniques. A key difference in the dynamic meta-analysis process, however, is the study structure and data extraction. In the following sub-sections of the chapter we provide the details necessary to perform each step of dynamic meta-analysis: determining the study scope, performing literature searches and study inclusion/excusion, developing structure, extracting data, aggregating extracted data, implementing dynamic meta-analysis, and analyzing dynamic meta-analysis results.

2.4 Defining the study scope

Just as in traditional meta-analysis, defining the scope is an important step. There are several things to consider, including the outcome goals of the project, the measures and timepoints to be included, the statistical weight, and the desired timeline of the project. There is no methodological limit on the number of studies, measures, and timepoints that can be included in dynamic meta-analysis. Rather, the researcher must impose those limits. There is a balance between including enough studies to obtain statistically significant results and the amount of man-hours it takes to perform dynamic meta-analysis. The one drawback of meta-analysis is it is by no means a completely automated process. Rather, humans must be involved at each step, to search and more importantly extract the data from included studies.

To assist in balancing workload and the time it takes to get preliminary results from dynamic meta-analysis, we divide dynamic meta-analysis into two parts: a feasibility study and a full study. A full study, as the name implies, encompasses all of the primary articles that meet the inclusion criteria. In contrast, a feasibility study can potentially have the same number and breadth of outcome measures as the full study, but utilizes a lesser number of included primary studies for each metric (i.e. a lower "n"). That is, the statistical weight is decreased. The advantage of performing an initial feasibility study goes beyond simply obtaining preliminary results more quickly. The initial results of the feasibility study also provide insight and direction, which can be used to fine tune the targeting of the full study (e.g. determining if more or less measures are needed or if the scope of the study needs revised, etc.).

2.5 Literature searches, inclusion and exclusion criteria

Literature searches are performed in a semi-automated manner, similar to a systematic review (see Cochrane Review instructions for a full description of this method). Here, we utilize keyword searches in PubMed. Our strategy is not to be over-limiting in our resulting study selection. Rather, we limit the size of our dynamic meta-analysis by decreasing the study scope instead of using highly selective inclusion/exclusion criteria.

For the dynamic meta-analysis presented in this chapter, we perform two different literature searches, Phase I and Phase II. The first literature search (Phase I) is an all-encompassing literature search for primary research studies/articles. Phase I inclusion results in ~1,803 papers, while Phase I exclusion leaves a remainder of 1,144 papers. These 1,144 articles are the studies/data sets for dynamic meta-analysis. The second literature search (Phase II) is for ALS review articles. Phase II inclusion results in ~200 reviews, while Phase II exclusion reduces the number to 52. The review articles are utilized for the purposes of structure and aggregation (to be discussed in the following sub-sections).

Phase I Inclusion Criteria:

- All studies must be from peer-reviewed journals, which are indexed in the United States National Library of Medicine and National Institute of Health PubMed database.
- Amyotrophic Lateral Sclerosis" or "ALS" in title/abstract
- "G93A" or "transgenic mouse" in title/abstract
- Most Recent 15 years
- Primary research artciles

Phase I Exclusion Criteria:

- articles without verifiable controls for each experimental metric utilized
- articles without quantitative, statistically significant results
- studies not measured at two or more time points

Phase II Inclusion Criteria:

- all studies must be from peer-reviewed journals, which are indexed in the United States National Library of Medicine and National Institute of Health PubMed database.
- "Amytrophic Lateral Sclerosis" or "ALS" in title/abstract
- clinical or experimental review articles
- most recent 5 years

Phase II Exclusion Criteria:

- articles focused on human case studies
- articles focused on assessment metrics
- articles focused on ALS variants with dementia
- articles focused on disease management
- articles focused on non-mechanistic based therapies

2.6 Structure: Outcome measures, interactions, and categories

Similar to traditional meta-analysis, dynamic meta-analysis utilizes outcome measures (measures that are calculated or derived from the included studies) as a means of prediction. Unlike traditional meta-analysis, dynamic meta-analysis also includes *interactions* between the outcome measures. However, due to the larger scope of dynamic meta-analysis compared to traditional meta-analysis, it is helpful to combine individual experimental metrics or outcome metrics into aggregates we refer to as *categories*. The outcome measures, interactions, and their respective categories, together, make up the dynamic meta-analysis structure (Figure 1).

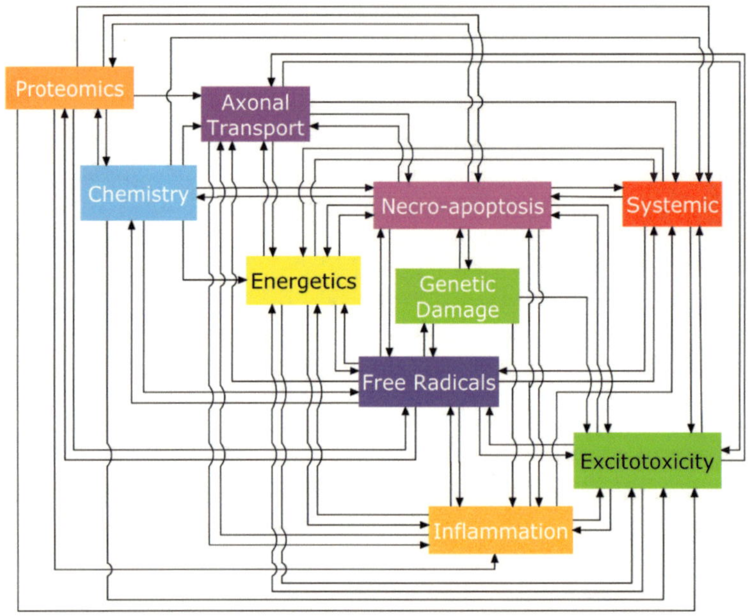

Fig. 1. Dynamic Meta-Analysis Feasibility Study Structure. Boxes represent the ten categories of outcome measures. Lines represent the 72 one-way interactions between categories of outcome measures. Systemics is shown in red as it represents the functional outcome metrics measured the in vivo G93A SOD1 mouse, and is used as the primary outcome for treatment evaluation (see Results). Categories are derived from the Phase II literature reviews. The outcome measures and their interactions are derived from the primary studies obtained from the Phase I literature search.

2.6.1 Category definitions

Aggregation of primary study metrics into categories balances the number and specificity of dynamic meta-analysis outcome measures with statistical weight. Too little aggregation will result in too disparate of a collection of very specific experimental mesasures or outcomes and will reduce the statistical weight of their predictions. In contrast, too much aggregation will result in outcome measures that are too broad; while this will increase their stasticial weight, it will also ultimately reduce the specificity of the dynamic meta-analysis predictions. Thus, the level, type, and implementation of aggregation will depend on the scope of the study, the number or primary studies utilized, as well as the desired statistical weight.

If the quantitative outcome metrics and their measured interactions come from the primary studies of Phase I, where do their categories come from? Categories are derived from the review articles of Phase II. Reviews do a nice job of providing key topics that are being researched by the field. For this feasibility study, reviews were analyzed for common research topics, based on broad categories of related physiological measures. For example, all measures of dynein, kinesin, mitochondrial transport, neurofilament transport, and neurofilament transport, etc, were grouped into the category outcome measure "Axonal Transport". Key terms were then extracted from these topics and used to sort the primary studies, and their respective outcome measures, into the following categories (definitions follow at the end of this sub-section): axonal transport, chemistry, energetics, excitotoxicity, free radicals, genetics, inflammation, necro-apoptosis, proteomics, and systemics. Reviews were also used to preliminarily determine which categories are inter-related (without having to examine each and every primary article). This is extremely helpful for development of the feasibility study. The quantitative specifics of the data aggregation process are discussed in Data Aggregation, while the category definitions are given below.

Excitotoxicity: encompasses measures of electrophysiology; ion, neurotransmitter, and buffer concentrations; activation of ionotropic/metabotropic receptors (Ikonomidou, Qin Qin et al. 1996; Dunlop, Beal McIlvain et al. 2003; Van Damme, Leyssen et al. 2003); altered excitability related to sodium (Kuo, Schonewille et al. 2004; Kuo, Siddique et al. 2005); and transport and pump capacity (Guatteo, Carunchio et al. 2007), causing toxic over-activation.

Axonal transport: encompasses measures of the anterograde and retrograde transport of cargos, such as mitochondria, neurotransmitters, neurofilaments, and endosomes/ lysosomes, as well as the measures of the involved machinery, such as the molecular motors kinesin and dynein. The most recognized impairments and their measures include mutations to cargos (Meyer and Potter 1995; Wong, He et al. 2000) and molecular motor cargo carriers (Hafezparast, Ahmad-Annuar et al. 2003; Teuchert, Fischer et al. 2006; Mitchell and Lee, 2009) that prevent the cargo from be appropriately bound to either dynein or kinesin. Other deficits include correlations to energetics, such as decreased mitochondrial transport or a decrease in overall transport due to a drop in mitochondrial potential (Ackerley, Grierson et al. 2004).

Energetics: encompasses measures of all machinery and processes related to cellular respiration and production of cellular ATP (Echaniz-Laguna, Zoll et al. 2002). Energetic contributors include impairments to the cellular machinery responsible for the production of ATP, especially mitochondria (Kong and Xu 1998; Sumi, Nagano et al. 2006), whose dysfunction also leads to accumulation of free radicals and calcium. Overburdened energetic capabilities because of increased homeostatic and transport demands from excitotoxicity (Dupuis, Oudart et al. 2004) have also been observed.

Genetic damage: encompasses measures of an extremely diverse spectrum of either inherited or sporadic mutations resulting in cellular dysfunction (Tanaka, Niwa et al. 2006). The most widely known genetic mutation, accounting for 2% of all ALS cases, is superoxide dismutase-1 (SOD1), which has over 100 known different mutations (Banci, Bertini et al. 2008) (for list, see www.alsod.org) that result in a gain of one or more toxic properties that are independent of the levels of SOD1 activity (Stathopulos, Rumfeldt et al. 2003).

Proteomics: encompasses measures of protein folding, degradation, and translation, which become impaired, resulting in defective essential proteins, toxic accumulation of aggregates or aggresomes, and inhibition of organelle function (Watanabe, Dykes-Hoberg et al. 2001; Urushitani, Kurisu et al. 2002; Rumfeldt, Lepock et al. 2009).

Chemistry: encompasses measures of aberrant cellular chemistry, enzymatics, or catalysis (Tiwari, Xu et al. 2005; Tokuda, Ono et al. 2008) that results in oxidative damage and metal mishandling that can be seen alone or in conjunction with SOD1 mutations.

Inflammation: encompasses measures of immune-induced inflammation, including astrocyte (Nagai, Re et al. 2007) and microglia (Hall, Andrus et al. 1998) counts, gliosis and the release of nitric oxide and proinflammatory cytokines, which in combination with impaired growth factors/trophic support (Narai, Nagano et al. 2005; Kadoyama, Funakoshi et al. 2007), further inhibit the neural environment.

Free radicals: encompasses measures of oxidation or inflammation-induced nitric oxide, but particularly the accumulation of reactive oxygen species, such as the superoxides and peroxides that are associated with mitochondrial dysfunction or failure. Free radicals initiate reactions that damage DNA (Pehar, Vargas et al. 2007).
Necro-apoptosis: encompasses the measures of cell death, including the signaling cascades, their constituents, and machinery, which promote cell death. The final destination of an ALS affected motoneuron is cell death either through inflammation-induced necrosis or more likely through apoptosis (Mattson and Duan 1999) via the activation of stress response and caspase pathways (Beere 2004; Gifondorwa, Robinson et al. 2007).
Systemic: encompasses invivo measures of function in the G93A mouse model (Derave, Van Den Bosch et al. 2003). It includes measures of muscle weakness, atrophy, fasiculations, denervation and ultimately loss of function that decreases essential stimulatory retrograde signaling, causing further progression of the diseased state.

2.6.2 G93A feasibility study structure

The dynamic meta-analysis structure is best illustrated like an engineering process flow diagram. Here we show in Figure 1 the categories of outcome measures (boxes) and their interactions (lines). Based on the presented study structure, we determined that there are minimally 72 interactions between the 10 categories of outcome measures. Thus, the minimum number of primary studies to be included in the feasibility study is 72, one for each interaction. Note that we define a primary study as an experiment that measures the interaction between two outcome measures. Therefore, a single published primary experimental article can, and often does, contain more than one primary study. However, it is easier to think of each interaction as needing at least one primary article, and thus, approximately 72 primary articles are need for data extraction to complete a minimalistic feasibility study. The differences between the full and feasibility study structure are shown in Figure 2.
Even for a feasibility study, an "n" of one for each interaction may not sound like meta-analysis, but keep in mind that there are multiple interactions contributing to the effect and prediction of each category. For example, in the structure presented in Figure 1, there are 3-10 interactions for each category. Therefore, 3-10 primary studies contribute to the prediction of each category of outcome measures. That range is in line with the number of primary studies per outcome measure that we might expect for a traditional meta-analysis.

2.7 Extracting data

Quantifiable data is extracted from included primary study figures and tables. Figure 3 shows a hypothetical example of the type of data figure one typically seen in the G93A literature. The Y-axis is typically the affected measure (in this case, percent of cargos travelling retrogradely) and the X-axis is typically the controlled measure (glutamate concentration in our hypothetical example). Additionally, the measure is usually quantified in both the wild-type and G93A mice populations.
Upon extraction, data is normalized to make it unitless. That is, we only look at the relative changes between measures. In this example data, the wild-type retrograde transport went down by ~20% with a 40% increase in glutamate concentration, whereas the SOD1 retrograde transport went down by ~25% with a 40% increase in glutamate concentration.

Therefore, the slope or gain (dY/dX) for wild-type is -0.2 for the interaction from glutamate to retrograde transport. Correspondingly, the gain, for SOD1, is -0.25. Because we only calculate relative changes in dynamic meta-analysis, the magnitude of the gain utilized is actually the relative difference between the wild-type and SOD1 gain magnitudes, (|SOD1| - |wild-type|)/|wild-type|, or [(0.25) - (0.20)]/(0.25) = 0.25, and the sign of this final gain value for this example is net negative (-). Applying the gain of the experimental outcome measures to the category measures, the interaction *from* the category outcome measure of excitotoxicity *to* the category outcome measure of axonal transport is -0.25. Finally, we divide the gain by the time point (or in the case of a feasibility study, the *to* category time constant) to obtain the interaction coefficient (B) used in Equation 2.

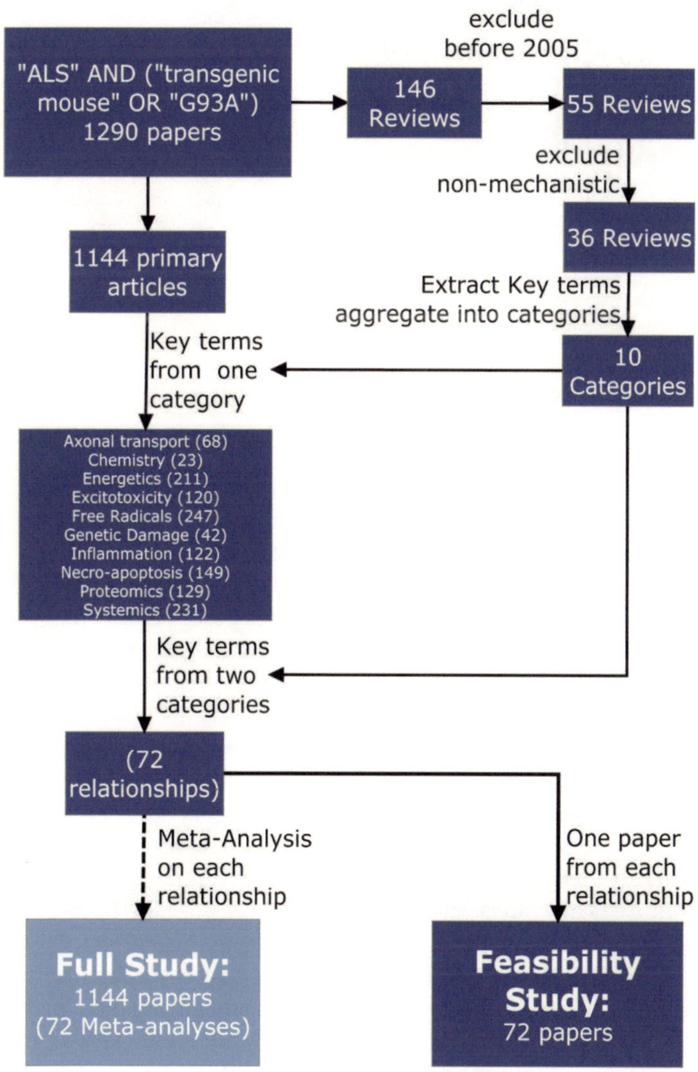

Fig. 2. Scope of dynamic meta-analysis study for the G93A SOD1 mouse model of ALS: feasibility study versus a full study.

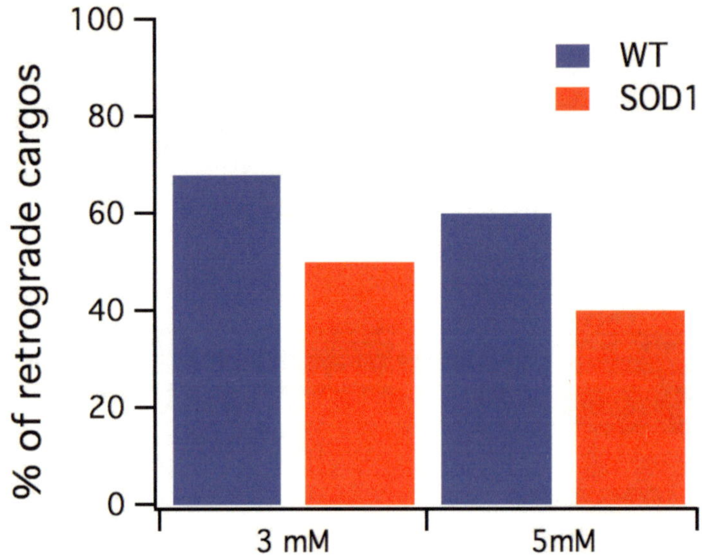

Fig. 3. Example data from a prototypical primary study.

2.8 Quantified data aggregation

For a category-level feasiblity study, such as presented here, it is appropriate to take a non-parametric approach to aggregating the quantitative experimental measures, as the aggregated relationships too disparate to make normalization practical. Consequently, gains were first qualitatively grouped into "small," "medium," or "large". Based on the overall range and resolution of the quantified category interaction magnitudes obtained from the primary studies, numerical gain values for small, medium, and large were set to 0.33, 1, and 3, respectively. However, other values were also explored (e.g. 0.5, 1, and 2; 0.25, 0.5, and 1 etc.) with no qualitative change in result. Table 1 lists the relative magnitude and sign of the category relationships and the primary references from which data was extracted.

Additionally, the corresponding time points for each category utilize a qualitative grouping of small, medium, and large. Based on our mathematical implementaiton of the time points, which is analagous to that used with time constants, we refer to the time points as time constants. Their numerical values and scaling are chosen based on the average onset of associated changes documented for a particular category using the G93A SOD1 mouse model time course. For example, measurable changes are occurring by day 40 in axonal transport, such as the appearance of aggregates and changes in cargo distribution (Kieran, Hafezparast et al. 2005; Teuchert, Fischer et al. 2006); thus, 40 days is used as the time constant for that category. Using the range and resolution of documented changes in G93A over all of the categories, the small, medium, and large time constants are set to 40, 80, and 120 days, respectively (Table 2).

From	To	Size	Sign	Primary Reference(s)
Axonal Transport	Axonal Transport	M	-	(Kieran, 2005; De Vos, 2007; Zhang, Strom 2007)
	Energetics	S	-	(Sakama, 2003; Miller , 2004; De Vos, 2007)
	Excitotoxicity	S	-	(Hiruma, 2003; Stevenson, 2009; Tateno, Kato, 1999)
	Necro-Apoptosis	M	+	(Collard, 1995; Ackerley, 2004)
	Inflammation	S	-	(Brooks,1991; Sasaki, 1996)
Chemistry	Systemic	M	+	(Tiwari, 2005; Ludolph, 2006; Watanabe, 2007; Hozumi, 2008)
	Axonal Transport	S	-	(LaMonte, 2002; Strom, 2008)
	Excitotoxicity	S	+	(Kawahara, 2004; Sasabe, 2007)
	Energetics	S	-	(Wendt, 2002; Lee, Shin, 2008)
	Free Radicals	S	+	(Poon, 2005; Furukawa, 2006)
	Necro-Apoptosis	M	+	(Elam, 2003; Kiaei, 2007; Lee, Shin, 2008)
	Proteomics	M	+	(Lindberg, 2002; Bergemalm, 2006; Rumfeldt, Stathopulos,2006)
Excitotoxicity	Axonal Transport	S	-	(Hiruma, 2003; Tateno, 2008; Stevenson, Yates. 2009)
	Excitotoxicity	M	+	(Rothstein, 1990; Rothstein, 1995; Kuo, 2004; Damiano, Starkov, 2006; Kuwabara, 2007)
	Energetics	L	-	(Beal, 1992; Nicholls, 1998; Jabaudon, 2000; Ellis, 2003)
	Free Radicals	L	+	(Kruman, 1999; Kruman, 1999; Carriedo, 2000; Ellis, 2003)
	Inflammation	L	+	(Hewett, 1994; Cholet, 2002; Barbeito, 2004)
	Necro-Apoptosis	L	+	(Liu, 1999; Sun, 2006; Gibb, 2007; Boutahar, 2008)
	Systemic	S	+	(Bittigau, 1997; Corona, 2007)
Energetics	Axonal Transport	M	+	(Sickles, 1990; Magrane, 2009)
	Excitotoxicity	L	+	(Beal, 1992; Agrawal, 1996; Ellis, 2003; Nicholls, 2003)
	Energetics	M	+	(Mattson, 1999; Mattiazzi, 2002)
	Free Radicals	L	+	(Mattson, 1999; Liu, 2002; Cassina, 2008)
	Inflammation	M	+	(Levine, 1999; Bilsland, 2008)
	Necro-Apoptosis	L	+	(Kruman, 1999; Kaal, 2000; Guegan, 2001; Dupuis, Gonzalez de Aguilar, 2004; Ilzecka, 2007; Knudson, 2008)
	Systemic	M	+	(Verstreken, 2005)
Free Radicals	Axonal Transport	S	-	(Chou, 1996; Chou, 1996; Ferrante, 1997)
	Chemistry	S	+	(Poon, 2005; Furukawa, 2006)
	Excitotoxicity	S	+	(Kruman,1999; Kruman, 1999; Ellis, 2003)
	Energetics	L	-	(Liu, 1996; Liu, 1999; Mattson, 1999; Liu, 2002; Cassina, 2005)
	Free Radicals	M	-	(Liu 1996; Liu. 1999; Cookson, 2002; Cassina, Pehar 2005; Pehar 2007)

From	To	Size	Sign	Primary Reference(s)
	Genetic Damage	M	+	(Aguirre, 2005; Mitsumoto, 2008)
	Inflammation	M	+	(Hensley, 2006; Liu, 2008; Nagai, 2007; Pehar, 2005)
	Necro-Apoptosis	L	+	(Chen, 2009; Estevez, 1999; Pehar, 2005; Pehar, 2007; Wood, 1995)
	Proteomics	S	+	(Dalle-Donne, 2007; Poon, 2005)
	Systemic	S	+	(Dalle-Donne, 2007; Poon, 2005; Kato, 2005; Mahoney, 2006; Mitsumoto, 2008; Sohmiya, 2005)
Genetic Damage	Excitotoxicity	M	+	(Kawahara, 2004; Ignacio, Moore, 2005; Kawahara, 2006)
	Free Radicals	S	+	(Armon, 2005; Wiedau-Pazos, 1996)
	Genetic Damage	M	-	(Armon, 2005; Jiang, 2005; Muller, 2008)
	Inflammation	S	-	(Puttaparthi, 2005; Di Giorgio, 2007; Puttaparthi, 2007)
	Necro-Apoptosis	M	+	(Locatelli, 2007; Lu, 2000)
Inflammation	Axonal Transport	S	-	(Chou, 1996; Kaasik, 2007; King, 2009; Morimoto, 2007)
	Excitotoxicity	M	+	(Hewett, 1994; Cholet, 2002; Pehar, 2004)
	Energetics	S	-	(Cassina, 2008; Cassina, 2005; Takeuchi, 2005; Bilsland, 2008)
	Free Radicals	L	+	(Hensley, 2006; Nagai, 2007; Pehar, 2007)
	Inflammation	M	-	(Gowing, 2008; Puttaparthi, 2005; Schiffer, 1996)
	Necro-Apoptosis	L	+	(Collard, 1995; Ackerley, 2004)
	Systemic	S	+	(Hall, 1998; Cassina, 2005; Cho, 1999)
Necro-Apoptosis	Axonal Transport	S	+	(Ackerley, 2004; Collard, 1995)
	Chemistry	S	-	(Kiaei, 2007; Elam, 2003; Lee, 2009)
	Excitotoxicity	L	+	(Gibb, 2007; Sun, 2002; Liu, 1999)
	Energetics	L	-	(Guegan, 2001; Guegan, 2002)
	Free Radicals	M	+	(Raoul, 2002; Raoul, 2005)
	Genetic Damage	S	+	(Muller, 2007; Raoul, 2006)
	Inflammation	L	+	(Hall, 1998; Cassina, 2005)
	Necro-Apoptosis	L	-	(Gonzalez de Aguilar, 2000; Gonzalez de Aguilar, 1999)
	Proteomics	M	+	(Gal, 2007; Gal, 2009; Yamashita, 2007)
	Systemic	M	+	(Li, 2007; Narai, 2005)
Proteomics	Axonal Transport	M	+	(Eaton, 2005; De Vos, 2007; Sasaki, 2005)
	Chemistry	M	+	(Rumfeldt, 2009; Atkin, 2006)
	Excitotoxicity	S	+	(Rothstein, 2005; Vanoni, 20040
	Free Radicals	S	+	(Aquilano, Rotilio et al. 2003; Clement, 2003)
	Inflammation	M	+	(Stieber, 2000)
	Necro-Apoptosis	M	+	(Urushitani, 2008; Atkin, 2008; Gal, 2007)

From	To	Size	Sign	Primary Reference(s)
	Proteomics	S	-	(Puttaparthi, 2007; Morimoto, 2007; Cheroni, 2009)
	Systemic	M	+	(Turner, 2005; Bucher, 2007)
Systemic	Excitotoxicity	S	+	(Kuner, 2005 ; Pieri, 2008)
	Energetics	S	-	(Wendt, 2002; Zhao, 2006)
	Free Radicals	S	+	(Mahoney, 2006; Pierce, 2008)
	Necro-Apoptosis	S	+	(Martin, 2000; Patel, 2010)
	Systemic	S	-	(Nagano, 2005; Deforges, 2009)

Table 1. Parametric gains for category interactions. Interactions are listed directionally-oriented *from* the category imposing the effected *to* the category being affected. The sign indicates whether the interaction is increasing or decreasing the category, and size (small, medium, large) qualitatively represents the gain magnitude (see Extracted Data Aggregation).

Category	Time Point (days)
Axonal Transport	40
Chemistry	40
Excitotoxicity	80
Energetics	80
Free Radicals	80
Genetic Damage	40
Inflammation	120
Necro-Apoptosis	120
Proteomics	40
Systemic	120

Table 2. Feasibility study time constants utilized for the calculation of the interaction term (B), as shown in Equation 2. Time points are aggregated from primary studies.

2.9 Implementation

Differential equations, in the form shown in Equation 2, are use to construct the dynamic meta-analysis computations. Thus, each category has its own first order differential equation, which includes the effects of each interaction as well as the category time point (or in the case of a feasibility study, a time constant). Each interaction gain coefficient (B) in Equation 2 is simply the change in the affected interaction measure divided by the time point (or in the case of a feasibility study, the category time constant). Because the effect of time is included, the dynamic meta-analysis can predict outcome measures at multiple time points over the entire disease course. Thus, a dynamic meta-analysis can be "simulated" much like a traditional mechanistic model. Because the time-based differential equation computations of dynamic meta-analysis are inherently more complicated than the algebraic regression equations of traditional meta-analysis, the use of a computer simulator assists in its implementation. For this feasibility study, the dynamic meta-analysis was coded, simulated, and analyzed in Matlab (Mathworks, Inc.).

2.10 Post-result analysis and prediction

The basic results of dynamic meta-analysis are quantitative predictions of each outcome measure or category outcome measure changes over time. Additional, higher level results can be obtained by performing sensitivity analyses, which perturb the system and measure the resulting affects. Perturbation can include varying the initial conditions of each category individually or en masse, or varying the interaction gain coefficients (B). Changing initial conditions provides an assessment of the effect size whereas varying specific or category gains provides an assessment of their sensitivity/specificity. For more detail on sensitivity analyses, see (Mitchell, Feng et al. 2007; Mitchell and Lee 2007; Mitchell and Lee 2009).

Traditional meta-analysis analytical tools, such as statistical linear regression and effect size prediction, are still useful to analyze dynamic meta-analysis results. However, the dynamic and multi-variate nature of dynamic meta-analysis also provides possibilities for richer analyses like those typically seen in the analysis of complex or dynamical systems. Given that the two greatest advantages of dynamic analysis are the implicit inclusion of interactions and explicit inclusion of time, analyses that examine how relationships change over time are particularly telling. Analyses such as cross-correlation (or landscapes) of outcome measures or category outcome measures at specific disease time points, such was done in (Mitchell and Lee 2008) and (Mitchell and Lee 2007), provide a overview of what the system is doing without becoming mired in detail.

Finally, the implicit inclusion of interactions allows combination treatments to be examined. All clinical treatments, in some form, exploit a cellular interaction at some level. For example, pharmaceutical modulators typically exploit the interaction between a receptor and its ligand. Thus, every potential interaction within the dynamic meta-analysis structure can be evaluated as a hypothetical treatment possibility. Furthermore, the structure of dynamic meta-analysis allows every single interaction (whether between outcome measures or between categories of outcome measures) to be varied and simulated individually and in combination. Measuring the resultant effect size of an interaction or combination of interactions predicts its potential treatment efficacy. For more methodological detail on simulating combination therapies, see our previous work with combination treatments and spinal cord injury (Mitchell and Lee 2008).

3. Results of a G93A SOD1 feasibility study

We begin by examing the effect size of each category, an analysis that is typically seen with traditional meta-analysis. Table 3 reveals the average, standard deviation, maximum, and minimum effect size of each category based on a sensitivity analysis that perturbed the intial conditions. Note that "N" is the connectivity, or number of interactions (as shown in Figure 1), affecting the category measure. This examination reveals that the average effect of, for example, treating energetics is a relatively unimpressive 19% outcome change for a 100% treatment effect on energetics itself. (Note that a "real" treatment would have effects substantially smaller than 100%, often only 10% or so.). However, this type of analysis misses the potential for interactions completely and to some extent even minimizes the potential significance of targeted treatments by averaging.

Category	Avg	Stdev	Min	Max	N
Axon Transport	-1%	12%	-21%	16%	6
Chemistry	11%	27%	-6%	71%	7
Energetics	-19%	71%	-98%	102%	7
Excitotoxicity	0%	39%	-80%	36%	7
Free Radical	2%	24%	-53%	44%	10
Genetics	3%	6%	-3%	12%	5
Inflammation	14%	21%	-6%	49%	7
Necro-Apoptosis	16%	26%	-35%	59%	10
Proteomics	13%	24%	-17%	56%	8
Systemic	-2%	5%	-10%	2%	5

Table 3. Standard meta-analysis result table illustrating the effect of each category on disease outcome measures (survival and function).

3.1 Dynamics of the G93A SOD1 mouse pathology

Next, we examine the relative changes in the category outcome measures over time in order to get a better feel of the system dynamics. As shown in Figure 4, initially, the system exhibits a period of relative quiescence (days 0-80) in which there appears to be little variation from the baseline operating point. However, closer examination reveals a few fluctuations, which appear as small oscillations from baseline (Figure 5). Over time each oscillation grows in magnitude, with the first notable oscillation starting around day 40. However, the component trajectories do eventually explode at approximately day 150.

These qualitative system features of ALS align well with the characterization of the G-93A SOD-1 experimental paradigm. In fact, the first large oscillation corresponds to the average onset of measurable functional deficits and the final explosion aligns with the average time of death for the G-93A SOD-1 mouse model (Xu, Jung et al. 2004; Kieran, Hafezparast et al. 2005; Gould, Buss et al. 2006; Teuchert, Fischer et al. 2006). It should be noted that the oscillations of this system do not necessarily represent the relapsing and remitting of functional deficits, such as is seen with multiple sclerosis, but rather the oscillations of individual mechanisms and pathways. In fact, such oscillations could be responsible for small fluctuations sometimes seen within and among mechanistic studies, such as those examining axonal transport (De Vos, Chapman et al. 2007) and protein aggregation (Stieber, Gonatas et al. 2000; Gould, Buss et al. 2006). How oscillations correlating with specific losses in muscle function remains to be seen. It is likely that the overall loss of systemic control aligns with what is typically seen as continuously degenerating function or degenerative function with intermixed plateaus.

From a system dynamics point of view, it is likely that the exploding oscillations of ALS are the result of an unstable system. Initially, the regulatory systems, including excitability, ionic and axonal transport, cellular energetics and others, are able to maintain partial control, as evidenced by the smaller oscillations, which are an attempt to regulate. However, as the disease progresses the control mechanisms simply fail to keep up.

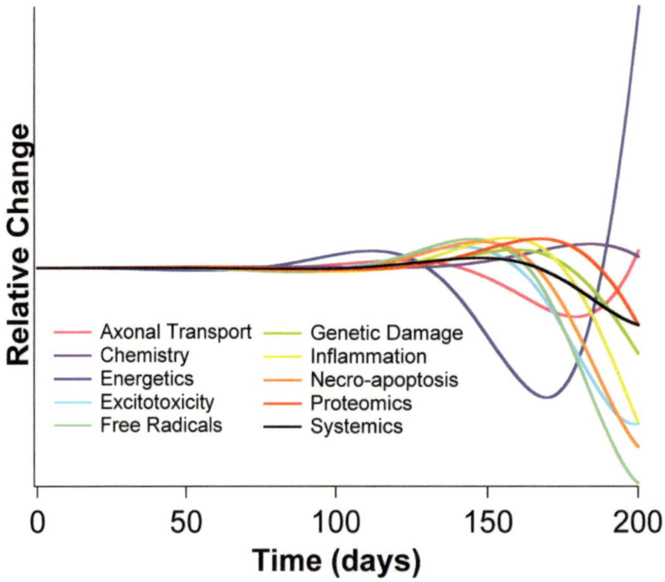

Fig. 4. Unstable, oscillatory dynamics of ALS predicted by dynamic meta-analysis .

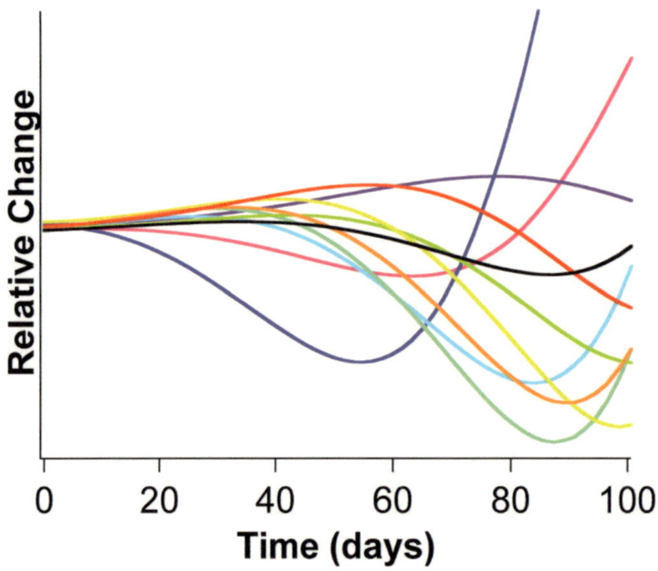

Fig. 5. Expansion of oscillations initiating during the pre-symptomatic quiescent period.

3.2 Combination therapy predictions

We examine how hypothetical therapeutics that exploit single and multi-category interactions can potentially "treat" the system. We utilize the systemic category as our primary outcome measure since it includes known functional metrics. Two different combination treatment types are examined: 1.) combination treatments that stabilize the system (e.g. dampen the oscillations) and 2.) synergistic combination treatments.

Stabilizing Treatments: If pathological progression is driven by, or is the result of, system instability, then one potential therapeutic strategy is to develop treatments that rectify the instability. We tested single treatments that targeted individual category interactions as well as combination treatments that simultaneously targeted up to 3 category interactions. A small percentage of the over 44,000 different combinations treatments investigated rectified the system instability (See example in Figure 6), thereby preventing the "explosion" typically seen between days 150-200 at the average time of death. That is, these treatments have the potential to greatly extend the life span of the typical G-93A mouse.

Of note is that many of the most successful treatment combinations did not include the component that was responsible for the initiating perturbation. Also in some cases, the directions (sign of the relationship) that components best treated the system could be non-intuitive, again likely owing to the highly interactive nature of the ALS system.

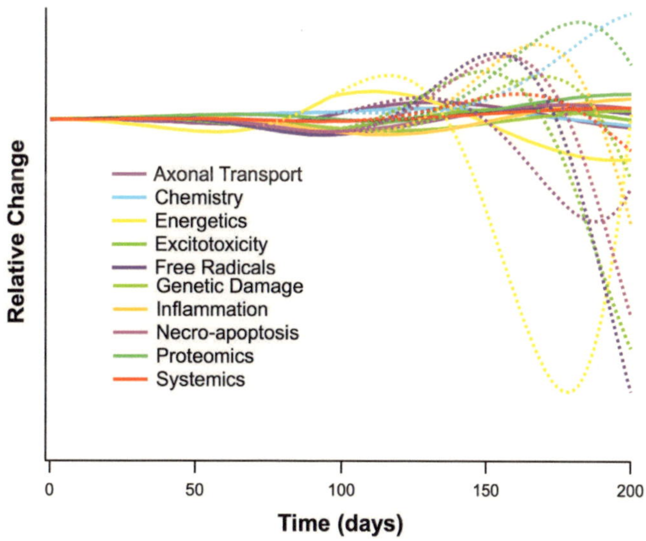

Fig. 6. Dynamics of ALS predicted by dynamic analysis of the G93A SOD1 mouse model. ALS dynamics are unstable, (dashed lines) characterized by growing oscillations that "explode" near the average time of death. Dynamic meta-analysis of potential treatment combinations predicts that a small percentage of 3-way treatment combinations can assist in re-stabilization of the system (solid lines).

Treatment synergism: Whether stabilizing or not, or just purely interaction-based, many of the ALS treatments have a synergistic effect. That is, their combined effects are substantially greater than the sum of their individual effects. For two-way treatments (treatments addressing two category interactions), 16% of the total possible 10,000 combinations are synergistic. (Note that treatment direction was made in the more favorable direction.) For three-way combinations, approximately 22% of the possible 900,000 combinations are synergistic (Figure 7).

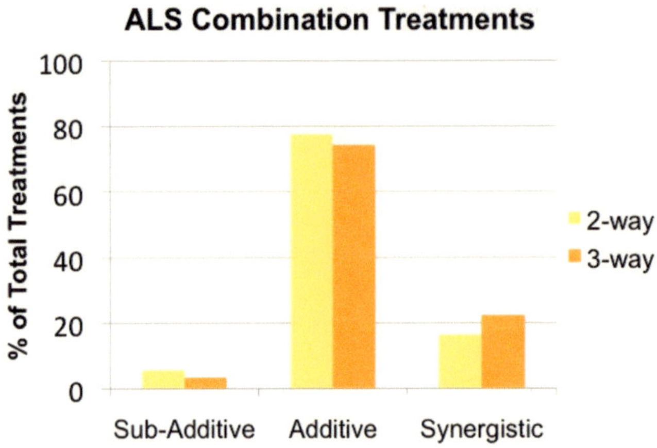

Fig. 7. Percentage of total treatment combinations belonging to each efficacy type.

Tables 4 and 5, show the efficacies of 2-way and 3-way synergistic combination treatments. A linearly additive treatment (combination A&B effect = A effect + B effect) was assigned an efficacy factor of 1.0. Thus, synergistic treatments have efficacy factors >1 and sub-additive treatments have efficacy factors <1. Therefore, categories with higher average and maximum efficacy factors have a tendency to produce greater synergistic effects in combination.

Category	Avg	Stdev	Max	Count
Axonal Transport	1.08	0.16	1.74	59
Chemistry	1.02	0.05	1.39	107
Energetics	1.23	0.32	2.44	229
Excitotoxicity	1.09	0.24	2.33	160
Free Radical	1.06	0.14	1.93	311
Genetics	1.01	0.02	1.21	86
Inflammation	1.03	0.07	1.66	195
Necro-Apoptosis	1.10	0.23	2.35	327
Proteomics	1.04	0.15	2.05	154
Systemic	1.05	0.07	1.23	22

Table 4. Synergistic two-way combination treatment predictions.

Category	Avg	Stdev	Max	Count
Axonal Transport	1.08	0.17	2.82	17395
Chemistry	1.19	0.26	4.85	23101
Energetics	1.09	0.19	2.82	22332
Excitotoxicity	1.05	0.13	2.13	33020
Free Radical	1.04	0.12	2.01	12929
Genetics	1.05	0.12	3.26	22589
Inflammation	1.09	0.19	2.67	35586
Necro-Apoptosis	1.09	0.20	2.60	22603
Proteomics	1.06	0.14	2.05	11322
Systemic	1.00	0.00	1.00	0

Table 5. Synergistic three-way combination treatment predictions.

4. Conclusions

System dynamics revealed. Conventional wisdom in ALS research has been that there is a single, specific root cause. However, dynamic meta-analysis predicts that a system-level instability is the actual problem (see oscillations in Figure 4). Lending credence to the predictions of dynamic meta-analysis is the mounting evidence from recent studies that indicates that multiple mutations or underlying mechanisms can result in the symptoms characterized as ALS (Rothstein 2009).

Novel treatment strategies identified. In this small scale feasibility study of ALS, dynamic meta-analysis predicts that reducing the overall feedback gain will be more effective than identifying and ameliorating a single "source" or point of initiation (Mitchell and Lee 2010). That is, inducing small changes across multiple categories of mechanisms is more effective than inducing a large change in a single category. Additionally, treatments that target the underyling system dyanmics, such as stabilizing oscillations, could be another potentially effective path.

Combination treatment prediction enabled. Another key opportunity afforded by dynamic meta-analysis is an innovative approach to predicting combination treatment effectiveness in a high-throughput manner. The interacting differential equations of dynamic meta-analysis implicitly include all possible treatment interactions. Thus, potential synergistic combinations can be identified before they are explicitly examined experimentally. For example, in spinal cord injury, a sweep of all possible combinations of virtual treatments revealed that none were synergistic (Mitchell and Lee 2008). While disappointing, we were at least able to discover treatments that combined linearly. On the other hand, in our initial evaluation of ALS, a small percentage of treatment combinations show very profound synergism! It appears that in ALS, the broader the treatment the more effective it becomes. (Figure 6 illustrates an example of a 3-way combination that appears to arrest the oscillatory explosion observed in the control case.) Finally, dynamic meta-analysis is not only well suited to identify promising combinations but can be used to prioritize them as well.

5. Acknowledgments

This work was supported by the National Institute of Health (NS069616 and NS062200).

6. References

Ackerley, S., A. J. Grierson, et al. (2004). "p38alpha stress-activated protein kinase phosphorylates neurofilaments and is associated with neurofilament pathology in amyotrophic lateral sclerosis." *Mol Cell Neurosci* 26(2): 354-364.

Banci, L., I. Bertini, et al. (2008). "SOD1 and amyotrophic lateral sclerosis: mutations and oligomerization." *PLoS One* 3(2): e1677.

Beere, H. M. (2004). ""The stress of dying": the role of heat shock proteins in the regulation of apoptosis." *J Cell Sci* 117(Pt 13): 2641-2651.

Bilsland, L. G., E. Sahai, et al. "Deficits in axonal transport precede ALS symptoms in vivo." *Proc Natl Acad Sci U S A.*

Bogdanov, M. B., L. E. Ramos, et al. (1998). "Elevated "hydroxyl radical" generation in vivo in an animal model of amyotrophic lateral sclerosis." *J Neurochem* 71(3): 1321-1324.

De Vos, K. J., A. L. Chapman, et al. (2007). "Familial amyotrophic lateral sclerosis-linked SOD1 mutants perturb fast axonal transport to reduce axonal mitochondria content." *Hum Mol Genet* 16(22): 2720-2728.
Derave, W., L. Van Den Bosch, et al. (2003). "Skeletal muscle properties in a transgenic mouse model for amyotrophic lateral sclerosis: effects of creatine treatment." *Neurobiol Dis* 13(3): 264-272.
Dobrowolny, G., M. Aucello, et al. (2008). "Skeletal muscle is a primary target of SOD1G93A-mediated toxicity." *Cell Metab* 8(5): 425-436.
Dunlop, J., H. Beal McIlvain, et al. (2003). "Impaired spinal cord glutamate transport capacity and reduced sensitivity to riluzole in a transgenic superoxide dismutase mutant rat model of amyotrophic lateral sclerosis." *J Neurosci* 23(5): 1688-1696.
Dupuis, L., H. Oudart, et al. (2004). "Evidence for defective energy homeostasis in amyotrophic lateral sclerosis: benefit of a high-energy diet in a transgenic mouse model." *Proc Natl Acad Sci U S A* 101(30): 11159-11164.
Echaniz-Laguna, A., J. Zoll, et al. (2002). "Mitochondrial respiratory chain function in skeletal muscle of ALS patients." *Ann Neurol* 52(5): 623-627.
Gifondorwa, D. J., M. B. Robinson, et al. (2007). "Exogenous delivery of heat shock protein 70 increases lifespan in a mouse model of amyotrophic lateral sclerosis." *J Neurosci* 27(48): 13173-13180.
Gould, T. W., R. R. Buss, et al. (2006). "Complete dissociation of motor neuron death from motor dysfunction by Bax deletion in a mouse model of ALS." *J Neurosci* 26(34): 8774-8786.
Guatteo, E., I. Carunchio, et al. (2007). "Altered calcium homeostasis in motor neurons following AMPA receptor but not voltage-dependent calcium channels' activation in a genetic model of amyotrophic lateral sclerosis." *Neurobiol Dis* 28(1): 90-100.
Hafezparast, M., A. Ahmad-Annuar, et al. (2003). "Paradigms for the identification of new genes in motor neuron degeneration." *Amyotroph Lateral Scler Other Motor Neuron Disord* 4(4): 249-257.
Hall, E. D., P. K. Andrus, et al. (1998). "Relationship of oxygen radical-induced lipid peroxidative damage to disease onset and progression in a transgenic model of familial ALS." *J Neurosci Res* 53(1): 66-77.
Hayward, L. J., J. A. Rodriguez, et al. (2002). "Decreased metallation and activity in subsets of mutant superoxide dismutases associated with familial amyotrophic lateral sclerosis." *J Biol Chem* 277(18): 15923-15931.
Ikonomidou, C., Y. Qin Qin, et al. (1996). "Motor neuron degeneration induced by excitotoxin agonists has features in common with those seen in the SOD-1 transgenic mouse model of amyotrophic lateral sclerosis." *J Neuropathol Exp Neurol* 55(2): 211-224.
Kadoyama, K., H. Funakoshi, et al. (2007). "Hepatocyte growth factor (HGF) attenuates gliosis and motoneuronal degeneration in the brainstem motor nuclei of a transgenic mouse model of ALS." *Neurosci Res* 59(4): 446-456.
Kieran, D., M. Hafezparast, et al. (2005). "A mutation in dynein rescues axonal transport defects and extends the life span of ALS mice." *J Cell Biol* 169(4): 561-567.
King, A. E., T. C. Dickson, et al. (2009). "Neuron-glia interactions underlie ALS-like axonal cytoskeletal pathology." *Neurobiol Aging*.
Kong, J. and Z. Xu (1998). "Massive mitochondrial degeneration in motor neurons triggers the onset of amyotrophic lateral sclerosis in mice expressing a mutant SOD1." *J Neurosci* 18(9): 3241-3250.

Kuo, J. J., M. Schonewille, et al. (2004). "Hyperexcitability of cultured spinal motoneurons from presymptomatic ALS mice." *J Neurophysiol* 91(1): 571-575.

Kuo, J. J., T. Siddique, et al. (2005). "Increased persistent Na(+) current and its effect on excitability in motoneurones cultured from mutant SOD1 mice." *J Physiol* 563(Pt 3): 843-854.

Mattson, M. P. and W. Duan (1999). "Apoptotic" biochemical cascades in synaptic compartments: roles in adaptive plasticity and neurodegenerative disorders." *J Neurosci Res* 58(1): 152-166.

Meyer, M. A. and N. T. Potter (1995). "Sporadic ALS and chromosome 22: evidence for a possible neurofilament gene defect." *Muscle Nerve* 18(5): 536-539.

Miller, R. G., J. D. Mitchell, et al. (2007). "Riluzole for amyotrophic lateral sclerosis (ALS)/motor neuron disease (MND)." *Cochrane Database Syst Rev*(1): CD001447.

Mitchell, C. S. (2009). Viewpoint aggregation via relational modeling and analysis: A new approach to systems physiology. *Wallace H. Coulter Department of Biomedical Engineering*. Atlanta, GA, Georgia Institute of Technology and Emory University.

Mitchell, C. S., S. S. Feng, et al. (2007). "An analysis of glutamate spillover on the N-methyl-D-aspartate receptors at the cerebellar glomerulus." *J Neural Eng* 4(3): 276-282.

Mitchell, C. S. and R. H. Lee (2007). "Output-based comparison of alternative kinetic schemes for the NMDA receptor within a glutamate spillover model." *J Neural Eng* 4(4): 380-389.

Mitchell, C. S. and R. H. Lee (2008). "Pathology dynamics predict spinal cord injury therapeutic success." *J Neurotrauma* 25(12): 1483-1497.

Mitchell, C. S. and R. H. Lee (2009). "A quantitative examination of the role of cargo-exerted forces in axonal transport." *J Theor Biol* 257(3): 430-437.

Mitchell, C. S. and R. H. Lee (2010). *Dynamic Meta-Analysis of the G93A SOD1 mouse model: Pathology dynamics and combination treatment predictions*. 21st International Symposium on ALS/MND, Orlando, FL.

Nagai, M., D. B. Re, et al. (2007). "Astrocytes expressing ALS-linked mutated SOD1 release factors selectively toxic to motor neurons." *Nat Neurosci* 10(5): 615-622.

Nagano, I., T. Murakami, et al. (2002). "Early decrease of survival factors and DNA repair enzyme in spinal motor neurons of presymptomatic transgenic mice that express a mutant SOD1 gene." *Life Sci* 72(4-5): 541-548.

Narai, H., I. Nagano, et al. (2005). "Prevention of spinal motor neuron death by insulin-like growth factor-1 associating with the signal transduction systems in SODG93A transgenic mice." *J Neurosci Res* 82(4): 452-457.

Pastula, D. M., D. H. Moore, et al. (2010). "Creatine for amyotrophic lateral sclerosis/motor neuron disease." *Cochrane Database Syst Rev*(6): CD005225.

Pehar, M., M. R. Vargas, et al. (2007). "Mitochondrial superoxide production and nuclear factor erythroid 2-related factor 2 activation in p75 neurotrophin receptor-induced motor neuron apoptosis." *J Neurosci* 27(29): 7777-7785.

Peviani, M., I. Caron, et al. "Unraveling the complexity of amyotrophic lateral sclerosis: recent advances from the transgenic mutant SOD1 mice." *CNS Neurol Disord Drug Targets* 9(4): 491-503.

Rothstein, J. D. (2009). "Current hypotheses for the underlying biology of amyotrophic lateral sclerosis." *Ann Neurol* 65 Suppl 1: S3-9.

Roy, J., S. Minotti, et al. (1998). "Glutamate potentiates the toxicity of mutant Cu/Zn-superoxide dismutase in motor neurons by postsynaptic calcium-dependent mechanisms." *J Neurosci* 18(23): 9673-9684.

Rumfeldt, J. A., J. R. Lepock, et al. (2009). "Unfolding and folding kinetics of amyotrophic lateral sclerosis-associated mutant Cu,Zn superoxide dismutases." *J Mol Biol* 385(1): 278-298.

Shi, P., J. Gal, et al. "Mitochondrial dysfunction in amyotrophic lateral sclerosis." *Biochim Biophys Acta* 1802(1): 45-51.

Stathopulos, P. B., J. A. Rumfeldt, et al. (2003). "Cu/Zn superoxide dismutase mutants associated with amyotrophic lateral sclerosis show enhanced formation of aggregates in vitro." *Proc Natl Acad Sci U S A* 100(12): 7021-7026.

Stieber, A., J. O. Gonatas, et al. (2000). "Aggregation of ubiquitin and a mutant ALS-linked SOD1 protein correlate with disease progression and fragmentation of the Golgi apparatus." *J Neurol Sci* 173(1): 53-62.

Sumi, H., S. Nagano, et al. (2006). "Inverse correlation between the formation of mitochondria-derived vacuoles and Lewy-body-like hyaline inclusions in G93A superoxide-dismutase-transgenic mice." *Acta Neuropathol* 112(1): 52-63.

Tanaka, F., J. Niwa, et al. (2006). "Gene expression profiling toward understanding of ALS pathogenesis." *Ann N Y Acad Sci* 1086: 1-10.

Teuchert, M., D. Fischer, et al. (2006). "A dynein mutation attenuates motor neuron degeneration in SOD1(G93A) mice." *Exp Neurol* 198(1): 271-274.

Tiwari, A., Z. Xu, et al. (2005). "Aberrantly increased hydrophobicity shared by mutants of Cu,Zn-superoxide dismutase in familial amyotrophic lateral sclerosis." *J Biol Chem* 280(33): 29771-29779.

Trelle, S., S. Reichenbach, et al. (2011). "Cardiovascular safety of non-steroidal anti-inflammatory drugs: network meta-analysis." *BMJ* 342: c7086.

Tokuda, E., S. Ono, et al. (2008). "Ammonium tetrathiomolybdate delays onset, prolongs survival, and slows progression of disease in a mouse model for amyotrophic lateral sclerosis." *Exp Neurol* 213(1): 122-128.

Urushitani, M., J. Kurisu, et al. (2002). "Proteasomal inhibition by misfolded mutant superoxide dismutase 1 induces selective motor neuron death in familial amyotrophic lateral sclerosis." *J Neurochem* 83(5): 1030-1042.

Van Damme, P., M. Leyssen, et al. (2003). "The AMPA receptor antagonist NBQX prolongs survival in a transgenic mouse model of amyotrophic lateral sclerosis." *Neurosci Lett* 343(2): 81-84.

Vukosavic, S., M. Dubois-Dauphin, et al. (1999). "Bax and Bcl-2 interaction in a transgenic mouse model of familial amyotrophic lateral sclerosis." *J Neurochem* 73(6): 2460-2468.

Watanabe, M., M. Dykes-Hoberg, et al. (2001). "Histological evidence of protein aggregation in mutant SOD1 transgenic mice and in amyotrophic lateral sclerosis neural tissues." *Neurobiol Dis* 8(6): 933-941.

Wong, N. K., B. P. He, et al. (2000). "Characterization of neuronal intermediate filament protein expression in cervical spinal motor neurons in sporadic amyotrophic lateral sclerosis (ALS)." *J Neuropathol Exp Neurol* 59(11): 972-982.

Wood, J. D., T. P. Beaujeux, et al. (2003). "Protein aggregation in motor neurone disorders." *Neuropathol Appl Neurobiol* 29(6): 529-545.

Xu, Z., C. Jung, et al. (2004). "Mitochondrial degeneration in amyotrophic lateral sclerosis." *J Bioenerg Biomembr* 36(4): 395-399.

4

In Vivo and *In Vitro* Models to Study Amyotrophic Lateral Sclerosis

François Berthod and François Gros-Louis
Centre LOEX de l'Université Laval,
Centre de recherche FRSQ du Centre hospitalier affilié universitaire de Québec,
Département de Chirurgie, Faculté de Médecine, Université Laval, Québec,
Canada

1. Introduction

Amyotrophic Lateral Sclerosis (ALS) is the most common adult-onset neurodegenerative disorder characterized by the death of large motor neurons in the cerebral cortex and spinal cord (Tandan and Bradley, 1985). Dysfunction and death of these cell populations lead to progressive muscle weakness, atrophy, fasciculations, spasticity and ultimately, paralysis and death usually within 3 to 5 years after disease onset (Mulder, 1982). The estimated worldwide incidence for this disease is around 2 per 100,000 in the general population and the life-long risk to develop ALS is approximately 1:2000. The disease occurs in sporadic (90%) and familial forms (10%) (Gros-Louis, et al., 2006). With the exception of few FALS cases in which other neurodegenerative disorders can simultaneously occur, FALS and SALS are clinically indistinguishable. To date, mutations in the Cu/Zn superoxide dismutase 1 (*SOD1*) gene have remained the major known genetic causes associated with ALS. However, the mechanism whereby mutant SOD1 causes specific degeneration of motor neurons remains unclear. Nonetheless, many neuronal death pathways have been revealed through studies with transgenic mice expressing SOD1 mutants. Other vertebrate, invertebrate and *in vitro* models of ALS have also been described. Here, we will review various animal and cellular models that have been used to study the toxicity of ALS-linked gene mutations and also to investigate pathological hallmarks of the disease.

1.1 Familial ALS

Though most cases of ALS are sporadic, 10% of cases have affected relatives, some with clear Mendelian inheritance and high penetrance (Gros-Louis, et al., 2006). The landmark discovery in 1993 of missense mutations in the *SOD1* gene in subsets of familial cases directed most ALS research to elucidate the mechanism of SOD1-mediadted disease (Rosen, et al., 1993). More recently, mutations in two other genes, *TARDBP* and *FUS/TLS* have been found in ALS patients (Kabashi, et al., 2008; Sreedharan, et al., 2008; Vance, et al., 2009). Rare mutations in other genes such as *ANG, ALS2, DCTN1, MAPT, SETX* and *VAPB* have also been described (for reviews see (Gros-Louis, et al., 2006)). Various other genetic mutations in the *ELP3* ((Simpson, et al., 2009), *FIG4* (Chow, et al., 2009), *DAO* (Mitchell, et al., 2010), *OPTN* (Maruyama, et al., 2010) and *CHGB* (Gros-Louis, et al., 2009a) genes have also been associated with the disease through several candidate gene-based association studies. Given the high degree of genetic and clinical heterogeneity seen in ALS patients, along with population-specific genetic risk factors for ALS, independent replication of these genetic association studies would be crucial in order to better understand the different mechanisms involved in these disease. As there are several excellent reviews in the literature describing these genes and their relevance to ALS, we will mainly describe the most recent and exciting advances involving *SOD1*, *TARDBP* and *FUS* in this area.

To date, family-based linkage studies and positional cloning have led to the identification of fifteen ALS-associated genes in which mutations have been identified in familial ALS cases (Table 1). Different research groups or consortiums have replicated these results in several populations. To date, a number of genes have been discovered as causative for the classical adult onset form of familial ALS with typical symptoms, namely *SOD1*, *TARDBP*, *FUS/TLS*, and *C9ORF72* (DeJesus-Hernandez, et al., 2011; Kabashi, et al., 2008; Kwiatkowski, et al., 2009; Renton, et al., 2011; Rosen, et al., 1993; Sreedharan, et al., 2008). These genes cumulatively account for about 25% of familial cases, indicating that other causative genes remain to be identified. The difficulties to identify gene responsible for FALS arise in part because large families with sufficient statistical power for linkage analysis are hard to come by, due to the late-onset and age-dependant penetrance of the disease, and the relative short survival time of affected ALS patients. Furthermore, the high degree of genetic heterogeneity, i.e. many rare variants in many different genes individually having a modest effect on the total number of ALS cases, is also certainly a limiting factor for the identification of causative ALS-predisposing genes. Four other genes, namely *DAO*, *OPTN*, *ATAX2* and *VCP* have also been included in this category, but the evidence for their role in predisposing to classical ALS needs to be confirmed in replication studies, and more families linked to these genes also need to be described (Elden, et al., 2010; Johnson, et al., 2010; Maruyama, et al., 2010; Mitchell, et al., 2010).

FALS-associated known genes (gene symbol)	Inheritance	Onset	Mutation types	References
Superoxyde dismutase 1 (SOD1)	AD	Adult	Missense and truncation mutation	Rosen et al., 1993
TAR DNA-binding protein (TARDBP)	AD	Adult	Missense and nonsense mutations	Kabashi et al., 2008; Sreedharan et al., 2008
Fused in sarcoma/translated in liposarcoma (FUS/TL	AD and AR	Adult	Missense mutations, indels	Kwiatkowski et al., 2009; Vance et al., 2009
Chromosome 9 opend reading frame 72 (C9ORF72)	AD	Adult	lexanucleotide GGGGCC expansion repe	enton et al., 2011, DeJesus-Hernandez et al., 201
Ataxin 2 (ATAX2)	AD	Adult	Trinucleotide CAG expansion repeat	Elden et al., 2010
Ubiquitin-like protein ubiquilin2 (UBQLN2)	X-linked	Adult	Missense mutations	Deng et al., 2011
Optineurin (OPTN)	AD	Adult	Missense and nonsense mutations	Maruyama et al., 2010
D-amino acid oxidase (DAO)	AD	Adult	One R199W missense mutation	Mitchell et al., 2010
Amyotrophic lateral sclerosis 2 (ALS2)	AR	Juvenile	Missense and nonsense mutations	Hadano et al., 2002, Yang et al., 2002
Valosin-containing protein (VCP)	AD	Adult	Missense mutations	Johnson et al., 2010
Vesicle-associated membrane protein B (VAPB)	AD	Adult	Missense mutations	Nishimura et al., 2004
Microtubule-associated protein tau (MAPT)	AD	Adult	Missense and 5'-splice-site mutations	Hutton et al., 1998
Dynactin 1 (DCTN1)	AD	Adult	Missense mutations	Puls et al., 2003
Angiogenin	AD	Adult	Missense mutations	Chen et al., 2004
Senataxin (SETX)	AD	Juvenile	Missense mutations	Greeway et al., 2006

Table 1. Identified genes predisposing for familial ALS and/or ALS-FTLD
FALS: Familial ALS, ALS-FTLD: ALS with frontotemporal lobar degeneration,
AD: autosomal dominant, AR: autosomal recessive, Indels: insertions, deletions

The identification of other genes responsible for the disease and the understanding of the molecular pathways involved will bring some new insights into the mechanisms of disease pathogenesis, and may also elucidate the underlying mechanism(s) for specific motor neuron degeneration observed in ALS.

1.2 Sporadic ALS

For most cases of ALS, the causes are unknown. A genetic component is also thought to contribute to the pathogenesis of sporadic ALS, which accounts for the majority of ALS cases. However, identification of gene mutations associated with SALS has met with limited success so far. Several groups have reported on gene variants and association studies found in individuals with sporadic ALS, each accounting for a small number of the total cases reflecting a complex pattern of inheritance with very low penetrance, a high degree of heterogeneity and/or the existence of environmental factors predisposing to ALS. Because familial and sporadic forms of the disease are clinically and pathologically similar, understanding the familial form will shed light on possible epidemiological and pathophysiological mechanisms in SALS.

Many divergent data generated by different research groups who have studied different populations around the world have been published. The use of an adequate size population with appropriate control individuals is needed in order to reach enough statistical power and to observe any significant results. Homogeneity regarding ethnical origin, age, age of onset, disease duration, site of the first symptoms and gender among the studied populations is essential to design a good and robust genetic study. The requirement for larger sample sizes and possibly more sensitive and efficient analytic tools allowing for reliable detection across studied populations are now becoming more and more available as non cost-effective genotyping strategies are being developed.

The identifications of different genes and genetic risk factors associated with ALS over the past years have highlighted common molecular pathways mainly involving intracellular cell trafficking and RNA metabolism. To what extent these pathways are implicated in ALS remain to be determined and studied further. However, it is interesting to note that genes such as *ALS2, VAPB, MAPT, DCTN1, EAAT2, NEFH, PRPH, FIG4, CNTF, CHGB* and *OPTN* in which mutations have been found in a subset of FALS and/or SALS patients, are all related to intracellular trafficking either via axonal transport, vesicle docking and transport, or microtubule and neurofilament stabilization. Furthermore, this common theme is also seen in other motor neuron diseases and neurodegenerative disorders such as hereditary spastic paraplegia, Parkinson's disease, spinal muscular atrophy and Charcot-Marie-tooth disease. It is also noteworthy that RNA metabolism via alternative splicing abnormalities or RNA binding is also a common theme observed amongst the different ALS related genes such as *ALS2, MAPT, EAAT2, PRPH, GluR2, CNTF, SETX, SMN1, SMN2, TARDBP and FUS/TLS.* The high degree of genetic heterogeneity observed in ALS suggests that an individual phenotype could result from the sum of several contributing gene defects and/or epigenetic influences, which individually do not cause disease, and may explain the difficulties in identifying genes associated with SALS. The identification of other genes associated with motor neuron disease, as well as the determination of genetic and/or environmental factors that predispose to SALS is crucial in the development of novel therapies for ALS. The generation of cellular or animal models to study SALS, in which the disease can be closely replicated, would also be the utmost importance to reach a full understanding of the molecular mechanisms and environmental factors associated with SALS.

1.3 ALS with cognitive impairments

In recent years, key developments have revealed a novel neurodegenerative disease spectrum with clinical symptoms overlapping between ALS and frontotemporal lobar degeneration (FTLD) (Strong and Yang, 2011). Cognitive and behavioral impairment is well described in ALS with a significant proportion of patients meeting strict diagnostic criteria for FTLD. Neuroimaging and pathological studies have shown clear involvement of non-motor areas of the brain. More recently, distinct subtypes of frontotemporal lobar dysfunction have been identified in ALS and further work to distinguish these phenotypes and their correlate neuropathology is under way. Attention has been devoted lately to a gene coding for a DNA/RNA binding protein, which have been implicated in the pathogenesis of ALS with cognitive impairments. Indeed, dominant mutations in the *TARDBP* gene, encoding for TDP-43, were reported by several groups as a primary cause of ALS in about 3% familial cases and 1.5% sporadic cases (Chio, et al., 2011; Corrado, et al., 2009; Daoud, et al., 2009; Gitcho, et al., 2008; Kabashi, et al., 2008; Millecamps, et al., 2010; Sreedharan, et al., 2008; Van Deerlin, et al., 2008). The discovery of gene mutations linked to human ALS has provided plethora opportunities to develop model systems for investigating mechanisms of TDP-43 associated disease.

Motor neuron degeneration can also occasionally occurs in patients with Parkinson's disease and frontotemporal dementia (FTD). This disease is also called Disinhibition-dementia-parkinsonism-amyotrophy complex (DDPAC) or FTDP17 (Lynch, et al., 1994). The pathologic features distinguish this disease from the ALS-parkinsonism-dementia complex of Guam seen in the peninsula of Japan and from ALS-FTD linked to chromosome 9. Mutations in the *microtubule-associated protein tau* gene (*MAPT*) have been shown to be associated with FTD and Parkinsonism (Hutton, et al., 1998). Tau is a member of the microtubule-associated protein family, which have the principal function stabilizing microtubules and promoting their assembly by binding to tubulin. As a number of reviews (Gros-Louis, et al., 2006; Julien and Kriz, 2006) have already described the relationship between MAPT and ALS, the following sections will not discuss in details about this gene and FTDP17 models that have been generated.

2. In vivo models to study ALS

The exact mechanisms by which all the above-described gene products are involved in ALS pathogenesis are the subject of many ongoing researches. Current thinking about ALS pathogenesis revolves around the interplay between pre-existing genetic susceptibility and environmental factors that may trigger disease. The search for putative environmental factors has remained elusive however; transgenic animal studies have yielded the greatest wealth of information to date. Through these studies, multiple cellular pathways have been identified including, protein misfolding, RNA processing, oxidative stress, excitotoxicity, axonal transport, mitochondrial dysfunction and abnormal secretion of proteins. Nevertheless, how accurately these animal models replicate all ALS clinical symptoms of the human illness remains an unanswered and troublesome question. This section will include the complete description of all published invertebrate and vertebrate models of ALS. Other considerations such as advantages, disadvantages, cost and availability of each model will also be discussed. Each model organism has its own advantages and disadvantages. Choosing an appropriate model depends on the question being asked. Many laboratories find it useful to perform parallel experiments in two or more model systems to understand different aspects of a biochemical process.

2.1 Invertebrate models

Invertebrate model organisms include systems such as the simple yeast (fungi), fly, and nematode. The study of these experimental systems began with genetics and development, moved into molecular and cellular biology prior to most recently propelled into functional genomics and proteomics. These model organisms have highly manipulable genomes allowing for rapid generation of transgenic lines to provide insight on gene functions and protein network interactions. In 2002, Sydner Brenner, Robert Horvitz and John Sulston received the Nobel Prize in Physiology and Medicine for their establishment of the nematode *Caenorhadditis elegans* as a novel model organism to explore the molecular bases of organ development and cell death. Their discoveries identified key genes involved in cell division, differentiation and apoptosis. They determined that these genes were in fact highly conserved both structurally and functionally with higher organisms, including humans. Their studies provided the framework in which simpler organisms can be used to define key pathways and processes of relevance with the important benefit that the results are often directly applicable to understand human diseases.

The key points into generating models for human disease using smaller invertebrate organisms should encompass high degree of conservation with mammals in order for the model to be useful for the identification of the molecular components implicated in disease pathogenesis. A fully sequenced genome of the studied organism should ideally be also easily accessible for genome comparison with higher vertebrates and mammals in order to facilitate evolutionary genomics studies and to quickly generate transgenic animals through DNA transformation. The model organism should also provide significant experimental advantages over their mammalian counterparts, including a short generation time, small size, ease and reasonable cost of maintenance. It should be also amenable to both forward (phenotype to gene) and reverse (gene to phenotype) genetic approaches, which are essential molecular tools to dissect out and understand gene function. Classic forward genetic characteristics allow for the identification of novel molecules or pathways involved in a particular cellular process. This can be one of the most powerful attributes of invertebrate models. Forward-genetic screens using chemical mutagens are one of the most universal ways to generate mutants to elucidate gene function. On the other side, reverse genetics allows the quick identification of pathways on which a particular gene acts. Genetic knockdown mutants, using RNA interference (RNAi) technology in which a gene product is dramatically reduced by introducing double-stranded RNA (dsRNA) into the organism, can also provide invaluable information on the role a gene plays in a biological process.

The obvious disadvantage of using invertebrate model organisms such as fly or worm models is that there are evolutionarily far from mammals and that many physiological functions are not conserved, e.g. the immune system. Furthermore, their organs are extremely undeveloped and simple compared to other animals. The limited cellular diversity also represents a major disadvantage.

2.1.1 Caenorhabditis elegans

Yet, for the vast majority of neurodegenerative disorders including ALS, the mechanisms underlying neuronal dysfunction and death remain poorly understood despite the identification of relevant disease genes. Given the fact that molecular conservation in neuronal signaling pathways across vertebrate and invertebrate is relatively high and since the *Caenorhabditis elegans* nervous system contains almost all of the known signaling and neurotransmitter systems found in mammals (Bargmann, 1998), many researchers have turned to this model organism to identify the mechanisms underlying neurodegenerative disease pathology.

Research in *C. elegans* has been instrumental, especially over the last decade, for the elucidation of molecular pathways implicated in many human diseases. This is highly related to the fact that the *C. elegans* genome was the first multicellular organism to be completely sequenced in 1998 (Anonymous, 1998). The worm genome contains approximately 20,000 genes, compared with 25,000 in the human genome highlighting that *C. elegans* is a powerful model system for genetic analysis and for exploring the molecular mechanisms of neuron development, function, and disease. Furthermore, at least 42% of human disease related genes have a *C. elegans* ortholog, suggesting that most biochemical pathways are conserved across evolution (Culetto and Sattelle, 2000).

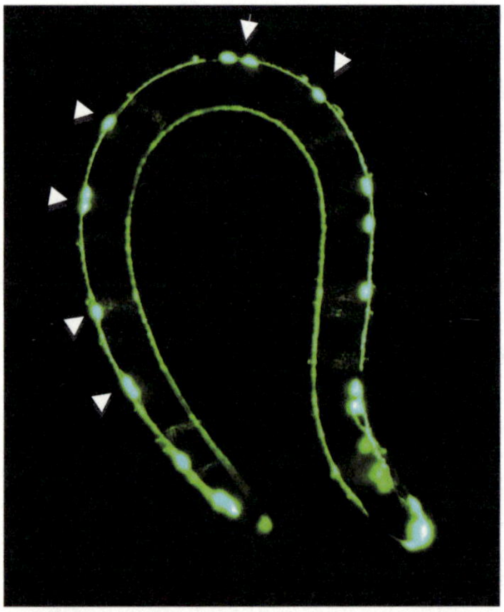

Fig. 1. Transgenic UNC-47:GFP *C. elegans*

In *C. elegans*, 26 neurons of 5 different classes express the neurotransmitter Gamma-Aminobutyric Acid (GABA) (McIntire, et al., 1993). Nineteen of these GABAergic neurons, known as the type D neurons, are required for normal locomotion by providing dorsoventral cross-inhibition to body wall muscles (McIntire, et al., 1993; White, et al., 1986). Therefore, this transgenic worm would be a good model to depict pathological changes associated with locomotor dysfunction. Arrowheads point to type D neurons (only some of the D neurons are indicated). *Courtesy of Dr Alex J. Parker from the Centre of Excellence in Neuromics, University of Montreal, Quebec, Canada.*

C. elegans is a free-living nematode of about 1 millimeter in length with a short generation cycle (3 days) and lifespan (around 3 weeks), large brood size (approximately 300 progeny from a single hermaphrodite), and a transparent anatomically simple body that allows for the visualization of all cell types at all stages of development (Brenner, 1974). This last feature allows researchers to easily detect and quantify neuronal cell death and protein inclusions using optical techniques. The complete *C. elegans* embryonic cell-lineage is also known, making it possible to follow organogenesis from the earliest stages of embryos formation to the terminal steps of differentiation and morphogenesis (Sulston, et al., 1983). Additionally, *C. elegans* have a simple nervous system of 302 neurons out of 959 cells in the adult hermaphrodite, in which each neuron has a unique position (Sulston, 1983). Twenty of these neurons are located inside the pharynx, which has its own nervous system. The remaining 282 neurons are located in various ganglia in the head and tail and also along the ventral cord, the main longitudinal axon tract (Fig. 1). The majority of the neurons develop during embryogenesis. However, 80 of them, mainly motor neurons, develop post-embryonically. The structure of the nervous system is highly reproducible from animal to animal and has been described in detail by electron microscopic reconstruction (White, et al., 1986) This technique allowed White and colleague to obtain high-resolution images to identify all the synapses formed in *C. elegans* (about 5000 chemical synapses, 2000 neuromuscular junctions and some 500 gap junctions) and to map all the connections in order to work out the entire neuronal circuit of this model organism.

In addition, gene knockdown by RNA interference can be relatively easily achieved in most cell types *in vivo* or *in vitro* by injecting the double stranded RNA for a specific gene of interest, by simply soaking the animals in dsRNA, or by feeding the animals with bacteria expressing the desired dsRNA (Fire, et al., 1998; Maeda, et al., 2001). Primary neuronal and muscular cell cultures obtained by dissecting this animal have also been optimized to allow for stable growth of embryonic cells (Christensen, et al., 2002).

For all these reasons, *C. elegans* has emerged as an attractive and powerful *in vivo* model system for studying pathological mechanisms in several major neurodegenerative disorders, including ALS, providing clear leads towards the identification of potential targets for the development of new therapeutic interventions against human diseases.

2.1.1.1 C. Elegans SOD1 models

A number of *C. elegans* models have been developed that recapitulate many aspects of ALS pathogenesis. These transgenic models mainly expressed either the SOD1 or the TDP-43 protein under the control of various gene promoters. The first *C. elegans* ALS model was first generated in 2001 (Oeda, et al., 2001). This transgenic *C. elagans* model has been generated by introducing human wild type and various human FALS *SOD1*-linked mutations (A4V, G37R and G93A) under the control of hsp16-2 heat shock and myo-3 muscle-specific promoters. The heat inducible hsp16-2 promoter allows expression of mutant SOD1 in almost all tissues, including neurons, while the myo-3 muscle-specific promoter allows high level of protein expression in all of the muscle tissues except for the pharynx. Unfortunately, no morphological abnormalities and no discernable changes in survival or behavior were observed. However, the authors reported some interesting findings. The mutant SOD1 expressing nematodes showed a reduced resistance to paraquat-induced oxidative stress. Furthermore, oxidative stress significantly reduced the degradation rate of mutant SOD1 protein, and finally aberrant accumulation of mutant human SOD1 proteins was also observed when expressed in muscle cells. Interestingly, this later pathological phenotype is in line with the pathology observed in human post-mortem ALS tissues.

In a subsequent study, pan-neuronal expression of the G85R ALS-linked mutant form of human SOD1, using the *C. elegans* syntobrevin gene promoter (*snb-1*), coupled to a yellow fluorescent protein (YFP) produces strong locomotor defects and paralysis in this transgenic snb-1/G85RSOD1-YFP *C. elegans* model (Wang, et al., 2009a). Interestingly, the observed phenotype correlated with intra-neuronal SOD1 aggregation. Another SOD1 mutant *C. elegans* model in which aggregation, toxicity, and cellular interactions can be directly compared between different SOD1 mutants was also reported. This mutant SOD1-YFP model, expressing various SOD1 mutants (G85R, G93A, 127X) in *C. elegans* muscle cells by the use of the muscle specific *unc-54* gene promoter resulted in mild cellular dysfunction (Gidalevitz, et al., 2009). However, when mutant SOD1 was introduced into genetic backgrounds harboring destabilizing temperature-sensitive mutations, the toxicity was enhanced significantly and a variety of toxic phenotypes were observed. Based on theses results, the authors concluded that the specific toxic phenotypes may not be simply due to aggregation toxicity of the causative mutant proteins, but may be modulated by the genetic interactions with cellular pathways harboring mildly destabilizing polymorphisms in the genetic background.

2.1.1.2 C. Elegans TDP-43 models

In order to study TDP-43 function and neurotoxicity, transgenic *C. elegans* model was generated allowing pan-neuronal expression of the wild-type TDP-43 human protein (Ash, et al., 2010). This was done using the *snb-1* gene promoter driving the expression of human TDP-43 cDNA in all neurons. The transgenic snb-1/hTDP-43 worms displayed a distinctive uncoordinated phenotype characterized by non-sinusoidal, slow movement and inappropriate responses to stimulus. Transgenic worms first display this phenotype during larval stages, and the phenotype remains constant throughout the adulthood. The authors have also found that this uncoordinated phenotype correlated with abnormal motor neuron synapses. The mechanism by which nuclear TDP-43 activity leads to abnormal synapses is still unknown, but the authors hypothesized that excessive TDP-43 activity may alters some component of RNA metabolism (e.g. alternative splicing), subsequently leading to altered production of specific proteins required for proper synaptic function. In another study, also describing a *C. elegans* model of TDP-43 proteinopathy, Liachko and colleagues similarly found that overexpression of normal human TDP-43 in all *C. elegans* neurons causes motor defects (Liachko, et al., 2010). However, they also found that overexpression of various human ALS-associated TDP-43 mutants (G290A, A315T, or M337V) cause a more severe motor dysfunction phenotype. Interestingly, the authors also demonstrated that the observed motor phenotype worsen over time and that the described mutant TDP-43 *C. elegans* model recapitulates some characteristic features seen in ALS and FTLD-U patients including progressive paralysis, reduced lifespan, and degeneration of motor neurons accompanied by hyperphosphorylation, truncation, and ubiquitination of the TDP-43 protein that accumulates in detergent insoluble protein deposits.

All the above described *C. elegans* models provide a good *in vivo* system to further dissect cellular and molecular mechanisms underlying disease. Further investigations using these models may reveal insights into SOD1 and TDP-43 functions, potentially reveal neurotoxic mechanisms relevant to ALS and other neurodegenerative diseases, and ultimately lead to the development of novel therapeutic targets.

2.1.2 Drosophila melanogaster

The fruit fly *Drosophila melanogaster* is a powerful genetic tool to study neurodegenerative diseases. *Drosophila* is a complex organism, with a functioning brain and nervous system, capable of many behaviors like learning, motility, and visual acuity. This model organism is one of the oldest multi cellular eukaryotic genetic models and has been used for almost a century to examine a variety of basic biological principles, including genetic inheritance, behavioral and developmental processes, and the first experimental description of the gene as a functional unit. Its importance for human health was recognized by the award of the Nobel Prize in Physiology and Medicine to Ed Lewis, Christiane Nusslein-Volhard and Eric Wieschaus in 1995 for their discoveries concerning the genetic control of early embryonic development using *D. melanogaster* as a model.

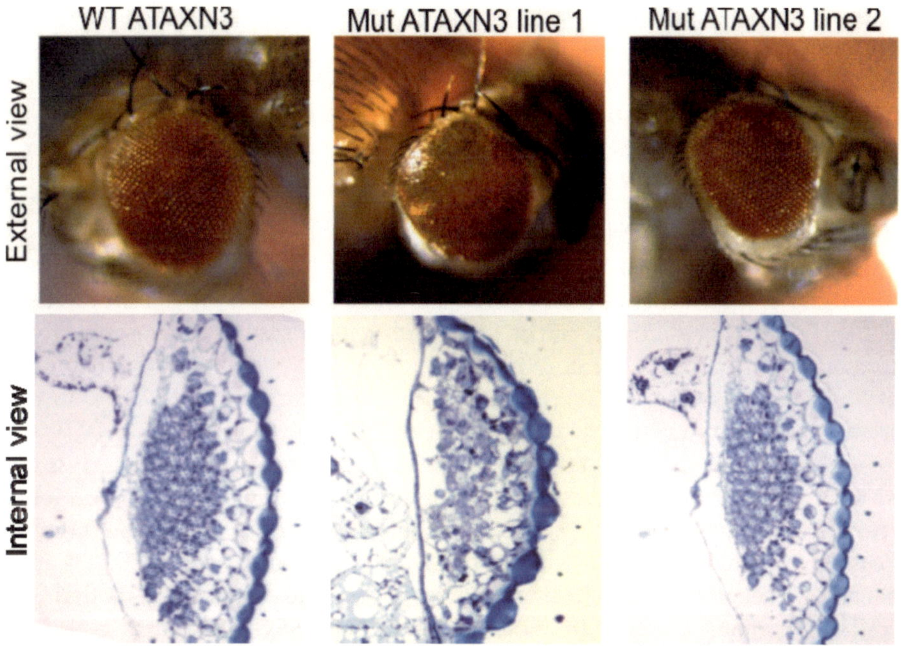

Fig. 2. Expression of human *Ataxin3* gene in the compound eye of transgenic flies using the GAL4/UAS system.
Transgenic *drosophila* expressing human full-length WT or mutated Ataxin 3 (ATXN3) gene in the compound eye. Only mutant ATAXN3 flies showed an external and internal degeneration, which is characterized by cell death and irregular ommatidia and photoreceptor distribution. *Courtesy of Dr Guy A. Rouleau from the Centre of Excellence in Neuromics, University of Montreal, Quebec, Canada.*

Drosophila is cheap, of small size (approximately 2.5mm) and easy to maintain in the laboratory. One of the most attractive aspects of *Drosophila* for use as a model organism is its short reproductive cycle and large number of genetically identical progeny. Adult females can lay, following a circadian pattern, over 400 eggs within 10 days and their short 2-week generation time allows for quick analysis of mutant animals. The fly has only four pairs of chromosomes, including three autosomal chromosomes and one set of sexual X/Y chromosomes which can be directly visualized in the giant polytene chromosome of the larval salivary gland. The *Drosophila* genome has been completely sequenced (Adams, et al., 2000). Its entire genome is encoded by roughly 13,600 genes as compared to 25,000 human genes. Another interesting feature of the fly is that it is relatively easy to drive time- and tissue-specific expression of any gene of interest using the yeast transcription activator protein Gal4 in combination with the Upstream Activation Sequence (UAS) to which Gal4 specifically binds to activate gene transcription (Brand and Perrimon, 1993). To study neurodegenerative diseases, the compound eye is predominantly used because it allows the

generation of a neurodegenerative phenotype (rough eye phenotype) that can be easily appreciated under a standard light microscope (Fig. 2). In turn, the Gal4/UAS system can be also used to screen for genetic modifier (enhancer or suppressor) genes.
Based on these observations, it is obvious that *Drosophila melanogaster* can offer unique opportunities in the study of human neurodegeneration. Nonetheless, the major disadvantage of using *D. melanogaster* as a model is that forward genetic screen using RNA interference technology is more tedious than in the *C.elegans* model. For instance, at the moment, knockdown of genes by RNAi cannot be carried out by simply feeding flies with double-stranded RNA (as in the worm model); it has to be injected into the embryo. Although very laborious, this problem could be overcome by generating transgenic constructs expressing dsRNA for each transcript.

2.1.2.1 Drosophila SOD1 models

Initial ALS studies in *Drosophila* showed either reduced longevity and fertility, increased susceptibility to oxidative stress, motor deficits and/or necrotic cell death in the fly eye of *Sod* null flies (Phillips, et al., 1989). Surprisingly, subsequent studies in transgenic fly model, overexpressing human WT SOD1 only in motor neurons, showed an extension of lifespan, without affecting locomotion or motor neuron survival (Parkes, et al., 1998). In contrast, another study showed that selective expression of WT or human SOD1 (hSOD1) disease-linked (A4V, G85R) mutants in motor neurons induced progressive motor dysfunctions, coupled with electrophysiological defects and abnormal accumulation of the protein and a stress response in surrounding glial cells (Watson, et al., 2008). These effects were accompanied by synaptic transmission deficits, focal accumulation of hSOD1 in motor neurons, and up-regulation of heat shock protein in glia. This work suggests that SOD can cause cell-autonomous damage to motor neurons, and highlights that motor neuron selective expression of hSOD1 can induces change in glial cells. These results are in line with findings that disease is not strictly autonomous to motor neurons and that toxicity can propagate from one cell to another (Boillee, et al., 2006; Clement, et al., 2003). Expression of a human *SOD1* transgene in *Drosophila* motor neurons was achieved by using the yeast GAL4/UAS system. Interestingly, Mocket and colleagues showed that human WT SOD1 expression, placed in a *Drosophila* Cu-Zn Sod null background, at very low levels was sufficient to rescue the life-span reduction, increased oxidative stress, and impaired physiological function associated with the *Drosophila* Sod null model described above (Mockett, et al., 2003). However, the introduction of FALS-linked SOD1 alleles (A4V, G37R, G41D, G93C, and I113T) only partly reversed these effects. These results, in conjunction with earlier findings from FALS SOD1 expression restricted to motor neurons, suggest that the introduction of FALS mutant SOD1 alleles in *Drosophila* does not result in a dominant gain-of-function, as it is observed in human patients.

2.1.2.2 Drosophila TDP-43 models

A number of models for TDP-43 toxicity in flies have also been generated, revealing that the protein shows toxicity *in vivo*. Mainly, these independent studies have examined phenotypes associated with manipulation of both endogenous *Drosophila* TDP-43 ortholog (dTDP) and transgenic expression of human TDP-43. The major findings of these complementary studies were largely consistent with one other. Flies lacking dTDP appeared externally normal but presented deficient locomotive behaviors, reduced life span, anatomical defects at the neuromuscular junctions and decreased dendritic branching

(Feiguin, et al., 2009; Lin, et al., 2011; Lu, et al., 2009). These phenotypes were rescued by expression of the human TDP-43 protein in a restricted group of neurons including motor neurons (Feiguin, et al., 2009). These findings support the notion that loss of normal TDP-43 function may contribute to the pathogenesis of ALS and FTLD. On the other hand, ubiquitous or tissue-specific overexpression of either dTDP or human TDP-43 also recapitulated key hallmark features of ALS pathology including premature lethality, neuronal loss, neuromuscular junctions architecture defects and locomotor deficits (Elden, et al., 2010; Estes, et al., 2011; Hanson, et al., 2010; Li, et al., 2010; Lu, et al., 2009; Miguel, et al., 2011; Ritson, et al., 2010; Voigt, et al., 2010). Furthermore, TDP-43 expression appears to be independent of ALS/FTLD-linked mutations (Elden, et al., 2010; Estes, et al., 2011; Ritson, et al., 2010; Voigt, et al., 2010). These results also support the view of a toxic dominant gain-of-function mechanism(s) associated with TDP-43 proteinopathies.

To further explore the role of TDP-43 pathogenesis and identify pathogenic mechanisms, several independent research groups have used different genetic approaches to identify modifier genes that could suppress or enhance TDP-43 toxicity (Elden, et al., 2010; Hanson, et al., 2010; Ritson, et al., 2010). Interestingly, upregulation of Pab1-binding protein 1 (Pbp1), an ortholog of the human *ATXN2* gene, in a transgenic model of TDP-43 enhanced TDP-43 toxicity and led to a more severe TDP-43 associated phenotypes (Elden, et al., 2010). Similarly, overexpression of ubiquilin 1, a previously identified TDP- 43 interacting partner (Kim, et al., 2009), reduced steady-state TDP-43 expression but enhanced the severity of TDP-43 phenotypes (Hanson, et al., 2010). Another study also showed that the TDP-43 associated phenotypes observed in a transgenic *Drosophila* TDP-43 model was modulated by coexpression of valosin-containing protein (VCP), a member of the ATPases associated with multiple cellular activities (AAA+) family of proteins regulating a wide array of cellular processes (Ritson, et al., 2010). Further investigations on these interesting findings may enable the development of novel therapeutics targets that can regulate TDP-43 expression in patients and hopefully delay or cure TDP-43-linked patients.

2.1.2.3 Drosophila FUS models

The pathogenic mechanisms underlying FUS proteinopathy remain largely unknown, although it is clear that *FUS* mutations affects motor neurons and other neuronal populations such as cortical neurons. In order to study FUS related function *in vivo*, a FUS/TLS Drosophila model was generated in which targeted expression of mutant human FUS/TLS (R518K, R521C and R521H) caused severe neurodegeneration in Drosophila eyes, whereas expression of WT human FUS/TLS resulted in very mild eye degeneration (Lanson, et al., 2011). Locomotor dysfunction and premature lethality was also observed in the mutant FUS/TLS transgenic flies. In addition, overexpression of mutant FUS/TLS caused an accumulation of ubiquitinated proteins, a pathological hallmark feature of ALS. Similarly, a pathogenic role of human ALS-associated FUS/TLS mutations (R524S and P525L) using Drosiphila has been described (Chen, et al., 2011). In this model overexpression of either Wt or ALS-mutant in different neuronal subpopulations, including photoreceptors, mushroom bodies and motor neurons led to an age-dependent progressive neuronal degeneration, including axonal loss, morphological changes and functional impairment in motor neurons. The human FUS/TLS drosophila ortholog (*caz*) has been also disrupted in order to study FUS function. The *caz* deficient fly exhibited reduced life span and locomotor deficits as compared with controls. Interestingly, these phenotypes were fully rescued by WT human FUS, but not ALS-associated mutant FUS proteins suggesting that ALS-associated FUS/TLS mutations are toxics (Walker, et al., 2011). Through cross-rescue analysis, it has been demonstrated that FUS acted together with and downstream of TDP-43 in a common genetic pathway in neurons. Furthermore, the authors found that these proteins associated with each other in an RNA-dependent complex. These results establish that FUS and TDP-43 function together *in vivo* and suggest that molecular pathways requiring the combined activities of both of these proteins may be disrupted in ALS and FTD.

2.2 Vertebrate models

Projecting the human genome sequence into our understanding of human health and disease has been a new challenge faced in the post-genomic era. As described above, unicellular and invertebrate model systems can be of great value in defining the molecular components of pathways or processes that depend on the function of several interacting proteins. However, vertebrate models offer the best opportunity for defining landmarks of disease progression and for understanding the functional consequences of gene mutations. The great advantage of using vertebrates to model human diseases is clearly the possibility they offer for evaluation of new treatments. Indeed, testing new drugs on mice or other vertebrate models is often mandatory and asked by the Food and Drug Administration, for safety reasons, prior to approve new drug treatments. This step is also fundamental for paving the way towards human clinical trials, with both larger and smaller vertebrate model organisms.

Other advantages of using vertebrate models include: the ability to make efficient targeted gene knockouts by homologous recombination, they are evolutionary closer to human, the developmental overview is similar for all mammals, the availability of material at all stages of development, their brains are more similar to human, they respond to injury and can be conditioned (great advantages to study learning, neuronal connectivity and plasticity) and they provide a valuable source of primary cells for culture. The later feature will be discussed in more details in the next section of this book chapter.

On the contrary, the high maintenance cost, a relatively slow life cycle development, lower number of progeny, genetically identical offspring more difficult to obtain and the difficulty to manipulate embryos (intrauterine development) represent the major disadvantages of using vertebrate as disease model organisms.

2.2.1 Mice

Over the past century, the laboratory mouse (*Mus musculus*) has become the premier mammalian model organism for experimental studies and genetic research. Scientists from a wide range of biomedical fields have used the mouse because of its close genetic and physiological similarities to humans, as well as the ease with which its genome can be manipulated and analyzed, ease of handling and it's relatively high reproductive rate. Although yeasts, worms and flies are excellent models for studying many developmental processes, mice are far better models for studying diverse physiological systems such as the immune system, the endocrine system, the nervous system, the cardiovascular system, the skeletal system and other complex physiological systems that mammals share. Like humans and many other mammals, mice naturally develop diseases that affect these systems, including cancer, atherosclerosis, hypertension, diabetes, osteoporosis and glaucoma. In addition, manipulating the mouse genome and environment can induce certain diseases that afflict humans but normally do not strike mice, such as cystic fibrosis, obesity, blindness, anxiety, aggressive behavior, alcoholism, drug addiction and neurodegenerative disorders such as Alzheimer's disease, Parkinson's disease, Huntington's disease and ALS. Immunodeficient mice can also be used as hosts to facilitate cancer and AIDS research.

Researchers have used a collection of innovative genetic technologies to produce custom-made mouse models for a broad array of specific diseases, as well as to study the function of targeted genes. One of the most important technological advances has been the ability to produce transgenic mice, in which a new gene (cloned from human or other various species, wild-type or mutated) is inserted into the mouse's germline. Indeed, the 2007 Nobel Prize in Physiology and Medicine was awarded to Drs Mario R. Capecchi, Martin J. Evans and Oliver Smithies for their discoveries of principles for introducing specific gene modifications in mice by the use of embryonic stem cells. Even more potent approaches, it is now possible to knockout or to artificially drive the expression of an inserted gene in specific tissue or at various time during development or adulthood using the Cre/Loxp system (Sauer, 1998). There are many mouse models commercially available for genetic research including thousands of unique inbred strains and genetically engineered mutants.

Researches using the laboratory mouse led to major advances in our ability to treat a number of serious diseases and conditions. Genetically, mice are more closely related to humans than invertebrates in the sense that most human genes have functional mouse counterparts and the mouse genome is organized in a very similar manner to the human genome. The mouse and human genomes are approximately the same size. They most likely contain the same number of genes and show extensive synteny and conserved gene order. Importantly, mice have also genes that are often not represented in other models, such as *C. elegans* and *Drosophila*. All these advantages make the laboratory mouse the model organism of choice to study human diseases. Although mice are widely used in research, questions remain however about their reliability as a model for human diseases. In occurrence, how to explain that many drugs worked well during preclinical trials in mice, but turned out to be ineffective when used in clinical trials on humans? Here, we will review the mouse studies that contributed toward understanding the pathogenic pathways of motor neuron disease and the testing of therapeutic approaches.

2.2.1.1 Mice SOD1 models

The use of mouse models has been of particular importance in studying the pathogenesis of Amyotrophic Lateral Sclerosis. The initial description of *SOD1* gene mutations in familial ALS patients, in 1993, first led to the hypothesis that the disease resulted from compromised enzymatic activity due to the loss of the enzyme function (Rosen, et al., 1993). However, this loss of function hypothesis was rapidly refuted, as *Sod1* KO mice in which the murine *Sod1* gene was disrupted, do not develop disease (Reaume, et al., 1996). To date, over 150 different *SOD1* missense mutations have been reported. In contrast, transgenic mice ubiquitously overexpressing various *SOD1* gene mutations with different biochemical properties, even in the presence of endogenous mouse *Sod1* gene, develop a neurodegenerative disease that is quite similar to the human illness. Of particular interest, transgenic mice overexpressing WT human SOD1 or specifically expressing mutant SOD1 only in neurons or only in glial cells do not develop disease (Bruijn, et al., 1998; Gong, et al., 2000; Pramatarova, et al., 2001). A toxic gain-of-function rather than a loss-of-function of mutant *SOD1* gene is therefore believe to be involved in ALS-linked SOD1 patients. All published mouse models have used the endogenous murine *Sod1* promoter resulting in high levels of expression of the mutant transgene in all tissues. Although these models implicate mutant SOD1 in the development of motor neuron degeneration, many questions regarding the mechanism of pathogenesis remain unanswered. One of the central mysteries in ALS research is why an ubiquitously expressed gene such as *SOD1* causes selective devastation to motor neurons in the absence of pathology in other tissues. One possible explanation is that expression of the mutant protein in motor neurons may not be sufficient to lead to the development of a neurodegenerative disease in mice, suggesting that mutant *SOD1* expression in other cells may be necessary for the development of the disease. Although there are indications that neurodegeneration in ALS may not strictly result from a cell-autonomous process, the selective motor neuron vulnerability observed in the disease pathogenesis remains enigmatic.

The favored hypothesis at this time of SOD1-mediated disease is that toxicity of SOD1 mutants is related to the misfolding and aggregation of SOD1 species (Gros-Louis, et al., 2009b). However, it is not clear which conformational SOD1 species and oligomers cause ALS and the exact mechanism of toxicity of the misfolded SOD1 species remains unknown. Deleterious effects could result from the interaction of misfolded SOD1 species with essential cellular components such as Bcl-2 (Pasinelli, et al., 2004), from their recruitment to outer membrane of mitochondria or from overwhelming the capacity of the protein folding chaperones and/or of ubiquitin proteasome pathway to degrade important cellular regulatory factors (Turner, et al., 2005; Urushitani, et al., 2008; Urushitani, et al., 2002). The misfolded SOD1 protein may also form aggregates that might sequester important cellular components causing cytotoxicity. Recent studies demonstrated that a fraction of SOD1 could be translocated via the ER-Golgi network and that chromogranins, which are abundant proteins in motor neurons, interneurons and activated astrocytes, may act as chaperone-like proteins to promote secretion of misfolded SOD1 mutants (Urushitani, et al., 2008; Urushitani, et al., 2006). Moreover, it has been reported that extracellular mutant SOD1 can induce microgliosis and motor neuron death (Urushitani, et al., 2006). Such ALS pathogenic mechanism based on toxicity of secreted SOD1 mutant is in line with findings that disease is not strictly autonomous to motor neurons and that toxicity can propagate from one cell to another. Interestingly, it has been proposed that endoplasmic reticulum (ER) stress response might exert a critical role in the disease pathogenesis. The ER is the site of synthesis and folding of secretory and membrane bound proteins. The capacity of the ER to process proteins is limited and the accumulation of misfolded proteins may activate different ER stress pathways. The challenges in the future are to find out which somatic insults are causing the initial protein change, and to discover ways of preventing the misfolded proteins from spreading through the nervous system.

The overexpression of either G37R, G85R, G86R, D90A, G93A, H46R/H48Q or H46R/H48Q/H63G/H120G, L126Z and G127X mutant SOD1 protein in mice leads to motor neuron degeneration (Borchelt, et al., 1994; Bruijn, et al., 1997; Gurney, et al., 1994; Jonsson, et al., 2004; Jonsson, et al., 2006; Ripps, et al., 1995; Tu, et al., 1996; Wang, et al., 2003; Wang, et al., 2002; Wong, et al., 1995). In all of these mouse models, massive death of motor neurons in the ventral horn of the spinal cord and loss of myelinated axons in ventral motor roots ultimately leads to paralysis and muscle atrophy. Histopathological findings observed in these transgenic animals include progressive accumulation of detergent-resistant aggregates containing SOD1 and ubiquitin, aberrant neurofilament accumulations in degenerating motor neurons. In addition to neuronal degeneration, similar to that observed in ALS patients, Golgi fragmentation and neuroinflammation noted by the presence of reactive astroglia and microglia in diseased tissue are also observed. However, the severity of the phenotype (in term of age of onset, disease progression and disease duration) varies from one model to another and may be dependant on mouse genetic background (Heiman-Patterson, et al., 2005) and gene dosage. In deed, the life span of these ALS mice is inversely proportional to gene dosage, i.e. the number of transgene insertion within the mouse genome, leading to different steady state level of mutant SOD1 protein in the central nervous system. Such variation in the steady state protein levels must reflect different stabilities and degradation of the various human SOD1 mutants.

The G93A-SOD1 mouse line is currently the most widely used experimental model in ALS research and drug testing. Unfortunately, several pharmacological approaches tested so far have produced only modest beneficial effects. Riluzole, a glutamate antagonist, extended the life span of G93A-SOD1 mice by 10 to 15 days without affecting disease onset (Gurney, et al., 1996). Today, riluzole is the only drug currently approved for ALS treatment. This treatment only produces modest beneficial effect in some ALS patients. Interestingly, is has been shown that treatment with the ER stress-protective agent salubrinal attenuated disease manifestations and delayed progression in a G93A-SOD1 mouse model (Saxena, et al., 2006). This result suggests a role of ER stress in ALS. Furthermore, it has been also shown that immunization therapy, using specific anti-misfolded SOD1 monoclonal antibodies, succeeded in reducing the level of mutant SOD1 by 23% in the spinal cord of immunized animals, in delaying disease onset and in prolonging the lifespan of G93A-SOD1 mice in proportion to the duration of treatment (Gros-Louis, et al., 2010). These results suggest that accumulation of misfolded SOD1 species is toxic, and reducing the burden of these toxic species leads to beneficial effect. Interestingly, it has been recently reported that WT SOD1 can acquire properties of ALS-linked mutant SOD1 species possibly implying a shared pathophysiological pathway between SALS and FALS (Bosco, et al., 2010b; Ezzi, et al., 2007). Another study also demonstrated that WT SOD1 may acquire toxic properties upon oxidative damage and that WT SOD1 expression dramatically exacerbated disease in transgenic mice expressing mutant SOD1 forms such as A4V, G85R, L126Z, and G93A SOD1 mutants (Wang, et al., 2009b). It is noteworthy that overexpression of WT SOD1 conferred ALS disease to unaffected A4V SOD1 mice. Based on these results, the possibility that WT SOD1 may be a contributor of pathogenesis in sporadic ALS must be considered.

2.2.1.2 Mice TDP-43 models

As previously mentioned, several research groups have reported that dominant mutations in the *TARDBP* gene, which encodes for TDP-43, cause ALS (Kabashi, et al., 2008; Sreedharan, et al., 2008; Van Deerlin, et al., 2008). Following these initials studies, a number of TDP-43 ALS mouse model has been described. Embryonic lethality is observed in homozygous mouse knockouts for TDP-43 (Kraemer, et al., 2010; Sephton, et al., 2010; Wu, et al., 2010). The TDP-43 deficient embryos die at embryonic day 7.5 thereby demonstrating the essential function of TDP-43 protein in development. Mice heterozygous for TDP-43 disruption only exhibit subtle muscle weakness with no evidence of motor neuron pathology.

Many of the transgenic mouse lines overexpressing WT or mutant TDP-43 reported to date have showed some ALS features including early paralysis leading to premature death (Stallings, et al., 2010; Wegorzewska, et al., 2009; Wils, et al., 2010). These pan-neuronal TDP-43 transgenic mouse models expressing high-level of either WT or mutant (A315T and

M337V) TDP-43 transgene in neurons both showed aggressive paralysis accompanied by increased ubiquitination in specific neuronal populations (Stallings, et al., 2010; Wegorzewska, et al., 2009; Wils, et al., 2010; Xu, et al., 2010). However, many concerns have been raised regarding the biological validity of these models, as they do not completely mimics disease. Since TDP-43 is a moderately and ubiquitously expressed protein, restricted non-physiological neuronal expression of TDP-43 is one of them, along with the use of the TDP-43 cDNA as transgene and the lack of cytoplasmic ubiquitinated TDP-43 inclusions. In order to better mimic the ubiquitous and moderate levels of TDP-43 expression seen in humans, another transgenic mouse models have been generated allowing the expression of genomic TDP-43 fragments (Swarup, et al., 2011). This TDP-43 mouse model exhibited age-related phenotypic defects as seen in the human condition including both cognitive and motor deficits. Other pathological features as seen in human patients were also observed including, cytoplasmic TDP-43-positive ubiquitinated inclusions, intermediate filament abnormalities, axonopathy and neuroinflammation. These phenotypes were more severe in the transgenic TDP-43 mutant (G348C and A315T) models than the transgenic TDP-43 WT model.

2.2.1.3 Mice intermediate filament models

Several transgenic mouse lines and knockout mice implicating different neurofilament subunits have been extensively studied over the past years (for complete review, see: (Julien and Kriz, 2006; Lariviere and Julien, 2004)). Even though genetic mutations in intermediate filament (IF) genes are not major causes of ALS, it is of potential relevance to ALS that transgenic mice with altered stoichiometry of neuronal intermediate filament develop pathological features of the disease (Beaulieu, et al., 2000; Beaulieu and Julien, 2003; Cote, et al., 1993; Millecamps, et al., 2006). Of particular interest was the finding that overexpression of WT peripherin, a type III intermediate filament, in *NEFL* null background mice caused age-dependant selective motor neurons degeneration (Beaulieu, et al., 1999). This mouse model is also characterized by the formation of perikaryal and axonal intermediate filament inclusions resembling spheroids in motor neurons of human ALS. The precise mechanism by which accumulation of intermediate neurofilament leads to neurodegenerative disorders is not fully understood. Neurofilament and peripherin proteins are two types of intermediate filaments detected in the majority of axonal inclusion bodies, called spheroids, in motor neurons of ALS patients (Corbo and Hays, 1992). Multiple factors can potentially cause the accumulation of intermediate filament proteins including deregulation of intermediate filament protein synthesis, proteolysis, defective axonal transport, abnormal phosphorylation, and other protein modifications.

2.2.1.4 Mice ALS2 models

Truncating mutations were discovered in coding exons of a the *ALS2* gene encoding for Alsin, from patients with an autosomal recessive form of juvenile ALS, primary lateral sclerosis (PLS) and infantile-onset ascending hereditary spastic paralysis (IAHSP) (Devon, et al., 2003; Eymard-Pierre, et al., 2002; Eymard-Pierre, et al., 2006; Gros-Louis, et al., 2003; Hadano, et al., 2001; Kress, et al., 2005; Yang, et al., 2001). The pattern of inheritance and the nature of the mutations identified in this gene suggest that motor neuron degeneration seen in patients results from a loss of protein function. Six different groups have reported the generation of an alsin knockout mouse (Cai, et al., 2005; Deng, et al., 2007; Devon, et al., 2003; Gros-Louis, et al., 2008; Hadano, et al., 2006; Yamanaka, et al., 2006). Despite an age-dependent loss of motor coordination revealed by rotarod and grip strength performances of the Als2 KO mice, no major motor deficits consistent with ALS or other motor neuron diseases were present in these models. All Als2-deficient mice appear to be grossly normal, viable and fertile with lifespan expectancy similar to WT littermates. However, some differences are noteworthy and may explain the heterogeneity of the phenotype, ranging from ALS to less severe PLS or IAHSP. The diversity of the apparent phenotypes among different Als2 KO mouse models may be due in part by different gene targeting strategies used to generate each mice models, ES cell lines used leading to differences in the genetic background, housing conditions or approaches taken to evaluate the mice.

Interestingly, thorough molecular analysis of one of these *Als2* KO mouse model revealed the presence of a number of novel *Als2* isoforms expressed in the central nervous system of these animals (Gros-Louis, et al., 2008). These results suggest that other alternatively spliced *Als2* isoforms may exist and that some of these novel *Als2* mRNA species still can be transcribed in *Als2* null animals and may compensate for the loss of the full-length protein.

2.2.1.5 Mice models associated with other motor neuron diseases

Different other transgenic mice models overexpressing different human proteins either ubiquitously or specifically in neurons have been generated (for review see (Gros-Louis, et al., 2006; Julien and Kriz, 2006). These mice acquire age-dependent central nervous system pathology similar to other related motor neuron diseases such as FTDP17, progressive supranuclear palsy, spinal muscular atrophy or hereditary spastic paraplegia. Interesting pathological features, which are also associated with ALS, can be seen in these different mouse models including axonal degeneration in brain and spinal cord, progressive motor disturbance, behavioral impairment, and the presence of cellular aggregates and intermediate filament inclusions.

2.2.2 Rat

As a model of human disease, the laboratory rat (*Rattus norvegicus*) offers some advantages over the mouse and other organisms. The main advantage is in fact that rats are physiologically more similar to humans compare to mice. The size of the animal also confers a valuable advantage and enhances its use as a disease model. The later advantage is especially true when performing surgical procedures, microdialysis, intravenous cannulation and for pharmacodynamic drug studies as its size enables serial blood sampling. Thereby, the rat would be a better model than the mouse to study cardiovascular disease, hypertension, diabetes, arthritis, and many autoimmune, behavioral, and addiction disorders. The rat is also a good model in neurobehavioral and stereotaxic neurological studies. The size of the rat brain offers unique possibilities for the application of microsurgical techniques, intrathecal administration of drugs, stem cell transplantation, serial sampling of the cerebrospinal fluid (CSF), *in vivo* nerve recordings, and neuroimaging procedures.

However, even though its size is considered as an advantage over mice, the higher cost of maintenance (bigger cages, food, less animals can be housed per cages) and limited housing capacity in animal facilities directly related to its size also confers the principal limitation of using rats as a model.

2.2.2.1 Rat SOD1 models

Transgenic rat models of ALS have also been generated. In these models overexpression of G93A or H46R mutant SOD1 led to an ALS-like phenotype (Howland, et al., 2002; Nagai, et al., 2001). These transgenic rat models reproduce the major phenotypic features of human ALS, such as selective motor neuron loss, ubiquitination, hyaline inclusions, vacuolation, and neuroinflammation. However, several differences between the rat and mouse ALS models can be denoted including a more rapid progression of disease and the transient appearance of vacuoles in the transgenic SOD1 rats. As the CSF volume of a rat is 10- to 20-fold greater than that of a mouse (Nagai, et al., 2001), transgenic *SOD1* rats may facilitate to study the CSF proteome and to detect SOD1 activity or drug concentrations, even in an age-dependent manner. Therefore, ALS rat models may be useful to demonstrate therapeutic efficacy, blood-brain barrier filtration and to assess the toxicity of novel therapeutic compounds in drug development.

2.2.2.2 Rat TDP-43 models

In order to generate a TDP-43 rodent model that is more suitable for pharmacological studies, rat models ubiquitously overexpressing either WT TDP-43 or the M337V-associated *TARDBP* mutation were generated (Zhou, et al., 2010). In contrast to what it is observed in TDP-43 transgenic mouse models, overexpression of mutant TDP-43 only, but not the WT protein, caused widespread neurodegeneration. Despite the fact that this transgenic mutant TDP-43 rat model exhibited progressive degeneration of motor neurons, neurodegeneration was not only restricted to motor neurons. However, TDP-43 mutation affected motor neurons earlier and more severely than other neurons in the CNS at end stage of the disease. In some aspects, this rat model recapitulated TDP-43 pathological features both seen in the different mouse models and in ALS patients indicating that this model could be used in future pharmalogical studies in order to identify novel therapeutic avenues to treat TDP-43 related disorders.

2.2.3 Zebrafish

In the last decade, a new vertebrate model has emerged in the study of human diseases. The principal attraction of using zebrafish (*Danio renio*) as model organisms is that its genome can be much more easily manipulated and studied in terms of genetics and development than other vertebrate model organisms. As being a vertebrate with common organs and tissues with conserved organization such as brain and spinal cord, the attractiveness of zebrafish to model human diseases lies therefore in its biology and genetics. Although there are obvious differences in the physiology of fish and humans the zebrafish offers several advantages that make it an important complement to mouse models of disease. These advantages include the embryo and larvae optical clarity (which allows easy visualization of developmental processes), the external fertilization (which facilitates gene expression manipulation), high fecundity (adult female can lay hundreds of eggs per day), and rapid development (swimming behavior appears less than 48 hours post-fertilization). As in invertebrate models, it is also relatively easy to perform forward and reverse genetic screens for gene identification and to understand specific gene function.

Forward-genetic screens in zebrafish, using random mutagenesis, can be used to identify novel genes involved in embryogenesis, organogenesis or different specific biological processes. To generate mutants, male fish are exposed to the mutagen ethyl-nitroso-urea (ENU), which typically induces point mutations within zebrafish genome (Driever, et al., 1996; Haffter, et al., 1996; Henion, et al., 1996; Solnica-Krezel, et al., 1996). Random mutagenesis has also been successfully carried out in zebrafish using retroviral methods (Amsterdam, et al., 1999). Treated males are then crossed to wildtype females to produce the

F1 heterozygous progeny and so on so forth in order to generate homozygous progeny and to facilitate the identification of gene mutation by positional cloning. Forward-genetic screens in zebrafish are greatly facilitated by the transparency of embryos and larvae, simplifying phenotypic screening and allowing large scale screening without sophisticated expansive equipments. These features provide an advantage over other vertebrate models in which aspects of organogenesis and disease pathology cannot be examined without surgical interventions. Large-scale forward-genetic screens have allowed the identification of numerous mutations in zebrafish genes (Amsterdam and Hopkins, 2006). Comparative genomic can be then used in order to identify the corresponding orthologous gene in humans and, in some instances, the mutant phenotypes have been sufficiently similar to the human pathology to allow the identification of gene mutations by a candidate gene approach.

On the other hand, reverse genetics refers to the study of the phenotypic consequences following manipulation of gene expression. An essential tool for investigating gene function during development is the ability to perform gene knockdown, overexpression, and misexpression studies. The external egg fertilization in zebrafish enables microinjection of RNA, DNA, proteins, antisense oligonucleotides and other small molecules into the developing embryo thereby providing researchers a quick and robust assay for exploring gene function *in vivo*. Antisense morpholino oligonucleotides (AMO) are now widely used to modify gene expression by blocking translation of a targeted protein or by modifying pre-mRNA splicing (Nasevicius and Ekker, 2000)). The ability to examine the course of a pathological process *in vivo* and in real time using AMO reverse genetic is a particular strength of zebrafish models. In particular, AMO are powerful reverse genetic tools for the biological validation of genetic variants identified in human and for defining the pathological nature of a particular gene mutation (Amsterdam and Hopkins, 2006). Finally, high-throughput screening for small-molecule chemical able to modify disease pathogenesis, firmly establishing a role for zebrafish in the field of pharmaceutical drug discovery.

2.2.3.1 Zebrafish SOD1 models

In order to generate a SOD1 zebrafish model of ALS, transient overexpression of human SOD1 mutants (A4V, G37R and G93A) was achieved using mRNA microinjection into 2 to 4 cell stage blastulae (Lemmens, et al., 2007). Overexpression of mutant human SOD1 in zebrafish embryos induced a dose-dependant motor axonopathy in all studied mutations. Likewise in ALS patients, ubiquitous expression of the mutant protein produced motor neuron specific neuropathology, suggesting that this model may be useful to elucidate the mechanisms underlying specific vulnerability of motor neurons in *SOD1*-linked ALS. Interestingly, the observed motor neuron phenotype in this transient SOD1mutant zebrafish embryo expresser suggests that ALS may be a developmental disease.

With the goal of achieving constitutive mutant SOD1 expression in zebrafish, Ramesh and colleagues generated transgenic zebrafish models overexpressing either WT or mutant SOD1 (Ramesh, et al., 2010). Zebrafish overexpressing mutant SOD1 exhibited many hallmark phenotypes of ALS including neuromuscular junction defects, spinal motor neuron loss, muscle degeneration, decreased endurance to swim, partial paralysis and premature death. Interestingly, all of these pathological features are consistent with those seen in SOD1 transgenic mice and rats, supporting the idea that overexpression of SOD1 in vertebrate models results in the development of common pathologies. As zebrafish are highly amenable to chimeric analysis, this zebrafish model will offer a tool to hopefully address in future studies the cell autonomous hypothesis seen in SOD1-linked ALS.

2.2.3.2 Zebrafish TDP-43 models

In order to test the toxicity associated with various *TARDBP* mutations (A315T, G348C and A382T), transient overexpression of WT and mutant TDP-43 was achieved by *TARDBP* mRNA microinjection (Kabashi, et al., 2010). Mutant TDP-43 overexpression resulted in motor neuron defects, including shorter axons, abnormal axonal branching and swimming deficits in the absence of sensory deficits. These phenotypes were also observed in WT *TARDBP* overexpressing zebrafish, but were less severe. These results confirmed that the studied *TARDBP* mutations are toxic and suggested that TDP-43 linked mutations preferentially target motor neurons for degeneration. Interestingly, knocking down the zebrafish *Tardbp* gene (z*Tardbp*), using a specific AMO designed to block z*Tardbp* translation, led to a similar phenotype, which was rescued by co-expressing WT but not mutant human TDP-43 (Kabashi, et al., 2010). Together these two reverse genetic approaches showed that *TARDBP* mutations cause motor neuron defects and toxicity, suggesting that mutant TDP-43 contributes to disease pathogenesis by both a toxic gain-of-function and a loss-of-function molecular mechanisms.

2.2.3.3 Zebrafish FUS models

To test the FUS/TLS-linked mutations toxicity, transient expression of mRNAs encoding green fluorescent protein (GFP)-FUS (WT, H517Q, R521G, R495X or G515X) fused proteins was achieved by injecting these mRNA into zebrafish eggs at the 1 to 2 cells stage of development (Bosco, et al., 2010a). Interestingly, the expression of human FUS WT and the H517Q and R521G mutants each exhibited a predominantly nuclear pattern in the spinal cord, whereas the R495X and G515X truncation mutants accumulated in the cytoplasm. Noteworthy, abnormal accumulation of protein in the cytoplasm has been frequently observed in post-mortem tissues collected from ALS patients. This phenotype was exacerbated after heat shock treatment. These results suggest that the studied FUS-linked mutations induce toxicity and that multiple factors may influence the subcellular localization of GFP-FUS *in vivo*, including various cellular stresses. Similarly, upon transient overexpression of a FUS-linked ALS mutation (R521H) in zebrafish embryos, motor deficits characterized by abnormal touch-evoke escape response was observed in 57% of the mRNA injected zebrafish larvae as compared to 23% in controls (Kabashi, et al., 2011). These results, from both studies, indicate that ALS-linked FUS/TLS mutants can cause motor neuron deficits by a toxic gain-of-function. On the other hand, loss-of-function cannot be totally excluded as knockdown of the zebrafish *Fus* (z*Fus*) gene, using antisense morpholino oligo, also yielded a motor phenotype characterized by a deficient touch-evoked escape response, reduced motor neuron outgrowth and axonal branching (Kabashi, et al., 2011). Interestingly, these phenotypes could be rescued upon co-expression of WT human FUS but not ALS-linked *FUS/TLS* mutations.

2.2.3.4 Zebrafish ALS2 models

To investigate *ALS2* gene function and to elucidate if the identified mouse Als2 splicing isoforms may compensate for the loss of the full length protein in Als2 KO mice described earlier, a knock-down of the zebrafish Als2 ortholog (z*Als2*) in zebrafish was performed using an AMO directed against the start codon of the z*Als2* gene (Gros-Louis, et al., 2008).

Consistent with this hypothesis, Gros-Louis and colleagues found that the zAls2 knocked down zebrafish led to both severe developmental abnormalities and an obvious behavioral phenotype, including swimming impairment and motor neuron disruption. This model is still the only ALS2 animal model mimicking the severe motor neuron degeneration observed in ALS2 patients. Interestingly, some of these Als2 splice variants rescued the zebrafish phenotype suggesting that these identified spliced variants, observed in Als2 null mice and in ALS2 patients, prevented the Als2 KO mice from developing severe neurodegenerative disease. These findings may also explain the variable phenotype observed in ALS2-linked patients.

2.2.4 Dog

The domestic dog (*Canis familiaris*), with over 450 naturally-occurring hereditary diseases, is a valuable model organism for the study of human genetic diseases and complex traits. In humans, common diseases show complex modes of inheritance, and as a result, genetic analysis and gene mapping could be tedious. Rodent systems are more tractable genetically, but studies using transgenic mouse models represent an induction of a particular mutation rather than naturally arising alleles, and results are often of limited direct relevance to human disease because of profound differences in physiology. In contrast, the physiology, disease presentation and clinical response of dogs to drugs often mimic human diseases closely. The dog genome is similar in size to the human genome; containing an estimated 2.8 billion DNA base pairs (Lindblad-Toh, et al., 2005). Canine models have played an important role in advancing biomedical knowledge and techniques. Due to a long history of selective breeding, many breeds of dogs are naturally prone to genetic diseases including cancer, autoimmune and neurological disorders afflicting humans. These dog models, in which naturally occurring mutations in different genes was described, may help the study of genetic diseases difficult to study in humans. The structure of the canine population offers specific advantages for genetic mapping studies. The dog enjoys a genetic diversity unrivaled by any other mammalian species. A thousand centuries of directed breeding by humans has been responsible for that diversity leading to an unequaled variety of morphologies and behaviors, and also into a number of inherited diseases. The top 10 diseases in dogs include cancer, epilepsy, allergy, retinal disease, cataracts, and heart disease. Several of these diseases constitute also a major health concerns to humans.
The disadvantages of using dog as a model are its size, cost of maintenance and housing limitations in order to provide adequate area for the dogs to run. Furthermore, there use in research has been more controversial and of public concerns than other animal models because of an obvious emotional tie toward dogs.

2.2.4.1 Dog SOD1 model

A genome-wide association analysis reveals a *SOD1* mutation in canine degenerative myelopathy (Awano, et al., 2009). This disease has been recognized for more than 35 years as a spontaneously occurring, adult-onset spinal cord disorder of dogs (Averill, 1973). The resequencing of the canine *Sod1* gene revealed a recessive E40K missense mutation. Pathological studies of spinal cords from affected dogs showed myelin and axonal loss, SOD1-positive neuronal cytoplasmic inclusions similar to those seen in patients. The disease is also fatal in dogs and, typically, presents with progressive upper motor neuron spasticity and general proprioceptive ataxia in the pelvic limbs leading to paraplegia. Dogs develop disease generally around 8 years of age or older and disease duration will not exceed, if euthanasia is delayed, 3 years. These findings suggest that this disease afflicting dogs is closely related to ALS and identify canine degenerative myelopathy to be the first recognized spontaneously occurring animal model for ALS. The canine ALS model may be particularly valuable for evaluating therapeutic interventions as the environmental conditions and the SOD1 level of expression mimic better the human ALS situation.

2.2.5 Pig

Pigs, although not easily kept for laboratory research, are readily available for biomedical research through the large-scale industrial production of pigs produced for human consumption. Recent research has facilitated the biological experimentation with pigs, and helped develop the pig into a novel model organism for biomedical research.

The domesticated pig (*Sus scrofa*) shares several similarities with human, in particular the size of organs and various aspects of anatomy and physiology. The development of somatic cloning technology and the merger with techniques of targeted genetic modification and conditional gene expression will enhance the possibilities for creating useful models for human diseases in pigs. The pig has also evolved as the major target species for producing xenografts in order to provide appropriate human organs. The sequencing of the domestic pig genome has not yet been fully completed. However, initial draft revealed that the size and composition of the porcine genome is comparable to that of humans; comprising about 2.7 billion base pairs (Hart, et al., 2007). Furthermore, both gene content and sequence are highly conserved between pig and human. Detailed information on the porcine genome together with emerging transgenic technologies, such as siRNA or conditional knockouts will enhance our possibilities to create useful pig models. Other advantages of using domestic pigs to model human diseases include high fertility, great abundance, rapid growth, anatomy and physiology not too different from human and the possibility to introduce genetic modifications in its genome. The pig has been an essential and very successful model in biomedical research and is particularly suited to close the gap between basic research in current models and clinical application. The future will certainly see several promising porcine models for human diseases.

The high resemblance between the central nervous systems of humans and pigs makes the pig an ideal model organism for studying human neurodegenerative diseases. For neurodegenerative disorders such as ALS, Parkinson's disease and Alzheimer's disease, the pig may represent a model superior to other models presently available. Large animals, including pigs and non-human primates in neuroscience enable the use of conventional clinical brain imaging and the direct testing of surgical procedures. The evaluation of novel therapeutic avenues in an animal model with higher brain complexity will allow a more direct translation to human diseases.

3. In vitro models to study ALS

In vitro models are extremely helpful to study human diseases because they allow to analyze different cell types independently from each other and to perform dynamic studies on isolated cells. Moreover, diseased cells can be combined with healthy ones to better understand which cell type is the most critical in the different stages of the disease.

Some of these *in vitro* models were developed using the ALS animal models previously discussed. However, neural cells are impossible to obtain from patients and their extraction

from post-mortem tissues is limited due to the difficulty to isolate living cells from adult brain or spinal cord, especially motor neurons.
Thus, such postmortem tissue biopsies are mostly used to perform histological and immunohistochemical, genetic as well as proteomic studies. More recently, they were also used to extract neural precursor cells that were further differentiated into motor neurons and glial cells to develop innovative models of the disease.

3.1 Organotypic cultures of spinal cord slices

The best way to preserve all the cellular content and the complex electrophysiological and biochemical organization of cells in the spinal cord is to maintain a whole tissue slice in an organotypic culture. In addition, organotypic slice cultures can be obtained from both embryos and postnatal animals, conferring a major advantage when using transgenic mice from which the disease genotype has to be ascertained after birth (Kosuge, et al., 2009; Mazzone and Nistri, 2011). After dissection of the lumbar spinal cord and removal of the meninges, 200 to 400µm-thick transversal sections are sectioned and transferred into membrane inserts fitting six-well or 12-well culture plates (Caldero, et al., 2010). These organotypic cultures can be used for more than 2 months (Delfs, et al., 1989). Various types of molecules can be added in the culture medium, such as kainate or lithium, to modulate neurotoxicity (Caldero, et al., 2010; Mazzone and Nistri, 2011).
These tissue sections can then be used to perform various analysis like recording the neuron rhythmic activity by placing the tissue on a multielectrode array (Tscherter, et al., 2001; Young, et al., 2007), or studying real-time glutamate release using a biosensor and redox reaction current using a multichannel potentiostat (Mazzone and Nistri, 2011), in addition to the conventional immunohistochemical staining and electrophysiological recordings (Caldero, et al., 2010; Young, et al., 2007). Neonatal brainstem slices can be used to analyze excitotoxicity on hypoglossal motor neurons that control the respiratory drive. These neurons are particularly useful for electrophysiological studies because they exhibit a range of rhythmic patterns that will be altered during early onset of ALS (Cifra, et al., 2011a; Cifra, et al., 2011b).
Organotypic culture is a convenient culture system that closely reproduces the *in vivo* situation and allows dynamic studies with various drugs and useful analysis systems. However, it does not always fully recapitulate what is happening *in vivo* (Tovar, et al., 2009). In addition, it does not easily allow the study of different mixed cell combinations by removing or by adding specific cell types to the tissue slices. These organotypic spinal cord slice cultures are difficult to obtain from postmortem patients due to limited availability and it is obviously impossible to study disease progression using human spinal cord biopsies as opposed to biopsies obtained from animal models.

3.2 Spinal cord cell cultures

The isolation of individual cells is extremely useful to study various intracellular mechanisms from proliferation to mRNA expression, mitochondrial function, protein aggregation, intermediate filament assembly or axonal transport. However, neurons cannot proliferate and are difficult to maintain in culture. In addition, adult nervous tissues are difficult to access and the viability of the cells extracted from them is very low. Actually, most of the cells that can be maintained in culture after extraction are neural precursor cells (Haidet-Phillips, et al., 2011).
To overcome this limitation, embryos are preferred for nervous tissue harvesting. Indeed, at the E12-13 embryonic developmental stage, the spinal cord of mice embryos is easy to access

and remove, and motor neurons, astrocytes and microglia can be extracted, purified and maintain in culture with high viability yields (Gingras, et al., 2007b; Sanelli, et al., 2007; Schnaar and Schaffner, 1981). These cells can be dissociated from the spinal cord and cultured together to facilitate motor neuron survival (Tradewell, et al., 2011; Tradewell and Durham, 2010). Motor neurons will be easy to identify because of their large cell body (>20μm in diameter) and dendritic trees, and can be stained for expression of the transcription factor Hb9 and choline acetyltransferase, specific molecular markers of motor neuron (Fig 3) (Gingras, et al., 2007b; Tradewell, et al., 2011).

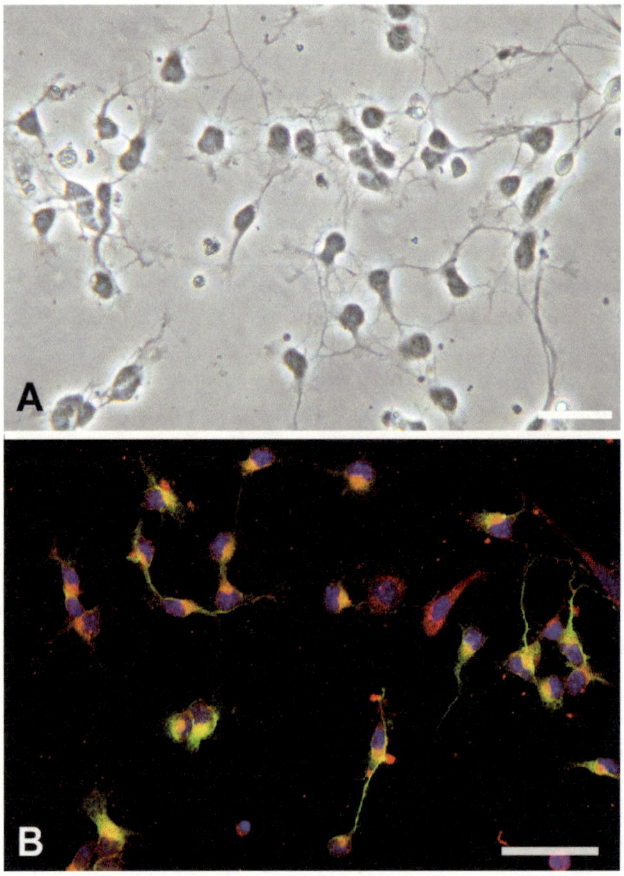

Fig. 3. E12 mouse embryo-purified motor neurons.
A: phase contrast microscopy of purified motor neurons 24h after seeding. B: Motor neurons were labeled in red with Hb9 and in green with MAP2. Bar represent 30 μm in A and 50μm in B. *Courtesy of Dr. Marie Gingras.*

Cultures of purified motor neurons without the trophic support of glial cells are difficult to maintain for more than 2 weeks (Bar, 2000; Lunn, et al., 2009). In order to perform studies on a chronic disease like ALS, especially while looking for long-term cell survival effects, dissociated spinal cord cell cultures constitute a better choice as they can be maintain in culture for up to 7 weeks (Tradewell, et al., 2011). Purified motor neurons can also be cultured on an astrocyte feeder layer for several weeks on which they display characteristics (neurite pattern) closer to adult motor neurons (Bar, 2000). To reproduce an ALS phenotype, motor neurons can be induced to express multiple copies of the gene of interest, for example, mutated human G93A SOD1, by microinjection of the vectors into the cells identified by their specific morphology (Tradewell, et al., 2011; Tradewell and Durham, 2010). Motor neurons can also be purified and cultured separately, to allow their adenoviral transduction with G93A SOD1 (Lunn, et al., 2009), and then, to enhance their survival, they can be plated on a glial cell feeder layer treated with arabinofuranosyl cytidine (AraC), to prevent cell proliferation (De Paola, et al., 2008). These *in vitro* cultures are particularly useful to study cellular morphometry (axon length), gene expression using RT-PCR (ideally with only one purified cell type), apoptosis, signaling pathways, calcium imaging, mitochondrial membrane potential, glutamate uptake, excitotoxicity, etc.

The major drawbacks of spinal cord cell cultures are the need to perform cell extraction from embryos for each new experiment. In addition, cells cultured on plastic dishes cannot recapitulate the *in vivo* environment and some results obtained *in vitro* may not be reproducible *in vivo* at least in part because the complex interactions developed in the nervous system are lost. Furthermore, another disadvantage to use primary cells from embryos is that some features of the adult phenotype may not be expressed at this early stage (Park, et al., 2004).

3.3 NCS-34 motor neuron cell line

To greatly facilitate *in vitro* studies, motor neuron-enriched embryonic mouse spinal cord cells were fused with mouse neuroblastoma to generate the hybrid cell line NCS-34 (Cashman, et al., 1992; Durham, et al., 1993; Hunter, et al., 1991). This cell line contains small proliferative and undifferentiated cells and larger multinucleate cells. These cells express properties of motor neurons such as choline acetyltransferase, acethylcholine synthesis and neurofilament expression. They respond to agents affecting voltage-gated ion channels, cytoskeletal organization and axonal transport similarly with primary motor neurons, but failed to reproduce synaptic connections (Durham, et al., 1993). This cell line is widely used in several studies related to ALS (Foran, et al., 2011; Tabata, et al., 2008; Vijayalakshmi, et al., 2009; Yang, et al., 2010). For example, NCS-34 cells were treated with the cerebrospinal fluid (CSF) collected from sporadic ALS patients. It induced intracellular aggregates formation, ubiquitin immunoreactivity, neurofilament phosphorylation and choline acetyl transferase expression through induction of endoplasmic reticular stress. This effect was attenuated by addition of VEGF prior to exposition to CSF (Kulshreshtha, et al., 2011; Vijayalakshmi, et al., 2011; Vijayalakshmi, et al., 2009). NCS-34 cells can also be used to screen antioxidant molecules capable of rescuing them from expression of mutated SOD1 (Barber, et al., 2009).

3.4 Xenopus oocyte model for electrophysiological recordings

The *Xenopus Laevi* is an African frog from which the oocyte (egg) is a commonly used model for electrophysiological recording because of its large size (about 1mm in diameter) which facilitates its handling. The oocyte has been used for decades to study various ion channels, transporters and receptors. This cell can be transduced with a molecules of interest for co-expression studies including the human glutamate transporter GLT1 (EAAT2) or NMDA receptors (Boehmer, et al., 2006; Texido, et al., 2011; Trotti, et al., 2001). This model has been used in some studies related to ALS, such as the analysis of the properties of the GLT1 transporter activities under controlled voltage clamp in presence or not of mutant SOD1 (Trotti, et al., 1999).

3.5 Neural precursor cells (NPCs) and induced pluripotent stem cells (iPS)

One important advantage of *in vitro* cell cultures could gain over animal models would be to collect neural precursor cells directly from patients. These cells can be differentiated into all neural cell types, including motor neurons. As previously discussed, most of animal and cell culture models developed to study ALS so far were derived from known FALS-associated mutations in the *SOD1*, *TARDBP* or *FUS/TLS* genes. While these models are particularly useful to study FALS, they are not ideal for the study of SALS. Therefore, trying to understand the cause of the disease through the study of motor neurons and glial cells obtained from SALS patients would be challenging but potentially highly promising. However, motor neurons, and even glial cells are extremely difficult to isolate from brain and spinal cord samples obtained from post-mortem ALS patients.

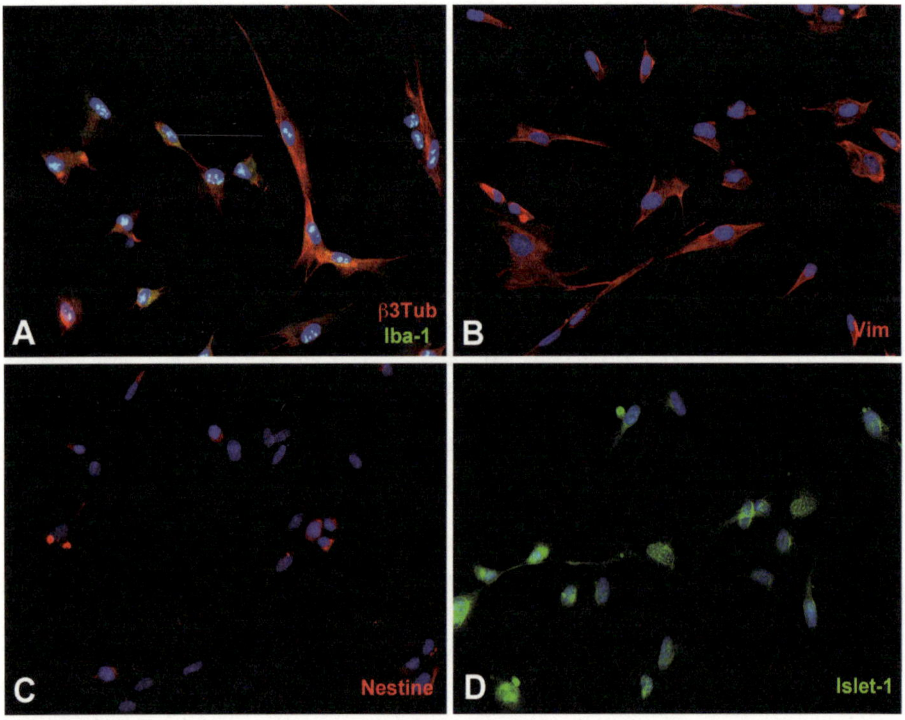

Fig. 4. Characterization of neural precursor cells (NPCs) extracted from postmortem ALS patient's spinal cord.
Cells express Iba1 (a marker of microglia) and β3-tubulin (early marker of neuronal differentiation) (A), Vimentin (transiently expressed in neuronal precursors) (B), Nestin (transiently expressed in neuronal precursors) (C) and Islet-1 (an early marker for motor neuron differentiation) (C) that highlight their NPC status when co-expressed together in the same cells. *Courtesy of Dr. Marie-Josée Beaulieu.*

One very promising alternative is to take advantage of the neural precursor cells that can be extracted from adult tissues. Indeed, in a first step, the potential of mouse embryonic stem cells (ESCs) to differentiate into motor neurons has been well established (Wichterle, et al., 2002) and applied to the development of *in vitro* ALS models using ALS-linked G93A *SOD1* gene mutation and WT SOD1 mouse embryos as source of stem cells (Di Giorgio, et al.,

2007). It was shown that G93A-SOD1 ESCs differentiated into motor neurons had a lower survival over 2 to 4 weeks in culture than their WT counterparts and showed ALS pathology hallmarks such as SOD1 protein aggregates and increase in activated caspase-3 expression after 21 days of culture (Di Giorgio, et al., 2007). Motor neurons have also been successfully differentiated from human ESCs (Hester, et al., 2011; Hu and Zhang, 2009). However, to obtain a source of multipotent stem cells from adult ALS patients, other approaches needed to be developed. These cells can be obtained from easily accessible tissues such as skin (Gingras, et al., 2007a; Toma, et al., 2001), but their limited proliferation capacity *in vitro* needs a relatively large amount of starting materials that up to now preclude their extraction from patients. Another possibility is to obtain postmortem biopsies of brain and spinal cord from ALS patients. It has been shown that if living glial cells and neurons are difficult to isolate from these tissues, neural precursor cells (NPCs) with a good proliferation rate are oppositely easy to purify and culture *in vitro*. These cells can then be differentiated in the cell type of interest. Neurons, astrocytes and oligodendrocytes were differentiated from NPCs purified from familial and sporadic ALS patient postmortem spinal cord samples (Fig 4) to study the toxic properties of patients-derived astrocytes on motor neurons (Haidet-Phillips, et al., 2011). Both FALS and SALS-derived astrocytes were shown to be toxic to motor neurons, and the knock-down of SOD1 in SALS-derived astrocytes was demonstrated to attenuate this toxicity (Haidet-Phillips, et al., 2011). But postmortem tissues are difficult to obtain.

A much more versatile technique to generate multipotent stem cells from adults is to generate induced pluripotent stem cells (iPS cells) starting from somatic cells. This technique only requires a small punch biopsy of a few millimeters in diameter collected from the patient's skin, which will heal spontaneously without scarring. From this biopsy, dermal fibroblasts will be extracted and expanded to generate iPS cells. Generation of IPs cells is possible via overexpression of a defined set of transcription factors (*c-Myc*, *Oct3/4*, *Klf4* and *SOX2*) (Takahashi, et al., 2007a; Takahashi, et al., 2007b). The genetic transduction of these oncogenes is usually achieved by using retroviral or lentiviral vectors. However, the use of integrating viral vectors represent a major obstacle to the therapeutic translation of iPS cells as this technology can produce insertional mutagenic lesions that are potentially tumorigenic. Other methods to reprogram cells are now being intensively tested, such as the use of secreted recombinant reprogramming factors present in the culture media. These iPS cells are morphologically and phenotypically similar to embryonic stem (ES) cells and thus offer exciting possibilities in stem cell research and regenerative medicine. This method has been successfully applied to ALS patients and allowed to study iPS-derived motor neurons *in vitro* (Dimos, et al., 2008; Mitne-Neto, et al., 2011). Since this technology is still recent, it is not clear whether motor neurons and glial cells derived from ALS patients-iPS cells will efficiently recapitulate the disease *in vitro*. However, these cells seem to behave like ESCs and even if they only partly mimic the ALS phenotype in culture, they certainly will be extremely interesting to use, especially for a better understanding of sporadic ALS.

3.6 Three-dimensional in vitro models

Now that iPS or NPCs ALS patient-derived motor neurons and glial cells will be available to develop better ALS *in vitro* models, their design could also be improved. The culture of neural cells in two dimensions on plastic does not mimic properly the *in vivo* situation. Building three-dimensional environment around ALS patient-derived neural cells could be a major improvement in the development of *in vitro* models of the disease. The culture of NPCs in methylcellulose scaffold enriched with laminin has been shown to reduce apoptosis and enhance survival, differentiation into neurons, astrocytes or oligodendrocytes and neurite extension (Cullen, et al., 2007; Stabenfeldt, et al., 2010). Motor neurons axonal migration can also be analyzed when these cells are cultured on the top of a three-dimensional reconstructed connective tissue made of a collagen sponge populated with fibroblasts. The addition of neurotrophic factors underneath the construct promotes neurite growth from the top to the bottom of the tissue. The main advantage of this model is to enable myelin sheath formation by Schwann cells around axons in the connective tissue and the possibility to add various glial cells (astrocytes, microglia) in the motor neuron layer (Fig 5) (Gingras, et al., 2008). In addition, it is possible to easily combine cells from different origin, like WT motor neurons with ALS glial cells, and vice-versa in order to further explore the non-cell autonomous effect observed in SOD1-linked ALS pathology. Such combinations could also be very informative in the study of sporadic ALS. Alternatively, a 3 dimensional reconstructed muscle model has been developed to study *in vitro* the effect of muscle stretching on mRNA expression of muscle cells. This model was prepared using primary muscle cultures from human control subjects and ALS patients. The cells were embedded in a collagen gel tethered to a Culture Force Monitor to analyze gel contraction (Cheema, et al., 2003; Evans, et al., 2010).

Finally, the combination of ALS patient NPC-derived neural cells in tissue-engineered reconstructed spinal cord models is a promising strategy to develop the next generation of *in vitro* models of ALS.

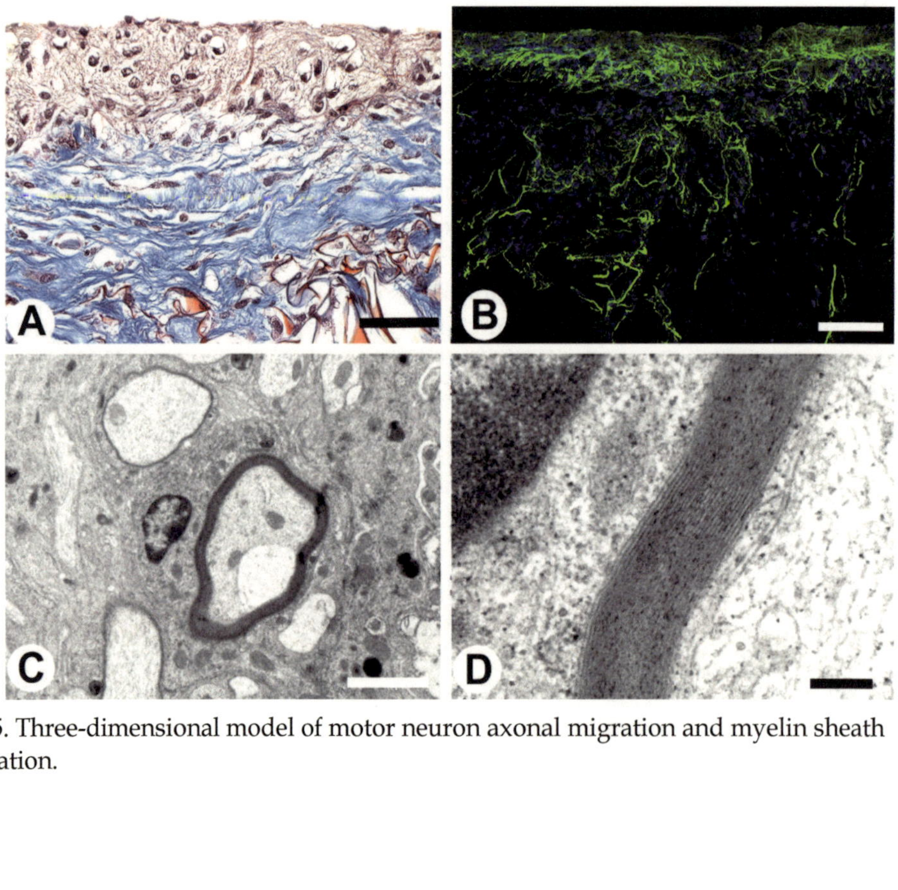

Fig. 5. Three-dimensional model of motor neuron axonal migration and myelin sheath formation.

In A, after the culture of fibroblasts and Schwann cells for 21 days in a collagen sponge (blue area), mouse motor neurons were seeded on top of the sponge (purple area) and cultured for an additional 14 days and observed by histology staining with Masson's trichrom. In B, axonal migration (stained in green with an antibody against Neurofilament-M) originating from the top layer was shown migrating through the connective tissue. In C, a transmission electron microscopic picture showed that some neurites were wrapped with thick myelin sheaths, observed at higher magnification in D. Bar in A, 60μm; bar in B, 100μm; bar in C, 2μm; bar in F, 0,2μm *(Modified from Gingras, et al., 2008).*

4. Conclusion

A very large body of knowledge has been built over the years with the development of various *in vivo* models to better understand ALS. Particularly, the generation of a large number of different transgenic mice has been extremely useful to study familial ALS, but has met with limited success so far to study SALS or to identify drugs alleviating the disease symptoms. This could be explained by the existence of redundant compensatory mechanisms present in higher vertebrates. The use of invertebrates together with higher animal models will hopefully allow the identification of novel pathogenic pathways and novel therapeutic avenues in order to cure this devastating disease.

In parallel, the development of *in vitro* models will give valuable information about the intracellular modulations induced by the disease. In addition, the promise of building sophisticated *in vitro* models using patient's cells will also be crucial to better understand the disease. However, the results obtained from *in vitro* models may not always be relevant because they are oversimplified compared to the *in vivo* situation. Therefore, the best strategy to reduce the limitations inherent to all these different models, and to benefit from their specific advantages is to combine both *in vivo* and *in vitro* models in order to better model the disease. Future work, focusing on different neuronal in vitro system and animal models, will certainly increases our knowledge in the biology of ALS and hopefully leads to more translational researches in order to find a cure or to slow down the course of this yet untreatable disease.

5. Acknowledgment

We would like to thank Dr. Alex J. Parker and Dr Guy A. Rouleau, from the Centre of Excellence in Neuromics, University of Montreal, Quebec, Canada, for having provided respectively the figure 1 and 2 of this book chapter. We also thank Marie Gingras and Marie-Josée Beaudet for their assistance in generating figure 3 to 5. Dr François Gros-Louis is supported by the Fond de la recherche en santé du Québec (FRSQ) and by the Fondation des hôpitaux Enfant-Jésus–St-Sacrement. Dr François Berthod is supported by the Muscular Dystrophy Association USA (www.mda.org). The authors declare no conflict of interest.

6. References

Adams, M. D., Celniker, S. E., Holt, R. A., Evans, C. A., Gocayne, J. D., Amanatides, P. G., Scherer, S. E., Li, P. W., Hoskins, R. A., Galle, R. F., George, R. A., Lewis, S. E., Richards, S., Ashburner, M., Henderson, S. N., Sutton, G. G., Wortman, J. R., Yandell, M. D., Zhang, Q., Chen, L. X., Brandon, R. C., Rogers, Y. H., Blazej, R. G., Champe,

M., Pfeiffer, B. D., Wan, K. H., Doyle, C., Baxter, E. G., Helt, G., Nelson, C. R., Gabor, G. L., Abril, J. F., Agbayani, A., An, H. J., Andrews-Pfannkoch, C., Baldwin, D., Ballew, R. M., Basu, A., Baxendale, J., Bayraktaroglu, L., Beasley, E. M., Beeson, K. Y., Benos, P. V., Berman, B. P., Bhandari, D., Bolshakov, S., Borkova, D., Botchan, M. R., Bouck, J., Brokstein, P., Brottier, P., Burtis, K. C., Busam, D. A., Butler, H., Cadieu, E., Center, A., Chandra, I., Cherry, J. M., Cawley, S., Dahlke, C., Davenport, L. B., Davies, P., de Pablos, B., Delcher, A., Deng, Z., Mays, A. D., Dew, I., Dietz, S. M., Dodson, K., Doup, L. E., Downes, M., Dugan-Rocha, S., Dunkov, B. C., Dunn, P., Durbin, K. J., Evangelista, C. C., Ferraz, C., Ferriera, S., Fleischmann, W., Fosler, C., Gabrielian, A. E., Garg, N. S., Gelbart, W. M., Glasser, K., Glodek, A., Gong, F., Gorrell, J. H., Gu, Z., Guan, P., Harris, M., Harris, N. L., Harvey, D., Heiman, T. J., Hernandez, J. R., Houck, J., Hostin, D., Houston, K. A., Howland, T. J., Wei, M. H., Ibegwam, C., Jalali, M., Kalush, F., Karpen, G. H., Ke, Z., Kennison, J. A., Ketchum, K. A., Kimmel, B. E., Kodira, C. D., Kraft, C., Kravitz, S., Kulp, D., Lai, Z., Lasko, P., Lei, Y., Levitsky, A. A., Li, J., Li, Z., Liang, Y., Lin, X., Liu, X., Mattei, B., McIntosh, T. C., McLeod, M. P., McPherson, D., Merkulov, G., Milshina, N. V., Mobarry, C., Morris, J., Moshrefi, A., Mount, S. M., Moy, M., Murphy, B., Murphy, L., Muzny, D. M., Nelson, D. L., Nelson, D. R., Nelson, K. A., Nixon, K., Nusskern, D. R., Pacleb, J. M., Palazzolo, M., Pittman, G. S., Pan, S., Pollard, J., Puri, V., Reese, M. G., Reinert, K., Remington, K., Saunders, R. D., Scheeler, F., Shen, H., Shue, B. C., Siden-Kiamos, I., Simpson, M., Skupski, M. P., Smith, T., Spier, E., Spradling, A. C., Stapleton, M., Strong, R., Sun, E., Svirskas, R., Tector, C., Turner, R., Venter, E., Wang, A. H., Wang, X., Wang, Z. Y., Wassarman, D. A., Weinstock, G. M., Weissenbach, J., Williams, S. M., WoodageT, Worley, K. C., Wu, D., Yang, S., Yao, Q. A., Ye, J., Yeh, R. F., Zaveri, J. S., Zhan, M., Zhang, G., Zhao, Q., Zheng, L., Zheng, X. H., Zhong, F. N., Zhong, W., Zhou, X., Zhu, S., Zhu, X., Smith, H. O., Gibbs, R. A., Myers, E. W., Rubin, G. M. and Venter, J. C. (2000). The genome sequence of Drosophila melanogaster. *Science*, 287, 2185-95.

Amsterdam, A., Burgess, S., Golling, G., Chen, W., Sun, Z., Townsend, K., Farrington, S., Haldi, M. and Hopkins, N. (1999). A large-scale insertional mutagenesis screen in zebrafish. *Genes Dev*, 13, 2713-24.

Amsterdam, A. and Hopkins, N. (2006). Mutagenesis strategies in zebrafish for identifying genes involved in development and disease. *Trends Genet*, 22, 473-8.

Anonymous (1998). Genome sequence of the nematode C. elegans: a platform for investigating biology. *Science*, 282, 2012-8.

Ash, P. E., Zhang, Y. J., Roberts, C. M., Saldi, T., Hutter, H., Buratti, E., Petrucelli, L. and Link, C. D. (2010). Neurotoxic effects of TDP-43 overexpression in C. elegans. *Hum Mol Genet*, 19, 3206-18.

Averill, D. R., Jr. (1973). Degenerative myelopathy in the aging German Shepherd dog: clinical and pathologic findings. *J Am Vet Med Assoc*, 162, 1045-51.

Awano, T., Johnson, G. S., Wade, C. M., Katz, M. L., Johnson, G. C., Taylor, J. F., Perloski, M., Biagi, T., Baranowska, I., Long, S., March, P. A., Olby, N. J., Shelton, G. D., Khan, S., O'Brien, D. P., Lindblad-Toh, K. and Coates, J. R. (2009). Genome-wide association analysis reveals a SOD1 mutation in canine degenerative myelopathy that resembles amyotrophic lateral sclerosis. *Proc Natl Acad Sci U S A*, 106, 2794-9.

Bar, P. R. (2000). Motor neuron disease in vitro: the use of cultured motor neurons to study amyotrophic lateral sclerosis. *Eur J Pharmacol*, 405, 285-95.

Barber, S. C., Higginbottom, A., Mead, R. J., Barber, S. and Shaw, P. J. (2009). An in vitro screening cascade to identify neuroprotective antioxidants in ALS. *Free Radic Biol Med*, 46, 1127-38.

Bargmann, C. I. (1998). Neurobiology of the Caenorhabditis elegans genome. *Science*, 282, 2028-33.

Beaulieu, J. M., Jacomy, H. and Julien, J. P. (2000). Formation of intermediate filament protein aggregates with disparate effects in two transgenic mouse models lacking the neurofilament light subunit. *J Neurosci*, 20, 5321-8.

Beaulieu, J. M. and Julien, J. P. (2003). Peripherin-mediated death of motor neurons rescued by overexpression of neurofilament NF-H proteins. *J Neurochem*, 85, 248-56.

Beaulieu, J. M., Nguyen, M. D. and Julien, J. P. (1999). Late onset of motor neurons in mice overexpressing wild-type peripherin. *J Cell Biol*, 147, 531-44.

Boehmer, C., Palmada, M., Rajamanickam, J., Schniepp, R., Amara, S. and Lang, F. (2006). Post-translational regulation of EAAT2 function by co-expressed ubiquitin ligase Nedd4-2 is impacted by SGK kinases. *J Neurochem*, 97, 911-21.

Boillee, S., Yamanaka, K., Lobsiger, C. S., Copeland, N. G., Jenkins, N. A., Kassiotis, G., Kollias, G. and Cleveland, D. W. (2006). Onset and progression in inherited ALS determined by motor neurons and microglia. *Science*, 312, 1389-92.

Borchelt, D. R., Lee, M. K., Slunt, H. S., Guarnieri, M., Xu, Z. S., Wong, P. C., Brown, R. H., Jr., Price, D. L., Sisodia, S. S. and Cleveland, D. W. (1994). Superoxide dismutase 1 with mutations linked to familial amyotrophic lateral sclerosis possesses significant activity. *Proc Natl Acad Sci U S A*, 91, 8292-6.

Bosco, D. A., Lemay, N., Ko, H. K., Zhou, H., Burke, C., Kwiatkowski, T. J., Jr., Sapp, P., McKenna-Yasek, D., Brown, R. H., Jr. and Hayward, L. J. (2010a). Mutant FUS proteins that cause amyotrophic lateral sclerosis incorporate into stress granules. *Hum Mol Genet*, 19, 4160-75.

Bosco, D. A., Morfini, G., Karabacak, N. M., Song, Y., Gros-Louis, F., Pasinelli, P., Goolsby, H., Fontaine, B. A., Lemay, N., McKenna-Yasek, D., Frosch, M. P., Agar, J. N., Julien, J. P., Brady, S. T. and Brown, R. H., Jr. (2010b). Wild-type and mutant SOD1 share an aberrant conformation and a common pathogenic pathway in ALS. *Nat Neurosci*, 13, 1396-403.

Brand, A. H. and Perrimon, N. (1993). Targeted gene expression as a means of altering cell fates and generating dominant phenotypes. *Development*, 118, 401-15.

Brenner, S. (1974). The genetics of Caenorhabditis elegans. *Genetics*, 77, 71-94.

Bruijn, L. I., Becher, M. W., Lee, M. K., Anderson, K. L., Jenkins, N. A., Copeland, N. G., Sisodia, S. S., Rothstein, J. D., Borchelt, D. R., Price, D. L. and Cleveland, D. W. (1997). ALS-linked SOD1 mutant G85R mediates damage to astrocytes and promotes rapidly progressive disease with SOD1-containing inclusions. *Neuron*, 18, 327-38.

Bruijn, L. I., Houseweart, M. K., Kato, S., Anderson, K. L., Anderson, S. D., Ohama, E., Reaume, A. G., Scott, R. W. and Cleveland, D. W. (1998). Aggregation and motor neuron toxicity of an ALS-linked SOD1 mutant independent from wild-type SOD1. *Science*, 281, 1851-4.

Cai, H., Lin, X., Xie, C., Laird, F. M., Lai, C., Wen, H., Chiang, H. C., Shim, H., Farah, M. H., Hoke, A., Price, D. L. and Wong, P. C. (2005). Loss of ALS2 function is insufficient to trigger motor neuron degeneration in knock-out mice but predisposes neurons to oxidative stress. *J Neurosci*, 25, 7567-74.

Caldero, J., Brunet, N., Tarabal, O., Piedrafita, L., Hereu, M., Ayala, V. and Esquerda, J. E. (2010). Lithium prevents excitotoxic cell death of motoneurons in organotypic slice cultures of spinal cord. *Neuroscience*, 165, 1353-69.

Cashman, N. R., Durham, H. D., Blusztajn, J. K., Oda, K., Tabira, T., Shaw, I. T., Dahrouge, S. and Antel, J. P. (1992). Neuroblastoma x spinal cord (NSC) hybrid cell lines resemble developing motor neurons. *Dev Dyn*, 194, 209-21.

Cheema, U., Yang, S. Y., Mudera, V., Goldspink, G. G. and Brown, R. A. (2003). 3-D in vitro model of early skeletal muscle development. *Cell Motil Cytoskeleton*, 54, 226-36.

Chen, Y., Yang, M., Deng, J., Chen, X., Ye, Y., Zhu, L., Liu, J., Ye, H., Shen, Y., Li, Y., Rao, E. J., Fushimi, K., Zhou, X., Bigio, E. H., Mesulam, M., Xu, Q. and Wu, J. Y. (2011). Expression of human FUS protein in Drosophila leads to progressive neurodegeneration. *Protein Cell*, 2, 477-86.

Chio, A., Borghero, G., Pugliatti, M., Ticca, A., Calvo, A., Moglia, C., Mutani, R., Brunetti, M., Ossola, I., Marrosu, M. G., Murru, M. R., Floris, G., Cannas, A., Parish, L. D., Cossu, P., Abramzon, Y., Johnson, J. O., Nalls, M. A., Arepalli, S., Chong, S., Hernandez, D. G., Traynor, B. J. and Restagno, G. (2011). Large proportion of amyotrophic lateral sclerosis cases in Sardinia due to a single founder mutation of the TARDBP gene. *Arch Neurol*, 68, 594-8.

Chow, C. Y., Landers, J. E., Bergren, S. K., Sapp, P. C., Grant, A. E., Jones, J. M., Everett, L., Lenk, G. M., McKenna-Yasek, D. M., Weisman, L. S., Figlewicz, D., Brown, R. H. and Meisler, M. H. (2009). Deleterious variants of FIG4, a phosphoinositide phosphatase, in patients with ALS. *Am J Hum Genet*, 84, 85-8.

Christensen, M., Estevez, A., Yin, X., Fox, R., Morrison, R., McDonnell, M., Gleason, C., Miller, D. M., 3rd and Strange, K. (2002). A primary culture system for functional analysis of C. elegans neurons and muscle cells. *Neuron*, 33, 503-14.

Cifra, A., Nani, F. and Nistri, A. (2011a). Respiratory motoneurons and pathological conditions: Lessons from hypoglossal motoneurons challenged by excitotoxic or oxidative stress. *Respir Physiol Neurobiol*, doi:10.1016/j.resp.2011.03.017.

Cifra, A., Nani, F. and Nistri, A. (2011b). Riluzole is a potent drug to protect neonatal rat hypoglossal motoneurons in vitro from excitotoxicity due to glutamate uptake block. *Eur J Neurosci*, 33, 899-913.

Clement, A. M., Nguyen, M. D., Roberts, E. A., Garcia, M. L., Boillee, S., Rule, M., McMahon, A. P., Doucette, W., Siwek, D., Ferrante, R. J., Brown, R. H., Jr., Julien, J. P., Goldstein, L. S. and Cleveland, D. W. (2003). Wild-type nonneuronal cells extend survival of SOD1 mutant motor neurons in ALS mice. *Science*, 302, 113-7.

Corbo, M. and Hays, A. P. (1992). Peripherin and neurofilament protein coexist in spinal spheroids of motor neuron disease. *J Neuropathol Exp Neurol*, 51, 531-7.

Corrado, L., Ratti, A., Gellera, C., Buratti, E., Castellotti, B., Carlomagno, Y., Ticozzi, N., Mazzini, L., Testa, L., Taroni, F., Baralle, F. E., Silani, V. and D'Alfonso, S. (2009). High frequency of TARDBP gene mutations in Italian patients with amyotrophic lateral sclerosis. *Hum Mutat*, 30, 688-94.

Cote, F., Collard, J. F. and Julien, J. P. (1993). Progressive neuronopathy in transgenic mice expressing the human neurofilament heavy gene: a mouse model of amyotrophic lateral sclerosis. *Cell*, 73, 35-46.

Culetto, E. and Sattelle, D. B. (2000). A role for Caenorhabditis elegans in understanding the function and interactions of human disease genes. *Hum Mol Genet*, 9, 869-77.

Cullen, D. K., Stabenfeldt, S. E., Simon, C. M., Tate, C. C. and LaPlaca, M. C. (2007). In vitro neural injury model for optimization of tissue-engineered constructs. *J Neurosci Res*, 85, 3642-51.

Daoud, H., Valdmanis, P. N., Kabashi, E., Dion, P., Dupre, N., Camu, W., Meininger, V. and Rouleau, G. A. (2009). Contribution of TARDBP mutations to sporadic amyotrophic lateral sclerosis. *J Med Genet*, 46, 112-4.

De Paola, M., Diana, V., Bigini, P. and Mennini, T. (2008). Morphological features and responses to AMPA receptor-mediated excitotoxicity of mouse motor neurons: comparison in purified, mixed anterior horn or motor neuron/glia cocultures. *J Neurosci Methods*, 170, 85-95.

DeJesus-Hernandez, M., Mackenzie, I. R., Boeve, B. F., Boxer, A. L., Baker, M., Rutherford, N. J., Nicholson, A. M., Finch, N. A., Flynn, H., Adamson, J., Kouri, N., Wojtas, A., Sengdy, P., Hsiung, G. R., Karydas, A., Seeley, W. W., Josephs, K. A., Coppola, G., Geschwind, D. H., Wszolek, Z. K., Feldman, H., Knopman, D. S., Petersen, R. C., Miller, B. L., Dickson, D. W., Boylan, K. B., Graff-Radford, N. R. and Rademakers, R. (2011). Expanded GGGGCC Hexanucleotide Repeat in Noncoding Region of C9ORF72 Causes Chromosome 9p-Linked FTD and ALS. *Neuron*.

Delfs, J., Friend, J., Ishimoto, S. and Saroff, D. (1989). Ventral and dorsal horn acetylcholinesterase neurons are maintained in organotypic cultures of postnatal rat spinal cord explants. *Brain Res*, 488, 31-42.

Deng, H. X., Zhai, H., Fu, R., Shi, Y., Gorrie, G. H., Yang, Y., Liu, E., Dal Canto, M. C., Mugnaini, E. and Siddique, T. (2007). Distal axonopathy in an alsin-deficient mouse model. *Hum Mol Genet*, 16, 2911-20.

Devon, R. S., Helm, J. R., Rouleau, G. A., Leitner, Y., Lerman-Sagie, T., Lev, D. and Hayden, M. R. (2003). The first nonsense mutation in alsin results in a homogeneous phenotype of infantile-onset ascending spastic paralysis with bulbar involvement in two siblings. *Clin Genet*, 64, 210-5.

Di Giorgio, F. P., Carrasco, M. A., Siao, M. C., Maniatis, T. and Eggan, K. (2007). Non-cell autonomous effect of glia on motor neurons in an embryonic stem cell-based ALS model. *Nat Neurosci*, 10, 608-14.

Dimos, J. T., Rodolfa, K. T., Niakan, K. K., Weisenthal, L. M., Mitsumoto, H., Chung, W., Croft, G. F., Saphier, G., Leibel, R., Goland, R., Wichterle, H., Henderson, C. E. and Eggan, K. (2008). Induced pluripotent stem cells generated from patients with ALS can be differentiated into motor neurons. *Science*, 321, 1218-21.

Driever, W., Solnica-Krezel, L., Schier, A. F., Neuhauss, S. C., Malicki, J., Stemple, D. L., Stainier, D. Y., Zwartkruis, F., Abdelilah, S., Rangini, Z., Belak, J. and Boggs, C. (1996). A genetic screen for mutations affecting embryogenesis in zebrafish. *Development*, 123, 37-46.

Durham, H. D., Dahrouge, S. and Cashman, N. R. (1993). Evaluation of the spinal cord neuron X neuroblastoma hybrid cell line NSC-34 as a model for neurotoxicity testing. *Neurotoxicology*, 14, 387-95.

Elden, A. C., Kim, H. J., Hart, M. P., Chen-Plotkin, A. S., Johnson, B. S., Fang, X., Armakola, M., Geser, F., Greene, R., Lu, M. M., Padmanabhan, A., Clay-Falcone, D., McCluskey, L., Elman, L., Juhr, D., Gruber, P. J., Rub, U., Auburger, G., Trojanowski, J. Q., Lee, V. M., Van Deerlin, V. M., Bonini, N. M. and Gitler, A. D. (2010). Ataxin-2 intermediate-length polyglutamine expansions are associated with increased risk for ALS. *Nature*, 466, 1069-75.

Estes, P. S., Boehringer, A., Zwick, R., Tang, J. E., Grigsby, B. and Zarnescu, D. C. (2011). Wild-type and A315T mutant TDP-43 exert differential neurotoxicity in a Drosophila model of ALS. *Hum Mol Genet*, 20, 2308-21.

Evans, R. M., Harridge, S. D., Velloso, C. P., Yang, S. Y., Goldspink, G. and Orrell, R. W. (2010). Investigation of MGF mRNA expression in patients with amyotrophic lateral sclerosis using parallel in vivo and in vitro approaches. *Amyotroph Lateral Scler*, 11, 172-7.

Eymard-Pierre, E., Lesca, G., Dollet, S., Santorelli, F. M., di Capua, M., Bertini, E. and Boespflug-Tanguy, O. (2002). Infantile-onset ascending hereditary spastic paralysis is associated with mutations in the alsin gene. *Am J Hum Genet*, 71, 518-27.

Eymard-Pierre, E., Yamanaka, K., Haeussler, M., Kress, W., Gauthier-Barichard, F., Combes, P., Cleveland, D. W. and Boespflug-Tanguy, O. (2006). Novel missense mutation in ALS2 gene results in infantile ascending hereditary spastic paralysis. *Ann Neurol*, 59, 976-80.

Ezzi, S. A., Urushitani, M. and Julien, J. P. (2007). Wild-type superoxide dismutase acquires binding and toxic properties of ALS-linked mutant forms through oxidation. *J Neurochem*, 102, 170-8.

Feiguin, F., Godena, V. K., Romano, G., D'Ambrogio, A., Klima, R. and Baralle, F. E. (2009). Depletion of TDP-43 affects Drosophila motoneurons terminal synapsis and locomotive behavior. *FEBS Lett*, 583, 1586-92.

Fire, A., Xu, S., Montgomery, M. K., Kostas, S. A., Driver, S. E. and Mello, C. C. (1998). Potent and specific genetic interference by double-stranded RNA in Caenorhabditis elegans. *Nature*, 391, 806-11.

Foran, E., Bogush, A., Goffredo, M., Roncaglia, P., Gustincich, S., Pasinelli, P. and Trotti, D. (2011). Motor neuron impairment mediated by a sumoylated fragment of the glial glutamate transporter EAAT2. *Glia*.

Gidalevitz, T., Krupinski, T., Garcia, S. and Morimoto, R. I. (2009). Destabilizing protein polymorphisms in the genetic background direct phenotypic expression of mutant SOD1 toxicity. *PLoS Genet*, 5, e1000399.

Gingras, M., Beaulieu, M. M., Gagnon, V., Durham, H. D. and Berthod, F. (2008). In vitro study of axonal migration and myelination of motor neurons in a three-dimensional tissue-engineered model. *Glia*, 56, 354-64.

Gingras, M., Champigny, M. F. and Berthod, F. (2007a). Differentiation of human adult skin-derived neuronal precursors into mature neurons. *J Cell Physiol*, 210, 498-506.

Gingras, M., Gagnon, V., Minotti, S., Durham, H. D. and Berthod, F. (2007b). Optimized protocols for isolation of primary motor neurons, astrocytes and microglia from embryonic mouse spinal cord. *J Neurosci Methods*, 163, 111-8.

Gitcho, M. A., Baloh, R. H., Chakraverty, S., Mayo, K., Norton, J. B., Levitch, D., Hatanpaa, K. J., White, C. L., 3rd, Bigio, E. H., Caselli, R., Baker, M., Al-Lozi, M. T., Morris, J. C., Pestronk, A., Rademakers, R., Goate, A. M. and Cairns, N. J. (2008). TDP-43 A315T mutation in familial motor neuron disease. *Ann Neurol*, 63, 535-8.

Gong, Y. H., Parsadanian, A. S., Andreeva, A., Snider, W. D. and Elliott, J. L. (2000). Restricted expression of G86R Cu/Zn superoxide dismutase in astrocytes results in astrocytosis but does not cause motoneuron degeneration. *J Neurosci*, 20, 660-5.

Gros-Louis, F., Andersen, P. M., Dupre, N., Urushitani, M., Dion, P., Souchon, F., D'Amour, M., Camu, W., Meininger, V., Bouchard, J. P., Rouleau, G. A. and Julien, J. P. (2009a). Chromogranin B P413L variant as risk factor and modifier of disease onset for amyotrophic lateral sclerosis. *Proc Natl Acad Sci U S A*.

Gros-Louis, F., Gaspar, C. and Rouleau, G. A. (2006). Genetics of familial and sporadic amyotrophic lateral sclerosis. *Biochim Biophys Acta*, 1762, 956-72.

Gros-Louis, F., Gowing, G. and Julien, J. P. (2009b). Development of immunotherapeutic approaches to amyotrophic lateral sclerosis. *Future Neurol*, 4, 435-47.

Gros-Louis, F., Kriz, J., Kabashi, E., McDearmid, J., Millecamps, S., Urushitani, M., Lin, L., Dion, P., Zhu, Q., Drapeau, P., Julien, J. P. and Rouleau, G. A. (2008). Als2 mRNA splicing variants detected in KO mice rescue severe motor dysfunction phenotype in Als2 knock-down zebrafish. *Hum Mol Genet*, 17, 2691-702.

Gros-Louis, F., Meijer, I. A., Hand, C. K., Dube, M. P., MacGregor, D. L., Seni, M. H., Devon, R. S., Hayden, M. R., Andermann, F., Andermann, E. and Rouleau, G. A. (2003). An ALS2 gene mutation causes hereditary spastic paraplegia in a Pakistani kindred. *Ann Neurol*, 53, 144-5.

Gros-Louis, F., Soucy, G., Lariviere, R. and Julien, J. P. (2010). Intracerebroventricular infusion of monoclonal antibody or its derived Fab fragment against misfolded forms of SOD1 mutant delays mortality in a mouse model of ALS. *J Neurochem*, 113, 1188-99.

Gurney, M. E., Cutting, F. B., Zhai, P., Doble, A., Taylor, C. P., Andrus, P. K. and Hall, E. D. (1996). Benefit of vitamin E, riluzole, and gabapentin in a transgenic model of familial amyotrophic lateral sclerosis. *Ann Neurol*, 39, 147-57.

Gurney, M. E., Pu, H., Chiu, A. Y., Dal Canto, M. C., Polchow, C. Y., Alexander, D. D., Caliendo, J., Hentati, A., Kwon, Y. W., Deng, H. X. and et al. (1994). Motor neuron degeneration in mice that express a human Cu,Zn superoxide dismutase mutation. *Science*, 264, 1772-5.

Hadano, S., Benn, S. C., Kakuta, S., Otomo, A., Sudo, K., Kunita, R., Suzuki-Utsunomiya, K., Mizumura, H., Shefner, J. M., Cox, G. A., Iwakura, Y., Brown, R. H., Jr. and Ikeda, J. E. (2006). Mice deficient in the Rab5 guanine nucleotide exchange factor ALS2/alsin exhibit age-dependent neurological deficits and altered endosome trafficking. *Hum Mol Genet*, 15, 233-50.

Hadano, S., Hand, C. K., Osuga, H., Yanagisawa, Y., Otomo, A., Devon, R. S., Miyamoto, N., Showguchi-Miyata, J., Okada, Y., Singaraja, R., Figlewicz, D. A., Kwiatkowski, T., Hosler, B. A., Sagie, T., Skaug, J., Nasir, J., Brown, R. H., Jr., Scherer, S. W., Rouleau, G. A., Hayden, M. R. and Ikeda, J. E. (2001). A gene encoding a putative GTPase regulator is mutated in familial amyotrophic lateral sclerosis 2. *Nat Genet*, 29, 166-73.

Haffter, P., Granato, M., Brand, M., Mullins, M. C., Hammerschmidt, M., Kane, D. A., Odenthal, J., van Eeden, F. J., Jiang, Y. J., Heisenberg, C. P., Kelsh, R. N., Furutani-Seiki, M., Vogelsang, E., Beuchle, D., Schach, U., Fabian, C. and Nusslein-Volhard, C. (1996). The identification of genes with unique and essential functions in the development of the zebrafish, Danio rerio. *Development*, 123, 1-36.

Haidet-Phillips, A. M., Hester, M. E., Miranda, C. J., Meyer, K., Braun, L., Frakes, A., Song, S., Likhite, S., Murtha, M. J., Foust, K. D., Rao, M., Eagle, A., Kammesheidt, A., Christensen, A., Mendell, J. R., Burghes, A. H. and Kaspar, B. K. (2011). Astrocytes from familial and sporadic ALS patients are toxic to motor neurons. *Nat Biotechnol*.

Hanson, K. A., Kim, S. H., Wassarman, D. A. and Tibbetts, R. S. (2010). Ubiquilin modifies TDP-43 toxicity in a Drosophila model of amyotrophic lateral sclerosis (ALS). *J Biol Chem*, 285, 11068-72.

Hart, E. A., Caccamo, M., Harrow, J. L., Humphray, S. J., Gilbert, J. G., Trevanion, S., Hubbard, T., Rogers, J. and Rothschild, M. F. (2007). Lessons learned from the initial sequencing of the pig genome: comparative analysis of an 8 Mb region of pig chromosome 17. *Genome Biol*, 8, R168.

Heiman-Patterson, T. D., Deitch, J. S., Blankenhorn, E. P., Erwin, K. L., Perreault, M. J., Alexander, B. K., Byers, N., Toman, I. and Alexander, G. M. (2005). Background and gender effects on survival in the TgN(SOD1-G93A)1Gur mouse model of ALS. *J Neurol Sci*, 236, 1-7.

Henion, P. D., Raible, D. W., Beattie, C. E., Stoesser, K. L., Weston, J. A. and Eisen, J. S. (1996). Screen for mutations affecting development of Zebrafish neural crest. *Dev Genet*, 18, 11-7.

Hester, M. E., Murtha, M. J., Song, S., Rao, M., Miranda, C. J., Meyer, K., Tian, J., Boulting, G., Schaffer, D. V., Zhu, M. X., Pfaff, S. L., Gage, F. H. and Kaspar, B. K. (2011). Rapid and Efficient Generation of Functional Motor Neurons From Human Pluripotent Stem Cells Using Gene Delivered Transcription Factor Codes. *Mol Ther*.

Howland, D. S., Liu, J., She, Y., Goad, B., Maragakis, N. J., Kim, B., Erickson, J., Kulik, J., DeVito, L., Psaltis, G., DeGennaro, L. J., Cleveland, D. W. and Rothstein, J. D. (2002). Focal loss of the glutamate transporter EAAT2 in a transgenic rat model of SOD1 mutant-mediated amyotrophic lateral sclerosis (ALS). *Proc Natl Acad Sci U S A*, 99, 1604-9.

Hu, B. Y. and Zhang, S. C. (2009). Differentiation of spinal motor neurons from pluripotent human stem cells. *Nat Protoc*, 4, 1295-304.

Hunter, D. D., Cashman, N., Morris-Valero, R., Bulock, J. W., Adams, S. P. and Sanes, J. R. (1991). An LRE (leucine-arginine-glutamate)-dependent mechanism for adhesion of neurons to S-laminin. *J Neurosci*, 11, 3960-71.

Hutton, M., Lendon, C. L., Rizzu, P., Baker, M., Froelich, S., Houlden, H., Pickering-Brown, S., Chakraverty, S., Isaacs, A., Grover, A., Hackett, J., Adamson, J., Lincoln, S., Dickson, D., Davies, P., Petersen, R. C., Stevens, M., de Graaff, E., Wauters, E., van Baren, J., Hillebrand, M., Joosse, M., Kwon, J. M., Nowotny, P., Che, L. K., Norton, J., Morris, J. C., Reed, L. A., Trojanowski, J., Basun, H., Lannfelt, L., Neystat, M., Fahn, S., Dark, F., Tannenberg, T., Dodd, P. R., Hayward, N., Kwok, J. B., Schofield, P. R., Andreadis, A., Snowden, J., Craufurd, D., Neary, D., Owen, F., Oostra, B. A., Hardy, J., Goate, A., van Swieten, J., Mann, D., Lynch, T. and Heutink, P. (1998). Association of missense and 5'-splice-site mutations in tau with the inherited dementia FTDP-17. *Nature*, 393, 702-5.

Johnson, J. O., Mandrioli, J., Benatar, M., Abramzon, Y., Van Deerlin, V. M., Trojanowski, J. Q., Gibbs, J. R., Brunetti, M., Gronka, S., Wuu, J., Ding, J., McCluskey, L., Martinez-Lage, M., Falcone, D., Hernandez, D. G., Arepalli, S., Chong, S., Schymick, J. C., Rothstein, J., Landi, F., Wang, Y. D., Calvo, A., Mora, G., Sabatelli, M., Monsurro, M. R., Battistini, S., Salvi, F., Spataro, R., Sola, P., Borghero, G., Galassi, G., Scholz, S. W., Taylor, J. P., Restagno, G., Chio, A. and Traynor, B. J. (2010). Exome sequencing reveals VCP mutations as a cause of familial ALS. *Neuron*, 68, 857-64.

Jonsson, P. A., Ernhill, K., Andersen, P. M., Bergemalm, D., Brannstrom, T., Gredal, O., Nilsson, P. and Marklund, S. L. (2004). Minute quantities of misfolded mutant superoxide dismutase-1 cause amyotrophic lateral sclerosis. *Brain*, 127, 73-88.

Jonsson, P. A., Graffmo, K. S., Andersen, P. M., Brannstrom, T., Lindberg, M., Oliveberg, M. and Marklund, S. L. (2006). Disulphide-reduced superoxide dismutase-1 in CNS of transgenic amyotrophic lateral sclerosis models. *Brain*, 129, 451-64.

Julien, J. P. and Kriz, J. (2006). Transgenic mouse models of amyotrophic lateral sclerosis. *Biochim Biophys Acta*, 1762, 1013-24.

Kabashi, E., Bercier, V., Lissouba, A., Liao, M., Brustein, E., Rouleau, G. A. and Drapeau, P. (2011). FUS and TARDBP but Not SOD1 Interact in Genetic Models of Amyotrophic Lateral Sclerosis. *PLoS Genet*, 7, e1002214.

Kabashi, E., Lin, L., Tradewell, M. L., Dion, P. A., Bercier, V., Bourgouin, P., Rochefort, D., Bel Hadj, S., Durham, H. D., Vande Velde, C., Rouleau, G. A. and Drapeau, P. (2010). Gain and loss of function of ALS-related mutations of TARDBP (TDP-43) cause motor deficits in vivo. *Hum Mol Genet*, 19, 671-83.

Kabashi, E., Valdmanis, P. N., Dion, P., Spiegelman, D., McConkey, B. J., Vande Velde, C., Bouchard, J. P., Lacomblez, L., Pochigaeva, K., Salachas, F., Pradat, P. F., Camu, W., Meininger, V., Dupre, N. and Rouleau, G. A. (2008). TARDBP mutations in individuals with sporadic and familial amyotrophic lateral sclerosis. *Nat Genet*, 40, 572-4.

Kim, S. H., Shi, Y., Hanson, K. A., Williams, L. M., Sakasai, R., Bowler, M. J. and Tibbetts, R. S. (2009). Potentiation of amyotrophic lateral sclerosis (ALS)-associated TDP-43 aggregation by the proteasome-targeting factor, ubiquilin 1. *J Biol Chem*, 284, 8083-92.

Kosuge, Y., Sekikawa-Nishida, K., Negi, H., Ishige, K. and Ito, Y. (2009). Characterization of chronic glutamate-mediated motor neuron toxicity in organotypic spinal cord culture prepared from ALS model mice. *Neurosci Lett*, 454, 165-9.

Kraemer, B. C., Schuck, T., Wheeler, J. M., Robinson, L. C., Trojanowski, J. Q., Lee, V. M. and Schellenberg, G. D. (2010). Loss of murine TDP-43 disrupts motor function and plays an essential role in embryogenesis. *Acta Neuropathol*, 119, 409-19.

Kress, J. A., Kuhnlein, P., Winter, P., Ludolph, A. C., Kassubek, J., Muller, U. and Sperfeld, A. D. (2005). Novel mutation in the ALS2 gene in juvenile amyotrophic lateral sclerosis. *Ann Neurol*, 58, 800-3.

Kulshreshtha, D., Vijayalakshmi, K., Alladi, P. A., Sathyaprabha, T. N., Nalini, A. and Raju, T. R. (2011). Vascular endothelial growth factor attenuates neurodegenerative changes in the NSC-34 motor neuron cell line induced by cerebrospinal fluid of sporadic amyotrophic lateral sclerosis patients. *Neurodegener Dis*, 8, 322-30.

Kwiatkowski, T. J., Jr., Bosco, D. A., Leclerc, A. L., Tamrazian, E., Vanderburg, C. R., Russ, C., Davis, A., Gilchrist, J., Kasarskis, E. J., Munsat, T., Valdmanis, P., Rouleau, G. A., Hosler, B. A., Cortelli, P., de Jong, P. J., Yoshinaga, Y., Haines, J. L., Pericak-Vance, M. A., Yan, J., Ticozzi, N., Siddique, T., McKenna-Yasek, D., Sapp, P. C., Horvitz, H. R., Landers, J. E. and Brown, R. H., Jr. (2009). Mutations in the FUS/TLS gene on chromosome 16 cause familial amyotrophic lateral sclerosis. *Science*, 323, 1205-8.

Lanson, N. A., Jr., Maltare, A., King, H., Smith, R., Kim, J. H., Taylor, J. P., Lloyd, T. E. and Pandey, U. B. (2011). A Drosophila model of FUS-related neurodegeneration reveals genetic interaction between FUS and TDP-43. *Hum Mol Genet*, 20, 2510-23.

Lariviere, R. C. and Julien, J. P. (2004). Functions of intermediate filaments in neuronal development and disease. *J Neurobiol*, 58, 131-48.

Lemmens, R., Van Hoecke, A., Hersmus, N., Geelen, V., D'Hollander, I., Thijs, V., Van Den Bosch, L., Carmeliet, P. and Robberecht, W. (2007). Overexpression of mutant superoxide dismutase 1 causes a motor axonopathy in the zebrafish. *Hum Mol Genet*, 16, 2359-65.

Li, Y., Ray, P., Rao, E. J., Shi, C., Guo, W., Chen, X., Woodruff, E. A., 3rd, Fushimi, K. and Wu, J. Y. (2010). A Drosophila model for TDP-43 proteinopathy. *Proc Natl Acad Sci U S A*, 107, 3169-74.

Liachko, N. F., Guthrie, C. R. and Kraemer, B. C. (2010). Phosphorylation promotes neurotoxicity in a Caenorhabditis elegans model of TDP-43 proteinopathy. *J Neurosci*, 30, 16208-19.

Lin, M. J., Cheng, C. W. and Shen, C. K. (2011). Neuronal function and dysfunction of Drosophila dTDP. *PLoS One*, 6, e20371.

Lindblad-Toh, K., Wade, C. M., Mikkelsen, T. S., Karlsson, E. K., Jaffe, D. B., Kamal, M., Clamp, M., Chang, J. L., Kulbokas, E. J., 3rd, Zody, M. C., Mauceli, E., Xie, X., Breen, M., Wayne, R. K., Ostrander, E. A., Ponting, C. P., Galibert, F., Smith, D. R., DeJong, P. J., Kirkness, E., Alvarez, P., Biagi, T., Brockman, W., Butler, J., Chin, C. W., Cook, A., Cuff, J., Daly, M. J., DeCaprio, D., Gnerre, S., Grabherr, M., Kellis, M., Kleber, M., Bardeleben, C., Goodstadt, L., Heger, A., Hitte, C., Kim, L., Koepfli, K. P., Parker, H. G., Pollinger, J. P., Searle, S. M., Sutter, N. B., Thomas, R., Webber, C., Baldwin, J., Abebe, A., Abouelleil, A., Aftuck, L., Ait-Zahra, M., Aldredge, T., Allen, N., An, P., Anderson, S., Antoine, C., Arachchi, H., Aslam, A., Ayotte, L., Bachantsang, P., Barry, A., Bayul, T., Benamara, M., Berlin, A., Bessette, D., Blitshteyn, B., Bloom, T., Blye, J., Boguslavskiy, L., Bonnet, C., Boukhgalter, B., Brown, A., Cahill, P., Calixte, N., Camarata, J., Cheshatsang, Y., Chu, J., Citroen, M., Collymore, A., Cooke, P., Dawoe, T., Daza, R., Decktor, K., DeGray, S., Dhargay, N., Dooley, K., Dorje, P., Dorjee, K., Dorris, L., Duffey, N., Dupes, A., Egbiremolen, O., Elong, R., Falk, J., Farina, A., Faro, S., Ferguson, D., Ferreira, P., Fisher, S., FitzGerald, M., Foley, K., Foley, C., Franke, A., Friedrich, D., Gage, D., Garber, M., Gearin, G., Giannoukos, G., Goode, T., Goyette, A., Graham, J., Grandbois, E., Gyaltsen, K., Hafez, N., Hagopian, D., Hagos, B., Hall, J., Healy, C., Hegarty, R., Honan, T., Horn, A., Houde, N., Hughes, L., Hunnicutt, L., Husby, M., Jester, B., Jones, C., Kamat, A., Kanga, B., Kells, C., Khazanovich, D., Kieu, A. C., Kisner, P., Kumar, M., Lance, K., Landers, T., Lara, M., Lee, W., Leger, J. P., Lennon, N., Leuper, L., LeVine, S., Liu, J., Liu, X., Lokyitsang, Y., Lokyitsang, T., Lui, A., Macdonald, J., Major, J., Marabella, R., Maru, K., Matthews, C., McDonough, S., Mehta, T., Meldrim, J., Melnikov, A., Meneus, L., Mihalev, A., Mihova, T., Miller, K., Mittelman, R., Mlenga, V., Mulrain, L., Munson, G., Navidi, A., Naylor, J., Nguyen, T., Nguyen, N., Nguyen, C., Nicol, R., Norbu, N., Norbu, C., Novod, N., Nyima, T., Olandt, P., O'Neill, B., O'Neill, K., Osman, S., Oyono, L., Patti, C., Perrin, D., Phunkhang, P., Pierre, F., Priest, M., Rachupka, A., Raghuraman, S., Rameau, R., Ray, V., Raymond, C., Rege, F., Rise, C., Rogers, J., Rogov, P., Sahalie, J., Settipalli, S., Sharpe, T., Shea, T., Sheehan, M., Sherpa, N., Shi, J., Shih, D., Sloan, J., Smith, C., Sparrow, T., Stalker, J., Stange-Thomann, N., Stavropoulos, S., Stone, C., Stone, S., Sykes, S., Tchuinga, P., Tenzing, P., Tesfaye, S., Thoulutsang, D., Thoulutsang, Y., Topham, K., Topping, I., Tsamla, T., Vassiliev, H., Venkataraman, V., Vo, A., Wangchuk, T., Wangdi, T., Weiand, M., Wilkinson, J., Wilson, A., Yadav, S., Yang, S., Yang, X., Young, G., Yu, Q., Zainoun, J., Zembek, L., Zimmer, A. and Lander, E. S. (2005). Genome sequence, comparative analysis and haplotype structure of the domestic dog. *Nature*, 438, 803-19.

Lu, Y., Ferris, J. and Gao, F. B. (2009). Frontotemporal dementia and amyotrophic lateral sclerosis-associated disease protein TDP-43 promotes dendritic branching. *Mol Brain*, 2, 30.

Lunn, J. S., Sakowski, S. A., Kim, B., Rosenberg, A. A. and Feldman, E. L. (2009). Vascular endothelial growth factor prevents G93A-SOD1-induced motor neuron degeneration. *Dev Neurobiol*, 69, 871-84.

Lynch, T., Sano, M., Marder, K. S., Bell, K. L., Foster, N. L., Defendini, R. F., Sima, A. A., Keohane, C., Nygaard, T. G., Fahn, S. and et al. (1994). Clinical characteristics of a family with chromosome 17-linked disinhibition-dementia-parkinsonism-amyotrophy complex. *Neurology*, 44, 1878-84.

Maeda, I., Kohara, Y., Yamamoto, M. and Sugimoto, A. (2001). Large-scale analysis of gene function in Caenorhabditis elegans by high-throughput RNAi. *Curr Biol*, 11, 171-6.

Maruyama, H., Morino, H., Ito, H., Izumi, Y., Kato, H., Watanabe, Y., Kinoshita, Y., Kamada, M., Nodera, H., Suzuki, H., Komure, O., Matsuura, S., Kobatake, K., Morimoto, N., Abe, K., Suzuki, N., Aoki, M., Kawata, A., Hirai, T., Kato, T., Ogasawara, K., Hirano, A., Takumi, T., Kusaka, H., Hagiwara, K., Kaji, R. and Kawakami, H. (2010). Mutations of optineurin in amyotrophic lateral sclerosis. *Nature*, 465, 223-6.

Mazzone, G. L. and Nistri, A. (2011). Electrochemical detection of endogenous glutamate release from rat spinal cord organotypic slices as a real-time method to monitor excitotoxicity. *J Neurosci Methods*, 197, 128-32.

McIntire, S. L., Jorgensen, E. and Horvitz, H. R. (1993). Genes required for GABA function in Caenorhabditis elegans. *Nature*, 364, 334-7.

Miguel, L., Frebourg, T., Campion, D. and Lecourtois, M. (2011). Both cytoplasmic and nuclear accumulations of the protein are neurotoxic in Drosophila models of TDP-43 proteinopathies. *Neurobiol Dis*, 41, 398-406.

Millecamps, S., Robertson, J., Lariviere, R., Mallet, J. and Julien, J. P. (2006). Defective axonal transport of neurofilament proteins in neurons overexpressing peripherin. *J Neurochem*, 98, 926-38.

Millecamps, S., Salachas, F., Cazeneuve, C., Gordon, P., Bricka, B., Camuzat, A., Guillot-Noel, L., Russaouen, O., Bruneteau, G., Pradat, P. F., Le Forestier, N., Vandenberghe, N., Danel-Brunaud, V., Guy, N., Thauvin-Robinet, C., Lacomblez, L., Couratier, P., Hannequin, D., Seilhean, D., Le Ber, I., Corcia, P., Camu, W., Brice, A., Rouleau, G., LeGuern, E. and Meininger, V. (2010). SOD1, ANG, VAPB, TARDBP, and FUS mutations in familial amyotrophic lateral sclerosis: genotype-phenotype correlations. *J Med Genet*, 47, 554-60.

Mitchell, J., Paul, P., Chen, H. J., Morris, A., Payling, M., Falchi, M., Habgood, J., Panoutsou, S., Winkler, S., Tisato, V., Hajitou, A., Smith, B., Vance, C., Shaw, C., Mazarakis, N. D. and de Belleroche, J. (2010). Familial amyotrophic lateral sclerosis is associated with a mutation in D-amino acid oxidase. *Proc Natl Acad Sci U S A*, 107, 7556-61.

Mitne-Neto, M., Machado-Costa, M., Marchetto, M. C., Bengtson, M. H., Joazeiro, C. A., Tsuda, H., Bellen, H. J., Silva, H. C., Oliveira, A. S., Lazar, M., Muotri, A. R. and Zatz, M. (2011). Downregulation of VAPB expression in motor neurons derived from induced pluripotent stem cells of ALS8 patients. *Hum Mol Genet.*

Mockett, R. J., Radyuk, S. N., Benes, J. J., Orr, W. C. and Sohal, R. S. (2003). Phenotypic effects of familial amyotrophic lateral sclerosis mutant Sod alleles in transgenic Drosophila. *Proc Natl Acad Sci U S A*, 100, 301-6.

Mulder, D. W. (1982). Clinical limits of amyotrophic lateral sclerosis. *Adv Neurol*, 36, 15-22.

Nagai, M., Aoki, M., Miyoshi, I., Kato, M., Pasinelli, P., Kasai, N., Brown, R. H., Jr. and Itoyama, Y. (2001). Rats expressing human cytosolic copper-zinc superoxide dismutase transgenes with amyotrophic lateral sclerosis: associated mutations develop motor neuron disease. *J Neurosci*, 21, 9246-54.

Nasevicius, A. and Ekker, S. C. (2000). Effective targeted gene 'knockdown' in zebrafish. *Nat Genet*, 26, 216-20.

Oeda, T., Shimohama, S., Kitagawa, N., Kohno, R., Imura, T., Shibasaki, H. and Ishii, N. (2001). Oxidative stress causes abnormal accumulation of familial amyotrophic lateral sclerosis-related mutant SOD1 in transgenic Caenorhabditis elegans. *Hum Mol Genet*, 10, 2013-23.

Park, K. S., Kim, H. J., Choi, W. J., Kim, M. and Lee, K. W. (2004). Detection method of the adjacent motor neuronal death in an in vitro co-culture model of familial ALS-associated Cu/Zn superoxide dismutase. *Biotechnol Lett*, 26, 1201-5.

Parkes, T. L., Elia, A. J., Dickinson, D., Hilliker, A. J., Phillips, J. P. and Boulianne, G. L. (1998). Extension of Drosophila lifespan by overexpression of human SOD1 in motorneurons. *Nat Genet*, 19, 171-4.

Pasinelli, P., Belford, M. E., Lennon, N., Bacskai, B. J., Hyman, B. T., Trotti, D. and Brown, R. H., Jr. (2004). Amyotrophic lateral sclerosis-associated SOD1 mutant proteins bind and aggregate with Bcl-2 in spinal cord mitochondria. *Neuron*, 43, 19-30.

Phillips, J. P., Campbell, S. D., Michaud, D., Charbonneau, M. and Hilliker, A. J. (1989). Null mutation of copper/zinc superoxide dismutase in Drosophila confers hypersensitivity to paraquat and reduced longevity. *Proc Natl Acad Sci U S A*, 86, 2761-5.

Pramatarova, A., Laganiere, J., Roussel, J., Brisebois, K. and Rouleau, G. A. (2001). Neuron-specific expression of mutant superoxide dismutase 1 in transgenic mice does not lead to motor impairment. *J Neurosci*, 21, 3369-74.

Ramesh, T., Lyon, A. N., Pineda, R. H., Wang, C., Janssen, P. M., Canan, B. D., Burghes, A. H. and Beattie, C. E. (2010). A genetic model of amyotrophic lateral sclerosis in zebrafish displays phenotypic hallmarks of motoneuron disease. *Dis Model Mech*, 3, 652-62.

Reaume, A. G., Elliott, J. L., Hoffman, E. K., Kowall, N. W., Ferrante, R. J., Siwek, D. F., Wilcox, H. M., Flood, D. G., Beal, M. F., Brown, R. H., Jr., Scott, R. W. and Snider, W. D. (1996). Motor neurons in Cu/Zn superoxide dismutase-deficient mice develop normally but exhibit enhanced cell death after axonal injury. *Nat Genet*, 13, 43-7.

Renton, A. E., Majounie, E., Waite, A., Simon-Sanchez, J., Rollinson, S., Gibbs, J. R., Schymick, J. C., Laaksovirta, H., van Swieten, J. C., Myllykangas, L., Kalimo, H., Paetau, A., Abramzon, Y., Remes, A. M., Kaganovich, A., Scholz, S. W., Duckworth, J., Ding, J., Harmer, D. W., Hernandez, D. G., Johnson, J. O., Mok, K., Ryten, M., Trabzuni, D., Guerreiro, R. J., Orrell, R. W., Neal, J., Murray, A., Pearson, J., Jansen, I. E., Sondervan, D., Seelaar, H., Blake, D., Young, K., Halliwell, N., Callister, J. B., Toulson, G., Richardson, A., Gerhard, A., Snowden, J., Mann, D., Neary, D., Nalls, M. A., Peuralinna, T., Jansson, L., Isoviita, V., Kaivorinne, A., Holtta-Vuori, M., Ikonen, E., Sulkava, R., Benatar, M., Wuu, J., Chio, A., Restagno, G., Borghero, G., Sabatelli, M., Consortium, T. I., Heckerman, D., Rogaeva, E., Zinman, L., Rothstein, J. D., Sendtner, M., Drepper, C., Eichler, E. E., Alkan, C., Abdullaev, Z., Pack, S. D., Dutra, A., Pak, E., Hardy, J., Singleton, A., Williams, N. M., Heutink, P., Pickering-Brown, S., Morris, H. R., P.J., T. and Traynor, B. J. (2011). A Hexanucleotide Repeat Expansion in C9ORF72 Is the Cause of Chromosome 9p21-Linked ALS-FTD. *Neuron*.

Ripps, M. E., Huntley, G. W., Hof, P. R., Morrison, J. H. and Gordon, J. W. (1995). Transgenic mice expressing an altered murine superoxide dismutase gene provide an animal model of amyotrophic lateral sclerosis. *Proc Natl Acad Sci U S A*, 92, 689-93.

Ritson, G. P., Custer, S. K., Freibaum, B. D., Guinto, J. B., Geffel, D., Moore, J., Tang, W., Winton, M. J., Neumann, M., Trojanowski, J. Q., Lee, V. M., Forman, M. S. and Taylor, J. P. (2010). TDP-43 mediates degeneration in a novel Drosophila model of disease caused by mutations in VCP/p97. *J Neurosci*, 30, 7729-39.

Rosen, D. R., Siddique, T., Patterson, D., Figlewicz, D. A., Sapp, P., Hentati, A., Donaldson, D., Goto, J., O'Regan, J. P., Deng, H. X. and et al. (1993). Mutations in Cu/Zn superoxide dismutase gene are associated with familial amyotrophic lateral sclerosis. *Nature*, 362, 59-62.

Sanelli, T., Ge, W., Leystra-Lantz, C. and Strong, M. J. (2007). Calcium mediated excitotoxicity in neurofilament aggregate-bearing neurons in vitro is NMDA receptor dependant. *J Neurol Sci*, 256, 39-51.

Sauer, B. (1998). Inducible gene targeting in mice using the Cre/lox system. *Methods*, 14, 381-92.

Saxena, S., Cabuy, E. and Caroni, P. (2006). A role for motoneuron subtype-selective ER stress in disease manifestations of FALS mice. *Nat Neurosci*, 12, 627-36.

Schnaar, R. I. and Schaffner, A. E. (1981). Separation of cell types from embryonic chicken and rat spinal cord: characterization of motoneuron-enriched fractions. *J Neurosci*, 1, 204-17.

Sephton, C. F., Good, S. K., Atkin, S., Dewey, C. M., Mayer, P., 3rd, Herz, J. and Yu, G. (2010). TDP-43 is a developmentally regulated protein essential for early embryonic development. *J Biol Chem*, 285, 6826-34.

Simpson, C. L., Lemmens, R., Miskiewicz, K., Broom, W. J., Hansen, V. K., van Vught, P. W., Landers, J. E., Sapp, P., Van Den Bosch, L., Knight, J., Neale, B. M., Turner, M. R., Veldink, J. H., Ophoff, R. A., Tripathi, V. B., Beleza, A., Shah, M. N., Proitsi, P., Van Hoecke, A., Carmeliet, P., Horvitz, H. R., Leigh, P. N., Shaw, C. E., van den Berg, L. H., Sham, P. C., Powell, J. F., Verstreken, P., Brown, R. H., Jr., Robberecht, W. and Al-Chalabi, A. (2009). Variants of the elongator protein 3 (ELP3) gene are associated with motor neuron degeneration. *Hum Mol Genet*, 18, 472-81.

Solnica-Krezel, L., Stemple, D. L., Mountcastle-Shah, E., Rangini, Z., Neuhauss, S. C., Malicki, J., Schier, A. F., Stainier, D. Y., Zwartkruis, F., Abdelilah, S. and Driever, W. (1996). Mutations affecting cell fates and cellular rearrangements during gastrulation in zebrafish. *Development*, 123, 67-80.

Sreedharan, J., Blair, I. P., Tripathi, V. B., Hu, X., Vance, C., Rogelj, B., Ackerley, S., Durnall, J. C., Williams, K. L., Buratti, E., Baralle, F., de Belleroche, J., Mitchell, J. D., Leigh, P. N., Al-Chalabi, A., Miller, C. C., Nicholson, G. and Shaw, C. E. (2008). TDP-43 mutations in familial and sporadic amyotrophic lateral sclerosis. *Science*, 319, 1668-72.

Stabenfeldt, S. E., Munglani, G., Garcia, A. J. and LaPlaca, M. C. (2010). Biomimetic microenvironment modulates neural stem cell survival, migration, and differentiation. *Tissue Eng Part A*, 16, 3747-58.

Stallings, N. R., Puttaparthi, K., Luther, C. M., Burns, D. K. and Elliott, J. L. (2010). Progressive motor weakness in transgenic mice expressing human TDP-43. *Neurobiol Dis*, 40, 404-14.

Strong, M. J. and Yang, W. (2011). The Frontotemporal Syndromes of ALS. Clinicopathological Correlates. *J Mol Neurosci*.

Sulston, J. E. (1983). Neuronal cell lineages in the nematode Caenorhabditis elegans. *Cold Spring Harb Symp Quant Biol*, 48 Pt 2, 443-52.

Sulston, J. E., Schierenberg, E., White, J. G. and Thomson, J. N. (1983). The embryonic cell lineage of the nematode Caenorhabditis elegans. *Dev Biol*, 100, 64-119.

Swarup, V., Phaneuf, D., Bareil, C., Robertson, J., Rouleau, G. A., Kriz, J. and Julien, J. P. (2011). Pathological hallmarks of amyotrophic lateral sclerosis/frontotemporal lobar degeneration in transgenic mice produced with TDP-43 genomic fragments. *Brain*, 134, 2610-26.

Tabata, R. C., Wilson, J. M., Ly, P., Zwiegers, P., Kwok, D., Van Kampen, J. M., Cashman, N. and Shaw, C. A. (2008). Chronic exposure to dietary sterol glucosides is neurotoxic to motor neurons and induces an ALS-PDC phenotype. *Neuromolecular Med*, 10, 24-39.

Takahashi, K., Okita, K., Nakagawa, M. and Yamanaka, S. (2007a). Induction of pluripotent stem cells from fibroblast cultures. *Nat Protoc*, 2, 3081-9.

Takahashi, K., Tanabe, K., Ohnuki, M., Narita, M., Ichisaka, T., Tomoda, K. and Yamanaka, S. (2007b). Induction of pluripotent stem cells from adult human fibroblasts by defined factors. *Cell*, 131, 861-72.

Tandan, R. and Bradley, W. G. (1985). Amyotrophic lateral sclerosis: Part 1. Clinical features, pathology, and ethical issues in management. *Ann Neurol*, 18, 271-80.

Texido, L., Hernandez, S., Martin-Satue, M., Povedano, M., Casanovas, A., Esquerda, J., Marsal, J. and Solsona, C. (2011). Sera from amyotrophic lateral sclerosis patients induce the non-canonical activation of NMDA receptors "in vitro". *Neurochem Int*, doi:10.1016/j.neuint.2011.07.006.

Toma, J. G., Akhavan, M., Fernandes, K. J., Barnabe-Heider, F., Sadikot, A., Kaplan, D. R. and Miller, F. D. (2001). Isolation of multipotent adult stem cells from the dermis of mammalian skin. *Nat Cell Biol*, 3, 778-84.

Tovar, Y. R. L. B., Santa-Cruz, L. D. and Tapia, R. (2009). Experimental models for the study of neurodegeneration in amyotrophic lateral sclerosis. *Mol Neurodegener*, 4, 31.

Tradewell, M. L., Cooper, L. A., Minotti, S. and Durham, H. D. (2011). Calcium dysregulation, mitochondrial pathology and protein aggregation in a culture model of amyotrophic lateral sclerosis: mechanistic relationship and differential sensitivity to intervention. *Neurobiol Dis*, 42, 265-75.

Tradewell, M. L. and Durham, H. D. (2010). Calpastatin reduces toxicity of SOD1G93A in a culture model of amyotrophic lateral sclerosis. *Neuroreport*, 21, 976-9.

Trotti, D., Aoki, M., Pasinelli, P., Berger, U. V., Danbolt, N. C., Brown, R. H., Jr. and Hediger, M. A. (2001). Amyotrophic lateral sclerosis-linked glutamate transporter mutant has impaired glutamate clearance capacity. *J Biol Chem*, 276, 576-82.

Trotti, D., Rolfs, A., Danbolt, N. C., Brown, R. H., Jr. and Hediger, M. A. (1999). SOD1 mutants linked to amyotrophic lateral sclerosis selectively inactivate a glial glutamate transporter. *Nat Neurosci*, 2, 427-33.

Tscherter, A., Heuschkel, M. O., Renaud, P. and Streit, J. (2001). Spatiotemporal characterization of rhythmic activity in rat spinal cord slice cultures. *Eur J Neurosci*, 14, 179-90.

Tu, P. H., Raju, P., Robinson, K. A., Gurney, M. E., Trojanowski, J. Q. and Lee, V. M. (1996). Transgenic mice carrying a human mutant superoxide dismutase transgene develop neuronal cytoskeletal pathology resembling human amyotrophic lateral sclerosis lesions. *Proc Natl Acad Sci U S A*, 93, 3155-60.

Turner, B. J., Atkin, J. D., Farg, M. A., Zang, D. W., Rembach, A., Lopes, E. C., Patch, J. D., Hill, A. F. and Cheema, S. S. (2005). Impaired extracellular secretion of mutant superoxide dismutase 1 associates with neurotoxicity in familial amyotrophic lateral sclerosis. *J Neurosci*, 25, 108-17.

Urushitani, M., Ezzi, S. A., Matsuo, A., Tooyama, I. and Julien, J. P. (2008). The endoplasmic reticulum-Golgi pathway is a target for translocation and aggregation of mutant superoxide dismutase linked to ALS. *Faseb J*, 22, 2476-87.

Urushitani, M., Kurisu, J., Tsukita, K. and Takahashi, R. (2002). Proteasomal inhibition by misfolded mutant superoxide dismutase 1 induces selective motor neuron death in familial amyotrophic lateral sclerosis. *J Neurochem*, 83, 1030-42.

Urushitani, M., Sik, A., Sakurai, T., Nukina, N., Takahashi, R. and Julien, J. P. (2006). Chromogranin-mediated secretion of mutant superoxide dismutase proteins linked to amyotrophic lateral sclerosis. *Nat Neurosci*, 9, 108-18.

Van Deerlin, V. M., Leverenz, J. B., Bekris, L. M., Bird, T. D., Yuan, W., Elman, L. B., Clay, D., Wood, E. M., Chen-Plotkin, A. S., Martinez-Lage, M., Steinbart, E., McCluskey, L., Grossman, M., Neumann, M., Wu, I. L., Yang, W. S., Kalb, R., Galasko, D. R., Montine, T. J., Trojanowski, J. Q., Lee, V. M., Schellenberg, G. D. and Yu, C. E. (2008). TARDBP mutations in amyotrophic lateral sclerosis with TDP-43 neuropathology: a genetic and histopathological analysis. *Lancet Neurol*, 7, 409-16.

Vance, C., Rogelj, B., Hortobagyi, T., De Vos, K. J., Nishimura, A. L., Sreedharan, J., Hu, X., Smith, B., Ruddy, D., Wright, P., Ganesalingam, J., Williams, K. L., Tripathi, V., Al-Saraj, S., Al-Chalabi, A., Leigh, P. N., Blair, I. P., Nicholson, G., de Belleroche, J., Gallo, J. M., Miller, C. C. and Shaw, C. E. (2009). Mutations in FUS, an RNA processing protein, cause familial amyotrophic lateral sclerosis type 6. *Science*, 323, 1208-11.

Vijayalakshmi, K., Alladi, P. A., Ghosh, S., Prasanna, V. K., Sagar, B. C., Nalini, A., Sathyaprabha, T. N. and Raju, T. R. (2011). Evidence of endoplasmic reticular stress in the spinal motor neurons exposed to CSF from sporadic amyotrophic lateral sclerosis patients. *Neurobiol Dis*, 41, 695-705.

Vijayalakshmi, K., Alladi, P. A., Sathyaprabha, T. N., Subramaniam, J. R., Nalini, A. and Raju, T. R. (2009). Cerebrospinal fluid from sporadic amyotrophic lateral sclerosis patients induces degeneration of a cultured motor neuron cell line. *Brain Res*, 1263, 122-33.

Voigt, A., Herholz, D., Fiesel, F. C., Kaur, K., Muller, D., Karsten, P., Weber, S. S., Kahle, P. J., Marquardt, T. and Schulz, J. B. (2010). TDP-43-mediated neuron loss in vivo requires RNA-binding activity. *PLoS One*, 5, e12247.

Walker, L. M., Huber, M., Doores, K. J., Falkowska, E., Pejchal, R., Julien, J. P., Wang, S. K., Ramos, A., Chan-Hui, P. Y., Moyle, M., Mitcham, J. L., Hammond, P. W., Olsen, O. A., Phung, P., Fling, S., Wong, C. H., Phogat, S., Wrin, T., Simek, M. D., Principal Investigators, P. G., Koff, W. C., Wilson, I. A., Burton, D. R. and Poignard, P. (2011). Broad neutralization coverage of HIV by multiple highly potent antibodies. *Nature*, 477, 466-70.

Wang, J., Farr, G. W., Hall, D. H., Li, F., Furtak, K., Dreier, L. and Horwich, A. L. (2009a). An ALS-linked mutant SOD1 produces a locomotor defect associated with aggregation and synaptic dysfunction when expressed in neurons of Caenorhabditis elegans. *PLoS Genet*, 5, e1000350.

Wang, J., Slunt, H., Gonzales, V., Fromholt, D., Coonfield, M., Copeland, N. G., Jenkins, N. A. and Borchelt, D. R. (2003). Copper-binding-site-null SOD1 causes ALS in transgenic mice: aggregates of non-native SOD1 delineate a common feature. *Hum Mol Genet*, 12, 2753-64.

Wang, L., Deng, H. X., Grisotti, G., Zhai, H., Siddique, T. and Roos, R. P. (2009b). Wild-type SOD1 overexpression accelerates disease onset of a G85R SOD1 mouse. *Hum Mol Genet*, 18, 1642-51.

Wang, L. J., Lu, Y. Y., Muramatsu, S., Ikeguchi, K., Fujimoto, K., Okada, T., Mizukami, H., Matsushita, T., Hanazono, Y., Kume, A., Nagatsu, T., Ozawa, K. and Nakano, I. (2002). Neuroprotective effects of glial cell line-derived neurotrophic factor mediated by an adeno-associated virus vector in a transgenic animal model of amyotrophic lateral sclerosis. *J Neurosci*, 22, 6920-8.

Watson, M. R., Lagow, R. D., Xu, K., Zhang, B. and Bonini, N. M. (2008). A drosophila model for amyotrophic lateral sclerosis reveals motor neuron damage by human SOD1. *J Biol Chem*, 283, 24972-81.

Wegorzewska, I., Bell, S., Cairns, N. J., Miller, T. M. and Baloh, R. H. (2009). TDP-43 mutant transgenic mice develop features of ALS and frontotemporal lobar degeneration. *Proc Natl Acad Sci U S A*, 106, 18809-14.

White, J., Southgate, E., Thomson, J. and Brenner, S. (1986). The structure of the nervous system of the nematode Caenorhabditis elegans. *Philos Trans R Soc Lond Biol*, 314, 1-340.

Wichterle, H., Lieberam, I., Porter, J. A. and Jessell, T. M. (2002). Directed differentiation of embryonic stem cells into motor neurons. *Cell*, 110, 385-97.

Wils, H., Kleinberger, G., Janssens, J., Pereson, S., Joris, G., Cuijt, I., Smits, V., Ceuterick-de Groote, C., Van Broeckhoven, C. and Kumar-Singh, S. (2010). TDP-43 transgenic mice develop spastic paralysis and neuronal inclusions characteristic of ALS and frontotemporal lobar degeneration. *Proc Natl Acad Sci U S A*, 107, 3858-63.

Wong, P. C., Pardo, C. A., Borchelt, D. R., Lee, M. K., Copeland, N. G., Jenkins, N. A., Sisodia, S. S., Cleveland, D. W. and Price, D. L. (1995). An adverse property of a familial ALS-linked SOD1 mutation causes motor neuron disease characterized by vacuolar degeneration of mitochondria. *Neuron*, 14, 1105-16.

Wu, L. S., Cheng, W. C., Hou, S. C., Yan, Y. T., Jiang, S. T. and Shen, C. K. (2010). TDP-43, a neuro-pathosignature factor, is essential for early mouse embryogenesis. *Genesis*, 48, 56-62.

Xu, Y. F., Gendron, T. F., Zhang, Y. J., Lin, W. L., D'Alton, S., Sheng, H., Casey, M. C., Tong, J., Knight, J., Yu, X., Rademakers, R., Boylan, K., Hutton, M., McGowan, E., Dickson, D. W., Lewis, J. and Petrucelli, L. (2010). Wild-type human TDP-43 expression causes TDP-43 phosphorylation, mitochondrial aggregation, motor deficits, and early mortality in transgenic mice. *J Neurosci*, 30, 10851-9.

Yamanaka, K., Miller, T. M., McAlonis-Downes, M., Chun, S. J. and Cleveland, D. W. (2006). Progressive spinal axonal degeneration and slowness in ALS2-deficient mice. *Ann Neurol*, 60, 95-104.

Yang, C., Tan, W., Whittle, C., Qiu, L., Cao, L., Akbarian, S. and Xu, Z. (2010). The C-terminal TDP-43 fragments have a high aggregation propensity and harm neurons by a dominant-negative mechanism. *PLoS One*, 5, e15878.

Yang, Y., Hentati, A., Deng, H. X., Dabbagh, O., Sasaki, T., Hirano, M., Hung, W. Y., Ouahchi, K., Yan, J., Azim, A. C., Cole, N., Gascon, G., Yagmour, A., Ben-Hamida, M., Pericak-Vance, M., Hentati, F. and Siddique, T. (2001). The gene encoding alsin, a protein with three guanine-nucleotide exchange factor domains, is mutated in a form of recessive amyotrophic lateral sclerosis. *Nat Genet*, 29, 160-5.

Young, K. C., McGehee, D. S. and Brorson, J. R. (2007). Glutamate receptor expression and chronic glutamate toxicity in rat motor cortex. *Neurobiol Dis*, 26, 78-85.

Zhou, H., Huang, C., Chen, H., Wang, D., Landel, C. P., Xia, P. Y., Bowser, R., Liu, Y. J. and Xia, X. G. (2010). Transgenic rat model of neurodegeneration caused by mutation in the TDP gene. *PLoS Genet*, 6, e1000887.

5

Advantages and Pitfalls in Experimental Models Of ALS

Marina Boido[1], Elisa Buschini[1], Antonio Piras[1], Giada Spigolon[1], Valeria Valsecchi[1], Letizia Mazzini[2] and Alessandro Vercelli[1]
[1]*Neuroscience Institute of the Cavalieri Ottolenghi Foundation, University of Turin,*
[2]*ALS Centre, Department of Neurology, Eastern Piedmont University, "Maggiore della Carità" Hospital, Novara*
Italy

1. Introduction

Amyotrophic lateral sclerosis (ALS) is a progressive neurodegenerative disease that targets upper and lower motoneurons (MN) and leads to death in 2-5 years. 5–10% ALS cases are familial (fALS) with a Mendelian pattern of inheritance. The remaining 90% ALS cases are classified as having sporadic disease (sALS). Only in about 30% of fALS mutations in specific genes have been identified, whereas for the others the etiology is unknown. The clinical phenotype of fALS is usually indistinguishable from sALS.

An effective therapy is still lacking, even though many clinical trials have been already conducted. In order to perform preclinical studies to study the etiology and the molecular mechanisms, to design and to test new therapeutic targets and molecules, several *in vitro* and *in vivo* experimental models have been identified, to reproduce the hallmarks of the disease. Such models include transgenic or spontaneously mutated animals as well as *in vitro* preparations, i.e. MN/spinal cord organotypic cultures. Unfortunately, all these models fail to reproduce the complexity of the human disease, even though they represent a very useful tool to investigate several features of the disease.

2. Genetic animal models

To date, at least 13 genes and loci of major effect in fALS have been identified. The most frequent mutations found in fALS consist in mutations in the gene encoding copper/zinc superoxide dismutase 1 (Cu/Zn SOD1), a ubiquitously expressed enzyme that plays a key role in oxygen free radical scavenging. SOD1 catalyzes the dismutation of superoxide (O_2^-) to hydrogen peroxide (Scozzafava & Viezzoli, 1993; Tainer et al., 1982). On average, SOD1 mutations are responsible for about 20% of fALS cases (Deng et al., 1993; Rosen et al., 1993) and 5% of apparently sALS (Andersen et al., 2007). Over 70 different mutations at more than 60 residues throughout SOD1 (153 amino acids) have been linked to fALS (Andersen, 2000). The vast majority of mutations are amino acid substitutions, but a few cause C-terminal truncations of the protein. A spontaneous mutation in SOD1 has also been found in a canine degenerative myelopathy which resembles ALS (Awano et al., 2009).

Recently, mutations in the genes encoding the TAR DNA/RNA-binding protein 43 (TDP-43) (Corrado et al., 2009; Gitcho et al., 2008; Kabashi et al., 2008; Sreedharan et al., 2008; Van Deerlin et al., 2008; Yokoseki et al., 2008) and Fused in sarcoma/Translocated in liposarcoma (FUS/TLS) (Corrado et al., 2010; Kwiatkowski et al., 2009; Vance et al., 2009) have also been identified in approximately 5%-10% typical fALS.

Other genetic causes of rare and/or atypical fALS include mutations in the genes encoding alsin (ALS2; Hadano et al., 2001) and senataxin (ALS4; Chen et al., 2004) in juvenile ALS, spatacsin (ALS5; Orlacchio et al., 2010), vescicle-associated membrane protein B (VAPB; ALS8; Nishimura et al., 2004), angiogenin (ALS9; Greenway et al., 2006), optineurin (ALS12; Maruyama et al., 2010) and dynactin (Puls et al., 2003). Looking for a genotype-phenotype correlation for the different genes, a significant correlation have been demonstrated only for single mutations and considerable intrafamilial phenotypic differences were observed in some families carrying various mutations in the SOD1, TARDBP and FUS genes (Millecamps et al., 2010).

Aiming to unravel the pathogenic mechanisms leading to ALS, several animal models based on genetic mutations in fALS have been created.

2.1 Typical ALS models

2.1.1 SOD1 mutations

The first transgenic mouse model of human fALS was realized by Gurney and colleagues (1994), consisting in overexpressing a dominant "gain-of-function" mutation of the human SOD1. The mutation is characterized by the amino acid substitution at position 93 from glycine to alanine (G93A), which has little effect on the activity of hSOD1. G93A mice express the largest amount of mutant SOD in the brain, and develop neurological changes reminiscent of human MN disorders: they become paralyzed in hindlimbs and die by 5 to 6 months of age. The severity of the disease, in terms of age of onset and death, depends on the number of copies of the transgene. Paralysis is due to spinal MN loss. The pre-symptomatic phase in these mice is characterized by vacuolar degeneration of MNs, leading to the atrophic, neuron-depleted appearance of the anterior horns at later time points (Dal Canto & Gurney, 1994). The end-stage pattern of disease most closely mimics the pathological changes which characterize human ALS, with filamentous inclusions in both neurons and axonal processes (Hirano, 1991). By and large, this is the most used experimental model of ALS. On the other hand, the expression level of mutated SOD1 can vary independently from the number of copies of the transgene, thus modifying the onset and progression of the disease. In fact, the appearance of the first symptoms varies among the animals, in a time window of 1/2 weeks. Afterwards, the progression of the disease is quite fast, and the animals die approximately in one month. In our experience, in order to determine the onset of the symptomatic phase in G93A mice and initiate experimental treatment, we use a battery of motor behavioral tests (Rotarod, Paw Grip Endurance and Neurological tests).

Alternatively, Ripps and coll. (1995) introduced a missense mutation in the mouse SOD1 gene, that switched the glycine at position 86 to an arginine (G86R). The same mutation has been observed in the corresponding amino acid residue (position 85) of some fALS patients (Deng et al., 1993; Rosen, 1993). High expression of this gene in the spinal cord, brain stem and neocortex of transgenic mice is associated with age-related progressive pathological changes of MNs. Moreover, biochemical studies indicate normal total SOD activity in transgenic mice tissues, suggesting that also G86R mutation has no effects on SOD activity. The early symptoms are variable, consisting in either a flaccid or a spastic paralysis of forelimbs/hindlimbs, whereas the time of the onset is very predictable and the progression of the disease extremely rapid: in fact, the disorder progresses from a mild gait abnormality to total paralysis within a 5-days period: animals are healthy at the age of 3 months and dye by 4 months.

The original G85R mutation observed in fALS was introduced in a mouse background by Bruijn and coll. (1997). Low levels of accumulated human G85R are sufficient to cause severe MN disease without altering the protein and activity levels of endogenous SOD1. After an 8 month-latency period, MN loss proceeds nearly synchronously with 40% of large spinal MN axons degenerating in 2 weeks. Moreover, prominent SOD1-containing inclusions in astrocytes appear prior to clinical signs and increase markedly during disease progression, indicating astrocytes as first players in mutant-SOD1 mediated damage. Furthermore, in this mouse model the presence of glial glutamate transporter, the major glutamate transporter in spinal cord, decreases in end-stage G85R mice. This finding is strikingly similar to that observed in patients with sALS (Rothstein et al., 1995), implicating glutamate mediated excitotoxicity as a mechanism to account for the nearly synchronous degeneration of MNs.

Wong and coll. (1995) produced multiple lines of transgenic mice expressing the human G37R SOD1 mutant. These mice, expressing 5 to 14 times normal SOD1 activity levels, develop the clinical phenotype of MN disease. At lower levels of mutant protein accumulation, the pathology is restricted to lower MNs, whereas higher levels cause more severe abnormalities and affect a variety of other neuronal populations (striatum, thalamus, hypothalamus, pyriform cortex), with conspicuous vacuolar degeneration of axons and dendrites even in pre-symptomatic mice. However, vacuolar degeneration is not a well recognized component of MN pathology in human G37R fALS patients. Furthermore, in these mice neurofilamentous accumulations in cell bodies and proximal axons are rarely present, although they are a constant feature of the pathology in SOD1-linked fALS and in sALS (Hirano et al., 1984; Kato et al., 1991).

Wang and coll. (2002) engineered the human SOD1 gene, to encode mutations at the first two of the four histidine residues (46, 48, 63 and 120) that coordinately bind Cu^{2+} in the active site of the enzyme (Parge et al., 1992), as found in a Japanese and an English families, respectively (Aoki et al., 1995; Enayat et al., 1995). The experimental juxtaposition of disease-linked mutations at histidine 46 and 48 (H46R/H48Q) in transgenic mice creates a mutant enzyme with little or no superoxide scavenging ability that induced MN disease (Wang et al., 2003). These mice develop MN disease before 1 year of age, proportionally to the expression level of the transgene. The most prominent pathological feature in the spinal cord from paralyzed mice consists in the accumulation of high molecular weight SOD1 aggregates, and non-native, detergent-insoluble species of mutant protein. Combining the two disease-causing mutations at histidines 46 and 48 with two experimental mutations at histidines 63 and 120 (H63G and H120G), a stable but inactive protein (H46G/H48Q/H63G/H120G or Quad) is obtained: its expression in mice results in a MN disease clinically and pathologically similar to the H46R/H48Q mouse model (Wang et al., 2003).

Among the reported mutations, the hSOD1-D90A is the milder. Homozygous mice develop a fatal MN disease, but the progression is slow. Mice display bladder disturbances similar to those found in human fALS homozygous for this mutation (Jonsson et al., 2006). Transgenic mice accumulate detergent-resistant hSOD1 aggregates in the spinal cord, and hSOD1 inclusions and vacuoles especially in the ventral horns.

In fALS Oki Family a 2 base pair deletion was found at codon 126 of SOD1 gene, causing a frame shift and a premature stop in the protein sequence at codon 131 (Leu126delTT; Nakashima et al., 1995; Pramatarova et al., 1994). The truncated protein lacks important parts for dimer contact and activity site loop (Watanabe et al., 1997). Transgenic mice expressing this mutation display loss of MNs, microglia activation and Lewy body-like hyaline (LBHIs) cytoplasmic inclusions, with a rapid progression to complete paralysis after initial hindlimb paraparesis (Watanabe et al., 2005).

Similarly, mice bearing other two mutations, consisting i) in the insertion of non-native sequence (TGGG) prior to premature termination (SOD1-G127X) (Jonsson et al., 2004) and ii) in a simple C-terminal deletion (SOD1-L126Z) (Wang et al., 2005), develop MN disease, and accumulation of relatively high levels of detergent-insoluble forms of the mutated variants in the spinal cord.

Taken together, transgenic mice bearing mutations on the SOD1 gene represent a good model for the study of human ALS, since they show several features of the disease: behaviorally, for the motor symptoms which can be assessed with standardized tests; morphologically, for the involvement of upper and lower MNs and the cellular alterations leading to death, together with the involvement of astroglia and microglia which make ALS a not cell-autonomous disease. Nevertheless, most clinical trials based on results obtained on SOD1 mice failed to obtain significant effects on disease (Benatar, 2007): it may be argued that SOD1 mice represent a good model for the only fALS, and even that most effective treatments are initiated in mice before the onset of the symptoms, which is not feasible in sALS.

Some experimental manipulations can be difficult to perform in mice for their innate size limitations, such as administration of compounds into the cerebrospinal fluid (CSF) or obtaining sufficient tissue to perform extensive biochemical analyses. Therefore, Nagai and coll. developed a rat model of ALS by expressing a human SOD1 transgene with two ALS-associated mutations: H46R and G93A (2001). Like the murine counterpart, these models reproduce the most common phenotypic features of human ALS. Rats with the highest transgene copy numbers and higher expression of the mutant protein develop a paralytic disorder characterized by MN death together with astrogliosis and microglia activation. In particular, H46R rat pathology is characterized by protein deposition and aggregation, as H46R/H48Q and G85R transgenic mice. Furthermore, H46R rats display a later onset of paralysis and a slower disease progression (24 days) than G93A rats (8 days). The rat model is ideal for drug administration via chronic intrathecal pumps, a strategy used in human ALS clinical trials. Rats can tolerate better than mice immunosuppressive therapy to allow survival of implanted cells. Moreover ALS rats allow CSF access, because their CSF volume is 10-20 fold greater than in the mouse (http://www.axon-neuroscience.at/rat_models_1.php).

ALS models have been engineered also in zebrafish (Lemmens et al., 2007) and in *Caenorhabditis elegans* (Wang et al., 2009). In particular, overexpression of hSOD1-G93A, hSOD1-G37R and hSOD1-A4V in zebrafish induces a very robust axonopathy in the embryos. The major advantages of this model in the zebrafish embryo are i) that spinal motor axons are easily identifiable, ii) that treatment of animals with small compound libraries is more feasible and iii) that drug testing can be performed within 2 days. The C.

elegans approach, instead, aims to reveal the primary target of the toxic effect of hSOD1 mutations. In fact, overexpression of the hSOD1-G85R mutant protein leads to severe locomotor defects, associated with macroscopic aggregation in neuronal cell bodies. The mutant protein is unable to fold properly producing neuronal dysfunction at the synaptic level and possibly causing a deficient trafficking of pre-synaptic vesicles.

2.1.2 TDP-43 mutations

Recently, great interest has been raised by studies on TDP-43, a protein implicated in regulation of alternative splicing of mRNA, mRNA stability and transcriptional control. Several different neurodegenerative diseases are characterized by TDP-43 proteinopathies (Wegorzewska et al., 2009; Zhou et al., 2010). For instance, abnormal levels of aggregated TDP-43 are detected in the majority of patients with ALS, frontotemporal lobar dementia (FTLD) and Alzheimer's disease (AD), with ALS and FTLD often associated. Mutations in the TARDBP gene result in neuronal aggregation of abnormal TDP-43 protein in patients dying of MN disease: TDP-43-positive inclusions are present in both sALS and in the syndrome affecting fALS patients with TARDBP mutations, although they are more frequent in the last ones (Sreedharan et al., 2008). The clinical course of patients with TARDBP mutations is similar to that of sALS. Elevated levels of TDP-43 has been found in ALS patients in which the lower MNs were mostly affected (Geser et al., 2011; Noto et al., 2011). Pathological TDP-43 seems to be a less consistent feature of other MN disease phenotypes, such as primary lateral sclerosis and progressive muscular atrophy (Dickson et al., 2007).

Therefore, TDP-43 has been targeted to create animal models of ALS in mice, rats and *Drosophila*. In *Drosophila melanogaster*, the depletion of the TDP homolog results in deficient locomotor activity and defects at neuromuscular junctions (NMJs) (Feiguin et al., 2009). On the other hand, wild-type (WT) TDP-43 overexpression exerts more severe effects on neuromuscular junction architecture, viability and MN vitality (Estes et al., 2011). The neurotoxicity is modulated by the proteasome, the chaperone Hsp70 and the apoptosis pathway (Estes et al., 2011).

Transgenic mice expressing the human mutated TDP-43 gene (A315T and M337V) or the human WT gene (hTDP-43), develop a severe early MN degeneration phenotype, that correlates with TDP-43 levels in spinal cord (Stallings et al., 2010). In particular, TDP-43-A315T mice develop later onset paralysis with cytoplasmic ubiquitin inclusions, gliosis and TDP-43 redistribution and fragmentation (Stallings et al., 2010). Moreover, *in vivo* and also *in vitro* the A315T mutant enhances neurotoxicity and the formation of aberrant TDP-43 species, including protease-resistant fragments (Guo et al., 2011).

Moderate overexpression of hTDP-43 results in TDP-43 truncation, increased cytoplasmic and nuclear ubiquitin levels, intranuclear and cytoplasmic aggregates immunopositive for phosphorylated TDP-43. Furthermore, abnormal juxtanuclear aggregates of mitochondria are observed, accompanied by enhanced levels of Fis1 and phosphorylated DLP1, the key components of the mitochondrial fission machinery. Conversely, a marked reduction in mitofusin 1 expression, which plays an essential role in mitochondrial fusion is observed. Furthermore, hTDP-43 mice show reactive gliosis, axonal and myelin degeneration, gait abnormalities, and early lethality (Xu et al., 2010). Wils and coworkers (2010) confirmed a dose dependent degeneration of cortical and spinal MNs and development of spastic quadriplegia, reminiscent of ALS.

Constitutive and conditional transgenic rat models, overexpressing the hTDP-43-M337V protein develop a widespread neurodegeneration, mostly affecting the motor system. Features of this proteinopathy include the formation of TDP-43 inclusions, cytoplasmic localization of phosphorylated TDP-43, and its fragmentation. The number of MNs is reduced, striated muscles are denervated, astrogliosis and microglial activation are present (Zhou et al., 2010).

Finally, depletion of TDP-43 with antisense oligonucleotide strategy in mouse adult brain alters the expression levels of 601 mRNA (including Fus, Tis, progranulin and other transcripts encoding neurodegenerative disease-associated proteins) and 965 splicing events (e.g. in sortilin, the receptor for progranulin) (Polymenidou et al., 2011). RNAs with the most depleted levels derive from genes with very long introns that encode proteins involved in synaptic activity. The same RNA are altered in ALS patients (Xiao et al., 2011).

Thus far, TDP-43 transgenic mice together with SOD1-G93A mice, represent the ALS model which more closely adheres to human ALS.

Another RNA binding protein, FUS, has been found mutated in both 5% fALS (Lagier-Tourenne & Cleveland, 2009) and 1% sALS (Mackenzie et al., 2010) patients: FUS interacts with TDP-43 (Strong & Volkening, 2011), as shown also in a model of FUS-related neuronal degeneration in *Drosophila* (Lanson et al., 2011). Knocking down either Tardbp or FUS in zebrafish causes a motor phenotype which can be rescued by wild type FUS expression (Kabashi et al., 2011). To our knowledge, there are no transgenic mouse models for studying FUS role in ALS, but studies on TDP-43 mice have shown that this protein and FUS are strictly correlated.

2.2 Rare ALS models

Sequence variants in a number of genes are reported to be associated with ALS. These variations are found in candidate genes or through genome wide association studies. In all cases, it is unclear whether these genes and/or variations play a role in ALS, and these associations remain to be confirmed.

2.2.1 Alsin mutation

Great expectancies have been raised by the discovery of ALS2/alsin, a guanine nucleotide exchange factor (GEF) for the small GTPase Rab5 (Rab5GEF). ALS2 is a novel Rac1 effector, involved in Rac1-activated macropinocytosis and in macropinocytosis-associated endosome fusion and trafficking, and in neurite outgrowth. Therefore, loss of ALS2 may perturb macropinocytosis and/or the following membrane trafficking, which gives rise to neuronal dysfunction in the ALS2-linked MN diseases (Devon et al., 2006; Kunita et al., 2007). In fact, ALS2 loss of function mutations in humans account for several juvenile recessive MN diseases: the juvenile ALS, the primary lateral sclerosis and the infantile-onset ascending hereditary spastic paralysis (Eymard-Pierre et al., 2006; Orban et al., 2007). Furthermore, alsin plays a role in AMPA receptor trafficking, thus providing a novel pathogenic link between ALS2-deficiency and MN degeneration, suggesting a protective role in maintaining the survival of MNs (Lai et al., 2006).

Knocking down of alsin by small interfering RNA in cultured MNs display a reduced apparent size of early endosomes and an increased intracellular accumulation of transferrin and L1 cell adhesion molecule. Moreover, it induces MN death and significantly inhibits axon growth in the surviving ones (Jacquier et al., 2006).

On the other hand, loss of ALS2 in mice does not have a dramatic effect on the survival or function of lower MNs (Cai et al., 2008). On the contrary, ALS2 deficiency causes an upper MN disease that closely resembles a severe form of hereditary spastic paralysis, that is quite distinct from ALS. The hereditary spastic paralysis is characterized by progressive axonal degeneration and slows movement without muscle weakness (Yamanaka et al., 2006). ALS2 -/- mice are more susceptible to oxidative stress compared to WT, although they fail to recapitulate clinical or neuropathological phenotypes consistent with MN disease by 20 months of age (Cai et al., 2005). In addition, the effects of ALS2 ablation strongly depend on the genetic background and sex (Hadano et al., 2010b). Loss of ALS2 in SOD1 mice exacerbates the pathology (Hadano et al., 2010a).

2.2.2 VAPB mutation

A mutation in the vesicle-associated membrane protein-associated protein-B (VAPB) is the cause of a fALS, ALS8 (Nishimura et al., 2004). This mutation is characterized by a proline to serine substitution at position 56 (P56S). The physiological function of VAPB is in part unclear, but it seems involved in bouton formation at the NMJ and in vesicle transport from the endoplasmic reticulum (ER) to the Golgi. Indeed, the protein mainly localizes to the ER compartment and to the junction between intracellular vesicles and cytoskeletal structures (Skehel et al., 2000; Soussan et al., 1999). Transgenic mice expressing the VAPBP56S mutation were created by Tudor and coworkers (2010). These mice develop cytoplasmic TDP-43 accumulations within spinal MNs at 18 months of age, pointing out a possible link between TDP-43 mislocalization and abnormalities in VAPB. Besides, both brain and spinal cord neurons, including MN, show an altered cellular distribution of VAPBP56S with ER-derived aggregates of this protein. Despite this pathological hallmark, the motor function and the MN number in spinal cord are not significantly affected by the mutation, indicating that these animals do not develop overt MN disease, in contrast to mutant SOD1 where low levels of expression can induce aggressive MN disease. The difference between these two ALS models could be related to the late-onset and slowly progressive atypical disease of the vast majority of ALS8 cases.

2.2.3 Cytoskeletal protein mutations: Dynactin, neurofilaments, peripherin, TAU

An increasing number of neurodegenerative diseases are being linked to mutations in genes encoding proteins required for axonal transport and intracellular trafficking (e.g., dynactin). Furthermore, one hallmark of MN degeneration in both affected ALS patients and transgenic mice expressing the SOD1 mutation consists in the accumulation of intermediate filaments (IFs), in particular, the neurofilaments (NFs, the major type of IFs), in the perikarya and axons of MNs.

A missense mutations in a dynactin gene (Dctn1) encoding the p150Glued subunit of dynactin complex has been associated to both fALS and sALS. The dynactin complex consists of at least 10 distinct components, including p150Glued that is the largest subunit: it binds directly to microtubules (MTs) and is required for coordinated anterograde and retrograde organelle movement (Haghnia et al., 2007). The missense mutation occurring in the glycine-rich cytoskeleton-associated protein (CAP-Gly) domain of the p150Glued polypeptide, results in the substitution of serine for glycine at position 59 (G59S), leading to a decreased binding to MTs (Puls et al., 2003). Other missense mutations in Dctn1 have been identified and are linked to ALS, but the specific role of these mutations in the pathogenesis of the disease is unclear (Munch et al., 2005; Munch et al., 2004).

The mouse model expressing human mutant p150Glued dynactin (Thy-1; G59 p150^{Glued}) exhibits clinical and pathological hallmarks of MN disease and is characterized phenotypically by slowly progressive muscle weakness. MN degeneration in these mice is associated with abnormalities in intracellular vesicular trafficking, axonal swelling and axon-terminal degeneration. Evidence suggests that autophagic cell death is implicated in the pathogenesis of these mice (Laird et al., 2008). A similar animal model to study the pathogenic mechanism of the G59S mutation *in vivo* is represented by p150Glued G59S knock-in mice. These mice develop a late-onset, slowly progressive MN disease characterized by abnormal accumulation of NFs and synaptic vesicle proteins at the NMJs, loss of MNs, and gait abnormalities (Lai et al., 2007).

LaMonte and coworkers (2002) engineered a targeted disruption of the dynein-dynactin complex in MNs of transgenic mice by overexpression of a subunit of dynactin (dynamitin, p50) that causes the disassembly of the whole complex. Mice overexpressing dynamitin demonstrate a late-onset, slowly progressive MN degenerative disease characterized by muscle weakness, spontaneous trembling, abnormal posture and gait, and deficits in strength and endurance. These mice show MN degeneration and muscle denervation/atrophy. NF accumulations and retrograde transport inhibition observed in these mice confirm the critical role of the axonal transport in the pathogenesis of MN degenerative disease. Whether NF (or more generally IF) accumulations contribute to pathogenesis of human ALS remains unknown; it could simply be the consequence of neuronal dysfunction. However, emerging evidence suggests that sometimes IF aggregates can have detrimental as well as protective effects in MN disease. Transgenic mouse models are used to address whether cytoskeletal changes may contribute to MN disease.

NFs in adult MNs are made by the copolymerization of three proteins, the light (NF-L, 61 kDa), medium (NF-M, 90 kDa) and heavy (NF-H, 115 KDa) NFs. Mice knockout for any of the three NF genes do not develop MN disease, although these deficiencies have several harmful effects: the formation of perikaryal NF accumulations resembling those found in human (Elder et al., 1998a; Elder et al., 1998b; Rao et al., 1998; Zhu et al., 1997). Transgenic mice accumulating NF-L (4-fold the normal level) in the sciatic nerve, also display huge accumulations of NFs in spinal MNs, swollen perikarya, and eccentrically localized nuclei. NF accumulation is associated with some neurodegenerative hallmarks, such as an increased frequency of axonal degeneration, proximal axon swelling, and severe skeletal muscle atrophy (Xu et al., 1993). Also transgenic mice expressing the human NF-H gene (up to 2-fold the levels of the endogenous protein) progressively develop neurological defects and abnormal neurofilamentous swellings by 3-4 months of age (Cote et al., 1993). Transgenic mice expressing a fusion protein in which the carboxyl terminus of the NF-H is replaced by beta-galactosidase accumulates such protein as large filamentous aggregates in perikarya. Axons are not invested with NFs but develop only small calibers (Eyer & Peterson, 1994). Increased expression of NF subunits in all these transgenic mouse models leads to MN dysfunction, in absence of the widespread MN death typical of human ALS.

However, a more severe phenotype is produced by the expression of an assembly-disrupting NF-L mutant having a leucine to proline substitution (NF-L L394P): this mutation causes massive degeneration of spinal MNs accompanied by abnormal accumulations of NFs and severe neurogenic atrophy of skeletal muscles (Lee et al., 1994).

Abnormal NF aggregates are observed in both fALS patients and in SOD1 mice, pointing out that NFs may contribute to SOD1-mediated disease. Mating experiments between SOD1 mice and transgenic mice with deregulated levels of NF proteins were carried out. The overexpression of human NF-H proteins confers an effective protection against the SOD1 mutation, a phenomenon probably due to the ability of NF proteins to chelate calcium. Therefore, these studies show that disorganized NFs can sometimes have noxious effects resulting in neuronopathy. However, there is emerging evidence that in the context of MN disease caused by mutant SOD1, NF proteins may play a protective role (Eyer et al., 1998; Williamson et al., 1998).

Among the IF proteins, also peripherin overexpression in mice determines ALS. Peripherin is a type III neuronal IF protein of 57 kD, found within NF in the majority of IF inclusions (89%) in MNs of ALS patients (Corbo & Hays, 1992; Migheli et al., 1993). In adult rats, peripherin is mostly expressed in autonomic nerves and in peripheral sensory neurons while is barely detectable in spinal MNs (Escurat et al., 1990; Parysek & Goldman, 1988). However, peripherin gene expression is increased up to 300% in spinal MNs after injury of the sciatic nerve (Troy et al., 1990), whereas expression of the other NF proteins is reduced (Muma et al., 1990). Inflammation occurred in injured neurons could explain peripherin upregulation. In fact, peripherin gene expression is upregulated by the inflammatory cytokines interleukin-6 (IL-6) and leukemia inhibitory factor (Djabali et al., 1993; Sterneck et al., 1996). This suggests that peripherin may be part of a general response of MNs to noxious stress and may explain peripherin inclusion bodies in MNs of ALS patients. Beaulieu and coll. (1999) generated two transgenic mice to investigate the potential detrimental effects of peripherin overexpression in MNs, in which the endogenous peripherin gene, inserted with its own promoter or under the control of the Thy1 gene promoters, was overexpressed. Both mouse strains display a late-onset and selective MN disease characterized by the formation of IF inclusions similar to those found in human ALS and in SOD1 mice. Moreover, a deficiency in NF-L protein exacerbates the formation of IF inclusion bodies and the onset of disease precipitates, probably through a deleterious action of the large NF subunits on peripherin organization (Beaulieu et al., 1999).

Cytoskeletal abnormalities reported in ALS involve also MT-associated proteins such as the tau protein, predominantly expressed in neurons. Since tau is required for neurite elaboration in different cell types, a central role in neuronal process outgrowth and integrity is proposed. To date, 30 different intronic and exonic pathogenic mutations have been identified in the human tau gene and have been correlated to several pathological conditions recognized as tauopathies. Among these, exonic tau gene mutations (i.e., P301L and R406W) impair the ability of tau to bind and stabilize MTs as well as to promote their assembly (Hasegawa et al., 1998; Hong et al., 1998). These mutations contribute to the formation of fibrillary tau aggregates (Crowther & Goedert, 2000; Delobel et al., 2002; Vogelsberg-Ragaglia et al., 2000). Transgenic mice expressing the human tau containing the P301L mutation exhibit motor behavioral deficits, with age- and gene-dose-dependent development of neurofibrillary tangles (NFT). This phenotype occurs as early as 6.5 months in hemizygous and 4.5 months in homozygous animals. The spinal cord of both these animals display axonal spheroids, anterior horn cell loss and axonal degeneration in anterior spinal roots. Counts of spinal MNs show a reduction of approximately 48% compared to control animals. Moreover, the expression of P301L mutation results in peripheral neuropathy and skeletal muscle with neurogenic atrophy (Gotz et al., 2001; Lewis et al.,

2000). The specific role of tau in the ALS pathogenesis remains unsettled, but the phenotypical and histological observations in P301L mutant mice suggests that it could be a key molecule in neurodegeneration occurring in ALS.

2.2.4 VEGF

Studies on the vascular endothelial growth factor (VEGF) suggest a novel function for VEGF in the pathogenesis of MN degeneration. VEGF may be involved in spinal cord neuropathy mainly by affecting vascular growth or function. However, VEGF might also affect neural cells directly, but the *in vivo* relevance of such a mechanism has been poorly investigated. To study the potential role of VEGF in MN degeneration, Oosthuyse and coll. (2001) generated a 'knock-in' mouse, in which the hypoxia-response element sequence in the Vegf promoter was deleted. Vegf $^{-/-}$ mice appear healthy until 5 months of age, when they develop symptoms of MN disease, i.e. severe adult-onset muscle weakness due to degeneration of lower MNs, reminiscent of the clinical symptoms and neuropathological signs of ALS. Similarly, VEGF replacement has beneficial effects in SOD1 G93A mice (Lunn et al., 2009). These findings indicate that reduced neural perfusion and maybe also insufficient VEGF-dependent neuroprotection cause MN degeneration (Oosthuyse et al., 2001).

3. Spontaneous mutation models

Since many years, several mouse models bearing spontaneous mutations leading to MN death have been identified: for instance, Wobbler (Duchen & Strich, 1968), Nmd (Cook et al., 1995), Pmn (Schmalbruch et al., 1991), Wasted (Newbery et al., 2005), Loa (Rogers et al., 2001) and Cra (Hrabe de Angelis et al., 2000) mice.

3.1 Wobbler mouse

The Wobbler mouse mutation spontaneously occurred in the breeding stock of Falconer (1956) and was later mapped to the proximal mouse chromosome (Kaupmann et al., 1992). It is the oldest known model of spontaneous MN disease, following a spontaneous recessive mutation in the wobbler (wr) gene, which encodes for the vacuolar-vesicular protein sorting 54 (Vps54) with a missense mutation L967Q. Vps54 mutation has been rarely described in ALS patients (Corrado et al., 2011). The protein is a subunit of the Golgi-associated retrograde protein (GARP) complex, used for fusion of endosome-derived transport vesicles to the trans-Golgi network. This model is considered a good model of MN degeneration, although the molecular mechanisms of the pathology in these mice are still unclear. Duchen and coll. (1968) showed that the progression of disease can be divided into three phases. i) The first, presymptomatic one, during the first 3 weeks after birth, ii) followed by the evolutionary one where the mice show alterations in motor behavior such as fine tremor of the head and slightly unsteady gait. iii) The third phase consists in the stabilization of the disease with the end of the neurodegenerative process. The progression of the disease is variable and leads to progressive denervation of skeletal muscles, determining muscle atrophy especially in the head, neck, shoulders and forelimbs. Limb muscles display different levels of atrophy: distally, atrophy is more severe than proximally, although in this model the hindlimbs are less severely affected. Moreover, there is a final progressive weight loss partially due to nutritional deprivation following muscle atrophy of the face and forelimbs (Boillee et al., 2003). Mice usually live up to 3-4 months, but sometimes the stabilization of the disease can delay their death for longer.

3.2 NMD mouse

Cox and coll. (1998) identified mice carrying 2 independent mutations in the neuromuscular degeneration (Nmd) gene on two alleles: nmd^{j} and nmd^{2j}, leading to a progressive degeneration of spinal MNs and muscular atrophy. The nmd gene produces a ubiquitously expressed DNA helicase/ATPase protein previously described as immunoglobulin S-mu binding protein-2 (Smbp2; Fukita et al., 1993), glial factor 1 (Gf1; Kerr & Khalili, 1991), rat insulin enhancer binding protein 1 (rip1; Shieh et al., 1995) and cardiac transcription factor 1 (Catf1; Sebastiani et al., 1995).

Mutant mice are characterized by a progressive paralysis that initially begins with the hindlimbs. The forelimbs are affected to a variable degree with paralysis, generally evident only toward the latest stages of the disease. Homozygous Nmd mutants can be easily distinguished from their littermate controls at 2 weeks of age by their dorsally contracted hindlimbs and impaired movement. Affected mice rarely survive beyond 4 weeks of age, but the exact cause of death is unclear.

3.3 PMN mouse

Bommel and colleagues (2002) identified animals suffering of a progressive motor neuronopathy (pmn), caused by an autosomal recessive mutation in the tubulin-specific chaperone e gene (tbce). The mutation results from a tryptophan to glycine substitution at position 524 (T524G; Martin et al., 2002). This protein is one of the main cofactors involved in MT stability or polymerization dynamics. These mice between P14 and P20 display a progressive caudal-cranial degeneration of motor axons leading to muscular atrophy, hindlimb paralysis and death in 4 to 6 weeks after birth (Schmalbruch et al., 1991).

Although the pathophysiology of MN death in pmn mice is mainly due to loss of neuromuscular integrity by distal axonopathy rather than alteration of neuron soma (which is instead a common feature in ALS), this model can be considered a good one for MN neurodegeneration.

3.4 WASTED mouse

Wasted (wst) mice bear a spontaneous autosomal mutation that results in the loss of gene encoding the translation factor eEF1A2. From the 3rd week of age they exhibit immunodeficiency and neurological disorders in terms of tremors and disturbance of gait. Subsequently these mice present MN degeneration and hindlimb paralysis.

Moreover, Newbery and coll. (2005) observed reactive gliosis at P19 in the cervical spinal cord with a rostrocaudal gradient, and retraction of MN fibers. Mice develop a rapid neurodegeneration and die around P28. Finally, several studies demonstrated that this model bears increased chromosomal breakage and DNA damage (Shultz et al., 1982).

3.5 LOA and CRA mice

"Legs at odd angles" (Loa) and "Cramping 1" (Cra) mice arose as the result of two independent N-ethyl-N-nitrosourea-(ENU) induced mutagenenesis experiments (Hrabe de Angelis et al., 2000; Rogers et al., 2001).

Loa mouse presents a point mutation that changes phenylalanine to tyrosine at position 580 (F580Y) in the gene encoding the heavy chain of dynein. On the other hand, Cra mice have a substitution from tyrosine to cytosine at position 1055 (Y1055C) in the same gene. Dynein is a motor protein which determines retrograde transport along MTs and this model has been partially used to evaluate the role of dynein in the neuronal migration. However, the disturbance in axonal transport leads to selective MN death, making these mice useful models in ALS studies. Particularly, Loa mice exhibit pathological features similar to human ones, as Lewy body-like inclusions containing SOD1, CDK5 and ubiquitin. However, Ilieva et al., (2008) found no α-MN loss at any age, but a sensory axon deficit of the large proprioceptive (type Ia) axons and the decrease of γ-motor axons innervating muscle spindles. Similarly, Cra mice do not show MN degeneration but rather peripheral sensory neuropathy due to loss of axons in dorsal roots and decrement of large proprioceptive axons (Dupuis et al., 2009).

In conclusion, the pathological features observed in both models do not properly correlate with hALS characteristics. Dynein mutation models will need further investigation, they better represent a model for sensory neuropathy rather than for MN disease.

3.6 Hereditary canine spinal muscular atrophy

Hereditary canine spinal muscular atrophy (HCSMA) is a lower motor neuron disease found in Brittany Spaniels. It shares clinical and pathological features with human ALS (Green et al., 2002). These animals show signs of oxidative stress (Green et al., 2001), but do not have mutations in the SOD1 gene (Green et al., 2002). From the histopathological point of view these animals are characterized by aberrant accumulation of extensively phosphorylated heavy (high molecular weight) neurofilament (NFH) and neurodegeneration (Green et al., 2005).

4. *In vitro* models

Despite *in vivo* models are extremely helpful for studying ALS, when the aim consists in studying the molecular mechanisms of MN death and the role and the involvement of the different cells in the pathological mechanisms, simplified *in vitro* models such as MN and organotypic cultures can be useful, allowing to control the experimental conditions.

4.1 Motoneuron and glia culture

Since the major feature of ALS consists in the progressive loss of upper and lower MNs, cultures of spinal MNs are a valuable tool for studying ALS pathomechanisms. Many authors have developed protocols to isolate MNs from newborn or embryonic murine spinal cord (Berg & Fischbach, 1978; Gingras et al., 2007; Schnaar & Schaffner, 1981), allowing to identify MNs for their size and their Choline Acetyl Transferase (ChAT) activity. However, more recently, Wiese and coll. (2010) have isolated embryonic spinal MNs from rodents using p75 neurotrophin receptor (NTR)-antibody panning step, a technique with low toxicity and high efficiency; in fact, at the embryonic stage, MNs are the only neurons expressing the p75 low-affinity nerve growth factor receptor (Camu & Henderson, 1992). Unlike most studies performed on cultured embryonic spinal MNs, those of cultures of spinal MNs from newborn rodents is less common. In 2004, Anderson and coworkers described a protocol for isolating and culturing neonatal spinal MNs positive to p75NTR and ChAT, in presence of a growth factor cocktail containing glial cell line-derived neurotrophic factor (GDNF), brain-derived neurotrophic factor (BDNF) and ciliary neurotrophic factor (CNTF) (Anderson et al., 2004).

In vitro preparations are age-dependent, since cells or tissues are generally obtained from animals at late embryonic or neonatal stages, but ALS related-alterations or neurodegenerative defects are not yet evident at this early stage. Indeed Avossa and coll. (2006) characterized the alterations in WT and G93A embryonic spinal cord cells analyzing MNs, glial cells, interneurons, distribution of hSOD1, mitochondria, MTs, NFs and synapses. They did not find any substantial difference in all these parameters, excepted for a significant increase in inhibitory synapses compared to excitatory ones in mutant cells. Therefore, it is necessary to use specific molecules or drugs to induce cell death mechanisms in these apparently normal cells.

Since in ALS an imbalance in the glutamatergic system has been described, leading to an excitotoxic environment around MNs (Boillee et al., 2006), an *in vitro* approach can be represented by NMDA exposure. Rothstein and coll. (1993) were the first to use this model, demonstrating that MN degeneration is prevented by non-NMDA glutamate receptor antagonists, consequently used as neuroprotective agents.

Similarly, some authors have proposed that spinal MNs are more vulnerable to AMPA receptor agonists than to NMDA, particularly in spinal cord cultures (Carriedo et al., 1996; Van Damme et al., 2002). In fact, microdialysis perfusion of AMPA agonists in spinal cord reveals a consistent loss of spinal MNs and the consequently paralysis of the hindlimbs, probably due to an increased cytoplasmic Ca^{2+} concentration (Corona & Tapia, 2007).

Finally, it is well-known that also the glia (astrocytes and microglial cells) actively contributes to the death of MNs (Philips & Robberecht, 2011). Glia can be easily obtained and cultured both from embryos/newborns and adults; the first method has been described in 1972 by Booher and Sensenbrenner (1972). Now, concerning astroglia culture, "primary culture", "subculture" and "shaken culture (once or twice)" can be performed (Du et al., 2010), each one with advantages and pitfalls relative to purity of astrocytes, cell viability, expression of glial fibrillary acidic protein (GFAP) and bystin, a protein potentially involved in embryo implantation, which is markedly up-regulated in reactive astrocytes (Fang et al., 2008). Similarly, protocols to isolate microglial cells are easy and reproducible (Ni & Aschner, 2010; Yip et al., 2009), and they have been recently improved by the column-free magnetic separation technology: the cells can be labeled and isolated on the strength of their expression of CD11b, a specific microglial marker, thus allowing to isolate an high number of cells and significantly reducing the animals needed (Gordon et al., 2011).

Cocultures of healthy hMNs with human astrocytes carrying either the WT or mutated SOD1 cDNA have demonstrated the role of astrocytes in ALS disease, since MN number decreased about 50% in the presence of mutant SOD1-expressing astrocytes (Marchetto et al., 2008). This neurotoxicity is probably mediated by the release of soluble factors from astrocytes, finally involving the Bax-dependent death machinery within MNs (Nagai et al., 2007).

4.2 Cell line culture

Due to the technical difficulties in establishing a MN culture for their poor proliferation ability when differentiated, an alternative is represented by the use of a neural hybrid cell line named NSC-34 (neuroblastoma spinal cord), derived from the fusion of neuroblastoma cells with MN enriched spinal cord. These cells perfectly show morphological and physiological properties of primary MNs: extending processes, contacts with cultured myotubes, synthesis and storage of acetylcholine, action potentials and NF proteins (Cashman et al., 1992).

NSC-34 can be transfected with vectors containing mutant forms of hSOD1, allowing to study specific neurodegenerative aspects such as mitochondrial degeneration, NF accumulation or Golgi apparatus disruption (Gomes et al., 2008; Menzies et al., 2002a; Menzies et al., 2002b). This model can also enlighten on the implicated cell death pathways in ALS, i.e. the involvement of MAP kinases (Guo & Bhat, 2007), the interaction between bcl2-A1 and pro-caspase-3 (Iaccarino et al., 2011) or the involvement of kynurenine pathway implicated in the regulatory mechanisms of the immune response (Chen et al., 2011).

In addition, different therapeutic agents have been tested in culture, such as the vascular endothelial growth factor (VEGF) (Kulshreshtha et al., 2011) or the semi-synthetic tetracycline called minocycline (Guo & Bhat, 2007), known for their neuroprotective effects in neurodegeneration models (Orsucci et al., 2009; Storkebaum et al., 2004).

Similarly, other cell lines have been transfected with WT or mutant (G93A) hSOD1 and used for the same purpose: N18TG2 neuroblastoma, the non-neuronal Madin–Darby Canine Kidney (MDCK) (Raimondi et al., 2006) or the mouse embryonic fibroblast NIH3T3 cell lines (Shinder et al., 2001).

The recent finding of human induced pluripotent stem cells (iPSCs) present a novel opportunity for *in vitro* disease modeling. iPSCs can be generated from readily accessible tissue from patients. iPSCs show similar capacity for directed MN differentiation as ESCs (Boulting et al., 2011). iPSCs can be generated from patients, thus carrying the actual mutations associated with the disease and allowing to correlate, any cellular phenotype with the patient's clinical characteristics such as onset, duration, and severity of disease at the time of tissue collection. In 2008, iPSCs were generated from a skin sample from an elderly patient with fALS displaying a SOD1 mutation (Dimos et al., 2008).

4.3 Organotypic cultures

Since ALS is a complex disease originating from an important crosstalk among MNs, glia and muscles (Strong, 2003), a step forward is represented by using organotypic cultures, where the *in vivo* architecture is maintained and MNs as well as neighboring cells (interneurons and glial cells) are preserved. However, this system presents an important limitation, due to the lack of correlation between morphological results and behavioral impairment (as well as for all the *in vitro* preparations) and the isolated slices undergo a series of little traumas (axotomy, deafferentation…) that can unintentionally originate a neuron selection.

Preparations of spinal cord organotypic culture from newborn animals is actually done according the Stoppini's procedure (1991): MNs survive more than 2 months, maintaining their structural and metabolic characteristics and allowing both morphological and electrophysiological experiments. Moreover, these experimental conditions stimulate glial proliferation, reproducing the glial activation observed *in vivo* in ALS patients/animal models (Hall et al., 1998; Vercelli et al., 2008).

As already mentioned, such model requires tissue obtained from embryos or pups, when ALS alterations are not full-blown (Avossa et al., 2006). Therefore, it is possible to use slice cultures obtained from normal animals and to add a glutamate transporter inhibitor (as threohydroxyaspartate (THA) or D,L-threo-B-benzyloxyaspartate), able to induce a chronic glutamate neurotoxicity. This treatment causes selective MNs death, simulating the human ALS neurodegeneration (Bilak et al., 2004; Rothstein et al., 1993). Some authors prepare organotypic spinal slice cultures directly from G93A SOD1 mice and expose them to THA in order to induce loss of MNs (Kosuge et al., 2009).

This *in vitro* model is helpful either for studying specific pathways/organelles or for testing treatments. Particularly, Tolosa and coll. (2008) studied the effects of VEGF on the survival and vulnerability to excitotoxicity of spinal cord MNs treated with THA, demonstrating that this growth factor plays an important role in neuroprotection by activating the phosphatidylinositol 3-kinase/Akt signal transduction pathway. Similarly Kosuge and coworkers (2009) tested the effect of GDNF, showing that threo-hydroxyaspartate -induced MN death was significantly inhibited in G93A mice slice. The pathway of caspase-12 was among the causes of MNs death. Also the anti-convulsant drugs topiramate (Maragakis et al., 2003), valproic acid (Sugai et al., 2004) and lithium (Caldero et al., 2010) were found to significantly prevent MN degeneration in this model.

5. Conclusion

ALS is a devastating neurodegenerative disease the etiology of which is still unclear. Even though the clinical hallmarks are similar, several different genetic and sporadic causes have been found or hypothesized. Experimental models of ALS have been created in transgenic animals, and spontaneously mutated animals affected by MN disease have been identified. Due to the multifactorial causes of the disease, all these models, even though they show motor impairment and neuropathological aspects typical of the human disease, cannot fully address the complexity of the human disease. Nevertheless, they represent useful tools to study the early and late development of the disease from a neuropathological point of view, and the molecular mechanisms involved. The major pitfall of the use of animals models thus far consists in the failure to translate the positive therapeutic outcome in human patients. This might be ascribed to mistakes in both preclinical and clinical research strategy: on one hand, animals, unlike patients, tend to be treated in the early phases of the disease and in any case represent a restricted, uniform population in terms of age, sex and genetic characteristics; on the other hand, patients represent a much more variable population. Therefore, an increasing collaboration between preclinical researchers and clinicians is needed to favor translation from benchside to clinics back and forth.

6. References

Andersen, P.M. (2000). Genetic factors in the early diagnosis of ALS. *Amyotroph Lateral Scler Other Motor Neuron Disord*, 1 Suppl 1, (Mar), pp. (S31-42), 1466-0822 (Print) 1466-0822 (Linking)

Andersen, P.M., Borasio, G.D., Dengler, R., Hardiman, O., Kollewe, K., Leigh, P.N., Pradat, P.F., Silani, V. & Tomik, B. (2007). Good practice in the management of amyotrophic lateral sclerosis: clinical guidelines. An evidence-based review with good practice points. EALSC Working Group. *Amyotroph Lateral Scler*, 8, 4, (Aug), pp. (195-213), 1748-2968 (Print) 1471-180X (Linking)

Anderson, K.N., Potter, A.C., Piccenna, L.G., Quah, A.K., Davies, K.E. & Cheema, S.S. (2004). Isolation and culture of motor neurons from the newborn mouse spinal cord. *Brain Res Brain Res Protoc*, 12, 3, (Feb), pp. (132-136), 1385-299X (Print) 1385-299X (Linking)

Aoki, M., Abe, K., Houi, K., Ogasawara, M., Matsubara, Y., Kobayashi, T., Mochio, S., Narisawa, K. & Itoyama, Y. (1995). Variance of age at onset in a Japanese family with amyotrophic lateral sclerosis associated with a novel Cu/Zn superoxide dismutase mutation. *Ann Neurol*, 37, 5, (May), pp. (676-679), 0364-5134 (Print) 0364-5134 (Linking)

Avossa, D., Grandolfo, M., Mazzarol, F., Zatta, M. & Ballerini, L. (2006). Early signs of motoneuron vulnerability in a disease model system: Characterization of transverse slice cultures of spinal cord isolated from embryonic ALS mice. *Neuroscience*, 138, 4, pp. (1179-1194), 0306-4522 (Print) 0306-4522 (Linking)

Awano, T., Johnson, G.S., Wade, C.M., Katz, M.L., Johnson, G.C., Taylor, J.F., Perloski, M., Biagi, T., Baranowska, I., Long, S., March, P.A., Olby, N.J., Shelton, G.D., Khan, S., O'Brien, D.P., Lindblad-Toh, K. & Coates, J.R. (2009). Genome-wide association analysis reveals a SOD1 mutation in canine degenerative myelopathy that resembles amyotrophic lateral sclerosis. *Proc Natl Acad Sci U S A*, 106, 8, (Feb 24), pp. (2794-2799), 1091-6490 (Electronic) 0027-8424 (Linking)

Beaulieu, J.M., Nguyen, M.D. & Julien, J.P. (1999). Late onset of motor neurons in mice overexpressing wild-type peripherin. *J Cell Biol*, 147, 3, (Nov 1), pp. (531-544), 0021-9525 (Print) 0021-9525 (Linking)

Benatar, M. (2007). Lost in translation: treatment trials in the SOD1 mouse and in human ALS. *Neurobiol Dis*, 26, 1, (Apr), pp. (1-13), 0969-9961 (Print) 0969-9961 (Linking)

Berg, D.K. & Fischbach, G.D. (1978). Enrichment of spinal cord cell cultures with motoneurons. *J Cell Biol*, 77, 1, (Apr), pp. (83-98), 0021-9525 (Print) 0021-9525 (Linking)

Bilak, M., Wu, L., Wang, Q., Haughey, N., Conant, K., St Hillaire, C. & Andreasson, K. (2004). PGE2 receptors rescue motor neurons in a model of amyotrophic lateral sclerosis. *Ann Neurol*, 56, 2, (Aug), pp. (240-248), 0364-5134 (Print) 0364-5134 (Linking)

Boillee, S., Peschanski, M. & Junier, M.P. (2003). The wobbler mouse: a neurodegeneration jigsaw puzzle. *Mol Neurobiol*, 28, 1, (Aug), pp. (65-106), 0893-7648 (Print) 0893-7648 (Linking)

Boillee, S., Vande Velde, C. & Cleveland, D.W. (2006). ALS: a disease of motor neurons and their nonneuronal neighbors. *Neuron*, 52, 1, (Oct 5), pp. (39-59), 0896-6273 (Print) 0896-6273 (Linking)

Bommel, H., Xie, G., Rossoll, W., Wiese, S., Jablonka, S., Boehm, T. & Sendtner, M. (2002). Missense mutation in the tubulin-specific chaperone E (Tbce) gene in the mouse mutant progressive motor neuronopathy, a model of human motoneuron disease. *J Cell Biol*, 159, 4, (Nov 25), pp. (563-569), 0021-9525 (Print) 0021-9525 (Linking)

Booher, J. & Sensenbrenner, M. (1972). Growth and cultivation of dissociated neurons and glial cells from embryonic chick, rat and human brain in flask cultures. *Neurobiology*, 2, 3, pp. (97-105), 0300-8819 (Print) 0300-8819 (Linking)

Boulting, G.L., Kiskinis, E., Croft, G.F., Amoroso, M.W., Oakley, D.H., Wainger, B.J., Williams, D.J., Kahler, D.J., Yamaki, M., Davidow, L., Rodolfa, C.T., Dimos, J.T., Mikkilineni, S., MacDermott, A.B., Woolf, C.J., Henderson, C.E., Wichterle, H. & Eggan, K. (2011). A functionally characterized test set of human induced pluripotent stem cells. *Nat Biotechnol*, 29, 3, (Mar), pp. (279-286), 1546-1696 (Electronic) 1087-0156 (Linking)

Bruijn, L.I., Becher, M.W., Lee, M.K., Anderson, K.L., Jenkins, N.A., Copeland, N.G., Sisodia, S.S., Rothstein, J.D., Borchelt, D.R., Price, D.L. & Cleveland, D.W. (1997). ALS-linked SOD1 mutant G85R mediates damage to astrocytes and promotes rapidly progressive disease with SOD1-containing inclusions. *Neuron*, 18, 2, (Feb), pp. (327-338), 0896-6273 (Print) 0896-6273 (Linking)

Cai, H., Lin, X., Xie, C., Laird, F.M., Lai, C., Wen, H., Chiang, H.C., Shim, H., Farah, M.H., Hoke, A., Price, D.L. & Wong, P.C. (2005). Loss of ALS2 function is insufficient to trigger motor neuron degeneration in knock-out mice but predisposes neurons to oxidative stress. *J Neurosci*, 25, 33, (Aug 17), pp. (7567-7574), 1529-2401 (Electronic) 0270-6474 (Linking)

Cai, H., Shim, H., Lai, C., Xie, C., Lin, X., Yang, W.J. & Chandran, J. (2008). ALS2/alsin knockout mice and motor neuron diseases. *Neurodegener Dis*, 5, 6, pp. (359-366), 1660-2862 (Electronic) 1660-2854 (Linking)

Caldero, J., Brunet, N., Tarabal, O., Piedrafita, L., Hereu, M., Ayala, V. & Esquerda, J.E. (2010). Lithium prevents excitotoxic cell death of motoneurons in organotypic slice cultures of spinal cord. *Neuroscience*, 165, 4, (Feb 17), pp. (1353-1369), 1873-7544 (Electronic) 0306-4522 (Linking)

Camu, W. & Henderson, C.E. (1992). Purification of embryonic rat motoneurons by panning on a monoclonal antibody to the low-affinity NGF receptor. *J Neurosci Methods*, 44, 1, (Aug), pp. (59-70), 0165-0270 (Print) 0165-0270 (Linking)

Carriedo, S.G., Yin, H.Z. & Weiss, J.H. (1996). Motor neurons are selectively vulnerable to AMPA/kainate receptor-mediated injury in vitro. *J Neurosci*, 16, 13, (Jul 1), pp. (4069-4079), 0270-6474 (Print) 0270-6474 (Linking)

Cashman, N.R., Durham, H.D., Blusztajn, J.K., Oda, K., Tabira, T., Shaw, I.T., Dahrouge, S. & Antel, J.P. (1992). Neuroblastoma x spinal cord (NSC) hybrid cell lines resemble developing motor neurons. *Dev Dyn*, 194, 3, (Jul), pp. (209-221), 1058-8388 (Print) 1058-8388 (Linking)

Chen, Y., Brew, B.J. & Guillemin, G.J. (2011). Characterization of the kynurenine pathway in NSC-34 cell line: implications for amyotrophic lateral sclerosis. *J Neurochem*, 118, 5, (Sep), pp. (816-825), 1471-4159 (Electronic) 0022-3042 (Linking)

Chen, Y.Z., Bennett, C.L., Huynh, H.M., Blair, I.P., Puls, I., Irobi, J., Dierick, I., Abel, A., Kennerson, M.L., Rabin, B.A., Nicholson, G.A., Auer-Grumbach, M., Wagner, K., De Jonghe, P., Griffin, J.W., Fischbeck, K.H., Timmerman, V., Cornblath, D.R. & Chance, P.F. (2004). DNA/RNA helicase gene mutations in a form of juvenile amyotrophic lateral sclerosis (ALS4). *Am J Hum Genet*, 74, 6, (Jun), pp. (1128-1135), 0002-9297 (Print) 0002-9297 (Linking)

Cook, S.A., Johnson, K.R., Bronson, R.T. & Davisson, M.T. (1995). Neuromuscular degeneration (nmd): a mutation on mouse chromosome 19 that causes motor neuron degeneration. *Mamm Genome*, 6, 3, (Mar), pp. (187-191), 0938-8990 (Print) 0938-8990 (Linking)

Corbo, M. & Hays, A.P. (1992). Peripherin and neurofilament protein coexist in spinal spheroids of motor neuron disease. *J Neuropathol Exp Neurol*, 51, 5, (Sep), pp. (531-537), 0022-3069 (Print) 0022-3069 (Linking)

Corona, J.C. & Tapia, R. (2007). Ca2+-permeable AMPA receptors and intracellular Ca2+ determine motoneuron vulnerability in rat spinal cord in vivo. *Neuropharmacology*, 52, 5, (Apr), pp. (1219-1228), 0028-3908 (Print) 0028-3908 (Linking)

Corrado, L., Del Bo, R., Castellotti, B., Ratti, A., Cereda, C., Penco, S., Soraru, G., Carlomagno, Y., Ghezzi, S., Pensato, V., Colombrita, C., Gagliardi, S., Cozzi, L., Orsetti, V., Mancuso, M., Siciliano, G., Mazzini, L., Comi, G.P., Gellera, C., Ceroni, M., D'Alfonso, S. & Silani, V. (2010). Mutations of FUS gene in sporadic amyotrophic lateral sclerosis. *J Med Genet*, 47, 3, (Mar), pp. (190-194), 1468-6244 (Electronic) 0022-2593 (Linking)

Corrado, L., Gagliardi, S., Carlomagno, Y., Mennini, T., Ticozzi, N., Mazzini, L., Silani, V., Cereda, C. & D'Alfonso, S. (2011). VPS54 genetic analysis in ALS Italian cohort. *Eur J Neurol*, 18, 4, (Apr), pp. (e41-42), 1468-1331 (Electronic) 1351-5101 (Linking)

Corrado, L., Ratti, A., Gellera, C., Buratti, E., Castellotti, B., Carlomagno, Y., Ticozzi, N., Mazzini, L., Testa, L., Taroni, F., Baralle, F.E., Silani, V. & D'Alfonso, S. (2009). High frequency of TARDBP gene mutations in Italian patients with amyotrophic lateral sclerosis. *Hum Mutat*, 30, 4, (Apr), pp. (688-694), 1098-1004 (Electronic) 1059-7794 (Linking)

Cote, F., Collard, J.F. & Julien, J.P. (1993). Progressive neuronopathy in transgenic mice expressing the human neurofilament heavy gene: a mouse model of amyotrophic lateral sclerosis. *Cell*, 73, 1, (Apr 9), pp. (35-46), 0092-8674 (Print) 0092-8674 (Linking)

Cox, G.A., Mahaffey, C.L. & Frankel, W.N. (1998). Identification of the mouse neuromuscular degeneration gene and mapping of a second site suppressor allele. *Neuron*, 21, 6, (Dec), pp. (1327-1337), 0896-6273 (Print) 0896-6273 (Linking)

Crowther, R.A. & Goedert, M. (2000). Abnormal tau-containing filaments in neurodegenerative diseases. *J Struct Biol*, 130, 2-3, (Jun), pp. (271-279), 1047-8477 (Print) 1047-8477 (Linking)

Dal Canto, M.C. & Gurney, M.E. (1994). Development of central nervous system pathology in a murine transgenic model of human amyotrophic lateral sclerosis. *Am J Pathol*, 145, 6, (Dec), pp. (1271-1279), 0002-9440 (Print) 0002-9440 (Linking)

Delobel, P., Flament, S., Hamdane, M., Delacourte, A., Vilain, J.P. & Buee, L. (2002). Modelling Alzheimer-specific abnormal Tau phosphorylation independently of GSK3beta and PKA kinase activities. *FEBS Lett*, 516, 1-3, (Apr 10), pp. (151-155), 0014-5793 (Print) 0014-5793 (Linking)

Deng, H.X., Hentati, A., Tainer, J.A., Iqbal, Z., Cayabyab, A., Hung, W.Y., Getzoff, E.D., Hu, P., Herzfeldt, B., Roos, R.P. & et al. (1993). Amyotrophic lateral sclerosis and structural defects in Cu,Zn superoxide dismutase. *Science*, 261, 5124, (Aug 20), pp. (1047-1051), 0036-8075 (Print) 0036-8075 (Linking)

Devon, R.S., Orban, P.C., Gerrow, K., Barbieri, M.A., Schwab, C., Cao, L.P., Helm, J.R., Bissada, N., Cruz-Aguado, R., Davidson, T.L., Witmer, J., Metzler, M., Lam, C.K., Tetzlaff, W., Simpson, E.M., McCaffery, J.M., El-Husseini, A.E., Leavitt, B.R. & Hayden, M.R. (2006). Als2-deficient mice exhibit disturbances in endosome trafficking associated with motor behavioral abnormalities. *Proc Natl Acad Sci U S A*, 103, 25, (Jun 20), pp. (9595-9600), 0027-8424 (Print) 0027-8424 (Linking)

Dickson, D.W., Josephs, K.A. & Amador-Ortiz, C. (2007). TDP-43 in differential diagnosis of motor neuron disorders. *Acta Neuropathol*, 114, 1, (Jul), pp. (71-79), 0001-6322 (Print) 0001-6322 (Linking)

Dimos, J.T., Rodolfa, K.T., Niakan, K.K., Weisenthal, L.M., Mitsumoto, H., Chung, W., Croft, G.F., Saphier, G., Leibel, R., Goland, R., Wichterle, H., Henderson, C.E. & Eggan, K. (2008). Induced pluripotent stem cells generated from patients with ALS can be differentiated into motor neurons. *Science*, 321, 5893, (Aug 29), pp. (1218-1221), 1095-9203 (Electronic) 0036-8075 (Linking)

Djabali, K., Zissopoulou, A., de Hoop, M.J., Georgatos, S.D. & Dotti, C.G. (1993). Peripherin expression in hippocampal neurons induced by muscle soluble factor(s). *J Cell Biol*, 123, 5, (Dec), pp. (1197-1206), 0021-9525 (Print) 0021-9525 (Linking)

Du, F., Qian, Z.M., Zhu, L., Wu, X.M., Qian, C., Chan, R. & Ke, Y. (2010). Purity, cell viability, expression of GFAP and bystin in astrocytes cultured by different procedures. *J Cell Biochem*, 109, 1, (Jan 1), pp. (30-37), 1097-4644 (Electronic) 0730-2312 (Linking)

Duchen, L.W. & Strich, S.J. (1968). An hereditary motor neurone disease with progressive denervation of muscle in the mouse: the mutant 'wobbler'. *J Neurol Neurosurg Psychiatry*, 31, 6, (Dec), pp. (535-542), 0022-3050 (Print) 0022-3050 (Linking)

Dupuis, L., Fergani, A., Braunstein, K.E., Eschbach, J., Holl, N., Rene, F., Gonzalez De Aguilar, J.L., Zoerner, B., Schwalenstocker, B., Ludolph, A.C. & Loeffler, J.P. (2009). Mice with a mutation in the dynein heavy chain 1 gene display sensory neuropathy but lack motor neuron disease. *Exp Neurol*, 215, 1, (Jan), pp. (146-152), 1090-2430 (Electronic) 0014-4886 (Linking)

Elder, G.A., Friedrich, V.L., Jr., Bosco, P., Kang, C., Gourov, A., Tu, P.H., Lee, V.M. & Lazzarini, R.A. (1998a). Absence of the mid-sized neurofilament subunit decreases axonal calibers, levels of light neurofilament (NF-L), and neurofilament content. *J Cell Biol*, 141, 3, (May 4), pp. (727-739), 0021-9525 (Print) 0021-9525 (Linking)

Elder, G.A., Friedrich, V.L., Jr., Kang, C., Bosco, P., Gourov, A., Tu, P.H., Zhang, B., Lee, V.M. & Lazzarini, R.A. (1998b). Requirement of heavy neurofilament subunit in the development of axons with large calibers. *J Cell Biol*, 143, 1, (Oct 5), pp. (195-205), 0021-9525 (Print) 0021-9525 (Linking)

Enayat, Z.E., Orrell, R.W., Claus, A., Ludolph, A., Bachus, R., Brockmuller, J., Ray-Chaudhuri, K., Radunovic, A., Shaw, C., Wilkinson, J. & et al. (1995). Two novel mutations in the gene for copper zinc superoxide dismutase in UK families with amyotrophic lateral sclerosis. *Hum Mol Genet*, 4, 7, (Jul), pp. (1239-1240), 0964-6906 (Print) 0964-6906 (Linking)

Escurat, M., Djabali, K., Gumpel, M., Gros, F. & Portier, M.M. (1990). Differential expression of two neuronal intermediate-filament proteins, peripherin and the low-molecular-mass neurofilament protein (NF-L), during the development of the rat. *J Neurosci*, 10, 3, (Mar), pp. (764-784), 0270-6474 (Print) 0270-6474 (Linking)

Estes, P.S., Boehringer, A., Zwick, R., Tang, J.E., Grigsby, B. & Zarnescu, D.C. (2011). Wild-type and A315T mutant TDP-43 exert differential neurotoxicity in a Drosophila model of ALS. *Hum Mol Genet*, 20, 12, (Jun 15), pp. (2308-2321), 1460-2083 (Electronic) 0964-6906 (Linking)

Eyer, J., Cleveland, D.W., Wong, P.C. & Peterson, A.C. (1998). Pathogenesis of two axonopathies does not require axonal neurofilaments. *Nature*, 391, 6667, (Feb 5), pp. (584-587), 0028-0836 (Print) 0028-0836 (Linking)

Eyer, J. & Peterson, A. (1994). Neurofilament-deficient axons and perikaryal aggregates in viable transgenic mice expressing a neurofilament-beta-galactosidase fusion protein. *Neuron*, 12, 2, (Feb), pp. (389-405), 0896-6273 (Print) 0896-6273 (Linking)

Eymard-Pierre, E., Yamanaka, K., Haeussler, M., Kress, W., Gauthier-Barichard, F., Combes, P., Cleveland, D.W. & Boespflug-Tanguy, O. (2006). Novel missense mutation in ALS2 gene results in infantile ascending hereditary spastic paralysis. *Ann Neurol*, 59, 6, (Jun), pp. (976-980), 0364-5134 (Print) 0364-5134 (Linking)

Falconer, D.S. (1956). Wobbler (wr). *Mouse News Letters*, 15, pp. (22),

Fang, D., Li, Z., Zhong-ming, Q., Mei, W.X., Ho, Y.W., Yuan, X.W. & Ya, K. (2008). Expression of bystin in reactive astrocytes induced by ischemia/reperfusion and chemical hypoxia in vitro. *Biochim Biophys Acta*, 1782, 11, (Nov), pp. (658-663), 0006-3002 (Print) 0006-3002 (Linking)

Feiguin, F., Godena, V.K., Romano, G., D'Ambrogio, A., Klima, R. & Baralle, F.E. (2009). Depletion of TDP-43 affects Drosophila motoneurons terminal synapsis and locomotive behavior. *FEBS Lett*, 583, 10, (May 19), pp. (1586-1592), 1873-3468 (Electronic) 0014-5793 (Linking)

Fukita, Y., Mizuta, T.R., Shirozu, M., Ozawa, K., Shimizu, A. & Honjo, T. (1993). The human S mu bp-2, a DNA-binding protein specific to the single-stranded guanine-rich sequence related to the immunoglobulin mu chain switch region. *J Biol Chem*, 268, 23, (Aug 15), pp. (17463-17470), 0021-9258 (Print) 0021-9258 (Linking)

Geser, F., Malunda, J.A., Hurtig, H.I., Duda, J.E., Wenning, G.K., Gilman, S., Low, P.A., Lee, V.M. & Trojanowski, J.Q. (2011). TDP-43 pathology occurs infrequently in multiple system atrophy. *Neuropathol Appl Neurobiol*, 37, 4, (Jun), pp. (358-365), 1365-2990 (Electronic)

Gingras, M., Gagnon, V., Minotti, S., Durham, H.D. & Berthod, F. (2007). Optimized protocols for isolation of primary motor neurons, astrocytes and microglia from embryonic mouse spinal cord. *J Neurosci Methods*, 163, 1, (Jun 15), pp. (111-118), 0165-0270 (Print) 0165-0270 (Linking)

Gitcho, M.A., Baloh, R.H., Chakraverty, S., Mayo, K., Norton, J.B., Levitch, D., Hatanpaa, K.J., White, C.L., 3rd, Bigio, E.H., Caselli, R., Baker, M., Al-Lozi, M.T., Morris, J.C., Pestronk, A., Rademakers, R., Goate, A.M. & Cairns, N.J. (2008). TDP-43 A315T mutation in familial motor neuron disease. *Ann Neurol*, 63, 4, (Apr), pp. (535-538), 1531-8249 (Electronic) 0364-5134 (Linking)

Gomes, C., Palma, A.S., Almeida, R., Regalla, M., McCluskey, L.F., Trojanowski, J.Q. & Costa, J. (2008). Establishment of a cell model of ALS disease: Golgi apparatus disruption occurs independently from apoptosis. *Biotechnol Lett*, 30, 4, (Apr), pp. (603-610), 0141-5492 (Print) 0141-5492 (Linking)

Gordon, R., Hogan, C.E., Neal, M.L., Anantharam, V., Kanthasamy, A.G. & Kanthasamy, A. (2011). A simple magnetic separation method for high-yield isolation of pure primary microglia. *J Neurosci Methods*, 194, 2, (Jan 15), pp. (287-296), 1872-678X (Electronic) 0165-0270 (Linking)

Gotz, J., Chen, F., van Dorpe, J. & Nitsch, R.M. (2001). Formation of neurofibrillary tangles in P301l tau transgenic mice induced by Abeta 42 fibrils. *Science*, 293, 5534, (Aug 24), pp. (1491-1495), 0036-8075 (Print) 0036-8075 (Linking)

Green, S.L., Bouley, D.M., Pinter, M.J., Cork, L.C. & Vatassery, G.T. (2001). Canine motor neuron disease: clinicopathologic features and selected indicators of oxidative stress. *J Vet Intern Med*, 15, 2, (Mar-Apr), pp. (112-119), 0891-6640 (Print) 0891-6640 (Linking)

Green, S.L., Tolwani, R.J., Varma, S., Quignon, P., Galibert, F. & Cork, L.C. (2002). Structure, chromosomal location, and analysis of the canine Cu/Zn superoxide dismutase (SOD1) gene. *J Hered*, 93, 2, (Mar-Apr), pp. (119-124), 0022-1503 (Print) 0022-1503 (Linking)

Green, S.L., Westendorf, J.M., Jaffe, H., Pant, H.C., Cork, L.C., Ostrander, E.A., Vignaux, F. & Ferrell, J.E., Jr. (2005). Allelic variants of the canine heavy neurofilament (NFH) subunit and extensive phosphorylation in dogs with motor neuron disease. *J Comp Pathol*, 132, 1, (Jan), pp. (33-50), 0021-9975 (Print) 0021-9975 (Linking)

Greenway, M.J., Andersen, P.M., Russ, C., Ennis, S., Cashman, S., Donaghy, C., Patterson, V., Swingler, R., Kieran, D., Prehn, J., Morrison, K.E., Green, A., Acharya, K.R., Brown, R.H., Jr. & Hardiman, O. (2006). ANG mutations segregate with familial and 'sporadic' amyotrophic lateral sclerosis. *Nat Genet*, 38, 4, (Apr), pp. (411-413), 1061-4036 (Print) 1061-4036 (Linking)

Guo, G. & Bhat, N.R. (2007). p38alpha MAP kinase mediates hypoxia-induced motor neuron cell death: a potential target of minocycline's neuroprotective action. *Neurochem Res*, 32, 12, (Dec), pp. (2160-2166), 0364-3190 (Print) 0364-3190 (Linking)

Guo, W., Chen, Y., Zhou, X., Kar, A., Ray, P., Chen, X., Rao, E.J., Yang, M., Ye, H., Zhu, L., Liu, J., Xu, M., Yang, Y., Wang, C., Zhang, D., Bigio, E.H., Mesulam, M., Shen, Y., Xu, Q., Fushimi, K. & Wu, J.Y. (2011). An ALS-associated mutation affecting TDP-43 enhances protein aggregation, fibril formation and neurotoxicity. *Nat Struct Mol Biol*, 18, 7, pp. (822-830), 1545-9985 (Electronic) 1545-9985 (Linking)

Gurney, M.E., Pu, H., Chiu, A.Y., Dal Canto, M.C., Polchow, C.Y., Alexander, D.D., Caliendo, J., Hentati, A., Kwon, Y.W., Deng, H.X. & et al. (1994). Motor neuron degeneration in mice that express a human Cu,Zn superoxide dismutase mutation. *Science*, 264, 5166, (Jun 17), pp. (1772-1775), 0036-8075 (Print) 0036-8075 (Linking)

Hadano, S., Hand, C.K., Osuga, H., Yanagisawa, Y., Otomo, A., Devon, R.S., Miyamoto, N., Showguchi-Miyata, J., Okada, Y., Singaraja, R., Figlewicz, D.A., Kwiatkowski, T., Hosler, B.A., Sagie, T., Skaug, J., Nasir, J., Brown, R.H., Jr., Scherer, S.W., Rouleau, G.A., Hayden, M.R. & Ikeda, J.E. (2001). A gene encoding a putative GTPase regulator is mutated in familial amyotrophic lateral sclerosis 2. *Nat Genet*, 29, 2, (Oct), pp. (166-173), 1061-4036 (Print) 1061-4036 (Linking)

Hadano, S., Otomo, A., Kunita, R., Suzuki-Utsunomiya, K., Akatsuka, A., Koike, M., Aoki, M., Uchiyama, Y., Itoyama, Y. & Ikeda, J.E. (2010a). Loss of ALS2/Alsin exacerbates motor dysfunction in a SOD1-expressing mouse ALS model by disturbing endolysosomal trafficking. *PLoS One*, 5, 3, pp. (e9805), 1932-6203 (Electronic) 1932-6203 (Linking)

Hadano, S., Yoshii, Y., Otomo, A., Kunita, R., Suzuki-Utsunomiya, K., Pan, L., Kakuta, S., Iwasaki, Y., Iwakura, Y. & Ikeda, J.E. (2010b). Genetic background and gender effects on gross phenotypes in congenic lines of ALS2/alsin-deficient mice. *Neurosci Res*, 68, 2, (Oct), pp. (131-136), 1872-8111 (Electronic) 0168-0102 (Linking)

Haghnia, M., Cavalli, V., Shah, S.B., Schimmelpfeng, K., Brusch, R., Yang, G., Herrera, C., Pilling, A. & Goldstein, L.S. (2007). Dynactin is required for coordinated bidirectional motility, but not for dynein membrane attachment. *Mol Biol Cell*, 18, 6, (Jun), pp. (2081-2089), 1059-1524 (Print) 1059-1524 (Linking)

Hall, E.D., Oostveen, J.A. & Gurney, M.E. (1998). Relationship of microglial and astrocytic activation to disease onset and progression in a transgenic model of familial ALS. *Glia*, 23, 3, (Jul), pp. (249-256), 0894-1491 (Print) 0894-1491 (Linking)

Hasegawa, M., Smith, M.J. & Goedert, M. (1998). Tau proteins with FTDP-17 mutations have a reduced ability to promote microtubule assembly. *FEBS Lett*, 437, 3, (Oct 23), pp. (207-210), 0014-5793 (Print) 0014-5793 (Linking)

Hirano, A. (1991). Cytopathology of amyotrophic lateral sclerosis. *Adv Neurol*, 56, pp. (91-101), 0091-3952 (Print) 0091-3952 (Linking)

Hirano, A., Nakano, I., Kurland, L.T., Mulder, D.W., Holley, P.W. & Saccomanno, G. (1984). Fine structural study of neurofibrillary changes in a family with amyotrophic lateral sclerosis. *J Neuropathol Exp Neurol*, 43, 5, (Sep), pp. (471-480), 0022-3069 (Print) 0022-3069 (Linking)

Hong, M., Zhukareva, V., Vogelsberg-Ragaglia, V., Wszolek, Z., Reed, L., Miller, B.I., Geschwind, D.H., Bird, T.D., McKeel, D., Goate, A., Morris, J.C., Wilhelmsen, K.C., Schellenberg, G.D., Trojanowski, J.Q. & Lee, V.M. (1998). Mutation-specific functional impairments in distinct tau isoforms of hereditary FTDP-17. *Science*, 282, 5395, (Dec 4), pp. (1914-1917), 0036-8075 (Print) 0036-8075 (Linking)

Hrabe de Angelis, M.H., Flaswinkel, H., Fuchs, H., Rathkolb, B., Soewarto, D., Marschall, S., Heffner, S., Pargent, W., Wuensch, K., Jung, M., Reis, A., Richter, T., Alessandrini, F., Jakob, T., Fuchs, E., Kolb, H., Kremmer, E., Schaeble, K., Rollinski, B., Roscher, A., Peters, C., Meitinger, T., Strom, T., Steckler, T., Holsboer, F., Klopstock, T., Gekeler, F., Schindewolf, C., Jung, T., Avraham, K., Behrendt, H., Ring, J., Zimmer, A., Schughart, K., Pfeffer, K., Wolf, E. & Balling, R. (2000). Genome-wide, large-scale production of mutant mice by ENU mutagenesis. *Nat Genet*, 25, 4, (Aug), pp. (444-447), 1061-4036 (Print) 1061-4036 (Linking)

Iaccarino, C., Mura, M.E., Esposito, S., Carta, F., Sanna, G., Turrini, F., Carri, M.T. & Crosio, C. (2011). Bcl2-A1 interacts with pro-caspase-3: Implications for amyotrophic lateral sclerosis. *Neurobiol Dis*, 43, 3, (Sep), pp. (642-650), 1095-953X (Electronic) 0969-9961 (Linking)

Ilieva, H.S., Yamanaka, K., Malkmus, S., Kakinohana, O., Yaksh, T., Marsala, M. & Cleveland, D.W. (2008). Mutant dynein (Loa) triggers proprioceptive axon loss that extends survival only in the SOD1 ALS model with highest motor neuron death. *Proc Natl Acad Sci U S A*, 105, 34, (Aug 26), pp. (12599-12604), 1091-6490 (Electronic) 0027-8424 (Linking)

Jacquier, A., Buhler, E., Schafer, M.K., Bohl, D., Blanchard, S., Beclin, C. & Haase, G. (2006). Alsin/Rac1 signaling controls survival and growth of spinal motoneurons. *Ann Neurol*, 60, 1, (Jul), pp. (105-117), 0364-5134 (Print) 0364-5134 (Linking)

Jonsson, P.A., Ernhill, K., Andersen, P.M., Bergemalm, D., Brannstrom, T., Gredal, O., Nilsson, P. & Marklund, S.L. (2004). Minute quantities of misfolded mutant superoxide dismutase-1 cause amyotrophic lateral sclerosis. *Brain*, 127, Pt 1, (Jan), pp. (73-88), 0006-8950 (Print) 0006-8950 (Linking)

Jonsson, P.A., Graffmo, K.S., Brannstrom, T., Nilsson, P., Andersen, P.M. & Marklund, S.L. (2006). Motor neuron disease in mice expressing the wild type-like D90A mutant superoxide dismutase-1. *J Neuropathol Exp Neurol*, 65, 12, (Dec), pp. (1126-1136), 0022-3069 (Print) 0022-3069 (Linking)

Kabashi, E., Bercier, V., Lissouba, A., Liao, M., Brustein, E., Rouleau, G.A. & Drapeau, P. (2011). FUS and TARDBP but Not SOD1 Interact in Genetic Models of Amyotrophic Lateral Sclerosis. *PLoS Genet*, 7, 8, (Aug), pp. (e1002214), 1553-7404 (Electronic) 1553-7390 (Linking)

Kabashi, E., Valdmanis, P.N., Dion, P., Spiegelman, D., McConkey, B.J., Vande Velde, C., Bouchard, J.P., Lacomblez, L., Pochigaeva, K., Salachas, F., Pradat, P.F., Camu, W., Meininger, V., Dupre, N. & Rouleau, G.A. (2008). TARDBP mutations in individuals with sporadic and familial amyotrophic lateral sclerosis. *Nat Genet*, 40, 5, (May), pp. (572-574), 1546-1718 (Electronic) 1061-4036 (Linking)

Kato, T., Hirano, A., Manaka, H., Sasaki, H., Katagiri, T., Kawanami, T., Shikama, Y. & Seino, T. (1991). Calcitonin gene-related peptide immunoreactivity in familial amyotrophic lateral sclerosis. *Neurosci Lett*, 133, 2, (Dec 9), pp. (163-167), 0304-3940 (Print) 0304-3940 (Linking)

Kaupmann, K., Simon-Chazottes, D., Guenet, J.L. & Jockusch, H. (1992). Wobbler, a mutation affecting motoneuron survival and gonadal functions in the mouse, maps to proximal chromosome 11. *Genomics*, 13, 1, (May), pp. (39-43), 0888-7543 (Print) 0888-7543 (Linking)

Kerr, D. & Khalili, K. (1991). A recombinant cDNA derived from human brain encodes a DNA binding protein that stimulates transcription of the human neurotropic virus JCV. *J Biol Chem*, 266, 24, (Aug 25), pp. (15876-15881), 0021-9258 (Print) 0021-9258 (Linking)

Kosuge, Y., Sekikawa-Nishida, K., Negi, H., Ishige, K. & Ito, Y. (2009). Characterization of chronic glutamate-mediated motor neuron toxicity in organotypic spinal cord culture prepared from ALS model mice. *Neurosci Lett*, 454, 2, (Apr 24), pp. (165-169), 0304-3940 (Print) 0304-3940 (Linking)

Kulshreshtha, D., Vijayalakshmi, K., Alladi, P.A., Sathyaprabha, T.N., Nalini, A. & Raju, T.R. (2011). Vascular endothelial growth factor attenuates neurodegenerative changes in the NSC-34 motor neuron cell line induced by cerebrospinal fluid of sporadic amyotrophic lateral sclerosis patients. *Neurodegener Dis*, 8, 5, pp. (322-330), 1660-2862 (Electronic) 1660-2854 (Linking)

Kunita, R., Otomo, A., Mizumura, H., Suzuki-Utsunomiya, K., Hadano, S. & Ikeda, J.E. (2007). The Rab5 activator ALS2/alsin acts as a novel Rac1 effector through Rac1-activated endocytosis. *J Biol Chem*, 282, 22, (Jun 1), pp. (16599-16611), 0021-9258 (Print) 0021-9258 (Linking)

Kwiatkowski, T.J., Jr., Bosco, D.A., Leclerc, A.L., Tamrazian, E., Vanderburg, C.R., Russ, C., Davis, A., Gilchrist, J., Kasarskis, E.J., Munsat, T., Valdmanis, P., Rouleau, G.A., Hosler, B.A., Cortelli, P., de Jong, P.J., Yoshinaga, Y., Haines, J.L., Pericak-Vance, M.A., Yan, J., Ticozzi, N., Siddique, T., McKenna-Yasek, D., Sapp, P.C., Horvitz, H.R., Landers, J.E. & Brown, R.H., Jr. (2009). Mutations in the FUS/TLS gene on chromosome 16 cause familial amyotrophic lateral sclerosis. *Science*, 323, 5918, (Feb 27), pp. (1205-1208), 1095-9203 (Electronic) 0036-8075 (Linking)

Lagier-Tourenne, C. & Cleveland, D.W. (2009). Rethinking ALS: the FUS about TDP-43. *Cell*, 136, 6, (Mar 20), pp. (1001-1004), 1097-4172 (Electronic) 0092-8674 (Linking)

Lai, C., Lin, X., Chandran, J., Shim, H., Yang, W.J. & Cai, H. (2007). The G59S mutation in p150(glued) causes dysfunction of dynactin in mice. *J Neurosci*, 27, 51, (Dec 19), pp. (13982-13990), 1529-2401 (Electronic) 0270-6474 (Linking)

Lai, C., Xie, C., McCormack, S.G., Chiang, H.C., Michalak, M.K., Lin, X., Chandran, J., Shim, H., Shimoji, M., Cookson, M.R., Huganir, R.L., Rothstein, J.D., Price, D.L., Wong, P.C., Martin, L.J., Zhu, J.J. & Cai, H. (2006). Amyotrophic lateral sclerosis 2-deficiency leads to neuronal degeneration in amyotrophic lateral sclerosis through altered AMPA receptor trafficking. *J Neurosci*, 26, 45, (Nov 8), pp. (11798-11806), 1529-2401 (Electronic) 0270-6474 (Linking)

Laird, F.M., Farah, M.H., Ackerley, S., Hoke, A., Maragakis, N., Rothstein, J.D., Griffin, J., Price, D.L., Martin, L.J. & Wong, P.C. (2008). Motor neuron disease occurring in a mutant dynactin mouse model is characterized by defects in vesicular trafficking. *J Neurosci*, 28, 9, (Feb 27), pp. (1997-2005), 1529-2401 (Electronic) 0270-6474 (Linking)

LaMonte, B.H., Wallace, K.E., Holloway, B.A., Shelly, S.S., Ascano, J., Tokito, M., Van Winkle, T., Howland, D.S. & Holzbaur, E.L. (2002). Disruption of dynein/dynactin inhibits axonal transport in motor neurons causing late-onset progressive degeneration. *Neuron*, 34, 5, (May 30), pp. (715-727), 0896-6273 (Print) 0896-6273 (Linking)

Lanson, N.A., Jr., Maltare, A., King, H., Smith, R., Kim, J.H., Taylor, J.P., Lloyd, T.E. & Pandey, U.B. (2011). A Drosophila model of FUS-related neurodegeneration reveals genetic interaction between FUS and TDP-43. *Hum Mol Genet*, 20, 13, (Jul 1), pp. (2510-2523), 1460-2083 (Electronic) 0964-6906 (Linking)

Lee, M.K., Marszalek, J.R. & Cleveland, D.W. (1994). A mutant neurofilament subunit causes massive, selective motor neuron death: implications for the pathogenesis of human motor neuron disease. *Neuron*, 13, 4, (Oct), pp. (975-988), 0896-6273 (Print) 0896-6273 (Linking)

Lemmens, R., Van Hoecke, A., Hersmus, N., Geelen, V., D'Hollander, I., Thijs, V., Van Den Bosch, L., Carmeliet, P. & Robberecht, W. (2007). Overexpression of mutant superoxide dismutase 1 causes a motor axonopathy in the zebrafish. *Hum Mol Genet*, 16, 19, (Oct 1), pp. (2359-2365), 0964-6906 (Print) 0964-6906 (Linking)

Lewis, J., McGowan, E., Rockwood, J., Melrose, H., Nacharaju, P., Van Slegtenhorst, M., Gwinn-Hardy, K., Paul Murphy, M., Baker, M., Yu, X., Duff, K., Hardy, J., Corral, A., Lin, W.L., Yen, S.H., Dickson, D.W., Davies, P. & Hutton, M. (2000). Neurofibrillary tangles, amyotrophy and progressive motor disturbance in mice expressing mutant (P301L) tau protein. *Nat Genet*, 25, 4, (Aug), pp. (402-405), 1061-4036 (Print) 1061-4036 (Linking)

Lunn, J.S., Sakowski, S.A., Kim, B., Rosenberg, A.A. & Feldman, E.L. (2009). Vascular endothelial growth factor prevents G93A-SOD1-induced motor neuron degeneration. *Dev Neurobiol*, 69, 13, (Nov), pp. (871-884), 1932-846X (Electronic) 1932-8451 (Linking)

Mackenzie, I.R., Rademakers, R. & Neumann, M. (2010). TDP-43 and FUS in amyotrophic lateral sclerosis and frontotemporal dementia. *Lancet Neurol*, 9, 10, (Oct), pp. (995-1007), 1474-4465 (Electronic) 1474-4422 (Linking)

Maragakis, N.J., Jackson, M., Ganel, R. & Rothstein, J.D. (2003). Topiramate protects against motor neuron degeneration in organotypic spinal cord cultures but not in G93A SOD1 transgenic mice. *Neurosci Lett*, 338, 2, (Feb 27), pp. (107-110), 0304-3940 (Print) 0304-3940 (Linking)

Marchetto, M.C., Muotri, A.R., Mu, Y., Smith, A.M., Cezar, G.G. & Gage, F.H. (2008). Non-cell-autonomous effect of human SOD1 G37R astrocytes on motor neurons derived from human embryonic stem cells. *Cell Stem Cell*, 3, 6, (Dec 4), pp. (649-657), 1875-9777 (Electronic)

Martin, N., Jaubert, J., Gounon, P., Salido, E., Haase, G., Szatanik, M. & Guenet, J.L. (2002). A missense mutation in Tbce causes progressive motor neuronopathy in mice. *Nat Genet*, 32, 3, (Nov), pp. (443-447), 1061-4036 (Print) 1061-4036 (Linking)

Maruyama, H., Morino, H., Ito, H., Izumi, Y., Kato, H., Watanabe, Y., Kinoshita, Y., Kamada, M., Nodera, H., Suzuki, H., Komure, O., Matsuura, S., Kobatake, K., Morimoto, N., Abe, K., Suzuki, N., Aoki, M., Kawata, A., Hirai, T., Kato, T., Ogasawara, K., Hirano, A., Takumi, T., Kusaka, H., Hagiwara, K., Kaji, R. & Kawakami, H. (2010). Mutations of optineurin in amyotrophic lateral sclerosis. *Nature*, 465, 7295, (May 13), pp. (223-226), 1476-4687 (Electronic) 0028-0836 (Linking)

Menzies, F.M., Cookson, M.R., Taylor, R.W., Turnbull, D.M., Chrzanowska-Lightowlers, Z.M., Dong, L., Figlewicz, D.A. & Shaw, P.J. (2002a). Mitochondrial dysfunction in a cell culture model of familial amyotrophic lateral sclerosis. *Brain*, 125, Pt 7, (Jul), pp. (1522-1533), 0006-8950 (Print) 0006-8950 (Linking)

Menzies, F.M., Grierson, A.J., Cookson, M.R., Heath, P.R., Tomkins, J., Figlewicz, D.A., Ince, P.G. & Shaw, P.J. (2002b). Selective loss of neurofilament expression in Cu/Zn superoxide dismutase (SOD1) linked amyotrophic lateral sclerosis. *J Neurochem*, 82, 5, (Sep), pp. (1118-1128), 0022-3042 (Print) 0022-3042 (Linking)

Migheli, A., Pezzulo, T., Attanasio, A. & Schiffer, D. (1993). Peripherin immunoreactive structures in amyotrophic lateral sclerosis. *Lab Invest*, 68, 2, (Feb), pp. (185-191), 0023-6837 (Print) 0023-6837 (Linking)

Millecamps, S., Salachas, F., Cazeneuve, C., Gordon, P., Bricka, B., Camuzat, A., Guillot-Noel, L., Russaouen, O., Bruneteau, G., Pradat, P.F., Le Forestier, N., Vandenberghe, N., Danel-Brunaud, V., Guy, N., Thauvin-Robinet, C., Lacomblez, L., Couratier, P., Hannequin, D., Seilhean, D., Le Ber, I., Corcia, P., Camu, W., Brice, A., Rouleau, G., LeGuern, E. & Meininger, V. (2010). SOD1, ANG, VAPB, TARDBP, and FUS mutations in familial amyotrophic lateral sclerosis: genotype-phenotype correlations. *J Med Genet*, 47, 8, (Aug), pp. (554-560), 1468-6244 (Electronic) 0022-2593 (Linking)

Muma, N.A., Hoffman, P.N., Slunt, H.H., Applegate, M.D., Lieberburg, I. & Price, D.L. (1990). Alterations in levels of mRNAs coding for neurofilament protein subunits during regeneration. *Exp Neurol*, 107, 3, (Mar), pp. (230-235), 0014-4886 (Print) 0014-4886 (Linking)

Munch, C., Rosenbohm, A., Sperfeld, A.D., Uttner, I., Reske, S., Krause, B.J., Sedlmeier, R., Meyer, T., Hanemann, C.O., Stumm, G. & Ludolph, A.C. (2005). Heterozygous

R1101K mutation of the DCTN1 gene in a family with ALS and FTD. *Ann Neurol*, 58, 5, (Nov), pp. (777-780), 0364-5134 (Print) 0364-5134 (Linking)

Munch, C., Sedlmeier, R., Meyer, T., Homberg, V., Sperfeld, A.D., Kurt, A., Prudlo, J., Peraus, G., Hanemann, C.O., Stumm, G. & Ludolph, A.C. (2004). Point mutations of the p150 subunit of dynactin (DCTN1) gene in ALS. *Neurology*, 63, 4, (Aug 24), pp. (724-726), 1526-632X (Electronic) 0028-3878 (Linking)

Nagai, M., Aoki, M., Miyoshi, I., Kato, M., Pasinelli, P., Kasai, N., Brown, R.H., Jr. & Itoyama, Y. (2001). Rats expressing human cytosolic copper-zinc superoxide dismutase transgenes with amyotrophic lateral sclerosis: associated mutations develop motor neuron disease. *J Neurosci*, 21, 23, (Dec 1), pp. (9246-9254), 1529-2401 (Electronic) 0270-6474 (Linking)

Nagai, M., Re, D.B., Nagata, T., Chalazonitis, A., Jessell, T.M., Wichterle, H. & Przedborski, S. (2007). Astrocytes expressing ALS-linked mutated SOD1 release factors selectively toxic to motor neurons. *Nat Neurosci*, 10, 5, (May), pp. (615-622), 1097-6256 (Print) 1097-6256 (Linking)

Nakashima, K., Watanabe, Y., Kuno, N., Nanba, E. & Takahashi, K. (1995). Abnormality of Cu/Zn superoxide dismutase (SOD1) activity in Japanese familial amyotrophic lateral sclerosis with two base pair deletion in the SOD1 gene. *Neurology*, 45, 5, (May), pp. (1019-1020), 0028-3878 (Print) 0028-3878 (Linking)

Newbery, H.J., Gillingwater, T.H., Dharmasaroja, P., Peters, J., Wharton, S.B., Thomson, D., Ribchester, R.R. & Abbott, C.M. (2005). Progressive loss of motor neuron function in wasted mice: effects of a spontaneous null mutation in the gene for the eEF1 A2 translation factor. *J Neuropathol Exp Neurol*, 64, 4, (Apr), pp. (295-303), 0022-3069 (Print) 0022-3069 (Linking)

Ni, M. & Aschner, M. (2010). Neonatal rat primary microglia: isolation, culturing, and selected applications. *Curr Protoc Toxicol*, Chapter 12, (Feb), pp. (Unit 12 17), 1934-9262 (Electronic) 1934-9254 (Linking)

Nishimura, A.L., Mitne-Neto, M., Silva, H.C., Richieri-Costa, A., Middleton, S., Cascio, D., Kok, F., Oliveira, J.R., Gillingwater, T., Webb, J., Skehel, P. & Zatz, M. (2004). A mutation in the vesicle-trafficking protein VAPB causes late-onset spinal muscular atrophy and amyotrophic lateral sclerosis. *Am J Hum Genet*, 75, 5, (Nov), pp. (822-831), 0002-9297 (Print) 0002-9297 (Linking)

Noto, Y., Shibuya, K., Sato, Y., Kanai, K., Misawa, S., Sawai, S., Mori, M., Uchiyama, T., Isose, S., Nasu, S., Sekiguchi, Y., Fujimaki, Y., Kasai, T., Tokuda, T., Nakagawa, M. & Kuwabara (2011)., S. Elevated CSF TDP-43 levels in amyotrophic lateral sclerosis: specificity, sensitivity, and a possible prognostic value. *Amyotroph Lateral Scler*, 12, 2, (Mar), pp. (140-143), 1471-180X (Electronic) 1471-180X (Linking)

Oosthuyse, B., Moons, L., Storkebaum, E., Beck, H., Nuyens, D., Brusselmans, K., Van Dorpe, J., Hellings, P., Gorselink, M., Heymans, S., Theilmeier, G., Dewerchin, M., Laudenbach, V., Vermylen, P., Raat, H., Acker, T., Vleminckx, V., Van Den Bosch, L., Cashman, N., Fujisawa, H., Drost, M.R., Sciot, R., Bruyninckx, F., Hicklin, D.J., Ince, C., Gressens, P., Lupu, F., Plate, K.H., Robberecht, W., Herbert, J.M., Collen, D. & Carmeliet, P. (2001). Deletion of the hypoxia-response element in the vascular endothelial growth factor promoter causes motor neuron degeneration. *Nat Genet*, 28, 2, (Jun), pp. (131-138), 1061-4036 (Print) 1061-4036 (Linking)

Orban, P., Devon, R.S., Hayden, M.R. & Leavitt, B.R. (2007). Chapter 15 Juvenile amyotrophic lateral sclerosis. *Handb Clin Neurol*, 82, pp. (301-312), 0072-9752 (Print) 0072-9752 (Linking)

Orlacchio, A., Babalini, C., Borreca, A., Patrono, C., Massa, R., Basaran, S., Munhoz, R.P., Rogaeva, E.A., St George-Hyslop, P.H., Bernardi, G. & Kawarai, T. (2010). SPATACSIN mutations cause autosomal recessive juvenile amyotrophic lateral sclerosis. *Brain*, 133, Pt 2, (Feb), pp. (591-598), 1460-2156 (Electronic) 0006-8950 (Linking)

Orsucci, D., Calsolaro, V., Mancuso, M. & Siciliano, G. (2009). Neuroprotective effects of tetracyclines: molecular targets, animal models and human disease. *CNS Neurol Disord Drug Targets*, 8, 3, (Jun), pp. (222-231), 1996-3181 (Electronic) 1871-5273 (Linking)

Parge, H.E., Hallewell, R.A. & Tainer, J.A. (1992). Atomic structures of wild-type and thermostable mutant recombinant human Cu,Zn superoxide dismutase. *Proc Natl Acad Sci U S A*, 89, 13, (Jul 1), pp. (6109-6113), 0027-8424 (Print) 0027-8424 (Linking)

Parysek, L.M. & Goldman, R.D. (1988). Distribution of a novel 57 kDa intermediate filament (IF) protein in the nervous system. *J Neurosci*, 8, 2, (Feb), pp. (555-563), 0270-6474 (Print) 0270-6474 (Linking)

Philips, T. & Robberecht, W. (2011). Neuroinflammation in amyotrophic lateral sclerosis: role of glial activation in motor neuron disease. *Lancet Neurol*, 10, 3, (Mar), pp. (253-263), 1474-4465 (Electronic) 1474-4422 (Linking)

Polymenidou, M., Lagier-Tourenne, C., Hutt, K.R., Huelga, S.C., Moran, J., Liang, T.Y., Ling, S.C., Sun, E., Wancewicz, E., Mazur, C., Kordasiewicz, H., Sedaghat, Y., Donohue, J.P., Shiue, L., Bennett, C.F., Yeo, G.W. & Cleveland, D.W. (2011). Long pre-mRNA depletion and RNA missplicing contribute to neuronal vulnerability from loss of TDP-43. *Nat Neurosci*, 14, 4, (Apr), pp. (459-468), 1546-1726 (Electronic) 1097-6256 (Linking)

Pramatarova, A., Goto, J., Nanba, E., Nakashima, K., Takahashi, K., Takagi, A., Kanazawa, I., Figlewicz, D.A. & Rouleau, G.A. (1994). A two basepair deletion in the SOD 1 gene causes familial amyotrophic lateral sclerosis. *Hum Mol Genet*, 3, 11, (Nov), pp. (2061-2062), 0964-6906 (Print) 0964-6906 (Linking)

Puls, I., Jonnakuty, C., LaMonte, B.H., Holzbaur, E.L., Tokito, M., Mann, E., Floeter, M.K., Bidus, K., Drayna, D., Oh, S.J., Brown, R.H., Jr., Ludlow, C.L. & Fischbeck, K.H. (2003). Mutant dynactin in motor neuron disease. *Nat Genet*, 33, 4, (Apr), pp. (455-456), 1061-4036 (Print) 1061-4036 (Linking)

Raimondi, A., Mangolini, A., Rizzardini, M., Tartari, S., Massari, S., Bendotti, C., Francolini, M., Borgese, N., Cantoni, L. & Pietrini, G. (2006). Cell culture models to investigate the selective vulnerability of motoneuronal mitochondria to familial ALS-linked G93ASOD1. *Eur J Neurosci*, 24, 2, (Jul), pp. (387-399), 0953-816X (Print) 0953-816X (Linking)

Rao, M.V., Houseweart, M.K., Williamson, T.L., Crawford, T.O., Folmer, J. & Cleveland, D.W. (1998). Neurofilament-dependent radial growth of motor axons and axonal organization of neurofilaments does not require the neurofilament heavy subunit (NF-H) or its phosphorylation. *J Cell Biol*, 143, 1, (Oct 5), pp. (171-181), 0021-9525 (Print) 0021-9525 (Linking)

Ripps, M.E., Huntley, G.W., Hof, P.R., Morrison, J.H. & Gordon, J.W. (1995). Transgenic mice expressing an altered murine superoxide dismutase gene provide an animal model of amyotrophic lateral sclerosis. *Proc Natl Acad Sci U S A*, 92, 3, (Jan 31), pp. (689-693), 0027-8424 (Print) 0027-8424 (Linking)

Rogers, D.C., Peters, J., Martin, J.E., Ball, S., Nicholson, S.J., Witherden, A.S., Hafezparast, M., Latcham, J., Robinson, T.L., Quilter, C.A. & Fisher, E.M. (2001). SHIRPA, a protocol for behavioral assessment: validation for longitudinal study of neurological dysfunction in mice. *Neurosci Lett*, 306, 1-2, (Jun 22), pp. (89-92), 0304-3940 (Print) 0304-3940 (Linking)

Rosen, D.R. (1993). Mutations in Cu/Zn superoxide dismutase gene are associated with familial amyotrophic lateral sclerosis. *Nature*, 364, 6435, (Jul 22), pp. (362), 0028-0836 (Print) 0028-0836 (Linking)

Rosen, D.R., Siddique, T., Patterson, D., Figlewicz, D.A., Sapp, P., Hentati, A., Donaldson, D., Goto, J., O'Regan, J.P., Deng, H.X. & et al. (1993). Mutations in Cu/Zn superoxide dismutase gene are associated with familial amyotrophic lateral sclerosis. *Nature*, 362, 6415, (Mar 4), pp. (59-62), 0028-0836 (Print) 0028-0836 (Linking)

Rothstein, J.D., Jin, L., Dykes-Hoberg, M. & Kuncl, R.W. (1993). Chronic inhibition of glutamate uptake produces a model of slow neurotoxicity. *Proc Natl Acad Sci U S A*, 90, 14, (Jul 15), pp. (6591-6595), 0027-8424 (Print) 0027-8424 (Linking)

Rothstein, J.D., Van Kammen, M., Levey, A.I., Martin, L.J. & Kuncl, R.W. (1995). Selective loss of glial glutamate transporter GLT-1 in amyotrophic lateral sclerosis. *Ann Neurol*, 38, 1, (Jul), pp. (73-84), 0364-5134 (Print) 0364-5134 (Linking)

Schmalbruch, H., Jensen, H.J., Bjaerg, M., Kamieniecka, Z. & Kurland, L. (1991). A new mouse mutant with progressive motor neuronopathy. *J Neuropathol Exp Neurol*, 50, 3, (May), pp. (192-204), 0022-3069 (Print) 0022-3069 (Linking)

Schnaar, R.I. & Schaffner, A.E. (1981). Separation of cell types from embryonic chicken and rat spinal cord: characterization of motoneuron-enriched fractions. *J Neurosci*, 1, 2, (Feb), pp. (204-217), 0270-6474 (Print) 0270-6474 (Linking)

Scozzafava, A. & Viezzoli, M.S. (1993). The role of the active site amino acid residues on the catalytic activity of Cu2Zn2SOD. *Mol Chem Neuropathol*, 19, 1-2, (May-Jun), pp. (193-204), 1044-7393 (Print) 1044-7393 (Linking)

Sebastiani, G., Durocher, D., Gros, P., Nemer, M. & Malo, D. (1995). Localization of the Catf1 transcription factor gene to mouse chromosome 19. *Mamm Genome*, 6, 2, (Feb), pp. (147-148), 0938-8990 (Print) 0938-8990 (Linking)

Shieh, S.Y., Stellrecht, C.M. & Tsai, M.J. (1995). Molecular characterization of the rat insulin enhancer-binding complex 3b2. Cloning of a binding factor with putative helicase motifs. *J Biol Chem*, 270, 37, (Sep 15), pp. (21503-21508), 0021-9258 (Print) 0021-9258 (Linking)

Shinder, G.A., Lacourse, M.C., Minotti, S. & Durham, H.D. (2001). Mutant Cu/Zn-superoxide dismutase proteins have altered solubility and interact with heat shock/stress proteins in models of amyotrophic lateral sclerosis. *J Biol Chem*, 276, 16, (Apr 20), pp. (12791-12796), 0021-9258 (Print) 0021-9258 (Linking)

Shultz, L.D., Sweet, H.O., Davisson, M.T. & Coman, D.R. (1982). 'Wasted', a new mutant of the mouse with abnormalities characteristic to ataxia telangiectasia. *Nature*, 297, 5865, (Jun 3), pp. (402-404), 0028-0836 (Print) 0028-0836 (Linking)

Skehel, P.A., Fabian-Fine, R. & Kandel, E.R. (2000). Mouse VAP33 is associated with the endoplasmic reticulum and microtubules. *Proc Natl Acad Sci U S A*, 97, 3, (Feb 1), pp. (1101-1106), 0027-8424 (Print) 0027-8424 (Linking)

Soussan, L., Burakov, D., Daniels, M.P., Toister-Achituv, M., Porat, A., Yarden, Y. & Elazar, Z. (1999). ERG30, a VAP-33-related protein, functions in protein transport mediated by COPI vesicles. *J Cell Biol*, 146, 2, (Jul 26), pp. (301-311), 0021-9525 (Print) 0021-9525 (Linking)

Sreedharan, J., Blair, I.P., Tripathi, V.B., Hu, X., Vance, C., Rogelj, B., Ackerley, S., Durnall, J.C., Williams, K.L., Buratti, E., Baralle, F., de Belleroche, J., Mitchell, J.D., Leigh, P.N., Al-Chalabi, A., Miller, C.C., Nicholson, G. & Shaw, C.E. (2008). TDP-43 mutations in familial and sporadic amyotrophic lateral sclerosis. *Science*, 319, 5870, (Mar 21), pp. (1668-1672), 1095-9203 (Electronic) 0036-8075 (Linking)

Stallings, N.R., Puttaparthi, K., Luther, C.M., Burns, D.K. & Elliott, J.L. (2010). Progressive motor weakness in transgenic mice expressing human TDP-43. *Neurobiol Dis*, 40, 2, (Nov), pp. (404-414), 1095-953X (Electronic) 0969-9961 (Linking)

Sterneck, E., Kaplan, D.R. & Johnson, P.F. (1996). Interleukin-6 induces expression of peripherin and cooperates with Trk receptor signaling to promote neuronal differentiation in PC12 cells. *J Neurochem*, 67, 4, (Oct), pp. (1365-1374), 0022-3042 (Print) 0022-3042 (Linking)

Stoppini, L., Buchs, P.A. & Muller, D. (1991). A simple method for organotypic cultures of nervous tissue. *J Neurosci Methods*, 37, 2, (Apr), pp. (173-182), 0165-0270 (Print) 0165-0270 (Linking)

Storkebaum, E., Lambrechts, D. & Carmeliet, P. (2004). VEGF: once regarded as a specific angiogenic factor, now implicated in neuroprotection. *Bioessays*, 26, 9, (Sep), pp. (943-954), 0265-9247 (Print) 0265-9247 (Linking)

Strong, M.J. (2003). The basic aspects of therapeutics in amyotrophic lateral sclerosis. *Pharmacol Ther*, 98, 3, (Jun), pp. (379-414), 0163-7258 (Print) 0163-7258 (Linking)

Strong, M.J. & Volkening, K. (2011). TDP-43 and FUS/TLS: Sending a complex message about messenger RNA in Amyotrophic Lateral Sclerosis? *FEBS J*, (Aug 2), 1742-4658 (Electronic) 1742-464X (Linking)

Sugai, F., Yamamoto, Y., Miyaguchi, K., Zhou, Z., Sumi, H., Hamasaki, T., Goto, M. & Sakoda, S. (2004). Benefit of valproic acid in suppressing disease progression of ALS model mice. *Eur J Neurosci*, 20, 11, (Dec), pp. (3179-3183), 0953-816X (Print) 0953-816X (Linking)

Tainer, J.A., Getzoff, E.D., Beem, K.M., Richardson, J.S. & Richardson, D.C. (1982). Determination and analysis of the 2 A-structure of copper, zinc superoxide dismutase. *J Mol Biol*, 160, 2, (Sep 15), pp. (181-217), 0022-2836 (Print) 0022-2836 (Linking)

Tolosa, L., Mir, M., Asensio, V.J., Olmos, G. & Llado, J. (2008). Vascular endothelial growth factor protects spinal cord motoneurons against glutamate-induced excitotoxicity via phosphatidylinositol 3-kinase. *J Neurochem*, 105, 4, (May), pp. (1080-1090), 1471-4159 (Electronic) 0022-3042 (Linking)

Troy, C.M., Muma, N.A., Greene, L.A., Price, D.L. & Shelanski, M.L. (1990). Regulation of peripherin and neurofilament expression in regenerating rat motor neurons. *Brain Res*, 529, 1-2, (Oct 8), pp. (232-238), 0006-8993 (Print) 0006-8993 (Linking)

Tudor, E.L., Galtrey, C.M., Perkinton, M.S., Lau, K.F., De Vos, K.J., Mitchell, J.C., Ackerley, S., Hortobagyi, T., Vamos, E., Leigh, P.N., Klasen, C., McLoughlin, D.M., Shaw, C.E. & Miller, C.C. (2010). Amyotrophic lateral sclerosis mutant vesicle-associated membrane protein-associated protein-B transgenic mice develop TAR-DNA-binding protein-43 pathology. *Neuroscience*, 167, 3, (May 19), pp. (774-785), 1873-7544 (Electronic) 0306-4522 (Linking)

Van Damme, P., Van Den Bosch, L., Van Houtte, E., Callewaert, G. & Robberecht, W. (2002). GluR2-dependent properties of AMPA receptors determine the selective vulnerability of motor neurons to excitotoxicity. *J Neurophysiol*, 88, 3, (Sep), pp. (1279-1287), 0022-3077 (Print) 0022-3077 (Linking)

Van Deerlin, V.M., Leverenz, J.B., Bekris, L.M., Bird, T.D., Yuan, W., Elman, L.B., Clay, D., Wood, E.M., Chen-Plotkin, A.S., Martinez-Lage, M., Steinbart, E., McCluskey, L., Grossman, M., Neumann, M., Wu, I.L., Yang, W.S., Kalb, R., Galasko, D.R., Montine, T.J., Trojanowski, J.Q., Lee, V.M., Schellenberg, G.D. & Yu, C.E. (2008). TARDBP mutations in amyotrophic lateral sclerosis with TDP-43 neuropathology: a genetic and histopathological analysis. *Lancet Neurol*, 7, 5, (May), pp. (409-416), 1474-4422 (Print) 1474-4422 (Linking)

Vance, C., Rogelj, B., Hortobagyi, T., De Vos, K.J., Nishimura, A.L., Sreedharan, J., Hu, X., Smith, B., Ruddy, D., Wright, P., Ganesalingam, J., Williams, K.L., Tripathi, V., Al-Saraj, S., Al-Chalabi, A., Leigh, P.N., Blair, I.P., Nicholson, G., de Belleroche, J., Gallo, J.M., Miller, C.C. & Shaw, C.E. (2009). Mutations in FUS, an RNA processing protein, cause familial amyotrophic lateral sclerosis type 6. *Science*, 323, 5918, (Feb 27), pp. (1208-1211), 1095-9203 (Electronic) 0036-8075 (Linking)

Vercelli, A., Mereuta, O.M., Garbossa, D., Muraca, G., Mareschi, K., Rustichelli, D., Ferrero, I., Mazzini, L., Madon, E. & Fagioli, F. (2008). Human mesenchymal stem cell transplantation extends survival, improves motor performance and decreases neuroinflammation in mouse model of amyotrophic lateral sclerosis. *Neurobiol Dis*, 31, 3, (Sep), pp. (395-405), 1095-953X (Electronic) 0969-9961 (Linking)

Vogelsberg-Ragaglia, V., Bruce, J., Richter-Landsberg, C., Zhang, B., Hong, M., Trojanowski, J.Q. & Lee, V.M. (2000). Distinct FTDP-17 missense mutations in tau produce tau aggregates and other pathological phenotypes in transfected CHO cells. *Mol Biol Cell*, 11, 12, (Dec), pp. (4093-4104), 1059-1524 (Print) 1059-1524 (Linking)

Wang, F.C., Bouquiaux, O., De Pasqua, V. & Delwaide, P.J. (2002). Changes in motor unit numbers in patients with ALS: a longitudinal study using the adapted multiple point stimulation method. *Amyotroph Lateral Scler Other Motor Neuron Disord*, 3, 1, (Mar), pp. (31-38), 1466-0822 (Print) 1466-0822 (Linking)

Wang, J., Farr, G.W., Hall, D.H., Li, F., Furtak, K., Dreier, L. & Horwich, A.L. (2009). An ALS-linked mutant SOD1 produces a locomotor defect associated with aggregation and synaptic dysfunction when expressed in neurons of Caenorhabditis elegans. *PLoS Genet*, 5, 1, (Jan), pp. (e1000350), 1553-7404 (Electronic) 1553-7390 (Linking)

Wang, J., Slunt, H., Gonzales, V., Fromholt, D., Coonfield, M., Copeland, N.G., Jenkins, N.A. & Borchelt, D.R. (2003). Copper-binding-site-null SOD1 causes ALS in transgenic mice: aggregates of non-native SOD1 delineate a common feature. *Hum Mol Genet*, 12, 21, (Nov 1), pp. (2753-2764), 0964-6906 (Print) 0964-6906 (Linking)

Wang, J., Xu, G., Li, H., Gonzales, V., Fromholt, D., Karch, C., Copeland, N.G., Jenkins, N.A. & Borchelt, D.R. (2005). Somatodendritic accumulation of misfolded SOD1-L126Z in motor neurons mediates degeneration: alphaB-crystallin modulates aggregation. *Hum Mol Genet*, 14, 16, (Aug 15), pp. (2335-2347), 0964-6906 (Print) 0964-6906 (Linking)

Watanabe, Y., Kuno, N., Kono, Y., Nanba, E., Ohama, E., Nakashima, K. & Takahashi, K. (1997). Absence of the mutant SOD1 in familial amyotrophic lateral sclerosis (FALS) with two base pair deletion in the SOD1 gene. *Acta Neurol Scand*, 95, 3, (Mar), pp. (167-172), 0001-6314 (Print) 0001-6314 (Linking)

Watanabe, Y., Yasui, K., Nakano, T., Doi, K., Fukada, Y., Kitayama, M., Ishimoto, M., Kurihara, S., Kawashima, M., Fukuda, H., Adachi, Y., Inoue, T. & Nakashima, K. (2005). Mouse motor neuron disease caused by truncated SOD1 with or without C-terminal modification. *Brain Res Mol Brain Res*, 135, 1-2, (Apr 27), pp. (12-20), 0169-328X (Print) 0169-328X (Linking)

Wegorzewska, I., Bell, S., Cairns, N.J., Miller, T.M. & Baloh, R.H. (2009). TDP-43 mutant transgenic mice develop features of ALS and frontotemporal lobar degeneration. *Proc Natl Acad Sci U S A*, 106, 44, (Nov 3), pp. (18809-18814), 1091-6490 (Electronic) 0027-8424 (Linking)

Wiese, S., Herrmann, T., Drepper, C., Jablonka, S., Funk, N., Klausmeyer, A., Rogers, M.L., Rush, R. & Sendtner, M. (2010). Isolation and enrichment of embryonic mouse motoneurons from the lumbar spinal cord of individual mouse embryos. *Nat Protoc*, 5, 1, pp. (31-38), 1750-2799 (Electronic) 1750-2799 (Linking)

Williamson, T.L., Bruijn, L.I., Zhu, Q., Anderson, K.L., Anderson, S.D., Julien, J.P. & Cleveland, D.W. (1998). Absence of neurofilaments reduces the selective vulnerability of motor neurons and slows disease caused by a familial amyotrophic lateral sclerosis-linked superoxide dismutase 1 mutant. *Proc Natl Acad Sci U S A*, 95, 16, (Aug 4), pp. (9631-9636), 0027-8424 (Print) 0027-8424 (Linking)

Wils, H., Kleinberger, G., Janssens, J., Pereson, S., Joris, G., Cuijt, I., Smits, V., Ceuterick-de Groote, C., Van Broeckhoven, C. & Kumar-Singh, S. (2010). TDP-43 transgenic mice develop spastic paralysis and neuronal inclusions characteristic of ALS and frontotemporal lobar degeneration. *Proc Natl Acad Sci U S A*, 107, 8, (Feb 23), pp. (3858-3863), 1091-6490 (Electronic) 0027-8424 (Linking)

Wong, P.C., Pardo, C.A., Borchelt, D.R., Lee, M.K., Copeland, N.G., Jenkins, N.A., Sisodia, S.S., Cleveland, D.W. & Price, D.L. (1995). An adverse property of a familial ALS-linked SOD1 mutation causes motor neuron disease characterized by vacuolar degeneration of mitochondria. *Neuron*, 14, 6, (Jun), pp. (1105-1116), 0896-6273 (Print) 0896-6273 (Linking)

Xiao, S., Sanelli, T., Dib, S., Sheps, D., Findlater, J., Bilbao, J., Keith, J., Zinman, L., Rogaeva, E. & Robertson, J. (2011). RNA targets of TDP-43 identified by UV-CLIP are deregulated in ALS. *Mol Cell Neurosci*, 47, 3, (Jul), pp. (167-180), 1095-9327 (Electronic) 1044-7431 (Linking)

Xu, Y.F., Gendron, T.F., Zhang, Y.J., Lin, W.L., D'Alton, S., Sheng, H., Casey, M.C., Tong, J., Knight, J., Yu, X., Rademakers, R., Boylan, K., Hutton, M., McGowan, E., Dickson,

D.W., Lewis, J. & Petrucelli, L. (2010). Wild-type human TDP-43 expression causes TDP-43 phosphorylation, mitochondrial aggregation, motor deficits, and early mortality in transgenic mice. *J Neurosci*, 30, 32, (Aug 11), pp. (10851-10859), 1529-2401 (Electronic) 0270-6474 (Linking)

Xu, Z., Cork, L.C., Griffin, J.W. & Cleveland, D.W. (1993). Increased expression of neurofilament subunit NF-L produces morphological alterations that resemble the pathology of human motor neuron disease. *Cell*, 73, 1, (Apr 9), pp. (23-33), 0092-8674 (Print) 0092-8674 (Linking)

Yamanaka, K., Miller, T.M., McAlonis-Downes, M., Chun, S.J. & Cleveland, D.W. (2006). Progressive spinal axonal degeneration and slowness in ALS2-deficient mice. *Ann Neurol*, 60, 1, (Jul), pp. (95-104), 0364-5134 (Print) 0364-5134 (Linking)

Yip, P.K., Kaan, T.K., Fenesan, D. & Malcangio, M. (2009). Rapid isolation and culture of primary microglia from adult mouse spinal cord. *J Neurosci Methods*, 183, 2, (Oct 15), pp. (223-237), 1872-678X (Electronic) 0165-0270 (Linking)

Yokoseki, A., Shiga, A., Tan, C.F., Tagawa, A., Kaneko, H., Koyama, A., Eguchi, H., Tsujino, A., Ikeuchi, T., Kakita, A., Okamoto, K., Nishizawa, M., Takahashi, H. & Onodera, O. (2008). TDP-43 mutation in familial amyotrophic lateral sclerosis. *Ann Neurol*, 63, 4, (Apr), pp. (538-542), 1531-8249 (Electronic) 0364-5134 (Linking)

Zhou, H., Huang, C., Chen, H., Wang, D., Landel, C.P., Xia, P.Y., Bowser, R., Liu, Y.J. & Xia, X.G. (2010). Transgenic rat model of neurodegeneration caused by mutation in the TDP gene. *PLoS Genet*, 6, 3, (Mar), pp. (e1000887), 1553-7404 (Electronic) 1553-7390 (Linking)

Zhu, Q., Couillard-Despres, S. & Julien, J.P. (1997). Delayed maturation of regenerating myelinated axons in mice lacking neurofilaments. *Exp Neurol*, 148, 1, (Nov), pp. (299-316), 0014-4886 (Print) 0014-4886 (Linking)

6

Electrophysiological Abnormalities in SOD1 Transgenic Models in Amyotrophic Lateral Sclerosis: The Commonalities and Differences

Sherif M. Elbasiouny[1], Katharina A. Quinlan[1],
Tahra L. Eissa[4] and Charles J. Heckman[1,2,3]
[1]*Departments of Physiology, Northwestern University*
[2]*Physical Medicine and Rehabilitation, Northwestern University*
[3]*Physical Therapy and Human Movement Sciences, Northwestern University*
[4]*Department of Biological and Environmental Engineering, Cornell University*
USA

1. Introduction

Since its first description in 1874 by Charcot, the hallmark feature of ALS is the progressive degeneration of upper and lower motoneurons (Charcot, 1874). In the spinal cord, motoneuron degeneration starts long before symptom onset and advances in a size-related fashion, in which large-size alpha-motoneurons degenerate first followed by small-size alpha-motoneurons (Pun et al., 2006; Hegedus et al., 2007; Hegedus et al., 2008). There are conflicting reports regarding the survival of the smallest-sized spinal motoneurons, the gamma-motoneurons (Swash and Fox, 1974; Sobue et al., 1981). Despite its original description, the neuronal degeneration in ALS is not limited to motoneurons. Recent reports have shown evidence for degeneration of neurons in the brain (Karim et al., 1998; Lloyd et al., 2000; Maekawa et al., 2004) and interneurons in the spinal cord (Konno et al., 1986; Williams et al., 1990; Takahashi et al., 1993; Stephens et al., 2006).

Before their degeneration, spinal motoneurons experience progressive changes in their properties. These changes result from the pathological actions of the disease and the compensatory mechanisms of the nervous system to mitigate the neuronal malfunction. In this chapter, we describe the changes in the anatomical and electrical properties of spinal motoneurons in various genetic mouse models of ALS and critically analyze literature for the common and different pathological features across these models. We also present data from computer simulations showing the consequences of the alterations in properties of mutant motoneurons on cell excitability and dendritic processing of synaptic inputs. The presented computational analysis allowed for the identification of motoneuron alterations undetectable using standard electrophysiological methods. This information is essential for understanding motoneuron pathophysiology in ALS.

2. The changes in motoneuron anatomical properties

One of the earliest abnormalities in transgenic mouse models of ALS is the change in anatomy of spinal motoneurons. In the G85R model, it has been shown that mutant motoneurons exhibit an increase in the overall cell size and branching pattern of dendrites (Amendola et al., 2007; Amendola and Durand, 2008). These changes appear in transgenic mice at 10 days after birth (P10), long before disease onset and life end-stage (225 and 240 days, respectively) (Bruijn et al., 1997). More specifically, in mutant motoneurons the total dendritic surface area and total dendritic length are increased by 58% and 65% relative to wild-type (WT) cells, respectively. For dendritic branching, the number of dendritic branches, terminal branches, branching nodes, and maximum branching order are increased by 93%, 89%, 97%, 37%, respectively (Fig. 1). On the other hand, the soma size (diameter and surface area) and primary dendrites properties (number, diameter, and cross-sectional area) are similar in WT and mutant motoneurons. Interestingly, the increase in number of branches occurs primarily in short branches (dendritic branches with path length < 100μm) and most of the anatomical changes take place over the middle dendrites (200μm - 500μm from the soma). Surprisingly, the longest dendritic length from the soma was not increased in mutant motoneurons, indicating that dendritic overbranching occurs mainly within the cell circumjacent. In other words, the cell does not swell into larger space in the cord but develops more branching within its dendritic spatial field.

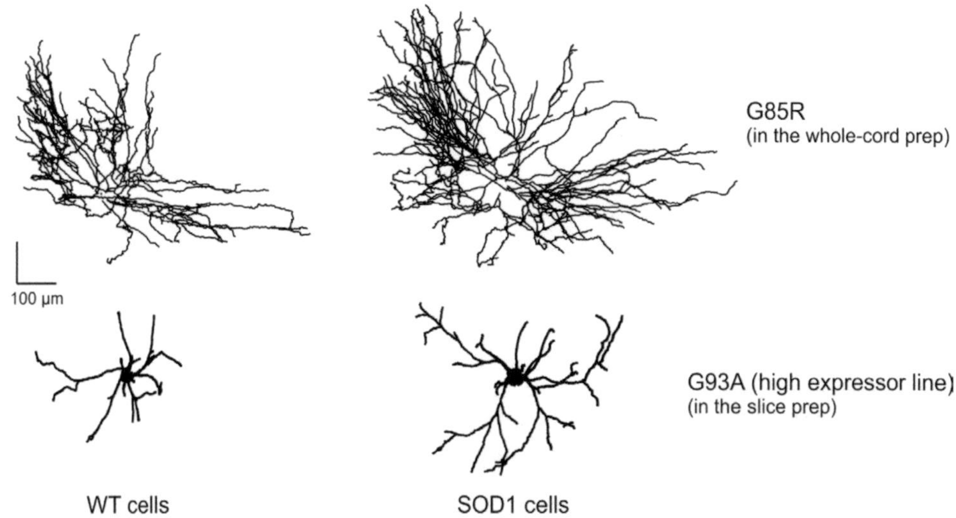

Fig. 1. Anatomical alterations in mutant motoneurons of the G85R (reconstructed from the whole-cord prep[1]) and G93A (high expressor line) (reconstructed from the slice prep.) transgenic models relative to WT cells. [1]: data from Amendola and Durand (2008).

Similar early abnormalities in the anatomical properties of motoneurons have been found in other transgenic mouse models of ALS. In the G93A (low expressor line), which expresses 8 copies of the human SOD1 gene, mutant motoneurons at P9 exhibit increased cell size, dendritic overbranching, and dendritic complexity (Filipchuk et al., 2010). The total dendritic length and number of branching nodes and terminal dendrites in mutant motoneurons were significantly increased relative to WT. Similar to the G85R transgenic model, these anatomical changes in the G93A (low expressor line) model occur early in the disease (at P9) way before symptom development (between 195 and 240 days) and end stage (between 240 and 270 days). Preliminary data from our laboratory obtained in the slice preparation show that neonatal mutant motoneurons (P7) of the G93A (high expressor line), which expresses 25 copies of the human SOD1 gene, experience analogous alterations in their morphology and dendritic branching (Fig. 1), in which the soma surface area, numbers of dendritic branches and terminal dendrites increase significantly relative to WT.

Post-mortem morphological analysis of large neurons in the ventral horn of spinal cord indicated an increase in the initial segment diameter, by 36%, in ALS patients (Sasaki and Maruyama, 1992). Conversely, the soma area of these neurons was smaller by 16% relative to control (Sasaki and Maruyama, 1992).

The similar findings on the anatomical alterations of neonatal motoneurons in various transgenic models of ALS indicate that the increase in cell size and dendritic overbranching are characteristic abnormalities in motoneuron pathophysiology in ALS. However, it is unclear whether the alteration in motoneuron anatomy is a disease mechanism or an adaptive response (see section 7 for discussion). Furthermore, it is important to understand the functional ramifications of the motoneuron anatomical alterations on the cell excitability and electrical properties and to what extent the anatomical alterations contribute to motoneuron degeneration in ALS (see section 6).

3. The changes in motoneuron electrical properties

3.1 The change in input resistance

Changes in a number of motoneuron electrical properties were reported in the transgenic mouse models of ALS. However, one challenge in the field of ALS is the large variability in data of mutant motoneuron electrical properties, which makes recording from a large number of cells is important to allow statistical tests to detect significant differences in electrophysiological properties between WT and mutant motoneuron samples. Table 1 summarizes the changes in electrical properties of mutant motoneurons observed in the various ALS transgenic mouse models. The summary shows that the changes in electrical properties involve the motoneuron passive properties (e.g., cell input resistance), the size and shape of the action potential spike and afterhyperpolarization, the amplitude of voltage-sensitive ionic currents, and the motoneuron excitability and firing activity. However, some of these changes were inconsistent (i.e., not observed consistently) across the ALS transgenic models, whereas others were contradictory (i.e., opposite changes were observed). For instance, the decrease in input resistance of mutant motoneurons relative to WT is an inconsistent finding in ALS transgenic models (see table 1, column 7). This observation was seen in some studies (Bories et al., 2007; ElBasiouny et al., 2010; Quinlan et al., 2011), whereas other studies did not find a statistically significant difference between the input resistance of WT and mutant motoneurons (Pieri et al., 2003; Kuo et al., 2004; Kuo et al., 2005; van Zundert et al., 2008; Pambo-Pambo et al., 2009; Pieri et al., 2009; Filipchuk et al., 2010; Meehan et al., 2010). The changes in action potential size and width in mutant motoneurons, on the other hand, is a conflicting finding in which some studies reported an increase in spike height (van Zundert et al., 2008) and duration (Fuchs et al., 2008, 2009; Pambo-Pambo et al., 2009) relative to WT, whereas others reported reduction in spike height (Kuo et al., 2004; Pambo-Pambo et al., 2009; Filipchuk et al., 2010) and duration (Pieri et al., 2003; Quinlan et al., 2011).

Publication	Model	Preparation	Age	Neuron Type	$[Ca^{2+}]_o$	R_{in} in mutant neurons	V_{rest} and AP properties in mutant neurons	AHP in mutant neurons	PIC properties in mutant neurons	F-I gain & firing properties in mutant neurons
(Pieri et al., 2003)	G93A (high)	Embryonic Culture	E15: 7-12 days	SMNs	2mM	No diff	↓AP duration ↑AP repol rate	No diff	n/a	↑firing freq
(Kuo et al., 2004)	G93A (high)	Organotypic slice culture	P7: 3 weeks	SMNs	2.4mM	No diff	No diff	No diff	n/a	↑F-I gain ↑max firing
	G93A (high)	Embryonic culture	E13: 12-14 days	SMNs	2.8mM	No diff	↓AP height	No diff	n/a	↑F-I gain
(Kuo et al., 2005)	G93A (high)	Embryonic Culture	E13: 10-30 days	SMNs	2.8mM	No diff	Depolarized Vrest in high conductance MNs	No diff	↑NaPIC (measured in VC)	↓rheobase ↑F-I gain ↑spontaneous firing in high conductance MNs
(Bories et al., 2007)	G85R	Whole-cord	P6-10	SMNs	4mM	↓by 30%	No diff	No diff	n/a	↓ F-I gain ↑rheobase
(van Zundert et al., 2008)	G93A (high)	Brainstem slice	P4-10	HGMNs & OINs	2mM	No diff	↑AP height	No diff	↑NaPIC (measured in VC)	↑firing freq
(Fuchs et al., 2008) (Fuchs et al., 2009)	G93A (high)	Brainstem slice	P80-120	HGMNs & OMNs	2mM	No diff	HGMNs (P120): ↑AP duration ↓AP repol rate	At P120: $\downarrow fAHP_{amp}$ $\uparrow mAHP_{amp}$	No diff	No diff
(Pambo-Pambo et al., 2009)	G93A (low)	Lumbar slice	P6-10	SMNs	2mM	No diff	↓AP height ↑AP half-width ↓AP rise & decay slopes Depolarized Vrest	No diff	No diff (measured in VC) ↓total PIC (estimated from ΔI data)	↑F-I gain (pulses)

Publication	Model	Preparation	Age	Neuron Type	$[Ca^{2+}]_o$	R_{in} in mutant neurons	V_{rest} and AP properties in mutant neurons	AHP in mutant neurons	PIC properties in mutant neurons	F-I gain & firing properties in mutant neurons
(Pambo-Pambo et al., 2009)	G85R	Lumbar slice	P6-10	SMNs	2mM	No diff	No diff	No diff	No diff (measured in VC) ↓total PIC (estimated from ΔI data)	↓F-I gain (ramp)
(Pieri et al., 2009)	G93A (high)	Cell culture	E15: 11-12 days	CNs	2mM	No diff	↓AP threshold	n/a	↑NaPIC (measured in VC)	↑firing freq ↓rheobase
(Meehan et al., 2010)	G127X	In-vivo lumbar cord	P240	SMNs	n/a	No diff	n/a	No diff	↑PIC (estimated from firing profiles)	No diff ↓Spike freq adaptation
(ElBasiouny et al., 2010)	G85R	Whole-cord	P8-10	SMNs	2mM	↓by 30%	No diff	No diff	n/a	No diff
(Filipchuk et al., 2010)	G93A (low)	Whole-cord	P8-9	SMNs	2mM	No diff	↓ AP height ↓AP rise and decay slopes	No diff	n/a	No diff
(Quinlan et al., 2011)	G93A (high)	Lumbar slice	P0-12	SMNs	2.5mM	↓by 19%	↓AP duration ↑AP rise and decay slopes	↓AHP time constant	↑Na & Ca PICs (measured in VC)	No diff

Table 1. Summary of the alterations in mutant motoneuron properties. SMNs: spinal motoneurons, CNs: cortical neurons, HGMNs: hypoglossal motoneurons, OMNs: ocular motoneurons, OINs: ocular interneurons. $[Ca2+]_o$: extracellular calcium concentration, R_{in}: input resistance, V_{rest}: resting membrane potential, AP: action potential, AHP: afterhyperpolarization, PIC: persistent inward current, F-I: frequency-current relationship. VC: voltage-clamp, ΔI: the difference in injected current at motoneuron recruitment and de-recruitment on a triangular current command, No diff: no difference.

3.1.1 Effect of tissue preparation

The discrepancy in the changes of electrical properties of mutant motoneurons probably results partially from the differences in transgenic model types (e.g., G85R, G93A high or low expressor lines) and is compounded by the variability in experimental conditions such as animal age (e.g., neonatal, pre- or post-symptomatic adult motoneurons) and tissue preparation (e.g., cell culture, slice, whole-cord, or in-vivo), in addition to the recording conditions (e.g., extracellular Ca^{2+} concentrations) and measurement methods (current- or voltage-clamp). However, critical analysis of the changes in electrical properties of mutant motoneurons shows that common pathological features could be identified across the various ALS transgenic models, whereas other features could be related to experimental conditions. For instance, the decrease in input resistance was detected mainly in studies conducted on the whole-cord preparation (in which the brainstem and spinal cord are intact), but was not observed in studies on motoneurons in cell culture or slice preparations (Table 1). Because input resistance is an indirect measure of cell size, it becomes reduced in mutant motoneurons to reflect the enlargement in motoneuron anatomy discussed in the previous section. In the whole-cord preparation, the motoneuron dendrites are completely intact and their effect on input resistance is more easily detected. In the slice preparation, conversely, the motoneuron dendrites are truncated at the surface of the slice. The lack of the middle and distal portions of dendrites could mask the anatomical differences between WT and mutant motoneurons and would explain the disappearance of input resistance differences between WT and mutant motoneurons in the slice preparation. Table 2 shows a comparison of the input resistance values of neonatal motoneurons in the various transgenic models of ALS. In the G85R and G93A (low expressor line) models, the input resistance values in the whole-cord preparation (ElBasiouny et al., 2010; Filipchuk et al., 2010) were on average half of those in the slice preparation (Pambo-Pambo et al., 2009), indicating that nearly half of the dendrites were severed in the slice preparation. Strikingly, the decrease in input resistance of mutant motoneurons of the G93A (high expressor line) model was still detected in the slice preparation in Quinlan et al. (2011). This could indicate that the motoneuron anatomical alterations in the G93A (high expressor line) model are so extensive that they were still substantial in the slice preparation and/or the motoneuron membrane biophysical properties change considerably in the G93A (high expressor line) model and contribute significantly to the decrease in input resistance (see section 4). For cell culture, given that the trigger signal for the alteration in motoneuron anatomy is poorly understood and could result from the alteration in motoneuron excitability and synaptic inputs (Duch et al., 2008), mutant motoneurons in the cell culture preparation might not experience anatomical alterations due to their isolation (in the cell culture) from the pathological neural circuit (in the transgenic mouse spinal cord), leading to absence of differences in input resistance between WT and mutant motoneurons.

3.1.2 Effect of extracellular Ca^{2+} concentration

The measurement of input resistance values, and other electrical properties, in mutant motoneurons also depends on the extracellular concentration of Ca^{2+} ions in the recording solution. For instance, the input resistance value of neonatal motoneurons of the G85R model measured in 4mM of extracellular Ca^{2+} concentration (Bories et al., 2007) was double of that measured in 2mM of extracellular Ca^{2+} concentration (ElBasiouny et al., 2010) (see table 2). Although 2mM is typical, the variability in extracellular Ca^{2+} concentration (ranging between 2mM and 4mM, see table 1) among the various ALS studies could contribute to the discrepancies in electrical properties of mutant motoneurons. This effect is produced because the level of extracellular Ca^{2+} concentration modulates the magnitude of the motoneuronal Ca^{2+}-gated (e.g., Cav 1.2, 1.3, and 2.2 channels) and Ca^{2+}-activated (e.g., SK and Ih channels) ionic currents, which regulate the motoneuron firing activity and affect the action potential and afterhyperpolarization properties.

Model	Publication	Preparation	$[Ca^{2+}]_o$	R_{in} WT/SOD1	Anatomical alterations
G93A (high)	Quinlan et al. (2011)	Slice	2mM	38.5/31.3 MΩ (↓ by 19%)*	Yes[1]
G85R	Bories et al. (2007)	Whole-cord	4mM	33.3/23.8 MΩ (↓ by 29%)*	Yes[2]
	ElBasiouny et al. (2010)	Whole-cord	2mM	16.2/11.4 MΩ (↓ by 30%)*	
	Pambo-Pambo et al. (2009)	Slice	2mM	34.5/33.1 MΩ ns	
G93A (low)	Pambo-Pambo et al. (2009)	Slice	2mM	34.5/37.2 MΩ ns	Yes[3]
	Filipchuk et al. (2010)	Whole-cord	2mM	18.5/16.1 MΩ ns	

Table 2. Comparison of the change in input resistance in mutant motoneurons (P6-P10) in the various ALS transgenic models. [1]: unpublished data, [2]: Amendola and Durand (2008), [3]: Filipchuk et al. (2010), *: statistically-significant ($p<0.05$), ns: not statistically-significant.

In sum, the reduction in input resistance of mutant motoneurons is a common, early pathological feature in the G93A (high expressor line) and G85R transgenic models, but not in the G93A (low expressor line). Also, this abnormality might sometimes not be evident depending on the tissue preparation used in the experiment.

3.2 The changes in action potential and afterhyperpolarization

A change in the action potential properties was frequently seen in mutant motoneurons relative to WT; however, these changes were conflicting across the transgenic models (Table 1, Fig. 2). In the G93A (high expressor line) model, neonatal spinal motoneurons frequently showed faster action potential rate of rise and decay and shorter action potential duration (Pieri et al., 2003; Quinlan et al., 2011), indicating an increase in transient and persistent Na^+ currents, which act to increase the excitability of mutant motoneurons. Signs of increased excitability were differently displayed in other studies as an increase in spike height (van Zundert et al., 2008), depolarization in resting membrane potential (Kuo et al., 2005), or reduction in action potential threshold (Pieri et al., 2009). Conversely, an increase in action potential duration and deceleration in rate of repolarization were observed in post-symptomatic adult hypoglossal motoneurons (Fuchs et al., 2009).

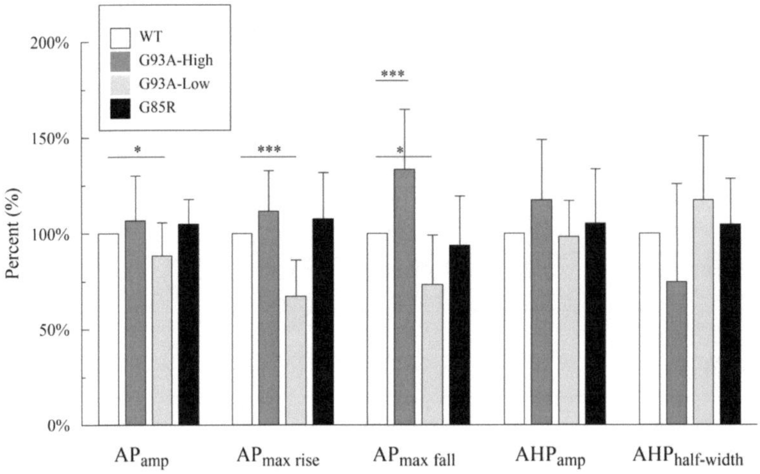

Fig. 2. The changes in action potential height (AP_{amp}), maximum rise ($AP_{max\ rise}$) and fall ($AP_{max\ fall}$) rates, and AHP amplitude (AHP_{amp}) and half-width ($AHP_{half\text{-}width}$) in mutant motoneurons of the G93A (high expressor line) [2nd bars][1], G93A (high expressor line) [3rd bars][2], and the G85R [last bars][2] transgenic models, relative to WT [1st bars]. All reported data from slice preparation. [1]: Quinlan et al. (2011), [2]: Pambo-Pambo et al. (2009).

In the G93A (low expressor line) model, neonatal spinal motoneurons exhibited a reduction in action potential height, increase in half-width, and deceleration in the rates of rise and decay (Pambo-Pambo et al., 2009; Filipchuk et al., 2010). In the G85R model, no changes were observed in the properties of the action potential regardless of the tissue preparation (whole-cord or slice) and extracellular Ca^{2+} concentration (2mM or 4mM) (Bories et al., 2007; Pambo-Pambo et al., 2009; ElBasiouny et al., 2010). Therefore, it appears that the alteration in action potential properties is not a common pathological characteristic, but depends on the ALS transgenic model type.
The after-spike afterhyperpolarization was not consistently altered in mutant motoneurons across the various transgenic models (Table 1, Fig. 2).

3.3 The change in persistent inward currents

Persistent inward currents are intrinsic Na^{+} and Ca^{2+} currents that depolarize the membrane potential when activated. Contrary to transient ionic currents, these currents do not inactivate with prolonged membrane depolarization (Schwindt and Crill, 1977). A change in the motoneuron persistent inward current was frequently observed in mutant motoneurons (Table 1, Fig. 3); however, conflicting data were reported on the nature of this change (i.e., increase or decrease). In the G93A (high expressor line) model, an increase in the Na^{+} persistent inward current of neonatal mutant motoneurons was consistently reported regardless of tissue preparation (cell culture and slice) or extracellular Ca^{2+} concentration (Table 1). In the G93A (low expressor line) and G85R models, persistent inward current measured in voltage-clamp protocols indicated no change in their amplitude between WT and mutant motoneurons, whereas persistent inward current estimated from the delta I (ΔI) technique indicated a reduction in their amplitude in mutant motoneurons relative to WT (Pambo-Pambo et al., 2009). The former is a more truthful result because voltage-clamp protocols allow direct measurement of the persistent inward current, whereas the ΔI technique (which is obtained from the difference in injected current at motoneuron recruitment and de-recruitment on a triangular current command) provides an indirect estimate of the persistent inward current amplitude (Bennett et al., 2001) and is sensitive to the inactivation of transient Na^+ channels (Miles et al., 2005) and activation of residual outward currents present in the motoneuron membrane (Hamm et al., 2010). However, it should be noted that the number of cells in which the voltage-clamp measurements were obtained was small. In the infrequently studied G127X transgenic model, an increase in the persistent inward current amplitude was estimated from the motoneuron firing profile (Meehan et al., 2010). However, this result is unconfirmed given that firing profile in mutant motoneurons would be also influenced by any differences in inward or outward currents and electrical properties of mutant motoneurons. Accordingly, the change in amplitude of persistent inward currents is not a common abnormality in the various ALS transgenic models. However, it appears that persistent inward currents are increased only in the G93A (high expressor line) transgenic model.

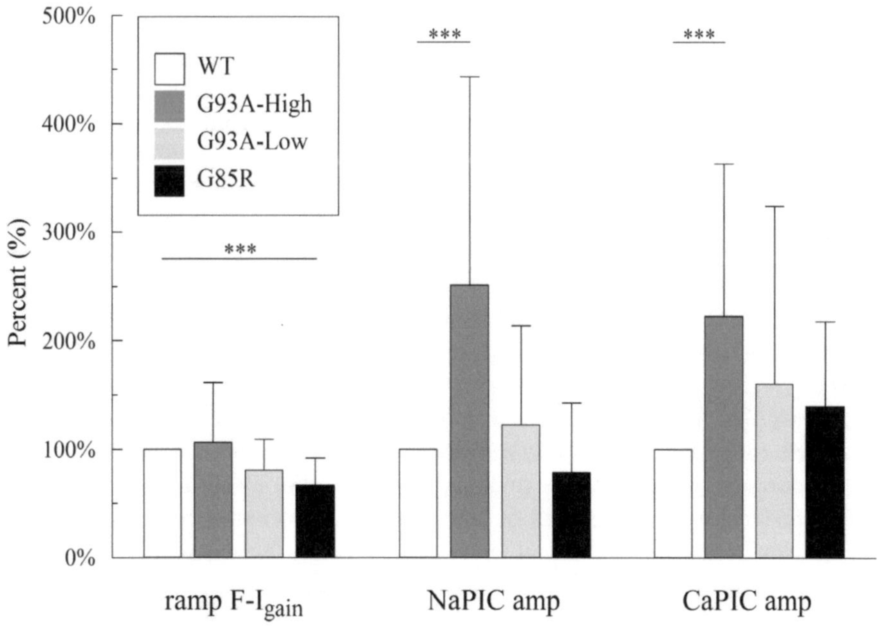

Fig. 3. The changes in ramp frequency-current relationship gain (ramp $F\text{-}I_{gain}$), sodium (NaPIC) and calcium (CaPIC) persistent inward currents in mutant motoneurons of the G93A (high expressor line) [2nd bars][1], G93A (high expressor line) [3rd bars][2], and the G85R [last bars][2] transgenic models, relative to WT [1st bars]. All reported data from slice preparation. [1]: Quinlan et al. (2011), [2]: Pambo-Pambo et al. (2009).

3.4 The change in motoneuron gain and firing activity

A change in the motoneuron gain (i.e., F-I relationship slope) or firing activity was commonly seen in mutant motoneurons, but conflicting observations were also reported. In the G93A (high expressor line) transgenic model, the firing activity and gain of mutant spinal motoneurons were consistently increased in cell culture (Pieri et al., 2003; Kuo et al.,

2004; Kuo et al., 2005; Zona et al., 2006; Pieri et al., 2009), but not in the slice (Quinlan et al., 2011) (Table 1). In the G85R transgenic model, the gain of mutant motoneurons was consistently reduced relative to WT (Bories et al., 2007; Pambo-Pambo et al., 2009). In the G93A (low expressor line) transgenic model, the gain of mutant motoneurons was increased in the slice preparation (Pambo-Pambo et al., 2009), but did not change in the whole-cord preparation (Filipchuk et al., 2010). The disagreement in reports on the change in motoneuron gain in the various transgenic models could be partially due to the variation in tissue preparation and extracellular Ca^{2+} concentration. Motoneuron dendrites have active conductances, which influence the motoneuron gain. Therefore, the portion of the motoneuron dendrites available during recording in the slice preparation would indirectly affect the measurement of the motoneuron gain in WT and mutant motoneurons. Also, the effect of extracellular Ca^{2+} concentration on the amplitude of Ca^{2+}-activated and Ca^{2+}-gated currents would influence the motoneuron gain measurement based on the degree of existence of these channels in WT and mutant motoneurons. Taken collectively, the change in gain and firing activity of mutant motoneurons is inconsistent within and across the various ALS transgenic models.

3.5 Motoneuron excitability in the various ALS transgenic models

Despite the discrepancy in data on the excitability of mutant motoneurons in the various ALS transgenic models, some insights could be attained from the trend in electrical properties change (Table 3). In the G93A (high expressor line) model, most changes in electrical properties push toward increased excitability of mutant motoneurons. For instance, the increases in action potential height and rise and decay rates and the reduction in action potential width are signs of elevated transient and persistent Na^+ currents that enhance the motoneuron excitability of mutant motoneurons. Also, the increase in persistent inward current amplitude further acts to enhance the motoneuron excitability. Collectively, these mechanisms push toward increased excitability of mutant motoneurons (i.e., excitability enhancement mechanisms). On the other hand, the increase in motoneuron size and reduction in input resistance are mechanisms that counteract increased excitability (i.e., excitability suppressive mechanisms) because the motoneuron becomes harder to recruit. It is unclear whether the excitability enhancement or suppressive mechanisms are disease or compensatory processes; however, the net effect of these mechanisms is increased excitability (i.e., hyperexcitability) of mutant motoneurons in the G93A (high expressor line) model (Table 3). This supposition is supported by the numerous reports on increased gain, although from cultured motoneurons, of mutant motoneurons in this transgenic model.

In the G93A (low expressor line) model, all changes in electrical properties indicate a reduction in the excitability of mutant motoneurons (i.e., hypoexcitability) (Table 3). These changes involve increase in motoneuron size, reduction in input resistance, smaller and broader action potential spikes, and slower rise rate (Table 3). The last two observations are indicative of a decrease in transient and persistent Na^+ currents in mutant motoneurons relative to WT. In contrast to these data, the gain of mutant motoneurons measured using long pulses was higher than that of WT motoneurons; however, the gain measured using current ramp was not different from WT motoneurons (Pambo-Pambo et al., 2009). Taken collectively, more evidence is available on reduced excitability of mutant motoneurons in the G93A (low expressor line).

Model	MN size	R_{in}	AP/AHP	PIC	Gain	Excitability
G93A (high)	↑↑	↓↓	Higher & briefer spikes Faster rise & decay rates	↑↑	↑↑/--	Hyperexcitability
G93A (low)	↑↑	--	Smaller & broader spikes Slower rise & decay rates	--	↑↑/--	More evidence on hypoexcitability
G85R	↑↑	↓↓	--	--	↓↓	Hypoexcitability

Table 3. Summary of changes in motoneuron properties in the various ALS transgenic models. MN: motoneuron, Rin: input resistance, AP/AHP: action potential and afterhyperpolarization, ↑↑: increase, ↓↓: decrease, --: no change.

In the G85R transgenic model, not many changes were reported in the electrical properties of mutant motoneurons; however, these changes were consistent with reduced excitability and are supported by the decrease in gain of mutant motoneurons (Table 3). In conclusion, motoneuron pathophysiology is different in the various transgenic mouse models of ALS and their excitability varies from hypo- to hyperexcitability. This disparity could be related to the number of copies of the human SOD1 gene or the severity of the disease (transgenic models with high copy number of SOD1 genes have more aggressive ALS than transgenic models with low copy number of SOD1 genes). Transgenic models with a low number of SOD1 copies (e.g., G85R and G93A-low expressor line) showed a tendency for reduced excitability of mutant motoneurons, whereas transgenic models with a high number of SOD1 copies (e.g., G93A-high expressor line) showed a tendency for increased excitability of mutant motoneurons. These differences should be considered when studying the motoneuron pathophysiology in these ALS transgenic models.

4. Effect of anatomical alterations on motoneuron electrical properties

The enlarged anatomy of mutant motoneurons has consequences for their electrical properties and firing behaviour. Computer simulations have been used to assess the effect of enlargement in motoneuron anatomy and its contribution to the changes in electrical properties (ElBasiouny et al., 2010). Realistic computer models were developed from the reconstructed morphologies of WT and mutant motoneurons of the G85R model and were optimized to replicate the electrophysiological recordings obtained from individual cells. For the 30% reduction in input resistance of mutant motoneurons relative to WT, computer simulations showed that one third of this reduction (i.e., input resistance decrease by 10%) is due to the enlargement of motoneuron anatomy, whereas two thirds of this reduction (i.e., input resistance decrease by additional 20%) is due to a decrease in the specific membrane resistance of the motoneuron membrane. The specific membrane resistance represents the number of leak channels available in a patch of cell membrane and its decrease means that there are more ion channels inserted into the membrane (i.e., the cell has higher conductance). Comparison of WT and mutant motoneuron models indicated a 25% decrease in the somatic and dendritic specific membrane resistance of the mutant models. Therefore, the simulation results indicate that the enlargement in motoneuron anatomy does not fully account for the reduction in input resistance as previously suggested by Bories et al. (2007). This is because the additional dendritic branches causing the increased surface area are electrotonically distant from the soma, the site of input resistance measurement. This electrotonic separation reduces the influence of the additional dendritic area at the soma. Thus, a 60% increase in total surface area of mutant motoneurons causes only a 10% decrease in cell input resistance (not 40% as would be predicted from the reciprocal of surface area increase of an electrotonically compact sphere). Secondly, the simulation results indicate that the reduction in input resistance of mutant motoneurons is a function of two factors: the enlargement in motoneuron anatomy and the decrease in specific membrane resistance; the weights of these factors determine the magnitude of input resistance reduction. This could explain why the enlargement of motoneuron anatomy was not always associated with reduction in input resistance as in the case of the G93A (low expressor line) model (see Table 2), suggesting an insignificant change in the membrane specific membrane resistance in this transgenic model. In contrast, the significant reduction in input resistance of mutant motoneurons of the G93A (high expressor line) model despite the truncation in motoneuron dendrites in the slice preparation in Quinlan et al. (2011) might indicate a substantial change in the specific membrane resistance in that transgenic model.

The effects of enlargement in mutant motoneuron anatomy are not only limited to cell input resistance, but also extend to cell firing properties. For instance, the enlargement in mutant motoneuron anatomy would be expected to cause reductions in the motoneuron F-I gain and initial and maximum firing rates and increases in rheobase current and total cell capacitance. Given that no change was seen in some of these properties of mutant motoneurons indicate that compensatory mechanisms have masked those effects (e.g., upregulation in motoneuron transient and persistent inward currents). Estimating the contribution of anatomy enlargement to the changes in mutant motoneurons firing activity and identifying potential ionic mechanisms for masking these changes using computer simulations would be an important step in revealing hidden alterations in motoneuron properties and improving our understanding of ALS pathogenesis.

5. The changes in synaptic inputs to motoneurons

In ALS patients and transgenic models, synaptic inputs converging onto motoneurons experience changes during disease progression. These changes involve loss of specific types of synaptic inputs, rearrangement of the synaptic contacts, and alteration in the size of synaptic boutons. For instance, it has been shown that cholinergic synapses on lumbar motoneurons are lost in ALS patients (Nagao et al., 1998). This loss starts before motoneuron degeneration. Given that cholinergic synapses provide inhibitory input to motoneurons (Nagy et al., 1993), their loss could alter the balance toward more excitatory inputs, leading to motoneurons overactivation. This prediction has been confirmed in G93A (high expressor line) transgenic mice in which the ratio of inhibitory to excitatory synapses was reduced due to the loss of inhibitory boutons (loss was mediated by nitric oxide) and increase in excitatory boutons (Sunico et al., 2011). Furthermore, residual inhibitory boutons exhibit shorter active zone length and smaller synaptic vesicle density (Sunico et al., 2011). Along the same line, there was a progressive increase in the

excitability of interneurons, through NMDA receptors, that starts in the presymptomatic stage of ALS (Jiang et al., 2009).
Computer simulations of mutant motoneuron models predicted a reduction in the efficacy of dendritic processing of synaptic inputs early in ALS (ElBasiouny et al., 2010). The amplitude of somatic excitatory postsynaptic potentials (EPSPs) was reduced in mutant motoneurons by 15%, relative to WT. This reduction was comparable to experimental measurements of EPSP amplitudes in the G85R transgenic model (Bories et al., 2007). The computer simulations showed that the reduction in EPSP amplitude resulted from the alteration in various motoneuron properties such as: the increase in motoneuron morphology, the decrease in specific membrane resistance, and the increase in dendritic active conductance activation. The changes in these properties counteract each other and produce the net reduction in EPSP amplitude. These changes were consistent in synaptic inputs with different dynamics (i.e., slow and fast inputs) (ElBasiouny et al., 2010).

6. The functional ramifications of the alteration in motoneuron properties

The combined changes in motoneuron properties (anatomical, electrical, biophysical) and synaptic inputs converging on them in ALS alter the input-output function of mutant motoneurons and affect their recruitment. For instance, the reduction in input resistance of mutant motoneurons makes them harder to recruit. Similarly, the enlargement in motoneuron anatomy and development of dendritic overbranching increase the attenuation of excitatory and inhibitory post synaptic potentials as they flow to the soma along the dendrites and reduce their efficacy. Computer simulations of reconstructed morphologies of WT and mutant motoneurons indicated a reduction in the efficacy of slow and fast synaptic inputs (by ≈20%) in mutant motoneurons (ElBasiouny et al., 2010). Half of this efficacy reduction was due to the dendritic overbranching, whereas the second half was due to the decrease in specific membrane resistance, leading to increased signal loss through leak conductances. The simulations demonstrated that reduction in synaptic efficacy was still present despite the upregulation in the dendritic active conductances mediating persistent inward current. These combined reductions in cell input resistance and synaptic input efficacy push toward reduced excitability of the cell. It is unclear whether these changes represent disease or protective mechanisms (see next section for discussion).

7. Anatomical alterations versus excitability changes: Disease versus neuroprotective mechanisms?

The individual changes seen in properties of mutant motoneurons could be a disease mechanism, which produces a physiological malfunction, or a neuroprotective (i.e., compensatory) mechanism of the nervous system, which mitigates the physiological malfunction caused by the disease. These mechanisms develop sequentially and act antagonistically. Given that ALS pathogenesis is still poorly understood (i.e., disease mechanisms are not identified yet), it is unfeasible to categorize the changes in mutant motoneurons to disease or compensatory mechanisms with assertion; however, some hypotheses could be formulated from available data regarding the nature of these changes. For instance, the relationship between the alterations in anatomy and excitability of mutant motoneurons is paradoxical. In the G93A (high expressor line) model, the enlargement in motoneuron anatomy and concomitant increase in persistent inward current have opposite actions on the excitability of motoneurons. Two hypotheses are described to infer the nature of these mechanisms. The first hypothesis is based on the effect of endurance training on healthy and transgenic mice. In healthy mice, endurance running exercise reduced the excitability of healthy motoneurons and increased their size, as suggested from their input resistance and cell capacitance measurements (Beaumont and Gardiner, 2002, 2003). In G93A mice, endurance running exercise reduced motor performance and shortened the life span of transgenic mice (Mahoney et al., 2004). Assuming that detrimental effects on transgenic mice would result from approaches that promote disease mechanisms, it is therefore plausible to suggest that anatomy enlargement of motoneurons is potentially an ALS disease mechanism. Consequently, the increase in motoneuron persistent inward current is potentially a compensatory mechanism to enhance the motoneuron excitability and offset the effect of enlarged anatomy. In this scenario, the additional dendrites would not possess active conductances and would reduce the motoneuron excitability by reducing the cell input resistance. However, this hypothesis is challenged by the beneficial effect of riluzole (the only FDA-approved drug available for ALS patients), which reduces motoneuron excitability and extends the life span of ALS patients (Bensimon et al., 1994; Miller et al., 1996) and transgenic mice (Gurney et al., 1998), suggesting increased excitability as the disease mechanism.

The second hypothesis is based on the relationship between the intrinsic motoneuron excitability and dendrite anatomy. When potassium channels were genetically manipulated to increase or decrease the motoneuron excitability, the overall motoneuron size was increased in both conditions with increased dendritic branch formation in the former case or dendritic branch elongation in the latter (Duch et al., 2008). Given that the anatomical alterations seen in mutant motoneurons resemble some features of those produced in response to increased excitability, this suggests that anatomy enlargement of mutant motoneurons is potentially a compensatory mechanism, whereas the increase in motoneuron excitability is potentially the disease mechanism. In this scenario, the pathologically-formed dendrites could contribute to the disease-state by having dendritic active conductances, which would dramatically increase the magnitude of persistent inward currents and enhance the motoneuronal excitability. The reduction in input resistance of mutant motoneurons would result from the increase in cell size. This hypothesis is supported by the beneficial effect of riluzole on mutant motoneurons survival by suppressing their excitability as explained above. Because motoneuron hyperexcitability is not a common feature of ALS transgenic models (hyperexcitability appears in models with high copy number of SOD1 gene, Table 3), riluzole's effect could be more pronounced in the more aggressive models of ALS that exhibit hyperexcitability, but less effective in the mild models of ALS (with less copy number of SOD1 gene) that exhibit hypoexcitability. This prediction might explain the discrepancy in studies on riluzole's efficacy in the various ALS transgenic models (for review see Bellingham, 2011). More data are needed to divulge the nature of these mechanisms.

In the G85R and G93A (low expressor line) models, alterations in anatomy and excitability of mutant motoneurons are observed, with no change in persistent inward current amplitude (Table 3). This disparity in the relationship between persistent inward current amplitude and motoneuron excitability in the various ALS transgenic models could be due to the difference in pace of disease progression in these models. In other words, disease and compensatory mechanisms advance at faster rates in aggressive ALS models (with high copy number of SOD1 genes) than in mild ALS models (with low copy number of SOD1 genes). This supposition is supported by the earlier disease onset and shorter life span in the G93A (high expressor line) than in the G85R and G93A (low expressor line) models (Turner and Talbot, 2008). Longitudinal studies in in-vivo mouse preparations in which the changes in motoneuron excitability, persistent inward currents, and anatomical properties in the various ALS transgenic models could be monitored at short time intervals during disease progression are needed to examine the development of these mechanisms.

8. Conclusion

Numerous alterations in the anatomical and electrical properties of mutant spinal motoneurons take place in the first two postnatal weeks, long before disease onset. Many of these alterations are inconsistent and sometimes contradictory; however, critical analysis of these alterations allowed for the identification of common pathological features within and across the various transgenic models of ALS. The enlargement in anatomy and reduction in input resistance of mutant motoneurons are characteristic features in the various transgenic models of ALS, whereas the alterations in motoneuron excitability and ionic currents (both transient and persistent) differ across transgenic models. To date, it is unfeasible to identify which of these alterations is an action of the disease (i.e., disease mechanism) or a reaction of the nervous system (i.e., compensatory mechanism) and more experiments are needed to elucidate the nature of these alterations. Computer simulations of realistic models of WT and mutant motoneurons allowed for the identification of hidden alteration in the biophysical properties of mutant motoneurons and demonstrated that synaptic efficacy is reduced in mutant motoneurons. It would be important to have extensive computational analysis of motoneuron properties in the various ALS transgenic models at various points in time during disease progression to identify and monitor the immeasurable changes in membrane properties of mutant motoneurons. This information would be expected to improve significantly our understanding of motoneuron pathophysiology in ALS.

9. Acknowledgment

This work was supported by grants to C.J.H. from the National Institutes of Health-National Institute of Neurological Disorders and Stroke (NS034382 and NS051462). S.M.E. was supported by the Tim E. Noel fellowship from the ALS Society of Canada and the Canadian Institutes of Health Research (CIHR). K.A.Q. was supported by the NRSA F32 fellowship (NS063535). T.L.E. was supported by the Joseph A. Blazek Foundation.

10. References

Amendola J, Durand J (2008) Morphological differences between wild-type and transgenic superoxide dismutase 1 lumbar motoneurons in postnatal mice. J Comp Neurol 511:329-341.

Amendola J, Gueritaud J, D'Incamps B, Bories C, Liabeuf S, Allene C, Pambo-Pambo A, Durand J (2007) Postnatal electrical and morphological abnormalities in lumbar motoneurons from transgenic mouse models of amyotrophic lateral sclerosis. Arch Ital Biol 145:311-323.

Beaumont E, Gardiner PF (2002) Effects of daily spontaneous running on the electrophysiological properties of hindlimb motoneurones in rats. J Physiol (Lond) 540:129-138.

Beaumont E, Gardiner PF (2003) Endurance training alters the biophysical properties of hindlimb motoneurons in rats. Muscle Nerve 27:228-236.

Bellingham MC (2011) A review of the neural mechanisms of action and clinical efficiency of riluzole in treating amyotrophic lateral sclerosis: what have we learned in the last decade? CNS Neurosci Ther 17:4-31.

Bennett DJ, Li Y, Siu M (2001) Plateau Potentials in Sacrocaudal Motoneurons of Chronic Spinal Rats, Recorded In Vitro. J Neurophysiol 86:1955-1971.

Bensimon G, Lacomblez L, Meininger V (1994) A controlled trial of riluzole in amyotrophic lateral sclerosis. ALS/Riluzole Study Group. N Engl J Med 330:585-591.

Bories C, Amendola J, Lamotte d'Incamps B, Durand J (2007) Early electrophysiological abnormalities in lumbar motoneurons in a transgenic mouse model of amyotrophic lateral sclerosis. Eur J Neurosci 25:451-459.

Bruijn LI, Becher MW, Lee MK, Anderson KL, Jenkins NA, Copeland NG, Sisodia SS, Rothstein JD, Borchelt DR, Price DL, Cleveland DW (1997) ALS-Linked SOD1 Mutant G85R Mediates Damage to Astrocytes and Promotes Rapidly Progressive Disease with SOD1-Containing Inclusions. Neuron 18:327-338.

Charcot J (1874) De la sclerose laterale amyotrophique. Prog Med 2:325-455.

Duch C, Vonhoff F, Ryglewski S (2008) Dendrite Elongation and Dendritic Branching Are Affected Separately by Different Forms of Intrinsic Motoneuron Excitability. J Neurophysiol 100:2525-2536.

ElBasiouny SM, Amendola J, Durand J, Heckman CJ (2010) Evidence from computer simulations for alterations in the membrane biophysical properties and dendritic processing of synaptic inputs in mutant superoxide dismutase-1 motoneurons. J Neurosci 30:5544-5558.

Filipchuk A, Pambo-Pambo A, Liabeuf S, Brocard C, Kulagina I, Korogod S, Gueritaud J, Durand J (2010) Evidence of early somato-dendritic alterations in lumbar motoneurons of sod1 juvenile mice. Amyotrophic Lat Scler 11:39-40.

Fuchs A, Schuetz B, Liss B, Roeper J (2008) Selective and disease-onset related action potential broadening in vulnerable brainstem motoneurons in the SOD1G93A ALS mouse model. Program No 44510 2008 Neuroscience Meeting Planner Washington, DC: Society for Neuroscience, 2008 Online

Fuchs A, Schuetz B, Liss B, Roeper J (2009) Persistent sodium currents are not altered at disease endstage in vulnerable brainstem motoneurons of the transgenic SOD1G93A ALS mouse model. Program No 6312 2009 Neuroscience Meeting Planner Chicago, IL: Society for Neuroscience, 2009 Online

Gurney ME, Fleck TJ, Himes CS, Hall ED (1998) Riluzole preserves motor function in a transgenic model of familial amyotrophic lateral sclerosis. Neurology 50:62-66.

Hamm TM, Turkin VV, Bandekar NK, O'Neill D, Jung R (2010) Persistent Currents and Discharge Patterns in Rat Hindlimb Motoneurons. J Neurophysiol 104:1566-1577.

Hegedus J, Putman CT, Gordon T (2007) Time course of preferential motor unit loss in the SOD1G93A mouse model of amyotrophic lateral sclerosis. Neurobiol Dis 28:154-164.

Hegedus J, Putman CT, Tyreman N, Gordon T (2008) Preferential motor unit loss in the SOD1G93A transgenic mouse model of amyotrophic lateral sclerosis. J Physiol:jphysiol.2007.149286.

Jiang M, Schuster JE, Fu R, Siddique T, Heckman CJ (2009) Progressive Changes in Synaptic Inputs to Motoneurons in Adult Sacral Spinal Cord of a Mouse Model of Amyotrophic Lateral Sclerosis. J Neuroscience 29:15031-15038.

Karim N, Kibble M, Everall I, Leigh N, Al-Sarraj S (1998) Extra motor neuronal loss in motor neuron disease. Neuropathol Appl Neurobiol 24:161-162.

Konno H, Yamamoto T, Iwasaki Y, Iizuka H (1986) Shy-Drager syndrome and amyotrophic lateral sclerosis. Cytoarchitectonic and morphometric studies of sacral autonomic neurons. J Neurol Sci 73:193-204.

Kuo JJ, Siddique T, Fu R, Heckman CJ (2005) Increased persistent Na+ current and its effect on excitability in motoneurones cultured from mutant SOD1 mice. J Physiol (Lond) 563:843-854.

Kuo JJ, Schonewille M, Siddique T, Schults ANA, Fu R, Bar PR, Anelli R, Heckman CJ, Kroese ABA (2004) Hyperexcitability of Cultured Spinal Motoneurons From Presymptomatic ALS Mice. J Neurophysiol 91:571-575.

Lloyd CM, Richardson MP, Brooks DJ, Al-Chalabi A, Leigh PN (2000) Extramotor involvement in ALS: PET studies with the GABA(A) ligand [(11)C]flumazenil. Brain 123 (Pt 11):2289-2296.

Maekawa S, Al-Sarraj S, Kibble M, Landau S, Parnavelas J, Cotter D, Everall I, Leigh PN (2004) Cortical selective vulnerability in motor neuron disease: a morphometric study. Brain 127:1237-1251.

Mahoney DJ, Rodriguez C, Devries M, Yasuda N, Tarnopolsky MA (2004) Effects of high-intensity endurance exercise training in the G93A mouse model of amyotrophic lateral sclerosis. Muscle Nerve 29:656-662.

Meehan CF, Moldovan M, Marklund SL, Graffmo KS, Nielsen JB, Hultborn H (2010) Intrinsic properties of lumbar motor neurones in the adult G127insTGGG superoxide dismutase-1 mutant mouse in vivo: evidence for increased persistent inward currents. Acta Physiol (Oxf) 200:361-376.

Miles GB, Dai Y, Brownstone RM (2005) Mechanisms underlying the early phase of spike frequency adaptation in mouse spinal motoneurones. J Physiol (Lond) 566:519-532.

Miller RG, Bouchard JP, Duquette P, Eisen A, Gelinas D, Harati Y, Munsat TL, Powe L, Rothstein J, Salzman P, Sufit RL (1996) Clinical trials of riluzole in patients with ALS. ALS/Riluzole Study Group-II. Neurology 47:S86-90; discussion S90-82.

Nagao M, Misawa H, Kato S, Hirai S (1998) Loss of cholinergic synapses on the spinal motor neurons of amyotrophic lateral sclerosis. J Neuropathol Exp Neurol 57:329-333.

Nagy JI, Yamamoto T, Jordan LM (1993) Evidence for the cholinergic nature of C-terminals associated with subsurface cisterns in alpha-motoneurons of rat. Synapse 15:17-32.

Pambo-Pambo AB, Durand J, Gueritaud JP (2009) Early excitability changes in lumbar motoneurons of transgenic SOD1G85R and SOD1G93A-Low mice. J Neurophysiol 102:3627-3642.

Pieri M, Carunchio I, Curcio L, Mercuri NB, Zona C (2009) Increased persistent sodium current determines cortical hyperexcitability in a genetic model of amyotrophic lateral sclerosis. Exp Neurol 215:368-379.

Pieri M, Albo F, Gaetti C, Spalloni A, Bengtson CP, Longone P, Cavalcanti S, Zona C (2003) Altered excitability of motor neurons in a transgenic mouse model of familial amyotrophic lateral sclerosis. Neurosci Lett 351:153-156.

Pun S, Santos AF, Saxena S, Xu L, Caroni P (2006) Selective vulnerability and pruning of phasic motoneuron axons in motoneuron disease alleviated by CNTF. 9:408-419.

Quinlan KA, Schuster JE, Fu R, Siddique T, Heckman CJ (2011) Altered postnatal maturation of electrical properties in spinal motoneurons in an ALS mouse model. J Physiol 589:2245-2260.

Sasaki S, Maruyama S (1992) Increase in diameter of the axonal initial segment is an early change in amyotrophic lateral sclerosis. J Neurol Sci 110:114-120.

Schwindt PC, Crill WE (1977) A persistent negative resistance in cat lumbar motoneurons. Brain Res 120:173-178.

Sobue G, Matsuoka Y, Mukai E, Takayanagi T, Sobue I, Hashizume Y (1981) Spinal and cranial motor nerve roots in amyotrophic lateral sclerosis and X-linked recessive bulbospinal muscular atrophy: morphometric and teased-fiber study. Acta Neuropathol 55:227-235.

Stephens B, Guiloff RJ, Navarrete R, Newman P, Nikhar N, Lewis P (2006) Widespread loss of neuronal populations in the spinal ventral horn in sporadic motor neuron disease. A morphometric study. J Neurol Sci 244:41-58.

Sunico CR, Dominguez G, Garcia-Verdugo JM, Osta R, Montero F, Moreno-Lopez B (2011) Reduction in the motoneuron inhibitory/excitatory synaptic ratio in an early-symptomatic mouse model of amyotrophic lateral sclerosis. Brain Pathol 21:1-15.

Swash M, Fox KP (1974) The pathology of the human muscle spindle: effect of denervation. J Neurol Sci 22:1-24.

Takahashi H, Oyanagi K, Ikuta F (1993) The intermediolateral nucleus in sporadic amyotrophic lateral sclerosis. Acta Neuropathol 86:190-192.

Turner BJ, Talbot K (2008) Transgenics, toxicity and therapeutics in rodent models of mutant SOD1-mediated familial ALS. Prog Neurobiol 85:94-134.

van Zundert B, Peuscher MH, Hynynen M, Chen A, Neve RL, Brown RH, Jr., Constantine-Paton M, Bellingham MC (2008) Neonatal Neuronal Circuitry Shows Hyperexcitable Disturbance in a Mouse Model of the Adult-Onset Neurodegenerative Disease Amyotrophic Lateral Sclerosis. J Neurosci 28:10864-10874.

Williams C, Kozlowski MA, Hinton DR, Miller CA (1990) Degeneration of spinocerebellar neurons in amyotrophic lateral sclerosis. Ann Neurol 27:215-225.

Zona C, Pieri M, Carunchio I (2006) Voltage-Dependent Sodium Channels in Spinal Cord Motor Neurons Display Rapid Recovery From Fast Inactivation in a Mouse Model of Amyotrophic Lateral Sclerosis. J Neurophysiol 96:3314-3322.

Molecular and Electrical Abnormalities in the Mouse Model of Amyotrophic Lateral Sclerosis

Katharina A. Quinlan[1], Sherif M. Elbasiouny[1] and C.J. Heckman[1,2,3]
[1]*Department of Physiology, Northwestern University Feinberg School of Medicine*
[2]*Department of Physical Medicine and Rehabilitation, Northwestern University Feinberg School of Medicine*
[3]*Department of Physical Therapy and Human Movement Sciences, Northwestern University Feinberg School of Medicine*
United States of America

1. Introduction

Amyotrophic lateral sclerosis (ALS) is a devastating, fast progressing and fatal disease for which there is little treatment. It is marked by loss of spinal and cortical motoneuron function. Many parameters are altered in the time leading up to this loss, including electrical properties, endoplasmic reticulum (ER) stress, glial functioning, glutamate signaling, protein degradation, mitochondrial functioning, axonal transport, and immune response. This chapter concentrates on the interplay between altered electrophysiological properties and molecular events. Emphasis is placed on the changes that precede overt symptom onset and results are mainly drawn from studies using the rodent models of ALS.

2. ALS animal models

Most cases of ALS are spontaneous (sALS), while the heritable form, familial ALS (fALS), represents about 5% of total ALS cases (Byrne et al., 2011). Of fALS patients, 20% have a mutation in the gene that encodes for the superoxide dismutase 1 (SOD1) copper/zinc enzyme (Rosen et al., 1993), 5% have a mutation in the TARDBP gene which encodes DNA-binding protein 43 (TDP-43), another 5% have a mutation in the FUS gene which encodes for the fused in sarcoma FUS/TLS protein (Mackenzie et al., 2010), some possess a mutation in the gene encoding vesicle-associated membrane protein (VAPB) (Nishimura et al., 2004), and a new study shows that some of those remaining have a mutation in the gene coding for the ubiquitin-like protein ubiquilin-2 (Deng et al., 2011). Transgenic mice expressing one of the various mutations of human SOD1, hereafter referred to as SOD1 mice; (Gurney et al., 1994, Bruijn et al., 1997, Zhang et al., 1997) are very common animal models of ALS; numerous other models of fALS are reviewed by Van Den Bosch (2011). It is not known how the SOD1 mutation leads to the degeneration of motoneurons, though it is probably not due to loss of its normal function converting superoxide into hydrogen peroxide. The mutant, misfolded protein likely possesses a toxic gain-of-function, as some mouse lines retain nearly normal levels of SOD1 enzymatic activity and still develop the disease, while SOD1 knockout mice, which do not possess any SOD1 enzymatic activity, do not develop the disease (Gurney et al., 1994, Reaume et al., 1996, Wong et al., 1995). Whatever the mechanism(s) leading to neurodegeneration, it is not immediate. The SOD1 enzyme is present throughout the nervous system (Pardo et al., 1995) starting embryonically, but does not lead to onset of overt symptoms until well into adulthood, even in mice that express high levels of the protein (Gurney et al., 1994). And within the nervous system, only certain neurons show susceptibility to the disease. This chapter will explore the earliest signs of malfunction in the neurons that are most vulnerable to the disease.

3. Timeline of deficits

In ALS, it is difficult to assess which of all the processes that have been found to be altered are causal to neurodegeneration and which are homeostatic, adaptive mechanisms that are actually allowing the maintenance function. Despite this, it is useful to map out the timing of the various altered properties collected from the mouse models, as presented in Figure 1. Depending on the particular SOD1 mouse model studied, the magnitude and timing of alterations observed does vary (reviewed in Elbasiouny et al, previous chapter). However, for this chapter, the deficits in these mice will be considered in their entirety and not separated based on the particular model from which the results were obtained.

Long before the onset of overt symptoms, within the first week after birth, electrical properties are altered. These properties include an increase in excitability (as measured by both the Na^{+}- and Ca^{2+}– mediated persistent inward current; PIC) and an increased neuronal size (including increased dendritic branching and increased specific input conductance). Significantly larger PICs first appear in cultured embryonic spinal and cortical motoneurons (Kuo et al., 2005, Pieri et al., 2009), persist at an age of about one week in spinal and hypoglossal motoneurons (van Zundert et al., 2008, Quinlan et al., 2011) and are likely still present in the spinal and cortical motoneurons of adults (Carunchio et al., 2010, Meehan et al., 2010). Interestingly, although the PIC is upregulated very early, what might otherwise be the beginning of motoneuron hyperexcitability is instead moderated by changes in size and specific input conductance (Amendola and Durand, 2008, Elbasiouny et al., 2010, Quinlan et al., 2011). In adulthood, but still well before the onset of symptoms, there are signs of defective protein degradation, endoplasmic reticulum (ER) stress, impaired axon transport, and deficiencies in mitochondrial function. Signs of aberrant protein clearance include increased expression of genes related to ubiquitination, UPR, and ER stress (Saxena et al., 2009). As these changes might suggest, there is a buildup of insoluble SOD1 proteins at this time (Johnston et al., 2000, Turner et al., 2003a), followed shortly by fragmentation of the Golgi (Mourelatos et al., 1996). The next signs of impairment appear in the mitochondria and in the cellular transport system (Zhang et al., 1997, Warita et al., 1999, Williamson and Cleveland, 1999, Mattiazzi et al., 2002, Kieran et al., 2005, Damiano et al., 2006, De Vos et al., 2007, Bilsland et al., 2008, Jaiswal et al., 2009, Nguyen et al., 2009, Bilsland et al., 2010, Li et al., 2010). The immune response is initiated next (Alexianu et al., 2001, Chiu et al., 2008, Gowing et al., 2008, Chiu et al., 2009). After this, denervation of the motor units and loss of maximal force begins (Kennel et al., 1996, Frey et al., 2000, Fischer et al., 2004, Hegedus et al., 2007, Hegedus et al., 2008), but the impairment of normal function in the mouse is subtle and onset of overt symptoms is several weeks off, even in the most severe models. Just before the impending functional loss, several of the

last changes before overt onset of symptoms involve the glia: activation of astrocytes, expression of different splice variants of EAAT2, decreased expression of the GluR2 subunit, and decreased number of glial K^+ channels (Bruijn et al., 1997, Bendotti et al., 2001, Sasaki et al., 2001, Munch et al., 2002, Warita et al., 2002, Fischer et al., 2004, Ignacio et al., 2005, Kaiser et al., 2006).
It is tempting to assume that the order of appearance of the altered parameters represents a chain reaction of events, but this is not necessarily the case. There is considerable interplay between these components within the neurons, such that one pathway cannot be altered without affecting any other aspect of cellular or synaptic function. These interactions will be considered next.

4. Calcium: No buffer for increased currents

Entry of Ca^{2+} occurs through voltage-gated Ca^{2+} channels and through ligand-gated channels activated by glutamate, particularly the NMDA-type glutamate receptors and those AMPA-type glutamate receptors which lack the Ca^{2+}-impermeable GluR2 subunit. Most voltage-gated Ca^{2+} channels open only when the cell depolarizes; however, the L-type $Ca_v1.3$ channels, which contribute to the PIC, open near the resting membrane potential (-40mV) and allow some Ca^{2+} influx even when the neuron is at rest (Xu and Lipscombe, 2001). There is very little expression of $Ca_v1.3$ channels in spinal motoneurons at birth, but $Ca_v1.3$ channels are increasingly present as the motoneurons mature, reaching adult levels by postnatal day 18 (P18) in mice, (Jiang et al., 1999, Quinlan et al., 2011). The PIC sets the level of excitability in neurons: PICs allow neurons to repetitively fire action potentials, and with large PICs, neurons can sustain firing long after the depolarizing stimulus is removed (Heckman et al., 2008). In addition, motoneurons from SOD1G93A-high-expressor mice show a significantly larger PIC during postnatal development, including significantly larger amplitudes of both Ca^{2+} and Na^+ currents (Quinlan et al., 2011). Larger PICs can increase the overall excitability of a neuron (though other factors, like size, can mitigate this), and the influx of Ca^{2+} could have many other consequences in cell-signaling. An increased PIC is found in cultured, embryonic, SOD1G93A-high motoneurons (both spinal and cortical), though at this point the PIC is completely Na^+-based (Kuo et al., 2005, Pieri et al., 2009). Postnatally, both spinal and brainstem SOD1 motoneurons show an increased PIC (van Zundert et al., 2008, Quinlan et al., 2011), and indirect evidence suggests larger PICs persist into adulthood in SOD1 cortical and spinal motoneurons (Carunchio et al., 2010, Meehan et al., 2010). In addition to the maturation of the PIC, there is an increase in AMPA-type glutamate receptors on motoneurons (Vinay et al., 2000). These receptors normally would not contribute to Ca^{2+} influx since, due to a single amino acid in the pore-forming GluR2 subunit they are impermeable to Ca^{2+}. However, in presymptomatic SOD1 motoneurons, there are fewer Ca^{2+}-impermeable GluR2 subunits; and more Ca^{2+}-permeable GluR3 subunits (Tortarolo et al., 2006). In sALS patients, AMPA receptors also are more Ca^{2+}-permeable, but through a different mechanism. Spinal motoneurons of symptomatic sALS patients, but not SOD1 rats, showed inefficient editing of the mRNA, resulting in mutant, GluR2Q subunits that are Ca^{2+}-permeable (Kawahara et al., 2004, Kwak and Kawahara, 2005, Kawahara et al., 2006). As motoneurons mature they must cope with an ever-increasing burden of Ca^{2+} influx through voltage-gated Ca^{2+} channels (as the Ca^{2+} PIC increases with age) and SOD1 motoneurons have a heavier burden due to potentiation of the Ca^{2+}PIC and altered AMPA receptors which are more Ca^{2+}-permeable.

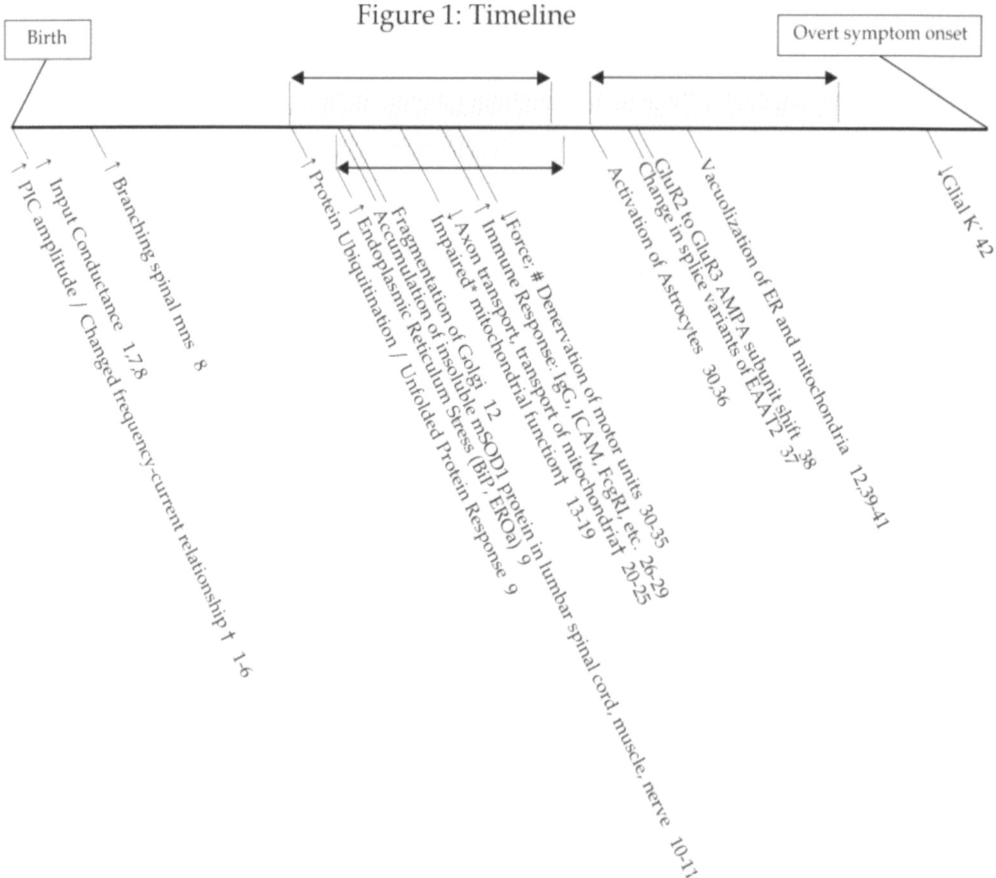

[1](Quinlan et al., 2011),[2](Kuo et al., 2005), [3](van Zundert et al., 2008), [4](Meehan et al., 2010), [5](Carunchio et al., 2010), [6](Pieri et al., 2009), [7](Bories et al., 2007), [8](Amendola and Durand, 2008), [9](Saxena et al., 2009), [10](Johnston et al., 2000), [11](Turner et al., 2003b), [12](Mourelatos et al., 1996), [13](Li et al., 2010), [14](Jaiswal and Keller, 2009),[15](Mattiazzi et al., 2002), [16](Nguyen et al., 2009), [17](Jaiswal et al., 2009), [18](Bilsland et al., 2008), [19](Damiano et al., 2006), [20](Bilsland et al., 2010), [21](De Vos et al., 2007), [22](Williamson and Cleveland, 1999), [23](Zhang et al., 1997), [24](Kieran et al., 2005), [25](Warita et al., 1999), [26](Alexianu et al., 2001), [27](Gowing et al., 2008), [28](Chiu et al., 2008), [29](Chiu et al., 2009), [30](Fischer et al., 2004), [31](Frey et al., 2000), [32](Pun et al., 2006), [33](Hegedus et al., 2007), [34](Hegedus et al., 2008), [35](Kennel et al., 1996), [36](Bruijn et al., 1997), [37](Munch et al., 2002), [38](Tortarolo et al., 2006), [39](Bendotti et al., 2001), [40](Dal Canto and Gurney, 1995), [41](Dal Canto and Gurney, 1994), [42](Kaiser et al., 2006).

Fig. 1. Timeline of deficits in mutant SOD1 mice. Earliest reported deficits in the above properties are used. Different SOD1 mutants were normalized to dates of overt symptom onset. When differences in timing between mouse lines were large (as it was for protein ubiquitination, stress of the ER, and activation of astrocytes), the range is indicated in the timeline with (///). † Also found in embryonic cultured motoneurons. * Different aspects of mitochondrial function were impaired at different time points. The first alteration in function is decreased Ca^{2+} storage capacity[19]. Another property, mitochondrial membrane potential, is not altered until just before symptom onset[17], while the function or regulation of the electron transport chain is impaired slightly before membrane potential[16].

While Ca^{2+} currents are increased in SOD1 motoneurons, large spinal and hypoglossal motoneurons do not have Ca^{2+}-binding proteins calbindin and parvalbumin and thus cannot quickly neutralize large influxes of Ca^{2+}. Instead, they depend heavily on mitochondrial uptake of Ca^{2+} (Ren and Ruda, 1994, Lips and Keller, 1998, Palecek et al., 1999, Bergmann and Keller, 2004). Small ocular motoneurons which have calbindin, parvalbumin and high Ca^{2+}-buffering capacities are unaffected by ALS (Vanselow and Keller, 2000, von Lewinski and Keller, 2005). Ca^{2+}-binding ratio, Ks, depends on Ca^{2+}-binding proteins, the intracellular $[Ca^{2+}]_i$, and the size and geometry of the cell (Neher, 1995). Although Ca^{2+} buffering at the soma of neonatal SOD1 and WT motoneurons was similar (von Lewinski et al., 2008), buffering has not been measured in adult motoneurons or in the processes, where Ca^{2+} channels are located (Sukiasyan et al., 2009). Ca^{2+} buffering could also change postnatally in motoneurons, as in rat Purkinje cells in which the Ca^{2+}-binding ratio more than doubles between P6 and P15 (Fierro and Llano, 1996). The increasing Ca^{2+} entry with postnatal maturation combined with the lack of Ca^{2+}-buffering proteins seems likely to contribute to motoneuronal vulnerability in adulthood.

5. Impaired transport, more places to go

The lack of Ca^{2+}-buffering proteins in vulnerable motoneurons make the mitochondria even more critical to their function. Mitochondria are normally highly mobile both in axons and dendrites (MacAskill et al., 2010). Mitochondrial movement can be halted by increased concentrations of ADP, so they tend to remain in compartments which are highly metabolically-active (Mironov, 2007). Mitochondrial movements are also regulated through Ca^{2+} signaling and synaptic activity (Rintoul et al., 2003, Yi et al., 2004, Macaskill et al., 2009). When glutamate binds NMDA- or certain AMPA-type receptor-channels, it allows the influx of Na^+ and Ca^{2+} into the cell. The Ca^{2+}-sensitive domain of Miro, the mitochondrial trafficking protein, then interacts with Ca^{2+} and the transport factors TRAK and KIF5, and pauses in its movement at active synapses (Rintoul et al., 2003, MacAskill et al., 2009). Postsynaptic NMDA receptors are also associated with PSD95 and with nitric oxide synthase (NOS) which, through nitric oxide (NO), also pauses mitochondrial movement (Rintoul et al., 2006). Once at a synapse, the mitochondria are probably tethered by neurofilaments, a process that depends both on the state of phosphorylation of the neurofilaments and a high mitochondrial membrane potential which indicates a high level of activity (Wagner et al., 2003).

In axons, but not in the soma of cultured SOD1 motoneurons, mitochondria are more sparsely distributed (De Vos et al., 2007), and *in vivo* mitochondria show more frequent pauses in their movements in pre-symptomatic SOD1 mice (Bilsland et al., 2010). Unfortunately, movement of mitochondria and other membrane-bound organelles has not yet been well studied in the dendrites of SOD1 motoneurons. If the mitochondria are similarly sparse in the dendrites, where most Ca^{2+} channels are located, this could have serious consequences for Ca^{2+} buffering. Spinal motoneurons of SOD1 mice show a significant proliferation in dendritic branches (Amendola and Durand, 2008) and an increased Ca^{2+} PIC (Quinlan et al., 2011), which could make mitochondrial motility in the dendrites more challenging. Without mitochondria to take up Ca^{2+} at the synapses, this would further exacerbate the low Ca^{2+} buffering in vulnerable motoneurons and any increased Ca^{2+} entry with synaptic inputs (Tortarolo et al., 2006). It is also worth noting that the motoneurons that are vulnerable are the largest: the fast, fatiguable alpha motoneurons (Pun et al., 2006, Hegedus et al., 2007, Hegedus et al., 2008). Evidence for further increases size in SOD1 motoneurons is reviewed in the previous chapter by Elbasiouny et al. Perhaps the size of the motoneuron and deficits in transport go hand in hand to produce vulnerability.

Axon transport has been extensively studied and is likely to contribute to ALS and to several neurodegenerative diseases, reviewed by (De Vos et al., 2008). In ALS, both slow and fast axon transport appear to be altered (Zhang et al., 1997, Warita et al., 1999, Williamson and Cleveland, 1999, Kieran et al., 2005, De Vos et al., 2007, Bilsland et al., 2010). Excessive glutamate could cause these deficiencies: high levels of glutamate activate a family of mitogen-activated protein kinases that phosphorylate neurofilaments, thereby decreasing transport (Ackerley et al., 2000, Hiruma et al., 2003, Stevenson et al., 2009). This process can be induced by NMDA or AMPA, blocked by removal of extracellular Ca^{2+}, or reduced by application of riluzole (Hiruma et al., 2003, Stevenson et al., 2009). The protein kinases JNKs, cdk/p35 and p38, which phosphorylate heavy and light chains of kinesin and medium and heavy neurofilament sidearms, may link glutamate neurotransmission and axon transport deficits (Kawasaki et al., 1997, Schwarzschild et al., 1997, Ackerley et al., 2000, Brownlees et al., 2000, Lee et al., 2000). Further suggesting this, p38 has been found to be activated in SOD1 mice and ALS patients (Raoul et al., 2002, Tortarolo et al., 2003, Ackerley et al., 2004). Axon transport deficiencies occur early, with reports of impaired axonal integrity and die-back from the neuromuscular junction occurring weeks in advance of onset of symptoms in SOD1 mice, and appearing in cultured embryonic neurons (Kennel et al., 1996, Zhang et al., 1997, Williamson and Cleveland, 1999, Frey et al., 2000, Fischer et al., 2004, Pun et al., 2006, De Vos et al., 2007, Hegedus et al., 2007, Hegedus et al., 2008, Bilsland et al., 2010). Strengthening these results, transgenic TDP-43 mice show significantly lower levels of expression of heavy and light neurofilaments, though axon transport itself has not yet been assessed (Swarup et al., 2011).

6. Mitochondrial deficiency and energy balance

In motoneurons under normal conditions, the mitochondrial membrane potential powers both the Ca^{2+} uniporter and ATP synthase, so in periods of heavy Ca^{2+} influx, ATP production could be impaired (Mattson et al., 2008, Nguyen et al., 2009). The increased Ca^{2+} influx in SOD1 motoneurons is likely to further impair the function of mitochondria under these conditions. In addition, SOD1 mitochondria appear to be impaired in function under basal conditions (Mattiazzi et al., 2002, Nguyen et al., 2009, Li et al., 2010). Before the onset of symptoms, SOD1 mitochondria show decreased protein import, altered Ca^{2+} sequestering, and an exaggerated response of the electrical gradient of the inner membrane to stimulation-induced Ca^{2+} influx (Damiano et al., 2006, Bilsland et al., 2008, Jaiswal et al., 2009, Nguyen et al., 2009, Li et al., 2010). By the time symptoms appear there is severe damage to mitochondrial membrane potentials, respiration, the electron transport chain and ATP synthesis (Mattiazzi et al., 2002, Jaiswal and Keller, 2009). Another impairment is misfolded SOD1 binding to VDAC1, the general diffusion pore for anions and cations, including Ca^{2+}. Both mitochondrial conductance and the uptake of ADP are thereby reduced, however, this is not observed until after the onset of symptoms (Israelson et al., 2010). Early alterations in SOD1 mitochondria must take place though another mechanism.

In summary, not only are there fewer mitochondria present in the processes of SOD1 neurons (De Vos et al., 2007, Bilsland et al., 2010), but those that are present are impaired in functioning. This is likely to have dire consequences for both Ca^{2+} buffering and ATP production in the large and metabolically-active SOD1 motoneurons.

7. Protein degradation and endoplasmic reticulum stress

Misfolded proteins are degraded through autophagy (Yang and Klionsky, 2010). When the capacity of the cellular machinery in the ER to properly fold proteins is exceeded, cells react with the unfolded protein response (UPR) and signs of ER stress (reviewed by Ron and Walter, 2007). The UPR decreases most protein synthesis in the cell while upregulating synthesis of some ER proteins that assist in proper folding and processing of proteins. Another pathway, known as ER-associated protein degradation (ERAD), helps to clear the ER of misfolded proteins by exporting them to proteasomes where they are broken down (Bernasconi and Molinari, 2011). Proteins to be exported and degraded are marked by ubiquitination, a process in which ubiquitin molecules bind to the protein, tagging it for destruction (Bingol and Sheng, 2011). Normal ER function can be disrupted by blocking the ER-resident proteins from folding properly, inadequate functioning of the ubiquitin-proteosome system, or failure to maintain a high level of Ca^{2+} inside the lumen of the ER (Paschen, 2003).

It is known that mice with the highest expression levels of mutant SOD1 protein have the earliest disease onset (Wong et al., 1995), and that markers for ER stress have been found in the spinal cords of sALS patients (Ilieva et al., 2007, Atkin et al., 2008, Ito et al., 2009). However, recent studies have shed more light on the role of protein degradation and ER stress in the pathology of ALS. In the first study, gene expression patterns from 3 different SOD1 mouse lines all showed an early increase in protein ubiquitination only in those motoneurons that are vulnerable to the disease. This is followed shortly by the UPR and signs of ER stress by P30 in SOD1G93A-high expressor mice (see Fig 1) (Saxena et al., 2009). In another study, cortical motoneurons from SOD1 mutant mice were compared to those from wild type mice that were fed a diet high in branched-chain amino acids (Carunchio et al., 2010). These branched chain amino acids are part of protein supplements that some athletes consume. Like mutant SOD1 neurons, cortical neurons from mice fed the high-protein diet were hyperexcitable compared with neurons from wild type mice on a normal diet. A return to normal levels of excitability after treatment with rapamycin was achieved for both the SOD1 and the amino- acid-supplement-treated cortical neurons (Carunchio et al., 2010). The protein kinase known as the mammalian target of rapamycin (mTOR) serves as an integration point for several cell signaling pathways. As its name suggests, mTOR is inhibited by rapamycin; it also inhibits protein degradation, and promotes increased cell size in some neurons (Lee et al., 2007). These results indicate that promoting autophagy with rapamycin can reduce abnormal excitability and could be beneficial for treatment of the disease (Carunchio et al., 2010). The third, most recent study described a mutation found in 5 different families, located in the gene encoding ubiquilin-2 as a novel genetic cause of fALS (Deng et al., 2011). The function of ubiquilin is to clear certain misfolded proteins during ERAD by shuttling ubiquitinated proteins from the ER to the proteasome, such that loss of ubiquilin leads to ER stress (Kim et al., 2008, Lim et al., 2009). The mutations in ubiquilin-2 found in ALS patients were also found to impair proteosome- mediated protein degradation *in vitro,* suggesting these mutations could be causing similar impairments in the families from whom they were isolated (Deng et al., 2011). Even in sALS patients, ubiquilin-2 was found in abnormal protein aggregates in degenerating neurons, indicating it could play a broad role in both fALS and sALS pathology (Deng et al., 2011). These studies suggest a key role for protein degradation and ER stress in ALS pathology.

In healthy neurons, the resting [Ca^{2+}] in the ER remains high. When ER [Ca^{2+}] drops, the Ca^{2+}-sensing STIM proteins promote Ca^{2+}-channel formation (Luik et al., 2008). Blocking this ER-mediated Ca^{2+}-entry affects neuronal activity and under conditions of chronic hyperexcitability, STIM proteins are upregulated (Steinbeck et al., 2011). Contributions to electrophysiological excitation-mediated Ca^{2+} transients from ER Ca^{2+} release have been documented in motoneurons (Scamps et al., 2004, Jahn et al., 2006). Supporting the possibility that neuronal excitability and neuronal protein processing and ER function could share common pathways, blocking L-type Ca^{2+} channels has been reported to increase autophagy (Williams et al., 2008). To summarize, due to the large role Ca^{2+} plays in cell signaling, (McCue et al., 2010, Pivovarova and Andrews, 2010), even small changes in electrophysiological properties could have broad consequences in cellular function.

8. Non-cell autonomous deficits: Astrocytes and glutamate excitotoxicity

Recent work has shown that the vulnerability of motoneurons is not cell autonomous, and that glia play critical roles in neurodegeneration in SOD1 mice. The involvement of astrocytes and microglia in the disease were elegantly demonstrated in a series of studies using mice with deletable mutant SOD1, mice with a selective knockdown of SOD1, and SOD1/WT chimera mice (Clement et al., 2003, Boillee et al., 2006, Yamanaka et al., 2008, Wang et al., 2009). Simply culturing WT motoneurons on mutant SOD1 astrocytes was sufficient to confer toxicity to motoneurons (Nagai et al., 2007). Glia have this effect on motoneurons through a variety of pathways, including activation of astrocytes, microglia, and T cells shortly after the first signs of pathology appear. The glial response is thought to influence the progression, but not the onset, of the disease (Beers et al., 2006, Boillee et al., 2006, Yamanaka et al., 2008, Wang et al., 2009, Philips and Robberecht, 2011). Presymptomatic involvement of the glia includes a reduction of glial K^{+} channel expression shortly before the onset of symptoms (Kaiser et al., 2006) and later in the course of the disease, a reduced expression of astroglial glutamate transporters, GLT1/EAAT2 which mediate glutamate reuptake at synapses and help prevent glutamate excitotoxicity (Bruijn et al., 1997, Bendotti et al., 2001, Warita et al., 2002). Earlier alterations in EAAT2 function are likely due to expression of different splice variants rather than decreased expressions levels (Sasaki et al., 2001, Munch et al., 2002, Ignacio et al., 2005). Some ALS patients also show abnormal splice variants of EAAT2, which could lead to decreased glutamate transport (Rothstein et al., 1992, Maragakis et al., 2004, Lauriat et al., 2007). Stimulation of the expression and transporter activity of EAAT2/GLT1 increases the lifespan of mutant SOD1 mice (Rothstein et al., 2005). An additional, critical function of the glia is regulation of the glutamate receptor's pore-forming GluR2 subunit (Van Damme et al., 2007). The challenges of Ca^{2+} buffering are exacerbated by alterations in the glutamate signaling across disease models of ALS. In SOD1 motoneurons, expression of subunits in the AMPA-type glutamate receptors is shifted from Ca^{2+}-impermeable to Ca^{2+}-permeable (Tortarolo et al., 2006). In TDP mice, levels of RNA that encode proteins involved in synaptic activity, including glutamate receptors, ion channels and voltage gated Ca2+ channels, are altered, with unknown consequences on synaptic transmission (Polymenidou et al., 2011). Lastly, in sALS patients, there is inefficient editing of AMPRA receptor GluR2Q subunit mRNA which also causes a shift from Ca^{2+}-impermeability of the receptors to Ca^{2+}-permeability (Kawahara et al., 2004, Kwak and Kawahara, 2005, Kawahara et al., 2006). Glutamatergic signaling is probably a significant factor in the onset of symptoms since reducing excitatory sensory input delayed the onset of disease in SOD1 mice (Ilieva et al., 2008), and intrathecal administration of the glutamate agonist kainic acid in normal rats produced slow, selective motoneuron death similar to ALS (Sun et al., 2006). If changes in the transmission of glutamate are taking place early enough, it could alter the activity of spinal networks during normal development (Blankenship and Feller, 2010, Landmesser and O'Donovan, 1984, Marder and Rehm, 2005, Gonzalez-Islas and Wenner, 2006). Some evidence for alterations in network activity has been shown in SOD1 hypoglossal motoneurons (van Zundert et al., 2008) and spinal motoneurons (Amendola et al., 2004, Bories et al., 2007) in juvenile mice. After symptom onset, increased network activity has also been shown in the spinal cord (Jiang et al., 2009). However, considering all the documented changes in glutamate-mediated neurotransmission, there has been surprisingly little research into the overall effects on cortical, brainstem and spinal network activity throughout the lifespan of the SOD1 mouse.

9. Future directions

There are many possibilities to explore for new treatments of ALS besides the now-standard drug riluzole (Bellingham, 2011). The neuroinflammation response is a promising approach (Philips and Robberecht, 2011); another could be to manipulate neuromodulatory input to the spinal cord. Serotonin (5HT) and norepinephrine (NE) have potent effects on motoneurons, including increasing PIC amplitude, decreasing input conductance, hyperpolarizing spike threshold, and depolarizing resting potential (Hounsgaard and Kiehn, 1989, Lee and Heckman, 1999, Powers and Binder, 2001, Alaburda et al., 2002, Hultborn et al., 2004, Perrier and Delgado-Lezama, 2005, Heckman et al., 2008). Furthermore, neuromodulators are constantly scaling the level of activation of motoneurons as needed (Heckman et al., 2004). Activation of $5HT_2$ receptors strongly depresses high-voltage-activated Ca^{2+} channels while probably increasing basal $[Ca^{2+}]_I$ by potentiating the Ca^{2+} PIC (Hounsgaard et al., 1988, Bayliss et al., 1995, Hsiao et al., 1998, Ladewig et al., 2004, Li et al., 2007). Both 5HT and dopamine (DA) modulate KIF-5-dependent cellular transport, including transport of mitochondria. Acting through the GSK3 regulator of KIF-5, 5HT is observed to increase transport, while DA decreases it (Chen et al., 2007, Chen et al., 2008). Other neuromodulators, such as nitric oxide, $GABA_B$, and adenosine, could also be worth investigating as modulators of motoneuron synaptic strength, reduction of the Ca^{2+} PIC, and modulation of both high-voltage-activated Ca^{2+} channels and input conductance, respectively (Marks et al., 1993, Mynlieff and Beam, 1994, Li et al., 2004, Moreno-Lopez et al., 2011). Another useful target of neuromodulators that modify Ca^{2+} influx is protein clearance; inhibition of L-type Ca^{2+} channels has been found to increase autophagy (Williams et al., 2008).

10. Conclusions

Factors causing neurodegeneration in ALS are present long before motor function is adversely affected. From research on the animal models of ALS, it is thought that excessive

Ca^{2+} entry, increased motoneuronal size, altered glutamate neurotransmission, astrocyte dysfunction, mitochondrial deficits, failures in axon transport, and problems in protein degradation act in concert and gradually push motoneurons outside the parameters under which they can function properly. The fact that motoneurons are able to remain functioning for as long as they do under adverse conditions suggests that there is a large window of time and intrinsic conditions within which motoneurons can maintain normal function. Hopefully future treatments can target these altered pathways to extend the time motoneuron properties remain within these parameters.

11. References

Ackerley S, Grierson AJ, Banner S, Perkinton MS, Brownlees J, Byers HL, Ward M, Thornhill P, Hussain K, Waby JS, Anderton BH, Cooper JD, Dingwall C, Leigh PN, Shaw CE, Miller CC (2004) p38alpha stress-activated protein kinase phosphorylates neurofilaments and is associated with neurofilament pathology in amyotrophic lateral sclerosis. Mol Cell Neurosci 26:354-364.

Ackerley S, Grierson AJ, Brownlees J, Thornhill P, Anderton BH, Leigh PN, Shaw CE, Miller CC (2000) Glutamate slows axonal transport of neurofilaments in transfected neurons. J Cell Biol 150:165-176.

Alaburda A, Perrier JF, Hounsgaard J (2002) Mechanisms causing plateau potentials in spinal motoneurones. Adv Exp Med Biol 508:219-226.

Alexianu ME, Kozovska M, Appel SH (2001) Immune reactivity in a mouse model of familial ALS correlates with disease progression. Neurology 57:1282-1289.

Amendola J, Durand J (2008) Morphological differences between wild-type and transgenic superoxide dismutase 1 lumbar motoneurons in postnatal mice. J Comp Neurol 511:329-341.

Amendola J, Verrier B, Roubertoux P, Durand J (2004) Altered sensorimotor development in a transgenic mouse model of amyotrophic lateral sclerosis. Eur J Neurosci 20:2822-2826.

Atkin JD, Farg MA, Walker AK, McLean C, Tomas D, Horne MK (2008) Endoplasmic reticulum stress and induction of the unfolded protein response in human sporadic amyotrophic lateral sclerosis. Neurobiol Dis 30:400-407.

Bayliss DA, Umemiya M, Berger AJ (1995) Inhibition of N- and P-type calcium currents and the after-hyperpolarization in rat motoneurones by serotonin. Journal of Physiology 485:635-647.

Beers DR, Henkel JS, Xiao Q, Zhao W, Wang J, Yen AA, Siklos L, McKercher SR, Appel SH (2006) Wild-type microglia extend survival in PU.1 knockout mice with familial amyotrophic lateral sclerosis. Proc Natl Acad Sci U S A 103:16021-16026.

Bellingham MC (2011) A review of the neural mechanisms of action and clinical efficiency of riluzole in treating amyotrophic lateral sclerosis: what have we learned in the last decade? CNS Neurosci Ther 17:4-31.

Bendotti C, Tortarolo M, Suchak SK, Calvaresi N, Carvelli L, Bastone A, Rizzi M, Rattray M, Mennini T (2001) Transgenic SOD1 G93A mice develop reduced GLT-1 in spinal cord without alterations in cerebrospinal fluid glutamate levels. J Neurochem 79:737-746.

Bergmann F, Keller BU (2004) Impact of mitochondrial inhibition on excitability and cytosolic Ca2+ levels in brainstem motoneurones from mouse. J Physiol 555:45-59.

Bernasconi R, Molinari M (2011) ERAD and ERAD tuning: disposal of cargo and of ERAD regulators from the mammalian ER. Curr Opin Cell Biol 23:176-183.

Bilsland LG, Nirmalananthan N, Yip J, Greensmith L, Duchen MR (2008) Expression of mutant SOD1 in astrocytes induces functional deficits in motoneuron mitochondria. J Neurochem 107:1271-1283.

Bilsland LG, Sahai E, Kelly G, Golding M, Greensmith L, Schiavo G (2010) Deficits in axonal transport precede ALS symptoms in vivo. Proc Natl Acad Sci U S A 107:20523-20528.

Bingol B, Sheng M (2011) Deconstruction for reconstruction: the role of proteolysis in neural plasticity and disease. Neuron 69:22-32.

Blankenship AG, Feller MB (2010) Mechanisms underlying spontaneous patterned activity in developing neural circuits. Nat Rev Neurosci 11:18-29.

Boillee S, Yamanaka K, Lobsiger CS, Copeland NG, Jenkins NA, Kassiotis G, Kollias G, Cleveland DW (2006) Onset and progression in inherited ALS determined by motor neurons and microglia. Science 312:1389-1392.

Bories C, Amendola J, Lamotte d'Incamps B, Durand J (2007) Early electrophysiological abnormalities in lumbar motoneurons in a transgenic mouse model of amyotrophic lateral sclerosis. Eur J Neurosci 25:451-459.

Brownlees J, Yates A, Bajaj NP, Davis D, Anderton BH, Leigh PN, Shaw CE, Miller CC (2000) Phosphorylation of neurofilament heavy chain side-arms by stress activated protein kinase-1b/Jun N-terminal kinase-3. J Cell Sci 113 (Pt 3):401-407.

Bruijn LI, Becher MW, Lee MK, Anderson KL, Jenkins NA, Copeland NG, Sisodia SS, Rothstein JD, Borchelt DR, Price DL, Cleveland DW (1997) ALS-linked SOD1 mutant G85R mediates damage to astrocytes and promotes rapidly progressive disease with SOD1-containing inclusions. Neuron 18:327-338.

Byrne S, Walsh C, Lynch C, Bede P, Elamin M, Kenna K, McLaughlin R, Hardiman O (2011) Rate of familial amyotrophic lateral sclerosis: a systematic review and meta-analysis. J Neurol Neurosurg Psychiatry 82:623-627.

Carunchio I, Curcio L, Pieri M, Pica F, Caioli S, Viscomi MT, Molinari M, Canu N, Bernardi G, Zona C (2010) Increased levels of p70S6 phosphorylation in the G93A mouse model of Amyotrophic Lateral Sclerosis and in valine-exposed cortical neurons in culture. Exp Neurol 226:218-230.

Chen S, Owens GC, Crossin KL, Edelman DB (2007) Serotonin stimulates mitochondrial transport in hippocampal neurons. Mol Cell Neurosci 36:472-483.

Chen S, Owens GC, Edelman DB (2008) Dopamine inhibits mitochondrial motility in hippocampal neurons. PLoS One 3:e2804.

Chiu IM, Chen A, Zheng Y, Kosaras B, Tsiftsoglou SA, Vartanian TK, Brown RH, Jr., Carroll MC (2008) T lymphocytes potentiate endogenous neuroprotective inflammation in a mouse model of ALS. Proc Natl Acad Sci U S A 105:17913-17918.

Chiu IM, Phatnani H, Kuligowski M, Tapia JC, Carrasco MA, Zhang M, Maniatis T, Carroll MC (2009) Activation of innate and humoral immunity in the peripheral nervous system of ALS transgenic mice. Proc Natl Acad Sci U S A 106:20960-20965.

Clement AM, Nguyen MD, Roberts EA, Garcia ML, Boillee S, Rule M, McMahon AP, Doucette W, Siwek D, Ferrante RJ, Brown RH, Jr., Julien JP, Goldstein LS, Cleveland DW (2003) Wild-type nonneuronal cells extend survival of SOD1 mutant motor neurons in ALS mice. Science 302:113-117.

Dal Canto MC, Gurney ME (1994) Development of central nervous system pathology in a murine transgenic model of human amyotrophic lateral sclerosis. The American journal of pathology 145:1271-1279.

Dal Canto MC, Gurney ME (1995) Neuropathological changes in two lines of mice carrying a transgene for mutant human Cu,Zn SOD, and in mice overexpressing wild type human SOD: a model of familial amyotrophic lateral sclerosis (FALS). Brain Res 676:25-40.

Damiano M, Starkov AA, Petri S, Kipiani K, Kiaei M, Mattiazzi M, Flint Beal M, Manfredi G (2006) Neural mitochondrial Ca2+ capacity impairment precedes the onset of motor symptoms in G93A Cu/Zn-superoxide dismutase mutant mice. J Neurochem 96:1349-1361.

De Vos KJ, Chapman AL, Tennant ME, Manser C, Tudor EL, Lau KF, Brownlees J, Ackerley S, Shaw PJ, McLoughlin DM, Shaw CE, Leigh PN, Miller CC, Grierson AJ (2007) Familial amyotrophic lateral sclerosis-linked SOD1 mutants perturb fast axonal transport to reduce axonal mitochondria content. Hum Mol Genet 16:2720-2728.

De Vos KJ, Grierson AJ, Ackerley S, Miller CC (2008) Role of axonal transport in neurodegenerative diseases. Annu Rev Neurosci 31:151-173.

Deng HX, Chen W, Hong ST, Boycott KM, Gorrie GH, Siddique N, Yang Y, Fecto F, Shi Y, Zhai H, Jiang H, Hirano M, Rampersaud E, Jansen GH, Donkervoort S, Bigio EH, Brooks BR, Ajroud K, Sufit RL, Haines JL, Mugnaini E, Pericak-Vance MA, Siddique T (2011) Mutations in UBQLN2 cause dominant X-linked juvenile and adult-onset ALS and ALS/dementia. Nature.

Elbasiouny SM, Amendola J, Durand J, Heckman CJ (2010) Evidence from computer simulations for alterations in the membrane biophysical properties and dendritic processing of synaptic inputs in mutant superoxide dismutase-1 motoneurons. J Neurosci In Press.

Fierro L, Llano I (1996) High endogenous calcium buffering in Purkinje cells from rat cerebellar slices. J Physiol 496 (Pt 3):617-625.

Fischer LR, Culver DG, Tennant P, Davis AA, Wang M, Castellano-Sanchez A, Khan J, Polak MA, Glass JD (2004) Amyotrophic lateral sclerosis is a distal axonopathy: evidence in mice and man. Exp Neurol 185:232-240.

Frey D, Schneider C, Xu L, Borg J, Spooren W, Caroni P (2000) Early and selective loss of neuromuscular synapse subtypes with low sprouting competence in motoneuron diseases. J Neurosci 20:2534-2542.

Gonzalez-Islas C, Wenner P (2006) Spontaneous network activity in the embryonic spinal cord regulates AMPAergic and GABAergic synaptic strength. Neuron 49:563-575.

Gowing G, Philips T, Van Wijmeersch B, Audet JN, Dewil M, Van Den Bosch L, Billiau AD, Robberecht W, Julien JP (2008) Ablation of proliferating microglia does not affect motor neuron degeneration in amyotrophic lateral sclerosis caused by mutant superoxide dismutase. J Neurosci 28:10234-10244.

Gurney ME, Pu H, Chiu AY, Dal Canto MC, Polchow CY, Alexander DD, Caliendo J, Hentati A, Kwon YW, Deng HX, et al. (1994) Motor neuron degeneration in mice that express a human Cu,Zn superoxide dismutase mutation. Science 264:1772-1775.

Heckman CJ, Johnson M, Mottram C, Schuster J (2008b) Persistent inward currents in spinal motoneurons and their influence on human motoneuron firing patterns. Neuroscientist 14:264-275.

Heckman CJ, Kuo JJ, Johnson MD (2004) Synaptic integration in motoneurons with hyper-excitable dendrites. Canadian journal of physiology and pharmacology 82:549-555.

Hegedus J, Putman CT, Gordon T (2007) Time course of preferential motor unit loss in the SOD1 G93A mouse model of amyotrophic lateral sclerosis. Neurobiol Dis 28:154-164.

Hegedus J, Putman CT, Tyreman N, Gordon T (2008) Preferential motor unit loss in the SOD1 G93A transgenic mouse model of amyotrophic lateral sclerosis. J Physiol 586:3337-3351.

Hiruma H, Katakura T, Takahashi S, Ichikawa T, Kawakami T (2003) Glutamate and amyloid beta-protein rapidly inhibit fast axonal transport in cultured rat hippocampal neurons by different mechanisms. J Neurosci 23:8967-8977.

Hounsgaard J, Hultborn H, Jespersen B, Kiehn O (1988) Bistability of alpha-motoneurones in the decerebrate cat and in the acute spinal cat after intravenous 5-hydroxytryptophan. J Physiol 405:345-367.

Hounsgaard J, Kiehn O (1989) Serotonin-induced bistability of turtle motoneurones caused by a nifedipine-sensitive calcium plateau potential. J Physiol Lond 414:265-282.

Hsiao CF, Del Negro CA, Trueblood PR, Chandler SH (1998) Ionic basis for serotonin-induced bistable membrane properties in guinea pig trigeminal motoneurons. J Neurophysiol 79:2847-2856.

Hultborn H, Brownstone RB, Toth TI, Gossard JP (2004) Key mechanisms for setting the input-output gain across the motoneuron pool. Prog Brain Res 143:77-95.

Ignacio S, Moore DH, Smith AP, Lee NM (2005) Effect of neuroprotective drugs on gene expression in G93A/SOD1 mice. Ann N Y Acad Sci 1053:121-136.

Ilieva EV, Ayala V, Jove M, Dalfo E, Cacabelos D, Povedano M, Bellmunt MJ, Ferrer I, Pamplona R, Portero-Otin M (2007) Oxidative and endoplasmic reticulum stress interplay in sporadic amyotrophic lateral sclerosis. Brain 130:3111-3123.

Ilieva HS, Yamanaka K, Malkmus S, Kakinohana O, Yaksh T, Marsala M, Cleveland DW (2008) Mutant dynein (Loa) triggers proprioceptive axon loss that extends survival only in the SOD1 ALS model with highest motor neuron death. Proc Natl Acad Sci U S A 105:12599-12604.

Israelson A, Arbel N, Da Cruz S, Ilieva H, Yamanaka K, Shoshan-Barmatz V, Cleveland DW (2010) Misfolded mutant SOD1 directly inhibits VDAC1 conductance in a mouse model of inherited ALS. Neuron 67:575-587.

Ito Y, Yamada M, Tanaka H, Aida K, Tsuruma K, Shimazawa M, Hozumi I, Inuzuka T, Takahashi H, Hara H (2009) Involvement of CHOP, an ER-stress apoptotic mediator, in both human sporadic ALS and ALS model mice. Neurobiol Dis 36:470-476.

Jahn K, Grosskreutz J, Haastert K, Ziegler E, Schlesinger F, Grothe C, Dengler R, Bufler J (2006) Temporospatial coupling of networked synaptic activation of AMPA-type glutamate receptor channels and calcium transients in cultured motoneurons. Neuroscience 142:1019-1029.

Jaiswal MK, Keller BU (2009) Cu/Zn superoxide dismutase typical for familial amyotrophic lateral sclerosis increases the vulnerability of mitochondria and perturbs Ca2+ homeostasis in SOD1G93A mice. Mol Pharmacol 75:478-489.

Jaiswal MK, Zech WD, Goos M, Leutbecher C, Ferri A, Zippelius A, Carri MT, Nau R, Keller BU (2009) Impairment of mitochondrial calcium handling in a mtSOD1 cell culture model of motoneuron disease. BMC Neurosci 10:64.

Jiang M, Schuster JE, Fu R, Siddique T, Heckman CJ (2009) Progressive changes in synaptic inputs to motoneurons in adult sacral spinal cord of a mouse model of amyotrophic lateral sclerosis. J Neurosci 29:15031-15038.

Jiang Z, Rempel J, Li J, Sawchuk MA, Carlin KP, Brownstone RM (1999) Development of L-type calcium channels and a nifedipine-sensitive motor activity in the postnatal mouse spinal cord. Eur J Neurosci 11:3481-3487.

Johnston JA, Dalton MJ, Gurney ME, Kopito RR (2000) Formation of high molecular weight complexes of mutant Cu, Zn-superoxide dismutase in a mouse model for familial amyotrophic lateral sclerosis. Proc Natl Acad Sci U S A 97:12571-12576.

Kaiser M, Maletzki I, Hulsmann S, Holtmann B, Schulz-Schaeffer W, Kirchhoff F, Bahr M, Neusch C (2006) Progressive loss of a glial potassium channel (KCNJ10) in the spinal cord of the SOD1 (G93A) transgenic mouse model of amyotrophic lateral sclerosis. J Neurochem 99:900-912.

Kawahara Y, Ito K, Sun H, Aizawa H, Kanazawa I, Kwak S (2004) Glutamate receptors: RNA editing and death of motor neurons. Nature 427:801.

Kawahara Y, Sun H, Ito K, Hideyama T, Aoki M, Sobue G, Tsuji S, Kwak S (2006) Underediting of GluR2 mRNA, a neuronal death inducing molecular change in sporadic ALS, does not occur in motor neurons in ALS1 or SBMA. Neurosci Res 54:11-14.

Kawasaki H, Morooka T, Shimohama S, Kimura J, Hirano T, Gotoh Y, Nishida E (1997) Activation and involvement of p38 mitogen-activated protein kinase in glutamate-induced apoptosis in rat cerebellar granule cells. J Biol Chem 272:18518-18521.

Kennel PF, Finiels F, Revah F, Mallet J (1996) Neuromuscular function impairment is not caused by motor neurone loss in FALS mice: an electromyographic study. Neuroreport 7:1427-1431.

Kieran D, Hafezparast M, Bohnert S, Dick JR, Martin J, Schiavo G, Fisher EM, Greensmith L (2005) A mutation in dynein rescues axonal transport defects and extends the life span of ALS mice. J Cell Biol 169:561-567.

Kim TY, Kim E, Yoon SK, Yoon JB (2008) Herp enhances ER-associated protein degradation by recruiting ubiquilins. Biochem Biophys Res Commun 369:741-746.

Kuo JJ, Siddique T, Fu R, Heckman CJ (2005) Increased persistent Na+ current and its effect on excitability in motoneurones cultured from mutant SOD1 mice. Journal of Physiology-London 563:843-854.

Kwak S, Kawahara Y (2005) Deficient RNA editing of GluR2 and neuronal death in amyotropic lateral sclerosis. J Mol Med (Berl) 83:110-120.

Ladewig T, Lalley PM, Keller BU (2004) Serotonergic modulation of intracellular calcium dynamics in neonatal hypoglossal motoneurons from mouse. Brain Res 1001:1-12.

Landmesser LT, O'Donovan MJ (1984) Activation patterns of embryonic chick hind limb muscles recorded in ovo and in an isolated spinal cord preparation. J Physiol 347:189-204.

Lauriat TL, Richler E, McInnes LA (2007) A quantitative regional expression profile of EAAT2 known and novel splice variants reopens the question of aberrant EAAT2 splicing in disease. Neurochemistry international 50:271-280.

Lee CH, Inoki K, Guan KL (2007) mTOR pathway as a target in tissue hypertrophy. Annual review of pharmacology and toxicology 47:443-467.

Lee MS, Kwon YT, Li M, Peng J, Friedlander RM, Tsai LH (2000) Neurotoxicity induces cleavage of p35 to p25 by calpain. Nature 405:360-364.

Lee RH, Heckman CJ (1999) Enhancement of bistability in spinal motoneurons in vivo by the noradrenergic alpha1 agonist methoxamine. Journal of neurophysiology 81:2164-2174.

Li Q, Vande Velde C, Israelson A, Xie J, Bailey AO, Dong MQ, Chun SJ, Roy T, Winer L, Yates JR, Capaldi RA, Cleveland DW, Miller TM (2010) ALS-linked mutant superoxide dismutase 1 (SOD1) alters mitochondrial protein composition and decreases protein import. Proc Natl Acad Sci U S A 107:21146-21151.

Li X, Murray K, Harvey PJ, Ballou EW, Bennett DJ (2007) Serotonin facilitates a persistent calcium current in motoneurons of rats with and without chronic spinal cord injury. J Neurophysiol 97:1236-1246.

Li Y, Li X, Harvey PJ, Bennett DJ (2004) Effects of baclofen on spinal reflexes and persistent inward currents in motoneurons of chronic spinal rats with spasticity. J Neurophysiol 92:2694-2703.

Lim PJ, Danner R, Liang J, Doong H, Harman C, Srinivasan D, Rothenberg C, Wang H, Ye Y, Fang S, Monteiro MJ (2009) Ubiquilin and p97/VCP bind erasin, forming a complex involved in ERAD. J Cell Biol 187:201-217.

Lips MB, Keller BU (1998) Endogenous calcium buffering in motoneurones of the nucleus hypoglossus from mouse. J Physiol 511 (Pt 1):105-117.

Luik RM, Wang B, Prakriya M, Wu MM, Lewis RS (2008) Oligomerization of STIM1 couples ER calcium depletion to CRAC channel activation. Nature 454:538-542.

MacAskill AF, Atkin TA, Kittler JT (2010) Mitochondrial trafficking and the provision of energy and calcium buffering at excitatory synapses. Eur J Neurosci 32:231-240.

Macaskill AF, Rinholm JE, Twelvetrees AE, Arancibia-Carcamo IL, Muir J, Fransson A, Aspenstrom P, Attwell D, Kittler JT (2009) Miro1 is a calcium sensor for glutamate receptor-dependent localization of mitochondria at synapses. Neuron 61:541-555.

Mackenzie IR, Rademakers R, Neumann M (2010) TDP-43 and FUS in amyotrophic lateral sclerosis and frontotemporal dementia. Lancet Neurol 9:995-1007.

Maragakis NJ, Dykes-Hoberg M, Rothstein JD (2004) Altered expression of the glutamate transporter EAAT2b in neurological disease. Ann Neurol 55:469-477.

Marder E, Rehm KJ (2005) Development of central pattern generating circuits. Curr Opin Neurobiol 15:86-93.

Marks JD, Donnelly DF, Haddad GG (1993) Adenosine-induced inhibition of vagal motoneuron excitability: receptor subtype and mechanisms. Am J Physiol 264:L124-132.

Mattiazzi M, D'Aurelio M, Gajewski CD, Martushova K, Kiaei M, Beal MF, Manfredi G (2002) Mutated human SOD1 causes dysfunction of oxidative phosphorylation in mitochondria of transgenic mice. J Biol Chem 277:29626-29633.

Mattson MP, Gleichmann M, Cheng A (2008) Mitochondria in neuroplasticity and neurological disorders. Neuron 60:748-766.

McCue HV, Haynes LP, Burgoyne RD (2010) The diversity of calcium sensor proteins in the regulation of neuronal function. Cold Spring Harb Perspect Biol 2:a004085.

Meehan CF, Moldovan M, Marklund SL, Graffmo KS, Nielsen JB, Hultborn H (2010) Intrinsic properties of lumbar motor neurones in the adult G127insTGGG superoxide dismutase-1 mutant mouse in vivo: evidence for increased persistent inward currents. Acta Physiol (Oxf) 200:361-376.

Mironov SL (2007) ADP regulates movements of mitochondria in neurons. Biophys J 92:2944-2952.

Moreno-Lopez B, Sunico CR, Gonzalez-Forero D (2011) NO orchestrates the loss of synaptic boutons from adult "sick" motoneurons: modeling a molecular mechanism. Mol Neurobiol 43:41-66.

Mourelatos Z, Gonatas NK, Stieber A, Gurney ME, Dal Canto MC (1996) The Golgi apparatus of spinal cord motor neurons in transgenic mice expressing mutant Cu,Zn superoxide dismutase becomes fragmented in early, preclinical stages of the disease. Proc Natl Acad Sci U S A 93:5472-5477.

Munch C, Ebstein M, Seefried U, Zhu B, Stamm S, Landwehrmeyer GB, Ludolph AC, Schwalenstocker B, Meyer T (2002) Alternative splicing of the 5'-sequences of the mouse EAAT2 glutamate transporter and expression in a transgenic model for amyotrophic lateral sclerosis. J Neurochem 82:594-603.

Mynlieff M, Beam KG (1994) Adenosine acting at an A1 receptor decreases N-type calcium current in mouse motoneurons. J Neurosci 14:3628-3634.

Nagai M, Re DB, Nagata T, Chalazonitis A, Jessell TM, Wichterle H, Przedborski S (2007) Astrocytes expressing ALS-linked mutated SOD1 release factors selectively toxic to motor neurons. Nat Neurosci 10:615-622.

Neher E (1995) The use of fura-2 for estimating Ca buffers and Ca fluxes. Neuropharmacology 34:1423-1442.

Nguyen KT, Garcia-Chacon LE, Barrett JN, Barrett EF, David G (2009) The Psi(m) depolarization that accompanies mitochondrial Ca2+ uptake is greater in mutant SOD1 than in wild-type mouse motor terminals. Proc Natl Acad Sci U S A 106:2007-2011.

Nishimura AL, Mitne-Neto M, Silva HC, Richieri-Costa A, Middleton S, Cascio D, Kok F, Oliveira JR, Gillingwater T, Webb J, Skehel P, Zatz M (2004) A mutation in the vesicle-trafficking protein VAPB causes late-onset spinal muscular atrophy and amyotrophic lateral sclerosis. American journal of human genetics 75:822-831.

Palecek J, Lips MB, Keller BU (1999) Calcium dynamics and buffering in motoneurones of the mouse spinal cord. J Physiol 520 Pt 2:485-502.

Pardo CA, Xu Z, Borchelt DR, Price DL, Sisodia SS, Cleveland DW (1995) Superoxide dismutase is an abundant component in cell bodies, dendrites, and axons of motor neurons and in a subset of other neurons. Proc Natl Acad Sci U S A 92:954-958.

Paschen W (2003) Endoplasmic reticulum: a primary target in various acute disorders and degenerative diseases of the brain. Cell calcium 34:365-383.

Perrier JF, Delgado-Lezama R (2005) Synaptic release of serotonin induced by stimulation of the raphe nucleus promotes plateau potentials in spinal motoneurons of the adult turtle. J Neurosci 25:7993-7999.

Philips T, Robberecht W (2011) Neuroinflammation in amyotrophic lateral sclerosis: role of glial activation in motor neuron disease. Lancet Neurol 10:253-263.

Pieri M, Carunchio I, Curcio L, Mercuri NB, Zona C (2009) Increased persistent sodium current determines cortical hyperexcitability in a genetic model of amyotrophic lateral sclerosis. Exp Neurol 215:368-379.

Pivovarova NB, Andrews SB (2010) Calcium-dependent mitochondrial function and dysfunction in neurons. The FEBS journal 277:3622-3636.

Polymenidou M, Lagier-Tourenne C, Hutt KR, Huelga SC, Moran J, Liang TY, Ling SC, Sun E, Wancewicz E, Mazur C, Kordasiewicz H, Sedaghat Y, Donohue JP, Shiue L, Bennett CF, Yeo GW, Cleveland DW (2011) Long pre-mRNA depletion and RNA missplicing contribute to neuronal vulnerability from loss of TDP-43. Nat Neurosci 14:459-468.

Powers RK, Binder MD (2001) Input-output functions of mammalian motoneurons. Rev Physiol Biochem Pharmacol 143:137-263.

Pun S, Santos AF, Saxena S, Xu L, Caroni P (2006) Selective vulnerability and pruning of phasic motoneuron axons in motoneuron disease alleviated by CNTF. Nat Neurosci 9:408-419.

Quinlan KA, Schuster JE, Fu R, Siddique T, Heckman CJ (2011) Altered postnatal maturation of electrical properties in spinal motoneurons in a mouse model of amyotrophic lateral sclerosis. J Physiol 589:2245-2260.

Raoul C, Estevez AG, Nishimune H, Cleveland DW, deLapeyriere O, Henderson CE, Haase G, Pettmann B (2002) Motoneuron death triggered by a specific pathway downstream of Fas. potentiation by ALS-linked SOD1 mutations. Neuron 35:1067-1083.

Reaume AG, Elliott JL, Hoffman EK, Kowall NW, Ferrante RJ, Siwek DF, Wilcox HM, Flood DG, Beal MF, Brown RH, Jr., Scott RW, Snider WD (1996) Motor neurons in Cu/Zn superoxide dismutase-deficient mice develop normally but exhibit enhanced cell death after axonal injury. Nat Genet 13:43-47.

Ren K, Ruda MA (1994) A comparative study of the calcium-binding proteins calbindin-D28K, calretinin, calmodulin and parvalbumin in the rat spinal cord. Brain Res Brain Res Rev 19:163-179.

Rintoul GL, Bennett VJ, Papaconstandinou NA, Reynolds IJ (2006) Nitric oxide inhibits mitochondrial movement in forebrain neurons associated with disruption of mitochondrial membrane potential. J Neurochem 97:800-806.

Rintoul GL, Filiano AJ, Brocard JB, Kress GJ, Reynolds IJ (2003) Glutamate decreases mitochondrial size and movement in primary forebrain neurons. J Neurosci 23:7881-7888.

Ron D, Walter P (2007) Signal integration in the endoplasmic reticulum unfolded protein response. Nat Rev Mol Cell Biol 8:519-529.

Rosen DR, Siddique T, Patterson D, Figlewicz DA, Sapp P, Hentati A, Donaldson D, Goto J, O'Regan JP, Deng HX, et al. (1993) Mutations in Cu/Zn superoxide dismutase gene are associated with familial amyotrophic lateral sclerosis. Nature 362:59-62.

Rothstein JD, Martin LJ, Kuncl RW (1992) Decreased glutamate transport by the brain and spinal cord in amyotrophic lateral sclerosis. N Engl J Med 326:1464-1468.

Rothstein JD, Patel S, Regan MR, Haenggeli C, Huang YH, Bergles DE, Jin L, Dykes Hoberg M, Vidensky S, Chung DS, Toan SV, Bruijn LI, Su ZZ, Gupta P, Fisher PB (2005) Beta-lactam antibiotics offer neuroprotection by increasing glutamate transporter expression. Nature 433:73-77.

Sasaki S, Warita H, Abe K, Komori T, Iwata M (2001) EAAT1 and EAAT2 immunoreactivity in transgenic mice with a G93A mutant SOD1 gene. Neuroreport 12:1359-1362.

Saxena S, Cabuy E, Caroni P (2009) A role for motoneuron subtype-selective ER stress in disease manifestations of FALS mice. Nat Neurosci 12:627-636.

Scamps F, Roig A, Boukhaddaoui H, Andre S, Puech S, Valmier J (2004) Activation of P-type calcium channel regulates a unique thapsigargin-sensitive calcium pool in embryonic motoneurons. Eur J Neurosci 19:977-982.

Schwarzschild MA, Cole RL, Hyman SE (1997) Glutamate, but not dopamine, stimulates stress-activated protein kinase and AP-1-mediated transcription in striatal neurons. J Neurosci 17:3455-3466.

Steinbeck JA, Henke N, Opatz J, Gruszczynska-Biegala J, Schneider L, Theiss S, Hamacher N, Steinfarz B, Golz S, Brustle O, Kuznicki J, Methner A (2011) Store-operated calcium entry modulates neuronal network activity in a model of chronic epilepsy. Exp Neurol.

Stevenson A, Yates DM, Manser C, De Vos KJ, Vagnoni A, Leigh PN, McLoughlin DM, Miller CC (2009) Riluzole protects against glutamate-induced slowing of neurofilament axonal transport. Neurosci Lett 454:161-164.

Sukiasyan N, Hultborn H, Zhang M (2009) Distribution of calcium channel Ca(V)1.3 immunoreactivity in the rat spinal cord and brain stem. Neuroscience 159:217-235.

Sun H, Kawahara Y, Ito K, Kanazawa I, Kwak S (2006) Slow and selective death of spinal motor neurons in vivo by intrathecal infusion of kainic acid: implications for AMPA receptor-mediated excitotoxicity in ALS. Journal of neurochemistry 98:782-791.

Swarup V, Phaneuf D, Bareil C, Robertson J, Rouleau GA, Kriz J, Julien JP (2011) Pathological hallmarks of amyotrophic lateral sclerosis/frontotemporal lobar degeneration in transgenic mice produced with TDP-43 genomic fragments. Brain.

Tortarolo M, Grignaschi G, Calvaresi N, Zennaro E, Spaltro G, Colovic M, Fracasso C, Guiso G, Elger B, Schneider H, Seilheimer B, Caccia S, Bendotti C (2006) Glutamate AMPA receptors change in motor neurons of SOD1G93A transgenic mice and their inhibition by a noncompetitive antagonist ameliorates the progression of amytrophic lateral sclerosis-like disease. J Neurosci Res 83:134-146.

Tortarolo M, Veglianese P, Calvaresi N, Botturi A, Rossi C, Giorgini A, Migheli A, Bendotti C (2003) Persistent activation of p38 mitogen-activated protein kinase in a mouse model of familial amyotrophic lateral sclerosis correlates with disease progression. Mol Cell Neurosci 23:180-192.

Turner BJ, Lopes EC, Cheema SS (2003a) Neuromuscular accumulation of mutant superoxide dismutase 1 aggregates in a transgenic mouse model of familial amyotrophic lateral sclerosis. Neurosci Lett 350:132-136.

Turner BJ, Rembach A, Spark R, Lopes EC, Cheema SS (2003b) Opposing effects of low and high-dose clozapine on survival of transgenic amyotrophic lateral sclerosis mice. J Neurosci Res 74:605-613.

Van Damme P, Bogaert E, Dewil M, Hersmus N, Kiraly D, Scheveneels W, Bockx I, Braeken D, Verpoorten N, Verhoeven K, Timmerman V, Herijgers P, Callewaert G, Carmeliet P, Van Den Bosch L, Robberecht W (2007) Astrocytes regulate GluR2 expression in motor neurons and their vulnerability to excitotoxicity. Proc Natl Acad Sci U S A 104:14825-14830.

Van Den Bosch L (2011) Genetic rodent models of amyotrophic lateral sclerosis. Journal of biomedicine & biotechnology 2011:348765.

van Zundert B, Peuscher MH, Hynynen M, Chen A, Neve RL, Brown RH, Jr., Constantine-Paton M, Bellingham MC (2008) Neonatal neuronal circuitry shows hyperexcitable disturbance in a mouse model of the adult-onset neurodegenerative disease amyotrophic lateral sclerosis. J Neurosci 28:10864-10874.

Vanselow BK, Keller BU (2000) Calcium dynamics and buffering in oculomotor neurones from mouse that are particularly resistant during amyotrophic lateral sclerosis (ALS)-related motoneurone disease. J Physiol 525 Pt 2:433-445.

Vinay L, Brocard F, Pflieger JF, Simeoni-Alias J, Clarac F (2000) Perinatal development of lumbar motoneurons and their inputs in the rat. Brain research bulletin 53:635-647.

von Lewinski F, Fuchs J, Vanselow BK, Keller BU (2008) Low Ca2+ buffering in hypoglossal motoneurons of mutant SOD1 (G93A) mice. Neurosci Lett 445:224-228.

von Lewinski F, Keller BU (2005) Mitochondrial Ca2+ buffering in hypoglossal motoneurons from mouse. Neurosci Lett 380:203-208.

Wagner OI, Lifshitz J, Janmey PA, Linden M, McIntosh TK, Leterrier JF (2003) Mechanisms of mitochondria-neurofilament interactions. J Neurosci 23:9046-9058.

Wang L, Sharma K, Grisotti G, Roos RP (2009) The effect of mutant SOD1 dismutase activity on non-cell autonomous degeneration in familial amyotrophic lateral sclerosis. Neurobiol Dis 35:234-240.

Warita H, Itoyama Y, Abe K (1999) Selective impairment of fast anterograde axonal transport in the peripheral nerves of asymptomatic transgenic mice with a G93A mutant SOD1 gene. Brain Res 819:120-131.

Warita H, Manabe Y, Murakami T, Shiote M, Shiro Y, Hayashi T, Nagano I, Shoji M, Abe K (2002) Tardive decrease of astrocytic glutamate transporter protein in transgenic mice with ALS-linked mutant SOD1. Neurological research 24:577-581.

Williams A, Sarkar S, Cuddon P, Ttofi EK, Saiki S, Siddiqi FH, Jahreiss L, Fleming A, Pask D, Goldsmith P, O'Kane CJ, Floto RA, Rubinsztein DC (2008) Novel targets for Huntington's disease in an mTOR-independent autophagy pathway. Nature chemical biology 4:295-305.

Williamson TL, Cleveland DW (1999) Slowing of axonal transport is a very early event in the toxicity of ALS-linked SOD1 mutants to motor neurons. Nat Neurosci 2:50-56.

Wong PC, Pardo CA, Borchelt DR, Lee MK, Copeland NG, Jenkins NA, Sisodia SS, Cleveland DW, Price DL (1995) An adverse property of a familial ALS-linked SOD1 mutation causes motor neuron disease characterized by vacuolar degeneration of mitochondria. Neuron 14:1105-1116.

Xu W, Lipscombe D (2001) Neuronal Ca(V)1.3alpha(1) L-type channels activate at relatively hyperpolarized membrane potentials and are incompletely inhibited by dihydropyridines. J Neurosci 21:5944-5951.

Yamanaka K, Chun SJ, Boillee S, Fujimori-Tonou N, Yamashita H, Gutmann DH, Takahashi R, Misawa H, Cleveland DW (2008) Astrocytes as determinants of disease progression in inherited amyotrophic lateral sclerosis. Nat Neurosci 11:251-253.

Yang Z, Klionsky DJ (2010) Eaten alive: a history of macroautophagy. Nat Cell Biol 12:814-822.

Yi M, Weaver D, Hajnoczky G (2004) Control of mitochondrial motility and distribution by the calcium signal: a homeostatic circuit. J Cell Biol 167:661-672.

Zhang B, Tu P, Abtahian F, Trojanowski JQ, Lee VM (1997) Neurofilaments and orthograde transport are reduced in ventral root axons of transgenic mice that express human SOD1 with a G93A mutation. J Cell Biol 139:1307-1315.

Part 2

Signalling Pathways and Molecular Pathophysiology

8

Role of Mitochondrial Dysfunction in Motor Neuron Degeneration in ALS

Luz Diana Santa-Cruz, Uri Nimrod Ramírez-Jarquín and Ricardo Tapia
División de Neurociencias, Instituto de Fisiología Celular, Universidad Nacional Autónoma de México, México, D.F., México

1. Introduction

Amyotrophic lateral sclerosis (ALS), which was described since 1869 by Jean Martin Charcot, is a devastating neurodegenerative disease characterized by the selective and progressive loss of upper and lower motor neurons of the cerebral cortex, brainstem and the spinal cord. Progressive motor neuron loss causes muscle weakness, spasticity and fasciculation, eventually paralysis and finally death by respiratory failure 3 to 5 years after diagnosis. ALS worldwide prevalence is about 2 to 8 people per 100,000, and presents two important differences with respect to other neurogenerative diseases: the cognitive process is not affected and is not merely the result of aging because may occur at young ages (Chancellor & Warlow, 1992; Huisman et al., 2011). Two forms of ALS are known, the familial type (FALS), associated with genetic mutations, mainly in the gene encoding superoxide dismutase 1 (SOD1, enzyme responsible for superoxide dismutation to oxygen and hydrogen peroxide), and the sporadic form (SALS), of unknown origin. FALS represents only about 5-10% of cases (Rosen et al., 1993; Rowland & Shneider, 2001), and SALS comprises the remaining 90%. Despite having different origins, both ALS types develop similar histopathological and clinical characteristics.

2. Mechanisms of motor neuron death in ALS

After one hundred fifty years since the first ALS description of the disease, the cause of motor neuron degeneration remains unknown, but progress in neuroscience and clinical research has identified several mechanisms that seem to be involved in the cell death process, such as glutamate-mediated excitotoxicity, inflammatory events, axonal transport deficits, oxidative stress, mitochondrial dysfunction and energy failure.

2.1 Excitotoxicity

Based on the reduction of glutamate transporter-1 (GLT1 in rodents and excitatory amino acid transporter 2 or EAAT2 in human) content detected post-mortem in motor cortex and spinal cord of ALS patients (Rothstein et al., 1992; Rothstein et al., 1995) and on the increase of glutamate concentration in the cerebrospinal fluid (CSF) of about 40% of ALS patients (Shaw et al., 1995b; Spreux-Varoquaux et al., 2002), one proposed mechanism to explain motor neuron death in ALS is glutamate-mediated excitotoxicity. This hypothesis has been generally accepted, although some data from our laboratory do not support it because a chronic increase in extracellular glutamate due to glutamate transport inhibition in the spinal cord in vivo was innocuous for motor neurons (Tovar-y-Romo et al., 2009b). However, overactivation of glutamate ionotropic receptors by agonists leads to neuronal death by augmenting the influx of Ca^{2+} into motor neurons. Experimental models in vivo have shown that of three major glutamate ionotropic receptor types, NMDA (N-methyl-D-aspartate), kainate and AMPA (α-amino-3-hydroxy-5-isoxazolepropionate), the Ca^{2+}-permeable AMPA receptor seems to be particularly involved in motor neuron death, because the selective blockade of Ca^{2+}-permeable AMPA receptors or the chelation of intracellular Ca^{2+} prevents the motor neuron loss and the consequent paralysis induced by the infusion of AMPA into the rat lumbar spinal cord (Corona & Tapia, 2004, 2007; Tovar-y-Romo et al., 2009a). The Ca^{2+} permeability of this receptor is governed by the presence of the GluR2 subunit and its edition in the Q/R (glutamine/arginine) site of the second transmembrane domain (Burnashev et al., 1992; Corona & Tapia, 2007; Hollmann et al., 1991; Hume et al., 1991).

Increases in cytoplasmic Ca^{2+} concentration can be buffered by mitochondria, but when maintained for prolonged periods can cause mitochondrial swelling and dysfunction. These alterations are associated with deficits in mitochondrial ATP synthesis and energetic failure (this topic will be discussed later). The energetic deficits have been mainly associated with cell death process similar to necrosis (Kroemer et al., 2009; Martin, 2010). On the other hand, mitochondrial damage has also been linked to the release of proapoptotic factors such as cytochrome c and apoptosis-inducing factor (Martin et al., 2009). Cytochrome c involvement has been stressed because of its role in triggering the caspases pathway, which leads to apoptotic cellular death. In the cytoplasm cytochrome c promotes the formation of the apoptosome complex and activates caspase-3. The necrosis and apoptosis pathways are illustrated in Fig. 1.

2.2 Axonal transport deficits

Because of the structural and functional characteristics of motor neuron axons, the role of axonal transport is essential for the communication between the neuronal soma and the periphery, as well as for the anterograde and retrograde dispersive distribution of cargo intracellular structures such as vesicles or organelles. Changes in the speed of anterograde and retrograde transport (Breuer & Atkinson, 1988; Breuer et al., 1987; Sasaki & Iwata, 1996), as well as neurofilament disorganization and accumulation of mitochondria, vesicles and smooth endoplasmic reticulum have been described in peripheral nerves of ALS patients (Hirano et al., 1984a, b; Sasaki & Iwata, 1996). These alterations in axonal transport have been observed also in transgenic models of FALS, which have allowed the study of their progression and the molecular machinery involved (Bilsland et al., 2010; Brunet et al., 2009; Collard et al., 1995; De Vos et al., 2007; Ligon et al., 2005; Perlson et al., 2009; Pun et al., 2006; Tateno et al., 2009; Warita et al., 1999; Williamson & Cleveland, 1999). In mutant SOD1 (mSOD1) rodents, some motor proteins such as: dynein, dynactin, kinesin, myosin, actin, and microtubules and neurofilaments are affected by mSOD1 aggregates (Breuer & Atkinson, 1988; Breuer et al., 1987; Collard et al., 1995; Ligon et al., 2005; Sasaki & Iwata, 1996; Williamson & Cleveland, 1999; Zhang et al., 2007).

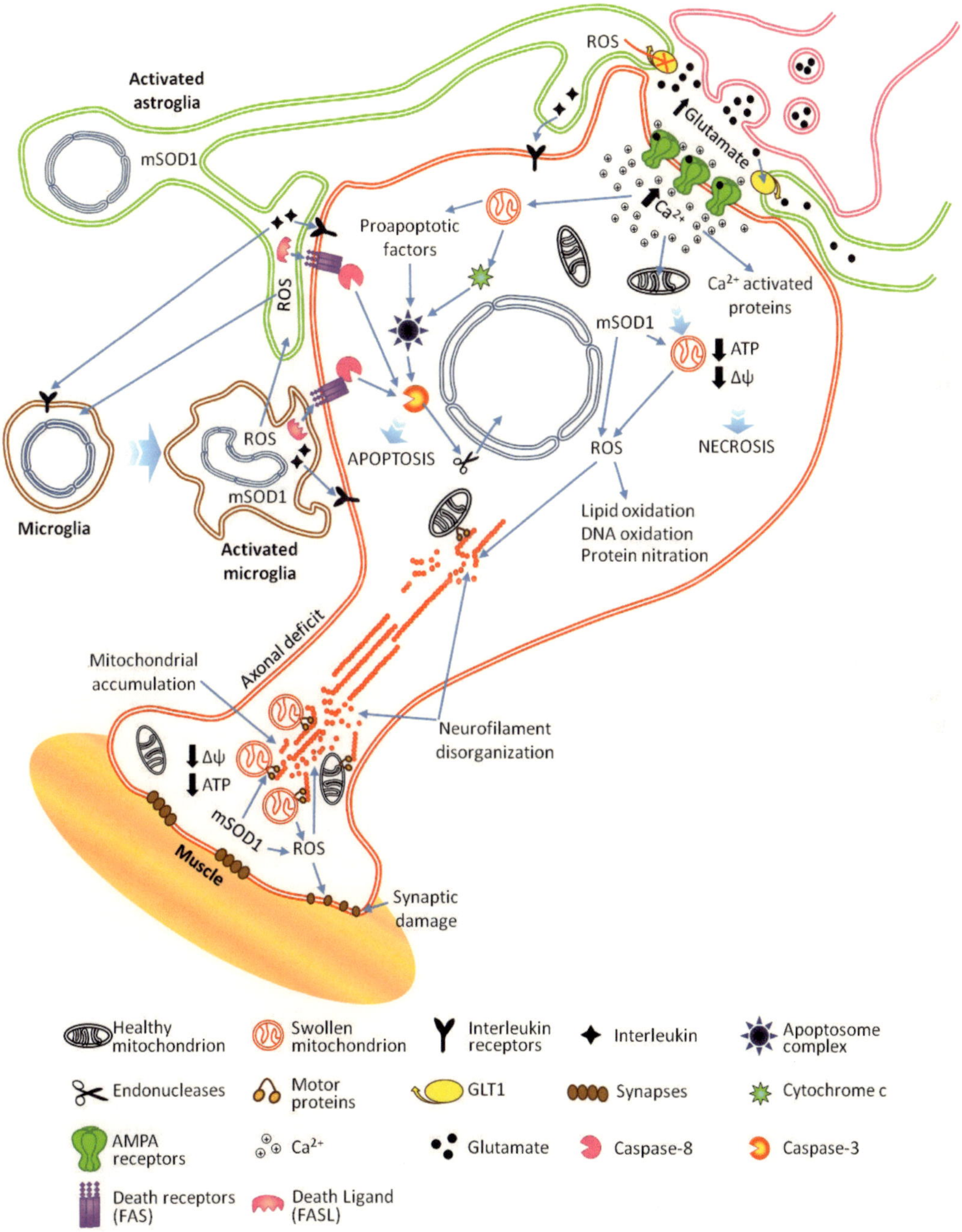

Fig. 1. Scheme of the main proposed mechanisms involved in motor neuron death. Description in the text.

These deficits may affect the renewal of organelles in the axon terminals of motor neurons, leading to accumulation of damaged mitochondria or autophagosomes, increased ROS production, disruption of microtubule formation and stability (Julien & Mushynski, 1998), as well as damage of presynaptic structure such as swelling of axon terminals (Komatsu et al., 2007). Accumulation of damaged mitochondria may result in energetic failure (Liu et al., 2004; Martin et al., 2009; Menzies et al., 2002a, b; Pasinelli et al., 2004; Wong et al., 1995; Zhu et al., 2002) and in the release of proapoptotic factors (Pasinelli et al., 2004) (Fig. 1, bottom left). These alterations may be involved in the distal neurophaty and impairment of muscular reinnervation observed in ALS.

2.3 Oxidative stress

Another mechanism implicated in motor neuron degeneration in ALS that involves both motor neurons and non-neuronal cells is oxidative stress. Reactive oxygen species (ROS) arise in cells as aerobic metabolism by-products, mostly due to the leakage of electrons from the mitochondrial respiratory chain, resulting in an incomplete reduction of molecular oxygen during the oxidative phosphorylation, generating the superoxide radical anion ($O_2^{\bullet -}$). The $O_2^{\bullet -}$ anion reacts quickly with the nitric oxide radical ($NO^{\bullet}$, produced by nitric oxide synthase, NOS) to form peroxynitrite ($ONOO^-$). Meanwhile, the product of $O_2^{\bullet -}$ dismutation, H_2O_2, slowly decomposes to form the highly reactive hydroxyl radical ($^{\bullet}OH$). Both $ONOO^-$ and $^{\bullet}OH$ are highly reactive and can damage proteins, membranes and DNA by oxidation. Cellular mechanisms to combat the constant production of free radicals are: 1) enzymes such as SOD, catalase and peroxidase, which catalytically remove reactive species; 2) reducing agents synthesized in vivo, such as glutathione, α-keto acids, lipoic acid and coenzyme Q, and compounds obtained from the diet, such as ascorbate (vitamin C) and α-tocopherol (vitamin E); and 3) chaperone heat shock proteins which remove or facilitate repair of damaged proteins. Oxidative stress arises from an imbalance between ROS production and its control mechanisms.

The involvement of oxidative stress in ALS pathogenesis is supported by abundant evidence that has been reported in both SALS and FALS patients, where several indicators of increased oxidative damage have been found: 1) In postmortem central nervous system (CNS) tissue samples (mainly spinal cord) these markers include oxidized DNA (Ferrante et al., 1997b; Fitzmaurice et al., 1996), lipid peroxidation (Siciliano et al., 2002), protein glycoxidation (Shibata et al., 2001), elevated protein carbonylation (Ferrante et al., 1997b; Shaw et al., 1995a), and increased protein tyrosine nitration; remarkably, nitrotyrosine immunoreactivity was more densely detected in motor neurons (Abe et al., 1995; Abe et al., 1997; Beal et al., 1997; Ferrante et al., 1997a). 2) Oxidation markers in CSF, plasma and blood from living ALS patients during the course of the disease have also been described. The most relevant are oxidized DNA (Bogdanov et al., 2000; Ihara et al., 2005), hydroxyl and ascorbate free radicals (Ihara et al., 2005), lipid peroxidation (Baillet et al., 2010; Bogdanov et al., 2000; Bonnefont-Rousselot et al., 2000; Ihara et al., 2005; Oteiza et al., 1997; Simpson et al., 2004; Smith et al., 1998), and a remarkable elevation of 3-nitrotyrosine levels in CSF (Tohgi et al., 1999). However, in other study, 3-nitroyrosine was not different between the CSF of ALS patients and control subjects (Ryberg et al., 2004). Increased oxidative damage to proteins, lipids and DNA has also been demonstrated in CNS tissue of transgenic mouse model of FALS expressing mSOD1 (Andrus et al., 1998; Casoni et al., 2005; Liu et al., 1999; Liu et al., 1998; Poon et al., 2005).

Mitochondria, ROS and glutamate-induced excitotoxicity are closely related and this is relevant in ALS, because the mitochondrion is the main oxygen consumer and it is also the main producer of ROS. These species can be produced in neurons and in non-neuronal cells and can cause failure in the glutamate uptake system of both motor neurons and astroglia (Rao et al., 2003; Trotti et al., 1996, 1998; Volterra et al., 1994; Zagami et al., 2009). This may contribute to an excitotoxic condition due to increased concentration of extracellular glutamate. ROS production and its effects on motor neurons and non-neuronal cells are illustrated in Fig. 1.

2.4 Inflammation

A mechanism of non-cell-autonomous death associated with motor neuron degeneration in both FALS and SALS is the participation of non-neuronal cells in inflammatory events (Boillee et al., 2006a; Boillee et al., 2006b; Hall et al., 1998; Yamanaka et al., 2008; Yang et al., 2011). The main histopathological feature of inflammation is the proliferation of reactive astrogliosis and of activated microglial cells, associated with alterations in their cellular functions, such as glutamate reuptake failure and release of proapoptotic and proinflammatory factors (Sanagi et al., 2010; Sargsyan et al., 2005; Sofroniew, 2005). Molecules associated with inflammatory process, such as interleukins 6, 12, 15, 17A, 23, C4d and C3d complement proteins, as well as tumor necrosis factor-alpha, have been found in blood and CSF from ALS patients (Almer et al., 2002; Fiala et al., 2010; Henkel et al., 2004; Kawamata et al., 1992; McGeer et al., 1991; Moreau et al., 2005; Rentzos et al., 2010a, b). The finding of increased levels of granzymes A, B in serum (Ilzecka, 2011) and decrease in cytochrome c levels in the CSF (Ilzecka, 2007), suggests an apoptotic process in human disease. The proliferation of activated non-neuronal cells has been associated with the disease severity (Clement et al., 2003). Nevertheless, alteration in their functions may be more important than their proliferation (Lepore et al., 2008). In experimental models of FALS (mSOD1) it has been attempted to prevent the motor neuron loss through the use of drugs with anti-inflammatory properties, such as minocycline (Keller et al., 2010; Kriz et al., 2002; Neymotin et al., 2009; Van Den Bosch et al., 2002; Zhu et al., 2002). This drug was effective in delaying the motor neurons loss when given prior to the symptoms onset, but when given at late stages it exaggerated the neuroinflammatory response and accelerated the progression of the symptoms (Keller et al., 2010). In this transgenic ALS model, apoptosis processes can be triggered by non-neuronal cells through the extrinsic apoptotic pathway, via the release from activated glial cells of several death ligands (for example FasL) that bind to their respective death receptor (Fas) and trigger the cleavage of caspase-8 (Locatelli et al., 2007; Petri et al., 2006; Raoul et al., 2006) (Fig. 1).

3. Mitochondrial dysfunction in ALS and in experimental motor neuron degeneration

A convergent point of the deleterious mechanisms discussed above is the mitochondrion. This organelle is the main energy producer in eukaryotic cells and plays a fundamental role in normal cell physiology. Among the functions mitochondria carry out, besides ATP synthesis, intracellular Ca^{2+}buffering has been recognized as another relevant factor for the protection against deleterious processes such as oxidative stress, excitotoxicity and necrotic and apoptotic death, thus playing a central role in neuronal survival.

Mitochondria are closely related to necrotic and apoptotic processes, which are the main cellular death mechanisms. During necrosis, mitochondria undergo rapid swelling and lysis. Although apoptosis is an energy-dependent active process, sometimes mitochondrial morphological alterations are associated with the intrinsic-apoptosis pathway. Furthermore, it is now recognized that apoptosis and necrosis are not two mutually exclusive processes, but they can occur simultaneously or one preceding the other (Kroemer et al., 2009; Martin, 2010; Martin et al., 2009; Shrivastava & Vivekanandhan, 2011).

As the organelle responsible for energy production in the cell, mitochondria possess the enzymatic machinery to catalyze the oxidation of various substrates generated inside and outside mitochondria, including pyruvate trough pyruvate dehydrogenase, fatty acids through β-oxidation, and carbon chains from amino acids. Energy is obtained by oxidation of all these biomolecules to finally CO_2 and H_2O through the tricarboxylic acid cycle and the respiratory chain. The tricarboxylic acid cycle is the converging point because the carbon skeletons of carbohydrates and fatty acids are metabolized to yield the acetyl group of acetyl-Coenzyme A, and many of the carbons of the amino acid skeleton also enter the cycle via its conversion to some cycle intermediates. The reducing equivalents generated in the tricarboxylic acid cycle reactions reduce pyridine and flavin nucleotides to NADH and $FADH_2$. These electron transporters enter the respiratory chain, where electron flux through various redox carriers and centers in the enzyme complexes located in the inner mitochondrial membrane finally reduces O_2 to H_2O; this flux is coupled to ATP synthesis through oxidative phosphorylation.

The energy released by the electron flux through respiratory chain complexes is used to pump protons through the inner mitochondrial membrane, producing an alkaline and negatively charged mitochondrial matrix, as compared to the intermembrane space, thus creating a proton gradient. This proton gradient generates an electrochemical potential called proton-motive force (Δp), which supplies the energy to ATP synthase for ATP synthesis from ADP and inorganic phosphate. The Δp depends mainly on the mitochondrial transmembrane potential ($\Delta\psi_m$), which is the electric potential (negative inside), but it also depends on the transmembrane pH gradient (ΔpH), which is the chemical potential (alkaline inside). Energy stored in the proton gradient can also transport solutes against concentration gradient across the membrane. The $\Delta\psi_m$ is a central parameter that controls three fundamental and highly relevant cellular processes for neuronal survival: ATP synthesis, mitochondrial Ca^{2+} sequestration, and mitochondrial ROS generation. On the other hand, $\Delta\psi_m$ is controlled by substrate availability, ATP demand, respiratory chain capacity, mitochondrial proton conductance, and mitochondrial Ca^{2+} sequestration (Nicholls & Budd, 2000). Therefore, mitochondrial bioenergetic status is crucial for controlling the susceptibility of neurons to chronic or acute stress and also in determining cellular fate (survival, apoptosis or necrosis).

Owing to the great relevance of mitochondria, their morphological, ultrastructural and functional characteristics have been studied in ALS patients. Deficits in respiratory chain complexes I and IV activities have been detected in the spinal cord and skeletal muscle (Borthwick et al., 1999; Crugnola et al., 2010; Vielhaber et al., 2000; Wiedemann et al., 2002; Wiedemann et al., 1998), and a temporal study of mitochondrial respiratory function in skeletal muscle in SALS demonstrated that respiratory complex IV activity is progressively altered as the disease develops (Echaniz-Laguna et al., 2006). Some cases of ALS have been described as a mitochondriopathy (Finsterer, 2002, 2003) including a mitochondrial DNA mutation in the gene encoding subunit I of the mitochondrial respiratory chain complex IV (Comi et al., 1998). The electron transport chain proteins FAD synthetase, riboflavin kinase, cytochrome C1, and succinate dehydrogenase complex subunit B expression were significantly decreased in some ALS patients (Lin et al., 2009).

In the mSOD1 mice or cell culture familial ALS model, complexes I, II and IV of the electron transport chain exhibit decreased enzyme activities, even at early stages of the disease (Jung et al., 2002; Mattiazzi et al., 2002; Menzies et al., 2002a,b). In G93A-SOD1 mice the association of cytochrome c with the inner mitochondrial membrane was reduced and there was a significant decrease in respiratory chain complex IV (Kirkinezos et al., 2005). SOD-containing aggregates (Higgins et al., 2002; Jaarsma et al., 2001; Pasinelli et al., 2004) and decreased oxygen consumption, lack of ADP-dependent respiratory control, and decreased membrane potential (Cassina et al., 2008), were observed in mitochondria from spinal cord of transgenic mSOD1 rodents.

In neuronal cultures, glutamate-mediated excitotoxicity caused significant changes in mitochondrial function, such as decline in ATP levels, mitochondrial transmembrane potential collapse, decreased mitochondrial and cellular oxygen consumption, and oxidative phosphorylation uncoupling, all these events preceding cell death (Ankarcrona et al., 1995; Atlante et al., 1996; Maus et al., 1999; Monje et al., 2001). There is a link between excitotoxicity-induced intracellular Ca^{2+} overload and the collapse of $\Delta\psi_m$, since intracellular Ca^{2+} increase and its accumulation in mitochondria are sufficient to induce prominent and persistent depolarization, leading to mitochondrial dysfunction and to neuronal death in vitro (Schinder et al., 1996; White & Reynolds, 1996).

Few studies on excitotoxicity have been carried out in vivo. In our laboratory we have developed two experimental models of spinal motor neurons degeneration by overactivation of AMPA receptors, both by infusing AMPA directly in the lumbar spinal cord of rats. In the first one AMPA is administered through microdialysis cannulas during short time periods (Corona & Tapia, 2004) and in the other AMPA is infused chronically during several days, using osmotic minipumps (Tovar-y-Romo et al., 2007). These models reproduce the main histopathological features of ALS: loss of lumbar motor neurons, astroglial activation and motor deficits that progresses to complete paralysis of the rear limbs. The main difference between the two models is the time required for the occurrence of motor neuron degeneration and the development of the paralysis. AMPA perfusion by microdialysis causes a rapid loss of motor neuron and paralysis, occurring within the initial 12 hours, while chronic AMPA infusion with osmotic minipumps triggers a progressive motor neuron loss and motor deficits throughout three to four days. For these reasons, the microdialysis model is defined as an acute model and the minipumps model as a chronic model of spinal motor neuron degeneration by excitotoxicity (Tovar-y-Romo et al., 2009a). The most important feature of both models is that motor neuron loss occurs without the influence of a genetic factor and thus presumably can be used to study the mechanisms that may be involved in motor neuron loss occurring in SALS, which accounts for over 90% of ALS cases.

We have recently assessed mitochondrial function in our acute model of spinal excitotoxic motor neuron degeneration, by studying mitochondrial oxygen consumption and transmembrane potential in mitochondria isolated from the lumbar spinal cord of rats perfused with AMPA. The AMPA-treated group showed decreased oxygen consumption, ADP-dependent respiratory control and transmembrane potential, as compared to control rats perfused only with Krebs-Ringer medium (Santa-Cruz and Tapia, in preparation). These results suggest that mitochondrial dysfunction plays a crucial role in spinal motoneuron degeneration induced by overactivation of AMPA receptors in vivo. These mechanisms could be involved in ALS motoneuron degeneration.

3.1 Ca^{2+}, mitochondria and motor neuron degeneration

Under physiological conditions, Ca^{2+} participates as intracellular messenger in many normal cellular functions, such as cell growth, differentiation, signal transduction, membrane excitability regulation, exocytosis and synaptic activity. Cytoplasmic Ca^{2+} concentration in resting neurons is maintained at low concentrations (~100 nM), 10,000 times lower than extracellular space concentration. To achieve this, neurons possess specialized homeostatic mechanisms, such as regulation of Ca^{2+} input and output, Ca^{2+} binding proteins, mitochondrial and endoplasmic reticulum storage, and Ca^{2+}-ATPases. Moreover, neurons not only control intracellular Ca^{2+} levels, but also its location in the cell by means of complex interactions among Ca^{2+} input, output, buffering and internal storage. Under physiological conditions, these processes maintain spatial and temporal location of Ca^{2+}, so that multiple Ca^{2+}-regulated signaling pathways can take place independently within the same cell.

Excessive intracellular Ca^{2+} concentration damages neurons through several mechanisms, including mitochondrial damage, energy metabolism deficit, toxic ROS generation, membrane depolarization, and activation of lytic enzymes such as proteases, lipases, phosphatases and endonucleases. Intracellular Ca^{2+} accumulation also stimulates ROS production through NOS activation and the conversion of xanthine dehydrogenase to xanthine oxidase through proteases activation. All these events eventually produce membrane destruction and neuronal death (Arundine & Tymianski, 2003; Shaw, 1999).

Intracellular Ca^{2+} regulation is an expensive process from the energy point of view. Ca^{2+} is extruded from the cell and sequestered into the endoplasmic reticulum through active transport using Ca^{2+}-ATPases, and it is also removed by secondary active transport using the Na^+/Ca^{2+} exchanger, which activates Na^+/K^+-ATPases to take out Na^+. Mitochondria also play a critical role in the regulation of cytosolic Ca^{2+} concentration, since they sequester this cation through a Ca^{2+} uniporter located in the inner mitochondrial membrane and driven by the electric potential (Nicholls, 1985). To prevent a potentially lethal Ca^{2+} accumulation in mitochondrial matrix, there is an output system that exchanges Na^+/Ca^{2+}, besides a mitochondrial Na^+/H^+ transporter that extrudes Na^+, so that ion flux under a constant Ca^{2+} entrance to mitochondria involves a sequential transfer of Ca^{2+}, Na^+ and H^+, the latter driven by the respiratory chain (Crompton & Heid, 1978; Nicholls & Budd, 2000). When Ca^{2+} concentration surpasses a certain critical point, under physiological phosphate concentration an osmotically inactive and rapidly dissociable Ca^{2+}-phosphate complex is formed in the mitochondrial matrix, so that mitochondria work as efficient buffers of extramitochondrial Ca^{2+} by accumulating this cation (Becker et al., 1980; Nicholls, 1978). Apparently, this organelle acts as a temporary Ca^{2+} store during high cytoplasmic concentrations peaks, as suggested by the kinetics of mitochondrial Ca^{2+} transport; because the Ca^{2+}-phosphate complex is rapidly dissociable, mitochondria can release Ca^{2+} back to the cytoplasm when its concentration decreases below the critical point. As long as mitochondria are polarized, cytosolic Ca^{2+} accumulates within the mitochondrial matrix through the Ca^{2+} uniporter. Mitochondrial Ca^{2+} uptake is driven by $\Delta\psi_m$, so it will compete with ATP synthase for proton gradient, in such a way that Ca^{2+} uptake could dominate due to the fact that ATP synthesis requires a thermodynamic threshold for $\Delta\psi_m$, while Ca^{2+} transport can proceed at much lower $\Delta\psi_m$ and excessive Ca^{2+} concentrations reduce $\Delta\psi_m$ dramatically. When Ca^{2+} concentration does not recover below the critical point, excessive Ca^{2+} overload in the mitochondrial matrix can lead to mitochondrial swelling, loss of respiratory control, increased mitochondrial ROS generation, $\Delta\psi_m$ collapse (depolarization) diminished ATP synthesis, and Ca^{2+} release from the mitochondrial matrix caused by inner mitochondrial membrane permeabilization through the mitochondrial permeability transition pore (MPTP, a large protein complex forming a non-selective pore through the inner mitochondrial membrane) (Al-Nasser & Crompton, 1986; Nicholls & Budd, 2000; Peng & Jou, 2010). When mitochondrion depolarizes, accumulated Ca^{2+} goes back into the cytoplasm, either through the Ca^{2+} uniporter, the Na^+/Ca^{2+} exchanger, or through the MPTP. Since Δp depends mainly on $\Delta\psi_m$, its collapse causes Δp collapse, which results not only in halting ATP synthesis but also in a rapid cytoplasmic ATP hydrolysis because ATP synthase catalytic function reverses in an attempt to restore Δp.

In motor neurons, the damage produced by these alterations may be enhanced because they do not have sufficient mitochondrial Ca^{2+}-buffering capacity, due in part to a lower mitochondrial density per volume compared to non-motor neurons (Grosskreutz et al., 2007). In addition, other buffering mechanisms are deficient in spinal and cortical motor neurons because they lack the Ca^{2+}-binding proteins calbindin D-28K and parvalbumin. This may explain why other motor neurons that express these proteins, such as those located in oculomotor and Onuf's nuclei, are not usually affected in ALS (Alexianu et al., 1994; Celio, 1990; Ince et al., 1993; Palecek et al., 1999). For all these reasons, mitochondrial Ca^{2+} overload plays a key role in glutamatergic excitotoxicity (Nicholls et al., 2003), given that overactivation of Ca^{2+}-permeable AMPA receptors, which are abundant in spinal motor neurons, confers to these cells a special vulnerability to AMPA receptor-mediated excitotoxicity (Corona & Tapia, 2007; Grosskreutz et al., 2010). AMPA exposure to spinal motor neuron cultures results in an intracellular Ca^{2+} concentration increase that triggers mitochondrial Ca^{2+} overload, depolarization and ROS generation (Carriedo et al., 2000). So, there is abundant evidence that suggest that mitochondrial damage, probably related to Ca^{2+} homeostasis disturbances, is involved in SALS and FALS (Manfredi & Xu, 2005; Menzies et al., 2002a; Swerdlow et al., 1998; von Lewinski & Keller, 2005).

3.2 Energy deficits

Due to the large size of motor neurons and their long processes reaching muscles, they have an expensive energy cost and this renders them very vulnerable to energy deficits. Much of the ATP demand in neurons is used in the ion pumping through plasma membrane to maintain membrane potential. Thus, Na^+/K^+-ATPase is the most demanding ATP process in neurons (Scott & Nicholls, 1980) in order to expel Na^+ excess resulting from excitation. Intracellular Ca^{2+} regulation by Ca-ATPases is also highly energy consuming, as previously discussed.

There is abundant evidence both in vitro and in vivo that any restriction in the ability of the cell to generate ATP can exacerbate or even induce glutamatergic excitotoxicity. The energy-linked excitotoxic hypothesis (Beal et al., 1993; Greene & Greenamyre, 1996; Novelli et al., 1988) proposes that the correlation between excitotoxic damage and energy restriction is due to plasma membrane depolarization. Diminished ATP levels cause a decrease in Na^+/K^+-ATPase and Ca^{2+}-ATPase functions, lessening Na^+ and Ca^{2+} removal. This triggers plasma membrane depolarization and as a consequence Ca^{2+} enters the cell through voltage-dependent Ca^{2+}channels and glutamate is released to the extracellular space by exocytosis. This in turn activates Ca^{2+} influx through the NMDA receptor, which is also voltage-dependent. Further, under energetic failure conditions, glutamate transporters operate in reverse because Na^{+}/K^{+} electrochemical gradient collapse due to ATP decrease, resulting in diminished glutamate uptake and non-vesicular glutamate release into extracellular space (Jabaudon et al., 2000; Longuemare & Swanson, 1995).

The observation that inhibition of mitochondrial respiratory chain complexes activity can induce pathological changes similar to those observed in some neurodegenerative diseases in specific CNS regions has generated great interest. Association among glutamatergic excitotoxicity and bioenergetic limitation has been proposed for Alzheimer, Parkinson, Huntington's disease and ALS (Beal, 1998), and in many cases specific respiratory chain complexes are involved. In organotypic spinal cord cultures, motor neurons are selectively vulnerable to chronic mitochondrial blockade by inhibitors of mitochondrial respiratory chain complex II and complex IV and this motor neuron degeneration displays structural changes similar to those seen following excitotoxicity (Brunet et al., 2009; Kaal et al., 2000).

In our acute model of excitotoxic motor neuron degeneration previously described (Corona & Tapia, 2004, 2007) we have demonstrated the importance of Ca^{2+}-permeable AMPA receptors and of intracellular Ca^{2+} overload in motor neuron death process. Using this model, we aimed to study the importance of energy deficits and oxidative stress in AMPA-induced degeneration. With this purpose, we assessed the potential neuroprotection of various energy substrates and antioxidants at different concentrations, co-perfusing them with AMPA in the rat lumbar spinal cord. We observed protection at different degrees depending on the concentration of each compound, but in general antioxidants only partially protected, while various energy substrates prevented the AMPA-induced motor impairment and the spinal motor neuron loss (Santa-Cruz and Tapia, in preparation). These findings suggest that intracellular Ca^{2+} overload in vivo disrupts mitochondrial energy metabolism. On the other hand, energy substrates can directly prevent $\Delta\psi_m$ collapse and thus prevent mitochondrial dysfunction. Because one of the factors that control $\Delta\psi_m$ is substrate availability, excess mitochondrial substrates administered exogenously can stimulate respiratory chain and increase oxidative phosphorylation, maintaining the electrochemical proton gradient and thus preventing the collapse of ATP synthesis.

3.3 Oxidative stress

Since mitochondria are the organelles where oxidative phosphorylation is accomplished, they consume about 98 % of the cell oxygen requirement and constitute a major site for intracellular ROS production. Some steps along mitochondrial oxygen reduction pathway have the potential to produce, and indeed generate free radicals, due to the fact that electron flux along respiratory chain may have leakage of electrons to oxygen. The intermediate radical ubisemiquinone, involved in the transfer of electrons through respiratory complexes III and I, can grant an electron to oxygen, forming the superoxide radical $O_2^{\bullet -}$, a powerful oxidant and a very reactive intermediate (Turrens et al., 1985) that must be rapidly removed by antioxidant enzymes to avoid its lethal effects. About 0.1-4% of the O_2 used by actively respiring mitochondria is converted to $O_2^{\bullet -}$. Nevertheless, respiratory chain enzymes defects or other mitochondrial perturbations could be responsible of an excessive mitochondrial

ROS production, triggering or increasing cellular injure. Among them, mitochondrial Ca^{2+} overload resulting from NMDA, AMPA or kainate receptor overactivation (Carriedo et al., 1998; Carriedo et al., 2000; Dugan et al., 1995) increases ROS production (Dykens, 1994; Peng & Jou, 2010); thus, an initial excitotoxic event might also contribute to increased oxidative stress.

In addition, it is important to consider that mitochondria are not only ROS producers but also that they are a susceptible target of them. Thereby, in a pathologic situation where an increased ROS production occurs initially, oxidative damage to mitochondrial lipids, nucleic acids and proteins can reduce mitochondrial respiration, disturb normal function and seriously damage this organelle (Lenaz et al., 2002). Furthermore, mitochondrial DNA is more susceptible to oxidative damage than nuclear DNA, due to its close location next to an important ROS production site, to the lack of protective histones and to less effective repair mechanisms, as compared to the nuclear DNA (Richter et al., 1988). Mitochondrial redox status also influences the opening of the MPTP, since it is enhanced by oxidative stress in isolated mitochondria (Saxena et al., 1995).

4. Mitochondrial structural damage in ALS and experimental motor neuron degeneration

The death process involved in the motor neuron loss characteristic of ALS is not yet fully understood. Several functional alterations present in both human disease and experimental models have been reviewed in the previous sections, but several studies have shown also morphological and ultrastructural changes in motor neurons that may be associated with apoptosis and/or necrosis.

Postmortem examination of ALS patients tissues has revealed morphological and ultrastructural abnormalities in mitochondria. Atypical mitochondrial aggregates were found in skeletal muscle subsarcolemmal region and in intramuscular axons (Afifi et al., 1966; Atsumi, 1981), and morphological abnormalities were also detected in proximal axons, as well as dense clusters of mitochondria in the ventral horn of spinal cord SALS patients (Hirano et al., 1984a; b; Sasaki & Iwata, 1996). Giant mitochondria with intramitochondrial inclusions were observed in the liver of some ALS patients and these alterations were disease specific (Nakano et al., 1987). Further, mitochondria with increased volume and with high Ca^{2+} concentration were found in motor nerve terminals in muscle biopsies of alive ALS patients, which were not observed in patients with other neuropathies or in control subjects (Siklos et al., 1996). Ultrastructural damage of mitochondria, characterized by swelling and rounding, was recently described in platelets of ALS patients (Shrivastava & Vivekanandhan, 2011; Shrivastava et al., 2011a,b).

The main problem with pathological studies in human ALS is the difficulty in determining whether the alterations observed are a cause or a consequence of the disease. This highlights the importance of developing experimental models of motor neuron death to study the temporal progress of the morphological changes, including the alterations of mitochondrial structure. With this objective, we have recently studied the ultrastructural changes of mitochondria in both our acute and chronic models of spinal motor neuron death described above. In the acute model we observed motor neurons with mitochondrial swelling as soon as 2 h after AMPA perfusion, followed in a few hours by the rupture of mitochondrial, nuclear and plasma membranes, which led to total neuronal disruption. These ultrastructural alterations are characteristic of a necrotic process. In contrast, in the chronic model we observed by day one swelling of the endoplasmic reticulum and only later progressive alterations in mitochondrial internal and external membranes that generated mitochondrial swelling. So, the initial mitochondrial integrity might indicate an apoptotic process, although motor neurons eventually probably die by a slow necrotic process (Fig. 2; Ramírez-Jarquín and Tapia, in preparation). The mitochondrial swelling observed in both models may be associated with energy failure, which as discussed above causes ATP depletion, oxidative stress and inflammatory events, leading to cell death.

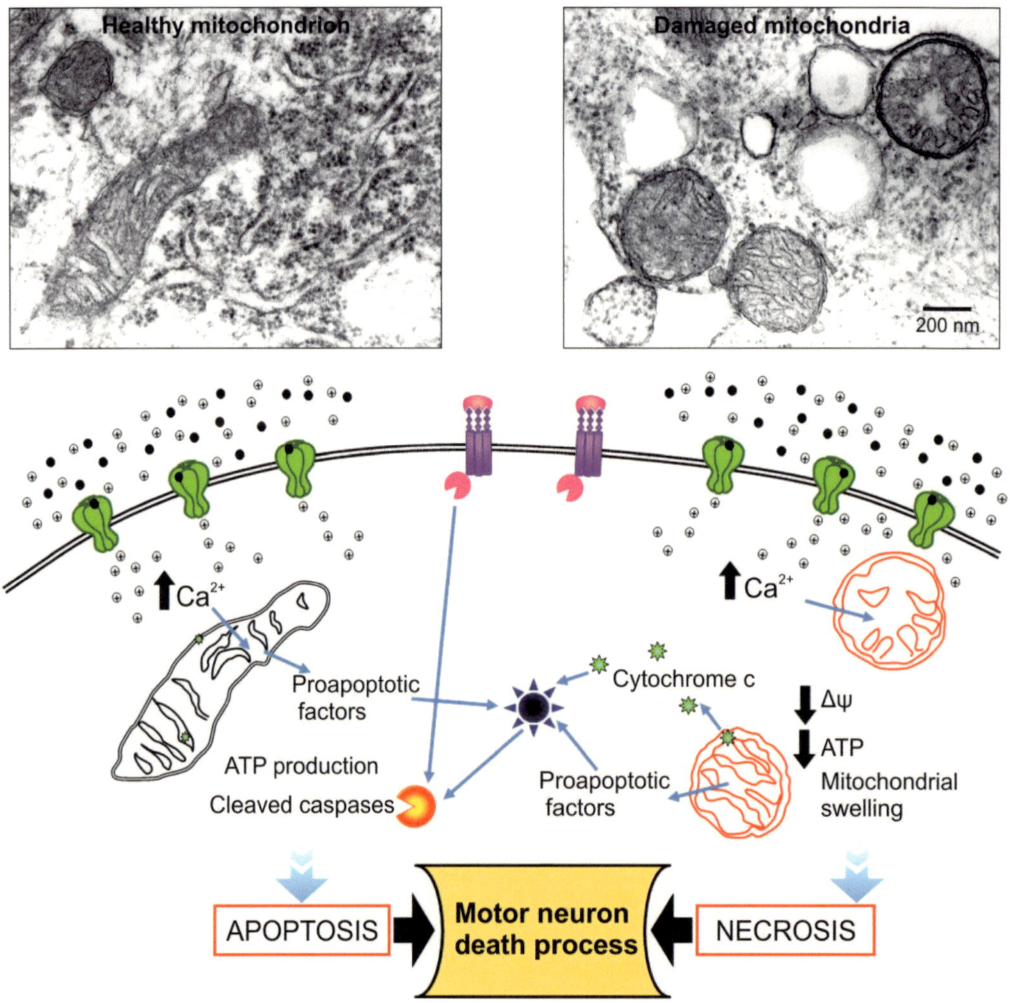

Fig. 2. Role of mitochondrial damage in motor neuron excitotoxicity. The electron-micrographs show normal mitochondria and endoplasmic reticulum in a spinal motor neuron of a control rat (left), and swollen mitochondria with altered cristae observed 2 h after perfusion of AMPA by microdialysis (right) (Ramírez-Jarquín and Tapia, unpublished). Bottom: proposal of the involvement of mitochondrial damage in the apoptosis and necrosis processes leading to motor neuron death. The symbols are the same as in Fig. 1. Description in the text.

The mitochondrial damage seen in our models is similar to those observed in the human disease and also in muscle and spinal cord of mSOD1 rodent models, namely mitochondrial fragmentation, enlargement, vacuolization, rearrangement of the cristae and swelling (Bendotti et al., 2001; Kong & Xu, 1998; Martin et al., 2009; Menzies et al., 2002b; Wong et al., 1995). The observed rearrangement of the inner membrane to form small vacuoles has been associated with an alteration in the MPTP permeability and also with the trigger of intrinsic-apoptosis pathway by release of proapoptotic factors, such as cytochrome c (Bendotti et al., 2001; Martin, 2010; Martin et al., 2009; Ohta et al., 2008) followed by the cleavage of caspases (Li et al., 2000; Pasinelli et al., 2000) Fig. 2 illustrates the ultrastructural mitochondrial damage and shows a schematic representation of the mechanisms associated with these alterations.

5. Conclusions

Altogether the foregoing data suggest that mitochondrial respiratory chain damage is a relevant event in ALS pathogenesis, although it is still unknown if mitochondrial abnormalities are the cause of the disease process or if they are consequence of neuronal degeneration, However, it is clear from the evidence reviewed here that mitochondria definitely play a central role in determining the fate of motor neurons and in their degeneration process. This evidence comes from studies in several tissues of ALS patients, both from biopsies or from postmortem observations, and from direct measurements of mitochondrial function in experimental models of motor neuron degeneration, both in vitro and in vivo. These experiments clearly point to energy deficits and disruption of Ca^{2+} homeostasis and axonal transport.

Integrity of the mitochondria morphology and structure is pivotal for their function and for cellular health. It is interesting that similar structural alterations have been observed in ALS tissues and in in vitro and in vivo models of motor neuron degeneration, including transgenic mSOD1 rodents and excitotoxicity. Clearly, this damage can be associated with the mitochondrial functional deficits, which trigger deleterious process resulting in cellular death by apoptosis, necrosis or a combination of these mechanisms. Although there is biochemical evidence of an apoptotic process involving the mitochondria, no ultrastructural evidence of classic apoptosis, such as apoptotic bodies, has been found. Rather, mitochondrial swelling and membrane disruption are frequently observed, suggesting the predominance of a necrotic process.

The evidence for a role of calcium homeostasis disruption in the induction of neuronal death is vast, and the involvement of mitochondria in this mechanism seems determinant. The advances in the elucidation of this process should help to understand the importance of the preservation of mitochondrial structure and function, which hopefully can lead to the design of preventive and therapeutic measures for ALS.

6. Acknowledgement

This work and the authors' experiments cited were supported by Dirección General del Personal Académico, Universidad Nacional Autónoma de México, (project IN215610) and Consejo Nacional de Ciencia y Tecnología (CONACYT), México (project 128229). L.D.S.C. and U.N.R.J. are recipients of a scholarship from CONACYT.

7. References

Abe, K., Pan, L. H., Watanabe, M., Kato, T. & Itoyama, Y. (1995). Induction of nitrotyrosine-like immunoreactivity in the lower motor neuron of amyotrophic lateral sclerosis. *Neuroscience letters,* Vol.199, No.2, (October 1995), pp. 152-154, ISSN 0304-3940.

Abe, K., Pan, L. H., Watanabe, M., Konno, H., Kato, T. & Itoyama, Y. (1997). Upregulation of protein-tyrosine nitration in the anterior horn cells of amyotrophic lateral sclerosis. *Neurological research,* Vol.19, No.2, (April 1997), pp. 124-128, ISSN 0161-6412.

Afifi, A. K., Aleu, F. P., Goodgold, J. & MacKay, B. (1966). Ultrastructure of atrophic muscle in amyotrophic lateral sclerosis. *Neurology,* Vol.16, No.5, (May 1996), pp. 475-481, ISSN 0028-3878.

Al-Nasser, I. & Crompton, M. (1986). The reversible Ca2+-induced permeabilization of rat liver mitochondria. *The Biochemical journal,* Vol.239, No.1, (October 1986), pp. 19-29, ISSN 0264-6021.

Alexianu, M. E., Ho, B. K., Mohamed, A. H., La Bella, V., Smith, R. G. & Appel, S. H. (1994). The role of calcium-binding proteins in selective motoneuron vulnerability in amyotrophic lateral sclerosis. *Annals of neurology,* Vol.36, No.6, (December 1994), pp. 846-858, ISSN 0364-5134

Almer, G., Teismann, P., Stevic, Z., Halaschek-Wiener, J., Deecke, L., Kostic, V. & Przedborski, S. (2002). Increased levels of the pro-inflammatory prostaglandin PGE2 in CSF from ALS patients. *Neurology,* Vol.58, No.8, (April 2002), pp. 1277-1279, ISSN 0028-3878.

Andrus, P. K., Fleck, T. J., Gurney, M. E. & Hall, E. D. (1998). Protein oxidative damage in a transgenic mouse model of familial amyotrophic lateral sclerosis. *Journal of neurochemistry,* Vol.71, No.5, (November 1998), pp. 2041-2048, ISSN 0022-3042.

Ankarcrona, M., Dypbukt, J. M., Bonfoco, E., Zhivotovsky, B., Orrenius, S., Lipton, S. A. & Nicotera, P. (1995). Glutamate-induced neuronal death: a succession of necrosis or apoptosis depending on mitochondrial function. *Neuron,* Vol.15, No.4, (October 1995), pp. 961-973, ISSN 0896-6273.

Arundine, M. & Tymianski, M. (2003). Molecular mechanisms of calcium-dependent neurodegeneration in excitotoxicity. *Cell calcium,* Vol.34, No.4-5, (October-November 2003), pp. 325-337, ISSN 0143-4160.

Atlante, A., Gagliardi, S., Minervini, G. M., Marra, E., Passarella, S. & Calissano, P. (1996). Rapid uncoupling of oxidative phosphorylation accompanies glutamate toxicity in rat cerebellar granule cells. *Neuroreport,* Vol.7, No.15-17, (November 1996), pp. 2519-2523, ISSN 0959-4965.

Atsumi, T. (1981). The ultrastructure of intramuscular nerves in amyotrophic lateral sclerosis. *Acta neuropathologica,* Vol.55, No.3, pp. 193-198, ISSN 0001-6322.

Baillet, A., Chanteperdrix, V., Trocme, C., Casez, P., Garrel, C. & Besson, G. (2010). The role of oxidative stress in amyotrophic lateral sclerosis and Parkinson's disease. *Neurochemical research,* Vol.35, No.10, (October 2010), pp. 1530-1537, ISSN 1573-6903 (Electronic), 0364-3190 (Linking).

Beal, M. F. (1998). Mitochondrial dysfunction in neurodegenerative diseases. *Biochimica et biophysica acta,* Vol.1366, No.1-2, (August 1998), pp. 211-223, ISSN 0006-3002.

Beal, M. F., Hyman, B. T. & Koroshetz, W. (1993). Do defects in mitochondrial energy metabolism underlie the pathology of neurodegenerative diseases? *Trends in neurosciences,* Vol.16, No.4, (April 1993), pp. 125-131, ISSN 0166-2236.

Beal, M. F., Ferrante, R. J., Browne, S. E., Matthews, R. T., Kowall, N. W. & Brown, R. H., Jr. (1997). Increased 3-nitrotyrosine in both sporadic and familial amyotrophic lateral sclerosis. *Annals of neurology,* Vol.42, No.4, (October 1997), pp. 644-654, ISSN 0364-5134.

Becker, G. L., Fiskum, G. & Lehninger, A. L. (1980). Regulation of free Ca2+ by liver mitochondria and endoplasmic reticulum. *The Journal of biological chemistry,* Vol.255, No.19, (October 1980), pp. 9009-9012, ISSN 0021-9258.

Bendotti, C., Calvaresi, N., Chiveri, L., Prelle, A., Moggio, M., Braga, M., Silani, V. & De Biasi, S. (2001). Early vacuolization and mitochondrial damage in motor neurons of FALS mice are not associated with apoptosis or with changes in cytochrome oxidase histochemical reactivity. *Journal of the neurological sciences,* Vol.191, No.1-2, (October 2001), pp. 25-33, ISSN 0022-510X.

Bilsland, L. G., Sahai, E., Kelly, G., Golding, M., Greensmith, L. & Schiavo, G. (2010). Deficits in axonal transport precede ALS symptoms in vivo. *Proceedings of the National Academy of Sciences of the United States of America,* Vol.107, No.47, (November 2010), pp. 20523-20528, ISSN 1091-6490 (Electronic), 0027-8424 (Linking).

Bogdanov, M., Brown, R. H., Matson, W., Smart, R., Hayden, D., O'Donnell, H., Flint Beal, M. & Cudkowicz, M. (2000). Increased oxidative damage to DNA in ALS patients. *Free radical biology & medicine,* Vol.29, No.7, (October 2000), pp. 652-658, ISSN 0891-5849.

Boillee, S., Vande Velde, C. & Cleveland, D. W. (2006a). ALS: a disease of motor neurons and their nonneuronal neighbors. *Neuron,* Vol.52, No.1, (October 2006), pp. 39-59, ISSN 0896-6273.

Boillee, S., Yamanaka, K., Lobsiger, C. S., Copeland, N. G., Jenkins, N. A., Kassiotis, G., Kollias, G. & Cleveland, D. W. (2006b). Onset and progression in inherited ALS determined by motor neurons and microglia. *Science (New York, N.Y,* Vol.312, No.5778, (June 2006), pp. 1389-1392, ISSN 1095-9203 (Electronic), 0036-8075 (Linking).

Bonnefont-Rousselot, D., Lacomblez, L., Jaudon, M., Lepage, S., Salachas, F., Bensimon, G., Bizard, C., Doppler, V., Delattre, J. & Meininger, V. (2000). Blood oxidative stress in amyotrophic lateral sclerosis. *Journal of the neurological sciences,* Vol.178, No.1, (September 2000), pp. 57-62, ISSN 0022-510X.

Borthwick, G. M., Johnson, M. A., Ince, P. G., Shaw, P. J. & Turnbull, D. M. (1999). Mitochondrial enzyme activity in amyotrophic lateral sclerosis: implications for the role of mitochondria in neuronal cell death. *Annals of neurology,* Vol.46, No.5, (November 1999), pp. 787-790, ISSN 0364-5134.

Breuer, A. C. & Atkinson, M. B. (1988). Fast axonal transport alterations in amyotrophic lateral sclerosis (ALS) and in parathyroid hormone (PTH)-treated axons. *Cell motility and the cytoskeleton,* Vol.10, No.1-2, pp. 321-330, ISSN 0886-1544.

Breuer, A. C., Lynn, M. P., Atkinson, M. B., Chou, S. M., Wilbourn, A. J., Marks, K. E., Culver, J. E. & Fleegler, E. J. (1987). Fast axonal transport in amyotrophic lateral sclerosis: an intra-axonal organelle traffic analysis. *Neurology,* Vol.37, No.5, (May 1987), pp. 738-748, ISSN 0028-3878.

Brunet, N., Tarabal, O., Esquerda, J. E. & Caldero, J. (2009). Excitotoxic motoneuron degeneration induced by glutamate receptor agonists and mitochondrial toxins in organotypic cultures of chick embryo spinal cord. *The Journal of comparative neurology,* Vol.516, No.4, (October 2009), pp. 277-290, ISSN 1096-9861 (Electronic), 0021-9967 (Linking).

Burnashev, N., Monyer, H., Seeburg, P. H. & Sakmann, B. (1992). Divalent ion permeability of AMPA receptor channels is dominated by the edited form of a single subunit. *Neuron,* Vol.8, No.1, (January 1992), pp. 189-198, ISSN 0896-6273.

Carriedo, S. G., Yin, H. Z., Sensi, S. L. & Weiss, J. H. (1998). Rapid Ca2+ entry through Ca2+-permeable AMPA/Kainate channels triggers marked intracellular Ca2+ rises and consequent oxygen radical production. *J Neurosci,* Vol.18, No.19, (October 1998), pp. 7727-7738, ISSN 0270-6474.

Carriedo, S. G., Sensi, S. L., Yin, H. Z. & Weiss, J. H. (2000). AMPA exposures induce mitochondrial Ca(2+) overload and ROS generation in spinal motor neurons in vitro. *J Neurosci,* Vol.20, No.1, (January 2000), pp. 240-250, ISSN 1529-2401 (Electronic), 0270-6474 (Linking).

Casoni, F., Basso, M., Massignan, T., Gianazza, E., Cheroni, C., Salmona, M., Bendotti, C. & Bonetto, V. (2005). Protein nitration in a mouse model of familial amyotrophic lateral sclerosis: possible multifunctional role in the pathogenesis. *The Journal of biological chemistry,* Vol.280, No.16, (April 2005), pp. 16295-16304, ISSN 0021-9258.

Cassina, P., Cassina, A., Pehar, M., Castellanos, R., Gandelman, M., de Leon, A., Robinson, K. M., Mason, R. P., Beckman, J. S., Barbeito, L. & Radi, R. (2008). Mitochondrial dysfunction in SOD1G93A-bearing astrocytes promotes motor neuron degeneration: prevention by mitochondrial-targeted antioxidants. *J Neurosci,* Vol.28, No.16, (April 2008), pp. 4115-4122, ISSN 1529-2401 (Electronic), 0270-6474 (Linking).

Celio, M. R. (1990). Calbindin D-28k and parvalbumin in the rat nervous system. *Neuroscience,* Vol.35, No.2, pp. 375-475, ISSN 0306-4522.

Chancellor, A. M. & Warlow, C. P. (1992). Adult onset motor neuron disease: worldwide mortality, incidence and distribution since 1950. *Journal of neurology, neurosurgery, and psychiatry,* Vol.55, No.12, (December 1992), pp. 1106-1115, ISSN 0022-3050 (Print), 0022-3050 (Linking).

Clement, A. M., Nguyen, M. D., Roberts, E. A., Garcia, M. L., Boillee, S., Rule, M., McMahon, A. P., Doucette, W., Siwek, D., Ferrante, R. J., Brown, R. H., Jr., Julien, J. P., Goldstein, L. S. & Cleveland, D. W. (2003). Wild-type nonneuronal cells extend survival of SOD1 mutant motor neurons in ALS mice. *Science (New York, N.Y,* Vol.302, No.5642, (October 2003), pp. 113-117, ISSN 1095-9203 (Electronic), 0036-8075 (Linking).

Collard, J. F., Cote, F. & Julien, J. P. (1995). Defective axonal transport in a transgenic mouse model of amyotrophic lateral sclerosis. *Nature,* Vol.375, No.6526, (May 1995), pp. 61-64, ISSN 0028-0836.

Comi, G. P., Bordoni, A., Salani, S., Franceschina, L., Sciacco, M., Prelle, A., Fortunato, F., Zeviani, M., Napoli, L., Bresolin, N., Moggio, M., Ausenda, C. D., Taanman, J. W. & Scarlato, G. (1998). Cytochrome c oxidase subunit I microdeletion in a patient with motor neuron disease. *Annals of neurology,* Vol.43, No.1, (January 1998), pp. 110-116, ISSN 0364-5134.

Corona, J. C. & Tapia, R. (2004). AMPA receptor activation, but not the accumulation of endogenous extracellular glutamate, induces paralysis and motor neuron death in rat spinal cord in vivo. *Journal of neurochemistry,* Vol.89, No.4, (May 2004), pp. 988-997, ISSN 0022-3042.

Corona, J. C. & Tapia, R. (2007). Ca2+-permeable AMPA receptors and intracellular Ca2+ determine motoneuron vulnerability in rat spinal cord in vivo. *Neuropharmacology,* Vol.52, No.5, (April 2007), pp. 1219-1228, ISSN 0028-3908.

Crompton, M. & Heid, I. (1978). The cycling of calcium, sodium, and protons across the inner membrane of cardiac mitochondria. *European journal of biochemistry / FEBS,* Vol.91, No.2, (November 1978), pp. 599-608, ISSN 0014-2956.

Crugnola, V., Lamperti, C., Lucchini, V., Ronchi, D., Peverelli, L., Prelle, A., Sciacco, M., Bordoni, A., Fassone, E., Fortunato, F., Corti, S., Silani, V., Bresolin, N., Di Mauro, S., Comi, G. P. & Moggio, M. (2010). Mitochondrial respiratory chain dysfunction in muscle from patients with amyotrophic lateral sclerosis. *Archives of neurology,* Vol.67, No.7, (July 2010), pp. 849-854, ISSN 1538-3687 (Electronic), 0003-9942 (Linking).

De Vos, K. J., Chapman, A. L., Tennant, M. E., Manser, C., Tudor, E. L., Lau, K. F., Brownlees, J., Ackerley, S., Shaw, P. J., McLoughlin, D. M., Shaw, C. E., Leigh, P. N., Miller, C. C. & Grierson, A. J. (2007). Familial amyotrophic lateral sclerosis-linked SOD1 mutants perturb fast axonal transport to reduce axonal mitochondria content. *Human molecular genetics,* Vol.16, No.22, (November 2007), pp. 2720-2728, ISSN 0964-6906 (Print), 0964-6906 (Linking).

Dugan, L. L., Sensi, S. L., Canzoniero, L. M., Handran, S. D., Rothman, S. M., Lin, T. S., Goldberg, M. P. & Choi, D. W. (1995). Mitochondrial production of reactive oxygen species in cortical neurons following exposure to N-methyl-D-aspartate. *J Neurosci,* Vol.15, No.10, (October 1995), pp. 6377-6388, ISSN 0270-6474.

Dykens, J. A. (1994). Isolated cerebral and cerebellar mitochondria produce free radicals when exposed to elevated CA2+ and Na+: implications for neurodegeneration. *Journal of neurochemistry,* Vol.63, No.2, (August 1994), pp. 584-591, ISSN 0022-3042.

Echaniz-Laguna, A., Zoll, J., Ponsot, E., N'Guessan, B., Tranchant, C., Loeffler, J. P. & Lampert, E. (2006). Muscular mitochondrial function in amyotrophic lateral sclerosis is progressively altered as the disease develops: a temporal study in man. *Experimental neurology,* Vol.198, No.1, (March 2006), pp. 25-30, ISSN 0014-4886.

Ferrante, R. J., Shinobu, L. A., Schulz, J. B., Matthews, R. T., Thomas, C. E., Kowall, N. W., Gurney, M. E. & Beal, M. F. (1997a). Increased 3-nitrotyrosine and oxidative damage in mice with a human copper/zinc superoxide dismutase mutation. *Annals of neurology,* Vol.42, No.3, (September 1997), pp. 326-334, ISSN 0364-5134.

Ferrante, R. J., Browne, S. E., Shinobu, L. A., Bowling, A. C., Baik, M. J., MacGarvey, U., Kowall, N. W., Brown, R. H., Jr. & Beal, M. F. (1997b). Evidence of increased oxidative damage in both sporadic and familial amyotrophic lateral sclerosis. *Journal of neurochemistry,* Vol.69, No.5, (November 1997), pp. 2064-2074, ISSN 0022-3042.

Fiala, M., Chattopadhay, M., La Cava, A., Tse, E., Liu, G., Lourenco, E., Eskin, A., Liu, P. T., Magpantay, L., Tse, S., Mahanian, M., Weitzman, R., Tong, J., Nguyen, C., Cho, T., Koo, P., Sayre, J., Martinez-Maza, O., Rosenthal, M. J. & Wiedau-Pazos, M. (2010). IL-17A is increased in the serum and in spinal cord CD8 and mast cells of ALS patients. *Journal of neuroinflammation,* Vol.7, pp. 76, ISSN 1742-2094.

Finsterer, J. (2002). Mitochondriopathy as a differential diagnosis of amyotrophic lateral sclerosis. *Amyotroph Lateral Scler Other Motor Neuron Disord,* Vol.3, No.4, (December 2002), pp. 219-224, ISSN 1466-0822.

Finsterer, J. (2003). Mitochondriopathy mimicking amyotrophic lateral sclerosis. *The neurologist,* Vol.9, No.1, (January 2003), pp. 45-48, ISSN 1074-7931.

Fitzmaurice, P. S., Shaw, I. C., Kleiner, H. E., Miller, R. T., Monks, T. J., Lau, S. S., Mitchell, J. D. & Lynch, P. G. (1996). Evidence for DNA damage in amyotrophic lateral sclerosis. *Muscle & nerve,* Vol.19, No.6, (June 1996), pp. 797-798, ISSN 0148-639X.

Greene, J. G. & Greenamyre, J. T. (1996). Bioenergetics and glutamate excitotoxicity. *Progress in neurobiology,* Vol.48, No.6, (April 1996), pp. 613-634, ISSN 0301-0082.

Grosskreutz, J., Van Den Bosch, L. & Keller, B. U. (2010). Calcium dysregulation in amyotrophic lateral sclerosis. *Cell calcium,* Vol.47, No.2, (February 2010), pp. 165-174, ISSN 1532-1991 (Electronic), 0143-4160 (Linking).

Grosskreutz, J., Haastert, K., Dewil, M., Van Damme, P., Callewaert, G., Robberecht, W., Dengler, R. & Van Den Bosch, L. (2007). Role of mitochondria in kainate-induced fast Ca2+ transients in cultured spinal motor neurons. *Cell calcium,* Vol.42, No.1, (July 2007), pp. 59-69, ISSN 0143-4160.

Hall, E. D., Oostveen, J. A. & Gurney, M. E. (1998). Relationship of microglial and astrocytic activation to disease onset and progression in a transgenic model of familial ALS. *Glia,* Vol.23, No.3, (July 1998), pp. 249-256, ISSN 0894-1491.

Henkel, J. S., Engelhardt, J. I., Siklos, L., Simpson, E. P., Kim, S. H., Pan, T., Goodman, J. C., Siddique, T., Beers, D. R. & Appel, S. H. (2004). Presence of dendritic cells, MCP-1, and activated microglia/macrophages in amyotrophic lateral sclerosis spinal cord tissue. *Annals of neurology,* Vol.55, No.2, (February 2004), pp. 221-235, ISSN 0364-5134.

Higgins, C. M., Jung, C., Ding, H. & Xu, Z. (2002). Mutant Cu, Zn superoxide dismutase that causes motoneuron degeneration is present in mitochondria in the CNS. *J Neurosci,* Vol.22, No.6, (March 2002), pp. RC215, ISSN 1529-2401 (Electronic), 0270-6474 (Linking).

Hirano, A., Donnenfeld, H., Sasaki, S. & Nakano, I. (1984a). Fine structural observations of neurofilamentous changes in amyotrophic lateral sclerosis. *Journal of neuropathology and experimental neurology,* Vol.43, No.5, (September 1984), pp. 461-470, ISSN 0022-3069.

Hirano, A., Nakano, I., Kurland, L. T., Mulder, D. W., Holley, P. W. & Saccomanno, G. (1984b). Fine structural study of neurofibrillary changes in a family with amyotrophic lateral sclerosis. *Journal of neuropathology and experimental neurology,* Vol.43, No.5, (September 1984), pp. 471-480, ISSN 0022-3069.

Hollmann, M., Hartley, M. & Heinemann, S. (1991). Ca2+ permeability of KA-AMPA--gated glutamate receptor channels depends on subunit composition. *Science (New York, N.Y,* Vol.252, No.5007, (May 1991), pp. 851-853, ISSN 0036-8075.

Huisman, M. H., de Jong, S. W., van Doormaal, P. T., Weinreich, S. S., Schelhaas, H. J., van der Kooi, A. J., de Visser, M., Veldink, J. H. & van den Berg, L. H. (2011). Population based epidemiology of amyotrophic lateral sclerosis using capture-recapture methodology. *Journal of neurology, neurosurgery, and psychiatry,* (May 2011), pp., ISSN 1468-330X (Electronic), 0022-3050 (Linking).

Hume, R. I., Dingledine, R. & Heinemann, S. F. (1991). Identification of a site in glutamate receptor subunits that controls calcium permeability. *Science (New York, N.Y,* Vol.253, No.5023, (August 1991), pp. 1028-1031, ISSN 0036-8075.

Ihara, Y., Nobukuni, K., Takata, H. & Hayabara, T. (2005). Oxidative stress and metal content in blood and cerebrospinal fluid of amyotrophic lateral sclerosis patients with and without a Cu, Zn-superoxide dismutase mutation. *Neurological research,* Vol.27, No.1, (January 2005), pp. 105-108, ISSN 0161-6412.

Ilzecka, J. (2007). Decreased cerebrospinal fluid cytochrome c levels in patients with amyotrophic lateral sclerosis. *Scandinavian journal of clinical and laboratory investigation,* Vol.67, No.3, pp. 264-269, ISSN 0036-5513.

Ilzecka, J. (2011). Granzymes A and B levels in serum of patients with amyotrophic lateral sclerosis. *Clinical biochemistry,* Vol.44, No.8-9, (June 2011), pp. 650-653, ISSN 1873-2933 (Electronic), 0009-9120 (Linking).

Ince, P., Stout, N., Shaw, P., Slade, J., Hunziker, W., Heizmann, C. W. & Baimbridge, K. G. (1993). Parvalbumin and calbindin D-28k in the human motor system and in motor neuron disease. *Neuropathology and applied neurobiology,* Vol.19, No.4, (August 1993), pp. 291-299, ISSN 0305-1846.

Jaarsma, D., Rognoni, F., van Duijn, W., Verspaget, H. W., Haasdijk, E. D. & Holstege, J. C. (2001). CuZn superoxide dismutase (SOD1) accumulates in vacuolated mitochondria in transgenic mice expressing amyotrophic lateral sclerosis-linked SOD1 mutations. *Acta neuropathologica,* Vol.102, No.4, (October 2001), pp. 293-305, ISSN 0001-6322.

Jabaudon, D., Scanziani, M., Gahwiler, B. H. & Gerber, U. (2000). Acute decrease in net glutamate uptake during energy deprivation. *Proceedings of the National Academy of Sciences of the United States of America,* Vol.97, No.10, (May 2000), pp. 5610-5615, ISSN 0027-8424.

Julien, J. P. & Mushynski, W. E. (1998). Neurofilaments in health and disease. *Progress in nucleic acid research and molecular biology,* Vol.61, pp. 1-23, ISSN 0079-6603.

Jung, C., Higgins, C. M. & Xu, Z. (2002). Mitochondrial electron transport chain complex dysfunction in a transgenic mouse model for amyotrophic lateral sclerosis. *Journal of neurochemistry,* Vol.83, No.3, (November 2002), pp. 535-545, ISSN 0022-3042.

Kaal, E. C., Vlug, A. S., Versleijen, M. W., Kuilman, M., Joosten, E. A. & Bar, P. R. (2000). Chronic mitochondrial inhibition induces selective motoneuron death in vitro: a new model for amyotrophic lateral sclerosis. *Journal of neurochemistry,* Vol.74, No.3, (March 2000), pp. 1158-1165, ISSN 0022-3042.

Kawamata, T., Akiyama, H., Yamada, T. & McGeer, P. L. (1992). Immunologic reactions in amyotrophic lateral sclerosis brain and spinal cord tissue. *The American journal of pathology,* Vol.140, No.3, (March 1992), pp. 691-707, ISSN 0002-9440.

Keller, A. F., Gravel, M. & Kriz, J. (2010). Treatment with minocycline after disease onset alters astrocyte reactivity and increases microgliosis in SOD1 mutant mice. *Experimental neurology,* Vol.228, No.1, (March 2010), pp. 69-79, ISSN 1090-2430 (Electronic), 0014-4886 (Linking).

Kirkinezos, I. G., Bacman, S. R., Hernandez, D., Oca-Cossio, J., Arias, L. J., Perez-Pinzon, M. A., Bradley, W. G. & Moraes, C. T. (2005). Cytochrome c association with the inner mitochondrial membrane is impaired in the CNS of G93A-SOD1 mice. *J Neurosci,* Vol.25, No.1, (January 2005), pp. 164-172, ISSN 1529-2401 (Electronic), 0270-6474 (Linking).

Komatsu, M., Wang, Q. J., Holstein, G. R., Friedrich, V. L., Jr., Iwata, J., Kominami, E., Chait, B. T., Tanaka, K. & Yue, Z. (2007). Essential role for autophagy protein Atg7 in the maintenance of axonal homeostasis and the prevention of axonal degeneration. *Proceedings of the National Academy of Sciences of the United States of America,* Vol.104, No.36, (September 2007), pp. 14489-14494, ISSN 0027-8424.

Kong, J. & Xu, Z. (1998). Massive mitochondrial degeneration in motor neurons triggers the onset of amyotrophic lateral sclerosis in mice expressing a mutant SOD1. *J Neurosci,* Vol.18, No.9, (May 1), pp. 3241-3250, ISSN 0270-6474.

Kriz, J., Nguyen, M. D. & Julien, J. P. (2002). Minocycline slows disease progression in a mouse model of amyotrophic lateral sclerosis. *Neurobiology of disease,* Vol.10, No.3, (August 2002), pp. 268-278, ISSN 0969-9961.

Kroemer, G., Galluzzi, L., Vandenabeele, P., Abrams, J., Alnemri, E. S., Baehrecke, E. H., Blagosklonny, M. V., El-Deiry, W. S., Golstein, P., Green, D. R., Hengartner, M., Knight, R. A., Kumar, S., Lipton, S. A., Malorni, W., Nunez, G., Peter, M. E., Tschopp, J., Yuan, J., Piacentini, M., Zhivotovsky, B. & Melino, G. (2009). Classification of cell death: recommendations of the Nomenclature Committee on Cell Death 2009. *Cell death and differentiation,* Vol.16, No.1, (January 2009), pp. 3-11, ISSN 1476-5403 (Electronic), 1350-9047 (Linking).

Lenaz, G., Bovina, C., D'Aurelio, M., Fato, R., Formiggini, G., Genova, M. L., Giuliano, G., Merlo Pich, M., Paolucci, U., Parenti Castelli, G. & Ventura, B. (2002). Role of mitochondria in oxidative stress and aging. *Annals of the New York Academy of Sciences,* Vol.959, (April 2002), pp. 199-213, ISSN 0077-8923.

Lepore, A. C., Dejea, C., Carmen, J., Rauck, B., Kerr, D. A., Sofroniew, M. V. & Maragakis, N. J. (2008). Selective ablation of proliferating astrocytes does not affect disease outcome in either acute or chronic models of motor neuron degeneration. *Experimental neurology,* Vol.211, No.2, (June 2008), pp. 423-432, ISSN 1090-2430 (Electronic), 0014-4886 (Linking).

Li, M., Ona, V. O., Guegan, C., Chen, M., Jackson-Lewis, V., Andrews, L. J., Olszewski, A. J., Stieg, P. E., Lee, J. P., Przedborski, S. & Friedlander, R. M. (2000). Functional role of caspase-1 and caspase-3 in an ALS transgenic mouse model. *Science (New York, N.Y,* Vol.288, No.5464, (April 2000), pp. 335-339, ISSN 0036-8075.

Ligon, L. A., LaMonte, B. H., Wallace, K. E., Weber, N., Kalb, R. G. & Holzbaur, E. L. (2005). Mutant superoxide dismutase disrupts cytoplasmic dynein in motor neurons. *Neuroreport,* Vol.16, No.6, (April 2005), pp. 533-536, ISSN 0959-4965.

Lin, J., Diamanduros, A., Chowdhury, S. A., Scelsa, S., Latov, N. & Sadiq, S. A. (2009). Specific electron transport chain abnormalities in amyotrophic lateral sclerosis. *Journal of neurology,* Vol.256, No.5, (May 2009), pp. 774-782, ISSN 1432-1459 (Electronic), 0340-5354 (Linking).

Liu, D., Wen, J., Liu, J. & Li, L. (1999). The roles of free radicals in amyotrophic lateral sclerosis: reactive oxygen species and elevated oxidation of protein, DNA, and membrane phospholipids. *Faseb J,* Vol.13, No.15, (December 1999), pp. 2318-2328, ISSN 0892-6638.

Liu, J., Lillo, C., Jonsson, P. A., Vande Velde, C., Ward, C. M., Miller, T. M., Subramaniam, J. R., Rothstein, J. D., Marklund, S., Andersen, P. M., Brannstrom, T., Gredal, O., Wong, P. C., Williams, D. S. & Cleveland, D. W. (2004). Toxicity of familial ALS-linked SOD1 mutants from selective recruitment to spinal mitochondria. *Neuron,* Vol.43, No.1, (July 2004), pp. 5-17, ISSN 0896-6273.

Liu, R., Althaus, J. S., Ellerbrock, B. R., Becker, D. A. & Gurney, M. E. (1998). Enhanced oxygen radical production in a transgenic mouse model of familial amyotrophic lateral sclerosis. *Annals of neurology,* Vol.44, No.5, (November 1998), pp. 763-770, ISSN 0364-5134.

Locatelli, F., Corti, S., Papadimitriou, D., Fortunato, F., Del Bo, R., Donadoni, C., Nizzardo, M., Nardini, M., Salani, S., Ghezzi, S., Strazzer, S., Bresolin, N. & Comi, G. P. (2007). Fas small interfering RNA reduces motoneuron death in amyotrophic lateral sclerosis mice. *Annals of neurology,* Vol.62, No.1, (July 2007), pp. 81-92, ISSN 0364-5134.

Longuemare, M. C. & Swanson, R. A. (1995). Excitatory amino acid release from astrocytes during energy failure by reversal of sodium-dependent uptake. *Journal of neuroscience research,* Vol.40, No.3, (February 1995), pp. 379-386, ISSN 0360-4012.

Manfredi, G. & Xu, Z. (2005). Mitochondrial dysfunction and its role in motor neuron degeneration in ALS. *Mitochondrion,* Vol.5, No.2, (April 2005), pp. 77-87, ISSN 1567-7249.

Martin, L. J. (2010). Mitochondrial and Cell Death Mechanisms in Neurodegenerative Diseases. *Pharmaceuticals (Basel, Switzerland),* Vol.3, No.4, pp. 839-915, ISSN 1424-8247.

Martin, L. J., Gertz, B., Pan, Y., Price, A. C., Molkentin, J. D. & Chang, Q. (2009). The mitochondrial permeability transition pore in motor neurons: involvement in the pathobiology of ALS mice. *Experimental neurology,* Vol.218, No.2, (August 2009), pp. 333-346, ISSN 1090-2430 (Electronic), 0014-4886 (Linking).

Mattiazzi, M., D'Aurelio, M., Gajewski, C. D., Martushova, K., Kiaei, M., Beal, M. F. & Manfredi, G. (2002). Mutated human SOD1 causes dysfunction of oxidative phosphorylation in mitochondria of transgenic mice. *The Journal of biological chemistry,* Vol.277, No.33, (August, 2002), pp. 29626-29633, ISSN 0021-9258.

Maus, M., Marin, P., Israel, M., Glowinski, J. & Premont, J. (1999). Pyruvate and lactate protect striatal neurons against N-methyl-D-aspartate-induced neurotoxicity. *The European journal of neuroscience,* Vol.11, No.9, (September 1999), pp. 3215-3224, ISSN 0953-816X.

McGeer, P. L., McGeer, E. G., Kawamata, T., Yamada, T. & Akiyama, H. (1991). Reactions of the immune system in chronic degenerative neurological diseases. *The Canadian journal of neurological sciences,* Vol.18, No.3 Suppl, (August 1991), pp. 376-379, ISSN 0317-1671.

Menzies, F. M., Ince, P. G. & Shaw, P. J. (2002a). Mitochondrial involvement in amyotrophic lateral sclerosis. *Neurochemistry international,* Vol.40, No.6, (May 2002), pp. 543-551, ISSN 0197-0186.

Menzies, F. M., Cookson, M. R., Taylor, R. W., Turnbull, D. M., Chrzanowska-Lightowlers, Z. M., Dong, L., Figlewicz, D. A. & Shaw, P. J. (2002b). Mitochondrial dysfunction in a cell culture model of familial amyotrophic lateral sclerosis. *Brain,* Vol.125, No.Pt 7, (July 2002), pp. 1522-1533, ISSN 0006-8950.

Monje, M. L., Phillips, R. & Sapolsky, R. (2001). Calbindin overexpression buffers hippocampal cultures from the energetic impairments caused by glutamate. *Brain research,* Vol.911, No.1, (August 2001), pp. 37-42, ISSN 0006-8993.

Moreau, C., Devos, D., Brunaud-Danel, V., Defebvre, L., Perez, T., Destee, A., Tonnel, A. B., Lassalle, P. & Just, N. (2005). Elevated IL-6 and TNF-alpha levels in patients with ALS: inflammation or hypoxia? *Neurology,* Vol.65, No.12, (December 2005), pp. 1958-1960, ISSN 1526-632X (Electronic), 0028-3878 (Linking).

Nakano, Y., Hirayama, K. & Terao, K. (1987). Hepatic ultrastructural changes and liver dysfunction in amyotrophic lateral sclerosis. *Archives of neurology,* Vol.44, No.1, (January 1987), pp. 103-106, ISSN 0003-9942.

Neymotin, A., Petri, S., Calingasan, N. Y., Wille, E., Schafer, P., Stewart, C., Hensley, K., Beal, M. F. & Kiaei, M. (2009). Lenalidomide (Revlimid) administration at symptom onset is neuroprotective in a mouse model of amyotrophic lateral sclerosis. *Experimental neurology,* Vol.220, No.1, (November 2009), pp. 191-197, ISSN 1090-2430 (Electronic), 0014-4886 (Linking).

Nicholls, D. G. (1978). The regulation of extramitochondrial free calcium ion concentration by rat liver mitochondria. *Biochem J,* Vol.176, No.2, (November 1978), pp. 463-474, ISSN 0264-6021.

Nicholls, D. G. (1985). A role for the mitochondrion in the protection of cells against calcium overload? *Progress in brain research,* Vol.63, pp. 97-106, ISSN 0079-6123.

Nicholls, D. G. & Budd, S. L. (2000). Mitochondria and neuronal survival. *Physiological reviews,* Vol.80, No.1, (January 2000), pp. 315-360, ISSN 0031-9333.

Nicholls, D. G., Vesce, S., Kirk, L. & Chalmers, S. (2003). Interactions between mitochondrial bioenergetics and cytoplasmic calcium in cultured cerebellar granule cells. *Cell calcium,* Vol.34, No.4-5, (October-November 2003), pp. 407-424, ISSN 0143-4160.

Novelli, A., Reilly, J. A., Lysko, P. G. & Henneberry, R. C. (1988). Glutamate becomes neurotoxic via the N-methyl-D-aspartate receptor when intracellular energy levels are reduced. *Brain research,* Vol.451, No.1-2, (June 1988), pp. 205-212, ISSN 0006-8993.

Ohta, Y., Kamiya, T., Nagai, M., Nagata, T., Morimoto, N., Miyazaki, K., Murakami, T., Kurata, T., Takehisa, Y., Ikeda, Y., Asoh, S., Ohta, S. & Abe, K. (2008). Therapeutic benefits of intrathecal protein therapy in a mouse model of amyotrophic lateral sclerosis. *Journal of neuroscience research,* Vol.86, No.13, (October 2008), pp. 3028-3037, ISSN 1097-4547 (Electronic), 0360-4012 (Linking).

Oteiza, P. I., Uchitel, O. D., Carrasquedo, F., Dubrovski, A. L., Roma, J. C. & Fraga, C. G. (1997). Evaluation of antioxidants, protein, and lipid oxidation products in blood from sporadic amyotrophic lateral sclerosis patients. *Neurochemical research,* Vol.22, No.4, (April 1997), pp. 535-539, ISSN 0364-3190.

Palecek, J., Lips, M. B. & Keller, B. U. (1999). Calcium dynamics and buffering in motoneurones of the mouse spinal cord. *The Journal of physiology,* Vol.520 Pt 2, (October 1999), pp. 485-502, ISSN 0022-3751.

Pasinelli, P., Houseweart, M. K., Brown, R. H., Jr. & Cleveland, D. W. (2000). Caspase-1 and -3 are sequentially activated in motor neuron death in Cu,Zn superoxide dismutase-mediated familial amyotrophic lateral sclerosis. *Proceedings of the National Academy of Sciences of the United States of America,* Vol.97, No.25, (December 2000), pp. 13901-13906, ISSN 0027-8424.

Pasinelli, P., Belford, M. E., Lennon, N., Bacskai, B. J., Hyman, B. T., Trotti, D. & Brown, R. H., Jr. (2004). Amyotrophic lateral sclerosis-associated SOD1 mutant proteins bind and aggregate with Bcl-2 in spinal cord mitochondria. *Neuron,* Vol.43, No.1, (July 2004), pp. 19-30, ISSN 0896-6273.

Peng, T. I. & Jou, M. J. (2010). Oxidative stress caused by mitochondrial calcium overload. *Annals of the New York Academy of Sciences,* Vol.1201, (July 2010), pp. 183-188, ISSN 1749-6632 (Electronic), 0077-8923 (Linking).

Perlson, E., Jeong, G. B., Ross, J. L., Dixit, R., Wallace, K. E., Kalb, R. G. & Holzbaur, E. L. (2009). A switch in retrograde signaling from survival to stress in rapid-onset neurodegeneration. *J Neurosci,* Vol.29, No.31, (August 2009), pp. 9903-9917, ISSN 1529-2401 (Electronic), 0270-6474 (Linking).

Petri, S., Kiaei, M., Wille, E., Calingasan, N. Y. & Flint Beal, M. (2006). Loss of Fas ligand-function improves survival in G93A-transgenic ALS mice. *Journal of the neurological sciences,* Vol.251, No.1-2, (December 2006), pp. 44-49, ISSN 0022-510X.

Poon, H. F., Hensley, K., Thongboonkerd, V., Merchant, M. L., Lynn, B. C., Pierce, W. M., Klein, J. B., Calabrese, V. & Butterfield, D. A. (2005). Redox proteomics analysis of oxidatively modified proteins in G93A-SOD1 transgenic mice--a model of familial amyotrophic lateral sclerosis. *Free radical biology & medicine,* Vol.39, No.4, (August 2005), pp. 453-462, ISSN 0891-5849.

Pun, S., Santos, A. F., Saxena, S., Xu, L. & Caroni, P. (2006). Selective vulnerability and pruning of phasic motoneuron axons in motoneuron disease alleviated by CNTF. *Nature neuroscience,* Vol.9, No.3, (March 2006), pp. 408-419, ISSN 1097-6256.

Rao, S. D., Yin, H. Z. & Weiss, J. H. (2003). Disruption of glial glutamate transport by reactive oxygen species produced in motor neurons. *J Neurosci,* Vol.23, No.7, (April 2003), pp. 2627-2633, ISSN 1529-2401 (Electronic), 0270-6474 (Linking).

Raoul, C., Buhler, E., Sadeghi, C., Jacquier, A., Aebischer, P., Pettmann, B., Henderson, C. E. & Haase, G. (2006). Chronic activation in presymptomatic amyotrophic lateral sclerosis (ALS) mice of a feedback loop involving Fas, Daxx, and FasL. *Proceedings of the National Academy of Sciences of the United States of America,* Vol.103, No.15, (April 2006), pp. 6007-6012, ISSN 0027-8424.

Rentzos, M., Rombos, A., Nikolaou, C., Zoga, M., Zouvelou, V., Dimitrakopoulos, A., Alexakis, T., Tsoutsou, A., Samakovli, A., Michalopoulou, M. & Evdokimidis, I. (2010a). Interleukin-15 and interleukin-12 are elevated in serum and cerebrospinal fluid of patients with amyotrophic lateral sclerosis. *European neurology,* Vol.63, No.5, pp. 285-290, ISSN 1421-9913 (Electronic), 0014-3022 (Linking).

Rentzos, M., Rombos, A., Nikolaou, C., Zoga, M., Zouvelou, V., Dimitrakopoulos, A., Alexakis, T., Tsoutsou, A., Samakovli, A., Michalopoulou, M. & Evdokimidis, J. (2010b). Interleukin-17 and interleukin-23 are elevated in serum and cerebrospinal fluid of patients with ALS: a reflection of Th17 cells activation? *Acta neurologica Scandinavica,* Vol.122, No.6, (December 2010), pp. 425-429, ISSN 1600-0404 (Electronic), 0001-6314 (Linking).

Richter, C., Park, J. W. & Ames, B. N. (1988). Normal oxidative damage to mitochondrial and nuclear DNA is extensive. *Proceedings of the National Academy of Sciences of the United States of America,* Vol.85, No.17, (September 1988), pp. 6465-6467, ISSN 0027-8424.

Rosen, D. R., Siddique, T., Patterson, D., Figlewicz, D. A., Sapp, P., Hentati, A., Donaldson, D., Goto, J., O'Regan, J. P., Deng, H. X. & et al. (1993). Mutations in Cu/Zn superoxide dismutase gene are associated with familial amyotrophic lateral sclerosis. *Nature,* Vol.362, No.6415, (March 1993), pp. 59-62, ISSN 0028-0836.

Rothstein, J. D., Martin, L. J. & Kuncl, R. W. (1992). Decreased glutamate transport by the brain and spinal cord in amyotrophic lateral sclerosis. *The New England journal of medicine,* Vol.326, No.22, (May 1992), pp. 1464-1468, ISSN 0028-4793.

Rothstein, J. D., Van Kammen, M., Levey, A. I., Martin, L. J. & Kuncl, R. W. (1995). Selective loss of glial glutamate transporter GLT-1 in amyotrophic lateral sclerosis. *Annals of neurology,* Vol.38, No.1, (July 1995), pp. 73-84, ISSN 0364-5134.

Rowland, L. P. & Shneider, N. A. (2001). Amyotrophic lateral sclerosis. *The New England journal of medicine,* Vol.344, No.22, (May 2001), pp. 1688-1700, ISSN 0028-4793.

Ryberg, H., Soderling, A. S., Davidsson, P., Blennow, K., Caidahl, K. & Persson, L. I. (2004). Cerebrospinal fluid levels of free 3-nitrotyrosine are not elevated in the majority of patients with amyotrophic lateral sclerosis or Alzheimer's disease. *Neurochemistry international,* Vol.45, No.1, (July 2004), pp. 57-62, ISSN 0197-0186.

Sanagi, T., Yuasa, S., Nakamura, Y., Suzuki, E., Aoki, M., Warita, H., Itoyama, Y., Uchino, S., Kohsaka, S. & Ohsawa, K. (2010). Appearance of phagocytic microglia adjacent to motoneurons in spinal cord tissue from a presymptomatic transgenic rat model of amyotrophic lateral sclerosis. *Journal of neuroscience research,* Vol.88, No.12, (September 2010), pp. 2736-2746, ISSN 1097-4547 (Electronic), 0360-4012 (Linking).

Sargsyan, S. A., Monk, P. N. & Shaw, P. J. (2005). Microglia as potential contributors to motor neuron injury in amyotrophic lateral sclerosis. *Glia,* Vol.51, No.4, (September 2005), pp. 241-253, ISSN 0894-1491.

Sasaki, S. & Iwata, M. (1996). Impairment of fast axonal transport in the proximal axons of anterior horn neurons in amyotrophic lateral sclerosis. *Neurology,* Vol.47, No.2, (August 1996), pp. 535-540, ISSN 0028-3878.

Saxena, K., Henry, T. R., Solem, L. E. & Wallace, K. B. (1995). Enhanced induction of the mitochondrial permeability transition following acute menadione administration. *Archives of biochemistry and biophysics,* Vol.317, No.1, (February 1995), pp. 79-84, ISSN 0003-9861.

Scott, I. D. & Nicholls, D. G. (1980). Energy transduction in intact synaptosomes. Influence of plasma-membrane depolarization on the respiration and membrane potential of internal mitochondria determined in situ. *Biochem J,* Vol.186, No.1, (January 1980), pp. 21-33, ISSN 0264-6021.

Schinder, A. F., Olson, E. C., Spitzer, N. C. & Montal, M. (1996). Mitochondrial dysfunction is a primary event in glutamate neurotoxicity. *J Neurosci,* Vol.16, No.19, (October 1996), pp. 6125-6133, ISSN 0270-6474.

Shaw, P. J. (1999). Calcium, glutamate, and amyotrophic lateral sclerosis: more evidence but no certainties. *Annals of neurology,* Vol.46, No.6, (December 1999), pp. 803-805, ISSN 0364-5134.

Shaw, P. J., Ince, P. G., Falkous, G. & Mantle, D. (1995a). Oxidative damage to protein in sporadic motor neuron disease spinal cord. *Annals of neurology,* Vol.38, No.4, (October 1995), pp. 691-695, ISSN 0364-5134.

Shaw, P. J., Forrest, V., Ince, P. G., Richardson, J. P. & Wastell, H. J. (1995b). CSF and plasma amino acid levels in motor neuron disease: elevation of CSF glutamate in a subset of patients. *Neurodegeneration,* Vol.4, No.2, (June 1995), pp. 209-216, ISSN 1055-8330.

Shibata, N., Nagai, R., Uchida, K., Horiuchi, S., Yamada, S., Hirano, A., Kawaguchi, M., Yamamoto, T., Sasaki, S. & Kobayashi, M. (2001). Morphological evidence for lipid peroxidation and protein glycoxidation in spinal cords from sporadic amyotrophic lateral sclerosis patients. *Brain research,* Vol.917, No.1, (October 2001), pp. 97-104, ISSN 0006-8993.

Shrivastava, M. & Vivekanandhan, S. (2011). An insight into ultrastructural and morphological alterations of platelets in neurodegenerative diseases. *Ultrastructural pathology,* Vol.35, No.3, (May 2011), pp. 110-116, ISSN 1521-0758 (Electronic), 0191-3123 (Linking).

Shrivastava, M., Das, T. K., Behari, M., Pati, U. & Vivekanandhan, S. (2011a). Ultrastructural variations in platelets and platelet mitochondria: a novel feature in amyotrophic lateral sclerosis. *Ultrastructural pathology,* Vol.35, No.2, (April 2011), pp. 52-59, ISSN 1521-0758 (Electronic), 0191-3123 (Linking).

Shrivastava, M., Vivekanandhan, S., Pati, U., Behari, M. & Das, T. K. (2011b). Mitochondrial perturbance and execution of apoptosis in platelet mitochondria of patients with amyotrophic lateral sclerosis. *The International journal of neuroscience,* Vol.121, No.3, (March 2011), pp. 149-158, ISSN 1563-5279 (Electronic), 0020-7454 (Linking).

Siciliano, G., D'Avino, C., Del Corona, A., Barsacchi, R., Kusmic, C., Rocchi, A., Pastorini, E. & Murri, L. (2002). Impaired oxidative metabolism and lipid peroxidation in exercising muscle from ALS patients. *Amyotroph Lateral Scler Other Motor Neuron Disord,* Vol.3, No.2, (June 2002), pp. 57-62, ISSN 1466-0822.

Siklos, L., Engelhardt, J., Harati, Y., Smith, R. G., Joo, F. & Appel, S. H. (1996). Ultrastructural evidence for altered calcium in motor nerve terminals in amyotropic lateral sclerosis. *Annals of neurology,* Vol.39, No.2, (February 1996), pp. 203-216, ISSN 0364-5134.

Simpson, E. P., Henry, Y. K., Henkel, J. S., Smith, R. G. & Appel, S. H. (2004). Increased lipid peroxidation in sera of ALS patients: a potential biomarker of disease burden. *Neurology,* Vol.62, No.10, (May 2004), pp. 1758-1765, ISSN 1526-632X (Electronic), 0028-3878 (Linking).

Smith, R. G., Henry, Y. K., Mattson, M. P. & Appel, S. H. (1998). Presence of 4-hydroxynonenal in cerebrospinal fluid of patients with sporadic amyotrophic lateral sclerosis. *Annals of neurology,* Vol.44, No.4, (October 1998), pp. 696-699, ISSN 0364-5134.

Sofroniew, M. V. (2005). Reactive astrocytes in neural repair and protection. *Neuroscientist,* Vol.11, No.5, (October 2005), pp. 400-407, ISSN 1073-8584.

Spreux-Varoquaux, O., Bensimon, G., Lacomblez, L., Salachas, F., Pradat, P. F., Le Forestier, N., Marouan, A., Dib, M. & Meininger, V. (2002). Glutamate levels in cerebrospinal fluid in amyotrophic lateral sclerosis: a reappraisal using a new HPLC method with coulometric detection in a large cohort of patients. *Journal of the neurological sciences,* Vol.193, No.2, (January 2002), pp. 73-78, ISSN 0022-510X.

Swerdlow, R. H., Parks, J. K., Cassarino, D. S., Trimmer, P. A., Miller, S. W., Maguire, D. J., Sheehan, J. P., Maguire, R. S., Pattee, G., Juel, V. C., Phillips, L. H., Tuttle, J. B., Bennett, J. P., Jr., Davis, R. E. & Parker, W. D., Jr. (1998). Mitochondria in sporadic amyotrophic lateral sclerosis. *Experimental neurology,* Vol.153, No.1, (September 1998), pp. 135-142, ISSN 0014-4886.

Tateno, M., Kato, S., Sakurai, T., Nukina, N., Takahashi, R. & Araki, T. (2009). Mutant SOD1 impairs axonal transport of choline acetyltransferase and acetylcholine release by sequestering KAP3. *Human molecular genetics,* Vol.18, No.5, (March 2009), pp. 942-955, ISSN 1460-2083 (Electronic), 0964-6906 (Linking).

Tohgi, H., Abe, T., Yamazaki, K., Murata, T., Ishizaki, E. & Isobe, C. (1999). Remarkable increase in cerebrospinal fluid 3-nitrotyrosine in patients with sporadic amyotrophic lateral sclerosis. *Annals of neurology,* Vol.46, No.1, (July 1999), pp. 129-131, ISSN 0364-5134.

Tovar-y-Romo, L. B., Zepeda, A. & Tapia, R. (2007). Vascular endothelial growth factor prevents paralysis and motoneuron death in a rat model of excitotoxic spinal cord neurodegeneration. *Journal of neuropathology and experimental neurology,* Vol.66, No.10, (October 2007), pp. 913-922, ISSN 0022-3069.

Tovar-y-Romo, L. B., Santa-Cruz, L. D. & Tapia, R. (2009a). Experimental models for the study of neurodegeneration in amyotrophic lateral sclerosis. *Molecular neurodegeneration,* Vol.4, pp. 31, ISSN 1750-1326.

Tovar-y-Romo, L. B., Santa-Cruz, L. D., Zepeda, A. & Tapia, R. (2009b). Chronic elevation of extracellular glutamate due to transport blockade is innocuous for spinal motoneurons in vivo. *Neurochemistry international,* Vol.54, No.3-4, (March-April 2009), pp. 186-191, ISSN 1872-9754 (Electronic), 0197-0186 (Linking).

Trotti, D., Danbolt, N. C. & Volterra, A. (1998). Glutamate transporters are oxidant-vulnerable: a molecular link between oxidative and excitotoxic neurodegeneration?

Trends in pharmacological sciences, Vol.19, No.8, (August 1998), pp. 328-334, ISSN 0165-6147.

Trotti, D., Rossi, D., Gjesdal, O., Levy, L. M., Racagni, G., Danbolt, N. C. & Volterra, A. (1996). Peroxynitrite inhibits glutamate transporter subtypes. *The Journal of biological chemistry,* Vol.271, No.11, (March 1996), pp. 5976-5979, ISSN 0021-9258.

Turrens, J. F., Alexandre, A. & Lehninger, A. L. (1985). Ubisemiquinone is the electron donor for superoxide formation by complex III of heart mitochondria. *Archives of biochemistry and biophysics,* Vol.237, No.2, (March 1985), pp. 408-414, ISSN 0003-9861.

Van Den Bosch, L., Tilkin, P., Lemmens, G. & Robberecht, W. (2002). Minocycline delays disease onset and mortality in a transgenic model of ALS. *Neuroreport,* Vol.13, No.8, (June 2002), pp. 1067-1070, ISSN 0959-4965.

Vielhaber, S., Kunz, D., Winkler, K., Wiedemann, F. R., Kirches, E., Feistner, H., Heinze, H. J., Elger, C. E., Schubert, W. & Kunz, W. S. (2000). Mitochondrial DNA abnormalities in skeletal muscle of patients with sporadic amyotrophic lateral sclerosis. *Brain,* Vol.123, (July 2000), pp. 1339-1348, ISSN 0006-8950.

Volterra, A., Trotti, D. & Racagni, G. (1994). Glutamate uptake is inhibited by arachidonic acid and oxygen radicals via two distinct and additive mechanisms. *Molecular pharmacology,* Vol.46, No.5, (November 1994), pp. 986-992, ISSN 0026-895X.

von Lewinski, F. & Keller, B. U. (2005). Ca2+, mitochondria and selective motoneuron vulnerability: implications for ALS. *Trends in neurosciences,* Vol.28, No.9, (September 2005), pp. 494-500, ISSN 0166-2236.

Warita, H., Itoyama, Y. & Abe, K. (1999). Selective impairment of fast anterograde axonal transport in the peripheral nerves of asymptomatic transgenic mice with a G93A mutant SOD1 gene. *Brain research,* Vol.819, No.1-2, (February 1999), pp. 120-131, ISSN 0006-8993.

White, R. J. & Reynolds, I. J. (1996). Mitochondrial depolarization in glutamate-stimulated neurons: an early signal specific to excitotoxin exposure. *J Neurosci,* Vol.16, No.18, (September 1996), pp. 5688-5697, ISSN 0270-6474.

Wiedemann, F. R., Manfredi, G., Mawrin, C., Beal, M. F. & Schon, E. A. (2002). Mitochondrial DNA and respiratory chain function in spinal cords of ALS patients. *Journal of neurochemistry,* Vol.80, No.4, (February 2002), pp. 616-625, ISSN 0022-3042.

Wiedemann, F. R., Winkler, K., Kuznetsov, A. V., Bartels, C., Vielhaber, S., Feistner, H. & Kunz, W. S. (1998). Impairment of mitochondrial function in skeletal muscle of patients with amyotrophic lateral sclerosis. *Journal of the neurological sciences,* Vol.156, No.1, pp. 65-72, ISSN 0022-510X.

Williamson, T. L. & Cleveland, D. W. (1999). Slowing of axonal transport is a very early event in the toxicity of ALS-linked SOD1 mutants to motor neurons. *Nature neuroscience,* Vol.2, No.1, (January 1999), pp. 50-56, ISSN 1097-6256.

Wong, P. C., Pardo, C. A., Borchelt, D. R., Lee, M. K., Copeland, N. G., Jenkins, N. A., Sisodia, S. S., Cleveland, D. W. & Price, D. L. (1995). An adverse property of a familial ALS-linked SOD1 mutation causes motor neuron disease characterized by vacuolar degeneration of mitochondria. *Neuron,* Vol.14, No.6, (June 1995), pp. 1105-1116, ISSN 0896-6273.

Yamanaka, K., Chun, S. J., Boillee, S., Fujimori-Tonou, N., Yamashita, H., Gutmann, D. H., Takahashi, R., Misawa, H. & Cleveland, D. W. (2008). Astrocytes as determinants of disease progression in inherited amyotrophic lateral sclerosis. *Nature neuroscience,* Vol.11, No.3, (March 2008), pp. 251-253, ISSN 1097-6256.

Yang, W. W., Sidman, R. L., Taksir, T. V., Treleaven, C. M., Fidler, J. A., Cheng, S. H., Dodge, J. C. & Shihabuddin, L. S. (2011). Relationship between neuropathology and disease progression in the SOD1(G93A) ALS mouse. *Experimental neurology,* Vol.227, No.2, (February 2011), pp. 287-295, ISSN 1090-2430 (Electronic), 0014-4886 (Linking).

Zagami, C. J., Beart, P. M., Wallis, N., Nagley, P. & O'Shea, R. D. (2009). Oxidative and excitotoxic insults exert differential effects on spinal motoneurons and astrocytic glutamate transporters: Implications for the role of astrogliosis in amyotrophic lateral sclerosis. *Glia,* Vol.57, No.2, (January 2009), pp. 119-135, ISSN 1098-1136 (Electronic), 0894-1491 (Linking).

Zhang, F., Strom, A. L., Fukada, K., Lee, S., Hayward, L. J. & Zhu, H. (2007). Interaction between familial amyotrophic lateral sclerosis (ALS)-linked SOD1 mutants and the dynein complex. *The Journal of biological chemistry,* Vol.282, No.22, (June 2007), pp. 16691-16699, ISSN 0021-9258.

Zhu, S., Stavrovskaya, I. G., Drozda, M., Kim, B. Y., Ona, V., Li, M., Sarang, S., Liu, A. S., Hartley, D. M., Wu, D. C., Gullans, S., Ferrante, R. J., Przedborski, S., Kristal, B. S. & Friedlander, R. M. (2002). Minocycline inhibits cytochrome c release and delays progression of amyotrophic lateral sclerosis in mice. *Nature,* Vol.417, No.6884, (May 2002), pp. 74-78, ISSN 0028-0836.

9

Role of Neuronal Mitochondrial Metabolic Phenotype in Pathogenesis of ALS

Alexander Panov[1,3], Nury Steuerwald[1], Valentin Vavilin[2],
Svetlana Dambinova[3] and Herbert L. Bonkovsky[1]
[1]*Cannon Research Center, Carolinas Medical Center, Charlotte, NC,*
[2]*Institute of Molecular Biology and Biophysics, Novosibirsk,*
[3]*Laboratory of Brain Biomarkers, WellStar College of Health & Human Services,*
Kennesaw State University, Kennesaw, GA,
[1,3]*USA*
[2]*Russia*

1. Introduction

Amyotrophic lateral sclerosis (ALS) is one of the group of diseases of the central nerve system (CNS), which are characterized by progressive loss of structure and function of neurons in different regions of brain or spinal cord. Therefore, these diseases are collectively designated as "Neurodegenerative Diseases" (NDDs). Usually the loss of specific functions precedes the death of affected neurons, and the related clinical features depend on localization and degree of neurodegeneration. NDDs include such diseases as Alzheimer's, Parkinson's, Huntington's, spinocerebellar ataxias, and ALS. In spite of differences in predominant localization of neurodegeneration and clinical features, there are many parallels among different neurodegenerative disorders. These include involvement of mitochondrial dysfunctions, increased oxidative stress, and atypical protein assemblies (Backman et al., 2006).

Amyotrophic lateral sclerosis (ALS) refers to several adult-onset conditions characterized by progressive degeneration of motor neurons. "Amyotrophic" refers to the muscle atrophy, weakness, and fasciculation (spontaneous contraction affecting a small number of muscle fibers) that signify disease of the lower motor neurons. There are two forms of this fatal disease: sporadic, with no known genetic component, and familial, which make up about 10% of all ALS cases (Rowland & Schneider, 2001; Martin et al., 2009). Among the familial cases, approximately 20% are caused by dominantly inherited mutations in the Cu/Zn superoxide dismutase (*SOD1*) gene, with more than 100 known mutations (reviewed in Bruijn et al., 2004). So far, there is very little information that links familial and sporadic cases of the disease. One established fact, based on studies of patients and transgenic animals, is that mitochondria dysfunction is an early manifestation. However, it is unclear whether mitochondrial dysfunctions are the primary pathogenic mechanism, or the result of some other proximate pathogenic mechanism.

Although the cases associated with mutations in the *SOD1* gene comprise only about 2% of all ALS cases, understandably, transgenic animals bearing mutated *SOD1* gene became the major targets for research on pathogenesis of ALS (Bendotti and Carri, 2004; Bruijn et al., 2004; Matsumoto et al., 2006). Of these, a transgenic mouse carrying the G93A (Gly-93 → Ala) mutant human *SOD1* gene was the first described (Gurney et al., 1994). This animal model of ALS was used all over the world because it closely recapitulates clinical and histopathological features of the human disease (Matsumoto et al., 2006).

Researchers from Wyeth, John Hopkins and Harvard in collaboration with ALS Association as part of its Lou Gehrig Challenge Initiative established the SOD1G93A mutant rat line. Taconic (Germantown, NY) established a production colony in 2002, which was sponsored by grant funding from ALS Association. The original publication on this strain (tgSOD1) reported disease onset around 115 days of age, with rapid disease progression thereafter (Howland et al., 2002). Taconic has maintained a colony since 2002. In our recent work (Panov et al., 2011b) we presented data obtained in 2007 on 45 tgSOD1 animals obtained from 9 separate simultaneous isolations of BM and SCM. We studied respiration and reactive oxygen species production by mitochondria isolated from the brains (tgBM) and spinal cords (tgSCM), of such rats and the results obtained were highly reproducible (Panov et al., 2011b). Beginning late in 2008 and in 2009 we encountered difficulties in reproducing the results obtained in 2007. Moreover, we have found that the transgenic rat line did not develop symptoms of the disease at age of more than 200 days even though the mutated gene was evident in DNA samples from tails and ears. In 2010 we received information from Taconic (Germantown, NY) that changes in features can be attributed to a variable phenotype in this model, "which may be due to in part to both the outbred nature of the background strain as well as to possible copy number variation of the transgene" (Information Letter from Taconic). Whether these phenotypic changes were associated with the decline of the level to which the transgene was expressed is impossible to conclude because, in the rats studied in 2007, neither Taconic company, nor our lab quantified the expression of the mutated SOD1 gene or protein. Nevertheless, our comparative studies of metabolic properties of BM and SCM suggest that potentially the loss of morbidity could be explained by different patterns of substrates metabolism and associated ROS generation in BM and SCM studied in 2007 and 2010.

In 2008 we found that BM and SCM isolated from the wild type Sprague Dawley rats began to show metabolic features that were different from those described earlier for the same strain of the wild type and tgSOD1 rats (Panov et al., 2009, 2011a). In this work we present a comparison of metabolic phenotypes and the substrate-dependent ROS generation in the wild type and transgenic rats with mutant G93A Cu/Zn-superoxide dismutase gene isolated in 2007 and 2010. We conclude that the shift in mitochondrial metabolic phenotype, which resulted in a dramatic decrease in ROS production by tgBM and tgSCM, may have contributed to the significant loss of morbidity of the established tgSOD1 rat line. This could result from the breeding method of the transgenic animals, when males bearing the dominant mutated *SOD1* gene were mated with the wild type females. Because mitochondrial DNA has maternal inheritance (Wallace, 2001), the resulting progeny has the mitochondrial phenotype of females, and thus the mutated SOD1 protein was acting on mitochondria with different metabolism that resulted in much lower rates of ROS production. We conclude that mitochondria are the key players in the pathogenesis of ALS.

We suggest a hypothesis, which links together pathogenic mechanisms of sporadic and familial forms of ALS. Our hypothesis is based on results obtained in experiments on animals, which showed that between species and even within one species there may exist different phenotypes of mitochondrial metabolism. Neuronal mitochondria of some phenotypes may produce very large amounts of superoxide radical, which is dismutated to hydrogen peroxide (H_2O_2). High levels of H_2O_2 may damage the extramitochondrial isoform of superoxide dismutase (SOD1). The oxidatively damaged proteins lose Cu and Zn from the hem centers, and the demetallated protein enters mitochondrial membranes, further increases ROS production by a mechanism similar to that described for cholesterol-β-D-glucoside and fitosterol glucosides (Panov et al., 2010b), causes mitochondrial dysfunctions, and finally the death of neurons. These are sporadic cases of ALS associated with disorders of mitochondrial metabolism. The familial cases with mutations in the *SOD1* gene have basically the same mechanism of motor neuron death, but, because mutated SOD1 protein is exceptionally sensitive to oxidative damage, the loss of Cu and Zn may occur at relatively low levels of H_2O_2 formation by neuronal mitochondria. The predominant involvement of spinal cord can be accounted for by metabolic and structural features of spinal cord and SCM, which were published elsewhere (Panov et al., 2011a, 2011b).

2. General characterization of mitochondria in ALS

Clinical features of ALS, a severe neuromuscular degenerative disease, were described by Charcot in 1874 (Rowland & Shneider, 2001). Since that time clinical definitions (Shook and Pioro, 2009) and pathological features of the disease have been greatly expanded, aided in no small measure by advances in genetics of the disease (Rowland & Shneider, 2001) and development of transgenic animal models of ALS (Bendotti & Carri, 2004; Matsumoto et al., 2006; Howland et al., 2002). However, the etiology and pathogenesis of the disease remain poorly understood.

Clinical and experimental evidence showed that ALS is a systemic disease, with particular vulnerability of motor neurons due to some unique properties (Martin et al., 2007; von Lewinski & Keller, 2005; Panov et al., 2011a). Many ALS patients are hypermetabolic, an early and persistent phenomenon (Bouteloup et al., 2009, Desport et al., 2005). Muscular mitochondrial function in amyotrophic lateral sclerosis is progressively altered in ALS patients (Echaniz-Laguna et al., 2006, Krasnianski et al., 2005), and subtle ultrastructural changes of hepatocytes and liver dysfunction have also been described in biopsy specimens from ALS patients (Nakano et al., 1987). Significant changes were also found in skeletal muscle mitochondria of transgenic SOD1 (tgSOD1) animals (Dupuis et al., 2009, Krasnianski et al., 2005). It was suggested that increased ROS generation by skeletal muscle mitochondria (Muller et al., 2007) or mitochondrial uncoupling (Dupuis et al., 2009) may be primarily responsible for the loss of neuromuscular junctions and secondary distal degeneration of motor neurons in SOD1 mice. This is an interesting and important alternative hypothesis, which requires a more detailed and critical discussion.

The paper by Muller et al. (2007) presents data on generation of ROS by skeletal muscle mitochondria (SMM) from two lines of transgenic mice bearing different mutations in SOD1 gene, SOD1 knockout mice, and mice with denervated muscle. The authors concluded that "enhanced generation of mitochondrial ROS may be a common factor in the mechanism underlying denervation-induced atrophy". The authors suggested also that increased ROS generation in ALS mutant model may also cause the loss of neuro-muscular junctions, and thus initiate the loss of motor neurons. There are, however, experimental facts, which oppose this conclusion. Muller et al (2007) isolated skeletal muscle mitochondria using a protease nagarse for digestion of the tissue. With the nagarse method, more than 90% of mitochondria are interfibrillar. Without the protease the yields of subsarcolemmal mitochondria are very low (A. Panov, unpublished observations). ROS generated *in situ* by interfibrillar mitochondria are unlikely to gain access to the sarcolemmal membrane where the neuro-muscular junctions are located. This is because superoxide radical has difficulty to leave mitochondria (Panov et al. 2005). Besides, both superoxide radicals and H_2O_2 are substrates for the antioxidant enzymes in the cytoplasm, such as SOD1, catalase, etc. Rather, it is more likely that increased ROS act locally to cause damage to interfibrillar mitochondria, particularly to mtDNA, and thus cause muscle atrophy. Data presented by Muller et al. (2007) do not show direct damage to neuromuscular junctions by increased ROS. Therefore this issue requires further study. There is also a quantitative aspect of ROS generation presented by Muller et al. (2007). A comparison of the rates of ROS production by skeletal muscle mitochondria (SMM) (Figure 1 in Muller et al., 2007) and brain (BM) and spinal cord mitochondria (SCM) (see Fig. 7 in Panov et al., 2011a) shows that BM and SCM generate several times more ROS than SMM. Therefore, it is more likely that the causes of degeneration of motor neurons in ALS are associated with primary pathological processes in neurons rather than in muscle.

Dupuis et al. (2009) also concluded that "a muscle restricted mitochondrial defect is sufficient to generate motor neuron degeneration". The authors based their conclusion on mitochondrial dysfunctions observed in animals with overexpression of uncoupling protein 1 (UCP1). Overexpression of UCP1 results in deenergization of the mitochondria due to increased conductivity of the inner membrane for protons. This condition results in complete inhibition of ROS production associated with the energy-dependent reverse electron transport. The major consequence of overexpression of UCP1 is inhibition of ATP production and suppression of functions, which depend on mitochondrial ATP levels. Because in neuronal tissue reverse electron transport is the major source of ROS production (Panov et al. 2007, 2009), and increased ROS generation is one of the leading pathogenic pathways in ALS, the mechanism proposed by Dupius et al. (2009), although interesting, probably has little to do with neurodegeneration in ALS.

It was hypothesized that sporadic and familial forms of ALS may share some final pathogenic mechanisms (Bendotti & Carri, 2004; von Lewinski & Keller, 2005). Several pathogenic factors have been proposed (reviewed in Bruijn et al., 2004): glutamate excitotoxicity (Heath & Shaw, 2002); mitochondrial dysfunction (Dupuis et al., 2009); increased production of reactive oxygen species (ROS) (reviewed in Barber & Shaw, 2010) and nitroxyradicals (NO^- and $ONOO^-$) (Martin et al., 2007); deregulation of Ca^{2+} homeostasis and triggering of permeability transition of mitochondria (von Lewinski and Keller, 2005; Martin et al., 2009; Morota et al., 2007); induction of pro-apoptotic pathways (Przedborski, 2004); misfolding and intracellular accumulation of mutant SOD1 (Tateno et al., 2004), including in brain and spinal mitochondria (Liu et al., 2004; Higgins et al., 2002); mutant SOD1-induced conformational changes in Bcl-2 (Pedrini et al., 2010) and VDAC1 (porin)

(Israelson et al., 2010); and abnormal axonal transport (Magrane & Manfredi, 2009). However, almost all of these proposed pathogenic mechanisms directly or indirectly involve mitochondria. The major problem in searching for alternative pathogenic mechanisms, in case of severe mitochondrial disability, is that practically all cellular and organ functions depend on energy and thus also become disturbed (Gershoni et al., 2009). Therefore, it is of paramount importance to precisely understand the nature and causes of mitochondrial dysfunctions, and whether they are early or late events in disease evolution.

In the majority of studies of ALS, the mitochondrial abnormalities were assessed using morphological methods, which showed swollen brain and spinal mitochondria with dilated cristae, and vacuoles in matrix (Sasaki et al., 2004, Jaarsma et al., 2006). It was suggested that vacuolization may depend on accumulation amount, rather than from toxic property, of mutant SOD1 (Jaarsma, 2006). Morphologic methods, including quantitative histochemistry, and immunological methods, showed that both in ALS patients and tgSOD1 animals, the activities of respiratory chain complexes were diminished (Jung et al., 2002), and that the spinal cord mitochondria are predisposed to opening of the Ca^{2+}-dependent permeability transition pores (mPTP), which trigger death of motor neurons (Martin et al., 2009). There is a large body of evidence that spinal cords in tgSOD1 animals are subjected to increased oxidative and nitrative stress, as indicated by accumulation of protein carbonyls and nitrated proteins (Martin et al., 2007, 2009). These data also demonstrated that mitochondria are involved early in the pathogenesis of ALS (Martin et al., 2007, 2009). Recently, Panov et al. (2011b) provided direct evidence that isolated mitochondria from the brain and spinal cord of tgSOD1 rats generate significantly more reactive oxygen species (ROS) as compared with mitochondria from wild type animals.

Morphological, histochemical and immunological methods provided important information about involvement of mitochondria in the pathology, however they do not tell us what caused the changes in mitochondrial morphology. Relatively few studies were performed on isolated BM and SCM mitochondria from control (Sullivan et al., 2004, Panov et al., 2011a), tgSOD1 animals (Kirkinezos et al., 2005, Damiano et al., 2006, Fischer et al., 2011, Panov et al., 2011b), Wobbler mice (Dave et al., 2003, Xu et al., 2001), or *mnd* mice, which spontaneously develop motor neuron pathology (Bertamini et al., 2002). In their pioneering work, Sullivan et al (2004) have shown that normal SCM have lower respiratory activity, lower threshold for calcium-induced mitochondrial permeability transition, and a higher degree of superoxide radical production (determined with dehydroethidium) and lipid peroxidation as compared with BM. However, the dehydroethidium method does not identify the origin of superoxide radical. Studies of isolated mitochondria from tgSOD1 mice showed that BM and SCM had decreased rates of respiration associated with the loss of complex IV activity (Kirkinezos et al., 2005). Very early in the course of the disease, the mitochondrial Ca^{2+} loading capacity was significantly diminished as compared with the age-matched control mice (Damiano et al., 2006). Respiratory activities were also diminished in SCM of Wobbler mice (Dave et al., 2003, Xu et al., 2001) and mice with motor neuron degeneration disease (Bertamini et al., 2002).

A comparative study of isolated normal and tgSOD1 brain and spinal cord mitochondria was published recently by Panov et al. (2011a, b), and the unique metabolic features of BM and SCM were described (see also Panov et al, 2009). Normal SCM produced significantly more ROS than BM, and this was associated with the succinate-dependent reverse electron transport (Panov et al. 2011a). A rather unexpected finding was that BM and SCM isolated from presymptomatic tgSOD1 rats showed almost normal rates of oxidative phosphorylation. Panov et all. (2011b) purified mitochondria in a Percoll gradient, and thus eliminated damaged mitochondria. This resulted in significantly lower yields of mitochondria per 1 gram of tissue of tgSOD1 rats: the yields were diminished by 27% for the brain and by 58% for spinal cord as compared with the normal Sprague Dawley rats (Panov et al., 2011b). Avossa et al. (2006) used immunocytochemistry and electron microscopy techniques to compare wild type and G93A spinal cord tissues after 14 days of growth under standard *in vitro* conditions. Wild type and mutant cultures displayed no differences in the analyzed parameters as well as in the number of motor neurons, and there were no signs of mitochondria vacuolization or protein aggregate formation in G93A ventral horns. Together, the results of Panov et al. (2011b) and Avossa et al. (2006) suggest that in tgSOD1 rats the BM and SCM are primarily normal but suffer from some pathological events, which rapidly deteriorate mitochondria and cause death of neurons.

In order to better understand the metabolic events involved in putative pathological mechanisms of neurodegeneration, we have to discuss the distinctive features of brain and spinal cord energy metabolism and their mitochondria.

3. General features of neuronal energy metabolism

Neuronal cells are strictly aerobic and require large quantities of ATP produced at high rate in order to function normally. Humans brain constitutes only 2% of the body's weight, but accounts for 20% of its resting O_2 metabolism (Attwell & Laughlin, 2001). However, even in humans, heart and kidney consume significantly more oxygen per unit of the organ's mass than the brain (Rolfe & Brown, 1997). In rats, liver, kidney and heart consume correspondingly 2, 3 and 3.9 times more oxygen than the brain (Rolfe & Brown, 1997). Thus it is not the necessity for the high rate of oxidative metabolism that is unique for the central nerve system, but how the oxidative metabolism is organized in neuronal cells.

Cortical tissue is composed mainly of two types of cells: the nerve cells (or neurons) and the neuroglial cells (or glia). Glial cells greatly outnumber the neurons (Abeles, 1991; Attwell & Laughlin, 2001; Stolzenburg et al., 1989). Glial cells do not directly take part in the interactions between neurons, but play an important role in maintaining neuronal metabolism and in directing the development and growth of the brain. The classical categorization of neurons was based mainly on morphology of the cell body and its dendritic tree, and to a lesser extent on the morphology of the axon and its branches (Abeles, 1991).

There are two main categories of the cortical cells according to their physiological effects on each other: excitatory and inhibitory cells. Excitatory cells release transmitters (glutamate) at their synaptic ends that, on contact with the postsynaptic membrane, create ion currents that depolarize the postsynaptic cell. Inhibitory cells release transmitters, such as γ-aminobutyric acid (GABA), that tend to hyperpolarize the postsynaptic cell or to increase the conductance of the postsynaptic membrane to chloride, thereby diminishing the effects of the depolarizing currents generated by the excitatory synapses. Excitatory synapses dominate the brain's grey matter because excitatory neurons outnumber inhibitory cells by a factor of 9 to 1, and 90% of synapses release glutamate (Abeles, 1991; Braitenberg & Schüz, 1998). The distribution of mitochondria points to these glutamatergic synapses as the major users of metabolic energy (Wong-Riley, 1989; Attwell & Laughlin, 2001).

More than 80% of neuronal mitochondria are located in the dendrites and axonal terminals (Wong-Riley, 1989; Attwell & Laughlin, 2001). With high synaptic density of 8×10^8 per 1

mm^3 in all cortices (the density of synapses is not very much different among species) it is clear that in the brain most energy expenditures are associated with synaptic activity, where most mitochondria are located (Abeles, 1991). The close spacing of terminals along axons (5 μm, implying a diffusion time of only 25 milliseconds) make terminal and axonal mitochondria functionally indistinguishable (Attwell & Laughlin, 2001).

Neurons communicate by means of signals that lead to depolarization of their excitable membranes. The degree of depolarization of the dendritic or soma membranes is determined by complex interactions between excitatory and inhibitory transmitters. The depolarization spreads to the axon, leading to release of an excitatory or inhibitory transmitter at the axonal endings of the cell, thus allowing information to be transferred to the next cell. When impulses are propagated, the cell loses K^+ and gains Na^+, and in order to preserve excitability the cell must extrude Na^+ and accumulate K^+, using metabolic energy derived from oxidative metabolism (Abeles, 1991). Postsynaptic ion fluxes (Na^+, K^+, Cl^-) and presynaptic Ca^{2+} influx consume in grey matter approximately 75% of the brain's energy (Abeles, 1991; Attwell & Laughlin, 2001). Because depolarization and restoration of ionic composition across the neuronal membrane occur in the millisecond scale, neuronal mitochondria must provide large quantities of ATP in a very short time. This distribution of energy use reflects the fact that a chemical synapse is an amplifier: for each glutamate released approximately 100 ions enter the postsynaptic terminal (Abeles, 1991). The rest (25%) of the brain's energy is used for the basic "housekeeping" functions, such as maintenance of pH gradients, asymmetrical distributions of phospholipids in membrane bilayers, protein synthesis (about 2%), anaplerotic functions and recycling of glutamate from synaptic clefts (Attwell & Laughlin, 2001). It was suggested that white and grey matter require similar amounts of energy on basic (nonsignaling) cellular activities (Attwell & Laughlin, 2001).

It is widely accepted that nerve tissues of adult mammals use glucose as the major source of energy. To fully understand the specifics of energy metabolism in brain, it is important to take into account that, in dendrites and synaptic terminals, there is limited space for glycolytic enzymes that would provide mitochondria with enough pyruvate derived from glucose. Therefore, neurons cannot be functionally and metabolically regarded without astroglia. Astrocytes provide neurons with lactate, as the major source of energy, replenish the neuronal pool of glutamine and recycle glutamate (Ebert et al., 2003; Pellerin et al., 2007; Suzuki et al., 2011). Of the total energy consumed by the brain, approximately 80% of energy expenditure is satisfied by oxidation of glucose and 20% by oxidation of fatty acids (Ebert et al., 2003). As we will see later, neurons also oxidize significant amounts of glutamate and GABA as a source of energy. The neurotransmitter GABA is formed from glutamate by the action of glutamate decarboxylase. It appears that glutamine serves as the precursor for glutamate and GABA. Therefore, the pool of glutamine must be constantly replenished in anaplerotic reactions, which occur predominantly in astroglia.

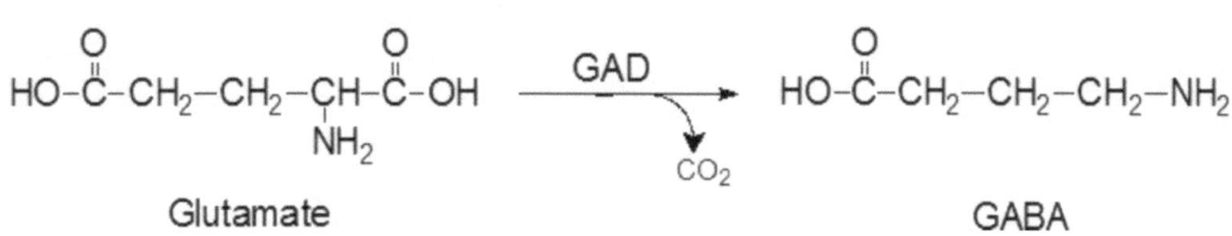

Fig. 1. Formation of GABA from glutamate. GAD – glutamate decarboxylase.

Because anaplerotic functions of astrocytes require energy, oxidation of fatty acids occurs in glial mitochondria (Ebert et al., 2003) providing energy and saving glucose for production of lactate in aerobic glycolysis and α-ketoglutarate for synthesis *de novo* neuromediators glutamate and GABA (Waagepetersen et al., 1999; Ebert et al., 2003). Glutamine synthetase is an astrocyte-specific enzyme (Norenberg & Martinez-Hernandez, 1979), and during octanoate oxidation in astrocytes most of the anaplerotic flux in brain is occurring in the TCA cycle associated with glutamine production (Ebert et al., 2003). In order to fulfill the task of metabolic provision of neuronal functions there are several mechanisms that ensure functional and metabolic compartmentalization and complementation between neurons and astroglia, which thus exclude competition for energy substrates. Neuronal mitochondria do not possess the full range activity of β-oxidation enzymes, whereas glial mitochondria readily oxidize fatty acids (Ebert et al., 2003). On the other hand, glial mitochondria do not have active glutamate-aspartate translocase (Berkich et al., 2007), which is the key enzyme of the malate aspartate shuttle and the major pathway for oxidation of glutamate by neuronal mitochondria. Thus astrocytes do not utilize glutamate as a respiratory substrate. The distribution of lactate dehydrogenase isoforms between glial cells and neurons promotes aerobic glycolysis in astroglia and utilization of lactate by neurons as the major respiratory substrate (Pellerin et al., 2007).

4. In activated neurons mitochondria utilize a mixture of substrates

Mitochondria are devices for burning hydrogen producing water and releasing energy, a large part of which is accumulated as electrochemical transmembrane potential ($\Delta\mu_H+$) (Mitchell, 1977; Nicholls, 2008). $\Delta\mu_H+$ is utilized for production of ATP, and other useful work in the mitochondria and cell. Therefore lactate, which has additional hydrogen, as compared with pyruvate, has higher energetic value for neuronal mitochondria. In the cytosol of a neuron, lactate is oxidized to pyruvate in the reaction catalyzed by lactate dehydrogenase (LDH): NAD^+ + Lactate → NADH + H^+ + Pyruvate. Pyruvate is transported into mitochondria and metabolized.

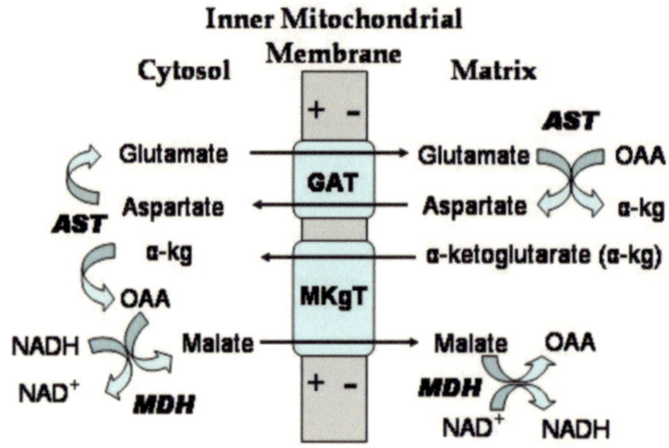

Abbreviations: AST - aspartate aminotransferase; GAT - glutamate-aspartate transporter, MDH - malate dehydrogenase; MKgT - malate- α -ketoglutarate transporter; OAA - oxaloacetate

Fig. 2. **The malate aspartate shuttle.** In a cell with respiring energized mitochondria the malate aspartate shuttle serves for transport and oxidation of hydrogen from cytosolic NADH to mitochondrial respiratory chain. The process is unidirectional because GAT is electrogenic and the matrix NADH is rapidly oxidized by respiratory chain.

In order to rapidly oxidize lactate to pyruvate, the cytosolic NADH must be oxidized back to NAD^+. In neurons the task of reoxidation of the cytosolic NADH and transport of hydrogen into mitochondria occur via a number of functionally coupled cytosolic and mitochondrial enzymes, which form the malate-aspartate shuttle (MAS) (Figure 2). Glutamate is a necessary component of MAS. Because nonsynaptic and presynaptic neuronal mitochondria effectively oxidize glutamate (Yudkoff et al. 1994), neuronal cells constantly have to replenish the cytosolic pool of glutamate.

Until recently, it was generally accepted that most of the glutamate is rapidly removed from the synaptic cleft by glutamate transporters EAAT1 (GLT-1) and EAAT2 (GLAST) located on presynaptic termini and glial cells (Furness et al., 2008). However, recent data show that a significant fraction of glutamate is rapidly bound and transported by the glutamate transporter isoform, EAAT4, located juxtasynaptically in the membranes of spines and dendrites (Auger & Attwell., 2000; Brasnjo& Otis., 2004). EAAT4 protein was found to be omnipresent throughout the fore- and midbrain (Massie et al., 2008). These data suggest that postsynaptic transport of glutamate into nerve terminals, where mitochondria are located (Abeles, 1991), may occur in all brain regions. According to calculations of Brasnjo and Otis (2004), in a single synapse EAAT4 bind and transport postsynaptically about $1.3 \pm 0.1 \times 10^6$ glutamate molecules. In the brain, on average, 1 mm^3 of tissue contains 1×10^8 synapses (Abeles, 1991; Nicholls, 1993). Because of the high density of synaptic contacts, the neuronal cells may be exposed to mediators released from hundreds of firing synapses. Thus in a narrow space of spines and dendrites several million glutamate molecules postsynaptically transported from synaptic boutons may create local cytosolic concentration of glutamate in a low mM range. Consequently, neuronal mitochondria, particularly those located at the axonal or dendritic synaptic junctions may temporarily metabolize, in addition to pyruvate, some amounts of glutamate (Yudkoff et al. 1994; Panov et al. 2009). Besides, GABA is also transported postsynaptically where it is catabolized in mitochondria to succinate (Tillakaratne et al., 1995).

As we have mentioned, for rapid conversion of lactate to pyruvate, postsynaptic neurons must receive a certain amount of glutamate to fuel MAS to recycle cytosolic NAD^+ (Berkich et al., 2007). Importantly, the activity of the brain mitochondrial isoform of aspartate glutamate transporter is controlled by Ca^{2+} (Pardo et al., 2006). Therefore increased neuronal activity through small changes in the extramitochondrial Ca^{2+} activates MAS, whereas increased mitochondrial Ca^{2+} activates mitochondrial respiration (Nicholls, 2009).

There is evidence (Yudkoff et al., 1994), that in the presence of glutamate + pyruvate, the tricarboxylic acid (TCA) cycle in brain mitochondria operates as two coupled cycles: one (cycle A) leads from α-KG to OAA, and another (cycle B) from OAA to a-KG that includes the citrate synthase reaction (see figure 3). According to Yudkoff et al. (1994), the flux of substrates through cycle A is 3-5-fold faster than that through the cycle B. Thus, with pyruvate + glutamate + malate, activation of α-ketoglutarate dehydrogenase complex (α-KGDHC) and succinate dehydrogenase (SDH) may significantly increase the rates of the tricarboxylic acid cycle (TCA) cycle and respiratory chain in state 3 and state 3U (Fig. 3). A high turnover of cycle A with activated SDH would increase reverse electron transport (RET) and the associated ROS production.

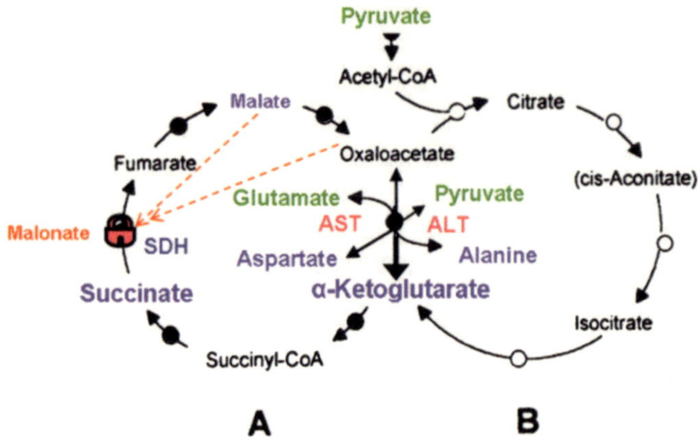

Abbreviations: ALT - alanine aminotransferase; AST -aspartate aminotransferase; SDH - succinate dehydrogenase (Complex II).

Fig. 3. **The tricarboxylic acid cycle in the presence of pyruvate and glutamate operates as two coupled cycles A and B**. In the presence of glutamate and/or pyruvate as substrates high activities of AST and ALT may "short-circuit" oxaloacetate and α-ketoglutarate, thus converting the "normal" TCA cycle into two independently operating cycles A and B. Malonate is a quasi-irreversible inhibitor of SDH, whereas oxaloacetate (OAA) is a competitive but strong inhibitor. SDH has similar affinities for succinate and malate, but oxidation of malate results in formation of OAA on the enzyme's active center, which makes malate a strong inhibitor of SDH.

Thus in activated neurons mitochondria may oxidize simultaneously glutamate, pyruvate, and metabolites of the TCA cycle, such as malate, and succinate. Postsynaptically transported GABA is catabolized in mitochondria to succinate (Tillakaratne et al., 1995). Under these conditions, brain (BM) and spinal cord (SCM) mitochondria significantly increase the rate of oxidative phosphorylation and the succinate-dependent production of ROS (Panov et al., 2009, 2011a). With glutamate + pyruvate + malate as substrates, increased production of ATP and ROS was associated with dramatic increase in the matrix concentration of α-ketoglutarate (Balasz, 1965a) due to increased activities of mitochondrial aminotransferases AST and ALT (Fig. 3). Under these conditions glutamate dehydrogenase (GLDH) does not participate in production of α-KG (Balasz, 1965b). Since AST and ALT are present in great excess, compared with the respiration rate, the oxaloacetate (OAA) formed is continuously removed by the transamination reactions. Balazs (1965b) concluded that a competition takes place between the α-KGDHC and GLDH, probably for NAD+, resulting in preferential oxidation of α-oxoglutarate.

5. Distinctive properties of ROS generation in brain and spinal cord mitochondria

In neuronal tissue mitochondria are the major source of ROS production (Stowe & Camara, 2009), which is indispensable feature of aerobic metabolism. It is generally accepted that during oxidation of the NAD-dependent substrates the limiting step is at the NADH-dehydrogenase site of Complex I (see Panov et al. 2007, 2009). With succinate as a substrate, production of ROS is significantly higher, because Complex II, which is also part of the TCA cycle - succinate dehydrogenase (SDH), feeds electrons into the mitochondrial pool of CoQ_{10} (ubiquinone, Q). The reduced ubiquinone (QH_2) in its turn reduces the sites on Complex I that can generate superoxide radicals at high rate. This process, known as reverse electron transport, is energy-dependent and inhibited by rotenone. Some researchers deny the significance of succinate in ROS production on the pretext that succinate concentration is too low in mitochondria (Starkov, 2008; Stowe & Camara, 2009; Zoccarato et al., 2007). As we have shown recently, however, brain and spinal cord mitochondria may produce succinate even in the presence of pyruvate + malate (Panov et al., 2009) , and as we show in this article (see Fig. 6) even with glutamate + malate a large part of ROS production may be associated with oxidation of succinate. However a particularly large production of the succinate-dependent ROS was observed in the presence of glutamate + pyruvate + malate (Panov et al., 2009, 2011a, 2011b). With these substrates the increased succinate oxidation was caused by a dramatic increase in mitochondrial α-ketoglutarate due to high activities of aminotransferases (Balasz, 1965a, 1965b). Besides, GABA is catabolized with formation of succinate in postsynaptic mitochondria (Tillakaratne et al. 1995). Thus, in the excited neurons succinate is an indispensable mitochondrial metabolite. In this paper we provide evidence that ROS generation associated with the succinate-dependent reverse electron transport is a subject for phenotypic variations.

Another objection to the importance of reverse electron transport (RET) in ROS generation argues that, because RET is energy-dependent, in the functioning cell the diminished mitochondrial energization will inhibit production of ROS (Starkov, 2008). The latter objection is valid for the most perpetually functioning organs, such as heart, kidney and liver. But it is only partially applicable to brain and spinal cord where a very large number of mitochondria are located at axonal and dendritic junctions (Wong-Riley, 1989). At the narrow spaces of synaptic junctions there is no other task for mitochondria beside provision of ATP for restoration of ionic composition in excited synapses. If the neurons are not excited, mitochondria become fully energized and produce ROS at high rate. Therefore axonal and synaptic junctions, including neuro muscular junctions, are particularly vulnerable to oxidative damage if neurons are not excited for some reason.

Another possible reason why the succinate-dependent ROS production was underrated could be the fact that most researchers use "classical" mixtures of substrates, such as glutamate + malate, pyruvate + malate, succinate alone, or, very often, in the presence of rotenone.

Figure 4 shows a representative experiment with the BM and SCM isolated in 2007 from tg SOD1 rats. One can see that with glutamate + malate, the rate of ROS production, measured as H_2O_2, there were no differences between tgBM and tgSCM, wtBM or wtSCM (not shown). With pyruvate + malate as substrates, tgSCM generated significantly more ROS than tgBM (see Fig. 5). This was because SCM in general oxidize succinate at higher rate than BM, presumably due to the lower intrinsic inhibition of SDH by oxaloacetate (Panov et al., 2011a). However, when tgBM and tgSCM oxidized a mixture of glutamate + pyruvate + malate, there was a several-fold increase in ROS production. TgSCM produced much more ROS than tgBM (Fig. 4, see also Fig. 6 in Panov et al., 2011b). Thus the usage of physiologically relevant mixtures of substrates is far more informative for understanding the role of mitochondria in pathogenesis of diseases, than the "classical" approach.

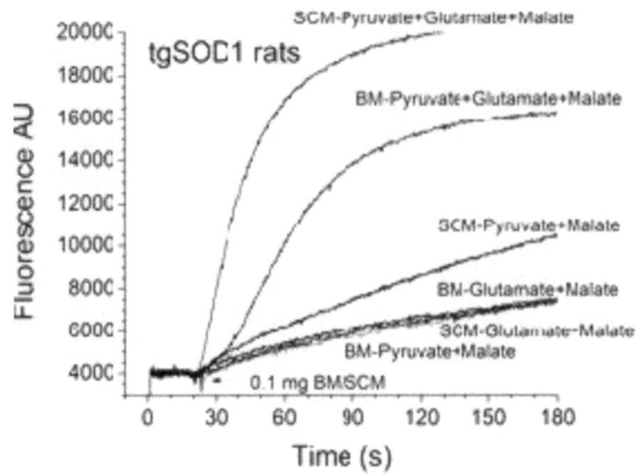

Fig. 4. **Production of ROS by brain and spinal cord mitochondria from tgSOD1 rats.** Mitochondrial production of ROS was registered as H_2O_2 by Amplex red method (Panov et al., 2009).

We suggested the following metabolic scenario for the neuronal mitochondria located at synaptic junctions. During neuronal activity, the postsynaptic mitochondria are exposed to increased levels of pyruvate and glutamate, which enhance ATP production due to specific interactions between the glutamate transforming enzymes and the TCA cycle enzymes. This effect of the substrate mixtures is specific for the BM, and SCM (Panov et al., 2009, 2011a). As soon as activation of a synapse comes to an end, transport of glutamate from the synaptic cleft would also stop. As a result, activation of respiration induced by the simultaneous presence of glutamate and pyruvate will also end because glutamate becomes exhausted. Thus the neuromediator glutamate controls energy metabolism in brain not only at the level of astrocytes by enhancing production of lactate, but also at the level of neurons by controlling the activity of MAS and specific interactions between aminotransferases.

In the absence of neuronal activation, SDH (Complex II) in the postsynaptic mitochondria is inhibited by OAA (Panov et al. 2010a). The physiological significance of this inhibition is to prevent excessive ROS production associated with reverse electron transport. This is particularly important for neurons because with pyruvate, which is the major mitochondrial substrate in resting neurons (Pellerin et al., 1994; Hertz, 2004), there is a substantial production of succinate and thus a possibility of increased RET-dependent ROS production (see Fig. 5A, 5B; Panov et al. 2009, 2011a, 2011b). During increased neuronal activity glutamate and pyruvate temporarily release the inhibition of SDH. Increased ATP production (state 3) prevents generation of ROS (Starkov, 2008; Votyakova & Reynolds, 2001). Because SCM in general oxidize succinate at higher rates than BM, due to lower intrinsic inhibition of SDH, they are more vulnerable to oxidative stress than BM (Panov et al., 2011a, 2011b).

Activation of oxidative phosphorylation and increased ROS generation with pyruvate + glutamate + malate was observed only with BM and SCM (Panov et al., 2009, 2011a). However, activation of succinate oxidation by pyruvate and glutamate may be a common phenomenon for mitochondria from many organs. Our experiments with mitochondria from different organs and different species of rats and mice, and with one species (Sprague Dawley) of rats over period of 6 years, have shown that mitochondrial metabolism is a subject to phenotypic variations between species and in one species with time (Panov et al., 2010). Below we describe how changes in mitochondrial metabolism of BM and SCM of wild type Sprague Dawley rats affected mitochondrial dysfunctions in tgSOD1 rats in 2007 and 2010.

6. Differences between BM and SCM isolated in 2007 and 2010 in the rates of ROS production with different substrates

ROS production by mitochondria strongly depends on the metabolic state of the mitochondria, type of substrates, and is also tissue-specific (Kwong, Sohal, 1998; Muller et al., 2008, Panov et al., 2007). There are two types of ROS production by mitochondria - energy-dependent and non-energy-dependent (Panov et al., 2007). The energy-dependent ROS production is associated with the reverse electron transport (Kwong, Sohal, 1998; Muller et al., 2008, Panov et al., 2007). ROS production, which does not depend on energization and the metabolic state of the mitochondria may occur on complexes I, II and III and depends on the presence of inhibitors of the electron transport (Kwong, Sohal, 1998; Panov et al., 2007; St-Pierre et al. 2002). In the absence of respiratory inhibitors the rate of the non-energy dependent ROS production is relatively slow (Panov et al., 2007). We have shown that in BM and SCM the major source of ROS correlates with the reverse electron transport, which occurs during oxidation of succinate (Kwong, Sohal, 1998; Panov et al., 2007, 2009, 2011a, b), fatty acids (Panov et al., 2010c), or α-glycerophosphate (Tretter et al., 2007). Thus respiration rates in State 4 in the well coupled mitochondria oxidizing succinate correlates with the rates of ROS production (Panov et al., 2007, 2011a). Therefore changes in the rates of ROS production presented in Figure 4 closely reflect metabolic pattern of the mitochondria. Another reason why we do not present respiratory data is that in 2010 we had limited number of tgSOD1 rats, which precluded obtaining statistically significant data with all substrates and their mixtures.

In our studies on mitochondrial dysfunctions in the rat model of ALS (tgSOD1), we used as a reference control Sprague Dawley rats from Taconic (Germantown, NY). In the years of 2005-2007 we have discovered, that in this strain both BM and SCM had a unique metabolic attribute, which was absent in mitochondria from other organs: during simultaneous oxidation of pyruvate + glutamate + malate the rates of oxidative phosphorylation and the State 4 ROS production were significantly higher than with either glutamate or pyruvate alone (Panov 2009, 2011a). This substrate mixture corresponded to the metabolic situation in activated neurons (Panov et al., 2009). Addition of malonate, a potent inhibitor of SDH, attenuated the rates of respiration and ROS production with pyruvate + malate and glutamate + pyruvate + malate to the level with glutamate + malate.

With succinate as a substrate, ROS production was several times higher than with glutamate + pyruvate + malate, and was further increased in the presence of glutamate + pyruvate (Fig. 5A, 5B). The stimulation of the succinate-supported State 4 respiration and ROS production by glutamate and pyruvate was attributed to removal of endogenous oxaloacetate, which inhibits succinate dehydrogenase (SDH) (Panov et al. 2009, 2010). SCM from the control rats produced significantly more ROS than BM, particularly with the succinate containing substrate mixtures (Figure 5A, 5B; see also Panov et al. 2009, 2011a). We have concluded that in BM the activity of SDH was primordially inhibited by endogenous oxaloacetate (Panov 2009, 2010). This intrinsic inhibition of SDH by oxaloacetate was less evident in SCM, and therefore SCM produced more ROS with substrate mixtures that produced or contained succinate (Panov 2011a). The described above metabolic features of BM and SCM were consistently observed in the wild type and tgSOD1 rats during period of 2005 - 2007 years (Panov et al. 2009, 2011a, 2011b).

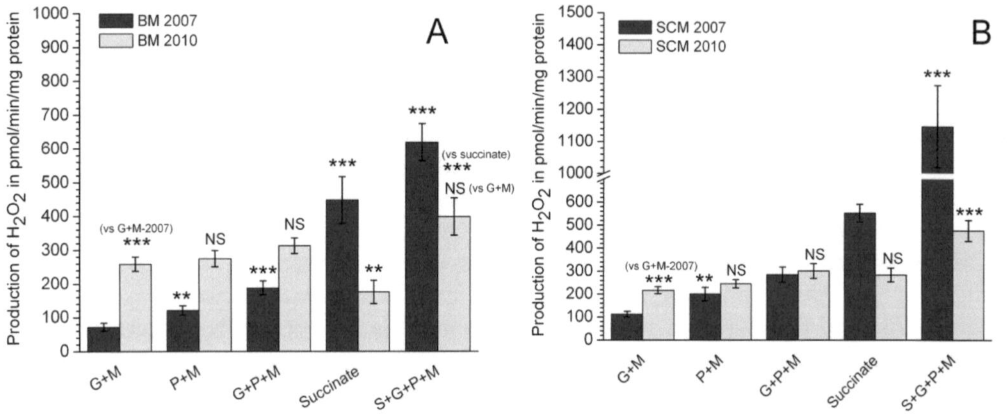

A. Brain mitochondria; **B.** Spinal cord mitochondria. Dark grey - wild type rats in 2007, light gray - wild type rats in 2010. Mitochondria were incubated in a medium containing: 125 mM KCl, 10 mM MOPS, pH 7.2, 2 mM $MgCl_2$, 2 mM KH_2PO_4, 10 mM NaCl, 1 mM EGTA, 0.7 mM $CaCl_2$. At a Ca^{2+}/EGTA ratio of 0.7, the free [Ca^{2+}] is close to 1 μM as determined using Fura-2. The substrate concentrations were: 5 mM succinate without rotenone, 5 mM glutamate, 2.5 mM pyruvate, and 2 mM malate. (Panov et al. 2009, 2011a, b). The results are presented as Mean ± SE, n = 3, and show the rates of ROS production in pmol H_2O_2 /minute/mg mitochondrial protein. Additions: 5 μM Amplex red, 1 U of horse radish peroxidase, 50 U of superoxide dismutase (Sigma), 0.05 mg mitochondria, glutamate 5 mM + malate 2 mM (G + M); pyruvate 2.5 mM + malate 2 mM (P + M); glutamate 5 mM + pyruvate 2.5 mM + malate 2 mM (G + P + M); succinate 5 mM (S); succinate 5 mM + glutamate 5 mM + pyruvate 2.5 mM + malate 2 mM (S + G + P + M). Statistics: ** $p < 0.01$; *** $p < 0.001$. For each year the data were compared with the rates of ROS production with glutamate + malate.

Fig. 5. **Comparison of ROS production by wild type brain and spinal cord mitochondria, isolated in 2007 and 2010, oxidizing different substrates and substrate mixtures.**

In 2008 we observed that BM and SCM from the wild type rats displayed a metabolic pattern that was different from the one described above. To highlight the differences in metabolic features of BM and SCM, we present data restricted to 2007, when significant mitochondrial dysfunctions in tgBM and tgSCM were observed as described in (Panov et al. 2011b), and 2010, when the tgSOD1 rat line failed to develop the disease features, and mitochondria showed little or no dysfunction as compared with the corresponding wild type animals. The related metabolic properties of the BM and SCM isolated from wild type animals in 2007 are presented and compared with those of 2010 in figures 5A and 5B.

Figure 5A compares ROS production by WT-BM isolated in 2007 and 2010. Of notice, the rate of ROS production by WT-BM isolated in 2010 was 3.5 fold higher than WT-BM isolated in 2007. However, in 2010 there was no differences in State 4 respiration (not shown) and ROS production (Fig. 5A) when BM oxidized glutamate + malate, pyruvate + malate or glutamate + pyruvate + malate. In contrast to WT-BM isolated in 2007, the much higher basic rate of ROS production supported by glutamate + malate in 2010 was inhibited by malonate to the level close to that in 2007 (Fig. 6). Similarly, in 2010 malonate inhibited ROS production in BM oxidizing glutamate + pyruvate + malate (Fig. 6) and pyruvate (not shown).

In contrast to WT-BM isolated in 2007, the WT-BM isolated in 2010 produced ROS supported by succinate at much lower rates than with glutamate + pyruvate + malate (Fig. 5A). Addition of glutamate + pyruvate + malate to the WT-BM -2010 oxidizing succinate stimulated ROS production only to the level with glutamate + malate (Fig. 5A). Similar metabolic features were also observed with the WT-SCM isolated in 2010, although the differences from 2007 WT-SCM were smaller than for the BM (Fig 5B). It is important to note that in 2010 WT-SCM generated ROS with different substrates at the same levels as WT-BM, whereas in 2007 the WT-SCM generated significantly more ROS than the corresponding WT-BM (Fig. 5A and 5B. Note the scale difference between the figures).

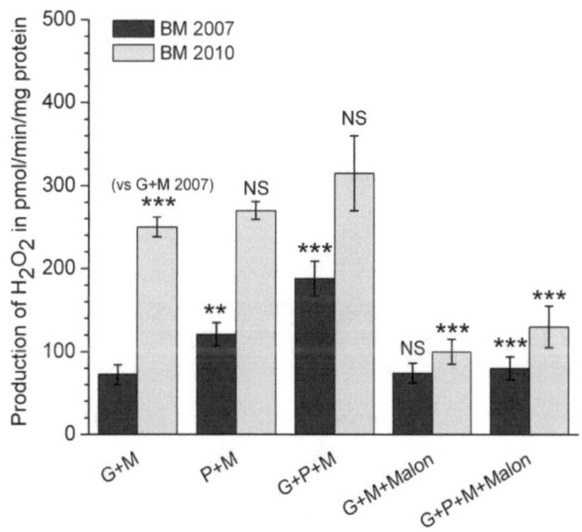

Incubation conditions and designations as described in Fig. 5. Malonate 5 mM was added before mitochondria. Dark gray - BM isolated in 2007, light gray columns - BM isolated in 2010. Statistics: *** $p < 0.001$, NS - not significant difference. The dark columns and grey columns were compared with the corresponding column representing ROS production with glutamate and malate, taken as 100%.

Fig. 6. Effect of malonate on ROS production by wild type brain mitochondria, isolated in 2007 and 2010, oxidizing glutamate + malate, pyruvate + malate, and glutamate + pyruvate + malate.

The sensitivity of the State 4 ROS production supported by either pyruvate or glutamate to malonate (Fig, 6; Panov et al. 2009) demonstrates that at least with BM and SCM both glutamate and pyruvate cannot be regarded as "pure complex I substrates", as is commonly accepted. In BM and SCM during oxidation of glutamate or pyruvate, and particularly when glutamate and pyruvate are present simultaneously, significant amounts of α-ketoglutarate can be formed in transaminase reactions, which is further converted to succinate (Balasz, 1965; Panov et al. 2009).

7. Effects of metabolic phenotype on ROS production by tgBM and tgSCM

Figure 7A shows generation of ROS by tgBM and tgSCM isolated from tgSOD1 rats in 2007, and figure 7B presents corresponding results for tgBM and tgSCM isolated from tgSOD1 rats in 2010. The figures clearly show that in spite of higher basic ROS production with glutamate and pyruvate by BM and SCM in 2010 (Fig. 5A and 5B), the overall rates of ROS generation with physiologically relevant substrate mixture - glutamate + pyruvate + malate were 5 times lower for tgBM and 10 times for tgSCM , when compared with transgenic mitochondria in 2007 (Fig. 7A and 7B).

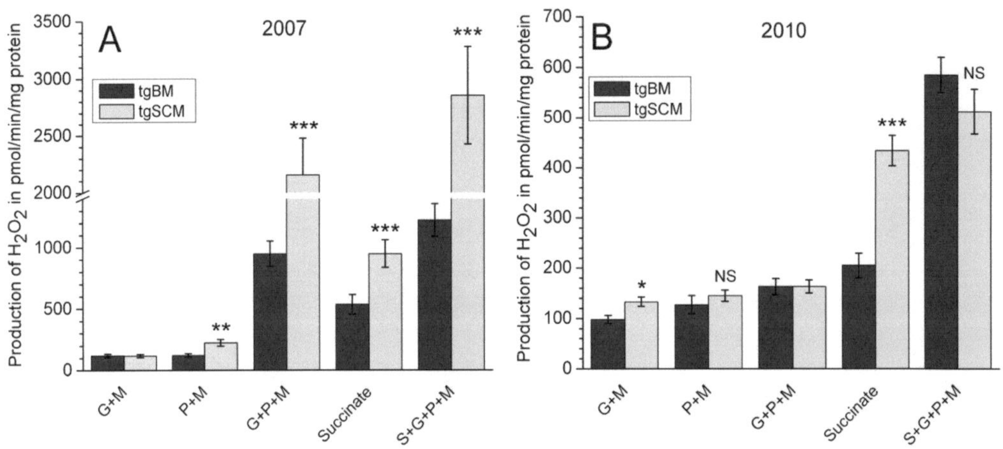

A. 2007; **B.** 2010. Dark grey – brain mitochondria, light gray – spinal cord mitochondria. Incubation conditions as in Fig. 5. Statistics: * $p < 0.05$; ** $p < 0.01$; *** $p < 0.001$. The data for tgSCM were compared with the corresponding results for tgBM.

Fig. 7. **Generation of ROS by brain and spinal cord mitochondria from tgSOD1 rats, isolated in 2007 and 2010, oxidizing various substrates.**

Similar multiple-fold differences in ROS production existed also with succinate and succinate containing substrate mixtures (Figs. 7A, 7B). In tgBM and tgSCM, the increases in ROS generation were substrate specific and depended on activity of SDH. These results led us to conclusion that changes in the metabolic phenotype of neuronal mitochondria, which occurred in 2008, resulted in a dramatic decrease in production of ROS in tgSOD1 rats.

8. Hydrogen peroxide is the major species to cause oxidative stress in tgSOD1 mitochondria

One of the distinctions of BM and SCM is a very high activity of MnSOD (SOD2) (Panov et al., 2009, 2011a, 2011b), which is distinct from the heart and skeletal muscle mitochondria (Muller et al., 2008). Even at very high rates of ROS production, such as shown in Figures 4 and 5A, 5B, addition of external SOD did not increase fluorescence of resorufin. The high activity of SOD2 means that BM and SCM effectively eliminate superoxide radicals from the matrix by converting them to H_2O_2. Therefore, we suggest that the major damaging factor in tgSOD1 motor neurons is H_2O_2. It was shown that H_2O_2 can interact with Cu,Zn-SOD (SOD1) resulting in peroxidase activity of SOD1 (Liochev, Fridovich, 2004), formation of strong oxidant $CO_3^{\bullet-}$ radical (reviewed in Valentine et al., 2005), enzyme inactivation, release of Cu^{2+}, protein oxidation and aggregation (Ramirez et al., 2009, Durer et al., 2009). At this point, the damaging effects of H_2O_2 will be increased dramatically because Cu^{2+} ions are several orders more active than Fe^{2+} in Fenton-like reaction with H_2O_2 (Dikalov et al., 2004), which will produce hydroxyl radical-like species and further drive lipid peroxidation, protein damage and promote mitochondrial dysfunction. Loss of metals by mutant SOD1 leads to formation of amyloid-like aggregates (Durer et al., 2009). Mutations in SOD1 amplify reactions with H_2O_2, increase the lifetime of incorrectly folded states, and if exposed to even mild oxidative stress, incorrect disulfide links form and stabilize larger aggregates that may be resistant to the degradation by the quality control machinery of the cell, and thus increase association with mitochondria (Field et al., 2003; Furukawa, O'Halloran, 2008).

9. Proposed mechanisms of increased ROS production in tgSOD1 mitochondria

There is strong evidence that tgSOD1 selectively binds to the outer (Vande Velde et al., 2008) and inner mitochondrial membranes (Liu et al., 2004; Ahtoniemi et al., 2008). Mutant SOD1 protein associated with mitochondria forms cross-linked oligomers and causes a shift in the redox state of respiratory components (Ferri et al., 2006). We propose a mechanism by which tgSOD1 might increase generation of ROS associated with reverse electron transport. The hypothesis is based on our recently published data on the effects of cholesterol β-D-glucoside and cycad phytosterol glucosides on ROS generation by BM (Panov et al., 2010b). These compounds are neurotoxic and suspected as the cause of the cluster of neurodegenerative disorders in the western Pacific termed amyotrophic lateral sclerosis-parkinsonism dementia complex (ALS-PDC) (Wilson et al., 2002). When added *in vitro* to mitochondria, cholesterol β-D-glucoside increased ROS production, which was specifically dependent on activity of SDH. Cholesterol β-D-glucoside is known to diminish the surface area of the membranes and thus affect the activity of the membrane's enzymes (Deliconstantinos et al., 1989). Here we suggest, that tgSOD1 upon its interaction with the mitochondria may change physical-chemical properties of the membranes and increase the rate of reverse electron transport in a way similar to that of cholesterol β-D-glucoside.

10. Oxidative stress increases sensitivity of mitochondria to Ca^{2+}-dependent excitotoxicity

Increased oxidative stress makes mitochondria more sensitive to the Ca^{2+}-induced permeability transition, which may initiate apoptotic or necrotic cell death (Halestrap et al., 2000; Nicholls, 2008b, 2009). Mitochondria from tgSOD1 animals have high sensitivity to the deleterious effects of calcium (Martin et al., 2009). SCM are particularly sensitive to calcium overload (Sullivan et al., 2004, Panov et al., 2011a). This scenario becomes very likely to occur in tgSOD1 animals in view of the fact that spinal cord tissue contains 8 times more calcium than brain tissue (Panov et al., 2011a). We estimated that when normalized for 1 gram of tissue, BM could sequester several times more Ca^{2+} than was available in the whole tissue. SCM, on the other hand, could sequester only approximately 20% of the total spinal cord tissue Ca^{2+} (Panov et al., 2011a). We suggest that the high content of Ca^{2+} is necessary to hold together the sheets of myelin, which protects the neurons. We have shown recently that increased oxidative stress promotes demyelination in brains of OXYS rats with genetically accelerated aging, which was ameliorated by feeding of animals with malate (Kolosova et al. 2011). Underwood et al. (2010), using magnetic resonance imaging, have shown signs of demyelination in the lumbar spinal cord of ALS-affected SOD1 mice, which were limited to white matter tracts arising from the motor neurons, whereas sensory white matter fibers were preserved. Damages to myelin sheets of motor neurons may evidently release large amounts of calcium. The tissue calcium content in the spinal cord from presymptomatic tgSOD1 rats was diminished by 26% (Panov et al., 2011b). Thus, oxidatively damaged mitochondria may encounter increased amounts of Ca^{2+} released during demyelination and undergo permeability transition. Halestrap (2005) has pointed out that when mitochondria massively undergo permeability transition, the cells will die by necrosis, which was documented Martin et al.(2009) for ALS animals.

11. Conclusions

The results presented by us in this and other papers (Panov et al., 2009, 20011a, 2011b) lead us to suggest the role of the brain and spinal cord mitochondria in the loss of motor neurons in ALS. We hypothesize that increased oxidative stress associated with specific metabolic phenotypes, which promote reverse electron transport due to reduction of the membrane pool of ubiquinone by succinate (Panov et al., 2009, 2011a, 2011b) or fatty acids (Panov et al., 2010c), is a prerequisite for cases of sporadic ALS. The energy-dependent reverse electron transport is a way of dissipation of the mitochondrial membrane potential, which increases the rate of resting mitochondrial respiration. In mammals, the standard metabolic rate depends on the intrinsic (in state 4) mitochondrial proton conductivity (Rolfe & Brown , 1997). Therefore in patients with ALS hypermetabolism could be associated with the systemically increased dissipation of mitochondrial membrane potential. The specific vulnerability of motor neurons in ALS is, more likely than not, associated with the specific features of spinal cord described in Panov et al. (2011a, 2011b).

Normally, SCM produce significantly more ROS than BM when oxidizing physiologically relevant mixture of neuromediator glutamate and the tricarboxylic acid cycle substrates pyruvate, succinate and malate. Mutated SOD1 is extremely sensitive to the damaging effect of H_2O_2, which in tgBM and tgSCM were dramatically increased. This results in demetallation of mSOD1 and association with mitochondria, thus changing the physical properties of the mitochondrial membranes and further enhancing production of ROS. Increased oxidative stress initiates damage to myelin and released the tissue calcium. Finally, oxidatively damaged mitochondria undergo the Ca^{2+}-induced permeability transition, and motor neurons die by apoptotic or necrotic pathway. Thus, mitochondria are early and directly involved in the pathogenesis of ALS. We suggest that sporadic ALS is preferentially acquired by individuals with the mitochondrial metabolic phenotype, that promotes very high levels of ROS production. In individuals with mutated SOD1 gene, the abnormal SOD1 protein has high sensitivity to deleterious effect of H_2O_2 and the disease may develop even at normal levels of ROS production.

12. Proposals for future studies

The results and the hypothesis presented in this article highlight the importance to consider determination of metabolic phenotypes together with the disease mechanisms when working with patients or animal models of the ALS.

13. Acknowledgements

The authors thank the Carolinas HealthCare Foundation and Carolinas ALS Research Fund for financial support of this study. The authors thank Dr. Richelle Hemendinger and Dr.

Nataliya Kubalik for testing in 2010 the tgSOD1 rats for the time of development of ALS symptoms.

14. References

Abeles, Moshe. *Corticonics: Neural Circuits of the Cerebral Cortex*. Cambridge Univ. Press, 1991 ISBN 0521374766

Ahtoniemi, T., Jaronen, M., Keksa-Goldsteine, V., Goldsteins, G., & Koistinaho, J. (2008) Mutant SOD1 from spinal cord of G93A rats is destabilized and binds to inner mitochondrial membrane. *Neurobiol. Dis.* 32 (3), 479-485

Attwell D., & Laughlin S.B. (2001) An energy budget for signaling in the grey matter of the brain. *J Cereb Blood Flow Metab.* 21, 1133-1145

Auger, C. & Attwell, D. (2000) Fast removal of synaptic glutamate by postsynaptic transporters. *Neuron.* 28 (2), 547-558

Avossa, D., Grandolfo, M., Mazzarol, F., Zatta, M. & Ballerini, L. (2006) Early signs of motoneuron vulnerability in a disease model system: Characterization of transverse slice cultures of spinal cord isolated from embryonic ALS mice. *Neuroscience.* 138 (4), 1179-1194

Bacman, S.R., Bradley, W.G. and Moraes, C.T. (2006) Mitochondrial involvement in amyotrophic lateral sclerosis: Trigger or target? *Mol. Neurobiol.* 33 (2), 113-131

Balazs, R. (1965) Control of glutamate metabolism. The effect of pyruvate. *J. Neurochem.* 12, 63-76

Balazs R. (1965) Control of glutamate oxidation in brain and liver mitochondrial systems. *Biochem. J.* 95, 497-508

Barber, S. C. & Shaw, P.J. (2010) Oxidative stress in ALS: key role in motor neuron injury and therapeutic target. *Free Radic. Biol. Med.* 48(5), 629-641

Bendotti, C., & Carri, M.T. (2004) Lessons from models of SOD1-linked familial ALS. *Trends Mol. Med.* 10 (8), 393-400

Berkich, D. A., Ola, M.S., Cole, J., Sweatt, A.J., Hutson, S.M., & LaNoue, K.F. (2007) Mitochondrial transport proteins of the brain. *J. Neurosci. Res.* 85 (15), 3367-3677

Bertamini, M., Marzani, B., Guarneri, R., Guarneri, P., Bigini, P., Mennini, T. & Curti, D. (2002) Mitochondrial oxidative metabolism in motor neuron degeneration (mnd) mouse central nervous system. *Eur. J. Neurosci.* 16 (12), 2291-2296

Bouteloup, C., Desport, J.C., Clavelou, P., Guy, N., Derumeaux-Burel, H., Ferrier, A. & Couratier, P. (2009) Hypermetabolism in ALS patients: an early and persistent phenomenon. *J. Neurol.* 256 (8), 1236-1242

Braitenberg, V., & Schüz, A. (1998) *Cortex: statistics and geometry of neuronal connectivity*, 2nd ed. Berlin: Springer.

Brasnjo, G., & Otis, T.S. (2004) Isolation of glutamate transport-coupled charge flux and estimation of glutamate uptake at the climbing fiber-purkinje cell synapse. *Proc. Natl. Acad. Sci. USA.* 101, 6273-6278

Bruijn, L.I., Miller, T.M., & Cleveland, D.W. (2004) Unraveling the mechanisms involved in motor neuron degeneration in ALS. *Annu. Rev. Neurosci.* 27, 723-749

Damiano, M., Starkov, A.A., Petri, S., Kipiani, K., Kiaei, M., Mattiazzi, M., Beal, F. M., & Manfredi, G. (2006) Neural mitochondrial Ca capacity impairment precedes the onset of motor symptoms in G93A Cu/Zn-superoxide dismutase mutant mice. *J. Neurochem.* 96, 1349-1361

Dave, K.R., Bradley, W.G., & Perez-Pinzon, M.A. (2003) Early mitochondrial dysfunction occurs in motor cortex and spinal cord at the onset of disease in the Wobbler mouse. *Exp Neurol.* 182, 412-420

Deliconstantinos, G, Kopeikina, L, &Villiotou, V. 1989. Evoked effects of cholesterol binding on integral proteins and lipid fluidity of dog brain synaptosomal plasma membranes. *Biochem. Cell. Biol.* 67 (1), 16-24

Desport, J. C., Torny, F., Lacoste, M., Preux, P.M. & Couratier, P. (2005). Hypermetabolism in ALS: correlations with clinical and paraclinical parameters. Neurodegener. Dis. 2 (3-4), 202-207

Dikalov, S. I., Vitek, M.P. & Mason, R.P. (2004). Cupric-amyloid beta peptide complex stimulates oxidation of ascorbate and generation of hydroxyl radical. *Free Radic. Biol. Med.* 36 (3), 340-347

Dupuis, L., Gonzalez de Aguilar, J.L., Echaniz-Laguna, A., Eschbach, J., Rene, F., Oudart, H., Halter, B., Huze, C., Schaeffer, L., Bouillaud, F., & Loeffler, J.P. (2009) Muscle mitochondrial uncoupling dismantles neuromuscular junction and triggers distal degeneration of motor neurons. *PLoS One.* 4 (4), e5390

Durer, Z.A.O., Cohlberg, J.A., Dinh, P., Padua, S., Ehrenclou, K., Downes, S., Tan, J.K., Nakano, Y., Bowman, C.J., Hoskins, J.L., Kwon, C., Mason, A.Z., Rodriguez, J.A., Doucette, P.A., Shaw, B.F., & Valentine, J.S. (2009) Loss of Metal Ions, Disulfide Reduction and Mutations Related to Familial ALS Promote Formation of Amyloid-Like Aggregates from Superoxide Dismutase. *PLoS One.* 4 (3), e5004

Ebert, D., Haller, R.G. & Walton, M.E. (2003) Energy contribution of octanoate to intact rat brain metabolism measured by 13C nuclear magnetic resonance spectroscopy. *J. Neurosci.* 23 (13), 5928-5935

Echaniz-Laguna, A., Zoll, J., Ponsot, E., N'Guessan, B., Tranchant, C., Loeffler, J.P. & Lampert, E. (2006) Muscular mitochondrial function in amyotrophic lateral sclerosis is progressively altered as the disease develops: a temporal study in man. *Exp. Neurol.* 198 (1), 25-30

Field, L. S., Y. Furukawa, T. V. O'Halloran and V. C. Culotta (2003). Factors controlling the uptake of yeast copper/zinc superoxide dismutase into mitochondria. *J. Biol. Chem.* 278 (30), 28052-28059

Fischer, L.R., Igoudjil, A., Magrané, J., Li, Y., Hansen, J.M., Manfredi, G., Glass, J.D. (2011) SOD1 targeted to the mitochondrial intermembrane space prevents motor neuropathy in the Sod1 knockout mouse. *Brain.* 134 (Pt 1),196-209

Furness, D. N., Dehnes, Y., Akhtar, A.Q., Rossi, D.J., Hamann, M., Grutle, N.J., Gundersen, V., Holmseth, S., Lehre, K.P., Ullensvang, K., Wojewodzic, M., Zhou, Y., Attwell, D. & Danbolt, D.C. (2008) A quantitative assessment of glutamate uptake into hippocampal synaptic terminals and astrocytes: New insights into a neuronal role for excitatory amino acid transporter 2 (EAAT2). *Neuroscience.* 157 (1), 80-94

Furukawa, Y. & O'Halloran, T.V. (2006) Posttranslational modifications in Cu,Zn-superoxide dismutase and mutations associated with amyotrophic lateral sclerosis. *Antioxid Redox Signal.* 8 (5-6), 847-867

Gershoni, M., Templeton, A.R. & Mishmar, D. (2009) Mitochondrial bioenergetics as a major motive force of speciation. *Bioessays.* 31 (6), 642-650

Gurney, M.E., Pu, H., Chiu, A.Y., Dal Canto, M.C., Polchow, C.Y., Alexander, D.D., Caliendo, J., Hentati, A., Kwon, Y.W., & Deng, H.X. (1994) Motor neuron degeneration in mice that express a human Cu,Zn superoxide dismutase mutation. *Science.* 264 (5166), 1772-1775

Halestrap, A.P., Doran, E., Gillespie, J,P.,b & O'Toole, A. (2000) Mitochondria and cell death. *Biochem. Soc. Trans.* 28 (2), 170-177.

Halestrap, H. A pore way to die. (2005) *Nature.* 434, 578-579

Heath P.R. & Shaw P.J. (2002) Update on the glutamatergic neurotransmitter system and the role of excitotoxicity in amyotrophic lateral sclerosis. *Muscle Nerve.* 26, 438-458

Hertz, L. (2004) Intercellular metabolic compartmentation in the brain: past, present and future. *Neurochem Int.* 45, (2-3), 285-296

Higgins C.M., Jung C., Ding H. & Xu Z. (2002) Mutant Cu, Zn superoxide dismutase that causes motoneuron degeneration is present in mitochondria in the CNS. *J. Neurosci.* 22, RC215

Howland, D.S., Liu, J., She, Y., Goad, B., Maragakis, N.J., Kim, B., Erickson, J., Kulik, J., DeVito, L., Psaltis, G., DeGennaro, L.J., Cleveland, D.W., Rothstein, J.D. (2002) Focal loss of the glutamate transporter EAAT2 in a transgenic rat model of SOD1 mutant-mediated amyotrophic lateral sclerosis (ALS). *Proc. Natl. Acad. Sci. USA.* 99, 1604-1609.

Israelson, A., Arbel, N., Da Cruz, S., Illeva, H., Yamanaka, K., Shoshan-Barmatz, V. & Cleveland, D.W. (2010) Misfolded mutant SOD1 directly inhibits VDAC1 conductance in a mouse model inherited ALS. *Neuron,* 67, 575-587

Jaarsma D. (2006) Swelling and vacuolisation of mitochondria in transgenic sod1-als mice: A consequence of supranormal sod1 expression? *Mitochondrion.* 6 (1), 48-49

Jung, C., Higgins, C.M.J. & Xu, Z. (2002) A quantitative histochemical assay for activities of mitochondrial electron transport chain complexes in mouse spinal cord sections. *J. Neurosci. Methods.* 114 (2), 165-172

Kirkinezos, I. G., Bacman, S.R., Hernandez, D., Oca-Cossio, J., Arias, L.J., Perez-Pinzon, M.A., Bradley, W.G. & Moraes, C.T. (2005) Cytochrome c association with the inner mitochondrial membrane is impaired in the CNS of G93A-SOD1 mice. *J. Neurosci.* 25, 164-172

Kolosova, N.G., Akulov, A.E., Stefanova, N.A., Moshkin, M.P., Savelov, A.A., Koptyug, I.V., Panov, A.V. & Vavilin, V.A. (2011) Effect of malate on development of rotenone-induced brain changes in Wistar and OXYS rats: An MRI study. *Doklady Biol. Sci.* 437, 1-4

Krasnianski, A., Deschauer, M., Neudecker, S., Gellerich, F.N., Muller, T., Schoser, B.G., Krasnianski, M. & Zierz, S. (2005) Mitochondrial changes in skeletal muscle in amyotrophic lateral sclerosis and other neurogenic atrophies. *Brain.* 128 (Pt 8), 1870-1876

Kwong, L.K. & Sohal, R.S. (1998) Substrate and site specificity of hydrogen peroxide generation in mouse mitochondria. *Arch. Biochem. Biophys.* 350 (1), 118-126

Liochev, S. I. & Fridovich, I. (2004) CO2 enhanced peroxidase activity of SOD1: the effects of pH. *Free Radic. Biol. Med.* 36 (11), 1444-1447

Liu, J., Lillo, C., Jonsson, P.A., Vande Velde, C., Ward, C.M., Miller, T.M., Subramaniam, J.R., Rothstein, J.D., Marklund, S., Andersen, P.M., Brannstrom, T., Gredal, O., Wong, P.C., Williams, D.S. & Cleveland, D.W. (2004) Toxicity of familial ALS-linked SOD1 mutants from selective recruitment to spinal mitochondria. *Neuron.* 43, 5-17

Magrane, J. & Manfredi, G. (2009) Mitochondrial function, morphology, and axonal transport in amyotrophic lateral sclerosis. *Antioxidants & Redox Signaling.* 11 (7), 1615-1626

Martin, L.J., Liu, Z., Chen, K., Price, A.C., Pan, Y., Swaby, J.A. & Golden, W.C. 2007. Motor neuron degeneration in amyotrophic lateral sclerosis mutant superoxide dismutase-1 transgenic mice: mechanisms of mitochondriopathy and cell death. *J. Comp. Neurol.* 500 (1), 20-46

Martin, L.J., Gertz, B., Pan, Y., Price, A.C., Molkentin, J.D. & Chang, Q. (2009) The mitochondrial permeability transition pore in motor neurons: Involvement in the pathobiology of ALS mice. *Experim. Neurol.* 218 (2), 333-346

Massie, A., Cnops, L., Smolders, I., McCullumsmith, R., Kooijman, R., Kwak, S., Arckens, L. & Michotte, Y. (2008) High-affinity Na+/K+-dependent glutamate transporter EAAT4 is expressed throughout the rat fore- and midbrain. *J Comp Neurol.* 511 (2), 155-172

Matsumoto, A., Okada, Y., Nakamichi, M., Nakamura, M., Toyama, Y., Sobue, G., Nagai, M., Aoki, M., Itoyama, Y. & Okano, H. (2006) Disease progression of human SOD1 (G93A) transgenic ALS model rats. *J. Neurosci. Res.* 83 (1), 119-133

Mitchell, P. (1977) Vectorial chemiosmotic processes. *Ann. Rev. Biochem.* 46, 996-1005

Morota, S.; Hansson, M.J.; Ishii, N.; Kudo, Y.; Elmer, E.; Uchino, H. (2007) Spinal cord mitochondria display lower calcium retention capacity compared with brain mitochondria without inherent differences in sensitivity to cyclophilin D inhibition. *J Neurochem.* 103 (5), 2066-2076, 2007

Muller, F.L., Liu, Y., Abdul-Ghani, M.A., Lustgarten, M.S., Bhattacharya, A., Jang, Y.C. & Van Remmen, H. (2008) High rates of superoxide production in skeletal-muscle mitochondria respiring on both complex I- and complex II-linked substrates. *Biochem. J.* 409 (2), 491-499.

Muller, F.L.; Song, W.; Jang, Y.C.; Liu, Y.; Sabia, M.; Richardson, A. & Van Remmen, H. (2007) Denervation-induced skeletal muscle atrophy is associated with increased mitochondrial ROS production. *Am. J. Physiol. Regul. Integr. Comp. Physiol.* 293, 3, R1159-R1168

Nakano, Y., Hirayama, K. & Terao, K. (1987) Hepatic ultrastructural changes and liver dysfunction in amyotrophic lateral sclerosis. *Arch. Neurol.* 44 (1), 103-106

Nicholls, D. G. (1993). The glutamatergic nerve terminal. *Eur. J. Biochem.* 212 (3), 613-631

Nicholls, D. G. (2008) Oxidative stress and energy crises in neuronal dysfunction. *Ann. N. Y. Acad. Sci.* 1147, 53-60

Nicholls, D. G. (2008) Forty years of Mitchell's proton circuit: From little grey books to little grey cells. *Biochim. Biophys. Acta.* 1777 (7-8), 550-556

Nicholls, D. G. (2009) Mitochondrial calcium function and dysfunction in the central nervous system. *Biochim. Biophys. Acta.* 1787 (11), 1416-142

Norenberg, M. D. & Martinez-Hernandez, A. (1979) Fine structural localization of glutamine synthetase in astrocytes of rat brain. *Brain Res.* 161 (2), 303-310

Panov, A., Dikalov, S., Shalbuyeva, N., Hemendinger, R., Greenamyre, J.T. & Rosenfeld, J. (2007) Species and tissue specific relationships between mitochondrial permeability transition and generation of ROS in brain and liver mitochondria of rats and mice. *Am. J. Physiol. Cell. Physiol.* 292 (2), C708-C718

Panov, A., Schonfeld, O., Dikalov, S., Hemendinger, R., Bonkovsky, H.L. & Brooks, B.R. (2009) The neuromediator glutamate, through specific substrate interactions, enhances mitochondrial ATP production and reactive oxygen species generation in nonsynaptic brain mitochondria. *J. Biol. Chem.* 284 (21), 14448-14456.

Panov, A.V., Vavilin, V.A., Lyalkhovich, V.V., Brooks, B.R., Bonkovsky, H.L. (2010a) Effects of defatted bovine serum albumin on respiratory activities of brain and liver mitochondria from C57Bl/6G mice and Sprague Dawley rats. *Bull. Exp. Biol. Med.* 149 (2), 187-190

Panov, A., Kubalik, N., Brooks, B.R. & Shaw, C.A. (2010b) In vitro effects of cholesterol β-D-glucoside, cholesterol and cycad phytosterol glucosides on respiration and reactive oxygen species generation in brain mitochondria. *J. Membr. Biol.* 237, 71-77

Panov, A., Kubalik, N., & Brooks, B.R. (2010c) Effects of palmitoyl carnitine on brain, spinal cord and heart mitochondria from wild type and transgenic SOD1 rats. 21st International Symposium on ALS/MND, Orlando 11-13 December, 2010. *Amyotrophic Lateral Sclerosis.* 11 (Suppl. 1), 115

Panov, A.V., Kubalik, N., Zinchenko, N., Hemendinger R., Brooks B.R. & Bonkovsky, H.L. (2011a) Metabolic and functional differences between brain and spinal cord mitochondria underlie different predisposition to pathology. *Am. J. Physiol. Regul. Integr. Comp. Physiol.* 300 (4), R844-R854

Panov, A., Kubalik, N., Zinchenko, N., Hemendinger, R., Dikalov, S. & Bonkovsky, H.L. (2011b) Respiration and ROS production in brain and spinal cord mitochondria of transgenic rats with mutant G93A Cu/Zn-Superoxide dismutase gene. *Neurobiol. Dis.* 44, 53-62

Pardo, B., Contreras, L., Serrano, A., Ramos, M., Kobayashi, K., Iijima, M., Saheki, T. & Satrustegui, J. (2006). Essential role of aralar in the transduction of small ca2+ signals to neuronal mitochondria. *J. Biol. Chem.* 281 (2), 1039-1047

Pedrini, S., Sau, D., Guareschi, S., Bogush, M., Brown, R.H., Jr., Naniche, N., Kia, A., Trotti, D. & Pasinelli, P. (2010) ALS-linked mutant SOD1 damages mitochondria by promoting conformational changes in Bcl-2. *Hum. Mol. Genet.* 19 (15), 2974-2986

Pellerin, L., Bouzier-Sore, A.K., Aubert, A., Serres, S., Merle, M., Costalat, R. & Magistretti, P.J. (2007) Activity-dependent regulation of energy metabolism by astrocytes: an update. *Glia.* 55 (12), 1251-1262

Przedborski S. (2004) Programmed cell death in amyotrophic lateral sclerosis: a mechanism of pathogenic and therapeutic importance. *Neurologist.* 10, 1-7

Ramirez, D.C., Gomez-Mejiba, S.E., Corbett, J.T., Deterding, L.J., Tomer, K.B. & Mason, R.P. (2009) Cu,Zn-superoxide dismutase-driven free radical modifications: copper- and carbonate radical anion-initiated protein radical chemistry. *Biochem. J.* 417 (1), 341-353

Rolfe, D.F.S. & Brown, G.C. (1997) Cellular energy utilization and molecular origin of standard metabolic rate in mammals. *Physiol. Rev.* 77, 731-758

Rowland, L.P. & Shneider, N.A. (2001) Amyotrophic lateral sclerosis. *N. Engl. J. Med.* 344 (22), 1688-1700

Shook, S.J. & Pioro, E.P. (2009) Racing against the clock: Recognizing differentiating, diagnosing, and referring the amyotrophic lateral sclerosis patient. *Ann. Neurol.*, 65 (suppl.), S10-S16

Starkov, A.A. (2008) The role of mitochondria in reactive oxygen species metabolism and signaling. *Ann. New York Acad. Sci.* 1147, 37-52

Stowe, D.F. & Camara, A.K. (2009) Mitochondrial reactive oxygen species production in excitable cells: Modulators of mitochondrial and cell function. *Antioxidants & Redox Signaling.* 11 (6), 1381-1414

St-Pierre, J., Buckingham, J.A., Roebuck, S.J. & Brand, M.D. (2002) Topology of superoxide production from different sites in the mitochondrial electron transport chain. *J. Biol. Chem.* 277 (47), 44784-44790

Stolzenburg, J.U., Reichenbach, A. & Neumann, M. (1989) Size and density of glial and neuronal cells within the cerebral neocortex of various insectivorian species. *Glia.* 2 (2), 78-84

Sullivan P.G., Rabchevsky, A.G., Keller, J.Y.N., Lovell, M., Sodhi, A., Hart, R.P. & Scheffer, S.W. (2004) Intrinsic differences in brain and spinal cord mitochondria: implication for therapeutic interventions. *J. Comparative Neurol.* 474, 524–534

Suzuki, A., Stern, S.A., Bozdagi, O., Huntley, G.W., Walker, R.H., Magistretti, P.J. & Alberini, C.M. (2011) Astrocyte-neuron lactate transport is required for long-term memory formation. *Cell.* 144 (5), 810-823

Tillakaratne N.J., Medina-Kauwe, L. & Gibson, K.M. (1995) Gamma-aminobutyric acid (gaba) metabolism in mammalian neural and nonneural tissues. *Comp. Biochem. Physiol. A Physiol.* 112 (2), 247-263

Tateno M., Sadakata H., Tanaka M., Itohara S., Shin R.M., Miura M., Masuda M., Aosaki T., Urushitani M., Misawa H. & Takahashi R. (2004) Calcium-permeable AMPA receptors promote misfolding of mutant SOD1 protein and development of amyotrophic lateral sclerosis in a transgenic mouse model. *Hum. Mol. Genet.* 13, 2183-2196

Tretter, L., Takacs, K., Hegedus, V. & Adam-Vizi, V. (2007) Characteristics of alpha-glycerophosphate-evoked H2O2 generation in brain mitochondria. *J. Neurochem.* 100 (3), 650-663

Valentine, J.S., Doucette, P.A. & Potter, S.Z. (2005) Copper-zinc superoxide dismutase and amyotrophic lateral sclerosis. *Annu. Rev. Biochem.* 74, 563-593

Vande Velde, C., Miller, T.M., Cashman, N.R. & Cleveland, D.W. (2008) Selective association of misfolded ALS-linked mutant SOD1 with the cytoplasmic face of mitochondria. *Proc. Natl. Acad. Sci. USA.* 105 (10), 4022-4027

Von Lewinski, F. & B. U. Keller (2005). Ca2+, mitochondria and selective motoneuron vulnerability: implications for ALS. *Trends Neurosci.* 28 (9), 494-500

Votyakova, T.V. & Reynolds, I.J. (2001) $\Delta\Psi$-dependent and independent production of reactive oxygen species by rat brain mitochondria. *J. Neurochem.* 79, 266-277

Waagepetersen, H.S., Sonnewald. U., Larsson, O.M. & Schousboe, A. (1999) Synthesis of vesicular GABA from glutamine involves TCA cycle metabolism in neocortical neurons. *J. Neurosci. Res.* 57 (3), 342-349

Wallace, D.C. (2001) Mouse models for mitochondrial disease. *Am. J. Med. Genet.* 106, 71-93

Wilson, J.M., Khabazian, I., Wong, M.C., Seyedalikhani, A., Bains, J.S., Pasqualotto, B.A., Williams, D.E., Andersen, R.J., Simpson, R.J., Smith, R., Craig, U.K., Kurland, L.T., & Shaw, C.A. (2002) Behavioral and neurological correlates of ALS-parkinsonism dementia complex in adult mice fed washed cycad flour. *Neuromolecular Med.* 1 (3), 207-221

Wong-Riley, M.T. (1989) Cytochrome oxidase: An endogenous metabolic marker for neuronal activity. *Trends Neurosci.* 12 (3), 94-101

Xu, G-P., Dave, K.R., Moraes, C.T., Busto, R., Sick, T.J., Bradley, W.G. & Perez-Pinzon, M.A. (2001) Dysfunctional mitochondrial respiration in the wobbler mouse brain. *Neurosci. Letters.* 300, 141-144

Yudkoff, M., Nelson, D., Daikhin, Y. & Erecinska, M. (1994). Tricarboxylic acid cycle in rat brain synaptosomes. Fluxes and interactions with aspartate aminotransferase and malate/aspartate shuttle. *J. Biol. Chem.* 269 (44), 27414-27420.

Zoccarato, F., Cavallini, L., Bortolami, S. & Alexandre, A. (2007) Succinate modulation of H_2O_2 release at NADH -ubiquinone oxidoreductase (Complex I) in brain mitochondria. *Biochem. J.* 406 (1), 125-129

10

Mutant Cu/Zn-Superoxide Dismutase Induced Mitochondrial Dysfunction in Amyotrophic Lateral Sclerosis

Jari Koistinaho and Gundars Goldsteins
A.I.Virtanen Institute for Molecular Sciences, University of Eastern Finland, Finland

1. Introduction

Mutations in Cu/Zn superoxide dismutase (SOD1) gene are linked to the motor neuron death in familial amyotrophic lateral sclerosis (FALS). More than 100 missense mutations have been described to cause the disease and are distributed throughout the whole 153 amino acid sequence of SOD1 molecule (Valentine et al., 2005; Boillée et al., 2006). Mutant SOD1 molecules can be grouped according to their biochemical characteristics into wild type-like proteins, that bind metal ions and possess enzymatic dismutase activity (e.g. G93A-SOD1 and G37R-SOD1), and mutant molecules with impaired metal binding capacity, which have significantly reduced dismutase activity (e.g. G85R-SOD1) (Valentine et al., 2005). Therefore, the toxicity of mutant SOD1 is not thought to be mediated by a lack of dismutase activity, but rather by gain of one or more detrimental functions.

The exact nature of the toxic gain of function for mutant SOD1 has not been identified yet. Most of the studies demonstrate a link between the disease pathology and increased oxidative stress. Augmented generation of free radicals and reactive oxygen species (ROS) is thought to be a major contributor to the destruction of motor neurons (Beckman et al., 1994; Wiedau-Pazos et al., 1996; Estévez et al., 1999).

The suggested toxic mechanisms include aberrant mutant SOD1 enzymatic activities (Beckman et al., 1993; Wiedau-Pazos et al., 1996) as well as destabilized SOD1 protein misfolding, causing enhanced aggregation of SOD1 or pathological interaction of SOD1 with other proteins (Stathopulos et al., 2003; Liu et al., 2004).

In a number of studies mitochondrial localization of mutant SOD1 has been implicated in ALS pathogenesis (Liu et al., 2004; Vijayvergiya et al., 2005; Bergemalm et al., 2006; Deng et al., 2006; Ferri et al., 2006) and increased recruitment of mutant SOD1 into mitochondria in the spinal cord might be a reason for death of motor neurons in some forms of familial ALS. However, the detailed mechanisms for toxicity of the mitochondria resident mutant SOD1 are not entirely clear yet. Here we review the current state of the art in the studies on mitochondrial toxicity of SOD1 in ALS.

2. Factors controlling SOD1 translocation to mitochondria and SOD1 activity in mitochondrial intermembrane space

Although the majority of SOD1 is present in the cytosol (Okado-Matsumoto & Fridovich, 2001), a fraction of SOD1 is translocated into the mitochondrial intermembrane space (IMS)

(Sturtz et al., 2001; Higgins et al., 2002). Since SOD1 does not contain mitochondrial targeting sequence, the true physiological function of SOD1 in the IMS remains mostly enigmatic.

In mammalian cells the mitochondrial localization of SOD1 is regulated by the folding state of this enzyme, depending on the intracellular distribution of copper chaperone for SOD1 (CCS), which in turn is regulated by oxygen concentration. Redox status of the cysteine residues in human SOD1 is critical for its retention in mitochondria. The cysteine residues form intramolecular disulphide bonds and interact with CCS (Kawamata & Manfredi, 2008). This regulation appears to be impaired for SOD1 mutants, which can lead to misfolding and aggregation of mutant SOD1 and eventually result in SOD1 accumulation inside the mitochondria. In animal models the mitochondrial association of mutant SOD1 is apparent even before the disease onset (Liu et al., 2004), indicating a causative link of mitochondrial SOD1 to the initiation of pathology.

Even though SOD1 has been suggested to be an important part of the mitochondrial superoxide scavenging system, as previously demonstrated in the yeast (Sturtz et al., 2001) and rat (Iñarrea et al., 2005) mitochondrion IMS, SOD1 activity is kept under redox control in this compartment and undergoes activation upon increased hydroperoxide concentration (Iñarrea et al., 2005).

There are 4 cysteines in the human SOD1 molecule, located at 6, 57, 111 and 144 position of the sequence. The intramolecular disulphide bridge between Cys57 and Cys146 is required for the proper tertiary and quaternary structure and enzymatic activity of SOD1 (Arnesano et al., 2004). Diminished copper loading and reduced intramolecular disulphide bound has been thought to be responsible for increased aggregation potential of G93A and D90A mutant SOD1 (Jonsson et al., 2006).

The maturation and activation of SOD1 in the cytosol is controlled by a number of factors and can be divided in several principal steps. Upon post-translational activation, an SOD1 monomer binds a Zn^{2+} ion. Next ,CCS transiently binds to SOD1 monomer and inserts a Cu^{2+} ion in the molecule (Culotta et al., 1997; Casareno et al., 1998). After the dissociation of SOD1 from CCS, oxidative formation of disulphide bounds takes place (Arnesano et al., 2004; Ding & Dokholyan, 2008), which is followed by dimerisation yielding an active SOD1 molecule (Vonk et al., 2010).

Active SOD1 dimers are not capable of entering mitochondria, in contrast to disulphide reduced apo-SOD1. According to the model proposed (Kawamata & Manfredi, 2008; Reddehase et al., 2009), CCS is first imported into mitochondria by interaction with Mia40, an IMS component critical for protein import to mitochondria. The CCS-Mia40 complex is formed through an intermolecular disulphide bound (Fig. 1.). Further disulphide rearrangement generates oxidized CCS, preventing its escape from the IMS. The activation of SOD1 in IMS is thought to be similar to the activation of SOD1 in cytosol, where SOD1 binds to CCS in the presence of Cu^{2+} ions and oxygen generating an active enzyme retained in IMS (Leitch et al., 2009).

Surprisingly, CCS overexpression in G93A-SOD1 mouse, a widely used transgenic mouse model of ALS, produces severe mitochondrial pathology and accelerates disease course (Son et al., 2007). According to the model above, the potentiation of mutant SOD1 toxicity by CCS overexpression can be explained by the CCS-mediated increase in SOD1 mitochondrial import, leading to enhanced SOD1 aggregation.

In contrast to the model of CCS-dependent activation of mitochondrial SOD1, a number of recent studies suggest that SOD1 in the IMS of intact mitochondria is mostly inactive and an oxidative modification of its critical thiol groups is necessary for the activation (Iñarrea et al., 2005, 2011; Goldsteins et al., 2008). This activation, at least partly, depends on protein disulphide isomerase (PDI) activity (Iñarrea et al., 2005). On the other hand, the toxicity of mutant SOD1 is not correlated with its aggregation potential but with the ability to form active dimeric molecules (Witan et al., 2008). These findings are in concert with a concept that mitochondrial dysfunction and cell damage are paradoxically induced by SOD1-mediated hydroperoxide production in the IMS (Goldsteins et al., 2008).

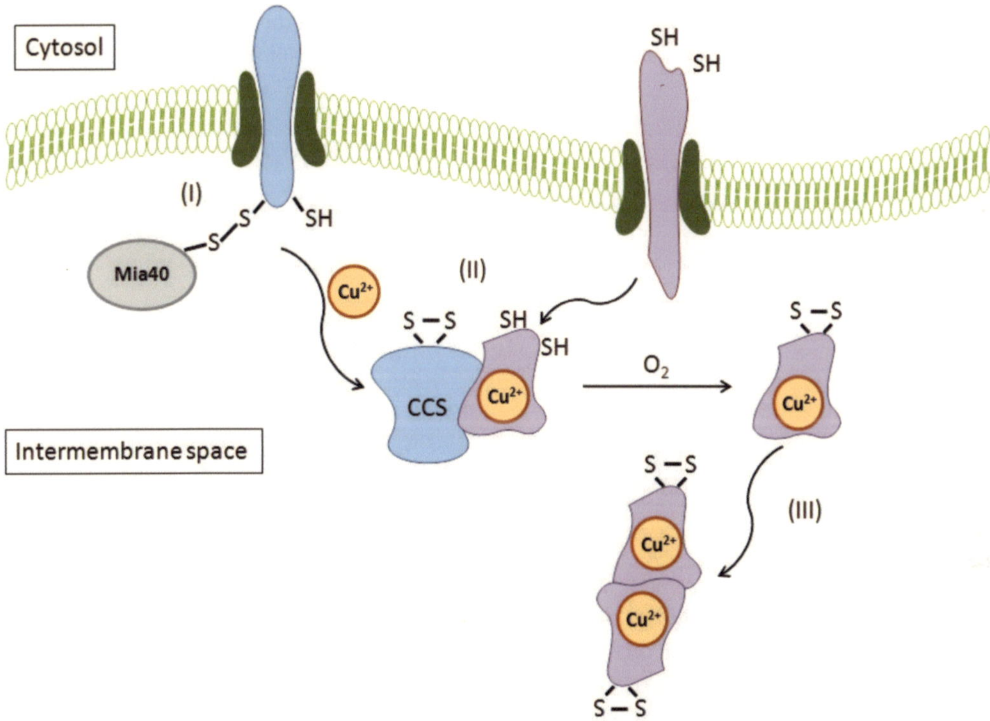

Fig. 1. Import and activation of SOD1 in IMS. CCS is imported into mitochondria through formation of a complex with Mia40 (I). Disulphide-reduced SOD1 monomer enters IMS and acquires copper ion (Cu^{2+}) with a help of CCS (II). Formation of intramolecular disulphide bound and dimerisation of SOD1 creates an active SOD1 molecule retained in IMS (III).

3. Proposed mechanisms for mutant SOD1 toxicity in mitochondria

Mitochondrial abnormalities and degeneration of motor neurons are early signs of ALS disease (Wong et al., 1995; Dal Canto & Gurney, 1997; Kong & Xu, 1998). They also represent pathological hallmarks in mutant SOD1 transgenic animal models for FALS as well as in patients with sporadic ALS (Kong & Xu, 1998; Mattiazzi et al., 2002; Manfredi & Xu, 2005). Mitochondrial toxicity may thus be an important factor in the degeneration of motor neurons. The pathology, demonstrated in sporadic ALS cases includes mitochondrial aggregates, mitochondrion swelling and increased calcium levels in mitochondria (Atsumi, 1981; Siklós et al., 1996). In G93A-SOD1 transgenic mice the disease onset is associated with a remarkable increase of vacuolated mitochondria in motor neurons (Kong & Xu, 1998). It has been proposed that formation of vacuoles originates from the expansion of mitochondrial IMS and degeneration of mitochondrial matrix (Jaarsma et al., 2001; Bendotti et al., 2001; Higgins et al., 2003; Xu et al., 2004).

Currently, there is no consensus on how mutant SOD1 causes mitochondrial pathology. The proposed mechanisms for mitochondrial toxicity of mutant SOD1 are summarized in Table 1. Among other toxic mechanisms reduced activities of respiratory complexes (Browne et al., 1998), mitochondrial depolarization and impaired calcium homeostasis (Kruman et al., 1999) have been demonstrated in the spinal cord of G93A-SOD1 mice. The observed dysfunctions of mitochondria might be caused by the recruitment of mutant SOD1, which has been shown to be selective to spinal cord mitochondria (Stathopulos et al., 2003; Liu et al., 2004; Pasinelli et al., 2004).

TOXIC MECHANISM	REFERENCES
Aggregate accumulation in mitochondria	(Higgins et al., 2002; Vande Velde et al., 2008)
Aberrant mutant SOD1 enzymatic activities, causing ROS production	(Estévez et al., 1999; Elliott, 2001)
Impaired energy metabolism	(Siciliano et al., 2001; Mattiazzi et al., 2002)
Impaired Ca^{2+} buffering	(Jaiswal & Keller, 2009; Grosskreutz et al., 2010)
Gain in pro-apoptotic function	(Pasinelli et al., 2004)
Interfering with mitochondrial protein import	(Liu et al., 2004)
Increased hydroperoxide production in IMS	(Goldsteins et al., 2008)

Table 1. Proposed mechanisms for mitochondrial toxicity of mutant SOD1

Among the proposed mechanisms, impairment of mitochondrial calcium buffering capacity has been shown in motor neurons of transgenic ALS mice (Damiano et al., 2006). On the other hand, ATP levels have been reported to be diminished in spinal cords of mutant SOD1 mouse model (Mattiazzi et al., 2002). Another view to the mitochondrial toxicity of mutant SOD1 was brought up by Vande Velde et al., who demonstrated that misfolded mutant SOD1 damages mitochondria by its deposition onto the cytoplasmic side of the outer membrane of spinal cord mitochondria (Vande Velde et al., 2008).

Other studies have demonstrated that the increased dismutase activity in rodent ALS models expressing mutant SOD1 paradoxically boosts the production of toxic ROS in the IMS (Goldsteins et al., 2008). It was shown that in a G93A-SOD1 rat model of ALS, the stability and quaternary structure of mutant SOD1 are lost most prominently in the spinal cord already several weeks before the onset of the disease (Ahtoniemi et al., 2008). These results suggest that destabilization of mutant SOD1 is associated with its increased binding to the inner mitochondrial membrane and elevated ROS production in the IMS. (Liu et al., 2004; Kirkinezos et al., 2005; Ahtoniemi et al., 2008).

Importantly, it was also recently demonstrated, that disulphide-reduced apo-SOD1 can rapidly initiate SOD1 fibrillation upon physiological conditions, suggesting that such disulphide-reduced apo-SOD1 may act as a seed for the amyloid like aggregates originating from the destabilized and folding intermediates of mutant SOD1 (Chattopadhyay et al., 2008).

Despite of rather different mechanisms proposed for the toxic properties of mutant SOD1 in mitochondria, most of the recent studies document that mitochondrial dysfunction results in increased ROS production (Beretta et al., 2003). Mitochondria isolated from the neural tissue (brain, spinal cord) have distinct metabolic properties regarding the extent of ROS produced upon oxidation of respiratory substrates (Panov et al., 2011). Especially in G93A-SOD1 transgenic rats, brain and spinal cord mitochondria generate 5-7 fold more ROS than mitochondria of corresponding wild-type tissues. Particularly, the spinal cord mitochondria produce two times more hydroperoxide than brain mitochondria of the same animals (Panov et al., n.d.)

Analysis of mitochondrial morphology in G37R and G85R-SOD1 transgenic mice has revealed that somal mitochondria become shorter and rounder in both dismutase active and inactive mutant SOD1 mouse lines. In contrast, axonal mitochondria in G37R-SOD1 animals shift from elongated tubular mitochondria to punctate mitochondria, while in G85R-SOD1 mice the mitochondria have been reported to show an increase in length (Vande Velde et al., 2011). These changes in mitochondrial shape and distribution were characteristic prior to ALS disease onset and support the notion of early mitochondrial pathology in ALS.

4. SOD1 catalyzes increased hydroperoxide production in IMS

The growing body of evidence provides support to the concept that superoxide dismutation in IMS may cause an increased hydroperoxide production with toxic consequences. Mitochondria are the major intracellular source of superoxide, the primary ROS, where superoxide anion radical is generated by one electron reduction of oxygen.

The two major pathways of superoxide production in mitochondria are autooxidation or complex III catalyzed oxidation of ubisemiquinone (Muller et al., 2004) and complex I catalyzed reduction of oxygen through reversed electron flow in the respiratory chain (Fig. 2.) (Liu et al., 2002). The produced superoxide anion radical has ability to actively react with a number of cellular targets leading to the loss of their proper function. The main detoxifying mechanism for superoxide instead of reverse oxidation of superoxide to oxygen, includes dismutation to hydroperoxide and oxygen.

Besides SOD1, there are other dedicated enzymes catalyzing this dismutation reaction. In mitochondria Mn-superoxide dismutase (SOD2), which is found in the mitochondrial matrix, scavenges superoxide in this compartment. Extracellular superoxide dismutase (SOD3) is secreted into the extracellular space and protects tissues against excess of superoxide (Zelko et al., 2002). In the IMS superoxide is produced presumably by complex III (Fig. 2.) (Muller et al., 2004). Unlike hydroperoxide, which freely diffuses through the membranes, superoxide cannot cross the mitochondrial inner membrane. In the matrix SOD2 converts superoxide to hydroperoxide, which in turn is reduced to water by the matrix glutathione peroxidase (Inoue et al., 2003). Homozygous SOD2 knockout mice are neonatally lethal (Li et al., 1995), whereas deletion of SOD1 gene does not have apparent motor neuron disease phenotype (Maier & Chan, 2002).

In IMS the fate of superoxide is determined by SOD1 and cytochrome c, which is present there in millimolar concentrations (Forman & Azzi, 1997; van Beek-Harmsen & van der Laarse, 2005). Cytochrome c is a heme containing protein, which functions as an electron carrier between complex III and cytochrome oxidase in the respiratory chain. Cytocrome c can also efficiently oxidize superoxide to oxygen. In this respect, cytochrome c can function as an efficient antioxidant, scavenging superoxide without production of secondary ROS (Fig. 2. reaction II), in contrast to SOD1, which produces hydroperoxide (Fig. 2, reaction III) (Pereverzev et al., 2003). However, cytochrome c has also a potential to catalyze oxidation by hydroperoxide. Upon this reaction, hydroperoxide oxidizes the prosthetic heme in the cytochrome c molecule to oxoferryl heme, forming so-called peroxidase compound I-type intermediate, a highly reactive oxidant that is able to react with a number of intracellular targets including proteins, nucleic acids and lipids, causing cell damage (Fig. 3) (Lawrence et al., 2003). Cytochrome c peroxidase activity is controlled by the coordination state of heme iron, particularly by the sulphur ligand of methionine-80 (Met-80), which can be easily displaced by hydroperoxide (Barr et al., 1996; Qian et al., 2002). The peroxidase activity of cytochrome c may increase by unfolding and post-translational modifications, such as proteolytic cleavage, nitration and oxidation (Diederix et al., 2002; Everse & Coates, 2005; Jang & Han, 2006).

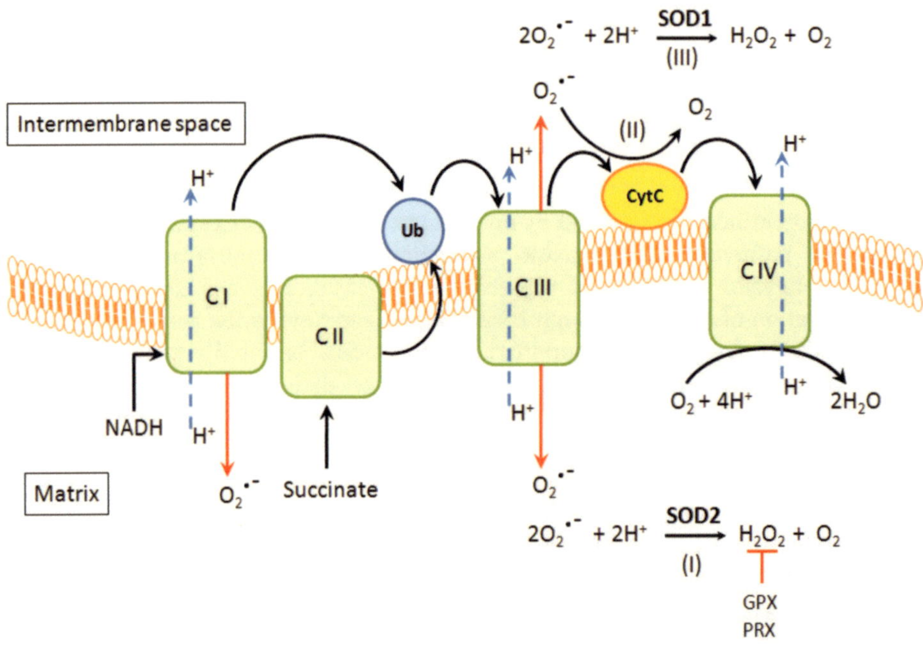

Fig. 2. Mitochondrial production and clearance of superoxide. Upon respiration superoxide is inevitably generated predominantly at respiratory complexes CI and CIII. The superoxide released to the matrix is dismutated by mitochondrial SOD2 (I) and the hydroperoxide produced is cleared by glutathione peroxidase and peroxyredoxins. Most of the superoxide released in IMS is generated at respiratory complex CIII. Oxidized form of cytochrome c, present in the IMS at high concentration can exercise clean clearance of superoxide by its oxidation to oxygen (II). An alternative dismutation catalyzed by SOD1 results in increased hydroperoxide generation in the IMS (III).

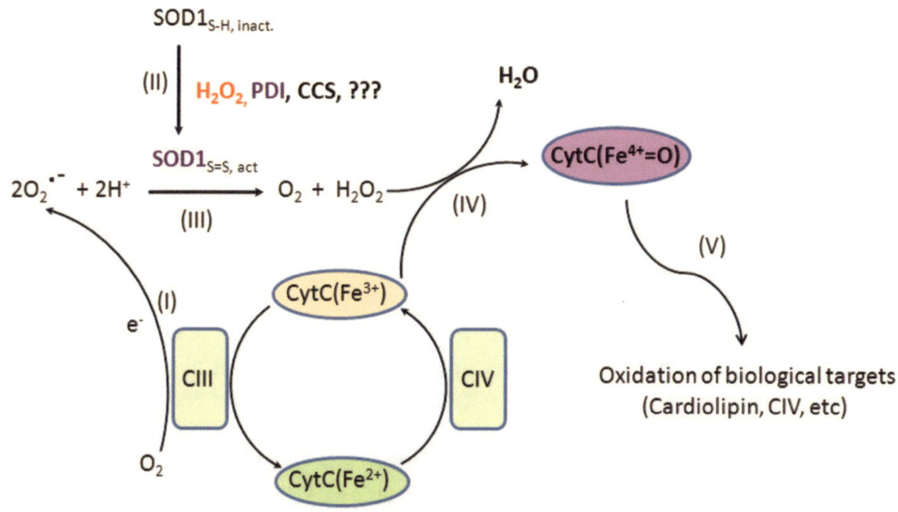

Fig. 3. Deleterious role of superoxide dismutase in the mitochondrial intermembrane space. Superoxide ($O2^{\cdot-}$) is released in IMS by one electron reduction of oxygen at a site in the inner membrane (I). Cu/Zn Superoxide dismutase (SOD1) in IMS is activated by oxidation of cysteine thiols, leading to formation of intramolecular S=S bounds (II). SOD1 produces hydroperoxide (H_2O_2) by dismutating superoxide (III). Hydroperoxide oxydizes cytochrome c (CytC) to oxoferryl-CytC (CytC(Fe^{4+}=O)), an exceptionally strong oxidant (IV), able to oxidize a number of vital biological targets (V).

We have recently proposed a model, where upon mitochondrial stress SOD1 may compete with cytochrome c for superoxide in the IMS and generate hydroperoxide, which then could react with cytochrome c and form peroxidase compound I-type intermediate, eventually leading to a deleterious increase in ROS production and cellular injury (Fig. 2) (Goldsteins et al., 2008). According to this model the SOD1-catalyzed superoxide dismutation in the IMS causes paradoxically augmented ROS production.

The data obtained demonstrate that inhibition of electron transfer at the level of complex III leads to SOD1 activation in the IMS, resulting in increased hydroperoxide production and, consequently, cytochrome c-catalyze peroxidation (Goldsteins et al., 2008). This could trigger a vicious circle where oxidative damage to mitochondrial respiratory components leads to further ROS production and peroxidation. Indeed, we have demonstrated that inhibition of mitochondrial respiration at the level of complex III causes SOD1-dependent ROS production and apoptotic death of isolated blood lymphocytes. In contrast, mitochondria isolated from SOD1 knockout mice do not show increased ROS production upon mitochondrial stress. Moreover, accumulation of mutant human G93A-SOD1 in the IMS that is observed in the tg animal models of ALS, leads to elevated SOD1 activity and increased cytochrome c-catalyzed oxidation in the IMS.

Our proposed model provides also an explanation for observations in other neurodegenerative disorders that elevated SOD1 activity worsens the pathology instead of the expected protective effect. For instance, immature mouse brains overexpressing SOD1 show an increased propensity for injury and accumulate more hydroperoxide after hypoxia-ischemia than wt mouse brains (Fullerton et al., 1998). Also, elevation of SOD1 increases acoustic trauma from noise exposure in some models (Endo et al., 2005). Impotantly, mice deficient in SOD1 have been reported to be resistant to acetaminophen toxicity (Lei et al., 2006). Even though SOD1 as a cytosolic antioxidant protects against mitochondrial dysfunction in a mouse model of transient focal cerebral ischemia (Fujimura et al., 2000), SOD1 deficiency, rather than overexpression, is associated with enhanced recovery and attenuated activation of NF-kappaB after brain trauma in mice (Beni et al., 2006).

This apparent discrepancy concerning the role of SOD1 in cellular injury can be explained by the model introduced, showing that increased SOD1 activity in the IMS paradoxically produces peroxides which are converted to highly toxic ROS. This view is further supported by an observation in mouse model of genetic disorder ataxia-telangiectasia, where elevated levels of SOD1 exacerbate the phenotype of neurodegeneration (Peter et al., 2001). It is also of interest that SOD1 overexpression and high tissue dismutase activity may potentiate atherogenesis in fat-fed atherosclerosis-susceptible mice (Tribble et al., 1997). The evidence about deleterious role of increased SOD1 expression has been most recently complemented by studies demonstrating that overexpression of SOD1 in retina leads to increased hydroperoxide levels and accelerated damage of cone cells (Usui et al., n.d.).

The key component for the SOD1-derived hydroperoxide toxicity in IMS is cytochrome c. Previous studies, including electron paramagnetic resonance (EPR) studies (Barr et al., 1996; Svistunenko, 2005; Belikova et al., 2006; Basova et al., 2007) have demonstrated that the reaction of cytochrome c with hydroperoxide results in formation of oxoferryl cytochrome c (peroxidase compound I-type intermediate) and corresponding protein-derived tyrosyl radical, which is highly reactive and has a potential to oxidize proteins, DNA, and lipids, as well as endogenous antioxidants such as glutathione, NADH, and ascorbate (Lawrence et al., 2003) (Fig. 3). In particular, oxidation of cardiolipin, a phospholipid which is in complex with cytochrome c on the surface of the inner mitochondrial membrane, causes the release of proapoptotic factors from mitochondria (Kagan et al., 2005; Belikova et al., 2006). This leads to a scenario where the hydroperoxide produced by increased SOD1 activity in the IMS, would thus serve as a substrate for cardiolipin-bound cytochrome c and consequently switch on very early proapoptotic processes, inducing consecutive programmed cell death. Additionally, upon increased hydroperoxide levels cytochrome c peroxidase activity may cause NADH oxidation producing a radical, which in turn donates an electron to oxygen augmenting superoxide formation (Velayutham et al., 2011).

The toxicity based on the dismutase activity of mutant SOD1 in the IMS might also be true even for dismutase inactive mutant SOD1 proteins. In human FALS SOD1 mutations are dominantly inherited resulting in the presence of both wild type and mutant SOD1 subunits in each cell. Thus, dismutase activity lacking G85R-SOD1 can form active heterodimers with wt SOD1 molecules. In mice the co-expression of human mutant and wt SOD1 accelerated disease (Jaarsma et al., 2000; Fukada et al., 2001; Deng et al., 2006). Importantly, unaffected A4V-SOD1 mutant mice developed the disease only when mated with human wt SOD1 overexpressing mice (Deng et al., 2006). It was also shown recently that the toxicity of mutant SOD1 dimers is not correlated with their capacity to form protein aggregates but rather with their dismutase activity (Witan et al., 2008).

5. Conclusion

Until now, several pathological mechanisms have been demonstrated how mutant SOD1 induces mitochondrial dysfunction in FALS models. Among them, the emerging evidence indicates that the SOD1-dependant hydroperoxide production in mitochondrial IMS may fuel the cytochrome c-catalyzed peroxidation and play a key role in oxidation of biological targets in the IMS. Thus, SOD1 activity and factors leading to its increase in this compartment can be regarded as deleterious mechanisms to the mitochondria and the cell. Increased SOD1 activity causing elevated hydroperoxide production in the IMS may be one of general mechanism in neurodegeneration.

At the moment it is not clear how mutations in SOD1 directly affect hydroperoxide production in IMS. One possibility may be the already demonstrated increased mitochondrial import for mutant molecules in neurons of ALS models. Another possible mechanism is linked to less strict dismutase activity control. Altogether, we hypothesize that the mutant SOD1 may gain toxic features because the proper control mechanism for its dismutase activity in mitochondrial IMS may be lost. In conclusion, we suggest that SOD1 activity in the IMS is a relevant therapeutic target for ALS and other neurodegenerative diseases involving mitochondrial pathogenesis.

6. Acknowledgment

For the construction of figures, elements from www.motifolio.com Free PowerPoint Diagrams were used.

The authors were supported by the Sigrid Juselius Foundation, Finland.

7. References

Ahtoniemi, T., Jaronen, M., Keksa-Goldsteine, V., Goldsteins, G. & Koistinaho, J. (2008). Mutant SOD1 from spinal cord of G93A rats is destabilized and binds to inner mitochondrial membrane. *Neurobiol Dis*, Vol.32, No.3, (December 2008), pp. 479-485.

Arnesano, F., Banci, L., Bertini, I., Martinelli, M., Furukawa, Y. & O'Halloran, T.V. (2004). The unusually stable quaternary structure of human Cu,Zn-superoxide dismutase 1 is controlled by both metal occupancy and disulfide status. *J Biol Chem*, Vol.279, No.46, (November 2004), pp. 47998-48003.

Atsumi, T. (1981). The ultrastructure of intramuscular nerves in amyotrophic lateral sclerosis. *Acta Neuropathol*, Vol.55, No.3, (1981), pp. 193-198.

Barr, D.P., Gunther, M.R., Deterding, L.J., Tomer, K.B. & Mason, R.P. (1996). ESR spin-trapping of a protein-derived tyrosyl radical from the reaction of cytochrome c with hydrogen peroxide. *J Biol Chem*, Vol.271, No.26, (1996), pp. 15498-503.

Basova, L.V., Kurnikov, I.V., Wang, L., Ritov, V.B., Belikova, N.A., Vlasova, I., Pacheco, A.A., Winnica, D.E., Peterson, J., Bayir, H., Waldeck, D.H. & Kagan, V.E. (2007). Cardiolipin switch in mitochondria: shutting off the reduction of cytochrome c and turning on the peroxidase activity. *Biochemistry*, Vol.46, No.11, (2007), pp. 3423-34.

Beckman, J.S., Carson, M., Smith, C.D. & Koppenol, W.H. (1993). ALS, SOD and peroxynitrite. *Nature*, Vol.364, No.6438, (August 1993), pp. 584.

Beckman, J.S., Chen, J., Crow, J.P. & Ye, Y.Z. (1994). Reactions of nitric oxide, superoxide and peroxynitrite with superoxide dismutase in neurodegeneration. *Prog Brain Res*, Vol.103, (1994), pp. 371-380.

van Beek-Harmsen, B.J. & van der Laarse, W.J. (2005). Immunohistochemical determination of cytosolic cytochrome C concentration in cardiomyocytes. *J Histochem Cytochem*, Vol.53, No.7, (2005), pp. 803-7.

Belikova, N.A., Vladimirov, Y.A., Osipov, A.N., Kapralov, A.A., Tyurin, V.A., Potapovich, M.V., Basova, L.V., Peterson, J., Kurnikov, I.V. & Kagan, V.E. (2006). Peroxidase Activity and Structural Transitions of Cytochrome c Bound to Cardiolipin-Containing Membranes. *Biochemistry*, Vol.45, No.15, (2006), pp. 4998-5009.

Bendotti, C., Calvaresi, N., Chiveri, L., Prelle, A., Moggio, M., Braga, M., Silani, V. & De Biasi, S. (2001). Early vacuolization and mitochondrial damage in motor neurons of FALS mice are not associated with apoptosis or with changes in cytochrome oxidase histochemical reactivity. *J Neurol Sci*, Vol.191, No.1-2, (October 2001), pp. 25-33.

Beni, S.M., Tsenter, J., Alexandrovich, A.G., Galron-Krool, N., Barzilai, A., Kohen, R., Grigoriadis, N., Simeonidou, C. & Shohami, E. (2006). CuZn-SOD deficiency, rather than overexpression, is associated with enhanced recovery and attenuated activation of NF-kappaB after brain trauma in mice. *J Cereb Blood Flow Metab*, Vol.26, No.4, (2006), pp. 478-90.

Beretta, S., Sala, G., Mattavelli, L., Ceresa, C., Casciati, A., Ferri, A., Carrì, M.T. & Ferrarese, C. (2003). Mitochondrial dysfunction due to mutant copper/zinc superoxide dismutase associated with amyotrophic lateral sclerosis is reversed by N-acetylcysteine. *Neurobiol Dis*, Vol.13, No.3, (August 2003), pp. 213-221.

Bergemalm, D., Jonsson, P.A., Graffmo, K.S., Andersen, P.M., Brännström, T., Rehnmark, A. & Marklund, S.L. (2006). Overloading of stable and exclusion of unstable human superoxide dismutase-1 variants in mitochondria of murine amyotrophic lateral sclerosis models. *J Neurosci*, Vol.26, No.16, (April 2006), pp. 4147-4154.

Boillée, S., Vande Velde, C. & Cleveland, D.W. (2006). ALS: a disease of motor neurons and their nonneuronal neighbors. *Neuron*, Vol.52, No.1, (October 2006), pp. 39-59.

Browne, S.E., Bowling, A.C., Baik, M.J., Gurney, M., Brown, R.H., Jr & Beal, M.F. (1998). Metabolic dysfunction in familial, but not sporadic, amyotrophic lateral sclerosis. *J Neurochem*, Vol.71, No.1, (July 1998), pp. 281-287.

Dal Canto, M.C. & Gurney, M.E. (1997). A low expressor line of transgenic mice carrying a mutant human Cu,Zn superoxide dismutase (SOD1) gene develops pathological changes that most closely resemble those in human amyotrophic lateral sclerosis. *Acta Neuropathol*, Vol.93, No.6, (June 1997), pp. 537-550.

Casareno, R.L.B., Waggoner, D. & Gitlin, J.D. (1998). The Copper Chaperone CCS Directly Interacts with Copper/Zinc Superoxide Dismutase. *Journal of Biological Chemistry*, Vol.273, No.37, (1998), pp. 23625 -23628.

Chattopadhyay, M., Durazo, A., Sohn, S.H., Strong, C.D., Gralla, E.B., Whitelegge, J.P. & Valentine, J.S. (2008). Initiation and elongation in fibrillation of ALS-linked superoxide dismutase. *Proc Natl Acad Sci U S A*, Vol.105, No.48, (December 2008), pp. 18663-18668.

Culotta, V.C., Klomp, L.W.J., Strain, J., Casareno, R.L.B., Krems, B. & Gitlin, J.D. (1997). The Copper Chaperone for Superoxide Dismutase. *Journal of Biological Chemistry*, Vol.272, No.38, (1997), pp. 23469 -23472.

Damiano, M., Starkov, A.A., Petri, S., Kipiani, K., Kiaei, M., Mattiazzi, M., Flint Beal, M. & Manfredi, G. (2006). Neural mitochondrial Ca2+ capacity impairment precedes the onset of motor symptoms in G93A Cu/Zn-superoxide dismutase mutant mice. *J Neurochem*, Vol.96, No.5, (March 2006), pp. 1349-1361.

Deng, H.-X., Shi, Y., Furukawa, Y., Zhai, H., Fu, R., Liu, E., Gorrie, G.H., Khan, M.S., Hung, W.-Y., Bigio, E.H., Lukas, T., Dal Canto, M.C., O'Halloran, T.V. & Siddique, T. (2006). Conversion to the amyotrophic lateral sclerosis phenotype is associated with intermolecular linked insoluble aggregates of SOD1 in mitochondria. *Proc Natl Acad Sci U S A*, Vol.103, No.18, (May 2006), pp. 7142-7147.

Diederix, R.E., Ubbink, M. & Canters, G.W. (2002). Peroxidase activity as a tool for studying the folding of c-type cytochromes. *Biochemistry*, Vol.41, No.43, (2002), pp. 13067-77.

Ding, F. & Dokholyan, N.V. (2008). Dynamical roles of metal ions and the disulfide bond in Cu, Zn superoxide dismutase folding and aggregation. *Proceedings of the National Academy of Sciences*, Vol.105, No.50, (December 2008), pp. 19696 -19701.

Elliott, J.L. (2001). Zinc and copper in the pathogenesis of amyotrophic lateral sclerosis. *Prog Neuropsychopharmacol Biol Psychiatry*, Vol.25, No.6, (August 2001), pp. 1169-1185.

Endo, T., Nakagawa, T., Iguchi, F., Kita, T., Okano, T., Sha, S.-H., Schacht, J., Shiga, A., Kim, T.-S. & Ito, J. (2005). Elevation of superoxide dismutase increases acoustic trauma from noise exposure. *Free Radic Biol Med*, Vol.38, No.4, (February 2005), pp. 492-498.

Estévez, A.G., Crow, J.P., Sampson, J.B., Reiter, C., Zhuang, Y., Richardson, G.J., Tarpey, M.M., Barbeito, L. & Beckman, J.S. (1999). Induction of nitric oxide-dependent apoptosis in motor neurons by zinc-deficient superoxide dismutase. *Science*, Vol.286, No.5449, (December 1999), pp. 2498-2500.

Everse, J. & Coates, P.W. (2005). Role of peroxidases in Parkinson disease: a hypothesis. *Free Radic Biol Med*, Vol.38, No.10, (2005), pp. 1296-310.

Ferri, A., Cozzolino, M., Crosio, C., Nencini, M., Casciati, A., Gralla, E.B., Rotilio, G., Valentine, J.S. & Carrì, M.T. (2006). Familial ALS-superoxide dismutases associate with mitochondria and shift their redox potentials. *Proc Natl Acad Sci U S A*, Vol.103, No.37, (September 2006), pp. 13860-13865.

Forman, H.J. & Azzi, A. (1997). On the virtual existence of superoxide anions in mitochondria: thoughts regarding its role in pathophysiology. *Faseb J*, Vol.11, No.5, (1997), pp. 374-5.

Fujimura, M., Morita-Fujimura, Y., Noshita, N., Sugawara, T., Kawase, M. & Chan, P.H. (2000). The cytosolic antioxidant copper/zinc-superoxide dismutase prevents the early release of mitochondrial cytochrome c in ischemic brain after transient focal cerebral ischemia in mice. *J Neurosci*, Vol.20, No.8, (2000), pp. 2817-24.

Fukada, K., Nagano, S., Satoh, M., Tohyama, C., Nakanishi, T., Shimizu, A., Yanagihara, T. & Sakoda, S. (2001). Stabilization of mutant Cu/Zn superoxide dismutase (SOD1) protein by coexpressed wild SOD1 protein accelerates the disease progression in familial amyotrophic lateral sclerosis mice. *Eur J Neurosci*, Vol.14, No.12, (December 2001), pp. 2032-2036.

Fullerton, H.J., Ditelberg, J.S., Chen, S.F., Sarco, D.P., Chan, P.H., Epstein, C.J. & Ferriero, D.M. (1998). Copper/zinc superoxide dismutase transgenic brain accumulates hydrogen peroxide after perinatal hypoxia ischemia. *Ann Neurol*, Vol.44, No.3, (September 1998), pp. 357-364.

Furukawa, Y. & O'Halloran, T.V. (2006). Posttranslational modifications in Cu,Zn-superoxide dismutase and mutations associated with amyotrophic lateral sclerosis. *Antioxid Redox Signal*, Vol.8, No.5-6, (June 2006), pp. 847-867.

Goldsteins, G., Keksa-Goldsteine, V., Ahtoniemi, T., Jaronen, M., Arens, E., Akerman, K., Chan, P.H. & Koistinaho, J. (2008). Deleterious role of superoxide dismutase in the mitochondrial intermembrane space. *J Biol Chem*, Vol.283, No.13, (March 2008), pp. 8446-8452.

Grosskreutz, J., Van Den Bosch, L. & Keller, B.U. (2010). Calcium dysregulation in amyotrophic lateral sclerosis. *Cell Calcium*, Vol.47, No.2, (February 2010), pp. 165-174.

Higgins, C.M.J., Jung, C. & Xu, Z. (2003). ALS-associated mutant SOD1G93A causes mitochondrial vacuolation by expansion of the intermembrane space and by involvement of SOD1 aggregation and peroxisomes. *BMC Neurosci*, Vol.4, (July 2003), pp. 16.

Higgins, C.M.J., Jung, C., Ding, H. & Xu, Z. (2002). Mutant Cu, Zn superoxide dismutase that causes motoneuron degeneration is present in mitochondria in the CNS. *J Neurosci*, Vol.22, No.6, (March 2002), pp. RC215.

Iñarrea, P., Casanova, A., Alava, M.A., Iturralde, M. & Cadenas, E. (2011). Melatonin and steroid hormones activate intermembrane Cu,Zn-superoxide dismutase by means of mitochondrial cytochrome P450. *Free Radic Biol Med*, Vol.50, No.11, (June 2011), pp. 1575-1581.

Iñarrea, P., Moini, H., Rettori, D., Han, D., Martínez, J., García, I., Fernández-Vizarra, E., Iturralde, M. & Cadenas, E. (2005). Redox activation of mitochondrial intermembrane space Cu,Zn-superoxide dismutase. *Biochem J*, Vol.387, No.Pt 1, (April 2005), pp. 203-209.

Inoue, M., Sato, E.F., Nishikawa, M., Park, A.M., Kira, Y., Imada, I. & Utsumi, K. (2003). Mitochondrial generation of reactive oxygen species and its role in aerobic life. *Curr Med Chem*, Vol.10, No.23, (2003), pp. 2495-505.

Jaarsma, D., Haasdijk, E.D., Grashorn, J.A., Hawkins, R., van Duijn, W., Verspaget, H.W., London, J. & Holstege, J.C. (2000). Human Cu/Zn superoxide dismutase (SOD1) overexpression in mice causes mitochondrial vacuolization, axonal degeneration, and premature motoneuron death and accelerates motoneuron disease in mice expressing a familial amyotrophic lateral sclerosis mutant SOD1. *Neurobiol Dis*, Vol.7, No.6 Pt B, (December 2000), pp. 623-643.

Jaarsma, D., Rognoni, F., van Duijn, W., Verspaget, H.W., Haasdijk, E.D. & Holstege, J.C. (2001). CuZn superoxide dismutase (SOD1) accumulates in vacuolated mitochondria in transgenic mice expressing amyotrophic lateral sclerosis-linked SOD1 mutations. *Acta Neuropathol*, Vol.102, No.4, (October 2001), pp. 293-305.

Jaiswal, M.K. & Keller, B.U. (2009). Cu/Zn superoxide dismutase typical for familial amyotrophic lateral sclerosis increases the vulnerability of mitochondria and perturbs Ca2+ homeostasis in SOD1G93A mice. *Mol Pharmacol*, Vol.75, No.3, (March 2009), pp. 478-489.

Jang, B. & Han, S. (2006). Biochemical properties of cytochrome c nitrated by peroxynitrite. *Biochimie*, Vol.88, No.1, (2006), pp. 53-8.

Jonsson, P.A., Graffmo, K.S., Andersen, P.M., Brännström, T., Lindberg, M., Oliveberg, M. & Marklund, S.L. (2006). Disulphide-reduced superoxide dismutase-1 in CNS of transgenic amyotrophic lateral sclerosis models. *Brain*, Vol.129, No.Pt 2, (February 2006), pp. 451-464.

Kagan, V.E., Tyurin, V.A., Jiang, J., Tyurina, Y.Y., Ritov, V.B., Amoscato, A.A., Osipov, A.N., Belikova, N.A., Kapralov, A.A., Kini, V., Vlasova, I., Zhao, Q., Zou, M., Di, P., Svistunenko, D.A., Kurnikov, I.V. & Borisenko, G.G. (2005). Cytochrome c acts as a cardiolipin oxygenase required for release of proapoptotic factors. *Nat Chem Biol*, Vol.1, No.4, (2005), pp. 223-32.

Kawamata, H. & Manfredi, G. (2008). Different regulation of wild-type and mutant Cu,Zn superoxide dismutase localization in mammalian mitochondria. *Hum Mol Genet*, Vol.17, No.21, (November 2008), pp. 3303-3317.

Kirkinezos, I.G., Bacman, S.R., Hernandez, D., Oca-Cossio, J., Arias, L.J., Perez-Pinzon, M.A., Bradley, W.G. & Moraes, C.T. (2005). Cytochrome c association with the inner mitochondrial membrane is impaired in the CNS of G93A-SOD1 mice. *J Neurosci*, Vol.25, No.1, (January 2005), pp. 164-172.

Kong, J. & Xu, Z. (1998). Massive mitochondrial degeneration in motor neurons triggers the onset of amyotrophic lateral sclerosis in mice expressing a mutant SOD1. *J Neurosci*, Vol.18, No.9, (May 1998), pp. 3241-3250.

Kruman, I.I., Pedersen, W.A., Springer, J.E. & Mattson, M.P. (1999). ALS-linked Cu/Zn-SOD mutation increases vulnerability of motor neurons to excitotoxicity by a mechanism involving increased oxidative stress and perturbed calcium homeostasis. *Exp Neurol*, Vol.160, No.1, (November 1999), pp. 28-39.

Lawrence, A., Jones, C.M., Wardman, P. & Burkitt, M.J. (2003). Evidence for the role of a peroxidase compound I-type intermediate in the oxidation of glutathione, NADH, ascorbate, and dichlorofluorescin by cytochrome c/H2O2. Implications for oxidative stress during apoptosis. *J Biol Chem*, Vol.278, No.32, (2003), pp. 29410-9.

Lei, X.G., Zhu, J.H., McClung, J.P., Aregullin, M. & Roneker, C.A. (2006). Mice deficient in Cu,Zn-superoxide dismutase are resistant to acetaminophen toxicity. *Biochem J*, Vol.399, No.3, (2006), pp. 455-61.

Leitch, J.M., Yick, P.J. & Culotta, V.C. (2009). The right to choose: multiple pathways for activating copper,zinc superoxide dismutase. *J Biol Chem*, Vol.284, No.37, (September 2009), pp. 24679-24683.

Li, Y., Huang, T.-T., Carlson, E.J., Melov, S., Ursell, P.C., Olson, J.L., Noble, L.J., Yoshimura, M.P., Berger, C., Chan, P.H., Wallace, D.C. & Epstein, C.J. (1995). Dilated cardiomyopathy and neonatal lethality in mutant mice lacking manganese superoxide dismutase. *Nat Genet*, Vol.11, No.4, (December 1995), pp. 376-381.

Liu, J., Lillo, C., Jonsson, P.A., Vande Velde, C., Ward, C.M., Miller, T.M., Subramaniam, J.R., Rothstein, J.D., Marklund, S., Andersen, P.M., Brännström, T., Gredal, O., Wong, P.C., Williams, D.S. & Cleveland, D.W. (2004). Toxicity of familial ALS-linked SOD1 mutants from selective recruitment to spinal mitochondria. *Neuron*, Vol.43, No.1, (July 2004), pp. 5-17.

Liu, Y., Fiskum, G. & Schubert, D. (2002). Generation of reactive oxygen species by the mitochondrial electron transport chain. *J Neurochem*, Vol.80, No.5, (2002), pp. 780-7.

Maier, C.M. & Chan, P.H. (2002). Role of superoxide dismutases in oxidative damage and neurodegenerative disorders. *Neuroscientist*, Vol.8, No.4, (August 2002), pp. 323-334.

Manfredi, G. & Xu, Z. (2005). Mitochondrial dysfunction and its role in motor neuron degeneration in ALS. *Mitochondrion*, Vol.5, No.2, (April 2005), pp. 77-87.

Mattiazzi, M., D'Aurelio, M., Gajewski, C.D., Martushova, K., Kiaei, M., Beal, M.F. & Manfredi, G. (2002). Mutated human SOD1 causes dysfunction of oxidative phosphorylation in mitochondria of transgenic mice. *J Biol Chem*, Vol.277, No.33, (August 2002), pp. 29626-29633.

Muller, F.L., Liu, Y. & Van Remmen, H. (2004). Complex III releases superoxide to both sides of the inner mitochondrial membrane. *J Biol Chem*, Vol.279, No.47, (2004), pp. 49064-73.

Okado-Matsumoto, A. & Fridovich, I. (2001). Subcellular distribution of superoxide dismutases (SOD) in rat liver: Cu,Zn-SOD in mitochondria. *J Biol Chem*, Vol.276, No.42, (October 2001), pp. 38388-38393.

Panov, A.V., Kubalik, N., Zinchenko, N., Ridings, D.M., Radoff, D.A., Hemendinger, R., Brooks, B.R. & Bonkovsky, H.L. (2011). Metabolic and functional differences between brain and spinal cord mitochondria underlie different predisposition to pathology. *Am J Physiol Regul Integr Comp Physiol*, Vol.300, No.4, (April 2011), pp. R844-854.

Panov, A., Kubalik, N., Zinchenko, N., Hemendinger, R., Dikalov, S. & Bonkovsky, H.L. (n.d.). Respiration and ROS production in brain and spinal cord mitochondria of transgenic rats with mutant G93a Cu/Zn-superoxide dismutase gene. *Neurobiology of Disease*, In Press

Pasinelli, P., Belford, M.E., Lennon, N., Bacskai, B.J., Hyman, B.T., Trotti, D. & Brown, R.H., Jr (2004). Amyotrophic lateral sclerosis-associated SOD1 mutant proteins bind and aggregate with Bcl-2 in spinal cord mitochondria. *Neuron*, Vol.43, No.1, (July 2004), pp. 19-30.

Pereverzev, M.O., Vygodina, T.V., Konstantinov, A.A. & Skulachev, V.P. (2003). Cytochrome c, an ideal antioxidant. *Biochem Soc Trans*, Vol.31, No.Pt 6, (2003), pp. 1312-5.

Peter, Y., Rotman, G., Lotem, J., Elson, A., Shiloh, Y. & Groner, Y. (2001). Elevated Cu/Zn-SOD exacerbates radiation sensitivity and hematopoietic abnormalities of Atm-deficient mice. *EMBO J*, Vol.20, No.7, (April 2001), pp. 1538-1546.

Qian, S.Y., Chen, Y.R., Deterding, L.J., Fann, Y.C., Chignell, C.F., Tomer, K.B. & Mason, R.P. (2002). Identification of protein-derived tyrosyl radical in the reaction of cytochrome c and hydrogen peroxide: characterization by ESR spin-trapping, HPLC and MS. *Biochem J*, Vol.363, No.Pt 2, (2002), pp. 281-8.

Reddehase, S., Grumbt, B., Neupert, W. & Hell, K. (2009). The disulfide relay system of mitochondria is required for the biogenesis of mitochondrial Ccs1 and Sod1. *J Mol Biol*, Vol.385, No.2, (January 2009), pp. 331-338.

Siciliano, G., Pastorini, E., Pasquali, L., Manca, M.L., Iudice, A. & Murri, L. (2001). Impaired oxidative metabolism in exercising muscle from ALS patients. *J Neurol Sci*, Vol.191, No.1-2, (October 2001), pp. 61-65.

Siklós, L., Engelhardt, J., Harati, Y., Smith, R.G., Joó, F. & Appel, S.H. (1996). Ultrastructural evidence for altered calcium in motor nerve terminals in amyotropic lateral sclerosis. *Ann Neurol*, Vol.39, No.2, (February 1996), pp. 203-216.

Son, M., Puttaparthi, K., Kawamata, H., Rajendran, B., Boyer, P.J., Manfredi, G. & Elliott, J.L. (2007). Overexpression of CCS in G93A-SOD1 mice leads to accelerated neurological deficits with severe mitochondrial pathology. *Proc Natl Acad Sci U S A*, Vol.104, No.14, (April 2007), pp. 6072-6077.

Stathopulos, P.B., Rumfeldt, J.A.O., Scholz, G.A., Irani, R.A., Frey, H.E., Hallewell, R.A., Lepock, J.R. & Meiering, E.M. (2003). Cu/Zn superoxide dismutase mutants associated with amyotrophic lateral sclerosis show enhanced formation of aggregates in vitro. *Proc Natl Acad Sci U S A*, Vol.100, No.12, (June 2003), pp. 7021-7026.

Sturtz, L.A., Diekert, K., Jensen, L.T., Lill, R. & Culotta, V.C. (2001). A fraction of yeast Cu,Zn-superoxide dismutase and its metallochaperone, CCS, localize to the intermembrane space of mitochondria. A physiological role for SOD1 in guarding against mitochondrial oxidative damage. *J Biol Chem*, Vol.276, No.41, (October 2001), pp. 38084-38089.

Svistunenko, D.A. (2005). Reaction of haem containing proteins and enzymes with hydroperoxides: the radical view. *Biochim Biophys Acta*, Vol.1707, No.1, (2005), pp. 127-55.

Tribble, D.L., Gong, E.L., Leeuwenburgh, C., Heinecke, J.W., Carlson, E.L., Verstuyft, J.G. & Epstein, C.J. (1997). Fatty streak formation in fat-fed mice expressing human copper-zinc superoxide dismutase. *Arterioscler Thromb Vasc Biol*, Vol.17, No.9, (September 1997), pp. 1734-1740.

Usui, S., Oveson, B.C., Iwase, T., Lu, L., Lee, S.Y., Jo, Y.-J., Wu, Z., Choi, E.-Y., Samulski, R.J. & Campochiaro, P.A. (n.d.). Overexpression of SOD in retina: Need for increase in H2O2-detoxifying enzyme in same cellular compartment. *Free Radical Biology and Medicine*, In Press

Valentine, J.S., Doucette, P.A. & Zittin Potter, S. (2005). Copper-zinc superoxide dismutase and amyotrophic lateral sclerosis. *Annu Rev Biochem*, Vol.74, (2005), pp. 563-593.

Vande Velde, C., McDonald, K.K., Boukhedimi, Y., McAlonis-Downes, M., Lobsiger, C.S., Bel Hadj, S., Zandona, A., Julien, J.-P., Shah, S.B. & Cleveland, D.W. (2011). Misfolded SOD1 Associated with Motor Neuron Mitochondria Alters Mitochondrial Shape and Distribution Prior to Clinical Onset. *PLoS ONE*, Vol.6, No.7, (2011), pp. e22031.

Vande Velde, C., Miller, T.M., Cashman, N.R. & Cleveland, D.W. (2008). Selective association of misfolded ALS-linked mutant SOD1 with the cytoplasmic face of mitochondria. *Proc Natl Acad Sci U S A*, Vol.105, No.10, (March 2008), pp. 4022-4027.

Velayutham, M., Hemann, C. & Zweier, J.L. (2011). Removal of H(2)O(2) and generation of superoxide radical: Role of cytochrome c and NADH. *Free Radic Biol Med*, Vol.51, No.1, (July 2011), pp. 160-170.

Wiedau-Pazos, M., Goto, J.J., Rabizadeh, S., Gralla, E.B., Roe, J.A., Lee, M.K., Valentine, J.S. & Bredesen, D.E. (1996). Altered reactivity of superoxide dismutase in familial amyotrophic lateral sclerosis. *Science*, Vol.271, No.5248, (January 1996), pp. 515-518.

Vijayvergiya, C., Beal, M.F., Buck, J. & Manfredi, G. (2005). Mutant superoxide dismutase 1 forms aggregates in the brain mitochondrial matrix of amyotrophic lateral sclerosis mice. *J Neurosci*, Vol.25, No.10, (March 2005), pp. 2463-2470.

Witan, H., Kern, A., Koziollek-Drechsler, I., Wade, R., Behl, C. & Clement, A.M. (2008). Heterodimer formation of wild-type and amyotrophic lateral sclerosis-causing mutant Cu/Zn-superoxide dismutase induces toxicity independent of protein aggregation. *Hum Mol Genet*, Vol.17, No.10, (May 2008), pp. 1373-1385.

Wong, P.C., Pardo, C.A., Borchelt, D.R., Lee, M.K., Copeland, N.G., Jenkins, N.A., Sisodia, S.S., Cleveland, D.W. & Price, D.L. (1995). An adverse property of a familial ALS-linked SOD1 mutation causes motor neuron disease characterized by vacuolar degeneration of mitochondria. *Neuron*, Vol.14, No.6, (June 1995), pp. 1105-1116.

Vonk, W.I.M., Wijmenga, C., Berger, R., van de Sluis, B. & Klomp, L.W.J. (2010). Cu,Zn Superoxide Dismutase Maturation and Activity Are Regulated by COMMD1. *Journal of Biological Chemistry*, Vol.285, No.37, (2010), pp. 28991 -29000.

Xu, Z., Jung, C., Higgins, C., Levine, J. & Kong, J. (2004). Mitochondrial degeneration in amyotrophic lateral sclerosis. *J Bioenerg Biomembr*, Vol.36, No.4, (August 2004), pp. 395-399.

Zelko, I.N., Mariani, T.J. & Folz, R.J. (2002). Superoxide dismutase multigene family: a comparison of the CuZn-SOD (SOD1), Mn-SOD (SOD2), and EC-SOD (SOD3) gene structures, evolution, and expression. *Free Radic Biol Med*, Vol.33, No.3, (2002), pp. 337-49.

11

Folding and Aggregation of Cu, Zn-Superoxide Dismutase

Helen R. Broom, Heather A. Primmer, Jessica A.O. Rumfeldt, Peter B. Stathopulos, Kenrick A. Vassall, Young-Mi Hwang and Elizabeth M. Meiering

Guelph-Waterloo Centre for Graduate Work in Chemistry and Biochemistry, University of Waterloo
Canada

1. Introduction

1.1 ALS and SOD1

In 1993, a genetic link was established between amyotrophic lateral sclerosis (ALS) and mutant forms of Cu,Zn superoxide dismutase (SOD1) (Deng et al. 1993; Rosen et al. 1993), an antioxidant enzyme that catalyzes the dismutation of the damaging free radical superoxide anion (O_2^-) to hydrogen peroxide (H_2O_2) and diatomic oxygen (O_2) via cyclic reduction and oxidation of a protein-bound Cu ion (Valentine et al. 2005). Today, over 150, predominantly missense mutations have been identified at ~75 sites spread throughout the protein (http://alsod.iop.kcl.ac.uk/). SOD1 mutations are found in ~15-20% of inherited or familial ALS (fALS) cases and in a small percentage of sporadic ALS (sALS) cases (Rosen et al. 1993; Kato et al. 2000; Liu et al. 2009; Forsberg et al. 2011). fALS accounts for ~10% of all ALS cases and so SOD1 mutations comprise ~1.5-2% of all ALS cases, but nevertheless represent a major known cause of the disease. The clinical symptoms of fALS and sALS are similar, yet fALS patients with SOD1 mutations have an earlier age of disease onset than sALS (by ~10 years) (Wijesekera and Leigh 2009). Furthermore, while the age of disease onset has not been identified as statistically different between different SOD1 mutations, disease duration for each mutation is often different, ranging from shorter (e.g. ~1 year for A4V, the most common mutation in North America) than the typical 3-5 years to longer (e.g. ~18 years for H46R) (Cudkowicz et al. 1997; Valentine et al. 2005; Wang et al. 2008). In humans and murine models of ALS, mutations in the gene encoding SOD1 are typically autosomal dominant and are associated with a toxic gain of function. Despite extensive research, the molecular basis for mutant SOD1 toxicity remains unclear (Valentine et al. 2005; Boillee et al. 2006; Ilieva et al. 2009). Extensive research has been conducted on SOD1-linked fALS, as understanding and treatment of this disease may be relevant to ALS in general. While ALS patients share many clinical symptoms, numerous genes have been linked to ALS, and there is evidence for differences in pathology related to both genetic and environmental factors; hence, ALS is a syndrome and not a single disease with unique pathology (Cozzolino et al. 2008).

Currently, there are two prevailing hypotheses for the toxic gain of SOD1 function that is observed in ALS: 1) new toxic enzymatic activity, and 2) protein misfolding resulting in formation of toxic aggregates (Valentine et al. 2005; Andersen 2006; Pasinelli and Brown 2006; Cozzolino et al. 2008; Turner and Talbot 2008). Since toxic enzymatic activity can damage the protein and cause aggregation, and conversely aggregation may result in toxic activity, these two hypotheses are not mutually exclusive. Theories involving gain of toxic activity involve altered metal binding by SOD1, resulting in the generation of reactive oxygen species, such as damaging hydroxyl and peroxynitrite radicals (Kurahashi et al. 2001; Alvarez et al. 2004). Alternatively, there is extensive evidence that ALS belongs to a growing group of protein misfolding diseases (Valentine et al. 2005; Chiti and Dobson 2006; Turner and Talbot 2008; Chiti and Dobson 2009; Deng et al. 2011). Protein inclusions, or aggregates, observed in the motor neurons and glial cells stain immunopositive for SOD1 in SOD1-linked fALS and some sALS patients (Kato et al. 2000; Liu et al. 2009; Forsberg et al. 2011) and are observed in mutant SOD1 animal models of ALS (Bruijn et al. 1998; Johnston et al. 2000). Thus, a major hypothesis in the field of ALS research is that SOD1 mutations decrease protein stability, alter protein folding and metal binding, and/or cause changes in other biophysical properties of the protein, resulting in an increased propensity of mutant SOD1 to form neurotoxic aggregates (Valentine et al. 2005).

Many reviews have summarized extensive investigations into the role of SOD1 in ALS, including *in vivo* mutant SOD1 models of ALS pathogenesis and their clinical implications (Bruijn et al. 2004; Boillee et al. 2006; Mitchell and Borasio 2007; Cozzolino et al. 2008), the numerous genetic elements and complex disease etiology associated with sALS and fALS (Boillee et al. 2006; Vucic and Kiernan 2009; Bastos et al. 2011), the various ALS rodent models used to study the underlying genetics and cause of motor neuron death in ALS (Van Den Bosch 2011), and the biophysical properties of mutant SOD1 in relation to possible disease mechanisms (Valentine et al. 2005). In this chapter we review recent research characterizing the stability, folding and misfolding, and the physical characteristics and mechanisms governing aggregation of mutant SOD1 *in vitro*. We describe in detail studies that reflect our own research and interests, but also include references to related work, to which we refer the interested reader. We will first review the general principles of protein stability and aggregation, which are pertinent to protein conformational diseases in general. Following this overview, we examine recent research that has characterized folding and aggregation of SOD1 and the relevance of this work to ALS.

1.2 Characteristics of protein aggregation

Protein aggregation is a common phenomenon observed in both normal and abnormal physiological processes, and has been studied extensively for more than 30 years (Chiti and Dobson 2006). While protein association reactions are highly regulated and essential for cellular function, unregulated protein association causes a wide range of diseases, such as sickle-cell anaemia, serpinopathies, and, in particular, many neurodegenerative diseases including prion, Parkinson's, Alzheimer's, and Huntington's diseases (Chiti and Dobson 2006; Eisenberg et al. 2006; Chiti and Dobson 2009). These protein misfolding diseases are characterized by the formation of insoluble proteinacious deposits (aggregates) (Chiti and Dobson 2006), and the mechanisms and biological effects of aggregation in different diseases are an area of active research. In some cases, toxicity may be caused by large protein aggregates; however, smaller oligomeric protein species are generally considered more neurotoxic (Caughey and Lansbury 2003). The harmful nature of these oligomers compared to larger protein aggregates may be due to their lower stability, higher degree of solvent accessible surface area, and an increased tendency to form non-native associations with essential cellular components (Bucciantini et al. 2002; Knowles et al. 2007). For example, aggregates of many disease-associated proteins, including mutant SOD1, have been found to interact with the ubiquitin-proteasome system (Mouradian 2002; Sakamoto 2002; Urushitani et al. 2002; Valentine et al. 2005), folding chaperones (Bruening et al. 1999; Wyttenbach et al. 2000; Shinder et al. 2001; Okado-Matsumoto and Fridovich 2002), and the outer mitochondrial membrane (Vande Velde et al. 2008). These cellular components play central roles in regulating many critical cellular events ranging from cell division to apoptosis, and their impairment may represent common mechanisms by which aggregates of different proteins can cause cellular dysregulation and cell death (Hol and Scheper 2008; Gidalevitz et al. 2010). Many factors are involved in modulating protein aggregation, and are surveyed in the following sections.

1.2.1 Protein folding, stability and aggregation

Globular protein folding begins on the ribosome, as newly synthesized, unstructured polypeptide chains start to make favourable intramolecular contacts (Dobson 2004). As it further folds into its mature, native state, a protein may populate multiple conformational or intermediate states, and undergo various co- and post-translational modifications (refer to Figure 1). The rate determining step of folding involves overcoming the major energetic barrier to folding by forming a transition state complex prior to attaining the native state. In more complex cases, protein folding can involve more than one energetic barrier (Dobson 2004). Other proteins are unable to adopt a stable, well folded structure and exist as an ensemble of fluctuating, poorly structured conformations (Uversky and Dunker 2010). Thermodynamic protein stability is defined as the difference in energy between the denatured, unfolded state and the native, folded state. If there is a large separation in energy between the unfolded and folded states, the protein has high global thermodynamic stability. Stability can also be assessed by the rate of native protein unfolding, which determines how long the polypeptide remains in the folded state. This is referred to as kinetic stability, defined as the difference in energy between the folded conformation and the transition state. The closer these species are in energy, the higher the rate of unfolding and the lower the kinetic stability (Figure 1A).

In general, both thermodynamic and kinetic destabilization of proteins by chemical modifications or by mutations favours global protein unfolding and exposure of the hydrophobic groups that are normally buried in the protein core. This can promote the formation of non-native intermolecular contacts between proteins and the formation of aggregates. However, even subtle decreases in global protein stability are often accompanied by local destabilization and recent investigations have provided evidence for aggregate formation from native-like species (N*, Figure 1) that have undergone much more restricted unfolding (Nelson and Eisenberg 2006; Chiti and Dobson 2009). Examples of aggregate formation from native-like states include various proteins associated with disease such as mutant lysozyme (Chiti and Dobson 2009), β2-microglobulin (Chiti and Dobson 2009), and SOD1 (Hwang et al. 2010). The propensity of a given globular protein to aggregate depends on how energetically feasible it is for the protein to access locally, partially or fully unfolded aggregation-prone state(s). Protein folding generally occurs in a cooperative fashion with minimal formation of partially folded species and this cooperativity generates a sufficiently large energy barrier between the unfolded and folded states, which decreases the likelihood of unfolding and aggregation (Dobson 1999; Dobson 2004; Tartaglia et al. 2008).

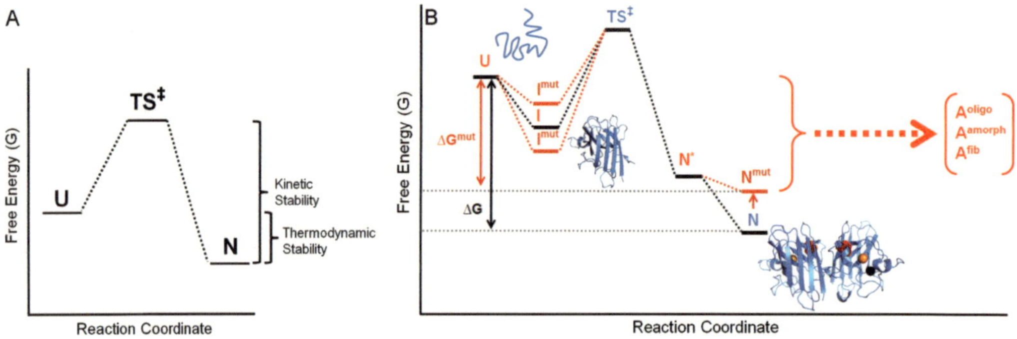

Fig. 1. Protein stability, misfolding and aggregation.
In panel A, the difference between thermodynamic and kinetic stability is shown. U, TS‡, and N refer to the unfolded, transition and native states of the protein, respectively. Refer to the main text for further explanation. In panel B, the effects of native state (N) destabilization by mutation on the population of locally unfolded, native-like (N*), partially folded intermediate (I) and fully unfolded (U) states is shown. Aggregation may occur from N*, I or U, and the morphology of the aggregates formed may depend on the conformation of the protein prior to aggregation. Mutations that destabilize N, decrease the energy difference between the N and the more unfolded states (N*, I or U), and thereby promote aggregation. Note that destabilization of N, does not necessarily imply destabilization of I. Mutations that destabilize N, may stabilize or destabilize I, resulting in a large increase or decrease, respectively, in the population of I compared to levels observed in the native folding pathway. Panel B was adapted from (Chiti and Dobson 2009).

1.2.2 Factors that modulate aggregation of polypeptides

In addition to protein stability and structure, many other factors, such as physicochemical properties of amino acids within a protein sequence and solution conditions, can affect protein aggregation. Hydrophobicity, β-sheet propensity, and charge of a polypeptide sequence have been shown to modulate the formation of amyloid aggregates (refer to section 1.2.3) by unfolded proteins (Chiti et al. 2003). Interestingly, these properties are also important for facilitating correct protein folding, suggesting that while similar forces contribute to both processes, different key residues are involved in forming the initial contacts that drive native protein folding and aggregation (Jahn and Radford 2008). In many cases, the overall aggregation propensity of a protein increases if the primary sequence contains short stretches of amino acids with properties that favour aggregation, for example, low net charge, extensive hydrophobicity, and/or a tendency to form a β-sheet over an α-helix (Tartaglia et al. 2008). Interestingly, many fALS-associated SOD1 mutations decrease the net charge of the protein, which may promote aggregation and explain why certain mutations give rise to a shorter disease duration (Sandelin et al. 2007; Shaw and Valentine 2007; Bystrom et al. 2010). Sequence hydrophobicity also plays a large role in modulating the aggregation propensity of a protein (Chiti et al. 2003). Several studies have suggested that SOD1 mutations promote exposure of hydrophobic regions that can promote aggregation (Tiwari et al. 2009; Munch and Bertolotti 2010). Taken together, these studies indicate that aggregation is at least partially controlled by the physicochemical properties of amino acid residues within a polypeptide sequence (Chiti et al. 2003; Tartaglia et al. 2008).

In addition, solution conditions can modulate the stability, conformation, and the intermolecular interactions of a protein in solution, and can thereby influence the rate of protein aggregation and the type of aggregate structure formed (Chi et al. 2003; Mahler et al. 2009). Importantly, variations in solution conditions can cause the same protein to aggregate by fundamentally different mechanisms (Goers et al. 2002; Vetri and Militello 2005; Necula et al. 2007). Temperature, pH, macromolecular crowding, agitation, and ionic strength are all variables that can influence aggregation (Chi et al. 2003; Munishkina et al. 2004; Mahler et al. 2009; Sicorello et al. 2009). A number of studies have used different solution conditions (increased temperature, decreased pH, increased ionic strength, sonication or agitation) to promote the formation of well-structured, fibrillar amyloid aggregates (see 1.2.3) by various forms of SOD1 (Stathopulos et al. 2004; Chattopadhyay et al. 2008; Chattopadhyay and Valentine 2009; Oztug Durer et al. 2009). Other studies have demonstrated soluble oligomer and small aggregate formation by various forms of SOD1 in quiescent, physiologically relevant solution conditions (Vassall, 2011, Hwang, 2010, Banci, 2008). Thus, it is evident that multiple factors can greatly influence protein folding and aggregation and these factors must be considered when investigating the molecular mechanisms of protein aggregation.

1.2.3 Amyloid formation

Protein aggregation is a general term that describes a number of diverse processes that culminate in the formation of non-native, multimeric complexes of varied conformations. These aggregates can range from small, soluble oligomers, to larger amorphous structures, and insoluble, well-structured fibrils (Uversky and Dunker 2010). Amyloid is a common, well characterized, type of aggregate formed by proteins associated with many diseases, including the neurodegenerative prion, Parkinson's, Alzheimer's, and Huntington's diseases (Chiti and Dobson 2006; Chiti and Dobson 2009). Extensive studies of amyloid have resulted in significant advances in understanding the underlying molecular basis of protein aggregation (Sipe and Cohen 2000; Chiti and Dobson 2006; Eisenberg et al. 2006; Chiti and Dobson 2009). Classically defined amyloid is characterized by an unbranched, fibrillar aggregate morphology, which exhibits green-gold birefringence upon binding Congo red (Sipe and Cohen 2000), a dye used in disease diagnosis, and a cross-β x-ray diffraction pattern due to the presence of β-strands oriented perpendicular to the long axis of the fibre (Serpell 2000). These large aggregates can be extremely stable and unaffected by cellular clearance machinery (Dobson 1999; Knowles et al. 2007). There is extensive evidence that most and perhaps all proteins can form amyloid under suitable, typically destabilizing, conditions (Dobson 1999; Munishkina et al. 2004; Stathopulos et al. 2004). Amyloid formation can arise from association of unstructured, partially folded, or native-like species, and can be prevented by factors that favour native folding (Chiti and Dobson 2009). These include such factors as: interactions with molecular chaperones that can stabilize partially folded conformations and increase the folding rate; and post-translational modifications or ligand binding that can stabilize the native state and prevent unfolding (Dobson 2004; Chiti and Dobson 2009). Protein size is also a factor that modulates the propensity of a protein to form amyloid fibrils, as it is less energetically favourable for large proteins to form an amyloid core, compared to smaller proteins (Baldwin et al. 2011; Ramshini et al. 2011).

It should be noted that ALS is not classified by pathologists as an amyloid disease (Kerman et al. 2010). Recent studies have reported the formation of SOD1 aggregates *in vitro* that exhibit some features of amyloid (Banci et al. 2008; Furukawa et al. 2008; Oztug Durer et al. 2009); however, the relevance of such studies to human disease is not known. Typically, there is considerable structural heterogeneity in amyloid (Platt and Radford 2009) and in other amorphous or ordered aggregate structures formed by many peptides and proteins (Fink 1998; Seshadri et al. 2009) (see 1.2.4). Careful analyses using multiple probes are required to distinguish between these different aggregate structures. Appropriately characterizing mixtures of aggregate structures is a major, ongoing challenge in the study of protein aggregation.

1.2.4 Protein aggregation heterogeneity and disease complexity

Neurodegenerative disorders characterized by protein misfolding and aggregation, including ALS, commonly display phenotypic diversity, such as variation in the age of onset, the rate of neuronal dysregulation, and the area of the nervous system affected (Armstrong et al. 2000; Goedert et al. 2001; Frost and Diamond 2009; Williamson et al. 2009). Although the molecular origins of such phenotypic diversity are complex and may differ between diseases, in recent years it has been shown that protein aggregates, including amyloid fibrils, exhibit extensive structural heterogeneity both *in vivo* and *in vitro* (Berryman et al. 2009; Frost and Diamond 2009). Not only do fibrils formed by different amino acid sequences adopt conformations that differ in length and twist, but the structure of fibrils formed by the *same* sequence can vary depending on solution conditions (Berryman et al. 2009). Fibres can vary in the number of amino acids that participate in forming the amyloid core, the arrangement of β-strands in a parallel or antiparallel conformation within each protofilament, and the alignment of β-sheets along the protofilament axis (Tycko 2006). The structure that a particular protein adopts prior to aggregation influences the structure of the aggregate formed and the conformational plasticity of a native protein may play a large role in determining the number of structurally different aggregates produced (Jones and Surewicz 2005; Natalello et al. 2008). Although aggregate structures formed from the same protein can be quite diverse (ie. amorphous versus amyloid structures), in many cases the formation of such structures is energetically favourable and therefore switching between aggregate conformations can require a large amount of energy. As a result, a particular fibril can become trapped in a single conformation (Berryman et al. 2009).

Structural heterogeneity of protein aggregates has been known for many years for amyloid fibrils derived from prion proteins, infectious protein agents that give rise to a number of neurodegenerative disorders known as spongiform encephalopathies or prionopathies. In these diseases, the infectious agent is a misfolded prion protein (PrP^{Sc}, S referring to Scrapie, the disease caused by this infectious agent), which once introduced into a host cell can bind to the native prion protein (PrP^{c}, c referring to cellular) and induce conversion to the PrP^{Sc} form, inevitably resulting in the spread of the disease phenotype (Tuite and Serio 2010). Because a prion protein can adopt a number of conformations, there is considerable heterogeneity in the structure of the amyloid fibrils that are formed from these proteins. Prion amyloid fibrils can differ in stability, surface charge and degree of polypeptide incorporation into the amyloid core, differences that may play a large role in determining rate of prion replication and the strength of the disease phenotype (Verges et al. 2011). In recent years, evidence for conformational diversity, or different strains, of protein aggregates has also been described for non-infectious protein conformational disorders such as Alzheimer's, Parkinson's, Frontal Temporal Dementia, and ALS (Frost and Diamond 2009; Furukawa et al. 2010). The proteins linked to many of these diseases are natively disordered, and so can easily sample different conformations, which may facilitate aggregation via multiple pathways. Mutations and/or post-translational modifications can greatly influence the population of different conformations of a protein, and thus can largely influence the aggregation process. This point may be particularly relevant to ALS toxicity, since SOD1, although natively folded, undergoes extensive post-translational modification *in vivo* (Valentine et al. 2005), and is increasingly malleable in its less stable, immature forms (refer to section 3). How different fALS-associated mutations modulate the stability of different forms of SOD1 may largely determine the ALS phenotype (Vassall et al. 2011).

2. Structure and function of Cu, Zn-superoxide dismutase (SOD1)

Before discussing SOD1 folding, misfolding and aggregation, we will give a brief description of the tertiary and quaternary structure of SOD1. Human SOD1 is a 32 kDa homodimeric metalloenzyme, with each subunit consisting of a 153 amino acid chain that is often N-terminally acetylated, contains a highly conserved, intrasubunit disulfide bond, and binds one Cu ion and one Zn ion (Figure 2A, C).

Each monomer folds into a Greek key β-barrel, comprised of two, four-stranded antiparallel β-sheets arranged at an angle with respect to one another. The β-barrel has a non-continuous topology such that strands 1 through 3 together with strand 6 form the first β-sheet, while strands 4, 5, 7 and 8 form the second β-sheet. The β-strands are connected by seven loops that differ greatly in length. Loop IV and loop VII are known as the metal binding and electrostatic loops, respectively, and play important roles in both stability and catalytic function by binding the metals and forming the catalytic site pocket. In addition to forming the Zn-binding site, Loop IV contains residues that are important for dimer interface and intrasubunit disulfide bond formation, which tethers Loop IV to β-strand 8 (Tainer et al. 1982). Thus, Zn binding, disulfide bond formation and dimerization together stabilize the native conformation of this long loop, greatly affecting the overall stability of the protein. Loop VII mainly plays a functional role, containing charged residues that shield the active site. These charged residues are important for guiding the superoxide anion from the surface of the protein into the active site where the redox active Cu ion is bound (Valentine et al. 2005).

SOD1 is abundant and ubiquitously expressed in the cytosol of aerobic organisms (Brown et al. 2004). Maturation of the protein involves a series of post-translational modifications, which are understood to varying extents. When it is initially synthesized in the reducing environment of the cytosol the protein is thought to adopt a marginally stable, folded, monomer structure with a reduced disulfide bond and no bound metals. How the protein acquires Zn is not known; however, Cu can be acquired by interaction with the copper chaperone for SOD1 (CCS) or by a CCS-independent mechanism that may involve glutathione, but that is not well understood (Leitch et al. 2009). CCS also catalyzes intrasubunit disulfide bond formation in the reducing cellular environment (Leitch et al. 2009). Although the most abundant form of SOD1 is usually the native, fully mature, dimeric protein (Valentine et al. 2005), there is also evidence for a significant pool of SOD1 that lacks bound Cu, and is activated in response to oxidative stress (Brown et al. 2004). From here we will refer to the various states of the protein in terms of disulfide and metallation status, with a focus on the disulfide reduced (2SH), disulfide oxidized (S-S), fully metallated (holo) and metal free (apo) states.

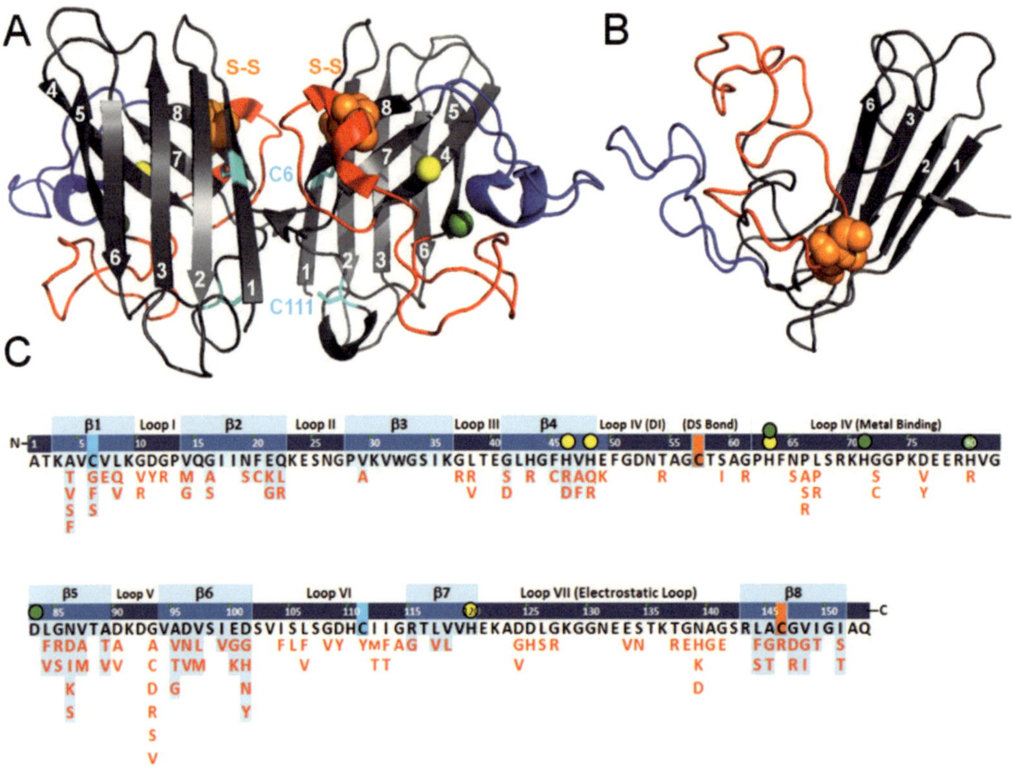

Fig. 2. The structural elements of SOD1.

The crystal structure of fully mature SOD1 is shown in panel A (pdb: 1HL5) (Strange et al. 2003). The β-strands are shown in gray and labelled in white starting from the N-terminus; the functional loops IV and VII are shown in red and blue, respectively; the conserved disulfide bond (S-S) between Cys57 and Cys146 is indicated by orange spheres, the non-conserved free Cys (6 and 111) are shown in cyan; and Cu and Zn are indicated by yellow and green spheres, respectively. The solution structure of the metal free SOD1 monomer variant (pWT*mon*, refer to the introduction of section 3) is shown in panel B (pdb: 1RK7) (Banci et al. 2003). In this structure, only β-strands 1-3 and 6 are well defined. The colour scheme in panel B is identical to panel A. The primary sequence of the SOD1 monomer is shown in panel C. The colours used to depict the secondary structure elements are identical to those used in panels A and B. The positions of known fALS-associated mutations are listed vertically in red below the naturally occurring amino acid in black. The yellow and green spheres indicate the metal binding residues and the secondary structure elements are listed above the primary sequence.

3. Folding, unfolding and misfolding of SOD1

A common and powerful approach to understanding the molecular basis for aggregate formation is to investigate the biophysical properties of mutant proteins in the native and unfolded states, as well as any equilibrium or kinetic intermediates that arise as the protein folds or unfolds (Dobson 2004). Equilibrium species refer to the most stable conformations that are significantly populated under specific steady-state conditions, while kinetic species refer to conformations that are transiently populated as an unfolded protein folds into its native conformation. Typically, kinetic folding intermediates have a relatively low energy barrier of formation, and therefore can form quickly, but they are generally not the most stable conformations. Before protein folding has reached equilibrium (ie. during kinetic conditions), it is not the stability of each state that determines the relative population of each species along the folding/unfolding pathway, but rather how rapidly these states can be accessed on the time scale of protein folding/unfolding. Investigating the molecular characteristics that govern the stability of different states and enable efficient folding of SOD1 can provide key insights into the cause of ALS (Rumfeldt et al. 2006; Stathopulos et al. 2006; Vassall et al. 2006; Rumfeldt et al. 2009; Vassall et al. 2011).

In recent years, systematic analyses of the effects of fALS-associated mutations on the stability and folding of various forms of SOD1, including holoS-S, apoS-S and apoSH, have been reported. Human SOD1 contains two free cysteine residues at amino acid positions 6 and 111 (Figure 2), and these free cysteine residues inhibit reversible unfolding of SOD1 *in vitro* by forming intramolecular and intermolecular non-native disulfide bonds, which promote SOD1 aggregation (Lepock et al. 1990; McRee et al. 1990). Reversible unfolding is a prerequisite for thermodynamic analysis, and so to overcome this limitation pseudo-wild type (pWT) constructs lacking these free cysteines have been used extensively for *in vitro* studies of SOD1. In the most widely used pWT construct, the free cysteines are mutated to alanine and serine at positions 6 and 111, respectively (Lepock et al. 1990; McRee et al. 1990; Stathopulos et al. 2003; Rumfeldt et al. 2006; Stathopulos et al. 2006; Vassall et al. 2006; Kayatekin et al. 2008; Rumfeldt et al. 2009; Vassall et al. 2011); however, other mutations at these positions have also been used (most notably C6A and C111A) (Lindberg et al. 2004; Nordlund and Oliveberg 2006; Nordlund et al. 2009). Not only are these chemically and structurally conservative mutations, a serine at position 111 is found in most other mammalian SOD1, and alanine at position 6 is observed in other non-mammalian organisms (Getzoff et al. 1989). Mutating the free cysteines results in highly reversible unfolding of pWT, while having very minimal effects on structure, function and stability (Lepock et al. 1990; McRee et al. 1990; Hallewell et al. 1991; Parge et al. 1992; Vassall et al. 2011). In addition, an engineered monomer construct (pWT*mon* SOD1) has been used to investigate the effects of ALS mutations on the stability and folding behaviour of individual SOD1 subunits (Nordlund and Oliveberg 2006; Hornberg et al. 2007; Kayatekin et al. 2008; Nordlund et al. 2009; Kayatekin et al. 2010). The monomer construct contains two glutamic acid residues in place of Phe50 and Gly51, and the presence of these charged residues in the dimer interface prevents SOD1 dimerization (Bertini et al. 1994; Banci et al. 1998). The use of both pWT and pWT*mon* SOD1 constructs has provided valuable insights into the mechanism of SOD1 folding and misfolding, which are described in the following sections, starting with the most immature to most mature form of SOD1.

SOD1 Form	t_m pWT (°C)	t_m WT (°C)	ΔG, 37°C pWT (kcal mol^{-1})
HoloS-S	**92.0[a] (81.7[b])**	**80.1[b]**	**33.0[a,c]**
ApoS-S	**59.0[a]**	**52.5[d]**	**13.2[a,c]**
Apo2SH	**47.6[e]**	**46.8[e]**	**1.8[e,f]**

Table 1. Stability parameters obtained from DSC measurements of different forms of wild type (WT) and pWT SOD1

[a](Stathopulos et al. 2006) The parameters were obtained using average fitted values determined using 0.5 mg mL^{-1} protein in 20 mM Hepes pH 7.8.

[b](Lepock et al. 1990) t_m defined as the temperature of half completion of the DSC profiles determined using 2-4 mg mL^{-1} protein in 100 mM phosphate.

[c]ΔG extrapolated to 37°C using methods described in (Stathopulos et al. 2006). Value is in units of per mol dimer.

[d](rodriguiz/valentine,2005,PNAS)determined using 2 mg mL^{-1} protein in 100 mM potassium phosphate pH 7.4.

[e](Vassal,2011,PNAS) parameters obtained using average fitted values determined using 0.5 mg mL^{-1} protein in 20 mM Hepes pH 7.4, 1mM TCEP.

[f]Value is in units of per mol monomer.

3.1 Equilibrium denaturation of apo2SH SOD1

In its most immature form, with no bound metals and reduced disulfide bond, apo2SH SOD1 adopts a marginally stable folded monomer structure. Chemical and thermal equilibrium denaturation of apo2SH SOD1 is well described by a 2-state unfolding transition between folded and unfolded monomers, denoted as M and U, respectively (M ↔ U) (Kayatekin et al. 2010; Vassall et al. 2011). At 37°C and neutral pH, this form of the protein has a low free energy of unfolding, 1.8 kcal mol^{-1} and 1.6 kcal mol^{-1} for pWT and WT, respectively (Vassall et al. 2011), indicating that ~95 % and 93 % of the protein is folded. Furthermore, the corresponding melting temperatures are 48 °C and 47 °C, respectively. This stability is relatively low compared to other globular proteins, which typically have unfolding free energies of ~5-15 kcal mol^{-1} (Jackson 1998) as well as to more mature forms of SOD1 (see sections 3.2-3.4, 3.6, 3.7, Table 1).

Structural investigations by x-ray crystallography and NMR have shown that without the bound metals and disulfide bond, the interface loop (Loop IV) is minimally structured and the dimer interface is disrupted (Arnesano et al. 2004; Hornberg et al. 2007). The NMR solution structure of monomeric (pWT*mon*) with no bound metals but intact disulfide bond, apoS-S (Banci et al. 2003) provides an interesting comparison (Figure 2B). pWT*mon* apoS-S SOD1 adopts an open β-barrel structure due to the flexibility of β-strands 4 and 5, and the inability of the two β-sheets to effectively pack against one another. Furthermore, Loops IV and VII are extensively disordered (Banci et al. 2003; Banci et al. 2010). Disulfide bond reduction promotes further disorder of the marginally stable Loop IV structure by releasing it from its anchor to β-strand 8 (Hornberg et al. 2007). Because Loop IV contains residues required for Zn binding, disulfide bond formation and dimerization, these modifications are thermodynamically coupled. When the disulfide bond is reduced, SOD1 has a much lower affinity for Zn (75 nM *verses* 100 pM for apoS-S SOD1) (Kayatekin et al. 2010), and dimer formation is energetically unfavourable (Arnesano et al. 2004).

Diverse fALS-associated mutations have markedly different effects on the stability and the folding reversibility of apo2SH SOD1 (Kayatekin et al. 2010; Vassall et al. 2011). Wild-type, pWT, and pWT*mon* apo2SH SOD1 are predominantly folded and can undergo reversible chemical and thermal denaturation, and hence resist aggregation from partially or fully unfolded states (Kayatekin et al. 2010; Vassall et al. 2011). Various fALS-associated mutations decrease the unfolding reversibility, which precludes determination of the free energy of unfolding, and suggests that these mutations increase the aggregation propensity of apo2SH SOD1 (Vassall et al. 2011). Interestingly, an increased tendency to aggregate is not observed for all fALS-associated mutants, in particular not for those with compromised metal binding (Kayatekin et al. 2010; Vassall et al. 2011). Although the free energy of unfolding could not be determined for all mutants studied, owing to the limited stability of this form of the protein, the effects of each mutation on stability could be estimated from their apparent melting temperatures. This revealed that fALS-associated mutations generally have the largest effect on the stability of this most immature form of SOD1 (Table 1), often decreasing the melting temperature of apoSH to below 37°C, and so markedly increasing the fraction of protein that is unfolded at physiological temperature (Furukawa and O'Halloran 2005; Kayatekin et al. 2010; Vassall et al. 2011). Of the mutant SOD1s that unfold reversibly, most show decreased thermodynamic stability, but some (e.g. those involved in metal binding) have little or even a stabilizing effect on stability (Valentine et al. 2005; Kayatekin et al. 2010; Vassall et al. 2011). These findings imply that in some cases the key effects of mutations in ALS may be manifested in more mature forms of SOD1.

3.2 Kinetic unfolding and refolding of apo2SH

Relatively little is known about the kinetic folding mechanism of apo2SH SOD1. Initial studies of engineered reduced monomer variants have reported 2-state (U $\leftrightarrow$ M) folding kinetics, which resembles the behaviour of monomeric apoS-S SOD1s (Lindberg et al. 2004; Kayatekin et al. 2010) (see section 3.4). A study using a monomeric C6A/C111A/C57A/C146A construct that resembles the apo2SH form, due to its inability to form a disulfide bond and dimerize, showed that disulfide bond formation was not required to facilitate the early contacts made in the monomer folding pathway (Lindberg et al. 2004). Thus, the transition state between unfolded and folded monomers in both the apo2SH and the apoS-S monomer folding pathways may be similar. However, the disulfide bond stabilizes the folded monomer by decreasing the rate of unfolding, thereby increasing the population of folded monomer (Lindberg et al. 2004) (see section 3.4).

3.3 Equilibrium denaturation of apoS-S SOD1

Formation of a disulfide bond between Cys57 and Cys146 greatly diminishes the conformational freedom of Loop IV (Hornberg et al. 2007), and gives rise to energetically favourable dimer formation (Lindberg et al. 2004; Vassall et al. 2006; Ding and Dokholyan 2008; Kayatekin et al. 2010; Vassall et al. 2011). The observed equilibrium folding mechanism of the pWT apoS-S SOD1 dimer depends on the method of inducing denaturation (i.e. chemical denaturant *versus* heat). Spectroscopically-monitored chemical denaturation of pWT apoS-S SOD1 can be described by a 3-state mechanism in which dimer dissociation is followed by monomer unfolding ($N_2 \leftrightarrow 2M \leftrightarrow 2U$) (Vassall et al. 2006). Due to mass action, however, at increased protein concentrations there is little population of the folded monomer and the mechanism appears 2-state ($N_2 \leftrightarrow 2U$) (Lindberg et al. 2004; Svensson et al. 2006; Vassall et al. 2006). Similarly, due to the higher stability of the apoS-S dimer compared to the apoS-S monomer and the high protein concentration requirement, thermal denaturation by differential scanning calorimetry (DSC) of apoS-S pWT SOD1 appears 2-state ($N_2 \leftrightarrow 2U$) and so does not provide direct information about the energetics of dimer dissocation ($N_2 \leftrightarrow 2M$) (Stathopulos et al. 2006; Vassall et al. 2006). Thermal denaturation does reveal, however, that the melting temperatures of wild-type and pWT apoS-S SOD1 are approximately 53°C (Rodriguez et al. 2005) and 60°C (Stathopulos et al. 2006), respectively; therefore, the oxidized form of the protein is predominantly folded at physiological temperature. The differences in the reported melting temperatures may be related to different buffer conditions used as well as the folding irreversibility of wild-type SOD1 (Lepock et al. 1992; Chrunyk and Wetzel 1993; Stathopulos et al. 2003). The changes in melting temperatures caused by fALS mutations generally range from -15°C to +2°C; thus, apoS-S SOD1 mutants are also mainly folded at physiological temperature (Rodriguez et al. 2005; Vassall et al. 2006; Kayatekin et al. 2010).

The stability as well as the conformational dynamics of a protein can be assessed using hydrogen-deuterium (H/D) exchange measurements, which can identify regions of the protein undergoing structural opening (Bai et al. 1995). Interestingly, a number of fALS-associated mutants, in particular those that compromise metal binding, display a similar exchange rate as wild type (Rodriguez et al. 2005). However, others increase the rate of structural fluctuations of apoS-S SOD1 (Rodriguez et al. 2005; Prudencio et al. 2009). In particular, some mutants show pronounced opening of the β-barrel around the edge strands at physiological temperatures (Prudencio et al. 2009). Thus, both equilibrium denaturation and H/D exchange experiments reveal that fALS-associated mutations have diverse effects on the stability of apoS-S SOD1, ranging from destabilizing to stabilizing.

Highly reversible chemical denaturation behaviour has enabled accurate measurements of the energetics of both dimer dissociation and monomer unfolding for pWT and mutant apoS-S. Determining how mutations affect the energy, and thus the population, of each species formed along the (un)folding pathway, provides insight into the mechanisms of apoS-S aggregation. Chemical denaturation experiments have revealed that for structurally and chemically diverse mutations, fALS-associated mutations generally decrease the stability of apoS-S SOD1 by destabilizing both the monomer and the dimer interface, with a larger affect on monomer stability compared to the dimer stability (Vassall et al. 2006). Remarkably, the effects of the mutations appear to propagate extensively through the apoS-S form of the protein, inevitably destabilizing the dimer interface (Vassall, K.A. et al. unpublished data) (Khare et al. 2006; Bystrom et al. 2010). Structurally, the apoS-S SOD1 dimer interface is small compared to the amount of solvent exposed surface area (Tainer et al. 1982; Parge et al. 1992); consequently, the dimer interface may be more easily perturbed in the apoS-S state. Moreover, metal loss induces asymmetry in the dynamics of the apoS-S SOD1 monomers, indicative of a structure that is less compact than the holoS-S dimer (Strange et al. 2007). The conformation of both the β-barrel core, in particular β-strand 5, and the functional Loops IV and VII are less rigid in the absence of bound metal (Banci et al. 2009; Teilum et al. 2009). It has been proposed that metal binding is important for shielding the charged residues in Loops IV and VII, which contain too few hydrophobic residues to facilitate close packing with the β-barrel core in the absence of bound metal (Nordlund et al. 2009). Similarly, metal binding may protect against conformational changes in SOD1 that increase hydrophobic exposure (Tiwari et al. 2009).

Therefore, it seems reasonable that many fALS-associated mutations have a large effect on the global stability of apoS-S SOD1. Structural perturbations in one region of the apoS-S SOD1 structure are likely to result in structural perturbations in another region. However, it is clear that fALS-associated mutations have differing effects on the global stability of apoS-S SOD1. In particular, both the apoS-S and apo2SH forms of the metal-binding mutants appear to possess similar stability compared to the wild-type protein (Rodriguez et al. 2005; Vassall et al. 2011). In fact, some fALS-associated mutations increase the stability of apo2SH and apoS-S forms compared to pWT SOD1 (Vassall et al. unpublished data) (Vassall et al. 2011). For example, the mutation H46R increases the stability of both apo2SH and apoS-S SOD1 and the reason for this increase in stability may be due to the introduction of a positively charged side chain into the metal binding pocket of the protein, effectively mimicking the stabilizing effects of the charged metals.

3.4 Kinetic unfolding and refolding of apoS-S SOD1

The kinetic unfolding mechanism of pWT apoS-S SOD1 can be described by the same 3-state mechanism previously outlined for equilibrium denaturation of the wild-type and pWT apoS-S form, where dimer dissociation is followed by the unfolding of two monomers (Figure 3) (Svensson et al. 2006). The overall observed rate of unfolding depends on four microscopic rate constants: the rate constant for folding (k_f), unfolding (k_u), monomer association (k_a), and dimer dissociation (k_d) (Figure 3B); however, under highly denaturing conditions (ie. high denaturant concentration), the marginally stable monomer unfolds rapidly and the rate of the entire unfolding pathway is determined by the rate of dimer dissociation (k_d) (Lindberg et al. 2004; Svensson et al. 2006). In contrast, the overall rate of the refolding pathway of wild-type and pWT apoS-S is limited only by the rate of monomer folding. Therefore, once the monomer has folded the rate of monomer association is extremely rapid (Lindberg et al. 2004; Svensson et al. 2006). The transition state for monomer association is similar to the native dimer with respect to the amount of buried surface area (Svensson et al. 2006). This is similar to the transition state between unfolded and folded monomer, which represents the major energetic barrier of the unfolding/refolding pathway. It has been observed that ~70% of the structure that is buried in the monomer intermediate is also buried in the transition state between the unfolded and folded monomer, suggesting that considerable structural rearrangements must occur before that transition state can form (Svensson et al. 2006). Interestingly, under both equilibrium and kinetic conditions, the population of monomer intermediate remains below 0.5% at physiologically relevant protein concentrations, suggesting that the folding pathway of SOD1 has evolved to limit accumulation of marginally stable monomer intermediates (Svensson et al. 2006). Equilibrium denaturation analyses of fALS-associated mutant apoS-S SOD1 demonstrate a decreased stability of both the monomer intermediate and the dimer interface, increasing the population of monomeric intermediate as well as the unfolded monomer (Lindberg et al. 2004; Vassall et al. 2006), which enhances the accessibility of partially folded, high energy states that may give rise to aggregation.

Kinetic unfolding/refolding studies of the monomeric apoS-S SOD1 (pWT*mon*) and the apo2SH forms of SOD1 can be compared to gain an understanding of how disulfide bond formation modulates the SOD1 folding pathway. Both the pWT apo2SH and the pWT*mon* apoS-S forms of SOD1 fold via a 2-state mechanism, whereby the unfolded monomer adopts a folded conformation in one step ($U \leftrightarrow M$) (Lindberg et al. 2004; Nordlund and Oliveberg

2006; Kayatekin et al. 2010). Owing to the similar folding/unfolding mechanism of apo2SH and pWT*mon* apoS-S, disulfide bond formation is probably not requisite in the early monomer folding events. Consistent with this notion, the topology of the β-barrel brings Cys57 and Cys146 close in space, promoting disulfide bond formation. Although reduction of the disulfide bond does not prevent formation of the necessary contacts that facilitate monomer folding, the maintenance of the disulfide bond modulates the stability of the SOD1 monomer by decreasing the rate of unfolding and to a smaller extent increasing the rate of folding (Lindberg et al. 2004; Kayatekin et al. 2010).

Removal of Loops IV and VII has little effect on the structure and dynamics of the core apoS-S β-barrel (Nordlund et al. 2009). Additionally, the folding behaviour of pWT*mon* apoS-S SOD1 in the absence of these functional loops remains 2-state; however, this SOD1 construct has a 10-fold increase in the rate of folding, while the rate of unfolding is less affected (Nordlund et al. 2009). Removing the Zn-binding site has little effect on the rate of folding, but decreases the rate of unfolding, stabilizing the folded apoS-S SOD1 monomer (Nordlund et al. 2009). These results suggest that while the β-barrel can fold independently of Loop IV and VII, these critical functional loops endow the protein with a less than optimal folding mechanism and may increase the aggregation propensity of the immature forms of the protein.

The overall rate of both apo2SH and apoS-S SOD1 folding appears to be dictated largely by the structural determinants of the monomer folding nucleus. Furthermore, regions extraneous to this folding nucleus are the more labile regions of the protein that unfold first, and thus have been suggested to play a role in SOD1 aggregation. It has been shown that β-strands 1-3 of the first β-sheet must make contact with β-strands 4 and 7 in the second β-sheet to overcome the monomer folding energy barrier. The other strands (β5, β6 and β8) remain disordered in the transition state between unfolded and folded monomers (Nordlund and Oliveberg 2006). By attaching Loop IV to β-strand 8 and forming the dimer interface the disulfide bond may prevent the structural fluctuations that lead to the unravelling of the more dynamic strands of the β-barrel.

3.5 Are the metal free forms of SOD1 the common denominator in fALS toxicity?

Taken together, equilibrium and kinetic folding studies of apo2SH and apoS-S SOD1 suggest that a number of factors may contribute to an increased tendency to aggregate. Many fALS-associated mutations increase the fraction of partially folded monomers, while a few mutations remain wild-type-like in their folding behaviour and aggregation propensity. Because the β-strands display differences in conformational freedom, the location of each fALS-associated mutation and the physicochemical properties of the amino acid introduced seem to greatly affect SOD1 stability and accessibility to partially folded species that may bridge the gap between productive folding and aggregation pathways. These differences may also change the structural properties of the aggregates formed. In recent years, many studies have focused on characterizing a common underlying cause of toxicity in all SOD1-associated fALS cases. Thus a great deal of attention has been directed towards studying the biophysical properties of the more immature forms of SOD1, since fALS-associated mutations have a greater effect on the stability of these forms compared to the fully mature holoS-S form (Lindberg et al. 2004; Furukawa and O'Halloran 2005; Furukawa and O'Halloran 2006; Khare et al. 2006; Nordlund and Oliveberg 2006; Svensson et al. 2006; Smith et al. 2007; Furukawa et al. 2008; Nordlund et al. 2009; Oztug Durer et al. 2009; Tiwari et al. 2009; Kayatekin et al. 2010; Vassall et al. 2011). Despite this recent focus, the form of SOD1 that is most relevant to ALS pathogenesis remains unknown. It is clear that some fALS-associated mutations minimally affect the stability and folding kinetics of apo2SH and apoS-S SOD1, which suggests that it is necessary to look beyond the immature forms of SOD to uncover the cause of ALS.

3.6 Equilibrium denaturation of holoS-S SOD1

Similar to the equilibrium denaturation pathway of apoS-S SOD1, the observed equilibrium denaturation mechanism of holoS-S SOD1 depends on the mode of denaturation and protein concentration. For pWT SOD1, holoS-S equilibrium denaturation curves fit a reversible 3-state model in which the folded holo native dimer transitions to the unfolded monomer through a folded, metallated, monomeric intermediate (Rumfeldt et al. 2006). The presence of bound metal stabilizes the monomer intermediate far more than the dimer interface. Thus, the dimer is only slightly stronger in holoS-S compared to apoS-S, while the free energy of monomer folding is much higher for holoS-S SOD1 compared to apoS-S SOD1 (Rumfeldt et al. 2006; Vassall et al. 2006). At high protein concentrations, the population of the monomer intermediate is significantly reduced and the equilibrium denaturation mechanism approaches 2-state (Rumfeldt et al. 2006). Similarly, in thermal denaturation by DSC, the monomeric intermediate is not significantly populated and the unfolding appears 2-state (Stathopulos et al. 2006). In both chemical and thermal denaturation of holoS-S SOD1, metals remain bound throughout the transition, although binding is weakened in the monomer intermediate and unfolded state compared to the dimer (Rumfeldt et al. 2006; Stathopulos et al. 2006; Kayatekin et al. 2008). Equilibrium denaturation of holoS-S SOD1 reveals that metal binding significantly increases the free energy of unfolding (Table 1). Consistent with this, the melting temperature of holoS-S SOD1 is ~30°C higher than apoS-S SOD1. Thus, it is likely that the stabilizing effects of metallation as well as disulfide bond formation are intrinsic inhibitors of SOD1 aggregation. Mutations therefore may exert toxicity to the cell by inhibiting SOD1 maturation and/or by promoting metal loss, dimer dissociation and/or disulfide reduction (Tiwari and Hayward 2003; Lindberg et al. 2004; Furukawa and O'Halloran 2005; Furukawa and O'Halloran 2006; Banci et al. 2007; Hornberg et al. 2007; Ding and Dokholyan 2008; Furukawa et al. 2008; Tiwari et al. 2009).

Comparable to apoS-S SOD1, the equilibrium denaturation mechanism of fALS-associated mutant holoS-S SOD1 remains the same as pWT. In a number of cases mutations have been shown to decrease the stability of holoS-S, by decreasing the stability of the monomer, with less effect on dimerization (Rumfeldt et al. 2006; Stathopulos et al. 2006; Vassall et al. 2006). This decreased stability of the holoS-S monomer can often be attributed to weakened metal binding (Hayward et al. 2002), as metal dissociation results in an increased population of the less stable apo state. Thus, in most cases mutations appear to have a more local effect on the stability of holoS-S SOD1 compared to apoS-S SOD1 (Rumfeldt et al. 2006; Vassall et al. 2006); yet, structural perturbations due to mutation may propagate further if metal binding is compromised since loop dynamics and interface stability are greatly affected by the presence of metals (Valentine et al. 2005; Smith et al. 2007; Museth et al. 2009). The overwhelming majority of fALS-associated mutations destabilize the holo state, but because of its extremely high thermodynamic stability the absolute increase in the amount of unfolded species will still be very small, and thus unlikely to affect aggregation. What seems more likely to impact disease is increased local structural fluctuations that can arise from metal loss and/or dimer dissociation, exposing regions of the SOD1 structure that can make favourable contacts with other SOD1 molecules, and thereby give rise to aggregation from native-like states (Elam et al. 2003; Hwang et al. 2010).

3.7 Kinetic unfolding and refolding of holoS-S SOD1

Analyzing the kinetics of holoS-S SOD1 folding and unfolding provides a method for further characterizing the marginally stable intermediates that form along the folding pathway as these are not always detected at equilibrium where only the most stable species are measurably populated. These kinetic intermediates nevertheless may play significant roles in holoS-S SOD1 aggregation. Both pWT and wild-type holoS-S kinetically unfold slowly *in vitro* via a monomeric intermediate species which has somewhat weaker metal binding affinity relative to the native dimer (Rumfeldt et al. 2006; Kayatekin et al. 2008; Mulligan et al. 2008; Rumfeldt et al. 2009). The overall rate of holoS-S unfolding is dependent on the microscopic rate constants that define each equilibrium transition (Figure 3A).

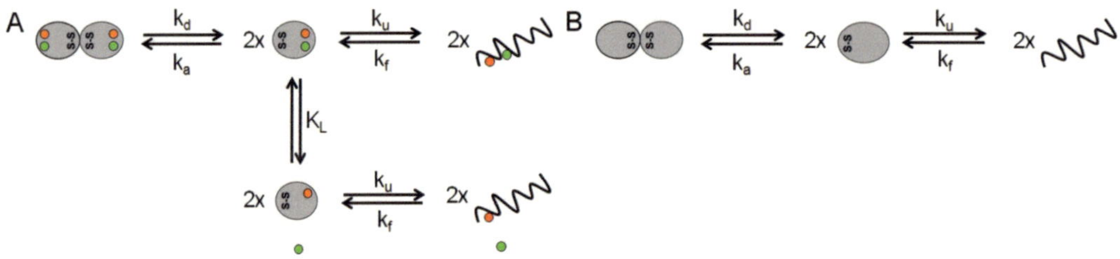

Fig. 3. The kinetic unfolding mechanism of holoS-S and apoS-S SOD1.
In panel A, the kinetic unfolding mechanism of holoS-S SOD1 is shown. The overall rate of unfolding is dependent on the microscopic rate constants k_d, k_a, k_u, k_f, and protein and metal concentration, as well as the equilibrium constant for Zn dissociation from the monomeric intermediate. For a more detailed description refer to (Rumfeldt et al. 2009). In panel B, the simpler kinetic unfolding mechanism of apoS-S SOD1 is shown. The overall rate of unfolding depends only on the microscopic rate constants k_d, k_a, k_u, k_f and protein concentration.

The observed unfolding kinetics therefore depend on the rate of dimer dissociation, which occurs rapidly, and the rate of monomer unfolding, a much slower process (Lynch et al. 2004; Rumfeldt et al. 2009). Under high protein concentration conditions, or in the presence of excess metals, pWT holoS-S SOD1 remains fully metallated as it unfolds, with metals remaining bound to the unfolded state, while at low protein concentrations, Zn can dissociate from both the monomeric intermediate and unfolded monomer (Rumfeldt et al. 2009). Similar results were obtained in kinetic unfolding studies of wild-type holoS-S SOD1 in the presence of a metal chelator, where dimer dissociation and Zn loss were found to occur simultaneously, followed by a conformational change in the β-barrel that precedes and facilitates Cu loss (Mulligan et al. 2008).

The differences in Cu and Zn binding as holoS-S SOD1 unfolds can be rationalized by considering the structural differences in the Cu and Zn binding sites, as follows. While SOD1 binds both metals with extremely high affinity, Cu binds with higher affinity than Zn, with dissociation constants (K_d) estimated as 10^{-18} M and 10^{-14} M (Crow et al. 1997), respectively. In principal, structural differences between the transition state resembling the free energy barrier between the folded and unfolded monomer, compared to the structure of the folded monomer, determine the regions of the protein that, if changed, will have the largest effect on the rate of unfolding. If a particular region is structured in both the monomer and the transition state, then alterations in the stability of that region, either by metal binding or mutation, will affect the free energy of the monomer and its unfolding transition state in a similar way. As a result, the difference in free energy between the folded monomer and transition state and therefore the rate of monomer unfolding will be unaffected. Alternatively, if a particular region of the protein is structured in the folded monomer, but not in the transition state, then changes in the stability of that region will affect the energetics of the folded monomer and transition state differently. In this case the rate of unfolding will be affected. The Cu binding site is formed by residues in β-strands 4 and 7, which are thought to be structured in the transition state, while the Zn binding site is formed mainly by residues in Loop IV and β-strand 5, which are thought to be disordered in the transition state (Nordlund and Oliveberg 2006). Therefore, the rate of unfolding should be affected more by Zn binding than Cu binding and indeed there is some experimental evidence that suggests this to be the case (Rumfeldt et al. 2009).

It has been shown that fALS-associated mutant holoS-S SOD1s increase the unfolding rates of holoS-S SOD1 (Rumfeldt et al. 2009; Ip et al. 2010). Increased unfolding rates and accessibility of either on or off-folding pathway intermediates may increase the accessibility of transient protein species that can initiate aggregation (Dobson 2003; Wang et al. 2008). Furthermore, it has been proposed that fALS-associated mutations, even those far from the metal binding sites, promote increased levels of Cu-deficient intermediates along the holoS-S SOD1 unfolding pathway (Ip et al. 2010). Cu-deficient intermediates are lower in stability and therefore may have a higher tendency to aggregate.

The *in vitro* refolding mechanism of holoS-S SOD1 is more complex than apoS-S SOD1 due to the presence of metal (Figure 3). While the apoS-S form folds via a simple 3-state (2-step) mechanism, with a rate constant that is limited by the rate of monomer folding (see section 3.4), holoS-S refolding occurs through parallel pathways that differ with respect to the fraction of metal bound to the unfolded and transition states (Rumfeldt et al. 2009). However, in the presence of excess Cu and Zn and at high protein concentrations, conditions that favour metal binding to the unfolded state, the refolding kinetics can be described as a simple 2-step process, as each unfolded SOD1 monomer is saturated with metal. Zn coordination in the native binding site stabilizes the monomer intermediate and folded dimer more than the unfolded monomer, accelerating refolding of apoS-S 100 fold (Kayatekin et al. 2008). However, Zn can also bind to non-native sites on the protein (Kayatekin et al. 2008; Nordlund et al. 2009). The Cu-coordinating residues are capable of binding Zn with micromolar affinity in the denatured state after mutation of the native Zn coordinating residues (Nordlund et al. 2009). This non-native coordination of Zn augments the stability of apoS-S SOD1 by increasing the rate of folding and decreasing the rate of unfolding, but forces SOD1 to adopt a non-native conformation. Thus misligation of Zn can cause misfolding and decrease the efficiency of folding (Nordlund et al. 2009). However, with intact Cu and Zn binding sites, Zn may be coordinated by the Cu-binding site first, helping to overcome the main energy barrier of folding, before moving to the Zn-binding site (Nordlund et al. 2009). Other studies have demonstrated that Zn-binding is required to pre-organize the Cu-binding site (Banci et al. 2003). Together these studies show that metal binding significantly modulates the efficiency of the SOD1 folding pathway by stabilizing both the monomer and dimer and decreasing the rate of unfolding. However, non-native metal binding may force the protein to be kinetically trapped in a partially folded, aggregation prone conformation that is more stable than the unfolded state (Nordlund et al. 2009). Together these results show that the kinetic unfolding and refolding mechanism of SOD1 is highly dependent on metal binding.

3.8 fALS mutations and modifications have complex effects on the folding and stability of SOD1

It is evident that fALS-associated mutants have different and complex effects on the stability of SOD1, and these effects depend on the form of SOD1 being studied. For example, mutations that have a large effect on holoS-S SOD1 stability, such as metal binding mutants, tend to have a much smaller effect on the more immature forms of the protein (Valentine et al. 2005). Also, the effects of mutations are more pronounced, but to varying extents for different mutations, with decreasing stability in immature forms of SOD1 (Vassall et al. 2006; Vassall et al. 2011). It is important to understand how both the equilibrium and kinetic folding pathways of all forms of SOD1 are altered by fALS-associated mutations to untangle the complexity of SOD1 aggregation. Certain mutations may have a large effect on the thermodynamic stability of the protein, through weakened metal binding or by decreasing the stability of the dimer interface, while having a smaller effect on the kinetic stability of SOD1. Other mutations may only subtly alter the thermodynamic stability of the native state, exerting their effects by altering the kinetic stability of SOD1 by decreasing the rate of folding, or by increasing the rate of unfolding (Rumfeldt et al. 2006). These effects can increase the equilibrium and/or transient population of folded or unfolded monomeric species that are prone to aggregate (see section 4).

In addition, fALS mutations may alter the susceptibility of SOD1 to post-translational modifications which will tend to decrease protein stability. These include not only enhanced metal loss and disulfide reduction (resulting in higher population of immature species), but also other modifications, in particular ones that are enhanced under oxidizing cellular conditions, which may occur late in disease. Examples include cysteine oxidation (Gruzman et al. 2007; Karch et al. 2009; Bosco et al. 2010), glutathionylation (Proctor et al. 2011), tryptophan oxidation (Elam et al. 2003), and glycation (Meiering 2008). While there is relatively little quantitative data on the effects of these modifications on stability, there is evidence that they can be destabilizing. Such modifications may play different roles at different disease stages; for example, oxidative modifications may become more pronounced as the disease progresses and contribute to rapid disease progression by enhancing formation of toxic aggregates (Karch et al. 2009).

4. SOD1 aggregation

Numerous experimental studies have characterized the aggregation of multiple forms of SOD1. These are described below, focussing mainly on *in vitro* studies, and their implications for disease. It is important to note, however, that it is not yet known what forms of SOD1 are involved in human disease: neither the disulfide bond status nor metal content of SOD1 in aggregates is known. Evidence supports the population of multiple forms of SOD1 *in vivo* (see section 2). Collectively, experimental findings provide support for contributions from many forms of SOD1 to toxic aggregation in ALS.

4.1 Aggregation of Apo2SH SOD1

4.1.1 Evidence of Apo2SH SOD1 aggregation

Aggregation of the marginally stable apoSH form of SOD1 has been suggested in a number of studies to be particularly important in ALS pathogenesis. Studies from multiple groups have reported that wild-type, pWT and fALS-associated mutant apoSH SOD1 are all predisposed to aggregate (Lindberg et al. 2004; Furukawa and O'Halloran 2005; Hornberg et al. 2007; Chattopadhyay et al. 2008; Furukawa et al. 2008; Oztug Durer et al. 2009; Vassall et al. 2011). Additional support for the biological significance of apoSH aggregation is that fALS-associated mutants expressed in insect cells tend to be more metal deficient and disulfide reduced compared to wild type; this finding was proposed to be a consequence of enhanced opening of the mutant SOD1 structures, exposing the disulfide bond to the reducing environment of the cytosol (Tiwari and Hayward 2003). Furthermore, murine models of fALS have revealed the presence of aggregated disulfide reduced SOD1 species (Jonsson et al. 2006; Zetterstrom et al. 2007). Based on what is known about the relationship between protein stability and aggregation propensity (see section 1.2.1), and on the relatively low stability and the expanded, fluctuating structure of apoSH SOD1 (see section 3.1), it appears that aggregation of this form of SOD1 could be significant under cellular conditions (Furukawa et al. 2008). Consistent with this idea, *in vitro* agitation of apo2SH SOD1 results in amyloid fibril formation (Chattopadhyay et al. 2008; Oztug Durer et al. 2009; Furukawa et al. 2010). Although the agitation phenomenon is poorly understood at a molecular level it may favour amyloid fibril formation over pathways to other morphologies. Agitation may enhance aggregation in general by promoting the formation of aggregation-prone species at air-solution or solid-solution interfaces, as well as increase the rate of aggregation by distributing aggregation nuclei more efficiently and causing preformed aggregates to break and create new nucleation sites (Sicorello et al. 2009). Again, it should be noted that since agitation can promote aggregation of many proteins (Rousseau et al. 2008; Mahler et al. 2009; Sicorello et al. 2009), and ALS is not classified as an amyloid disease (Kerman et al. 2010), it is not yet clear how agitation-induced aggregation *in vitro* is related to aggregation in disease.

4.1.2 Mechanisms of Apo2SH SOD1 aggregation

Intriguing structural variations in apoSH amyloid and non-amyloid aggregates have been reported and may be related to the different disease durations for different SOD1 mutants. Structural diversity has been observed in the amyloid fibrils formed by different SOD1 mutants (Furukawa et al. 2010). In addition, *in vitro* aggregation experiments without agitation showed that different apo2SH SOD1 mutants may form different sized, small (~40 nm - 1000 nm), soluble, non-amyloid aggregates (Vassall et al. 2011). These soluble species may be particularly relevant to fALS toxicity, as oligomeric protein aggregates have been implicated as key neurotoxic species in many other neurodegenerative diseases (Caughey and Lansbury 2003; Soto and Estrada 2008). The variations in structural characteristics for apo2SH SOD1s aggregates may indicate that different mutants favour distinct aggregation pathways, depending on the aggregation-prone conformations that mutants may adopt.

Another factor in the heterogeneity of aggregate structures formed may be that apo2SH is appreciably unfolded at physiological temperatures, and therefore may sample multiple aggregation-prone conformations.

4.2 Aggregation of ApoS-S SOD1

4.2.1 Evidence of ApoS-S SOD1 aggregation

Aggregation of the apo S-S form of SOD1 has been studied extensively *in vitro*. This is likely related to the reasonable ease of preparation and aggregation of this quite stable form of the protein (Table 1) (see section 3.3 and 3.4). A role for apoS-S in disease is supported by various *in vitro* and *in vivo* evidence for aggregation of metal-deficient SOD1 as well as evidence that mutations can promote loss of bound metals (Valentine et al. 2005; Molnar et al. 2009; Oztug Durer et al. 2009; Hwang et al. 2010; Lelie et al. 2011). Both wild-type and fALS mutant apoS-S SOD1s are predominantly folded, but mutations can significantly increase the population of folded and unfolded monomeric species (Lindberg et al. 2004; Svensson et al. 2006; Vassall et al. 2006), and increase structural fluctuations (Ding and Dokholyan 2008; Teilum et al. 2009), both of which can promote aggregation. The formation of the disulfide bond decreases the propensity of apoS-S to aggregate compared to apoSH (see section 4.1), while the absence of bound metals in apoS-S SOD1 increases its aggregation propensity compared to holoS-S (see also section 4.3).

Several studies have described the *in vitro* formation of amyloid-like soluble or fibrillar aggregates for wild-type and fALS-associated apoS-S SOD1 mutants (Furukawa and O'Halloran 2005; Banci et al. 2007; Banci et al. 2008; Oztug Durer et al. 2009). Aggregation of mutant SOD1 in these studies was often accelerated by agitation, resulting in the formation of aberrant disulfide bonds between Cys6 and Cys111 (Figure 2) and removal of the free thiol groups by mutation (Banci et al. 2007; Cozzolino et al. 2008) generally diminished aggregation. The role of aberrant disulfide bond formation has been investigated extensively using fALS mutant SOD1 mice models of ALS where it appears that such bonds are observed mainly late in disease (Cozzolino et al. 2008; Karch and Borchelt 2008). These results highlight an important question: does the role of SOD1 differ at different stages of disease? Considerable evidence suggests that the answer is yes; in particular, soluble oligomers may be particularly important early in disease, whereas larger aggregates become prominent after the onset of disease symptoms (Boillee et al. 2006; Cozzolino et al. 2008; Turner and Talbot 2008). Many questions on the roles of different aggregate species and their targets remain unanswered.

A number of studies have reported aggregation of apoS-S SOD1 in the absence of aberrant disulfide bond formation. Formation of such amyloid-like aggregates by pWT and mutant SOD1 can be induced by agitation at neutral pH; however, in these studies the observed ease of aggregation was not correlated with disease duration (Chattopadhyay et al. 2008; Furukawa et al. 2008; Oztug Durer et al. 2009; Furukawa et al. 2010). Also, soluble, reversible aggregates induced by heat were detected by DSC (Vassall et al. unpublished data) (Stathopulos et al. 2006; Vassall et al. 2006). In these studies, mutations in a pWT background generally increased aggregate formation. Furthermore, decreased stability of fALS-associated mutant apoS-S SOD1 was correlated with increased formation of amorphous aggregates that mature into fibril structures that resemble those found in fALS patients (Stathopulos et al. 2003).

4.2.2 Mechanisms of ApoS-S Aggregation

A number of studies have focussed on possible molecular mechanisms of apoS-S SOD1 aggregation, often based on various structural and dynamic data. In the absence of bound metal, there is still extensive disorder in the functional Loops IV and VII, and this disorder may promote exposure of the β-barrel core and deprotection of the β-barrel edge strands (β-strands 5 and 6) (Strange et al. 2007). With these edge strands exposed, H-bonding ligands within the strands are free to interact with the edge strands of other SOD1 molecules and these aberrant contacts can lead to fibril formation (Elam et al. 2003; Nordlund and Oliveberg 2006). As an evolutionary strategy to avoid this fibrillation mechanism, the edge strands of β-proteins often contain charged "gatekeeper" residues, advantageously positioned to disfavour β-sheet extension (Otzen et al. 2000). Protection of the β-barrel edge strands in SOD1 is facilitated both by charged residues in β-strands 5 and 6 and by Loops IV and VII, which block the edge of the β-barrel in the holoS-S form (Nordlund and Oliveberg 2006). The other edge of the β-barrel is buried within the dimer interface. Therefore, the dynamics of Loop IV and VII that cause exposure of either β-strands 5 and 6, or the dimer interface, may lead to fibrillation. Solution NMR experiments of wild-type apoS-S SOD1 suggest that disorder in Loops IV and VII allows stretches of amino acids within these functional loops to form additional β-strands, thereby initiating oligomerization (Banci et al. 2010).

In addition, β-strands 4 and 5 are connected by Loop IV and β-strands 7 and 8 by Loop VII, and the disorder in these long loops appears to propagate to the flanking β-strands. Consequently, the β-sheet formed by strands 4, 5, 7 and 8 is less defined in apoS-S SOD1 compared to the β-sheet formed by strands 1-3 and 6 (Banci et al. 2003; Banci et al. 2010). Thus, metal loss and increased mobility of Loops IV and VII may result in exposure of hydrophobic residues in the β-barrel core (Tiwari et al. 2009). In addition, β-strands 1-3 have been proposed to be a nucleation site for aggregation of apoS-S as they form a continuous patch of hydrophobic residues (Nordlund and Oliveberg 2006). These 3 strands form early in the monomer folding pathway (Lindberg et al. 2004; Nordlund and Oliveberg 2006) and therefore may become exposed by partial unfolding of the apoS-S protein.

The destabilizing effects of fALS-associated mutations appear to propagate significantly in apoS-S SOD1, in particular generally weakening the dimer interface (see section 3.3) (Vassall et al. unpublished data) (Khare et al. 2006; Bystrom et al. 2010). Destabilization of the apoS-S dimer interface can increase the levels of marginally stable, apoS-S monomers. Furthermore, it was demonstrated recently that breathing motions of the wild-type apoS-S monomer result in transient formation of a higher energy species with weakened packing and a partially exposed hydrophobic core (Teilum et al. 2009). fALS-mutations induce further perturbations in this higher energy state that open up the structure of the mutant apoS-S SOD1 monomer more compared to wild type (Teilum et al. 2009) and so may further promote aggregation.

The increased structural dynamics observed for metal-free SOD1 described above, suggests that apoS-S may be predisposed to aggregate compared to the holoS-S state. Several studies have demonstrated that apoS-S SOD1 can aggregate by a variety of different mechanisms that give rise to different aggregate morphologies, including both disulphide cross-linked and non cross-linked species, amyloid-like fibrils and non-amyloid amorphous aggregates.

4.3 Aggregation of SOD1 from the holoS-S state

4.3.1 Evidence of aggregation from the holoS-S state

While the highly stable, native holoS-S form of SOD1 (see section 3.5) generally appears to be much less susceptible to aggregation than other forms of the protein (Stathopulos et al. 2003; Valentine et al. 2005), there is evidence that a number of SOD1 mutants can give rise to aggregation from the holoS-S form. Hwang et al. found that prolonged incubation of both pWT and fALS-associated holoS-S SOD1 mutants at physiological temperature and pH results in changes in metal binding and/or dimerization, diminished specific dismutase activity, and the nucleated formation of low levels of amorphous aggregates (Hwang et al. 2010). Furthermore, these experiments show that, although the aggregated SOD1 demonstrated some metal loss, there was still a significant amount of metal bound, indicating that complete metal loss was not essential for aggregation. Although both pWT and mutant holoS-S SOD1 were observed to aggregate, in general the holoS-S SOD1 mutants lose specific activity quicker, and aggregate more rapidly, and to a greater extent, than pWT. Importantly, the aggregates formed from holoS-S SOD1 in this study exhibited similar structural, dye-binding, and immunological characteristics as the aggregates found in fALS patients (Hwang et al. 2010). In contrast, other studies have reported that SOD1 does not aggregate from the holoS-S form (Chattopadhyay et al. 2008), or requires extremely destabilizing conditions with agitation to promote fibrilization (Oztug Durer et al. 2009). The differences between these findings may be related to the different experimental conditions for studying SOD1 aggregation, such as length of incubation, frequency of sampling, and methods for monitoring aggregation.

4.3.2 Mechanisms of holoS-S aggregation

Immature forms of SOD1 can form amyloid fibrils far more readily than holoS-S (Banci et al. 2007; Furukawa et al. 2008; Oztug Durer et al. 2009), and this difference in aggregation tendency is likely related to the very high stability and rigidity of holoS-S compared to the less mature forms (Stathopulos et al. 2003; Rumfeldt et al. 2006; Stathopulos et al. 2006; Svensson et al. 2006; Vassall et al. 2006; Furukawa et al. 2008; Kayatekin et al. 2008; Kayatekin et al. 2010; Vassall et al. 2011). Highly disordered, predominantly unfolded, proteins tend to favour the formation of amyloid (as may be the case for apo forms of SOD1), whereas more structured proteins favour formation of amorphous aggregates (as for holoS-S) (Munishkina et al. 2004). Measurements of global thermodynamic stability have shown that, owing to the high stability of the holo form, destabilizing mutations will in general cause very small increases in the population of unfolded protein (Rumfeldt et al. 2006; Stathopulos et al. 2006); these increases are unlikely to account for SOD1 aggregation in ALS. Aggregation may alternatively arise from native-like, locally unfolded states (Chiti and Dobson 2009; Hwang et al. 2010) (Figure 1B) which appear to be enhanced in holoS-S SOD1 by some fALS-associated mutations (Shipp et al. 2003; Hough et al. 2004; Banci et al. 2005; Museth et al. 2009). Ultimately, it is likely that some sort of relatively rare/slow structural change is required to bring about aggregation from holoS-S SOD1 (Hwang et al. 2010), in contrast to the apo2SH form, which aggregates readily for some fALS-associated mutant SOD1s (Vassall et al. 2011).

SOD1 aggregation arising from the holoS-S form appears to occur through a nucleation-dependent mechanism that is characterized by a lag phase (i.e. slow nucleation) followed by fast aggregate growth (Hwang et al. 2010). The lag phase corresponds to the time required for holoS-S SOD1 to arrange into an aggregation-prone state and/or form the necessary contacts required for aggregation. It is likely that dimer dissociation and/or metal loss from SOD1 occur during this lag phase and may be important triggers of aggregation (Hwang et al. 2010). Furthermore, various fALS-associated mutations appear to decrease the length of the lag phase, perhaps due to weakened metal binding and/or a weakened dimer interface, (Crow et al. 1997; Khare et al. 2004; Tiwari et al. 2009).

These results suggest that fully mature SOD1 is not devoid of the ability to aggregate, as it could give rise to native-like aggregation-prone species via loss of metal, dimer dissociation, or local structural openings, promoted by mutation. Such aggregation may be highly relevant to fALS toxicity, since holo S-S is generally the most highly abundant form of SOD1 *in vivo* (Valentine et al. 2005).

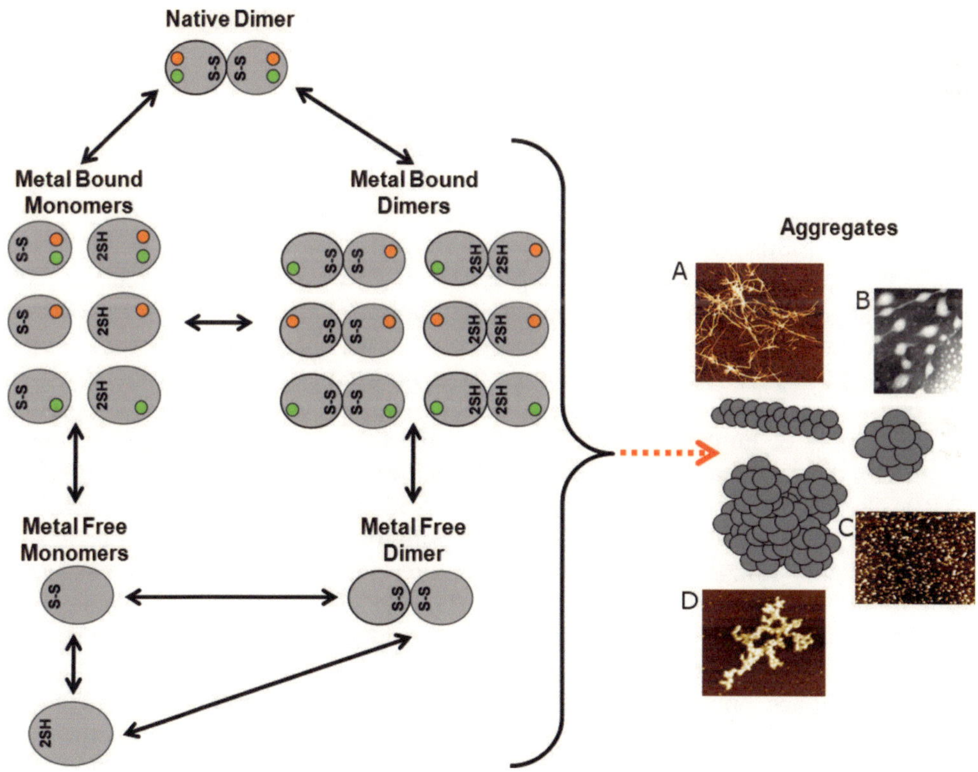

Fig. 4. Many forms of SOD1 may be relevant to ALS toxicity.

SOD1 can exist in many forms *in vivo*, which is illustrated in Figure 4. Each monomer is depicted as a grey sphere that is smaller when metals are bound and/or the disulfide is formed. The presence of Cu and Zn is shown by orange and green spheres, respectively; and S-S and 2SH indicate disulfide oxidized and reduced species, respectively. The difference in SOD1 conformation prior to aggregation may largely influence the morphology of the aggregates formed. Images and schematic representation of possible aggregate morphologies are shown in the centre on the right. Panels A, C and D are Atomic Force Microscopy images of SOD1 aggregates formed *in vitro* (Broom et al, unpublished data) (Hwang et al. 2010) and panel B is an electron microscopy image obtain from of SOD1 aggregates formed *in vitro* (Stathopulos et al. 2003).

5. Conclusion

Numerous studies have revealed that the effects of fALS-associated mutations on the folding, unfolding and aggregation of different forms of SOD1 are highly complex. Mutations can alter both equilibrium stability, in terms of the energetics of dimer dissociation, monomer intermediate stability, and metal binding, and kinetic stability, in terms of the rates of interconversion between various SOD1 species (Section 3). As a consequence, the populations of various aggregation prone species may be increased for different mutations, and this may give rise to different aggregate structures.

There have been a number of attempts to identify the relationships between the effects of the mutations and ALS disease characteristics. In particular, disease duration, which is characteristic for patients carrying a given SOD1 mutation, has been used as a measure of the toxicity of each fALS-associated SOD1 mutation. Early work focused on the loss of superoxide dismutase activity, and increased oxidative stress as the common underlying cause of disease (Valentine et al. 2005). Subsequently, the focus shifted to the toxic gain of function for mutant SOD1, both aberrant enzymatic SOD1 activity, or increased SOD1 aggregation, the latter being the predominant focus of this review. Owing to the high stability and lower aggregation propensity of the holoS-S form, many studies have focused on characterizing the stability and aggregation mechanisms of the more immature, metal deficient SOD1 forms. However, recent work suggests that disease duration does not correlate strongly with the stability of the apoS-S form of mutant SOD1 (Bystrom et al. 2010). This observation was rationalized by considering the role of factors beyond destabilization in modulating aggregation, such as changes in protein net charge and hydrogen bonding. An interesting study by Wang et al. reported that predicted aggregation propensity, based on the physicochemical properties of the polypeptide sequence (Chiti et al. 2003) combined with the stability of mutant apoS-S SOD1 in a summative score and weighted towards mutants with more patient data, correlated fairly well with fALS disease durations (Wang et al. 2008). On the other hand, recent work by Vassall et al. demonstrated that observed aggregation of the apo2SH form is not correlated with disease duration (Vassall et al. 2011). Collectively, these studies demonstrate that multiple factors including protein stability, dynamics, and biophysical characteristics are likely to play a role in modulating SOD1 aggregation, and that fALS phenotypic characteristics are not likely to be fully explained by the aggregation behaviour of any one form of SOD1.

Aggregation studies on holoS-S, apoS-S, and apo2SH SOD1 mutants have identified multiple mechanisms and aggregate morphologies (Section 4 and Figure 4). HoloS-S SOD1, widely thought believed to be much less susceptible to aggregation, has nevertheless been shown to form amorphous aggregates in a nucleation-dependent manner where the lag phase may involve metal loss or monomerization (Hwang et al. 2010). ApoS-S SOD1 may form amyloid- or non-amyloid-like aggregates with or without disulphide cross-linking depending on the solution conditions, and apo2SH SOD1 has been found to adopt the most diverse range of aggregate morphologies, including soluble aggregates under physiologically relevant conditions which may be particularly neurotoxic (Caughey and Lansbury 2003). Considering the influence of SOD1 mutations on the stability, unfolding and folding patterns of all forms of SOD, together with the diverse mechanisms of aggregation, different mutations may be influencing the protein in variable ways, resulting in a wide spectrum of effects. This diversity is likely to play a significant role in the variable disease courses for fALS patients with SOD1 mutations. Ultimately, the role of SOD1 in ALS may be similar to the roles of other globular, oligomeric proteins in misfolding diseases such as: transthyretin in familial amyloidotic polyneuropathy and senile systemic amyloidosis, lysozyme in hereditary non-neuropathic systemic amyloidosis, immunoglobulin light chain in monoclonal protein systemic amyloidosis, prion protein in Kreutzfeld Jakob, and serpins in serpinopathies (Ohnishi and Takano 2004; Harrison et al. 2007). In these diseases mutations are generally destabilizing, but the extent of destabilization of monomer versus subunit interfaces varies widely. The role of SOD1 in disease may be further complicated by the potential aberrant enzymatic activity of misfolded and/or aggregated species which could cause oxidative damage. In addition, it is worth considering the different roles of various types of SOD1 aggregate structures, or contributions of aberrant activity and the effects of these on other cellular components, at different stages throughout the disease course of ALS. For these reasons, it is important that future studies continue to consider the possible roles of multiple forms of SOD1 mutants in modulating the formation of different aggregate structures (Figure 4). A combination of further *in vitro* and *in vivo* studies of folding and aggregation will be critical for untangling the role of toxic aggregation in the syndrome of ALS.

6. Acknowledgements

We thank the ALS Society of Canada, Muscular Dystrophy Canada, and Canadian Institutes of Health Research for their financial support. Furthermore, we would like to express our appreciation to all the members of the Meiering group for their insightful and meaningful discussions, in particular Aron Broom, Martin Smith, Ming Sze Tong and Sarah M. Sullivan.

7. References

Alvarez, B., Demicheli, V., Duran, R., Trujillo, M., Cervenansky, C., Freeman, B. A. and Radi, R. (2004). "Inactivation of human Cu,Zn superoxide dismutase by peroxynitrite and formation of histidinyl radical." *Free Radic Biol Med* 37(6): 813-22.

Andersen, P. M. (2006). "Amyotrophic lateral sclerosis associated with mutations in the CuZn superoxide dismutase gene." *Curr Neurol Neurosci Rep* 6(1): 37-46.

Armstrong, R. A., Nochlin, D. and Bird, T. D. (2000). "Neuropathological heterogeneity in Alzheimer's disease: a study of 80 cases using principal components analysis." *Neuropathology* 20(1): 31-7.

Arnesano, F., Banci, L., Bertini, I., Martinelli, M., Furukawa, Y. and O'Halloran, T. V. (2004). "The unusually stable quaternary structure of human Cu,Zn-superoxide dismutase 1 is controlled by both metal occupancy and disulfide status." *J Biol Chem* 279(46): 47998-8003.

Bai, Y., Englander, J. J., Mayne, L., Milne, J. S. and Englander, S. W. (1995). "Thermodynamic parameters from hydrogen exchange measurements." *Methods Enzymol* 259: 344-56.

Baldwin, A. J., Knowles, T. P., Tartaglia, G., Fitzpatrick, A., Devlin, G., Shammas, S., Waudby, C. A., Mossuto, M. F., Gras, S. L., Christodoulou, J., Anthony-Cahill, S. J., Barker, P. D., Vendruscolo, M. and Dobson, C. M. (2011). "Metastability of Native Proteins and the Phenomenon of Amyloid Formation." *J Am Chem Soc.*

Banci, L., Benedetto, M., Bertini, I., Del Conte, R., Piccioli, M. and Viezzoli, M. S. (1998). "Solution structure of reduced monomeric Q133M2 copper, zinc superoxide dismutase (SOD). Why is SOD a dimeric enzyme?" *Biochemistry* 37(34): 11780-91.

Banci, L., Bertini, I., Blazevits, O., Cantini, F., Lelli, M., Luchinat, C., Mao, J. and Vieru, M. (2010). "NMR Characterization of a "Fibril-Ready" State of Demetalated Wild-Type Superoxide Dismutase." *J Am Chem Soc.*

Banci, L., Bertini, I., Boca, M., Calderone, V., Cantini, F., Girotto, S. and Vieru, M. (2009). "Structural and dynamic aspects related to oligomerization of apo SOD1 and its mutants." *Proc Natl Acad Sci U S A* 106(17): 6980-5.

Banci, L., Bertini, I., Boca, M., Girotto, S., Martinelli, M., Valentine, J. S. and Vieru, M. (2008). "SOD1 and amyotrophic lateral sclerosis: mutations and oligomerization." *PLoS One* 3(2): e1677.

Banci, L., Bertini, I., Cramaro, F., Del Conte, R. and Viezzoli, M. S. (2003). "Solution structure of Apo Cu,Zn superoxide dismutase: role of metal ions in protein folding." *Biochemistry* 42(32): 9543-53.

Banci, L., Bertini, I., D'Amelio, N., Gaggelli, E., Libralesso, E., Matecko, I., Turano, P. and Valentine, J. S. (2005). "Fully metallated S134N Cu,Zn-superoxide dismutase displays abnormal mobility and intermolecular contacts in solution." *J Biol Chem* 280(43): 35815-21.

Banci, L., Bertini, I., Durazo, A., Girotto, S., Gralla, E. B., Martinelli, M., Valentine, J. S., Vieru, M. and Whitelegge, J. P. (2007). "Metal-free superoxide dismutase forms soluble oligomers under physiological conditions: a possible general mechanism for familial ALS." *Proc Natl Acad Sci U S A* 104(27): 11263-7.

Bastos, A. F., Orsini, M., Machado, D., Mello, M. P., Nader, S., Silva, J. G., da Silva Catharino, A. M., de Freitas, M. R., Pereira, A., Pessoa, L. L., Sztajnbok, F. R., Leite, M. A., Nascimento, O. J. and Bastos, V. H. (2011). "Amyotrophic lateral sclerosis: one or multiple causes?" *Neurol Int* 3(1): e4.

Berryman, J. T., Radford, S. E. and Harris, S. A. (2009). "Thermodynamic description of polymorphism in Q- and N-rich peptide aggregates revealed by atomistic simulation." *Biophys J* 97(1): 1-11.

Bertini, I., Piccioli, M., Viezzoli, M. S., Chiu, C. Y. and Mullenbach, G. T. (1994). "A spectroscopic characterization of a monomeric analog of copper, zinc superoxide dismutase." *Eur Biophys J* 23(3): 167-76.

Boillee, S., Vande Velde, C. and Cleveland, D. W. (2006). "ALS: a disease of motor neurons and their nonneuronal neighbors." *Neuron* 52(1): 39-59.

Bosco, D. A., Morfini, G., Karabacak, N. M., Song, Y., Gros-Louis, F., Pasinelli, P., Goolsby, H., Fontaine, B. A., Lemay, N., McKenna-Yasek, D., Frosch, M. P., Agar, J. N., Julien, J. P., Brady, S. T. and Brown, R. H., Jr. (2010). "Wild-type and mutant SOD1 share an aberrant conformation and a common pathogenic pathway in ALS." *Nat Neurosci* 13(11): 1396-403.

Brown, N. M., Torres, A. S., Doan, P. E. and O'Halloran, T. V. (2004). "Oxygen and the copper chaperone CCS regulate posttranslational activation of Cu,Zn superoxide dismutase." *Proc Natl Acad Sci U S A* 101(15): 5518-23.

Bruening, W., Roy, J., Giasson, B., Figlewicz, D. A., Mushynski, W. E. and Durham, H. D. (1999). "Up-regulation of protein chaperones preserves viability of cells expressing toxic Cu/Zn-superoxide dismutase mutants associated with amyotrophic lateral sclerosis." *J Neurochem* 72(2): 693-9.

Bruijn, L. I., Houseweart, M. K., Kato, S., Anderson, K. L., Anderson, S. D., Ohama, E., Reaume, A. G., Scott, R. W. and Cleveland, D. W. (1998). "Aggregation and motor neuron toxicity of an ALS-linked SOD1 mutant independent from wild-type SOD1." *Science* 281(5384): 1851-4.

Bruijn, L. I., Miller, T. M. and Cleveland, D. W. (2004). "Unraveling the mechanisms involved in motor neuron degeneration in ALS." *Annu Rev Neurosci* 27: 723-49.

Bucciantini, M., Giannoni, E., Chiti, F., Baroni, F., Formigli, L., Zurdo, J., Taddei, N., Ramponi, G., Dobson, C. M. and Stefani, M. (2002). "Inherent toxicity of aggregates implies a common mechanism for protein misfolding diseases." *Nature* 416(6880): 507-11.

Bystrom, R., Andersen, P. M., Grobner, G. and Oliveberg, M. (2010). "SOD1 mutations targeting surface hydrogen bonds promote amyotrophic lateral sclerosis without reducing apo-state stability." *J Biol Chem* 285(25): 19544-52.

Caughey, B. and Lansbury, P. T., Jr. (2003). "Protofibrils, Pores, Fibrils, and Neurodegeneration: Separating the Responsibility Protein Aggregates from The Innocent Bystanders." *Annual Review of Neuroscience* 26: 267-298.

Chattopadhyay, M., Durazo, A., Sohn, S. H., Strong, C. D., Gralla, E. B., Whitelegge, J. P. and Valentine, J. S. (2008). "Initiation and elongation in fibrillation of ALS-linked superoxide dismutase." *Proc Natl Acad Sci U S A* 105(48): 18663-8.

Chattopadhyay, M. and Valentine, J. S. (2009). "Aggregation of Copper-Zinc Superoxide Dismutase in Familial and Sporadic ALS." *Antioxid Redox Signal.*

Chi, E. Y., Krishnan, S., Randolph, T. W. and Carpenter, J. F. (2003). "Physical stability of proteins in aqueous solution: mechanism and driving forces in nonnative protein aggregation." *Pharm Res* 20(9): 1325-36.

Chiti, F. and Dobson, C. M. (2006). "Protein misfolding, functional amyloid, and human disease." *Annu Rev Biochem* 75: 333-66.

Chiti, F. and Dobson, C. M. (2009). "Amyloid formation by globular proteins under native conditions." *Nat Chem Biol* 5(1): 15-22.

Chiti, F., Stefani, M., Taddei, N., Ramponi, G. and Dobson, C. M. (2003). "Rationalization of the effects of mutations on peptide and protein aggregation rates." *Nature* 424(6950): 805-8.

Chrunyk, B. A. and Wetzel, R. (1993). "Breakdown in the relationship between thermal and thermodynamic stability in an interleukin-1 beta point mutant modified in a surface loop." *Protein Eng* 6(7): 733-8.

Cozzolino, M., Ferri, A. and Carri, M. T. (2008). "Amyotrophic lateral sclerosis: from current developments in the laboratory to clinical implications." *Antioxid Redox Signal* 10(3): 405-43.

Crow, J. P., Sampson, J. B., Zhuang, Y., Thompson, J. A. and Beckman, J. S. (1997). "Decreased zinc affinity of amyotrophic lateral sclerosis-associated superoxide dismutase mutants leads to enhanced catalysis of tyrosine nitration by peroxynitrite." *J Neurochem* 69(5): 1936-44.

Cudkowicz, M. E., McKenna-Yasek, D., Sapp, P. E., Chin, W., Geller, B., Hayden, D. L., Schoenfeld, D. A., Hosler, B. A., Horvitz, H. R. and Brown, R. H. (1997).

"Epidemiology of mutations in superoxide dismutase in amyotrophic lateral sclerosis." *Ann Neurol* 41(2): 210-21.

Deng, H. X., Chen, W., Hong, S. T., Boycott, K. M., Gorrie, G. H., Siddique, N., Yang, Y., Fecto, F., Shi, Y., Zhai, H., Jiang, H., Hirano, M., Rampersaud, E., Jansen, G. H., Donkervoort, S., Bigio, E. H., Brooks, B. R., Ajroud, K., Sufit, R. L., Haines, J. L., Mugnaini, E., Pericak-Vance, M. A. and Siddique, T. (2011). "Mutations in UBQLN2 cause dominant X-linked juvenile and adult-onset ALS and ALS/dementia." *Nature.*

Deng, H. X., Hentati, A., Tainer, J. A., Iqbal, Z., Cayabyab, A., Hung, W. Y., Getzoff, E. D., Hu, P., Herzfeldt, B., Roos, R. P. and et al. (1993). "Amyotrophic lateral sclerosis and structural defects in Cu,Zn superoxide dismutase." *Science* 261(5124): 1047-51.

Ding, F. and Dokholyan, N. V. (2008). "Dynamical roles of metal ions and the disulfide bond in Cu, Zn superoxide dismutase folding and aggregation." *Proc Natl Acad Sci U S A* 105(50): 19696-701.

Dobson, C. M. (1999). "Protein misfolding, evolution and disease." *Trends Biochem Sci* 24(9): 329-32.

Dobson, C. M. (2003). "Protein folding and misfolding." *Nature* 426(6968): 884-90.

Dobson, C. M. (2004). "Principles of protein folding, misfolding and aggregation." *Semin Cell Dev Biol* 15(1): 3-16.

Eisenberg, D., Nelson, R., Sawaya, M. R., Balbirnie, M., Sambashivan, S., Ivanova, M. I., Madsen, A. O. and Riekel, C. (2006). "The structural biology of protein aggregation diseases: Fundamental questions and some answers." *Acc Chem Res* 39(9): 568-75.

Elam, J. S., Taylor, A. B., Strange, R., Antonyuk, S., Doucette, P. A., Rodriguez, J. A., Hasnain, S. S., Hayward, L. J., Valentine, J. S., Yeates, T. O. and Hart, P. J. (2003). "Amyloid-like filaments and water-filled nanotubes formed by SOD1 mutant proteins linked to familial ALS." *Nat Struct Biol* 10(6): 461-7.

Fink, A. L. (1998). "Protein aggregation: folding aggregates, inclusion bodies and amyloid." *Fold Des* 3(1): R9-23.

Forsberg, K., Andersen, P. M., Marklund, S. L. and Brannstrom, T. (2011). "Glial nuclear aggregates of superoxide dismutase-1 are regularly present in patients with amyotrophic lateral sclerosis." *Acta Neuropathol.*

Frost, B. and Diamond, M. I. (2009). "The expanding realm of prion phenomena in neurodegenerative disease." *Prion* 3(2): 74-7.

Furukawa, Y., Kaneko, K., Yamanaka, K. and Nukina, N. (2010). "Mutation-dependent polymorphism of Cu,Zn-superoxide dismutase aggregates in the familial form of amyotrophic lateral sclerosis." *J Biol Chem* 285(29): 22221-31.

Furukawa, Y., Kaneko, K., Yamanaka, K., O'Halloran, T. V. and Nukina, N. (2008). "Complete loss of post-translational modifications triggers fibrillar aggregation of SOD1 in the familial form of amyotrophic lateral sclerosis." *J Biol Chem* 283(35): 24167-76.

Furukawa, Y. and O'Halloran, T. V. (2005). "Amyotrophic lateral sclerosis mutations have the greatest destabilizing effect on the apo- and reduced form of SOD1, leading to unfolding and oxidative aggregation." *J Biol Chem* 280(17): 17266-74.

Furukawa, Y. and O'Halloran, T. V. (2006). "Posttranslational modifications in Cu,Zn-superoxide dismutase and mutations associated with amyotrophic lateral sclerosis." *Antioxid Redox Signal* 8(5-6): 847-67.

Getzoff, E. D., Tainer, J. A., Stempien, M. M., Bell, G. I. and Hallewell, R. A. (1989). "Evolution of CuZn superoxide dismutase and the Greek key beta-barrel structural motif." *Proteins* 5(4): 322-36.

Gidalevitz, T., Kikis, E. A. and Morimoto, R. I. (2010). "A cellular perspective on conformational disease: the role of genetic background and proteostasis networks." *Curr Opin Struct Biol* 20(1): 23-32.

Goedert, M., Spillantini, M. G., Serpell, L. C., Berriman, J., Smith, M. J., Jakes, R. and Crowther, R. A. (2001). "From genetics to pathology: tau and alpha-synuclein assemblies in neurodegenerative diseases." *Philos Trans R Soc Lond B Biol Sci* 356(1406): 213-27.

Goers, J., Permyakov, S. E., Permyakov, E. A., Uversky, V. N. and Fink, A. L. (2002). "Conformational prerequisites for alpha-lactalbumin fibrillation." *Biochemistry* 41(41): 12546-51.

Gruzman, A., Wood, W. L., Alpert, E., Prasad, M. D., Miller, R. G., Rothstein, J. D., Bowser, R., Hamilton, R., Wood, T. D., Cleveland, D. W., Lingappa, V. R. and Liu, J. (2007). "Common molecular signature in SOD1 for both sporadic and familial amyotrophic lateral sclerosis." *Proc Natl Acad Sci U S A* 104(30): 12524-9.

Hallewell, R. A., Imlay, K. C., Lee, P., Fong, N. M., Gallegos, C., Getzoff, E. D., Tainer, J. A., Cabelli, D. E., Tekamp-Olson, P., Mullenbach, G. T. and et al. (1991). "Thermostabilization of recombinant human and bovine CuZn superoxide dismutases by replacement of free cysteines." *Biochem Biophys Res Commun* 181(1): 474-80.

Harrison, R. S., Sharpe, P. C., Singh, Y. and Fairlie, D. P. (2007). "Amyloid peptides and proteins in review." *Rev Physiol Biochem Pharmacol* 159: 1-77.

Hayward, L. J., Rodriguez, J. A., Kim, J. W., Tiwari, A., Goto, J. J., Cabelli, D. E., Valentine, J. S. and Brown, R. H., Jr. (2002). "Decreased metallation and activity in subsets of mutant superoxide dismutases associated with familial amyotrophic lateral sclerosis." *J Biol Chem* 277(18): 15923-31.

Hol, E. M. and Scheper, W. (2008). "Protein quality control in neurodegeneration: walking the tight rope between health and disease." *J Mol Neurosci* 34(1): 23-33.

Hornberg, A., Logan, D. T., Marklund, S. L. and Oliveberg, M. (2007). "The coupling between disulphide status, metallation and dimer interface strength in Cu/Zn superoxide dismutase." *J Mol Biol* 365(2): 333-42.

Hough, M. A., Grossmann, J. G., Antonyuk, S. V., Strange, R. W., Doucette, P. A., Rodriguez, J. A., Whitson, L. J., Hart, P. J., Hayward, L. J., Valentine, J. S. and Hasnain, S. S. (2004). "Dimer destabilization in superoxide dismutase may result in disease-causing properties: structures of motor neuron disease mutants." *Proc Natl Acad Sci U S A* 101(16): 5976-81.

http://alsod.iop.kcl.ac.uk/.

Hwang, Y. M., Stathopulos, P. B., Dimmick, K., Yang, H., Badiei, H. R., Tong, M. S., Rumfeldt, J. A., Chen, P., Karanassios, V. and Meiering, E. M. (2010). "Nonamyloid aggregates arising from mature copper/zinc superoxide dismutases resemble those observed in amyotrophic lateral sclerosis." *J Biol Chem* 285(53): 41701-11.

Ilieva, H., Polymenidou, M. and Cleveland, D. W. (2009). "Non-cell autonomous toxicity in neurodegenerative disorders: ALS and beyond." *J Cell Biol* 187(6): 761-72.

Ip, P., Mulligan, V. K. and Chakrabartty, A. (2010). "ALS-causing SOD1 mutations promote production of copper-deficient misfolded species." *J Mol Biol* 409(5): 839-52.

Jackson, S. E. (1998). "How do small single-domain proteins fold? ." *Folding and Design* 3(4): R81-R91.

Jahn, T. R. and Radford, S. E. (2008). "Folding versus aggregation: polypeptide conformations on competing pathways." *Arch Biochem Biophys* 469(1): 100-17.

Johnston, J. A., Dalton, M. J., Gurney, M. E. and Kopito, R. R. (2000). "Formation of high molecular weight complexes of mutant Cu, Zn-superoxide dismutase in a mouse model for familial amyotrophic lateral sclerosis." *Proc Natl Acad Sci U S A* 97(23): 12571-6.

Jones, E. M. and Surewicz, W. K. (2005). "Fibril conformation as the basis of species- and strain-dependent seeding specificity of mammalian prion amyloids." *Cell* 121(1): 63-72.

Jonsson, P. A., Graffmo, K. S., Andersen, P. M., Brannstrom, T., Lindberg, M., Oliveberg, M. and Marklund, S. L. (2006). "Disulphide-reduced superoxide dismutase-1 in CNS of transgenic amyotrophic lateral sclerosis models." *Brain* 129(Pt 2): 451-64.

Karch, C. M. and Borchelt, D. R. (2008). "A limited role for disulfide cross-linking in the aggregation of mutant SOD1 linked to familial amyotrophic lateral sclerosis." *J Biol Chem* 283(20): 13528-37.

Karch, C. M., Prudencio, M., Winkler, D. D., Hart, P. J. and Borchelt, D. R. (2009). "Role of mutant SOD1 disulfide oxidation and aggregation in the pathogenesis of familial ALS." *Proc Natl Acad Sci U S A* 106(19): 7774-9.

Kato, S., Horiuchi, S., Liu, J., Cleveland, D. W., Shibata, N., Nakashima, K., Nagai, R., Hirano, A., Takikawa, M., Kato, M., Nakano, I. and Ohama, E. (2000). "Advanced glycation endproduct-modified superoxide dismutase-1 (SOD1)-positive inclusions are common to familial amyotrophic lateral sclerosis patients with SOD1 gene mutations and transgenic mice expressing human SOD1 with a G85R mutation." *Acta Neuropathol* 100(5): 490-505.

Kayatekin, C., Zitzewitz, J. A. and Matthews, C. R. (2008). "Zinc binding modulates the entire folding free energy surface of human Cu,Zn superoxide dismutase." *J Mol Biol* 384(2): 540-55.

Kayatekin, C., Zitzewitz, J. A. and Matthews, C. R. (2010). "Disulfide-reduced ALS variants of Cu, Zn superoxide dismutase exhibit increased populations of unfolded species." *J Mol Biol* 398(2): 320-31.

Kerman, A., Liu, H. N., Croul, S., Bilbao, J., Rogaeva, E., Zinman, L., Robertson, J. and Chakrabartty, A. (2010). "Amyotrophic lateral sclerosis is a non-amyloid disease in which extensive misfolding of SOD1 is unique to the familial form." *Acta Neuropathol* 119(3): 335-344.

Khare, S. D., Caplow, M. and Dokholyan, N. V. (2004). "The rate and equilibrium constants for a multistep reaction sequence for the aggregation of superoxide dismutase in amyotrophic lateral sclerosis." *Proc Natl Acad Sci U S A* 101(42): 15094-9.

Khare, S. D., Caplow, M. and Dokholyan, N. V. (2006). "FALS mutations in Cu, Zn superoxide dismutase destabilize the dimer and increase dimer dissociation propensity: a large-scale thermodynamic analysis." *Amyloid* 13(4): 226-35.

Knowles, T. P., Fitzpatrick, A. W., Meehan, S., Mott, H. R., Vendruscolo, M., Dobson, C. M. and Welland, M. E. (2007). "Role of intermolecular forces in defining material properties of protein nanofibrils." *Science* 318(5858): 1900-3.

Kurahashi, T., Miyazaki, A., Suwan, S. and Isobe, M. (2001). "Extensive investigations on oxidized amino acid residues in H(2)O(2)-treated Cu,Zn-SOd protein with LC-ESI-Q-TOF-MS, MS/MS for the determination of the copper-binding site." *J Am Chem Soc* 123(38): 9268-78.

Leitch, J. M., Yick, P. J. and Culotta, V. C. (2009). "The right to choose: multiple pathways for activating copper,zinc superoxide dismutase." *J Biol Chem* 284(37): 24679-83.

Lelie, H. L., Liba, A., Bourassa, M. W., Chattopadhyay, M., Chan, P. K., Gralla, E. B., Miller, L. M., Borchelt, D. R., Valentine, J. S. and Whitelegge, J. P. (2011). "Copper and zinc metallation status of copper-zinc superoxide dismutase from amyotrophic lateral sclerosis transgenic mice." *J Biol Chem* 286(4): 2795-806.

Lepock, J. R., Frey, H. E. and Hallewell, R. A. (1990). "Contribution of conformational stability and reversibility of unfolding to the increased thermostability of human and bovine superoxide dismutase mutated at free cysteines." *J Biol Chem* 265(35): 21612-8.

Lepock, J. R., Ritchie, K. P., Kolios, M. C., Rodahl, A. M., Heinz, K. A. and Kruuv, J. (1992). "Influence of transition rates and scan rate on kinetic simulations of differential scanning calorimetry profiles of reversible and irreversible protein denaturation." *Biochemistry* 31(50): 12706-12.

Lindberg, M. J., Normark, J., Holmgren, A. and Oliveberg, M. (2004). "Folding of human superoxide dismutase: disulfide reduction prevents dimerization and produces marginally stable monomers." *Proc Natl Acad Sci U S A* 101(45): 15893-8.

Liu, H. N., Sanelli, T., Horne, P., Pioro, E. P., Strong, M. J., Rogaeva, E., Bilbao, J., Zinman, L. and Robertson, J. (2009). "Lack of evidence of monomer/misfolded superoxide dismutase-1 in sporadic amyotrophic lateral sclerosis." *Ann Neurol* 66(1): 75-80.

Lynch, S. M., Boswell, S. A. and Colon, W. (2004). "Kinetic stability of Cu/Zn superoxide dismutase is dependent on its metal ligands: implications for ALS." *Biochemistry* 43(51): 16525-31.

Mahler, H. C., Friess, W., Grauschopf, U. and Kiese, S. (2009). "Protein aggregation: pathways, induction factors and analysis." *J Pharm Sci* 98(9): 2909-34.

McRee, D. E., Redford, S. M., Getzoff, E. D., Lepock, J. R., Hallewell, R. A. and Tainer, J. A. (1990). "Changes in crystallographic structure and thermostability of a Cu,Zn superoxide dismutase mutant resulting from the removal of a buried cysteine." *J Biol Chem* 265(24): 14234-41.

Meiering, E. M. (2008). "The threat of instability: neurodegeneration predicted by protein destabilization and aggregation propensity." *PLoS Biol* 6(7): e193.

Mitchell, J. D. and Borasio, G. D. (2007). "Amyotrophic lateral sclerosis." *Lancet* 369(9578): 2031-41.

Molnar, K. S., Karabacak, N. M., Johnson, J. L., Wang, Q., Tiwari, A., Hayward, L. J., Coales, S. J., Hamuro, Y. and Agar, J. N. (2009). "A common property of amyotrophic lateral sclerosis-associated variants: destabilization of the copper/zinc superoxide dismutase electrostatic loop." *J Biol Chem* 284(45): 30965-73.

Mouradian, M. M. (2002). "Recent advances in the genetics and pathogenesis of Parkinson disease." *Neurology* 58(2): 179-85.

Mulligan, V. K., Kerman, A., Ho, S. and Chakrabartty, A. (2008). "Denaturational stress induces formation of zinc-deficient monomers of Cu,Zn superoxide dismutase: implications for pathogenesis in amyotrophic lateral sclerosis." *J Mol Biol* 383(2): 424-36.

Munch, C. and Bertolotti, A. (2010). "Exposure of hydrophobic surfaces initiates aggregation of diverse ALS-causing superoxide dismutase-1 mutants." *J Mol Biol* 399(3): 512-25.

Munishkina, L. A., Henriques, J., Uversky, V. N. and Fink, A. L. (2004). "Role of protein-water interactions and electrostatics in alpha-synuclein fibril formation." *Biochemistry* 43(11): 3289-300.

Museth, A. K., Brorsson, A. C., Lundqvist, M., Tibell, L. A. and Jonsson, B. H. (2009). "The ALS-associated mutation G93A in human copper-zinc superoxide dismutase selectively destabilizes the remote metal binding region." *Biochemistry* 48(37): 8817-29.

Natalello, A., Prokorov, V. V., Tagliavini, F., Morbin, M., Forloni, G., Beeg, M., Manzoni, C., Colombo, L., Gobbi, M., Salmona, M. and Doglia, S. M. (2008). "Conformational plasticity of the Gerstmann-Straussler-Scheinker disease peptide as indicated by its multiple aggregation pathways." *J Mol Biol* 381(5): 1349-61.

Necula, M., Breydo, L., Milton, S., Kayed, R., van der Veer, W. E., Tone, P. and Glabe, C. G. (2007). "Methylene blue inhibits amyloid Abeta oligomerization by promoting fibrillization." *Biochemistry* 46(30): 8850-60.

Nelson, R. and Eisenberg, D. (2006). "Structural models of amyloid-like fibrils." *Adv Protein Chem* 73: 235-82.

Nordlund, A., Leinartaite, L., Saraboji, K., Aisenbrey, C., Grobner, G., Zetterstrom, P., Danielsson, J., Logan, D. T. and Oliveberg, M. (2009). "Functional features cause misfolding of the ALS-provoking enzyme SOD1." *Proc Natl Acad Sci U S A* 106(24): 9667-72.

Nordlund, A. and Oliveberg, M. (2006). "Folding of Cu/Zn superoxide dismutase suggests structural hotspots for gain of neurotoxic function in ALS: parallels to precursors in amyloid disease." *Proc Natl Acad Sci U S A* 103(27): 10218-23.

Ohnishi, S. and Takano, K. (2004). "Amyloid fibrils from the viewpoint of protein folding." *Cell Mol Life Sci* 61(5): 511-24.

Okado-Matsumoto, A. and Fridovich, I. (2002). "Amyotrophic lateral sclerosis: a proposed mechanism." *Proc Natl Acad Sci U S A* 99(13): 9010-4.

Otzen, D. E., Kristensen, O. and Oliveberg, M. (2000). "Designed protein tetramer zipped together with a hydrophobic Alzheimer homology: a structural clue to amyloid assembly." *Proc Natl Acad Sci U S A* 97(18): 9907-12.

Oztug Durer, Z. A., Cohlberg, J. A., Dinh, P., Padua, S., Ehrenclou, K., Downes, S., Tan, J. K., Nakano, Y., Bowman, C. J., Hoskins, J. L., Kwon, C., Mason, A. Z., Rodriguez, J. A., Doucette, P. A., Shaw, B. F. and Selverstone Valentine, J. (2009). "Loss of metal ions, disulfide reduction and mutations related to familial ALS promote formation of amyloid-like aggregates from superoxide dismutase." *PLoS One* 4(3): e5004.

Parge, H. E., Hallewell, R. A. and Tainer, J. A. (1992). "Atomic structures of wild-type and thermostable mutant recombinant human Cu,Zn superoxide dismutase." *Proc Natl Acad Sci U S A* 89(13): 6109-13.

Pasinelli, P. and Brown, R. H. (2006). "Molecular biology of amyotrophic lateral sclerosis: insights from genetics." *Nat Rev Neurosci* 7(9): 710-23.

Platt, G. W. and Radford, S. E. (2009). "Glimpses of the molecular mechanisms of beta2-microglobulin fibril formation in vitro: aggregation on a complex energy landscape." *FEBS Lett* 583(16): 2623-9.

Proctor, E. A., Ding, F. and Dokholyan, N. V. (2011). "Structural and thermodynamic effects of post-translational modifications in mutant and wild type Cu, Zn superoxide dismutase." *J Mol Biol* 408(3): 555-67.

Prudencio, M., Durazo, A., Whitelegge, J. P. and Borchelt, D. R. (2009). "Modulation of mutant superoxide dismutase 1 aggregation by co-expression of wild-type enzyme." *J Neurochem* 108(4): 1009-18.

Ramshini, H., Parrini, C., Relini, A., Zampagni, M., Mannini, B., Pesce, A., Saboury, A. A., Nemat-Gorgani, M. and Chiti, F. (2011). "Large proteins have a great tendency to aggregate but a low propensity to form amyloid fibrils." *PLoS One* 6(1): e16075.

Rodriguez, J. A., Shaw, B. F., Durazo, A., Sohn, S. H., Doucette, P. A., Nersissian, A. M., Faull, K. F., Eggers, D. K., Tiwari, A., Hayward, L. J. and Valentine, J. S. (2005). "Destabilization of apoprotein is insufficient to explain Cu,Zn-superoxide dismutase-linked ALS pathogenesis." *Proc Natl Acad Sci U S A* 102(30): 10516-21.

Rosen, D. R., Siddique, T., Patterson, D., Figlewicz, D. A., Sapp, P., Hentati, A., Donaldson, D., Goto, J., O'Regan, J. P., Deng, H. X. and et al. (1993). "Mutations in Cu/Zn superoxide dismutase gene are associated with familial amyotrophic lateral sclerosis." *Nature* 362(6415): 59-62.

Rousseau, F., Schymkowitz, J. and Oliveberg, M. (2008). "ALS precursor finally shaken into fibrils." *Proc Natl Acad Sci U S A* 105(48): 18649-50.

Rumfeldt, J. A., Lepock, J. R. and Meiering, E. M. (2009). "Unfolding and folding kinetics of amyotrophic lateral sclerosis-associated mutant Cu,Zn superoxide dismutases." *J Mol Biol* 385(1): 278-98.

Rumfeldt, J. A., Stathopulos, P. B., Chakrabarrty, A., Lepock, J. R. and Meiering, E. M. (2006). "Mechanism and thermodynamics of guanidinium chloride-induced denaturation of ALS-associated mutant Cu,Zn superoxide dismutases." *J Mol Biol* 355(1): 106-23.

Sakamoto, K. M. (2002). "Ubiquitin-dependent proteolysis: its role in human diseases and the design of therapeutic strategies." *Mol Genet Metab* 77(1-2): 44-56.

Sandelin, E., Nordlund, A., Andersen, P. M., Marklund, S. S. and Oliveberg, M. (2007). "Amyotrophic lateral sclerosis-associated copper/zinc superoxide dismutase mutations preferentially reduce the repulsive charge of the proteins." *J Biol Chem* 282(29): 21230-6.

Serpell, L. C. (2000). "Alzheimer's amyloid fibrils: structure and assembly." *Biochim Biophys Acta* 1502(1): 16-30.

Seshadri, S., Oberg, K. A. and Uversky, V. N. (2009). "Mechanisms and consequences of protein aggregation: the role of folding intermediates." *Curr Protein Pept Sci* 10(5): 456-63.

Shaw, B. F. and Valentine, J. S. (2007). "How do ALS-associated mutations in superoxide dismutase 1 promote aggregation of the protein?" *Trends Biochem Sci* 32(2): 78-85.

Shinder, G. A., Lacourse, M. C., Minotti, S. and Durham, H. D. (2001). "Mutant Cu/Zn-superoxide dismutase proteins have altered solubility and interact with heat shock/stress proteins in models of amyotrophic lateral sclerosis." *J Biol Chem* 276(16): 12791-6.

Shipp, E. L., Cantini, F., Bertini, I., Valentine, J. S. and Banci, L. (2003). "Dynamic properties of the G93A mutant of copper-zinc superoxide dismutase as detected by NMR spectroscopy: implications for the pathology of familial amyotrophic lateral sclerosis." *Biochemistry* 42(7): 1890-9.

Sicorello, A., Torrassa, S., Soldi, G., Gianni, S., Travaglini-Allocatelli, C., Taddei, N., Relini, A. and Chiti, F. (2009). "Agitation and high ionic strength induce amyloidogenesis of a folded PDZ domain in native conditions." *Biophys J* 96(6): 2289-98.

Sipe, J. D. and Cohen, A. S. (2000). "Review: history of the amyloid fibril." *J Struct Biol* 130(2-3): 88-98.

Smith, M. I., Sharp, J. S. and Roberts, C. J. (2007). "Nucleation and growth of insulin fibrils in bulk solution and at hydrophobic polystyrene surfaces." *Biophys J* 93(6): 2143-51.

Soto, C. and Estrada, L. D. (2008). "Protein misfolding and neurodegeneration." *Arch Neurol* 65(2): 184-9.

Stathopulos, P. B., Rumfeldt, J. A., Karbassi, F., Siddall, C. A., Lepock, J. R. and Meiering, E. M. (2006). "Calorimetric analysis of thermodynamic stability and aggregation for apo and holo amyotrophic lateral sclerosis-associated Gly-93 mutants of superoxide dismutase." *J Biol Chem* 281(10): 6184-93.

Stathopulos, P. B., Rumfeldt, J. A., Scholz, G. A., Irani, R. A., Frey, H. E., Hallewell, R. A., Lepock, J. R. and Meiering, E. M. (2003). "Cu/Zn superoxide dismutase mutants associated with amyotrophic lateral sclerosis show enhanced formation of aggregates in vitro." *Proc Natl Acad Sci U S A* 100(12): 7021-6.

Stathopulos, P. B., Scholz, G. A., Hwang, Y. M., Rumfeldt, J. A., Lepock, J. R. and Meiering, E. M. (2004). "Sonication of proteins causes formation of aggregates that resemble amyloid." *Protein Sci* 13(11): 3017-27.

Strange, R. W., Antonyuk, S., Hough, M. A., Doucette, P. A., Rodriguez, J. A., Hart, P. J., Hayward, L. J., Valentine, J. S. and Hasnain, S. S. (2003). "The structure of holo and metal-deficient wild-type human Cu, Zn superoxide dismutase and its relevance to familial amyotrophic lateral sclerosis." *J Mol Biol* 328(4): 877-91.

Strange, R. W., Yong, C. W., Smith, W. and Hasnain, S. S. (2007). "Molecular dynamics using atomic-resolution structure reveal structural fluctuations that may lead to polymerization of human Cu-Zn superoxide dismutase." *Proc Natl Acad Sci U S A* 104(24): 10040-4.

Svensson, A. K., Bilsel, O., Kondrashkina, E., Zitzewitz, J. A. and Matthews, C. R. (2006). "Mapping the folding free energy surface for metal-free human Cu,Zn superoxide dismutase." *J Mol Biol* 364(5): 1084-102.

Tainer, J. A., Getzoff, E. D., Beem, K. M., Richardson, J. S. and Richardson, D. C. (1982). "Determination and analysis of the 2 A-structure of copper, zinc superoxide dismutase." *J Mol Biol* 160(2): 181-217.

Tartaglia, G. G., Pawar, A. P., Campioni, S., Dobson, C. M., Chiti, F. and Vendruscolo, M. (2008). "Prediction of aggregation-prone regions in structured proteins." *J Mol Biol* 380(2): 425-36.

Teilum, K., Smith, M. H., Schulz, E., Christensen, L. C., Solomentsev, G., Oliveberg, M. and Akke, M. (2009). "Transient structural distortion of metal-free Cu/Zn superoxide dismutase triggers aberrant oligomerization." *Proc Natl Acad Sci U S A* 106(43): 18273-8.

Tiwari, A. and Hayward, L. J. (2003). "Familial amyotrophic lateral sclerosis mutants of copper/zinc superoxide dismutase are susceptible to disulfide reduction." *J Biol Chem* 278(8): 5984-92.

Tiwari, A., Liba, A., Sohn, S. H., Seetharaman, S. V., Bilsel, O., Matthews, C. R., Hart, P. J., Valentine, J. S. and Hayward, L. J. (2009). "Metal deficiency increases aberrant hydrophobicity of mutant superoxide dismutases that cause amyotrophic lateral sclerosis." *J Biol Chem* 284(40): 27746-58.

Tuite, M. F. and Serio, T. R. (2010). "The prion hypothesis: from biological anomaly to basic regulatory mechanism." *Nat Rev Mol Cell Biol* 11(12): 823-33.

Turner, B. J. and Talbot, K. (2008). "Transgenics, toxicity and therapeutics in rodent models of mutant SOD1-mediated familial ALS." *Prog Neurobiol* 85(1): 94-134.

Tycko, R. (2006). "Solid-state NMR as a probe of amyloid structure." *Protein Pept Lett* 13(3): 229-34.

Urushitani, M., Kurisu, J., Tsukita, K. and Takahashi, R. (2002). "Proteasomal inhibition by misfolded mutant superoxide dismutase 1 induces selective motor neuron death in familial amyotrophic lateral sclerosis." *J Neurochem* 83(5): 1030-42.

Uversky, V. N. and Dunker, A. K. (2010). "Understanding protein non-folding." *Biochim Biophys Acta* 1804(6): 1231-64.

Valentine, J. S., Doucette, P. A. and Zittin Potter, S. (2005). "Copper-zinc superoxide dismutase and amyotrophic lateral sclerosis." *Annu Rev Biochem* 74: 563-93.

Van Den Bosch, L. (2011). "Genetic rodent models of amyotrophic lateral sclerosis." *Journal of biomedicine & biotechnology* 348765.

Vande Velde, C., Miller, T. M., Cashman, N. R. and Cleveland, D. W. (2008). "Selective association of misfolded ALS-linked mutant SOD1 with the cytoplasmic face of mitochondria." *Proc Natl Acad Sci U S A* 105(10): 4022-7.

Vassall, K. A., Stathopulos, P. B., Rumfeldt, J. A., Lepock, J. R. and Meiering, E. M. (2006). "Equilibrium thermodynamic analysis of amyotrophic lateral sclerosis-associated mutant apo Cu,Zn superoxide dismutases." *Biochemistry* 45(23): 7366-79.

Vassall, K. A., Stubbs, H. R., Primmer, H. A., Tong, M. S., Sullivan, S. M., Sobering, R., Srinivasan, S., Briere, L. A., Dunn, S. D., Colon, W. and Meiering, E. M. (2011). "Decreased stability and increased formation of soluble aggregates by immature superoxide dismutase do not account for disease severity in ALS." *Proc Natl Acad Sci U S A* 108(6): 2210-5.

Verges, K. J., Smith, M. H., Toyama, B. H. and Weissman, J. S. (2011). "Strain conformation, primary structure and the propagation of the yeast prion [PSI+]." *Nat Struct Mol Biol* 18(4): 493-9.

Vetri, V. and Militello, V. (2005). "Thermal induced conformational changes involved in the aggregation pathways of beta-lactoglobulin." *Biophys Chem* 113(1): 83-91.

Vucic, S. and Kiernan, M. C. (2009). "Pathophysiology of neurodegeneration in familial amyotrophic lateral sclerosis." *Curr Mol Med* 9(3): 255-72.

Wang, Q., Johnson, J. L., Agar, N. Y. and Agar, J. N. (2008). "Protein aggregation and protein instability govern familial amyotrophic lateral sclerosis patient survival." *PLoS Biol* 6(7): e170.

Wijesekera, L. C. and Leigh, P. N. (2009). "Amyotrophic lateral sclerosis." *Orphanet J Rare Dis* 4: 3.

Williamson, J., Goldman, J. and Marder, K. S. (2009). "Genetic aspects of Alzheimer disease." *Neurologist* 15(2): 80-6.

Wyttenbach, A., Carmichael, J., Swartz, J., Furlong, R. A., Narain, Y., Rankin, J. and Rubinsztein, D. C. (2000). "Effects of heat shock, heat shock protein 40 (HDJ-2), and proteasome inhibition on protein aggregation in cellular models of Huntington's disease." *Proc Natl Acad Sci U S A* 97(6): 2898-903.

Zetterstrom, P., Stewart, H. G., Bergemalm, D., Jonsson, P. A., Graffmo, K. S., Andersen, P. M., Brannstrom, T., Oliveberg, M. and Marklund, S. L. (2007). "Soluble misfolded subfractions of mutant superoxide dismutase-1s are enriched in spinal cords throughout life in murine ALS models." *Proc Natl Acad Sci U S A* 104(35): 14157-62.

12

Oxidative Modifications of Cu, Zn-Superoxide Dismutase (SOD1) – The Relevance to Amyotrophic Lateral Sclerosis (ALS)

Seiichi Nagano
Department of Peripheral Nervous System Research, National Institute of Neuroscience, National Center of Neurology and Psychiatry
Japan

1. Introduction

Amyotrophic lateral sclerosis (ALS) is a fatal degenerative disease of motor neurons. About 10 % of ALS cases are affected in a familial trait, a subset of which is caused by the mutation of *Cu, Zn-superoxide dismutase (SOD1)* gene (Rosen et al., 1993). Since the identification of the gene for familial ALS, research emphasis for ALS has been placed on uncovering the pathogenic mechanism of motor neuronal death by the disease-causing mutant SOD1. So far over 150 different mutations of *SOD1* gene have been found in familial ALS patients, and they are scattered throughout the entire sequence of the gene regardless of specific functional domains. Transgenic mice that express mutant SOD1, but not wild type SOD1 nor SOD1 knockout mice, develop motor neuron disease, often while retaining normal dismutase activity (Gurney et al., 1994; Reaume et al., 1996). It means that mutant SOD1 gains a new aberrant toxic function apart from the primary enzymatic function of the protein, which has remained uncertain to date. Although the nature of mutant SOD1 toxicity has not been fully determined, conformational abnormalities of mutant SOD1 protein are deeply involved in the pathogenesis of familial ALS (Chattopadhyay & Valentine, 2009). Moreover, recent studies suggest that the phenotype of sporadic ALS also might be regulated by the conformational change of wild type SOD1 (Bosco et al., 2010). I review the recent concept of neuronal toxicity by oxidatively-modified SOD1, which is closely related to its conformational change, in ALS pathogenesis.

2. Cu-mediated oxidative toxicity by mutant SOD1

SOD1 is a major metal-binding enzyme expressed constitutively in tissues, and converts pro-oxidant superoxide radicals to hydrogen peroxide and oxygen (Valentine et al., 2005). In a metal-coordinated state, SOD1 forms homodimer to accomplish its full enzymatic activity. Each subunit coordinates one atom each of Cu and Zn. Cu is necessary for the enzymatic activity, whereas Zn mainly works to maintain the stable structure of the protein. Because Cu is catalytically redox-active and has a potential to oxidize proteins including SOD1 itself, inappropriate reactivity of Cu coordinated in SOD1 can underlie the conformational change of mutant SOD1. Inversely, conformational change in mutant SOD1 may increase the accessibility of substrates to Cu in the protein to generate reactive oxygen or nitrogen species. There is direct evidence that mutant SOD1 can promote abnormal pro-oxidant reactions cooperated with Cu. Mutant SOD1, unlike wild type SOD1, has a potential to generate hydroxyl radicals (Wiedau-Pazos et al., 1996; Yim et al., 1996) or peroxynitrite (Estevez et al., 1999) by Cu-dependent reaction *in vitro*, which can be inhibited by Cu chelators in cultured cells (Ghadge et al., 1997). Cu-mediated toxicity in mutant SOD1 is also reinforced with the reports that decreasing intracellular Cu, by treatment with Cu chelators or genetic reduction of Cu uptake, alleviates ALS phenotype in mutant SOD1 transgenic mice (Hottinger et al., 1997; Kiaei et al., 2004 ; Nagano et al., 2003; Tokuda et al., 2008). Moreover, metallothioneins, which bind Cu to prevent it from being pro-oxidant, are increased in the spinal cord of mutant SOD1 mice to attenuate the disease expression (Hashimoto et al., 2011; Nagano et al., 2001; Tokuda et al., 2007). These facts suggest that Cu-mediated oxidative chemistry underlies the pathogenesis of familial ALS linked to mutations of *SOD1* gene.

On the other hand, the phenotype of mutant SOD1 mice was not rescued by genetic removal of the Cu chaperone for SOD1 (CCS), which incorporates Cu into the buried active site of SOD1 (Subramaniam et al., 2002). Furthermore, mutant SOD1 still induces the disease in transgenic mice even when the active copper-binding site is totally disrupted by multiple mutations (Wang et al., 2003). These findings had been taken as evidence against the hypothesis of aberrant Cu chemistry in the toxicity of mutant SOD1. However, the theory implicating Cu toxicity cannot be excluded since ectopic binding of Cu away from the active site, for example, could contribute to the pathogenesis. In fact, H46R mutant SOD1, which disrupts Cu binding at the active site, still has the ectopic binding of Cu (Liu et al., 2000).

3. Increased affinity for Cu in mutant SOD1

To clarify a possible aberrant interaction of mutant SOD1 with Cu outside the active site in the context of familial ALS, we characterized the affinity for Cu of the mutants by immobilized metal affinity chromatography (IMAC), a method that separates proteins based on their affinities with an immobilized metal such as Cu (Watanabe et al., 2007). Mutant SOD1 commonly exhibited an aberrant fraction with **h**igh **a**ffinity for **C**u (SOD1HAC), in addition to that with **l**ow **a**ffinity for **C**u (SOD1LAC) seen in wild type SOD1 as well. SOD1HAC was detected whether the mutants were expressed in yeasts, mammalian cells or spinal cords of transgenic mice, while an unknown cellular factor(s) other than SOD1 was needed for its generation (Nagano, unpublished data). We observed SOD1HAC even in H46R or G85R mutant SOD1, the mutants that do not efficiently incorporate Cu into the active site, and therefore the immobilized Cu is likely to interact with SOD1 outside the active site, on a solvent-facing surface of the protein. Considering that mutant SOD1 is separated into two distinct fractions (SOD1LAC and HAC) and the interaction of proteins on IMAC is determined by topology of metal-coordinating residues on solvent-facing surfaces (Porath et al., 1975), conformational transition from the native to non-native state is implied to be critical for the increased affinity for Cu in SOD1HAC.

4. Monomerization of SOD1 by cysteine oxidation

Then what is the determinant of conformational transition for SOD1HAC in mutant SOD1? Human SOD1 has four cysteine residues—Cys6, Cys57, Cys111 and Cys146—in a subunit.

Two of them (Cys57 and Cys146) form an intramolecular disulfide bond that maintains the rigid structure and enzymatic activity of SOD1 protein, whereas the remaining two (Cys6 and Cys111) are present as cysteines having free sulfhydryl groups. Of the latter, Cys6 is deeply buried in the protein molecule and less accessible by substrates, while Cys111 is located on the surface of the protein near the dimer interface. Substitution of serine for Cys111 (C111S) is known to increase the structural stability and resistance to heat inactivation of wild type SOD1 (Lepock et al., 1990), implying that the mode of Cys111 may regulate the conformational state of mutant SOD1. H46R mutant SOD1, which has an ectopic binding to Cu as mentioned above, has been reported to bind the metal at Cys111 (Liu et al., 2000). We hypothesized that Cys111 might be a candidate site in human SOD1 that could enhance the coordination of the protein with immobilized Cu. Indeed, C111S substitution eliminated the increase of Cu binding in mutant SOD1. Moreover, the protein degradation assay in cell culture indicated that the decrease of SOD1HAC by C111S substitution well correlated with the stability of each mutant protein. That is, the stability was lower, the affinity for Cu was higher in mutant SOD1. In agreement with our findings, a previous report indicated that the decreased stability of mutant SOD1 correlated with its toxicity and the disease progression rate in familial ALS patients (Sato et al., 2005).

Next, to examine whether other cysteine residues play the same role as Cys111 in mutant SOD1, we introduced C57S substitution into the protein. In contrast to the effect of C111S, C57S substitution rather increased Cu binding, and did not rescue the instability of the mutant. C57S substitution prevents the disulfide bond between Cys57 and Cys146, which is supposed to make SOD1 protein difficult to keep its structure and stabilize. Although the function of the disulfide bond in SOD1 is not fully elucidated, it could be related to either the dimerization of SOD1 or the metal binding process at the active site or both. Thus, mutant SOD1 with C57S may become conformationally further destabilized, exposing Cu-interaction sites to enhance Cu affinity of the protein.

We performed further biochemical characterization of SOD1HAC and determined what properties could cause its formation and toxicity. Since mutant SOD1 is known to susceptible to intramolecular disulfide reduction (Tiwari & Hayward, 2003), we employed a cysteine-modifying reagent to estimate the redox status of cysteine residues in SOD1HAC. We found that sulfhydryl groups of free cysteine residues, especially of Cys111, were oxidized in SOD1HAC while the residues remained reduced in SOD1LAC (Kishigami et al., 2010). The intramolecular disulfide bond between Cys57 and Cys146 was unchanged in both components.

The dimeric structure of SOD1 is destabilized in pathogenic SOD1 mutants (Furukawa & O'Halloran, 2005). We therefore investigated the dimer/monomer status of SOD1LAC and SOD1HAC using gel filtration chromatography. SOD1HAC eluted predominantly as a monomer, whereas SOD1LAC consisted of a dimer structure. It means that SOD1HAC formation is concordant with the loss of dimeric stability to form a monomer.

We further employed nitrosoglutathione or hydrogen peroxide, cysteine-oxidizing reagents, in wild type SOD1 to mimic the sulfhydryl oxidation of Cys111 in SOD1HAC. We observed that the reaction actually modified Cys111, and engendered SOD1HAC. Moreover, we saw that Cys111-modified wild type SOD1 lost its dimeric conformation and mainly consisted of a monomer in SOD1HAC. Conversely, intersubunit crosslinking between Cys111 of each subunit prevented mutant SOD1 from monomerizing and developing SOD1HAC. These results mean that Cys111 is labile to be oxidized by endogenous agents such as nitrosoglutathione or hydrogen peroxide in familial ALS-linked mutant SOD1, which is the first step for the substantial monomerization of the protein and increase of the Cu affinity probably by exposing a Cu-accessible interface of the dimer.

5. Oxidative stress by cysteine-oxidized SOD1

In case that SOD1 is monomerized through conformational destabilization mediated by Cys111 oxidation, Cu coordinated at the ectopic binding site can be redox-active. To see whether SOD1HAC causes an aberrant redox reaction, we measured thiol oxidase activity, a Cu-dependent activity that is reported in human SOD1 (Winterbourn et al., 2002). We found that mutant or Cys111-oxidized wild type SOD1 developed the thiol oxidase activity when it was loaded with Cu, and that the activity was decreased by C111S substitution or intermolecular crosslinking of Cys111. Because SOD1 modified at Cys111 possesses the thiol oxidase activity, it is unlikely that Cys111 itself is the direct binding site for Cu. These results indicate that cysteine-oxidized SOD1 may exert the potentially toxic pro-oxidant activity through ectopic binding of Cu to SOD1HAC at a site within the dimer interface, which becomes exposed upon the dissociation of SOD1. The thiol oxidase activity of mutant SOD1 can promote oxidative stress because of the exhaustion of glutathione, the major free thiol and antioxidant. The activity may also oxidize cysteine residues of other proteins, deteriorating various cell functions (Fig. 1).

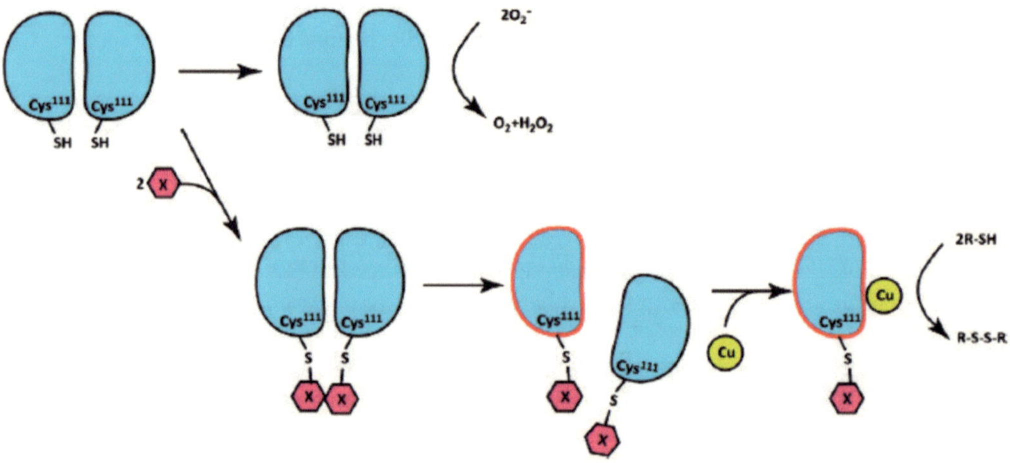

Fig. 1. Proposed model of mutant SOD1 toxicity. Modification of Cys111 leads to dissociation of SOD1 dimers into monomers. Cu, either resulting from rearrangement of the active site or from an external source, becomes ectopically bound to the former dimer interface surface, where it can now catalyze thiol oxidase activity (Kishigami et al., 2010).

6. Role of cysteine-oxidized mutant SOD1 in familial ALS

What is the role of Cys111 modification on the neuronal toxicity by mutant SOD1? In the spinal cords of familial ALS patients and mutant SOD1 transgenic mice, degenerating motor neurons contain SOD1-positive inclusion bodies, suggesting that mutant SOD1 is conformationally misfolded and subject to aggregate (Chattopadhyay & Valentine, 2009). As seen in other neurodegenerative diseases, abnormal protein accumulation in neurons can impair their cellular functions such as axonal transport (Tateno et al., 2009), oxidative phosphorylation in mitochondria and protein degradation machinery.

Various factors can cause conformational rearrangement or misfolding of mutant SOD1, including decreased metallation (Hayward et al., 2002), hydrophobicity (Tiwari et al., 2005) and reduction of repulsive charge (Sandelin et al., 2007). Modification of amino acid residues, especially by oxidative stress, can be a critical factor to enhance the misfolding of mutant SOD1 (Rakhit & Chakrabartty, 2006). Cysteine is in particular susceptible to oxidative modification, since its sulfhydryl moiety is readily attacked by redox active substrates such as glutathione or peroxides to form S-S or S-O covalent modification. Sulfhydryl groups also crosslink each other to form intra- or inter-molecular disulfide bond, which have important roles to maintain or disrupt physiological conformation of proteins. Oxidative reactivity and modification of Cys111, such as glutathionylation (Kajihara et al., 1988; Schinina et al., 1996) and peroxidation (Fujiwara et al., 2007), was documented with human or chick wild type SOD1, although the effect of which on the enzymatic activity or dimer stability had not been determined. Because Cys111 is located on the edge of the dimer interface of each subunit, the modification of Cys111, especially when a large molecule such as glutathione is adducted to the residue, can interrupt the dimer contact at the interface stereochemically and cause the dissociation of SOD1. Molecular dynamics simulations of SOD1 imply that the region including Cys111 is important for the residue interaction network in the protein, and likely to affect the dimer interface through the network and may disrupt their coupled motions (Khare & Dokholyan, 2006). In fact, glutathionylation of Cys111 has been confirmed with native human SOD1 in erythrocytes (Nakanishi et al., 1998; Wilcox et al., 2009), and it was noted that the modification caused SOD1 liable to monomerize and decrease its enzymatic activity (Wilcox et al., 2009). The SOD1 monomer is prone to form aggregates that might be the origin of intracellular inclusions found in motor neurons with SOD1-linked familial ALS. Supporting that, Cys111-peroxidized SOD1 was detected in the neuronal inclusions of mutant SOD1 mice (Fujiwara et al., 2007).

Oxidative modification of cysteine residues, including Cys111, is also possible to be involved in the aggregation process of mutant SOD1. High molecular weight dimers and multimers of mutant SOD1 can be detected in the spinal cords of transgenic mice in parallel to the disease onset (Deng et al., 2006; Furukawa et al., 2006). They are detergent-insoluble and reversed by reductants, supposing that disulfide-mediated crosslinking at cysteine residues is a major factor for mutant SOD1 to form aggregates and ALS phenotype. Cysteines forming the intramolecular disulfide bond (Cys57 and Cys146) are possibly involved in the crosslinking, since the disulfide bond between the residues is labile to be reduced (Tiwari & Hayward, 2003) and cause aberrant oxidation in mutant SOD1. The disulfide-reduced mutant SOD1 is actually enriched in the spinal cord of transgenic mice (Jonsson et al., 2006). The reduced form of mutant SOD1 can also translocate into the intermembrane space of mitochondria cooperated by CCS (Field et al., 2003), which may be components of aggregates in mitochondria (Deng et al., 2006; Ferri et al., 2006) and harmful to the mitochondrial function. However, intermolecular disulfide bonds mediated at free cysteines (Cys6 and Cys111) can also be components of the detergent-insoluble SOD1 aggregates (Banci et al., 2007; Niwa et al., 2007). In either case, apo SOD1 is more prone to the disulfide-linked oxidative aggregation than holo SOD1 (Banci et al., 2007; Furukawa & O'Halloran, 2005). That is in concert with the notion that immature SOD1 is the pathogenic species in familial ALS (Seetharaman et al., 2009).

It is still controversial whether the cysteine-mediated misfolding or aggregation of mutant SOD1 is the origin of the protein's toxicity. Removal of free cysteines, especially of Cys111, strongly reduced the ability of mutant SOD1 to form disulfide crosslinking and aggregates, and improved cell viability in cultured cells (Cozzolino et al., 2008; Niwa et al., 2007). Moreover, glutaredoxins, which specifically catalyze the reduction of protein-SSG-mixed disulfides, significantly increased the solubility of mutant SOD1 and protected neuronal cells (Cozzolino et al., 2008; Ferri et al., 2010). On the other hand, the intermolecular disulfide binding at cysteines is shown to have a limited effect on the aggregation of mutant SOD1 (Karch & Borchelt, 2008). Even in this case, Cys111-modified mutant SOD1 may cause neuronal toxicity independently of the aggregation, by oxidative stress such as thiol oxidase activity we have shown (Kishigami et al., 2010).

7. Role of cysteine-oxidized wild type SOD1 in sporadic ALS

In sporadic ALS, there had been no direct evidence that SOD1 was involved in the pathogenesis of the disease, except that some mutations of *SOD1* gene expressed familial ALS in a low penetration rate with seemingly 'sporadic' cases. The link between SOD1 and sporadic ALS was first introduced by the detection of SOD1 specifically modifiable with a chemical compound commonly in familial and sporadic ALS, although the molecular basis for it has not been determined in detail (Gruzman et al., 2007). It indicates that a similar conformational change in mutant and wild type SOD1 can trigger the phenotype of familial and sporadic ALS in common. In *in vitro* study, wild type SOD1 acquires toxic properties of mutant SOD1 through oxidation by hydrogen peroxide (Ezzi et al., 2007), implying that cysteine-oxidized wild type SOD1 may be a contributor to motor neuronal death in sporadic ALS.

Recently, a conformation-specific antibody generated against misfolded mutant SOD1 has been shown to recognize wild type SOD1 only when the protein was sulfonylated ($-SO_3H$) at Cys111, and the antibody immunostained motor neurons in the spinal cords of sporadic ALS patients, but not of SOD1-unrelated familial ALS patients or controls (Bosco et al., 2010). Chemically oxidized or purified wild type SOD1 from sporadic ALS spinal cords inhibited kinesin-based fast axonal transport as did mutant SOD1, supposing that Cys111-mediated conformational change or misfolding of SOD1 is a shared pathological denominator of familial and sporadic ALS. Interestingly, most of the sporadic ALS-derived toxic SOD1 was soluble and non-aggregated, meaning that misfolding or monomerization is sufficient for SOD1 to gain the toxic property such as oxidative insult we have shown in mutant and wild type SOD1 (Kishigami et al., 2010). Further studies *in vivo* will be required to clarify the detailed mechanism of SOD1 toxicity mediated by oxidation of cysteine residues including Cys111.

8. Conclusion

The findings mentioned above indicate that oxidative modification of SOD1 at cysteine residues is a critical factor to contribute to the oxidative stress, inclusion pathology and degeneration of motor neurons commonly to familial and sporadic ALS. Based on them, steric inhibition of cysteine oxidation, monomerization or exposure of the dimer interface can be the first-line treatment strategy of this incurable disease.

9. References

Banci, L.; Bertini, I.; Durazo, A.; Girotto, S.; Gralla, E.B.; Martinelli, M.; Valentine, J.S.; Vieru, M. & Whitelegge, J.P. (2007). Metal-free superoxide dismutase forms soluble oligomers under physiological conditions: A possible general mechanism for familial ALS. *Proceedings of the National Academy of Sciences of the United States of America,* Vol.104, No.27, pp. 11263-11267

Bosco, D.A.; Morfini, G.; Karabacak, N.M.; Song, Y.; Gros-Louis, F.; Pasinelli, P.; Goolsby, H.; Fontaine, B.A.; Lemay, N.; McKenna-Yasek, D.; Frosch, M.P.; Agar, J.N.; Julien, J.P.; Brady, S.T. & Brown R.H.J. (2010). Wild-type and mutant SOD1 share an aberrant conformation and a common pathogenic pathway in ALS. *Nature Neuroscience,* Vol.13, No.11, pp. 1396–1403

Chattopadhyay, M. & Valentine, J.S. (2009). Aggregation of copper-zinc superoxide dismutase in familial and sporadic ALS. *Antioxidants & Redox Signaling,* Vol.11, No.7, pp. 1603-1614

Deng, H.X.; Shi, Y.; Furukawa, Y.; Zhai, H.; Fu, R.; Liu, E.; Gorrie, G.H.; Khan, M.S.; Hung, W.Y.; Bigio, E.H.; Lukas, T.; Dal Canto, M.C.; O'Halloran, T.V. & Siddique, T. (2006). Conversion to the amyotrophic lateral sclerosis phenotype is associated with intermolecular linked insoluble aggregates of SOD1 in mitochondria. *Proceedings of the National Academy of Sciences of the United States of America,* Vol.103, No.18, pp. 7142-7147

Cozzolino, M.; Amori, I.; Pesaresi, M.G.; Ferri, A.; Nencini, M. & Carri, M.T. (2008). Cysteine 111 affects aggregation and cytotoxicity of mutant Cu,Zn-superoxide dismutase associated with familial amyotrophic lateral sclerosis. *Journal of Biological Chemistry,* Vol.283, No.2, pp. 866–874

Estevez, A.G.; Crow, J.P.; Sampson, J.B.; Reiter, C.; Zhuang, Y.; Richardson, G.J.; Tarpey, M.M.; Barbeito, L. & Beckman, J.S. (1999). Induction of nitric oxide-dependent apoptosis in motor neurons by zinc-deficient superoxide dismutase. *Science,* Vol.286, No.5449, pp. 2498–2500

Ezzi, S.A.; Urushitani, M. & Julien, J.P. (2007). Wild-type superoxide dismutase acquires binding and toxic properties of ALS-linked mutant forms through oxidation. *Journal of Neurochemistry,* Vol.102, No.1, pp. 170–178

Ferri, A.; Cozzolino, M.; Crosio, C.; Nencini, M.; Casciati, A.; Gralla, E.B.; Rotilio, G.; Valentine, J.S. & Carri, M.T. (2006). Familial ALS-superoxide dismutases associate with mitochondria and shift their redox potentials. *Proceedings of the National Academy of Sciences of the United States of America,* Vol.103, No.37, pp. 13860–13865

Ferri, A.; Fiorenzo, P.; Nencini, M.; Cozzolino, M.; Pesaresi, M.G.; Valle, C.; Sepe, S.; Moreno, S. & Carri, M.T. (2010). Glutaredoxin 2 prevents aggregation of mutant SOD1 in mitochondria and abolishes its toxicity. *Human Molecular Genetics,* Vol.19, No.22, pp. 4529-4542

Field, L.S.; Furukawa, Y.; O'Halloran, T.V. & Culotta, V.C. (2003). Factors controlling the uptake of yeast copper/zinc superoxide dismutase into mitochondria. *Journal of Biological Chemistry,* Vol.278, No.30, pp. 28052–28059

Fujiwara, N.; Nakano, M.; Kato, S.; Yoshihara, D.; Ookawara, T.; Eguchi, H.; Taniguchi, N. & Suzuki, K. (2007). Oxidative modification to cysteine sulfonic acid of Cys111 in human copper-zinc superoxide dismutase. *Journal of Biological Chemistry,* Vol.282, No.49, pp. 35933–35944

Furukawa, Y. & O'Halloran, T.V. (2005). Amyotrophic lateral sclerosis mutations have the greatest destabilizing effect on the apo- and reduced form of SOD1, leading to unfolding and oxidative aggregation. *Journal of Biological Chemistry,* Vol.280, No.17, pp. 17266-17274

Furukawa, Y.; Fu, R.; Deng, H.X.; Siddique, T. & O'Halloran, T.V. (2006). Disulfide cross-linked protein represents a significant fraction of ALS-associated Cu, Zn-superoxide dismutase aggregates in spinal cords of model mice. *Proceedings of the National Academy of Sciences of the United States of America,* Vol.103, No.18, pp. 7148-7153

Ghadge, G.D.; Lee, J.P.; Bindokas, V.P.; Jordan, J.; Ma, L.; Miller, R.J. & Roos, R.P. (1997). Mutant superoxide dismutase-1-linked familial amyotrophic lateral sclerosis: molecular mechanisms of neuronal death and protection. *Journal of Neuroscience,* Vol.17, No.22, pp. 8756-8766

Gruzman, A.; Wood, W.L.; Alpert, E.; Prasad, M.D.; Miller, R.G.; Rothstein, J.D.; Bowser, R.; Hamilton, R.; Wood, T.D.; Cleveland, D.W.; Lingappa, V.R. & Liu, J. (2007). Common molecular signature in SOD1 for both sporadic and familial amyotrophic lateral sclerosis. *Proceedings of the National Academy of Sciences of the United States of America,* Vol.104, No.30, pp. 12524-12529

Gurney, M.E.; Pu, H.; Chiu, A.Y.; Dal Canto, M.C.; Polchow, C.Y.; Alexander, D.D.; Caliendo, J.; Hentati, A.; Kwon, Y.W.; Deng, H.X.; Chen, W.; Zhai, P.; Sufit, R.L. & Siddique, T. (1994). Motor neuron degeneration in mice that express a human Cu,Zn superoxide dismutase mutation. *Science,* Vol.264, No.5166, pp. 1772-1775

Hashimoto, K; Hayashi, Y; Watabe, K; Inuzuka, T & Hozumi, I. (2011). Metallothionein-III prevents neuronal death and prolongs life span in amyotrophic lateral sclerosis model mice. *Neuroscience,* Vol.189, No.1, pp. 293-298

Hayward, L.J.; Rodriguez, J.A.; Kim, J.W.; Tiwari, A.; Goto, J.J.; Cabelli, D.E.; Valentine, J.S. & Brown, R.H.J. (2002). Decreased metallation and activity in subsets of mutant superoxide dismutases associated with familial amyotrophic lateral sclerosis. *Journal of Biological Chemistry,* Vol.277, No.18, pp. 15923-15931

Hottinger, A.F.; Fine, E.G.; Gurney, M.E.; Zurn, A.D. & Aebischer, P. (1997). The copper chelator d-penicillamine delays onset of disease and extends survival in a transgenic mouse model of familial amyotrophic lateral sclerosis. *European Journal of Neuroscence,* Vol.9, No.7, pp. 1548-1551

Jonsson, P.A.; Graffmo, K.S.; Andersen, P.M.; Brannstrom, T,; Lindberg, M.; Oliveberg, M. & Marklund, S.L. (2006). Disulphide-reduced superoxide dismutase-1 in CNS of transgenic amyotrophic lateral sclerosis models. *Brain,* Vol.129, No.2, pp. 451–464

Kajihara, J.; Enomoto, M.; Seya, K.; Sukenaga, Y. & Katoh, K. (1988). Physicochemical properties of charge isomers of recombinant human superoxide dismutase. *Journal of Biochemistry,* Vol.104, No.4, pp. 638-642

Karch, C.M. & Borchelt, D.R. (2008). A limited role for disulfide cross-linking in the aggregation of mutant SOD1 linked to familial amyotrophic lateral sclerosis. *Journal of Biological Chemistry,* Vol.283, No.20, pp. 13528–13537

Khare, S.D. & Dokholyan, N.V. (2006). Common dynamical signatures of familial amyotrophic lateral sclerosis-associated structurally diverse Cu, Zn superoxide dismutase mutants. *Proceedings of the National Academy of Sciences of the United States of America,* Vol.103, No.9, pp. 3147-3152

Kiaei, M.; Bush, A.I.; Morrison, B.M.; Morrison, J.H.; Cherny, R.A.; Volitakis, I.; Beal, M.F. & Gordon, J.W. (2004). Genetically decreased spinal cord copper concentration prolongs life in a transgenic mouse model of amyotrophic lateral sclerosis. *Journal of Neuroscience,* Vol.24, No.36, pp. 7945-7950

Kishigami, H.; Nagano, S.; Bush, A.I. & Sakoda, S. (2010). Monomerized Cu,Zn-superoxide dismutase induces oxidative stress through aberrant Cu binding. *Free Radical Biology & Medicine,* Vol.48, No.7, pp. 945–952

Lepock, J.R.; Frey, H.E. & Hallewell, R.A. (1990). Contribution of conformational stability and reversibility of unfolding to the increased thermostability of human and bovine superoxide dismutase mutated at free cysteines. *Journal of Biological Chemistry,* Vol.265, No.35, pp. 21612-21618

Liu, H.; Zhu, H.; Eggers, D.K.; Nersissian, A.M.; Faull, K.F.; Goto, J.J.; Ai, J.; Sanders-Loehr, J.; Gralla, E.B. & Valentine, J.S. (2000). Copper(2+) binding to the surface residue cysteine 111 of His46Arg human copper–zinc superoxide dismutase, a familial amyotrophic lateral sclerosis mutant. *Biochemistry,* Vol.39, No.28, pp. 8125–8132

Nagano, S.; Satoh, M.; Sumi, H.; Fujimura, H.; Tohyama, C.; Yanagihara, T. & Sakoda, S. (2001). Reduction of metallothioneins promotes the disease expression of familial amyotrophic lateral sclerosis mice in a dose-dependent manner. *European Journal of Neuroscience,* Vol.13, No.7, pp. 1363-1370

Nagano, S.; Fujii, Y.; Yamamoto, T.; Taniyama, M.; Fukada, K.; Yanagihara, T. & Sakoda, S. (2003). The efficacy of trientine or ascorbate alone compared to that of the combined treatment with these two agents in familial amyotrophic lateral sclerosis model mice. *Experimental Neurology,* Vol.179, No.2, pp. 176-180

Nakanishi, T.; Kishikawa, M.; Miyazaki, A.; Shimizu, A.; Ogawa, Y.; Sakoda, S.; Ohi, T. & Shoji, H. (1998). Simple and defined method to detect the SOD-1 mutants from patients with familial amyotrophic lateral sclerosis by mass spectrometry. *Journal of Neuroscience Methods,* Vol.81, No.1-2, pp. 41-44

Niwa, J.; Yamada, S.; Ishigaki, S.; Sone, J.; Takahashi, M.; Katsuno, M.; Tanaka, F.; Doyu, M. & Sobue, G. (2007). Disulfide bond mediates aggregation, toxicity, and ubiquitylation of familial amyotrophic lateral sclerosis-linked mutant SOD1. *Journal of Biological Chemistry,* Vol.282, No.38, pp. 28087-28095

Porath, J.; Carlsson, J.; Olsson, I. & Belfrage, G. (1975). Metal chelate affinity chromatography, a new approach to protein fractionation. *Nature,* Vol.258, No.5536, pp. 598–599

Rakhit, R. & Chakrabartty, A. (2006). Structure, folding, and misfolding of Cu,Zn superoxide dismutase in amyotrophic lateral sclerosis. *Biochimica et Biophysica Acta,* Vol.1762, No.11-12, pp. 1025-1037

Reaume, A.G.; Elliott, J.L.; Hoffman, E.K.; Kowall, N.W.; Ferrante, R.J.; Siwek, D.F.; Wilcox, H.M.; Flood, D.G.; Beal, M.F.; Brown R.H.J.; Scott, R.W. & Snider, W.D. (1996). Motor neurons in Cu/Zn superoxide dismutase-deficient mice develop normally but exhibit enhanced cell death after axonal injury. *Nature Genetics,* Vol.13, No.1, pp. 43–47

Rosen, D.R.; Siddique, T.; Patterson, D.; Figlewicz, D.A.; Sapp, P.; Hentati, A.; Donaldson, D.; Goto, J.; O'Regan, J.P.; Deng, H.X.; Rahmani, Z.; Krizus, A.; Mckenna-Yasek, D.; Cayabyab, A.; Gaston, S.M.; Berger, R.; Tanzi, R.E.; Halperin, J.J.; Herzfeldt, B.;Van Den Bergh, R.; Hung, W.Y.; Bird, T.; Deng, G.; Mulder, D.W.; Smyth, C.; Laing, N.G.; Soriano, E.; Pericak–Vance, M.A.; Haines, J.; Rouleau, G.A.; Gusella, J.S.; Horvitz, H.R. & Brown, R.H.J. (1993). Mutations in Cu/Zn superoxide dismutase gene are associated with familial amyotrophic lateral sclerosis. *Nature,* Vol.362, No.6415, pp. 59–62

Sandelin, E.; Nordlund, A.; Andersen, P.M.; Marklund, S.S. & Oliveberg, M. (2007). Amyotrophic lateral sclerosis-associated copper/zinc superoxide dismutase mutations preferentially reduce the repulsive charge of the proteins. *Journal of Biological Chemistry,* Vol.282, No.29, pp. 21230-21236

Seetharaman, S.V.; Prudencio, M.; Karch, C.; Holloway, S.P.; Borchelt, D.R. & Hart, P.J. (2009). Immature copper-zinc superoxide dismutase and familial amyotrophic lateral sclerosis. *Experimental Biology and Medicine,* Vol.234, No.10, pp. 1140–1154

Sato, T.; Nakanishi, T.; Yamamoto, Y.; Andersen, P.M.; Ogawa, Y.; Fukada, K.; Zhou, Z.; Aoike, F.; Sugai, F.; Nagano, S.; Hirata, S.; Ogawa, M.; Nakano, R.; Ohi, T.; Kato, T.; Nakagawa, M.; Hamasaki, T.; Shimizu, A. & Sakoda, S. (2005). Rapid disease progression correlates with instability of mutant SOD1 in familial ALS. *Neurology,* Vol.65, No.12, pp. 1954-1957

Schinina, M.E.; Carlini, P.; Polticelli, F.; Zappacosta, F.; Bossa, F. & Calabrese L. (1996). Amino acid sequence of chicken Cu, Zn-containing superoxide dismutase and identification of glutathionyl adducts at exposed cysteine residues. *European Journal of Biochemistry,* Vol.237, No.2, pp. 433–439

Subramaniam, J.R.; Lyons, W.E.; Liu, J.; Bartnikas, T.B.; Rothstein, J.; Price, D.L.; Cleveland, D.W.; Gitlin, J.D. & Wong, P.C. (2002). Mutant SOD1 causes motor neuron disease independent of copper chaperone-mediated copper loading. *Nature Neuroscience,* Vol.5, No.4, pp. 301–307

Tateno, M.; Kato, S.; Sakurai, T.; Nukina, N.; Takahashi, R. & Araki, T. (2009). Mutant SOD1 impairs axonal transport of choline acetyltransferase and acetylcholine release by sequestering KAP3. *Human Molecular Genetics,* Vol.18, No.5, pp. 942-955

Tiwari, A. & Hayward, L.J. (2003). Familial amyotrophic lateral sclerosis mutants of copper/zinc superoxide dismutase are susceptible to disulfide reduction. *Journal of Biological Chemistry,* Vol.278, No.8, pp. 5984–5992

Tiwari, A.; Xu, Z. & Hayward, L.J. (2005). Aberrantly increased hydrophobicity shared by mutants of Cu,Zn-superoxide dismutase in familial amyotrophic lateral sclerosis. *Journal of Biological Chemistry,* Vol.280, No.33, pp. 29771-29779

Tokuda, E.; Ono, S.; Ishige, K.; Naganuma, A.; Ito, Y. & Suzuki, T. (2007). Metallothionein proteins expression, copper and zinc concentrations, and lipid peroxidation level in a rodent model for amyotrophic lateral sclerosis. *Toxicology,* Vol.229, No.1-2, pp. 33-41

Tokuda, E.; Ono, S.; Ishige, K.; Watanabe, S.; Okawa, E.; Ito, Y. & Suzuki, T. (2008). Ammonium tetrathiomolybdate delays onset, prolongs survival, and slows progression of disease in a mouse model for amyotrophic lateral sclerosis. *Experimental Neurology,* Vol.213, No.1, pp. 122-128.

Valentine, J.S.; Doucette, P.A. & Zittin Potter, S. (2005). Copper-zinc superoxide dismutase and amyotrophic lateral sclerosis. *Annual Review of Biochemistry,* Vol.74, No.1, pp. 563-593

Wang, J.; Slunt, H.; Gonzales, V.; Fromholt, D.; Coonfield, M.; Copeland, N.G.; Jenkins, N.A. & Borchelt, D.R. (2003). Copper-binding-site-null SOD1 causes ALS in transgenic mice: aggregates of non-native SOD1 delineate a common feature. *Human Molecular Genetics,* Vol.12, No.21, pp. 2753-64

Watanabe, S.; Nagano, S.; Duce, J.; Kiaei, M.; Li, Q.X.; Tucker, S.M.; Tiwari, A.; Brown, R.H.J.; Beal, M.F.; Hayward, L.J.; Culotta, V.C.; Yoshihara, S.; Sakoda, S. & Bush, A.I. (2007). Increased affinity for copper mediated by cysteine 111 in forms of mutant superoxide dismutase 1 linked to amyotrophic lateral sclerosis. *Free Radical Biology & Medicine,* Vol.42, No.10, pp. 1534–1542

Wiedau-Pazos, M.; Goto, J.J.; Rabizadeh, S.; Gralla, E.B.; Roe, J.A.; Lee, M.K.; Valentine, J.S. & Bredesen, D.E. (1996). Altered reactivity of superoxide dismutase in familial amyotrophic lateral sclerosis. *Science,* Vol.271, No.5248, pp. 515–518

Wilcox, K.C.; Zhou, L.; Jordon, J.K.; Huang, Y.; Yu, Y.; Redler, R.L.; Chen, X.; Caplow, M. & Dokholyan, N.V. (2009). Modifications of superoxide dismutase (SOD1) in human erythrocytes: a possible role in amyotrophic lateral sclerosis. *Journal of Biological Chemistry,* Vol.284, No.20, pp. 13940-13947

Winterbourn, C.C.; Peskin, A.V. & Parsons-Mair, H.N. (2002). Thiol oxidase activity of copper, zinc superoxide dismutase. *Journal of Biological Chemistry,* Vol.277, No.3, pp. 1906-1911

Yim, M.B.; Kang, J.H.; Yim, H.S.; Kwak, H.S.; Chock, P.B. & Stadtman, E.R. (1996). A gain-of-function of an amyotrophic lateral sclerosis-associated Cu,Zn-superoxide dismutase mutant: an enhancement of free radical formation due to a decrease in Km for hydrogen peroxide. *Proceedings of the National Academy of Sciences of the United States of America,* Vol.93, No.12, pp. 5709–5714

13

Reactive Nitrogen Species in Motor Neuron Apoptosis

María Clara Franco and Alvaro G. Estévez
Burnett School of Biomedical Sciences, College of Medicine, University of Central Florida, Orlando, USA

1. Introduction

Nitric oxide is a cellular messenger produced by different cell types in an organism, both in physiological and pathological conditions (Snyder 1993; Beckman and Koppenol 1996; Beckman and Koppenol 1996; Beckman 1996; Colasanti and Suzuki 2000; Pacher, Beckman, and Liaudet 2007). Nitric oxide was first described in biology as the endothelium-derived relaxation factor for its effects on vasodilatation (Ignarro 1990), but soon become evident it have other important physiological functions such as a retrograde messenger in the nervous systems, and during the immune response (Moncada, Palmer, and Higgins 1991). Nitric oxide can also regulate mitochondria respiration (Carreras and Poderoso 2007; Ramachandran et al. 2002), and reacts with oxygen and reactive oxygen species to form reactive nitrogen species, which in turn can damage the cells. The reactivity of nitric oxide and the metabolic state of the cell or tissue are determining factors on the specific actions mediated by nitric oxide. It is not our intention to examine the biochemistry and physiology of nitric oxide, which has been cover in several excellent reviews (Beckman and Crow 1993; Beckman 1996; Pacher, Beckman, and Liaudet 2007), but to concentrate in those nitric oxide-derivate species relevant to the regulation of motor neuron apoptosis. However, some relevant aspects of the biochemistry of nitric oxide will be reviewed as the necessary background to understand the biology of reactive nitrogen species in motor neurons.

2. Peroxynitrite

One important reaction of nitric oxide is with superoxide (another free radical) to produce the strong oxidant peroxynitrite (Beckman et al. 1990). The importance of this reaction is highlighted by its diffusion-limited rate (between 6.7×10^9 and 2×10^{10} $M^{-1}s^{-1}$)(Padmaja and Huie 1993; Nauser and Koppenol 2002), meaning that every collision of a molecule of nitric oxide with a molecule of superoxide results in the formation of peroxynitrite (Fig 1). In other words, peroxynitrite will be formed when superoxide and nitric oxide are formed simultaneously. The reason peroxynitrite is not formed in large amounts in normal metabolic conditions is the high intracellular concentration of the enzyme superoxide dismutase (SOD)(Rae et al. 1999), which competes for the superoxide with a rate of 2×10^9 $M^{-1}s^{-1}$ (Pacher, Beckman, and Liaudet 2007) (Fig 1). Briefly, when the concentration of nitric oxide is 5 times lower than the concentration of SOD, approximately 50% of the superoxide produced would react with nitric oxide to form peroxynitrite. In normal conditions, the intracellular concentration of SOD is in large excess of the concentrations of nitric oxide (Beckman and Koppenol 1996). However, the prediction from the rates is that a small amount of peroxynitrite will always be formed, allowing the speculation that the oxidant may have a physiological function (Go et al. 1999), or otherwise it is efficiently scavenged by small molecular weight antioxidants such as glutathione with rates in the order of 10^3-10^4 $M^{-1}s^{-1}$ (Radi et al. 1991; Alvarez et al. 1999). Other important aspect of the competition between SOD and nitric oxide for superoxide is the presence of membrane cellular compartments, which limit the diffusion of SOD and superoxide but not nitric oxide. SOD can only compete with nitric oxide when the enzyme is in the same compartment than superoxide is being produced, indicating that peroxynitrite can be formed with relatively high efficiency even at low nitric oxide concentrations if superoxide is formed in a compartment SOD cannot access or where the enzyme has been inactivated (Fig 1).

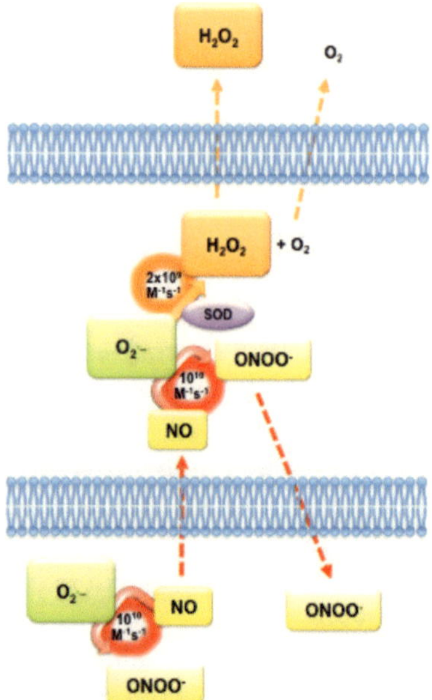

Fig. 1. In the cells, peroxynitrite formation depends on the levels of SOD that competes with nitric oxide for superoxide. Because cellular membranes (in blue) limit the diffusion of SOD and superoxide but not nitric oxide, peroxynitrite formation is also limited by the subcellular localization of the superoxide sources.

In pathological conditions, not only low micromolar concentrations of nitric oxide can be produced, but production of superoxide can also be boosted, increasing the probability for peroxynitrite formation at levels that may overwhelm the intracellular antioxidant defenses (Beckman and Crow 1993; Beckman and Koppenol 1996). Peroxynitrite affects normal cell metabolism by inducing lipid peroxidation (Radi et al. 1991), damage of the DNA (Groves and Marla 1995), and alteration of the mitochondrial function (Radi et al. 2002). In addition, it has been shown that peroxynitrite inhibits the activity in some proteins such as the tyrosine hydroxylase (Ara et al. 1998), mitochondrial manganese SOD, and tyrosine phosphatases (Takakura et al. 1999), activates src kinase (MacMillan-Crow et al. 2000) and alters the functionality of structural proteins such as neurofilament L, synuclein, actin, and tubulin (Aslan et al. 2003; Cappelletti et al. 2003; Eiserich et al. 1999; Chang et al. 2002; Crow et al. 1997; Paxinou et al. 2001). Changes in protein function are caused by oxidative modifications of amino acid residues by peroxynitrite (Alvarez et al. 1999). In the case of phosphatases and zinc-thiolate-containing proteins the oxidation of methionine and cysteine residues is critical for the loss of function of the enzymes (Takakura et al. 1999; Crow, Beckman, and McCord 1995). One particular modification of amino acids by peroxynitrite that has driven much attention is the nitration of tyrosine residues (Beckman et al. 1992). The interest is driven by the fact that nitrotyrosine seems to be a universal marker for inflammation and has been detected in a large number of pathological conditions (Ischiropoulos 1998; Greenacre and Ischiropoulos 2001; Ischiropoulos and Beckman 2003; Schopfer, Baker, and Freeman 2003; Radi 2004). It is accepted that nitration by the formation of the decomposition products of peroxynitrite is a major source of biological nitration, in spite that other mechanisms for tyrosine nitration have been described (Ischiropoulos 1998; Radi 2004; Schopfer, Baker, and Freeman 2003) (Fig 2).

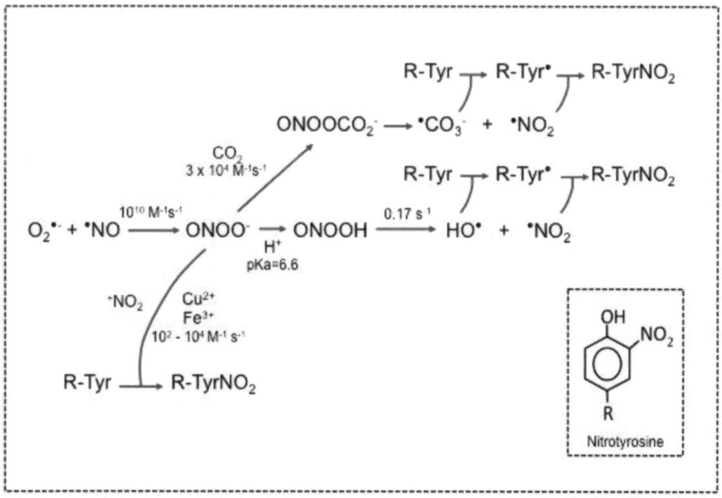

Fig. 2. Mechanisms for tyrosine nitration by the nitrative products of decomposition of peroxynitrite in the cells.

3. Peroxynitrite and apoptosis

Unsurprisingly, peroxynitrite induces apoptosis or necrosis depending on the concentration of the oxidant (Bonfoco et al. 1995; Estévez et al. 1995), and it has become the accepted mechanism for the toxic effects of nitric oxide in biological systems (Dawson and Dawson 1996; Dawson and Dawson 1996; Dawson and Dawson 1996; Beckman and Koppenol 1996). Although growing evidence suggests that peroxynitrite induces apoptosis by interacting with specific cellular signaling pathways (Estévez et al. 1995; Shin et al. 1996; Spear, Estévez, Barbeito, et al. 1997; Spear, Estévez, Radi, et al. 1997; Shacka et al. 2006; Ye et al. 2007) (Fig 3), the cellular targets responsible for peroxynitrite-induced apoptosis remain unknown. In addition, most studies were performed using exogenously applied stock solutions of pure peroxynitrite or peroxynitrite donors (Bonfoco et al. 1995; Estévez et al. 1995).

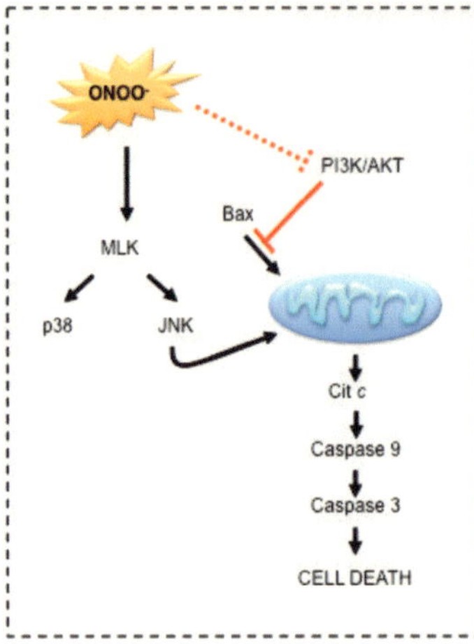

Fig. 3. Cell death-pathway induced by peroxynitrite in PC12 cells.

4. Motor neuron death and peroxynitrite *in vivo*

More recently, cultured motor neurons have become one of the best-described models for apoptosis induced by endogenous peroxynitrite (Estévez, Spear, Manuel, Radi, et al. 1998; Estévez, Spear, Manuel, Barbeito, et al. 1998; Estévez et al. 2000; Sendtner et al. 2000; Raoul et al. 2002; Raoul, Pettmann, and Henderson 2000; Kaal et al. 2000; Bar 2000). Motor neurons are large neurons located in the ventral spinal cord and brain stem responsible for the stimulation of muscle contraction. Motor neuron survival is highly dependent on trophic factors (Oppenheim 1991; Oppenheim 1996; Sendtner et al. 2000). Chronic administration of trophic factors prevents avian and mammalian motor neurons death during the period of programmed cell death (Neff et al. 1993) and motor neuron apoptosis induced by axon injury in mammals (Yan, Elliott, and Snider 1992; Li et al. 1994; Novikov, Novikova, and Kellerth 1995; Pennica et al. 1996). Remarkably, motor neurons induce the expression of neuronal NOS and the p75 neurotrophin receptor after injury (Wu 1993). Trophic factors such as BDNF, and nerve grafts prevent the induction of neuronal NOS and motor neuron death (Wu et al. 1994; Novikov, Novikova, and Kellerth 1995). Furthermore, inhibition of NOS activity prevents motor neuron death induced by axonal injury (Wu and Li 1993; Casanovas et al. 1996), suggesting that induction of motor neuron death after axonal injury may result from trophic factor deprivation leading to the induction of neuronal NOS as well as nitric oxide and peroxynitrite production, evidenced by the increase levels of nitrotyrosine in motor neurons after axotomy (Martin, Kaiser, and Price 1999).

5. Motor neuron apoptosis *in vitro*

Motor neuron survival in culture can be supported by a large number of trophic factors (Oppenheim 1996; Hughes, Sendtner, and Thoenen 1993), which also induce the extension of long and branched neurites. As many other cells in culture, trophic factor-deprived motor neurons undergo protein synthesis and caspase-dependent apoptosis (Milligan, Oppenheim, and Schwartz 1994; Milligan et al. 1995; Estévez, Spear, Manuel, Radi, et al. 1998; Estévez et al. 2000) (Fig 4).

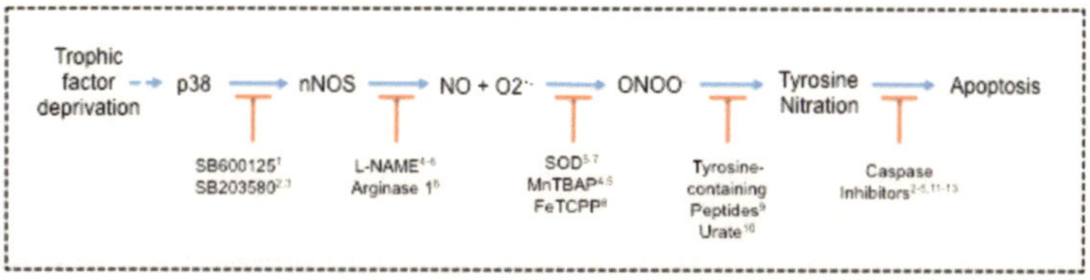

Fig. 4. Motor neuron apoptosis induced by trophic factor deprivation. Induction of motor neuron apoptosis by trophic factor deprivation is prevented by inhibition of JNK and p38 MAP kinases. The induction of neuronal NOS (nNOS) is regulated by the activation of p38 and responsible for the production of nitric oxide. Nitric oxide reacts with superoxide to form peroxynitrite. Inhbition of tyrosine nitration by peroxynitrite using tyrosine-containing peptides is enough to prevent apoptosis induced by trophic factor deprivation. Caspase inhbitors also prevented apoptosis mediated by trophic factors deprivation. [1](Ricart et al., 2006); [2](Raoul et al., 1999b); [3](Raoul et al., 2002); [4](Estévez et al., 1998); [5](Estévez et al., 2000); [6](Estevez et al., 2006); [7](Estévez et al., 1999); [8](Peluffo et al., 2004); [9](Ye et al., 2007); [10](Cassina et al., 2002); [11](Milligan et al., 1995); [12](Li et al., 1998); [13](Li et al., 2001)

Apoptosis induced by trophic factor deprivation is preceded by the induction of Fas ligand expression and prevented, at least in part, by inhibition of Fas and caspase 8 (Raoul, Henderson, and Pettmann 1999). In the presence of trophic factors, Fas activates two parallel pathways leading to motor neuron apoptosis by a mechanism similar to trophic factor deprivation (Raoul et al. 2002)(Fig 5).

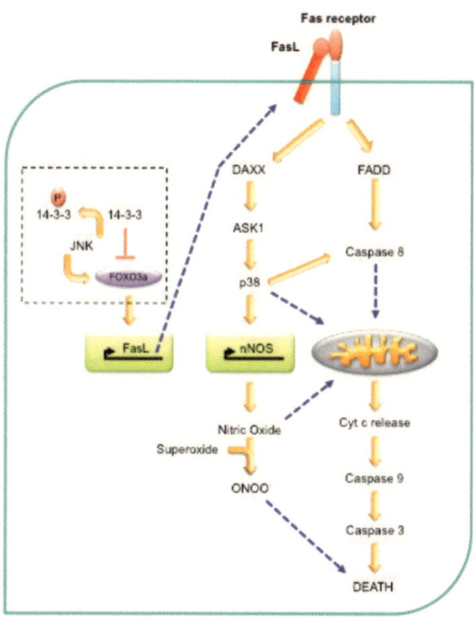

Fig. 5. In motor neurons, the activation of the Fas pathway leads to the simultaneous activation of the FADD and DAXX components of the pathway. Downstream of DAXX, p38 induces the expression of nNOS leading to the formation of peroxynitrite while activation of FADD leads to activation of caspases. Upon activation of Fas, both pathways participate simoultaneously in the induction of cell death. Inhibition of JNK may be upstream of the Fas pathway through activation of the transcription factor FOXO3a and transcription of FasL.

Motor neuron apoptosis induced by trophic factor deprivation is also dependent on the expression of neuronal NOS and the production of nitric oxide (Estévez, Spear, Manuel, Radi, et al. 1998; Estévez, Spear, Manuel, Barbeito, et al. 1998; Estévez et al. 2000; Raoul et al. 2002; Raoul et al. 2005). Either inhibition of nitric oxide production or scavenging of superoxide with Cu,Zn SOD prevents motor neuron apoptosis induced by trophic factor deprivation up to seven days after plating (Estévez et al. 2000). The protective effects of NOS inhibition are reverted by steady state concentrations of exogenous nitric oxide as low as 80 nM (Estévez et al. 2000). Remarkably, 7 days old motor neuron cultures undergo apoptosis when deprived of trophic factors by a mechanism indistinguishably from the cell death induced by plating motor neurons in the absence of trophic factors (Estévez et al. 2000). These results reveal that production of nitric oxide or superoxide alone is not sufficient for the induction of motor neuron apoptosis by trophic factor deprivation (Estévez et al. 2000; Estévez, Spear, Manuel, Radi, et al. 1998; Raoul et al. 2002; Raoul et al. 2005). In addition, an increase in nitrotyrosine immunoreactivity is detected in motor neurons deprived of trophic factors suggesting peroxynitrite formation (Estévez, Spear, Manuel, Radi, et al. 1998; Raoul et al. 2002)(Fig 4).

Inhibition of the JNK MAP kinase activity blocks trophic factor deprivation-induced apoptosis, but has not effect on motor neuron apoptosis induced by Fas activation (Raoul et al. 2002; Ricart et al. 2006; Li, Oppenheim, and Milligan 2001; Newbern et al. 2007). Activation of JNK leads to the phosphorylation of transcription factors and the induction of protein synthesis and might induce the expression of Fas ligand (Le-Niculescu et al. 1999; Morishima et al. 2001), suggesting that JNK activation may be upstream of Fas activation (Barthelemy, Henderson, and Pettmann 2004). JNK phosphorylation of 14-3-3 proteins can stimulate the translocation of Bad to the mitochondria and the activation of FOXO3a (Sunayama et al. 2005; Vogt, Jiang, and Aoki 2005). In turn, FOXO3a regulates the expression of Fas ligand in motor neurons (Barthelemy, Henderson, and Pettmann 2004), which suggests a pathway integrating the dependence of both JNK and FOXO3a in the induction of motor neuron apoptosis.

Inhibition of p38 MAP kinase prevents apoptosis induced by Fas pathway activation but has no effect on trophic factor deprivation-induced apoptosis, further suggesting the activation of more than one apoptotic pathway by trophic factor deprivation. In fact, motor neuron apoptosis induced by Fas activation occurs by an atypical mechanism involving the two parallel pathways (Raoul et al. 2002; Raoul et al. 2006)(Fig 5). One of the pathways is the classical caspase 8-mediated mitochondrial apoptotic pathway. The other pathway is responsible for the induction of neuronal NOS by a mechanism involving sequential activation of DAXX, ASK1 and p38 MAP kinase (Raoul et al. 2002). Activation of either pathway seems to be able to induce apoptosis by itself, but when activated together the process occurs faster. The original discussion on a possible mechanism for peroxynitrite and nitric oxide to enhance the caspase 8-mitochondria apoptotic pathway was based in the literature indicating that both peroxynitrite and nitric oxide affect the mitochondrial function. On the other hand, activation of caspase 8 by Fas occurs by means of the DISC complex recruitment (Medema et al. 1997). Another possible explanation is that peroxynitrite may be able to induce the activation of caspase 8 by interacting with some of the components of the DISC, which also could make the Fas activation of this complex easier, resulting in a faster induction of motor neuron apoptosis.

On the other hand, although formation of nitrotyrosine can be catalyzed from nitrite and hydrogen peroxide by peroxidases and transition metals (van der Vliet et al. 1997; Eiserich et al. 1998; Schopfer, Baker, and Freeman 2003), incubation of motor neurons with micromolar concentrations of nitrite and/or hydrogen peroxide has no effect on the survival of motor neurons in culture (Estévez et al. 2000) or tyrosine nitration (Ye et al. 2007), further supporting peroxynitrite formation. Together these results suggest that peroxynitrite formation is necessary for the induction of motor neuron apoptosis by trophic factor deprivation and after Fas pathway activation. In addition, scavenging the nitrating radical products of peroxynitrite by tyrosine-containing peptides does not affect thiol oxidation but prevents nitrotyrosine formation and motor neuron death (Ye et al. 2007)(Fig 6). These results suggest that tyrosine nitration has a causal role in the induction of motor neurons apoptosis by peroxynitrite and it is not only a marker for the formation of reactive nitrogen species.

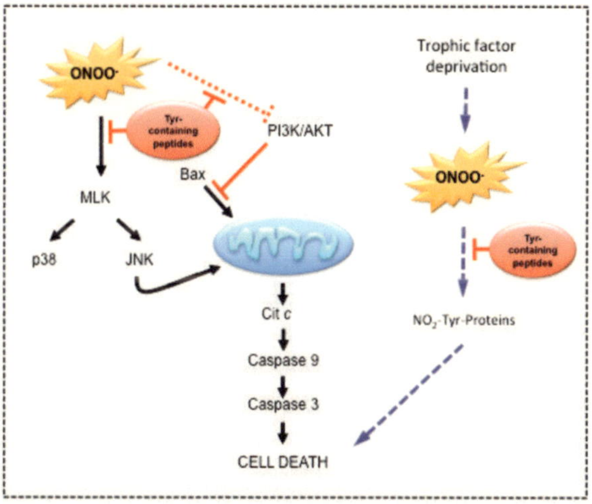

Fig. 6. Peptides that scavenge the nitrating products derived from peroxynitrite decomposition prevent cell death induced by the pure oxidant or endogenously produced peroxynitrite.

6. Extrinsic apoptotic pathway and motor neuron apoptosis *in vivo*

The relevance of the Fas pathways in the regulation of motor neurons death *in vivo* was shown in studies on the effects of axonal injury in mice knockout for Fas and transgenic mice expressing a dominant negative form of FADD, where axotomy-induced motor neuron degeneration was blocked (Ugolini et al. 2003; Martin, Chen, and Liu 2005). Axonal injury is also associated with increased nitrotyrosine immunoreactivity (Martin, Kaiser, and Price 1999; Martin, Chen, and Liu 2005), reveling that in addition to the activation of the classical Fas pathway, peroxynitrite is also produced. These observations suggest that the atypical pathways involved in the induction of motor neuron apoptosis by Fas activation are also active *in vivo* and play a role in the degeneration of adult motor neurons. In addition, SOD deficiency increases motor neuron vulnerability to axotomy (Reaume et al. 1996), indicating that production of superoxide plays an important role in motor neuron degeneration *in vivo*. Even when the source of superoxide for the formation of peroxynitrite *in vivo* and in cultured motor neurons remains unknown, evidence from other neuronal types suggest that the induction and activation of NADPH oxidase might be responsible for the production of superoxide that makes nitric oxide toxic to motor neurons (Noh and Koh 2000; Tammariello, Quinn, and Estus 2000). In motor neurons, activation of the p75 neurotrophic receptor results in apoptosis in different conditions (Ricart et al. 2006; Pehar et al. 2004; Pehar et al. 2007; Wiese et al. 1999). At least in part this toxicity is mediated by induction of superoxide production by mitochondria (Pehar et al. 2007). In summary, inhibition of nitric oxide production blocks motor neuron death induced by ventral root avulsion, and deletion of SOD increases the sensitivity of motor neurons to the same noxious stimulus. Moreover, motor neuron degeneration after ventral root avulsion is preceded by increased tyrosine nitration and the activation of the death receptor pathways. In aggregate these results reveal that motor neuron death *in vitro* and *in vivo* occurs largely by the same mechanisms and through the activation of the same signaling pathways.

7. ALS and reactive nitrogen species

A pathological condition associated with an increased expression of neuronal NOS and nitrotyrosine in motor neurons is amyotrophic lateral sclerosis (ALS)(Abe et al. 1995; Beal et al. 1997; Chou, Wang, and Komai 1996; Chou, Wang, and Taniguchi 1996, , Barber, 2010 #1694). As for today more than 25 reports have found increased levels of nitrotyrosine immunoreactivity or free nitrotyrosine in tissue from patients and animal models of ALS. The definitive evidence for the presence of nitrotyrosine, at least in a transgenic mouse model of ALS, was provided by mass spectrometry studies identifying some of the nitrated proteins and the nitrated residues. Other studies confirmed the identity of the nitrated proteins showing that motor neurons in pre-symptomatic mutant SOD1 mice generate superoxide, NO and ONOO- at higher levels than control motor neurons. In addition, nitration of Cox-I, SOD2 and α-synuclein occurs in pre-symptomatic mutant SOD1 mice suggesting a role for peroxynitrite in the pathogenesis of the disease (Martin et al. 2007).
ALS is a neurodegenerative disease characterized by the death of pyramidal neurons in the motor cortex and motor neurons in the brain stem and ventral spinal cord. About 2% of all ALS cases are due to the presence of one of more than 100 mutations in the gene encoding Cu,Zn SOD (Cleveland and Rothstein 2001; Traub, Mitsumoto, and Rowland 2011). When expressed in mice and rats, some of the human ALS-linked SOD mutations produce a motor neuron disease reminiscent of ALS (Gurney et al. 1994; Dal Canto and Gurney 1995; Wong et al. 1995; Bruijn et al. 1997); these are currently the most widely accepted models for the disease. It is generally accepted that the toxic effect of the mutations is due to a gain-of-function (Cleveland and Rothstein 2001). Growing evidence implicates apoptosis as the mechanism of motor neuron death in the ALS. The fact that the morphological and biochemical characteristics of apoptosis only last upwards of 24 hours in conjunction with the slow progression of the disease, which implicate that only a few motor neurons are dying at a time, make the definitive detection of apoptosis in post mortem tissue from ALS patients challenging (Sathasivam, Ince, and Shaw 2001). However, a comprehensive analysis of degenerating motor neurons in ALS patients revealed their apoptotic morphology in the ventral horn of the spinal cord and motor cortex, combined with an increase in DNA fragmentation and caspase 3 activation (Martin 1999). Further analysis of the post mortem human tissue showed increased formation of Bax-Bax homodimers and a decrease in Bcl-2-Bax heterodimers in motor neurons, suggestive of an increased pro-apoptotic tone in the disease (Martin 1999).

Further evidence for the participation of apoptosis in ALS was provided by the use of transgenic models of the disease (Shibata 2001). Histological analysis of motor neurons from transgenic mice carrying G93A SOD mutant shows decreased expression of the anti-apoptotic proteins Bcl-2 and Bcl-xl and increased expression of the pro-apoptotic Bcl-2 family members Bax and Bad, which expression was attenuated following over-expression of Bcl-2 (Vukosavic et al. 1999; Vukosavic et al. 2000). Genetic deletion of Bax in transgenic mice for the G93A ALS-linked mutant SOD delays onset and extends the lifespan of the animals, but it does not prevent the disease in spite of preventing motor neuron death (Gould et al. 2006). These results are a clear testimony to the complexity of the disease process. Although motor neurons are protected against apoptosis, other abnormalities such as neuromuscular denervation and mitochondrial vacuolization are still occurring (Gould et al. 2006). Other studies suggest that alterations of the neuromuscular junction are between the first symptoms of the disease both in humans and animals models of the disease (Fischer et al. 2004). However, it is important to remember that in the human disease motor neurons do die. The artificial deletion of a gene that regulates apoptosis may just inhibit the final step in the death process, without affecting upstream pathways responsible for the death of the cells. In addition, these results suggest that reactive oxygen and nitrogen species formed during the disease process are not final effectors of cell death, but rather upstream triggers of the activation of signaling pathways resulting in motor neuron death.

Further evidence for the role of apoptosis in the pathogenesis of ALS comes from the delay in onset and progression of the disease due to over-expression of the anti-apoptotic protein Bcl-2 in a transgenic mouse model of ALS (Vukosavic et al. 2000). More recently it was reported that Bcl-2 binds both wild-type and mutant SOD1 *in vitro* and *in vivo*. Because Bcl-2 associated with mutant SOD1 is present in protein aggregates located in mitochondria from the spinal cord of ALS patient and animal models of the disease, it was suggested that entrapment of Bcl-2 by SOD1 leads to the depletion of the anti-apoptotic protein in motor neurons, increasing the vulnerability of these cells (Pasinelli et al. 2004). However, no evidence for the aggregates selectively located in motor neuron mitochondria has been reported. Conversely, BIM, a member of the pro-apoptotic family of Bcl-2 proteins, is upregulated in the $SOD1^{G93A}$ familial ALS mouse model during the symptomatic stage of the disease, and its expression is required to trigger cell death induced by SOD1 mutants *in vitro*. Genetic deletion of BIM in an animal model of ALS results in reduced cellular apoptosis in the spinal cord ventral horn and increases lifespan (Hetz et al. 2007).

The role of caspases in ALS is more controversial. While several authors have reported activation of caspases and a functional role for these activated proteases in animal models of the disease (Friedlander et al. 1997; Li et al. 2000; Pasinelli et al. 1998; Nagai et al. 2001; Pasinelli et al. 2000), others were unable to find a functional role for the enzymes and report that motor neuron death in the G93A mouse model is independent of caspase activation (Martin et al. 2007).

To study the role of mutant SOD1 in different cell types involved in the pathology of ALS, chimeric mice were developed with mixtures of normal and SOD1 mutant-expressing cells. Normal motor neurons in SOD1 mutant chimeras develop features of ALS pathology. However, non-neuronal cells that do not express mutant SOD1 delay degeneration and significantly extend survival of mutant expressing motor neurons (Clement et al. 2003). When primary mouse spinal motor neurons express mutant human SOD1, the cells are not triggered to degenerate, however when rodent astrocytes express mutated SOD1, they kill spinal primary and embryonic mouse stem cell-derived motor neurons (Nagai et al. 2007). In addition, when G93A mutant embryonic stem cells are cultured as motor neurons through *in vitro* differentiation, co-cultures with G93A mutant glial cells lead to a decrease in survival of the motor neurons (Di Giorgio et al. 2007). Using conditional knockout to delete the mutant SOD in specific cell types it was found that the expression of mutant SOD in motor neurons plays a key role on the onset of the disease and the early phases of disease progression. When the levels of mutant SOD were reduced in microglia, the onset and early phases of the disease were not affected, but the later stage of the disease was slowed down. Therefore, onset and progression of ALS are dependent on distinct cell types, indicating the occurrence of a non-cell-autonomous death of motor neurons (Boillee et al. 2006; Boillee, Vande Velde, and Cleveland 2006).

8. SOD1 toxicity

In spite of all the studies done to date on mutant SOD1 in ALS, the mechanism of SOD toxicity remains elusive and highly controversial. The devolpment of an antibody that recognizes the monomer misfolded forms of SOD1 showed the presence of the misfolded monomer in three ALS mouse models with G37R, G85R and G93A SOD1 mutations as well as in a human individual with an A4V SOD1 mutation (Rakhit et al. 2007). One of the hypotheses for mutant SOD toxicity proposes that an aberrant SOD chemistry, which allows small molecules such us peroxynitrite or hydrogen peroxide to produce damaging free radicals, is responsible for the toxic gain-of-function (Beckman and Crow 1993; Lyons et al. 1996). This aberrant chemistry could be the result of a reversal in SOD function caused by the loss of the structural zinc atom (Estévez et al. 1999; Beckman et al. 2001), since the mutant enzymes show a lower affinity for zinc than the wild type SOD, thus increasing the probability for the formation of Zn-deficient SOD (Lyons et al. 1996). There is great controversy about whether this proposed mechanism can take place and its relevance in the pathogenesis of ALS (Subramaniam et al. 2002), but the hypothesis also has its supporters (Liochev and Fridovich 2003).

The Zn-deficient hypothesis was tested using cultured motor neurons and liposomes for the intracellular release of the enzyme (Estévez et al. 1999). These experiments revealed that Zn-deficient human SOD, either mutant or wild type are equally toxic to motor neurons in culture by a mechanism requiring copper and the production of peroxynitrite (Estévez et al. 1999). On the other hand, Cu,Zn mutant and wild type SOD are equally protective for trophic factor deprived motor neurons (Estévez et al. 1999). Based on these results and the characteristics of the altered chemistry of the Zn-deficient SOD, the conclusion was that Zn-deficient SOD produces superoxide using intracellular reducing activities leading to the formation of peroxynitrite (Fig 7).

Further confirmation of an altered mutant SOD chemistry was found using cultured motor neurons isolated from a transgenic mice model of human ALS in conjunction with wild type SOD (Raoul et al. 2002). Nitric oxide is not toxic to non-transgenic mouse and rat motor neurons (Estévez, Spear, Manuel, Radi, et al. 1998; Estévez et al. 2000; Raoul et al. 2002). In contrast, motor neurons isolated from transgenic rats and mice carrying human ALS-linked SOD G85R and G93A die after exposure to nanomolar steady state concentrations of nitric oxide (Raoul et al. 2002; Sahawneh et al. 2010). Transgenic motor neurons carrying mutant SOD are also ten times more sensitive to Fas-induced apoptosis, while transgenic motor neurons carrying human wild type SOD are 100 times more resistant than non-transgenic motor neurons to Fas-mediated apoptosis (Raoul et al. 2002; Raoul et al. 2006). Nitric oxide toxicity in transgenic motor neurons can be reversed by copper chelators and scavenging of superoxide and peroxynitrite (Sahawneh et al. 2010), suggesting production of superoxide in transgenic motor neurons.

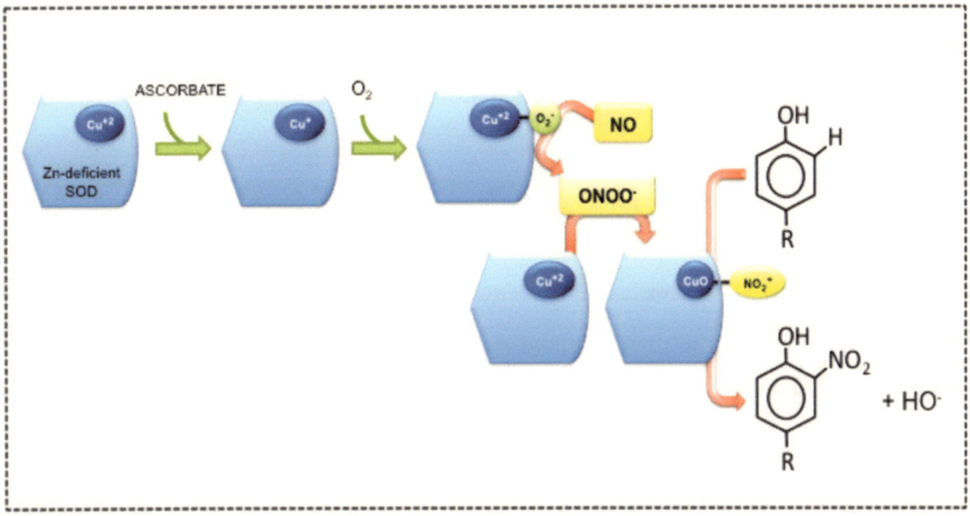

Fig. 7. Zn-deficient SOD as a catalyst for peroxynitrite formation and tyrosine nitration.

Intracellular delivery of wild type Cu,Zn-containing human SOD (Cu,Zn SOD) to motor neurons isolated from transgenic rats overexpressing G93A mutant SOD, has no effect on survival whether the cells are cultured in the presence or absence of trophic factors. However, these motor neurons carrying both, mutant and Cu,Zn-containing SOD are more sensitive to nitric oxide toxicity than transgenic motor neurons without intracellular delivered Cu,Zn SOD (Sahawneh et al. 2010). These *in vitro* results closely mimic the *in vivo* observations of acceleration of death when transgenic mice for mutant SOD are crossbreed with mice transgenic for wild type SOD (Jaarsma et al. 2000; Fukada et al. 2001; Deng et al. 2006). There is some controversy over the effects of wild type SOD on the survival of mice carrying the SOD^{G85R} were one group reported acceleration of disease (Wang et al. 2009) and other claims no effect in a different SOD^{G85R} line (Bruijn et al. 1998). The mechanism through which coexpression of Cu,Zn SOD wild type increases the toxicity of mutant SOD is controversial, with some groups arguing that aggregation plays a role (Deng et al. 2006; Furukawa et al. 2006), while others conclude that increased solubility of the enzyme contributes to the enhanced toxicity (Fig 8) (Fukada et al. 2001; Witan et al. 2008; Witan et al. 2009; Sahawneh et al. 2010).

The mechanisms of mutant SOD-induced motor neuron death in the presence of nitric oxide and Zn-deficient SOD stimulation of motor neuron apoptosis in culture seem identical (Estévez et al. 1999; Raoul et al. 2002; Sahawneh et al. 2010). The dependence on copper and the production of superoxide and peroxynitrite in both conditions indicate that nitrative stress plays a key role in the induction of cell death. In addition, Zn-deficient SOD toxicity is prevented by peptides that inhibit nitration (Ye et al. 2007; Sahawneh et al. 2010), as is the increased toxicity after the addition of Cu,Zn SOD (Sahawneh et al. 2010). Biochemical and biophysical studies indicate that the formation of a dimer between Zn-deficient SOD and Cu,Zn SOD increases the stability of the Zn-deficient SOD monomer (Beckman 1996; Roberts et al. 2007), in agreement with the *in vivo* and *in vitro* studies showing that wild type

SOD increases the stability and solubility of the mutant protein (Fukada et al. 2001; Witan et al. 2008; Witan et al. 2009).

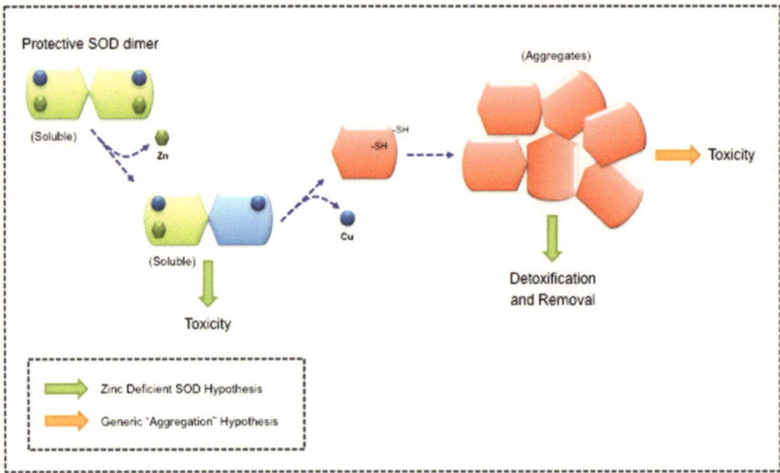

Fig. 8. Proposed mechanisms for the toxicity induced by mutant SOD.

Moreover, in spite of Cu,Zn SOD being a very stable enzyme, the half-life for exchange between this enzyme and Zn-deficient SOD at 37°C is surprisingly fast at 13-17 min when determined using differential mobility gel electrophoresis and 14 min by FRET (Roberts et al. 2007; Sahawneh et al. 2010). An important observation is that the reassociation of Cu,Zn SOD monomers is approximately 10,000 times slower than the reassociation of apoSOD monomers (Lindberg et al. 2004; Svensson et al. 2006), suggesting that the alterations of the dimer interface in the apoSOD are responsibly for the faster association of the monomers even though the stability of the dimer is diminished when compared with Cu,Zn SOD. It is possible that a similar mechanism occurs in the formation of the dimers between Cu,Zn and Zn-deficient SOD, which will explain the increased toxicity by a nitrative mechanism.

In addition, supporting the hypothesis that the increase in stability of Zn-deficient SOD is key in enhancing its toxicity, the substitution of the cysteine residues in positions 6 and 111 by alanine and serine in the human SOD increases its thermostability, and also increases the toxicity of the wild type SOD and $SOD1^{A4V}$ when they are Zn-deficient, but has no effect when the enzymes have the full content of metals (Sahawneh et al. 2010). Other studies reveal that mutation of these two cysteines decreases the stability of the SOD protein but prevents its aggregation (Lindberg et al. 2004; Svensson et al. 2006; Lepock, Frey, and Hallewell 1990). Zn-deficient enzyme with the double cysteine mutation shows more toxicity than the equivalent Zn-deficient SOD with the cysteine residues. In this model, the increased stability of the Zn-deficient form of the SOD is also responsible for the toxicity by a mechanism requiring the production of nitric oxide, superoxide and peroxynitrite followed by tyrosine nitration (Sahawneh et al. 2010).

In summary, reactive nitrogen species and some of their products, such as nitrotyrosine play a causal role in the activation of motor neuron death pathways rather than just having an effector activity. In addition, the abundant evidence indicating the formation of reactive nitrogen species and nitrotyrosine in pathological conditions also suggests that nitrotyrosine is more than a footprint in these conditions. In ALS is well documented the formation of reactive nitrogen species and tyrosine nitration. Most evidence indicates that the source of the toxic nitric oxide is the neuronal isoform of NOS. However, the knockdown of the exon 1 in neuronal NOS, which greatly decreases the enzyme levels, has no effect on the survival of transgenic mouse models of ALS (Facchinetti et al. 1999). On the other hand, inhibitors of neuronal NOS are equally protective to motor neurons isolated from wild type and mice deficient for neuronal NOS (Ricart and Estevez, unpublished observations). These results suggest that the beta isoform of the neuronal NOS, which lacks exon 1, is the responsible for the production of the toxic nitric oxide in motor neurons. If this is the case, then these results may explain why the partial neuronal NOS deficiency is not protective in ALS. The multiple controversies in the role of reactive nitrogen species in ALS are not likely to end soon and will stimulate much needed research to found a cure for this devastating disease.

9. Acknowledgements

This work was supported by the NIH/NIDNS (NS36761). We thanks the constructive criticism of Thong Ma and Mary Ann Sahawneh during the preparation of this manuscript.

10. References

Abe, K, L H Pan, M Watanabe, T Kato, and Y Itoyama. 1995. Induction of nitrotyrosine-like immunoreactivity in the lower motor neuron of amyotrophic lateral sclerosis. *Neurosci. Lett.* 199:152-154.

Alvarez, B, G Ferrer-Sueta, B A Freeman, and R Radi. 1999. Kinetics of peroxynitrite reaction with amino acids and human serum albumin. *J. Biol. Chem.* 274 (2):842-848.

Ara, J, S Przedborski, A B Naini, V Jackson-Lewis, R R Trifiletti, J Horwitz, and H Ischiropoulos. 1998. Inactivation of tyrosine hydroxylase by nitration following exposure to peroxynitrite and 1-methyl-4-phenyl-1,2,3,6-tetrahydropyridine(MPTP). *Proc Natl Acad Sci USA* 95 (13):7659-63.

Aslan, M., T. M. Ryan, T. M. Townes, L. Coward, M. C. Kirk, S. Barnes, C. B. Alexander, S. S. Rosenfeld, and B. A. Freeman. 2003. Nitric oxide-dependent generation of reactive species in sickle cell disease. Actin tyrosine induces defective cytoskeletal polymerization. *J Biol Chem* 278 (6):4194-204.

Bar, P. R. 2000. Motor neuron disease in vitro: the use of cultured motor neurons to study amyotrophic lateral sclerosis. *Eur J Pharmacol* 405 (1-3):285-95.

Barthelemy, C. Catherine, Christopher E. Henderson, and B. Brigitte Pettmann. 2004. Foxo3a induces motoneuron death through the Fas pathway in cooperation with JNK. *BMC neuroscience* 5 (1):48.

Beal, M F, L J Ferrante, S E Browne, R T Matthews, N W Kowall, and R H Brown. 1997. Increased 3-nitrotyrosine in both sporadic and familial amyotrophic lateral sclerosis. *Ann Neurol* 42:644-654.

Beckman, J S. 1996. Nitric oxide: Principles and actions. In *The Physiological and Pathological Chemistry of Nitric Oxide*, edited by J. R. Lanacaster. New York: Academic Press.

Repeated Author. 1996. The Physiological and Pathological Chemistry of Nitric Oxide. In *Nitric Oxide: Principles and Actions*, edited by J. L. Jr: Academic Press Inc.

Beckman, J S, T W Beckman, J Chen, P M Marshall, and B A Freeman. 1990. Apparent hydroxyl radical production by peroxynitrite: Implications for endothelial injury by nitric oxide and superoxide. *Proc. Natl. Acad. Sci. (USA)* 87 (4):1620-1624.

Beckman, J S, and J P Crow. 1993. Pathological implications of nitric oxide, superoxide and peroxynitrite formation. *Biochem. Soc. Trans.* 21 (2):330-334.

Beckman, J S, A G Estévez, J P Crow, and L Barbeito. 2001. Superoxide dismutase and the death of motoneurons in ALS. *TINS* 24 (11):S15-S20.

Beckman, J S, and W H Koppenol. 1996. Nitric oxide, superoxide, and peroxynitrite -- the good, the bad, and the ugly. *Am. J. Physiol.* 271 (Cell Physiol. 40):C1424-C1437.

Beckman, J. S., H. Ischiropoulos, L. Zhu, M. van der Woerd, C. Smith, J. Chen, J. Harrison, J. C. Martin, and M. Tsai. 1992. Kinetics of superoxide dismutase and iron- catalyzed nitration of phenolics by peroxynitrite. *Arch Biochem Biophys* 298 (2):438-445.

Beckman, J. S., and W. H. Koppenol. 1996. Nitric oxide, superoxide, and peroxynitrite: the good, the bad, and ugly. *Am J Physiol* 271 (5 Pt 1):C1424-37.

Boillee, Severine, Christine Vande Velde, and DonW Cleveland. 2006. ALS: A Disease of Motor Neurons and Their Nonneuronal Neighbors. *Neuron* 52 (1):39-59.

Boillee, Severine, Koji Yamanaka, Christian S. Lobsiger, Neal G. Copeland, Nancy A. Jenkins, George Kassiotis, George Kollias, and Don W. Cleveland. 2006. Onset and Progression in Inherited ALS Determined by Motor Neurons and Microglia. *Science* 312 (5778):1389-1392.

Bonfoco, E, D Krainc, M Ankarcrona, P Nicotera, and S A Lipton. 1995. Apoptosis and necrosis: Two distinct events induced, respectively, by mild and intense insults with *N*-methyl-D-aspartate or nitric oxide/superoxide in cortical cell cultures. *Proc. Natl. Acad. Sci. U.S.A.* 92 (16):7162-7166.

Bruijn, L I, M W Becher, M K Lee, K L Anderson, N A Jenkins, N G Copeland, S S Sisodia, J D Rothstein, D R Borchelt, D L Price, and D W Cleveland. 1997. ALS-Linked SOD1 Mutant G85R Mediates Damage to Astrocytes and Promotes Rapidly Progressive Disease with SOD1-Containing Inclusions. *Neuron* 18 (2):327-338.

Bruijn, L I, M K Houseweart, S Kato, K L Anderson, S D Anderson, E Ohama, A G Reaume, R W Scott, and D W Cleveland. 1998. Aggregation and Motor Neuron Toxicity of an ALS-Linked SOD1 Mutant Independent from Wild-Type SOD1. *Science* 281:1851-1854.

Cappelletti, G., M. G. Maggioni, G. Tedeschi, and R. Maci. 2003. Protein tyrosine nitration is triggered by nerve growth factor during neuronal differentiation of PC12 cells. *Exp Cell Res* 288 (1):9-20.

Carreras, Maria Cecilia, and Juan Jose Poderoso. 2007. Mitochondrial nitric oxide in the signaling of cell integrated responses. *Am J Physiol Cell Physiol* 292 (5):C1569-1580.

Casanovas, A., J. Ribera, M. Hukkanen, V. Riveros-Moreno, and J. E. Esquerda. 1996. Prevention by lamotrigine, MK-801 and N omega-nitro-L-arginine methyl ester of motoneuron cell death after neonatal axotomy. *Neuroscience* 71 (2):313-25.

Chang, W., D. R. Webster, A. A. Salam, D. Gruber, A. Prasad, J. P. Eiserich, and J. C. Bulinski. 2002. Alteration of the C-terminal amino acid of tubulin specifically inhibits myogenic differentiation. *Journal of Biological Chemistry* 277 (34):30690-30698.

Chou, S. M., H. S. Wang, and K. Komai. 1996. Colocalization of NOS and SOD1 in neurofilament accumulation within motor neurons of amyotrophic lateral sclerosis: an immunohistochemical study. *J Chem Neuroanat* 10 (3-4):249-58.

Chou, S. M., H. S. Wang, and A. Taniguchi. 1996. Role of SOD-1 and nitric oxide/cyclic GMP cascade on neurofilament aggregation in ALS/MND. *J Neurol Sci* 139 Suppl:16-26.

Clement, A. M., M. D. Nguyen, E. A. Roberts, M. L. Garcia, S. Boillee, M. Rule, A. P. McMahon, W. Doucette, D. Siwek, R. J. Ferrante, R. H. Brown, Jr., J. P. Julien, L. S. Goldstein, and D. W. Cleveland. 2003. Wild-type nonneuronal cells extend survival of SOD1 mutant motor neurons in ALS mice. *Science* 302 (5642):113-7.

Cleveland, D W, and J D Rothstein. 2001. From Charcot to Lou Gehrig: Deciphering Selective Motor Neuron Death in ALS. *Nature Neuroscience Review* 2 (11):806-819.

Colasanti, M., and H. Suzuki. 2000. The dual personality of NO. *Trends Pharmacol Sci* 21 (7):249-52.

Crow, J P, M J Strong, Y Zhuang, Y Ye, and J S Beckman 1997. Superoxide dimutase catalyzes nitration of tyrosines by peroxinitrite in the rod and head domains of neurofilament L. *J Neurochem* 69 (5):1945-1953.

Crow, J. P., J. S. Beckman, and J. M. McCord. 1995. Sensitivity of the essential zinc-thiolate moiety of yeast alcohol dehydrogenase to hypochlorite and peroxynitrite. *Biochemistry* 34 (11):3544-52.

Dal Canto, M.C. , and M.E. Gurney. 1995. Neuropathological changes in two lines of mice carrying a transgene for mutant human Cu, Zn SOD, and in mice overexpressing wild type human SOD: a model of familial amyotrophic lateral sclerosis (FALS). *Brain Res.* 676:25-40.

Dawson, V L, and T M Dawson. 1996. Nitric Oxide Toxicity in Central Nervous System Cultures. *Methods in Neurosciences* 30:26-43.

Dawson, V. L., and T. M. Dawson. 1996. Nitric oxide in neuronal degeneration. *Proc Soc Exp Biol Med* 211 (1):33-40.

Dawson, V.L., and T.M. Dawson. 1996. Nitric oxide neurotoxicity. *J Chem. Neuroanat* 10:179-190.

Deng, Han-Xiang, Yong Shi, Yoshiaki Furukawa, Hong Zhai, Ronggen Fu, Erdong Liu, George H. Gorrie, Mohammad S. Khan, Wu-Yen Hung, Eileen H. Bigio, Thomas Lukas, Mauro C. Dal Canto, Thomas V. O'Halloran, and Teepu Siddique. 2006. Conversion to the amyotrophic lateral sclerosis phenotype is associated with intermolecular linked insoluble aggregates of SOD1 in mitochondria. *PNAS* 103 (18):7142-7147.

Di Giorgio, Francesco Paolo, Monica A. Carrasco, Michelle C. Siao, Tom Maniatis, and Kevin Eggan. 2007. Non-cell autonomous effect of glia on motor neurons in an embryonic stem cell-based ALS model. *Nat Neurosci* 10 (5):608-614.

Eiserich, J P, A G Estévez, T V Bamberg, Y Z Ye, P H Chumley, J S Beckman, and B A Freeman. 1999. Microtubule dysfunction by posttranslational nitrotyrosination of a-tubulin: a nitric oxide-dependent mechanism of cellular injury. *Proc. Natl. Acad. Sci. USA* 96:6365-6370.

Eiserich, J. P., M. Hristova, C. E. Cross, A. D. Jones, B. A. Freeman, B. Halliwell, and A. van der Vliet. 1998. Formation of nitric oxide-derived inflammatory oxidants by myeloperoxidase in neutrophils. *Nature* 391 (6665):393-7.

Estévez, A G, J P Crow, J B Sampson, C Reiter, Y-X Zhuang, G J Richardson, M M Tarpey, L Barbeito, and J S Beckman. 1999. Induction of nitric oxide-dependent apoptosis in motor neurons by zinc-deficient superoxide dismutase. *Science* 286:2498-2500.

Estévez, A G, R Radi, L Barbeito, J T Shin, J A Thompson, and J S Beckman. 1995. Peroxynitrite-induced cytotoxicity in PC12 cells: evidence for an apoptotic mechanism differentially modulated by neurotrophic factors. *J. Neurochem.* 65 (4):1543-1550.

Estévez, A G, J B Sampson, Y-X Zhuang, N Spear, G J Richardson, J P Crow, M M Tarpey, L Barbeito, and J S Beckman. 2000. Liposome-delivered superoxide dismutase prevents nitric oxide-dependent motor neuron death induced by trophic factor withdrawal. *Free Rad. Biol. Med.* 28 (3):437-446.

Estévez, A G, N Spear, S Machelle Manuel, R Radi, C E Henderson, L Barbeito, and J S Beckman. 1998. Nitric oxide and superoxide contribute to motor neuron apoptosis induced by trophic factor deprivation. *J. Neurosci.* 18 (3):923-931.

Estévez, A. G. , N. Spear, S. Machelle Manuel, L. Barbeito, R. Radi, and J. S. Beckman. 1998. Role of endogenous nitric oxide and peroxinitrite formation in the survival and death of motor neurons in culture. *Progress in Brain Research* 118:269-280.

Facchinetti, F., M. Sasaki, F. B. Cutting, P. Zhai, J. E. MacDonald, D. Reif, M. F. Beal, P. L. Huang, T. M. Dawson, M. E. Gurney, and V. L. Dawson. 1999. Lack of involvement of neuronal nitric oxide synthase in the pathogenesis of a transgenic mouse model of familial amyotrophic lateral sclerosis. *Neuroscience* 90 (4):1483-92.

Fischer, Lindsey R., Deborah G. Culver, Philip Tennant, Albert A. Davis, Minsheng Wang, Amilcar Castellano-Sanchez, Jaffar Khan, Meraida A. Polak, and Jonathan D. Glass. 2004. Amyotrophic lateral sclerosis is a distal axonopathy: evidence in mice and man. *Experimental Neurology* 185 (2):232-240.

Friedlander, R M, J Wang, V Gagliardini, R H Jr Brown, and J Yuan. 1997. Inhibition of ICE slows ALS in mice. *Nature* 388:31.

Fukada, K., S. Nagano, M. Satoh, C. Tohyama, T. Nakanishi, A. Shimizu, T. Yanagihara, and S. Sakoda. 2001. Stabilization of mutant Cu/Zn superoxide dismutase (SOD1) protein by coexpressed wild SOD1 protein accelerates the disease progression in familial amyotrophic lateral sclerosis mice. *Eur J Neurosci* 14 (12):2032-6.

Furukawa, Yoshiaki, Ronggen Fu, Han-Xiang Deng, Teepu Siddique, and Thomas V. O'Halloran. 2006. From the Cover: Disulfide cross-linked protein represents a significant fraction of ALS-associated Cu, Zn-superoxide dismutase aggregates in spinal cords of model mice. *PNAS* 103 (18):7148-7153.

Go, Y. M., R. P. Patel, M. C. Maland, H. Park, J. S. Beckman, V. M. Darley-Usmar, and H. Jo. 1999. Evidence for peroxynitrite as a signaling molecule in flow-dependent activation of c-Jun NH(2)-terminal kinase. *Am J Physiol* 277 (4 Pt 2):H1647-53.

Gould, Thomas W., Robert R. Buss, Sharon Vinsant, David Prevette, Woong Sun, C. Michael Knudson, Carol E. Milligan, and Ronald W. Oppenheim. 2006. Complete Dissociation of Motor Neuron Death from Motor Dysfunction by Bax Deletion in a Mouse Model of ALS. *J. Neurosci.* 26 (34):8774-8786.

Greenacre, S A, and H Ischiropoulos. 2001. Tyrosine nitration: localisation, quantification, consequences for protein function and signal transduction. *Free Radical Research* 34 (6):541-581.

Groves, J T, and S S Marla. 1995. Peroxynitrite-induced DNA strand scission mediated by a manganese porphyrin. *J. Am. Chem. Soc.* 117:9578-9579.

Gurney, M E, H Pu, A Y Chiu, M C Dal Canto, C Y Polchow, D D Alexander, J Caliendo, A Hentati, Y W Kwon, H-X Deng, W Chen, P Zhai, R L Sufit, and T Siddique. 1994.

Motor neuron degeneration in mice that express a human Cu,Zn superoxide dismutase mutation. *Science* 264 (5166):1772-1775.

Hetz, C., P. Thielen, J. Fisher, P. Pasinelli, R. H. Brown, S. Korsmeyer, and L. Glimcher. 2007. The proapoptotic BCL-2 family member BIM mediates motoneuron loss in a model of amyotrophic lateral sclerosis. *Cell Death Differ* 14 (7):1386-1389.

Hughes, R A, M Sendtner, and H Thoenen. 1993. Members of several gene families influence survival of rat motoneurons *in vitro* and *in vivo*. *J. Neurosci. Res.* 36:663-671.

Ignarro, L. J. 1990. Biosynthesis and metabolism of endothelium-derived nitric oxide. *Annu Rev Pharmacol Toxicol* 30:535-60.

Ischiropoulos, H. 1998. Biological tyrosine nitration: A pathophysiological function of nitric oxide and reactive oxygen species. *Arch Biochem Biophys* 356:1-11.

Ischiropoulos, H., and J. S. Beckman. 2003. Oxidative stress and nitration in neurodegeneration: Cause, effect, or association? *Journal of Clinical Investigation* 111 (2):163-169.

Jaarsma, Dick, Elize D Haasdijk, J A C Grashorn, Richard Hawkins, Wim van Duijn, Hein W Verspaget, Jacqueline London, and Jan C Holstege. 2000. Human Cu/Zn superoxide dismutase (SOD1) overexpression in mice causes mitochondial vacuolization, axonal degeneration, and premature motor neuron death and accelerates motor neuron disease in mice expressing a familial amyotrophic lateral sclerosis mutant SOD1. *Neurobiol Disease* 7:623-643.

Kaal, E. C., A. S. Vlug, M. W. Versleijen, M. Kuilman, E. A. Joosten, and P. R. Bar. 2000. Chronic mitochondrial inhibition induces selective motoneuron death in vitro: a new model for amyotrophic lateral sclerosis. *J Neurochem* 74 (3):1158-65.

Le-Niculescu, H., E. Bonfoco, Y. Kasuya, F. X. Claret, D. R. Green, and M. Karin. 1999. Withdrawal of survival factors results in activation of the JNK pathway in neuronal cells leading to Fas ligand induction and cell death. *Mol Cell Biol* 19 (1):751-63.

Lepock, J. R., H. E. Frey, and R. A. Hallewell. 1990. Contribution of conformational stability and reversibility of unfolding to the increased thermostability of human and bovine superoxide dismutase mutated at free cysteines. *J Biol Chem* 265 (35):21612-8.

Li, L., R. W. Oppenheim, M. Lei, and L. J. Houenou. 1994. Neurotrophic agents prevent motoneuron death following sciatic nerve section in the neonatal mouse. *J Neurobiol* 25 (7):759-66.

Li, L., R. W. Oppenheim, and C. E. Milligan. 2001. Characterization of the execution pathway of developing motoneurons deprived of trophic support. *J Neurobiol* 46 (4):249-64.

Li, M., V. O. Ona, C. Guegan, M. Chen, V. Jackson-Lewis, L. J. Andrews, A. J. Olszewski, P. E. Stieg, J. P. Lee, S. Przedborski, and R. M. Friedlander. 2000. Functional role of caspase-1 and caspase-3 in an ALS transgenic mouse model. *Science* 288 (5464):335-9.

Lindberg, M. J., J. Normark, A. Holmgren, and M. Oliveberg. 2004. Folding of human superoxide dismutase: disulfide reduction prevents dimerization and produces marginally stable monomers. *Proc Natl Acad Sci U S A* 101 (45):15893-8.

Liochev, S. I., and I. Fridovich. 2003. Mutant Cu,Zn superoxide dismutases and familial amyotrophic lateral sclerosis: evaluation of oxidative hypotheses. *Free Radic Biol Med* 34 (11):1383-9.

Lyons, T J, H Liu, J J Goto, A Nersissian, J A Roe, J A Graden, C Café, L M Ellerby, D E Bredesen, E B Gralla, and J S Valentine. 1996. Mutations in copper-zinc superoxide dismutase that cause amyotrophic lateral sclerosis alter the zinc binding site and the redox behavior of the protein. *Proc. Natl. Acad. Sci. U.S.A.* 93:12240-12244.

MacMillan-Crow, L A, J S Greendorfer, S M Vickers, and J A Thompson. 2000. Tyrosine nitration of c-SRC tyrosine kinase in human pancreatic ductal adenocarcinoma. *Arch. Biochem. Biophys.* 377 (2):350-356.

Martin, L. J. 1999. Neuronal death in amyotrophic lateral sclerosis is apoptosis: possible contribution of a programmed cell death mechanism. *J Neuropathol Exp Neurol* 58 (5):459-71.

Martin, L. J., K. Chen, and Z. Liu. 2005. Adult motor neuron apoptosis is mediated by nitric oxide and Fas death receptor linked by DNA damage and p53 activation. *J Neurosci* 25 (27):6449-59.

Martin, L. J., A. Kaiser, and A. C. Price. 1999. Motor neuron degeneration after sciatic nerve avulsion in adult rat evolves with oxidative stress and is apoptosis. *J Neurobiol* 40 (2):185-201.

Martin, Lee J. , Zhiping Liu, Kevin Chen, Ann C. Price, Pan. Yan, Jason A. Swaby, and W. Christopher Golden. 2007. Motor neuron degeneration in amyotrophic lateral sclerosis mutant superoxide dismutase-1 transgenic mice: Mechanisms of mitochondriopathy and cell death. *The Journal of Comparative Neurology* 500 (1):20-46.

Medema, J. P., C. Scaffidi, F. C. Kischkel, A. Shevchenko, M. Mann, P. H. Krammer, and M. E. Peter. 1997. FLICE is activated by association with the CD95 death-inducing signaling complex (DISC). *Embo J* 16 (10):2794-804.

Milligan, C. E., R. W. Oppenheim, and L. M. Schwartz. 1994. Motoneurons deprived of trophic support in vitro require new gene expression to undergo programmed cell death. *J Neurobiol* 25 (8):1005-16.

Milligan, C. E., D. Prevette, H. Yaginuma, S. Homma, C. Cardwell, L. C. Fritz, K. J. Tomaselli, R. W. Oppenheim, and L. M. Schwartz. 1995. Peptide inhibitors of the ICE protease family arrest programmed cell death of motoneurons in vivo and in vitro. *Neuron* 15 (2):385-93.

Moncada, S , R M J Palmer, and E A Higgins. 1991. Nitric oxide: physiology, pathophysiology, phamacology. *Pharmacol Rev* 43 (2):109-142.

Morishima, Y., Y. Gotoh, J. Zieg, T. Barrett, H. Takano, R. Flavell, R. J. Davis, Y. Shirasaki, and M. E. Greenberg. 2001. Beta-amyloid induces neuronal apoptosis via a mechanism that involves the c-Jun N-terminal kinase pathway and the induction of Fas ligand. *J Neurosci* 21 (19):7551-60.

Nagai, M, M Aoki, I Miyoshi, M Kato, P Pasinelli, N Kasai, R H Jr. Brown, and Y Itoyama. 2001. Rats expressing human cytosolic copper-zinc superoxide dismutase transgenes with amyotrophic lateral sclerosis: associated mutations develop motor neuron disease. *J Neurosci* 21 (21):9246-9254.

Nagai, Makiko, Diane B. Re, Tetsuya Nagata, Alcmene Chalazonitis, Thomas M. Jessell, Hynek Wichterle, and Serge Przedborski. 2007. Astrocytes expressing ALS-linked mutated SOD1 release factors selectively toxic to motor neurons. *Nat Neurosci* 10 (5):615-622.

Nauser, T., and W. H. Koppenol. 2002. The rate constant of the reaction of superoxide with nitrogen monoxide: Approaching the diffusion limit. *Journal of Physical Chemistry A* 106 (16):4084-4086.

Neff, N. T., D. Prevette, L. J. Houenou, M. E. Lewis, M. A. Glicksman, Q. W. Yin, and R. W. Oppenheim. 1993. Insulin-like growth factors: putative muscle-derived trophic agents that promote motoneuron survival. *J Neurobiol* 24 (12):1578-88.

Newbern, J., A. Taylor, M. Robinson, M. O. Lively, and C. E. Milligan. 2007. c-Jun N-terminal kinase signaling regulates events associated with both health and degeneration in motoneurons. *Neuroscience* 147 (3):680-692.

Noh, K. M., and J. Y. Koh. 2000. Induction and activation by zinc of NADPH oxidase in cultured cortical neurons and astrocytes. *J Neurosci* 20 (23):RC111.

Novikov, L, L Novikova, and J-O Kellerth. 1995. Brain-derived neurotrophic factor promotes survival and blocks nitric oxide synthase expression in adult rat spinal motoneurons after ventral root avulsion. *Neurosci. Lett.* 200 (1):45-48.

Oppenheim, R W. 1996. Neurotrophic survival molecules for motoneurons: an embarrassment of riches. *Neuron* 17 (2):195-197.

Oppenheim, R. W. 1991. Cell death during development of the nervous system. *Annu Rev Neurosci* 14:453-501.

Pacher, Pal, Joseph S. Beckman, and Lucas Liaudet. 2007. Nitric Oxide and Peroxynitrite in Health and Disease. *Physiol. Rev.* 87 (1):315-424.

Padmaja, S, and R E Huie. 1993. The reaction of nitric oxide with organic peroxyl radicals. *Biochem. Biophys. Res. Commun.* 195:539-544.

Pasinelli, P , D R Borchelt, M K Houseweart, D W Cleveland, and R H Brown Jr. 1998. Caspase-1 is activated in neural cells and tissue with amyotrophic lateral sclerosis-associated mutations in copper-zinc superoxide dismutase. *Proc Natl Acad Sci USA* 95 (26):15763-8.

Pasinelli, P., M. E. Belford, N. Lennon, B. J. Bacskai, B. T. Hyman, D. Trotti, and R. H. Brown, Jr. 2004. Amyotrophic lateral sclerosis-associated SOD1 mutant proteins bind and aggregate with Bcl-2 in spinal cord mitochondria. *Neuron* 43 (1):19-30.

Pasinelli, P., M. K. Houseweart, R. H. Brown, and D. W. Cleveland. 2000. Caspase-1 and-3 are sequentially activated in motor neuron death in Cu,Zn superoxide dismutase-mediated familial amyotrophic lateral sclerosis. *Proceedings of the National Academy of Sciences of the United States of America* 97 (25):13901-13906.

Paxinou, E., Q. Chen, M. Weisse, B. I. Giasson, E. H. Norris, S. M. Rueter, J. Q. Trojanowski, V. M. Lee, and H. Ischiropoulos. 2001. Induction of alpha-synuclein aggregation by intracellular nitrative insult. *J Neurosci* 21 (20):8053-61.

Pehar, M., P. Cassina, M. R. Vargas, R. Castellanos, L. Viera, J. S. Beckman, A. G. Estevez, and L. Barbeito. 2004. Astrocytic production of nerve growth factor in motor neuron apoptosis: implications for amyotrophic lateral sclerosis. *J Neurochem* 89 (2):464-73.

Pehar, Mariana, Marcelo R. Vargas, Kristine M. Robinson, Patricia Cassina, Pablo J. Diaz-Amarilla, Tory M. Hagen, Rafael Radi, Luis Barbeito, and Joseph S. Beckman. 2007. Mitochondrial Superoxide Production and Nuclear Factor Erythroid 2-Related Factor 2 Activation in p75 Neurotrophin Receptor-Induced Motor Neuron Apoptosis. *J. Neurosci.* 27 (29):7777-7785.

Pennica, D, V Arce, T A Swanson, R Vejsada, R A Pollock, M Armanini, K Dudley, H S Phillips, A Rosenthal, A C Kato, and C E Henderson. 1996. Cardiotrophin-1, a cytokine present in embryonic muscle, supports long-term survival of spinal motoneurons. *Neuron* 17 (1):63-74.

Radi, R, J S Beckman, K M Bush, and B A Freeman. 1991. Peroxynitrite oxidation of sulfhydryls. The cytotoxic potential of superoxide and nitric oxide. *J. Biol. Chem.* 266 (7):4244-4250.

Repeated Author. 1991. Peroxynitrite-induced membrane lipid peroxidation: The cytotoxic potential of superoxide and nitric oxide. *Arch. Biochem. Biophys.* 288 (2):481-487.

Radi, R. 2004. Nitric oxide, oxidants, and protein tyrosine nitration. *Proc Natl Acad Sci U S A* 101 (12):4003-4008.

Radi, R., A. Cassina, R. Hodara, C. Quijano, and L. Castro. 2002. Peroxynitrite reactions and formation in mitochondria. *Free Radic Biol Med* 33 (11):1451-64.

Rae, T. D., P. J. Schmidt, R. A. Pufahl, V. C. Culotta, and T. V. O'Halloran. 1999. Undetectable intracellular free copper: the requirement of a copper chaperone for superoxide dismutase. *Science* 284 (5415):805-8.

Rakhit, R., J. Robertson, C. Vande Velde, P. Horne, D. M. Ruth, J. Griffin, D. W. Cleveland, N. R. Cashman, and A. Chakrabartty. 2007. An immunological epitope selective for pathological monomer-misfolded SOD1 in ALS. *Nature medicine* 13 (6):754-9.

Ramachandran, Anup, Anna-Liisa Levonen, Paul S. Brookes, Erin Ceaser, Sruti Shiva, Maria Cecilia Barone, and Victor Darley-Usmar. 2002. Mitochondria, nitric oxide, and cardiovascular dysfunction. *Free Radical Biology and Medicine* 33 (11):1465-1474.

Raoul, C, C E Henderson, and B Pettmann. 1999. Programmed cell death of embryonic motoneurons triggered though the Fas death receptor. *J Cell Biol* 147 (5):1049-1062.

Raoul, C, B Pettmann, and C E Henderson. 2000. Active killing of neurons during development and following stress: a role for $p75^{NTR}$ and Fas? *Curr Op Neurobiol* 10 (1):111-117.

Raoul, C., E. Buhler, C. Sadeghi, A. Jacquier, P. Aebischer, B. Pettmann, C. E. Henderson, and G. Haase. 2006. Chronic activation in presymptomatic amyotrophic lateral sclerosis (ALS) mice of a feedback loop involving Fas, Daxx, and FasL. *PNAS* 103 (15):6007-6012.

Raoul, Cedric, Catherine Barthelemy, Arnaud Couzinet, David Hancock, Brigitte Pettmann, and Anne-Odile Hueber. 2005. Expression of a dominant negative form of Daxx <I>in vivo</I> rescues motoneurons from Fas (CD95)-induced cell death. *Journal of Neurobiology* 62 (2):178-188.

Raoul, Cédric, Alvaro G Estévez, Hiroshi Nishimune, Don W Cleveland, Odile deLapeyrière, Chistopher E Henderson, Georg Haase, and Brigitte Pettmann. 2002. Motoneuron death triggered by a specific pathway downstream of Fas: potentiation by ALS-linked SOD1 mutations. *Neuron* 35:1067-1083.

Reaume, A G, J L Elliott, E K Hoffman, N W Kowall, R J Ferrante, D F Siwek, H M Wilcox, D G Flood, M F Beal, R H Jr Brown, R W Scott, and W D Snider. 1996. Motor neurons in Cu/Zn superoxide dimutase-deficient mice develop normally but exhibit enhanced cell death after axonal injury. *Nature Genetics* 13:43-47.

Ricart, Karina C., Richard J. Pearson, Liliana Viera, Patricia Cassina, Andrés Kamaid, Steven L Carroll, and Alvaro G Estévez. 2006. Interactions between b-neuregulin and neurotrophins in motor neuron apoptosis. *Journal of Neurochemistry* 97 (1):222-233.

Roberts, Blaine R., John A. Tainer, Elizabeth D. Getzoff, Dean A. Malencik, Sonia R. Anderson, Valerie C. Bomben, Kathrin R. Meyers, P. Andrew Karplus, and Joseph S. Beckman. 2007. Structural Characterization of Zinc-deficient Human Superoxide Dismutase and Implications for ALS. *Journal of Molecular Biology* 373 (4):877-890.

Sahawneh, M. A., K. C. Ricart, B. R. Roberts, V. C. Bomben, M. Basso, Y. Ye, J. Sahawneh, M. C. Franco, J. S. Beckman, and A. G. Estevez. 2010. Cu,Zn superoxide dismutase (SOD) increases toxicity of mutant and Zn-deficient superoxide dismutase by enhancing protein stability. *J Biol Chem* 285 (44):33885-97.

Sathasivam, S., P. G. Ince, and P. J. Shaw. 2001. Apoptosis in amyotrophic lateral sclerosis: a review of the evidence. *Neuropathology and Applied Neurobiology* 27 (4):257-274.

Schopfer, F. J., P. R. Baker, and B. A. Freeman. 2003. NO-dependent protein nitration: a cell signaling event or an oxidative inflammatory response? *Trends Biochem Sci* 28 (12):646-54.

Sendtner, M., G. Pei, M. Beck, U. Schweizer, and S. Wiese. 2000. Developmental motoneuron cell death and neurotrophic factors. *Cell Tissue Res* 301 (1):71-84.

Shacka, J. J., M. A. Sahawneh, J. D. Gonzalez, Y. Z. Ye, T. L. D'Alessandro, and A. G. Estévez. 2006. Two distinct signaling pathways regulate peroxynitrite-induced apoptosis in PC12 cells. *Cell Death Differ* 13:1506-1514.

Shibata, Noriyuki. 2001. Transgenic mouse model for familial amyotrophic lateral sclerosis with superoxide dismutase-1 mutation. *Neuropathology* 21 (1):82-92.

Shin, J T, L Barbeito, L A MacMillan-Crow, J S Beckman, and J A Thompson. 1996. Acidic fibroblast growth factor enhances peroxynitrite-induced apoptosis in primary murine fibroblasts. *Arch. Biochem. Biophys.* 335 (1):32-41.

Snyder, S. H. 1993. Janus faces of nitric oxide. *Nature* 364 (6438):577.

Spear, N, A G Estévez, L Barbeito, J S Beckman, and G V W Johnson. 1997. Nerve growth factor protects PC12 cells against peroxynitrite-induced apoptosis via a mechanism dependent on phosphatidylinositol-3 kinase. *J. Neurochem.* 69 (1):53-59.

Spear, N, A G Estévez, R Radi, and J S Beckman. 1997. Peroxynitrite and Cell signalling. In *Oxidative Stress and Signal Transduction*, edited by H. J. Forman and E. Cadenas. New york: Chapman&Hall.

Subramaniam, J R, W E Lyons, J Liu, T B Bartnikas, J Rothstein, D L Price, D W Cleveland, J D Gitlin, and P C Wong. 2002. Mutant SOD1 causes motor neuron disease independent of copper chaperone-mediated copper loading. *Nature Neurosci* 5 (4):301-307.

Sunayama, J., F. Tsuruta, N. Masuyama, and Y. Gotoh. 2005. JNK antagonizes Akt-mediated survival signals by phosphorylating 14-3-3. *The Journal of cell biology* 170 (2):295-304.

Svensson, A. K., O. Bilsel, E. Kondrashkina, J. A. Zitzewitz, and C. R. Matthews. 2006. Mapping the folding free energy surface for metal-free human Cu,Zn superoxide dismutase. *J Mol Biol* 364 (5):1084-102.

Takakura, K., J. S. Beckman, L. A. MacMillan-Crow, and J. P. Crow. 1999. Rapid and irreversible inactivation of protein tyrosine phosphatases PTP1B, CD45, and LAR by peroxynitrite. *Arch Biochem Biophys* 369 (2):197-207.

Tammariello, S. P., M. T. Quinn, and S. Estus. 2000. NADPH oxidase contributes directly to oxidative stress and apoptosis in nerve growth factor-deprived sympathetic neurons. *J Neurosci* 20 (1):RC53.

Traub, R., H. Mitsumoto, and L. P. Rowland. 2011. Research advances in amyotrophic lateral sclerosis, 2009 to 2010. *Current neurology and neuroscience reports* 11 (1):67-77.

Ugolini, G., C. Raoul, A. Ferri, C. Haenggeli, Y. Yamamoto, D. Salaun, C. E. Henderson, A. C. Kato, B. Pettmann, and A. O. Hueber. 2003. Fas/tumor necrosis factor receptor death signaling is required for axotomy-induced death of motoneurons in vivo. *J Neurosci* 23 (24):8526-31.

van der Vliet, A., J. P. Eiserich, B. Halliwell, and C. E. Cross. 1997. Formation of reactive nitrogen species during peroxidase-catalyzed oxidation of nitrite. A potential additional mechanism of nitric oxide-dependent toxicity. *J Biol Chem* 272 (12):7617-25.

Vogt, P. K., H. Jiang, and M. Aoki. 2005. Triple layer control: phosphorylation, acetylation and ubiquitination of FOXO proteins. *Cell cycle* 4 (7):908-13.

Vukosavic, S, M Dubois-Dauphin, N Romero, and S Przedborski. 1999. Bax and Bcl-2 interaction in a transgenic mouse model of familial amyotrophic lateral sclerosis. *J Neurochem* 73:2460-2468.

Vukosavic, S., L. Stefanis, V. Jackson-Lewis, C. Guegan, N. Romero, C. Chen, M. Dubois-Dauphin, and S. Przedborski. 2000. Delaying caspase activation by Bcl-2: A clue to disease retardation in a transgenic mouse model of amyotrophic lateral sclerosis. *J Neurosci* 20 (24):9119-25.

Wang, L., H. X. Deng, G. Grisotti, H. Zhai, T. Siddique, and R. P. Roos. 2009. Wild-type SOD1 overexpression accelerates disease onset of a G85R SOD1 mouse. *Hum Mol Genet* 18 (9):1642-51.

Wiese, S, F Metzger, B Holtmann, and M Sendtner. 1999. The role of $p75^{NTR}$ in modulating neurotrophin survival effects in developing motoneurons. *Eur. J. Neurosci.* 11 (5):1668-1676.

Witan, H., P. Gorlovoy, A. M. Kaya, I. Koziollek-Drechsler, H. Neumann, C. Behl, and A. M. Clement. 2009. Wild-type Cu/Zn superoxide dismutase (SOD1) does not facilitate, but impedes the formation of protein aggregates of amyotrophic lateral sclerosis causing mutant SOD1. *Neurobiol Dis* 36 (2):331-42.

Witan, Heidrun, Andreas Kern, Ingrid Koziollek-Drechsler, Rebecca Wade, Christian Behl, and Albrecht M. Clement. 2008. Heterodimer formation of wild-type and amyotrophic lateral sclerosis-causing mutant Cu/Zn-Superoxide dismutase induces toxicity independent of protein aggregation. *Hum. Mol. Genet.* 17 (10):1373-85.

Wong, P C, C A Pardo, D R Borchelt, M K Lee, N G Copeland, N A Jenkins, S S Sisodia, D W Cleveland, and D L Price. 1995. An adverse property of a familial ALS-Linked SOD1 mutation causes motor neuron disease characterised by vacuolar degeneration of mitochondria. *Neuron* 14:1105-1116.

Wu, W. 1993. Expression of nitric-oxide synthase (NOS) in injured CNS neurons as shown by NADPH diaphorase histochemistry. *Exp Neurol* 120 (2):153-9.

Wu, W., K. Han, L. Li, and F. P. Schinco. 1994. Implantation of PNS graft inhibits the induction of neuronal nitric oxide synthase and enhances the survival of spinal motoneurons following root avulsion. *Exp Neurol* 129 (2):335-9.

Wu, W., and L. Li. 1993. Inhibition of nitric oxide synthase reduces motoneuron death due to spinal root avulsion. *Neurosci Lett* 153 (2):121-4.

Yan, Q., J. Elliott, and W. D. Snider. 1992. Brain-derived neurotrophic factor rescues spinal motor neurons from axotomy-induced cell death. *Nature* 360 (6406):753-5.

Ye, Yaozu, Celia Quijano, Kristine M. Robinson, Karina C. Ricart, Amy L. Strayer, Mary Anne Sahawneh, John J. Shacka, Marion Kirk, Stephen Barnes, Mary Ann Accavitti-Loper, Rafael Radi, Joseph S. Beckman, and Alvaro G. Estevez. 2007. Prevention of peroxynitrite-induced apoptosis of motor neurons and PC12 cells by tyrosine-containing peptides. *J. Biol. Chem.* 282:6324-6337.

14

Protein Aggregates in Pathological Inclusions of Amyotrophic Lateral Sclerosis

Yoshiaki Furukawa
Department of Chemistry, Keio University
Japan

1. Introduction

Amyotrophic lateral sclerosis (ALS) is a neurodegenerative disorder that is characterized by a progressive loss of upper and/or lower motor neurons (Bruijn et al., 2004). Dysfunction and death of these neurons lead to muscle weakness, atrophy and spasticity. A fatal event for the majority of patients is a failure of the respiratory muscles, which generally occurs within one to five years of disease onset. The typical age of onset is between 50 and 60 years, and the prevalence rate is 5 - 10 cases per 100,000 populations (de Belleroche et al., 1996). No effective cures for this disease are currently available, and the pathomechanism still remains controversial. The majority of ALS cases have no genetic component (sporadic ALS, sALS), while about 10 % are inherited in a dominant manner (familial ALS, fALS).

Historically, ALS has been described by Charcot and Joffroy in 1869 (Charcot & Joffroy, 1869), and linkage analysis of fALS families was performed in 1991, by which the genetic locus was identified to be linked to chromosome 21q (Siddique et al., 1991). In 1993, Rosen et al. (Rosen et al., 1993) and Deng et al. (Deng et al., 1993) have found that mutations in the Cu,Zn-superoxide dismutase (SOD1) gene, which lies on chromosome 21q, are associated with fALS. Because SOD1-related fALS exhibited several clinicopathological similarities to sALS, various animal models including rodents, worms and flies have been constructed, in which mutant forms of SOD1 are expressed. Using these models, furthermore, various drugs have been continuingly tested to cure or alleviate ALS. In 2001, ALS2 (or called alsin) has been also identified as a new gene associated with a rare, recessively inherited and slowly progressed juvenile onset form of ALS, which is, however, significantly different from the disease phenotypes of sALS (Hadano et al., 2001; Yang et al., 2001). Accordingly, studies on mutant SOD1 have served as a "gold standard" for a long time and provided valuable insight into molecular pathomechanisms of ALS.

Recent progress on genetic analysis has fuelled the identification of other genes responsible for fALS: for example, **T**AR **D**NA-binding **p**rotein-43 (TDP-43) gene reported in 2008 (Gitcho et al., 2008; Kabashi et al., 2008; Sreedharan et al., 2008; Van Deerlin et al., 2008), **Fu**sed in **S**arcoma (FUS) gene in 2009 (Kwiatkowski et al., 2009; Vance et al., 2009). Each of TDP-43 and FUS mutations describes approximately 4 % of total fALS cases, which is a smaller number than that of SOD1 mutations (~20 % of total fALS cases). Unlike SOD1, however, TDP-43 and/or FUS pathologies are observed in many of sALS patients (Deng et al., 2011b; Mackenzie et al., 2007) and also in other neurodegenerative diseases (Lagier-

Tourenne et al., 2010); much attention has thus been increasingly paid on TDP-43/FUS genes. FALS cases with SOD1/TDP-43/FUS mutations exhibit distinct disease phenotypes such as site and age of onset (Millecamps et al., 2010), and the pathomechanism of fALS might be dependent upon which of the genes is mutated. Common to all ALS cases, nonetheless, inclusions can be found in motor neurons of the affected spinal cord; therefore, molecular characterization of such pathological inclusions will be important in understanding the ALS diseases.

2. Protein aggregates in pathological inclusions

Inclusions have been found in many neurodegenerative diseases and are formed by abnormal accumulation of protein aggregates (Ross & Poirier, 2004). Two types of protein aggregates generally constitute pathological inclusions: amorphous and fibrillar aggregates. Amorphous aggregates are assembled from unstructured protein molecules, while well-ordered protein aggregates often exhibit fibrillar morphologies. Among such fibrillar protein aggregates, amyloid constitutes an important structural entity; the amyloid-like aggregate *in vitro* and *in vivo* can be characterized by its fibrillar morphology with widths of approx. 10 nm (Soto, 2003). In a molecular level, amyloid is rich in β-sheet structures, which are maintained by hydrogen-bonding interactions between main chains of constituent proteins; therefore, all proteins seem to possess innate propensities of forming a common amyloid structure (Dobson, 2003). Fibrillar aggregates of amyloid-β peptides, which constitute the senile plaques in the Alzheimer disease patients, are the most famous example of amyloid-like aggregates (Serpell & Smith, 2000). It, however, remains controversial whether the pathological protein aggregates in ALS adopt amyloid-like structures. In all cases of ALS, two types of inclusions characterize the surviving motor neurons in a spinal cord; one is called skein-like inclusions, which are immunostained by anti-ubiquitin antibody, and the other, Bunina body, is eosinophilic but ubiquitin-negative (Piao et al., 2003). Pathogenic proteins such as SOD1, TDP-43 and FUS constitute the skein-like inclusions, while Bunina bodies have been shown to be immunoreactive for cystatin C and transferrin (Okamoto et al., 2008). In this chapter, therefore, I will overview recent studies on the *in vitro* and *in vivo* aggregates of ALS-pathogenic proteins, SOD1, TDP-43 and FUS as follows.

2.1 SOD1-positive inclusions in ALS patients

SOD1 is a copper and zinc-containing protein with 153 amino acids, and its physiological function is to detoxify superoxide radical by its dismutation into oxygen and hydrogen peroxide (McCord & Fridovich, 1969). As of now, approximately 150 pathogenic mutations have been reported (http://alsod.iop.kcl.ac.uk), and any preference is not found for the site and type of mutations.

A subset of these pathogenic mutations affects SOD1 activity, while some mutant SOD1s fully retain the catalytic activity (Hayward et al., 2002). Also, transgenic mice expressing mutant SOD1 reproduce disease-like symptoms (Turner & Talbot, 2008), which are absent in SOD1-knockout mice (Reaume et al., 1996). It has, therefore, been considered that pathogenic mutations in SOD1 cause fALS not through loss of an SOD1 physiological function but by gain of new toxic properties. One of such toxic properties proposed so far includes mutation-induced aggregation of SOD1 proteins, while it remains controversial whether SOD1 aggregation is really toxic or even protective. Neuronal hyaline inclusions in the spinal cord are pathological hallmark of mutant SOD1-linked fALS (Shibata et al., 1996b), and those inclusions are ultrastructurally composed of the granule-coated fibrils with a diameter of 15 - 25 nm that can be labeled by anti-SOD1 antibodies (Kato et al., 2000). Such fibrillar morphologies of protein aggregates are reminiscent of the amyloid formation observed in many neurodegenerative diseases (Ross & Poirier, 2004). Pathological inclusions containing mutant SOD1 seem, however, not fulfill some of the criteria for identification as amyloid; that is, neither Congo Red staining with apple-green birefringence nor Thioflavin T/S staining with significant enhancement of fluorescence has been observed in the fALS patient with SOD1^{A4V} (Kerman et al., 2010). Given that these staining methods for amyloid diagnosis have not been routinely performed in the tissue sections from fALS patients with SOD1 mutations, more investigations will be required on the tissue samples of fALS patients with several different types of SOD1 mutations.

Until recently, involvement of wild-type SOD1 (SOD1^{WT}) in pathogenesis of sALS had been considered to be limited (Shibata et al., 1994; Shibata et al., 1996a; Watanabe et al., 2001). Indeed, an antibody called SEDI (**S**OD1-**e**xposed-**d**imer-**i**nterface) that only labels monomer/misfolded forms of SOD1 were failed to immunostain the motor neurons from sALS patients (Liu et al., 2009). Nonetheless, novel antibodies raised against 4 - 20, 57 - 72, and 131 - 153 of an SOD1 amino acid sequence were found to specifically detect unfolded SOD1 and also immunostain inclusions in motor neurons of the spinal cord from all the 29 sporadic and 8 familial ALS patients (Forsberg et al., 2010). Furthermore, motor neurons in the spinal cord of sALS patients (four out of nine cases) are found to be immunoreactive to another monoclonal antibody called C4F6, which specifically recognizes the misfolded conformation of SOD1 (Bosco et al., 2010). The staining patterns of C4F6 in sALS are, however, diffusive, and solubility of SOD1^{WT} is also not different between sALS patients and controls. Pathological SOD1^{WT} in sALS would, therefore, be relatively soluble, compared to mutant SOD1 within the inclusions in fALS patients. Although it appears that SOD1 is not involved in fALS cases without SOD1 mutations (Bosco et al., 2010), more prevailing roles of SOD1 proteins in the pathogenesis of ALS have been recently considered.

2.1.1 SOD1 aggregates in mouse models

Transgenic mice expressing human SOD1 with several fALS-associated mutations have been published, and phenotypes in each model mouse have been concisely summarized in (Turner & Talbot, 2008). These transgenic mice well reproduce the formation of ubiquitin-positive SOD1 inclusions, which is the pathological hallmark of SOD1-related fALS diseases (Watanabe et al., 2001). Biochemical analysis on the inclusions has further suggested the ubiquitination of mutant SOD1, based upon which the molecular pathogenesis of ALS has been proposed to include the inhibition of intracellular ubiquitin-proteasome system clogged by insoluble SOD1 aggregates (Basso et al., 2006). Retardation of proteasomal activity thus decelerates degradation of misfolded mutant SOD1, which further promotes the SOD1 aggregation. Recent mass analysis on inclusions in SOD1^{G93A}, SOD1^{G37R}, and SOD1$^{H46R/H48Q}$ transgenic mice has, however, not supported any direct modifications on SOD1, and ubiquitinated mutant SOD1 may be a minor constituent of inclusions (Shaw et al., 2008). Immunohistochemical analysis has also shown that the inclusions in transgenic mice are immunostained with antibodies to a copper chaperone for SOD1 (see below) and several heat shock proteins such as Hsp70; however, the results are not always consistent with those in human fALS cases (Watanabe et al., 2001).

It is also important to note that amounts of inclusions in the transgenic mice depend upon the type of mutations in the SOD1 transgene. For example, transgenic mice expressing $SOD1^{G37R}$ and $SOD1^{G93A}$ exhibit prominent vacuolation of mitochondria with less amounts of inclusions; in contrast, significant amounts of inclusions are produced in $SOD1^{G85R}$ and $SOD1^{H46R}$ mice (Turner & Talbot, 2008). While such mutation-dependency of inclusion formation remains to be more characterized, H46R and G85R mutations notably reduce the affinity of SOD1 for copper/zinc ions (Hayward et al., 2002). In contrast, enzymatic activity of SOD1 is almost fully retained by G37R and G93A mutations, suggesting little effects on metal affinity/binding (Hayward et al., 2002). It is thus possible that SOD1 aggregation is facilitated by dissociation of metal ions from SOD1 (*vide infra*).

Ultrastructurally, both filamentous and amorphous aggregates that are immunoreactive to SOD1 and ubiquitin constitute the pathological inclusions in the transgenic mice. Unlike pathological inclusions in human fALS cases ($SOD1^{A4V}$) (Kerman et al., 2010), Thioflavin S does stain inclusions formed in $SOD1^{G37R}$ and $SOD1^{G93A}$ mice, suggesting the formation of amyloid-like protein aggregates (Furukawa et al., 2008; Wang et al., 2002). The apparent discrepancy in Thioflavin S staining between human and mouse needs to be described, but it remains unknown if this is due to the difference in the types of mutations (A4V in human vs. G37R/G93A in mouse). It is notable that SOD1 inclusions in $SOD1^{L126X}$ mice are not stained with Thioflavin S (Wang et al., 2005); therefore, tinctorial properties of SOD1 aggregates in pathological inclusions would depend upon the types of SOD1 mutations.

Disulfide cross-linking between SOD1 molecules is also an important feature of SOD1 aggregates in transgenic mice (Furukawa et al., 2006). A natively folded SOD1 possesses a highly conserved "intra"-molecular disulfide bond, but, in contrast, abnormal disulfide linkages "between" SOD1 molecules are detected in inclusions of the transgenic mice. Accumulation of disulfide-linked SOD1 aggregates occurs primarily in the later stages of the disease, concurrent with the appearance of rapidly progressing symptoms (Karch et al., 2009). Furthermore, the conserved intramolecular disulfide is found to be reduced in most of mutant SOD1 molecules constituting inclusions (Karch et al., 2009). Abnormalities in the thiol-disulfide chemistry of SOD1 would thus facilitate aggregation of mutant SOD1 proteins. These results of SOD1 transgenic mouse models strongly suggest the important roles of post-translational maturation of SOD1 polypeptides in the formation of pathological aggregates, which can be well reproduced by the following *in vitro* experiments.

2.1.2 SOD1 aggregates *in vitro*

Intracellular maturation of SOD1 requires several post-translational processes including copper and zinc binding and formation of an intramolecular disulfide bond (Furukawa & O'Halloran, 2006). These processes confer the significantly high structural stability to an SOD1 protein to the extent that the melting temperature of active SOD1 is around 90 °C (Forman & Fridovich, 1973). Many of ALS mutations have been shown to reduce the melting temperature of copper and/or zinc-bound form of SOD1 (Rodriguez et al., 2002), which is, however, still high enough to retain its structure at the physiological temperature (~37 °C). In general, aggregation associates with drastic conformational changes of protein molecules (Dobson, 2003); therefore, high structural (thermal) stability of fully mature SOD1 even in the presence of ALS mutations might not fit to the general aggregation mechanism. In contrast, immature forms of SOD1 have been shown to exhibit significantly reduced thermostability; the melting temperature of the most immature SOD1 (*i.e.* a metal-unbound (apo) and disulfide-reduced form ($SOD1^{SH}$)) is as low as 43 °C (Furukawa & O'Halloran, 2005). Very interestingly, furthermore, apo-$SOD1^{SH}$ with ALS mutations (A4V and G93A) starts to melt at the temperature below 37 °C, suggesting protein unfolding/misfolding under physiological conditions (Furukawa & O'Halloran, 2005). Although it has been claimed that apo-SOD1s are not universally destabilized by the ALS-causing mutations (Rodriguez et al., 2005), the majority of ALS mutations (18 out of 20 mutations they examined) have been shown to indeed decrease melting temperature of apo-SOD1 to some degrees. It is, therefore, possible that mutation-induced destabilization of SOD1 structures plays critical roles in the formation of pathological inclusions found in SOD1-related fALS.

2.1.3 A key role of a disulfide reduction in SOD1 aggregation

Indeed, I have shown for the first time that the SOD1 polypeptide without any post-translational modifications (*i.e.* apo-$SOD1^{SH}$) exhibits the highest propensities for the formation of amyloid-like fibrillar aggregates *in vitro* (Furukawa et al., 2008). Under physiological solution conditions (such as salt concentration and solution pH), *in vitro* aggregation of SOD1 is completely inhibited by addition of Zn^{2+} ion and/or introduction of an intramolecular disulfide bond. SOD1 is a very rare cytosolic protein that keeps a disulfide bond for its enzymatic activity (Furukawa et al., 2004). As described below, the intramolecular disulfide bond in SOD1 is introduced by its copper chaperone in the cell (Furukawa et al., 2004). Without this disulfide, SOD1 favors a monomeric state; but, once the disulfide forms, SOD1 adopts a dimeric structure (Arnesano et al., 2004). Dimerization of SOD1 appears to protect its disulfide from reduction by burying it in the dimer interface. In most of the mutant SOD1 proteins, however, presumably due to perturbation in the native tertiary structure, the affinity for copper and/or zinc ion is reduced (Hayward et al., 2002), and the susceptibility to a disulfide reduction is increased (Tiwari & Hayward, 2003). Given the reducing environment of the cytosol with high metal-chelating capacity (Rae et al., 1999), therefore, a molecular pathomechanism of SOD1-related fALS would involve increased concentration of aggregation-prone apo-$SOD1^{SH}$ state in neurons. Consistently, insoluble mutant SOD1 purified from inclusions in the transgenic mice appear to have no metal ions bound (Lelie et al., 2011). Although aggregation propensities of apo-$SOD1^{SH}$ were not consistently increased by all pathogenic mutations, the intracellular population of aggregation-prone apo-$SOD1^{SH}$ state is considered to increase by the fALS-causing mutations.

Consistent with these *in vitro* observations, intracellular formation of SOD1 aggregates has been shown to be inhibited by co-expression of a copper chaperone for SOD1 (CCS) in cultured cells (Furukawa et al., 2008). CCS is a metallochaperone that specifically loads a copper ion and introduces a disulfide bond into apo-$SOD1^{SH}$ (Culotta et al., 1997; Furukawa et al., 2004). Intracellular concentration of aggregation-prone apo-$SOD1^{SH}$ will thus be effectively reduced by CCS. Unlike the cultured cells, however, $SOD1^{G93A}$ transgenic mice exhibited accelerated progression of disease-like phenotypes with shortening of mean survival from 242 to 36 days upon overexpression of CCS (Son et al., 2007). In particular, the double transgenic mice presented severe mitochondrial pathologies. CCS has been known to regulate the mitochondrial import of SOD1 (Field et al., 2003; Kawamata & Manfredi, 2008);

therefore, in CCS/SOD1^{G93A} double transgenic mice, CCS overexpression would overload mitochondria with toxic SOD1^{G93A}. Because of such a short survival, it remains unclear whether CCS possesses a preventive role in SOD1 aggregation in rodent models. If CCS effectively protects SOD1 from aggregation by facilitating the post-translational maturation, knockout of the *CCS* gene is expected to increase the population of apo-SOD1^{SH} state and then aggravate the inclusion pathologies in ALS-model mice. Again, however, this is not the case; there are virtually no effects on the disease onset/progression, when the *CCS* gene is knocked out from SOD1^{G37R}, SOD1^{G85R}, and SOD1^{G93A} transgenic mice (Subramaniam et al., 2002). Notably, a significant level of SOD1 activity is confirmed in CCS-knockout mice, and this is in sharp contrast to the observations in *S. cerevisiae*, where SOD1 activity is completely vanished upon genetic removal of the *CCS* gene (Culotta et al., 1997). A CCS-independent pathway(s) of SOD1 activation has, therefore, been recently proposed in mammals, and the presence of a Pro residue in an SOD1 C-terminal region determines the dependency of its enzymatic activation on CCS (Leitch et al., 2009). It, therefore, remains difficult to test the potentially protecting role of CCS in SOD1 aggregation in animal models. Interestingly, *C.elegans* has no *CCS* gene and activates SOD1 in a CCS-independent mechanism (Jensen & Culotta, 2005). Worms may thus be able to use as a model to examine effects of fALS mutations on a CCS-independent pathway of SOD1 activation.

In vitro aggregates prepared from SOD1^{SH} have been recently found to exhibit mutation-dependent structural polymorphism (Furukawa et al., 2010). Three regions in an SOD1 amino acid sequence are resistant to be proteolyzed by proteases in the fibrillar SOD1^{SH} aggregates. These three regions can be regarded as building blocks in an SOD1 aggregate structure, and non-native interactions of these building blocks constitute a core in SOD1 aggregate. FALS-causing mutations are found to modulate non-native interactions of those three building blocks, leading to the formation of discrete core structures among SOD1 aggregates with different mutations. Such a mutation-dependent core structure, furthermore, determines morphological as well as biochemical properties of SOD1 aggregate, which may describe distinct disease phenotypes in patients with different mutations in SOD1 (Wang et al., 2008).

2.1.4 Aggregation of SOD1 with an intact disulfide under destabilizing conditions

Notably, apo-SOD1 with an intramolecular disulfide bond (apo-SOD1^{S-S}) is considered to be partially unfolded under physiological temperature, given the melting temperature of around 40 – 50 °C (Furukawa & O'Halloran, 2005). While partial unfolding of apo-SOD1^{S-S} could induce misfolding and aggregation, 10 μM apo-SOD1^{S-S} without free cysteines (C6S and C111S mutations) was not aggregated even with agitation in a physiological buffer (100 mM Na-Pi, 100 mM NaCl, 5 mM EDTA, pH 7.0) for at least 72 hours (Furukawa et al., 2008). In the same conditions, I have also confirmed no aggregation of wild-type apo-SOD1^{S-S} (with intact free cysteines, unpublished). Several other groups have nonetheless reported the aggregation of SOD1^{S-S}, which will be summarized below.

One of the conditions for triggering aggregation of non-reduced SOD1 is the addition of a chaotropic agent, guanidine hydrochloride (GdnHCl). Valentine and colleagues have performed agitation of 50 μM apo-SOD1^{S-S} with Teflon balls in a buffer (10 mM K-Pi, pH 7.4) containing 1 M GdnHCl and found the formation of Thioflavin-T (ThT)-positive aggregates after approximately 40 hours (Chattopadhyay et al., 2008; Oztug Durer et al., 2009). These apo-SOD1^{S-S} aggregates possess fibrillar morphologies, and its formation is accelerated when the solution pH becomes acidic (pH 3.0, 4.0, 5.0). Interestingly, aggregation of apo-$SOD1^{S-S}$ was accelerated by addition of sub-stoichiometric amounts of soluble apo-$SOD1^{SH}$, suggesting that apo-$SOD1^{SH}$ can initiate aggregation of apo-$SOD1^{S-S}$ by acting as nuclei. Thus, SOD1 with a disulfide bond would be aggregation-incompetent, but, once the disulfide is somehow reduced in a small fraction of $SOD1^{S-S}$ proteins during the *in vitro* aggregation reaction, the resultant $SOD1^{SH}$ might convert the residual $SOD1^{S-S}$ into aggregation-competent conformations. Chia et al. have also shown that aggregation of 10 μM $SOD1^{S-S}$ in the presence of 0.5 M GdnHCl at pH 4.0 is accelerated by addition of spinal cord homogenates from transgenic mice expressing $SOD1^{G93A}$ (120 days old) (Chia et al., 2010). Such a seeded aggregation was not observed by adding spinal cord homogenates of the non-transgenic littermates. Given that $SOD1^{G93A}$ mice contain pathological inclusions at 120 days of age (Gurney et al., 1994), the *in vitro* $SOD1^{S-S}$ aggregation is seeded by either pathological SOD1 aggregates, soluble $SOD1^{SH}$ or both.

Another aggregation-inducing condition is the addition of trifluoroethanol (TFE). TFE has been considered to stabilize secondary structures but disrupt the native tertiary structure of various intact proteins (Buck, 1998). Consistent with the high thermostability, a holo-form of $SOD1^{S-S}$ remains soluble in the presence of up to 80 % TFE; in contrast, apo-$SOD1^{S-S}$ readily forms visible aggregate in the presence of 15 % TFE (Stathopulos et al., 2003). Stathopulos et al. have further proposed the correlation of the melting temperature with the amount of TFE required for aggregation by using several fALS-causing mutant apo-$SOD1^{S-S}$ proteins (Stathopulos et al., 2003). Morphologies of TFE-induced $SOD1^{S-S}$ aggregates are fibrillar, but those aggregates exhibit 2- to 3-fold ThT fluorescence enhancement and small spectral changes upon addition of Congo Red. These tinctorial changes may be comparable to those in pathological SOD1 aggregates to the extent that inclusions in fALS patients are usually not stained by both Thioflavin S and Congo Red (Kato et al., 2000). Given that the typical amyloid aggregates lead to ~1000-fold increase in the intensity of ThT fluorescence and red-shift a spectrum of Congo Red (Klunk et al., 1999; LeVine, 1999), TFE-induced $SOD1^{S-S}$ aggregates will not be categorized as a typical amyloid.

It is also interesting to note that TFE-induced SOD1 aggregates act as seeds to trigger aggregation of endogenous SOD1 in cultured cells. Münch et al. have prepared the *in vitro* aggregates of $SOD1^{H46R}$ by adding 20 % TFE, although the thiol-disulfide status in the mutant SOD1 was not specified (Munch et al., 2011). These *in vitro* aggregates were found to penetrate inside neuronal cells, *Neuro2a*, by macropinocytosis, rapidly exit the macropinocytic compartment, and then nucleate aggregation of the transiently overexpressed $SOD1^{H46R}$-GFP in the cytosol. Intracellular $SOD1^{WT}$-GFP was not aggregated by exogenously added $SOD1^{H46R}$ aggregates. Importantly, the intracellularly seeded aggregates have been found to transfer from cell to cell; thereby, the phenotypes can be "infected" among cells. Such a seeded infection of protein aggregates is reminiscent of the prion phenomena and has been reported in several other pathogenic proteins for neurodegenerative diseases such as α-synuclein (Luk et al., 2009), Tau (Clavaguera et al., 2009), polyglutamine (Ren et al., 2009), and TDP-43 (Furukawa et al., 2011). Although it has not been confirmed if ALS is infectious, the seeding properties of TFE-induced aggregates may describe the propagation of pathological changes with the progression of diseases.

Metal-catalyzed oxidation of Zn-deficient SOD1 also leads to the protein aggregation (Rakhit et al., 2002; Rakhit et al., 2004). $CuCl_2$ with ascorbic acid generates reactive oxygen species, which then oxidize histidine residues in SOD1. This is consistent with the fact that the aggregation is significantly retarded at pH < 5.5. While SOD1 exists as a dimer, the oxidized SOD1 dissociates into monomers and then forms non-amyloid aggregates with amorphous and fibrillar morphologies. The oxidation-induced aggregation does not occur when SOD1 is in a holo state. Zinc-binding affinity of SOD1 has been known to decrease with fALS mutations (Hayward et al., 2002); therefore, mutant SOD1 is more susceptible to aggregation through the metal-catalyzed oxidation than the wild-type protein.

Incubation time will be another key factor to induce the aggregation of a mature SOD1 (*i.e.* a fully metallated SOD1 with an intramolecular disulfide bond). Usually, the aggregation kinetics of proteins has been monitored for at most 3 – 5 days, where either fully mature or even partially mature SOD1 does not aggregate in a physiological buffer without any chaotropic reagents. Nonetheless, Hwang et al. have extended the incubation time up to more than 300 hours (> 10 days) and found the fibrillar aggregation of fully mature SOD1 (with C6A/C111S mutations) under physiological conditions (~300 μM proteins, pH 7.8, 37 °C) (Hwang et al., 2010). The SOD1 aggregates after a prolonged incubation did not show apple-green birefringence upon binding Congo Red nor strong enhancement of ThT fluorescence, consistent with properties of inclusions in SOD1-related fALS patients (Kato et al., 2000). It remains unknown if SOD1 retains metal ions even in the aggregated state, it is possible that such a long incubation of SOD1 proteins somehow leads to the partial loss and/or the altered binding geometries of metal ions.

In summary, SOD1 can adopt theoretically 44 types of modified states when metal binding, disulfide formation and dimerization are taken into account (Furukawa & O'Halloran, 2006). Many papers point out the strengths of the SOD1 aggregation model for ALS; however, as mentioned above, there is still no consensus on which state of SOD1 is responsible for aggregation observed in fALS cases. Researchers including myself have thus continuingly pursued a mechanism describing why more than 100 ALS-causing mutations in SOD1 commonly facilitate the SOD1 aggregation process.

2.2 TDP-43-positive inclusions in ALS patients

TDP-43 is a DNA/RNA binding protein with 414 amino acids and contains two RNA recognition motifs (RRM1 and RRM2) and a C-terminal auxiliary region (Ayala et al., 2005). As of now, more than 40 mutations have been identified in the TDP-43 gene as being pathogenic, and most of the mutations are localized in the C-terminal region (http://alsod.iop.kcl.ac.uk). One of physiological functions of TDP-43 is to regulate an alternative splicing of several gene transcripts (Ayala et al., 2008a; Buratti & Baralle, 2001); usually, TDP-43 is localized at the nucleus but is also known to shuttle between nucleus and cytoplasm (Ayala et al., 2008b). Under pathological conditions, in contrast, TDP-43 is cleared from the nucleus and is mislocalized at the cytoplasm, where the ubiquitin- and TDP-43-positive inclusions are observed (Arai et al., 2006; Neumann et al., 2006). Formation of TDP-43 inclusions has been confirmed in sALS and SOD1-negative fALS but not in SOD1-linked fALS (Mackenzie et al., 2007). Actually, before identification of pathogenic mutations in the TDP-43 gene, proteomic analysis of ubiquitin-positive inclusions in sALS patients has revealed TDP-43 as a major component of inclusions (Arai et al., 2006; Neumann et al., 2006). TDP-43 immunoreactive inclusions have also been observed in many other neurodegenerative diseases such as frontotemporal lobar degeneration (FTLD), Huntington disease, and Alzheimer disease, which recently leads to a new disease category called TDP-43 proteinopathies (Geser et al., 2009).

In pathological inclusions, TDP-43 is abnormally hyper-phosphorylated and cleaved to generate C-terminal fragments (Arai et al., 2006; Neumann et al., 2006). Pathological TDP-43 is also distinct from its normal counterpart because it exhibits decreased solubility in a buffer containing a detergent, Sarkosyl. Ultrastructurally, inclusions observed in TDP-43 proteinopathies are characterized by bundles of straight fibrils with 10 - 20 nm diameter that are immunostained by anti-TDP-43 antibodies (Lin & Dickson, 2008). Similar to SOD1-positive inclusions, however, TDP-43 inclusions are also not stained by Thioflavin S and Congo Red (Kerman et al., 2010), implying less amyloid characters. Interestingly, the C-terminal fragments are enriched in the cytoplasmic inclusions in brain of ALS patients, but in the spinal cord, inclusions are composed of full-length TDP-43 (Igaz et al., 2008). Furthermore, Hasegawa et al. have found the immunoblot distinction of TDP-43 among different TDP-43 proteinopathies (Hasegawa et al., 2008); for example, Sarkosyl-insoluble fractions of ALS and FTLD brains exhibit different electrophoretic band patterns of the C-terminal fragments of phosphorylated TDP-43 in the Western blots. Depending upon the clinicopathological subtypes of TDP-43 proteinopathies, multiple pathways can thus be considered for the formation of TDP-43 inclusions; however, molecular mechanisms of truncation and phosphorylation in TDP-43 remain unknown.

2.2.1 TDP-43 aggregates in mouse models

Homozygous disruption of the TDP-43 gene is embryonic lethal in mice (Kraemer et al., 2010), and post-natal deletion of the TDP-43 gene by utilizing a Cre recombinase also produces lethality albeit without any ALS-like symptoms (Chiang et al., 2010). Expression of wild-type human TDP-43 has also been reported to be toxic in mice in a dose-dependent manner; indeed, TDP-43 transgenic mice exhibit a wide variety of motor dysfunctions, which appears to depend upon the promoter regulating the expression of the transgene (Da Cruz & Cleveland, 2011). More toxic effects of ALS-causing mutations (A315T and M337V examined so far) in the TDP-43 transgene has not been established yet. Surprisingly, any of the transgenic mice expressing wild-type and mutant TDP-43 have not reproduced the formation of ubiquitin- and TDP-43-positive inclusions. When human TDP-43 with A315T mutation is expressed in mice under the control of mouse prion promoter (Wegorzewska et al., 2009), the mice develop gait abnormality with an average survival of about 150 days, and ubiquitin-positive inclusions are observed in specific neuronal populations including spinal motor neurons. Despite this, those ubiquitin-positive inclusions are not immunostained with anti-TDP-43 antibodies, and very limited amounts of C-terminally truncated TDP-43 are confirmed. Furthermore, mutant TDP-43 exhibits similar solubility in a Sarkosyl-containing buffer to that of mouse endogenous wild-type TDP-43. Although truncation as well as insolubilization of TDP-43 characterizes the TDP-43 proteinopathies, both of these pathological processes may hence not be required for neurodegeneration.

In contrast, Wils et al. have constructed a mouse expressing wild-type human TDP-43 under the control of a neuronal murine Thy-1 promoter and found a dose-dependent degeneration of cortical and spinal motor neurons (Wils et al., 2010). Immunohistochemical analysis has further confirmed the formation of ubiquitin-positive inclusions, which are stained by an anti-TDP-43 antibody and also an antibody recognizing Ser409/410-phosphorylated TDP-43. Abnormal phosphorylation on TDP-43 is thus reproduced in this model mouse; furthermore, the C-terminal truncation of human TDP-43 is observed albeit much less amounts than that in ALS patients. Despite this, human TDP-43 in the affected mice remains soluble in a Sarkosyl-containing buffer, showing that the pathological processes of TDP-43 are not completely reproduced in the transgenic mouse model.

Transgenic rats expressing human wild-type and mutant (M337V) TDP-43 have also been made (Zhou et al., 2010). Soon after the birth, TDP-43^{M337V} transgenic rats become paralyzed at 20 - 30 days and die at postnatal ages; in contrast, TDP-43^{WT} transgenic rats exhibit no paralysis by the age of 200 days. Mutation-specific toxicity of TDP-43 has thus been reproduced in these rat transgenic models, but TDP-43 inclusions are rarely detected and present only in the cortex of paralyzed TDP-43^{M337V} transgenic rats. A very faint amount of truncated TDP-43 is detected, and phosphorylated TDP-43 is accumulated at the cytoplasm of spinal motor neurons. These molecular changes of TDP-43 are, however, confirmed in both TDP-43^{WT} and TDP-43^{M337V} transgenic rats, implying little roles of truncation and phosphorylation in expressing the mutant-specific toxicity of TDP-43. Accordingly, it still remains to be established in the rodent models how mutant TDP-43 exerts its toxicity and is involved in the inclusion formation under pathological conditions.

2.2.2 TDP-43 aggregates *in vitro*

Bacterially expressed TDP-43 normally forms insoluble inclusion bodies, which hampers biochemical characterization of TDP-43 proteins. Johnson et al. have nonetheless succeeded to obtain soluble full-length 6 x His-tagged TDP-43 by using a cold shock expression system in *E.coli* (Johnson et al., 2009) Agitation of 3 μM full-length TDP-43 in 40 mM HEPES/150 mM KCl/20 mM $MgCl_2$/1 mM DTT, pH 7.4 at 25 °C increases solution turbidity within an hour, supporting the high aggregation propensities of TDP-43. A TDP-43 truncate that is devoid of the C-terminal auxiliary domain does not increase its solution turbidity, suggesting an important role of the C-terminal domain in the aggregation *in vitro*. Aggregates of full-length TDP-43 exhibit both filament-like and thread-like morphologies but did not react with the amyloid-diagnostic dyes, Congo Red and ThT. A subset of fALS-linked mutations (M337V, Q331K) slightly facilitates the aggregation kinetics of full-length TDP-43. A high propensity for fibrillation has been also shown for the synthetic peptide fragment of a TDP-43 C-terminal region (Gly 287- Met 322) (Chen et al., 2010). Fibrillar aggregates of the C-terminal peptide did not increase the intensity of Thioflavin T fluorescence. Interestingly, an ALS-causing mutation, G294A, but not A315T renders the fibrillar aggregates ThT-positive. While fibrils of all C-terminal peptides (wild-type, A315T, G294A) possess β-sheet rich structures, ALS mutations would affect the biochemical/structural properties of TDP-43 aggregates.

I have recently reported that bacterially expressed full-length TDP-43 is resolubilized, purified in the presence of GdnHCl, and then refolded by dilution of GdnHCl (Furukawa et al., 2011). Such refolded TDP-43 proteins retain the physiological DNA binding function but forms fibrillar aggregates by agitation at 37 °C in 100 mM Na-Pi/100 mM NaCl/5 mM EDTA/5 mM DTT/10 % glycerol, pH 8.0. A C-terminal half of TDP-43 assumes a core in the fibrillar aggregates and reproduces the fibrillation propensities of full-length TDP-43 proteins. These *in vitro* TDP-43 fibrils are insoluble in a Sarkosyl-containing buffer, which is a consistent feature with the pathological inclusions. A seeding activity is also a notable feature of TDP-43 fibrils *in vitro*, where pre-formed fibrils (or called "seeds") function as a structural template to facilitate the recruitment of soluble proteins into insoluble fibrils. This seeding reaction has been found to also occur inside the cultured cells by transducing the cells with *in vitro* TDP-43 fibrils; thereby, the formation of Sarkosyl-insoluble and ubiquitinated TDP-43 inclusions is well reproduced in the cell. This is notable because simple overexpression of TDP-43 in the cultured cells has never generated the Sarkosyl-insoluble inclusions. It remains controversial whether the aggregation of TDP-43 is a cause or a result of the disease; however, as recently proposed in the other neurodegenerative diseases (Aguzzi & Rajendran, 2009; Brundin et al., 2010), a seeding activity of TDP-43 proteins may contribute to the propagation of pathological changes with the progression of diseases.

All recent *in vitro* studies on TDP-43 proteins have revealed its high propensities for aggregation, which are provided by the C-terminal auxiliary domain. Given that most of the fALS-causing mutations are located at this domain, the mutational alteration in the aggregation propensities of TDP-43 might be a part of the ALS pathomechanism. More *in vitro* experiments will, however, be required to reveal if the aggregation reactions of TDP-43 are affected by mutation, truncation, and phosphorylation.

2.3 FUS-positive inclusions in ALS patients

FUS was initially identified as the N-terminus of FUS-CHOP (CCAAT/enhancer binding protein homologous protein), a fusion oncoprotein expressed in human myxoid liposarcoma with the t(12;16) chromosomal translocation (Crozat et al., 1993). Like TDP-43, FUS is a DNA/RNA binding protein with 526 amino acids and comprised of multiple domains as follows (from N-terminal to C-terminal); a Q/G/S/Y-rich domain, a G-rich domain, an RNA-recognition motif (RRM), an R/G-rich domain, a Zn-finger motif, and a region containing a nuclear localization signal (NLS) (Dormann et al., 2010; Iko et al., 2004). Under physiological conditions, FUS has been proposed to be involved in transcription regulation (Uranishi et al., 2001), RNA splicing (Yang et al., 1998), and RNA transport including nucleo-cytoplasmic shuttling (Zinszner et al., 1997).

Late in 2007, which was before identification of pathological mutations in the *FUS* gene, FUS protein was found as one of major proteins recruited into neuronal intranuclear inclusions in patients of Huntington disease (Doi et al., 2008). In this neurodegenerative disease, a polyglutamine tract in a protein called huntingtin (HTT) is abnormally expanded, leading to fibrillar aggregation of mutant HTT in affected neurons (Zoghbi & Orr, 2000). FUS is sequestered by fibrillar HTT aggregates and then becomes insoluble and possibly dysfunctional (Doi et al., 2008). Loss of physiological functions of FUS would, therefore, contribute to neuronal cell death in Huntington's disease (Doi et al., 2008) as well as other polyglutamine diseases (Doi et al., 2010).

Then, fALS-causing mutations in the *FUS* gene have been identified in 2009 (Kwiatkowski et al., 2009; Vance et al., 2009), and, as of now, at least 40 mutations have been reported, most of which are localized at a G-rich domain and a C-terminal NLS-containing region (http://alsod.iop.kcl.ac.uk). Although neuropathological analysis of fALS patients with *FUS* mutations has been still limited, cytoplasmic mislocalization of nuclear FUS protein in motor neurons is a major pathological hallmark. Indeed, as shown by a recent study (Dormann et al., 2010), fALS-causing mutations at the C-terminal region of FUS result in the functional impairment of the NLS, facilitating the cytoplasmic mislocalization of mutant FUS. In FUS-related fALS, FUS-immunoreactive cytoplasmic inclusions are observed, which have been recently found to exhibit mutation-dependent heterogeneity (Mackenzie et al., 2011). For example, P525L mutation in FUS associates with a relatively early onset (twenties) of ALS, where round FUS-immunoreactive neuronal cytoplasmic inclusions are found. In contrast, late-onset (forties to sixties) ALS cases are linked to R521C mutation in FUS and have tangle-like FUS-immunoreative neuronal and glial cytoplasmic inclusions. Furthermore, it has been reported that FUS-immunoreactive inclusions are observed in spinall spinal anterior horn neurons in all sporadic and familial ALS cases tested, except for those with SOD1 mutations (Deng et al., 2011b). Although mutations in FUS account for only a small fraction of fALS and sALS cases, FUS proteins may be a common component of cytosolic inclusions in non-SOD1 ALS. In motor neurons of patients with juvenile ALS, FUS has been shown to form filamentous aggregates with a diameter of 15 - 20 nm, which are often associated with small granules (Baumer et al., 2010; Huang et al., 2011). Staining with Thioflavin T/S and Congo Red has not, however, been performed yet on the inclusions of FUS-linked ALS. It also remains unknown if pathological FUS decreases its solubility or is modified/truncated in inclusions.

2.3.1 FUS aggregates in a rat model

As of now, there is no mouse model of FUS-linked ALS, but a transgenic rat expressing wild-type or ALS-causing mutant (R521C) FUS has been published (Huang et al., 2011). Only the mutant FUS transgenic rats developed paralysis at an early age (1 - 2 mo) with a significant loss of neurons in the frontal cortex and dentate gyrus. These pathological changes are not observed in age-matched wild-type FUS transgenic rats, although, at the advanced age (> 1 yr), wild-type FUS transgenic rats display a deficit in spatial learning and memory with a moderate loss of neurons in the frontal cortex and dentate gyrus. Immunohistochemical analysis of the cortex and spinal cord has shown the appearance of ubiquitin-positive inclusions at the paralysis stages of both wild-type and mutant FUS rats; however, the inclusions are not immunostained with anti-FUS antibodies. Given that several different anti-FUS antibodies show distinct immunoreactivities toward FUS-containing inclusions in sALS cases (Deng et al., 2011b), more detailed investigations will be necessary to characterize the possible aggregation of FUS forming pathological inclusions.

2.3.2 FUS aggregates *in vitro*

There is only one paper published on the aggregation reaction of purified FUS proteins (Sun et al., 2011); Sun et al. have prepared GST-fused FUS proteins intervened with a TEV protease site and found that the cleavage of 2.5 - 5 μM GST-FUS with a TEV protease produces full-length FUS in 100 mM Tris/200 mM trehalose/0.5 mM EDTA/20 mM glutathione, pH 8.0, and starts aggregation without a lag-time at 22° C in the absence of agitation. The resultant *in vitro* aggregates of FUS do not increase the intensity of ThT fluorescence and are completely soluble in an SDS-containing buffer. They have further examined the aggregation reactions of several truncated FUS proteins and shown that the N-terminal region of FUS (1 - 422) is enough to reproduce the aggregation behavior of full-length FUS. Aggregates of both full-length FUS and truncated FUS (1 - 422) are fibrillar in the morphologies, which resemble to the FUS inclusions in the ALS patients. No effects of fALS-causing mutations (H517Q, R521H, R521C) are observed on the *in vitro* fibrillation kinetics of full-length FUS proteins.

3. Conclusion

In this chapter, recent progress has been reviewed on aggregation mechanisms of ALS pathogenic proteins, SOD1, TDP-43 and FUS. Common to all these three proteins, structural/biochemical characters of aggregates *in vitro* are much dependent upon experimental conditions, and it remains obscure which of aggregates *in vitro* reproduces the pathological inclusions in patients. In particular, post-translational processes such as metallation, disulfide formation, phosphorylation, and truncation appear to affect the aggregation pathway(s) of the pathogenic proteins. In future, therefore, it will become more important to correlate any abnormalities in these post-translational modifications with pathogenicity of ALS.

Very recently, mutations in another gene, optineurin (OPTN), have been linked to fALS cases, and hyaline inclusions in the anterior horn cells of spinal cord were immunoreactive for OPTN in patients with OPTN mutation (E478G) (Maruyama et al., 2010). Furthermore, albeit controversial, skein-like inclusions in all the sALS and non-SOD1 fALS have been reported to be immunostained with an anti-OPTN antibody (Deng et al., 2011a). Aggregation of an OPTN protein would thus be of relevance to describe the pathomechanism of both sporadic and familial ALS.

In spite of recent efforts to identify the causative genes for fALS, most of the cases are still genetically unidentified (Da Cruz & Cleveland, 2011). Given that the skein-like inclusions in the spinal anterior horn cells are characteristic of ALS, proteomic analysis of those inclusions will help to identify as-yet-unknown proteins pathogenic for ALS. In addition, the component analysis of skein-like inclusions will help to describe the common pathomechanism of sporadic and familial ALS cases.

4. References

Aguzzi, A. & Rajendran, L. (2009). The transcellular spread of cytosolic amyloids, prions, and prionoids. *Neuron*, Vol.64, No.6, pp. 783-790, ISSN 1097-4199

Arai, T.; Hasegawa, M.; Akiyama, H.; Ikeda, K.; Nonaka, T.; Mori, H.; Mann, D.; Tsuchiya, K.; Yoshida, M.; Hashizume, Y. & Oda, T. (2006). TDP-43 is a component of ubiquitin-positive tau-negative inclusions in frontotemporal lobar degeneration and amyotrophic lateral sclerosis. *Biochem Biophys Res Commun*, Vol.351, No.3, pp. 602-611, ISSN 0006-291X

Arnesano, F.; Banci, L.; Bertini, I.; Martinelli, M.; Furukawa, Y. & O'Halloran, T.V. (2004). The unusually stable quaternary structure of human SOD1 is controlled by both metal occupancy and disulfide status. *J Biol Chem*, Vol.279, pp. 47998-48003,

Ayala, Y.M.; Pantano, S.; D'Ambrogio, A.; Buratti, E.; Brindisi, A.; Marchetti, C.; Romano, M. & Baralle, F.E. (2005). Human, Drosophila, and C.elegans TDP43: nucleic acid binding properties and splicing regulatory function. *J Mol Biol*, Vol.348, No.3, pp. 575-588, ISSN 0022-2836

Ayala, Y.M.; Misteli, T. & Baralle, F.E. (2008a). TDP-43 regulates retinoblastoma protein phosphorylation through the repression of cyclin-dependent kinase 6 expression. *Proc Natl Acad Sci U S A*, Vol.105, No.10, pp. 3785-3789, ISSN 1091-6490

Ayala, Y.M.; Zago, P.; D'Ambrogio, A.; Xu, Y.F.; Petrucelli, L.; Buratti, E. & Baralle, F.E. (2008b). Structural determinants of the cellular localization and shuttling of TDP-43. *J Cell Sci*, Vol.121, No.Pt 22, pp. 3778-3785, ISSN 0021-9533

Basso, M.; Massignan, T.; Samengo, G.; Cheroni, C.; De Biasi, S.; Salmona, M.; Bendotti, C. & Bonetto, V. (2006). Insoluble mutant SOD1 is partly oligoubiquitinated in amyotrophic lateral sclerosis mice. *J Biol Chem*, Vol.281, No.44, pp. 33325-33335, ISSN 0021-9258

Baumer, D.; Hilton, D.; Paine, S.M.; Turner, M.R.; Lowe, J.; Talbot, K. & Ansorge, O. (2010). Juvenile ALS with basophilic inclusions is a FUS proteinopathy with FUS mutations. *Neurology*, Vol.75, No.7, pp. 611-618, ISSN 1526-632X

Bosco, D.A.; Morfini, G.; Karabacak, N.M.; Song, Y.; Gros-Louis, F.; Pasinelli, P.; Goolsby, H.; Fontaine, B.A.; Lemay, N.; McKenna-Yasek, D.; Frosch, M.P.; Agar, J.N.; Julien, J.P.; Brady, S.T. & Brown, R.H., Jr. (2010). Wild-type and mutant SOD1 share an aberrant conformation and a common pathogenic pathway in ALS. *Nat Neurosci*, Vol.13, No.11, pp. 1396-1403, ISSN 1546-1726

Bruijn, L.I.; Miller, T.M. & Cleveland, D.W. (2004). Unraveling the Mechanisms Involved in Motor Neuron Degeneration in ALS. *Annu Rev Neurosci*, Vol.27, pp. 723-749,

Brundin, P.; Melki, R. & Kopito, R. (2010). Prion-like transmission of protein aggregates in neurodegenerative diseases. *Nat Rev Mol Cell Biol*, Vol.11, No.4, pp. 301-307, ISSN 1471-0080

Buck, M. (1998). Trifluoroethanol and colleagues: cosolvents come of age. Recent studies with peptides and proteins. *Q Rev Biophys*, Vol.31, No.3, pp. 297-355, ISSN 0033-5835

Buratti, E. & Baralle, F.E. (2001). Characterization and functional implications of the RNA binding properties of nuclear factor TDP-43, a novel splicing regulator of CFTR exon 9. *J Biol Chem*, Vol.276, No.39, pp. 36337-36343, ISSN 0021-9258

Charcot, J.M. & Joffroy, A. (1869). Deux cas d'atrophie musculaire progressive avec lésions de la substance grise et des faisceaux antérolatéraux de la moelle épinière. *Arch. Physiol. Norm. Pathol.*, Vol.6, pp. 744-760,

Chattopadhyay, M.; Durazo, A.; Sohn, S.H.; Strong, C.D.; Gralla, E.B.; Whitelegge, J.P. & Valentine, J.S. (2008). Initiation and elongation in fibrillation of ALS-linked superoxide dismutase. *Proc Natl Acad Sci U S A*, Vol.105, No.48, pp. 18663-18668, ISSN 1091-6490

Chen, A.K.; Lin, R.Y.; Hsieh, E.Z.; Tu, P.H.; Chen, R.P.; Liao, T.Y.; Chen, W.; Wang, C.H. & Huang, J.J. (2010). Induction of amyloid fibrils by the C-terminal fragments of TDP-43 in amyotrophic lateral sclerosis. *J Am Chem Soc*, Vol.132, No.4, pp. 1186-1187, ISSN 1520-5126

Chia, R.; Tattum, M.H.; Jones, S.; Collinge, J.; Fisher, E.M. & Jackson, G.S. (2010). Superoxide dismutase 1 and tgSOD1 mouse spinal cord seed fibrils, suggesting a propagative cell death mechanism in amyotrophic lateral sclerosis. *PLoS One*, Vol.5, No.5, pp. e10627, ISSN 1932-6203

Chiang, P.M.; Ling, J.; Jeong, Y.H.; Price, D.L.; Aja, S.M. & Wong, P.C. (2010). Deletion of TDP-43 down-regulates Tbc1d1, a gene linked to obesity, and alters body fat metabolism. *Proc Natl Acad Sci U S A*, Vol.107, No.37, pp. 16320-16324, ISSN 1091-6490

Clavaguera, F.; Bolmont, T.; Crowther, R.A.; Abramowski, D.; Frank, S.; Probst, A.; Fraser, G.; Stalder, A.K.; Beibel, M.; Staufenbiel, M.; Jucker, M.; Goedert, M. & Tolnay, M. (2009). Transmission and spreading of tauopathy in transgenic mouse brain. *Nat Cell Biol*, Vol.11, No.7, pp. 909-913, ISSN 1476-4679

Crozat, A.; Aman, P.; Mandahl, N. & Ron, D. (1993). Fusion of CHOP to a novel RNA-binding protein in human myxoid liposarcoma. *Nature*, Vol.363, No.6430, pp. 640-644, ISSN 0028-0836

Culotta, V.C.; Klomp, L.W.J.; Strain, J.; Casareno, R.L.B.; Krems, B. & Gitlin, J.D. (1997). The copper chaperone for superoxide dismutase. *J Biol Chem*, Vol.272, No.38, pp. 23469-23472,

Da Cruz, S. & Cleveland, D.W. (2011). Understanding the role of TDP-43 and FUS/TLS in ALS and beyond. *Curr Opin Neurobiol*, pp. ISSN 1873-6882

de Belleroche, J.; Orrell, R.W. & Virgo, L. (1996). Amyotrophic lateral sclerosis: recent advances in understanding disease mechanisms. *J Neuropathol Exp Neurol*, Vol.55, No.7, pp. 747-757, ISSN 0022-3069

Deng, H.X.; Hentati, A.; Tainer, J.A.; Iqbal, Z.; Cayabyab, A.; Hung, W.Y.; Getzoff, E.D.; Hu, P.; Herzfeldt, B.; Roos, R.P. & et al. (1993). Amyotrophic lateral sclerosis and structural defects in Cu,Zn superoxide dismutase. *Science*, Vol.261, No.5124, pp. 1047-1051,

Deng, H.X.; Bigio, E.H.; Zhai, H.; Fecto, F.; Ajroud, K.; Shi, Y.; Yan, J.; Mishra, M.; Ajroud-Driss, S.; Heller, S.; Sufit, R.; Siddique, N.; Mugnaini, E. & Siddique, T. (2011a). Differential Involvement of Optineurin in Amyotrophic Lateral Sclerosis With or Without SOD1 Mutations. *Arch Neurol*, Vol.68, No.8, pp. 1057-1061, ISSN 1538-3687

Deng, H.X.; Zhai, H.; Bigio, E.H.; Yan, J.; Fecto, F.; Ajroud, K.; Mishra, M.; Ajroud-Driss, S.; Heller, S.; Sufit, R.; Siddique, N.; Mugnaini, E. & Siddique, T. (2011b). FUS-immunoreactive inclusions are a common feature in sporadic and non-SOD1 familial amyotrophic lateral sclerosis. *Ann Neurol*, Vol.67, No.6, pp. 739-748, ISSN 1531-8249

Dobson, C.M. (2003). Protein folding and misfolding. *Nature*, Vol.426, No.6968, pp. 884-890,

Doi, H.; Okamura, K.; Bauer, P.O.; Furukawa, Y.; Shimizu, H.; Kurosawa, M.; Machida, Y.; Miyazaki, H.; Mitsui, K.; Kuroiwa, Y. & Nukina, N. (2008). RNA-binding protein TLS is a major nuclear aggregate-interacting protein in huntingtin exon 1 with expanded polyglutamine-expressing cells. *J Biol Chem*, Vol.283, No.10, pp. 6489-6500, ISSN 0021-9258

Doi, H.; Koyano, S.; Suzuki, Y.; Nukina, N. & Kuroiwa, Y. (2010). The RNA-binding protein FUS/TLS is a common aggregate-interacting protein in polyglutamine diseases. *Neurosci Res*, Vol.66, No.1, pp. 131-133, ISSN 1872-8111

Dormann, D.; Rodde, R.; Edbauer, D.; Bentmann, E.; Fischer, I.; Hruscha, A.; Than, M.E.; Mackenzie, I.R.; Capell, A.; Schmid, B.; Neumann, M. & Haass, C. (2010). ALS-associated fused in sarcoma (FUS) mutations disrupt Transportin-mediated nuclear import. *EMBO J*, Vol.29, No.16, pp. 2841-2857, ISSN 1460-2075

Field, L.S.; Furukawa, Y.; O'Halloran, T.V. & Culotta, V.C. (2003). Factors controlling the uptake of yeast copper/zinc superoxide dismutase into mitochondria. *J Biol Chem*, Vol.278, pp. 28052-28059,

Forman, H.J. & Fridovich, I. (1973). On the stability of bovine superoxide dismutase. The effects of metals. *J Biol Chem*, Vol.248, No.8, pp. 2645-2649,

Forsberg, K.; Jonsson, P.A.; Andersen, P.M.; Bergemalm, D.; Graffmo, K.S.; Hultdin, M.; Jacobsson, J.; Rosquist, R.; Marklund, S.L. & Brannstrom, T. (2010). Novel antibodies reveal inclusions containing non-native SOD1 in sporadic ALS patients. *PLoS One*, Vol.5, No.7, pp. e11552, ISSN 1932-6203

Furukawa, Y.; Torres, A.S. & O'Halloran, T.V. (2004). Oxygen-induced maturation of SOD1: a key role for disulfide formation by the copper chaperone CCS. *EMBO J*, Vol.23, pp. 2872-2881,

Furukawa, Y. & O'Halloran, T.V. (2005). ALS mutations have the greatest destabilizing effect on the apo, reduced form of SOD1, leading to unfolding and oxidative aggregation. *J Biol Chem*, Vol.280, pp. 17266-17274,

Furukawa, Y.; Fu, R.; Deng, H.X.; Siddique, T. & O'Halloran, T.V. (2006). Disulfide cross-linked protein represents a significant fraction of ALS-associated Cu, Zn-superoxide dismutase aggregates in spinal cords of model mice. *Proc Natl Acad Sci U S A*, Vol.103, No.18, pp. 7148-7153, ISSN 0027-8424

Furukawa, Y. & O'Halloran, T.V. (2006). Posttranslational modifications in Cu,Zn-superoxide dismutase and mutations associated with amyotrophic lateral sclerosis. *Antioxid Redox Signal*, Vol.8, No.5-6, pp. 847-867, ISSN 1523-0864

Furukawa, Y.; Kaneko, K.; Yamanaka, K.; O'Halloran, T.V. & Nukina, N. (2008). Complete loss of post-translational modifications triggers fibrillar aggregation of SOD1 in familial form of ALS. *J Biol Chem*, Vol.283, No.35, pp. 24167-24176, ISSN 0021-9258

Furukawa, Y.; Kaneko, K.; Yamanaka, K. & Nukina, N. (2010). Mutation-dependent polymorphism of Cu,Zn-superoxide dismutase aggregates in the familial form of amyotrophic lateral sclerosis. *J Biol Chem*, Vol.285, No.29, pp. 22221-22231, ISSN 1083-351X

Furukawa, Y.; Kaneko, K.; Watanabe, S.; Yamanaka, K. & Nukina, N. (2011). A seeding reaction recapitulates intracellular formation of Sarkosyl-insoluble transactivation response element (TAR) DNA-binding protein-43 inclusions. *J Biol Chem*, Vol.286, No.21, pp. 18664-18672, ISSN 1083-351X

Geser, F.; Martinez-Lage, M.; Kwong, L.K.; Lee, V.M. & Trojanowski, J.Q. (2009). Amyotrophic lateral sclerosis, frontotemporal dementia and beyond: the TDP-43 diseases. *J Neurol*, Vol.256, No.8, pp. 1205-1214, ISSN 1432-1459

Gitcho, M.A.; Baloh, R.H.; Chakraverty, S.; Mayo, K.; Norton, J.B.; Levitch, D.; Hatanpaa, K.J.; White, C.L., 3rd; Bigio, E.H.; Caselli, R.; Baker, M.; Al-Lozi, M.T.; Morris, J.C.; Pestronk, A.; Rademakers, R.; Goate, A.M. & Cairns, N.J. (2008). TDP-43 A315T mutation in familial motor neuron disease. *Ann Neurol*, Vol.63, No.4, pp. 535-538, ISSN 1531-8249

Gurney, M.E.; Pu, H.; Chiu, A.Y.; Dal Canto, M.C.; Polchow, C.Y.; Alexander, D.D.; Caliendo, J.; Hentati, A.; Kwon, Y.W.; Deng, H.X. & et al. (1994). Motor neuron degeneration in mice that express a human Cu,Zn superoxide dismutase mutation. *Science*, Vol.264, No.5166, pp. 1772-1775,

Hadano, S.; Hand, C.K.; Osuga, H.; Yanagisawa, Y.; Otomo, A.; Devon, R.S.; Miyamoto, N.; Showguchi-Miyata, J.; Okada, Y.; Singaraja, R.; Figlewicz, D.A.; Kwiatkowski, T.; Hosler, B.A.; Sagie, T.; Skaug, J.; Nasir, J.; Brown, R.H., Jr.; Scherer, S.W.; Rouleau, G.A.; Hayden, M.R. & Ikeda, J.E. (2001). A gene encoding a putative GTPase regulator is mutated in familial amyotrophic lateral sclerosis 2. *Nat Genet*, Vol.29, No.2, pp. 166-173, ISSN 1061-4036

Hasegawa, M.; Arai, T.; Nonaka, T.; Kametani, F.; Yoshida, M.; Hashizume, Y.; Beach, T.G.; Buratti, E.; Baralle, F.; Morita, M.; Nakano, I.; Oda, T.; Tsuchiya, K. & Akiyama, H. (2008). Phosphorylated TDP-43 in frontotemporal lobar degeneration and amyotrophic lateral sclerosis. *Ann Neurol*, Vol.64, No.1, pp. 60-70, ISSN 1531-8249

Hayward, L.J.; Rodriguez, J.A.; Kim, J.W.; Tiwari, A.; Goto, J.J.; Cabelli, D.E.; Valentine, J.S. & Brown, R.H., Jr. (2002). Decreased metallation and activity in subsets of mutant superoxide dismutases associated with familial amyotrophic lateral sclerosis. *J Biol Chem*, Vol.277, No.18, pp. 15923-15931,

Huang, C.; Zhou, H.; Tong, J.; Chen, H.; Liu, Y.J.; Wang, D.; Wei, X. & Xia, X.G. (2011). FUS transgenic rats develop the phenotypes of amyotrophic lateral sclerosis and frontotemporal lobar degeneration. *PLoS Genet*, Vol.7, No.3, pp. e1002011, ISSN 1553-7404

Hwang, Y.M.; Stathopulos, P.B.; Dimmick, K.; Yang, H.; Badiei, H.R.; Tong, M.S.; Rumfeldt, J.A.; Chen, P.; Karanassios, V. & Meiering, E.M. (2010). Nonamyloid aggregates arising from mature copper/zinc superoxide dismutases resemble those observed in amyotrophic lateral sclerosis. *J Biol Chem*, Vol.285, No.53, pp. 41701-41711, ISSN 1083-351X

Igaz, L.M.; Kwong, L.K.; Xu, Y.; Truax, A.C.; Uryu, K.; Neumann, M.; Clark, C.M.; Elman, L.B.; Miller, B.L.; Grossman, M.; McCluskey, L.F.; Trojanowski, J.Q. & Lee, V.M. (2008). Enrichment of C-terminal fragments in TAR DNA-binding protein-43 cytoplasmic inclusions in brain but not in spinal cord of frontotemporal lobar degeneration and amyotrophic lateral sclerosis. *Am J Pathol*, Vol.173, No.1, pp. 182-194, ISSN 1525-2191

Iko, Y.; Kodama, T.S.; Kasai, N.; Oyama, T.; Morita, E.H.; Muto, T.; Okumura, M.; Fujii, R.; Takumi, T.; Tate, S. & Morikawa, K. (2004). Domain architectures and characterization of an RNA-binding protein, TLS. *J Biol Chem*, Vol.279, No.43, pp. 44834-44840, ISSN 0021-9258

Jensen, L.T. & Culotta, V.C. (2005). Activation of CuZn superoxide dismutases from Caenorhabditis elegans does not require the copper chaperone CCS. *J Biol Chem*, Vol.280, No.50, pp. 41373-41379, ISSN 0021-9258

Johnson, B.S.; Snead, D.; Lee, J.J.; McCaffery, J.M.; Shorter, J. & Gitler, A.D. (2009). TDP-43 is intrinsically aggregation-prone, and amyotrophic lateral sclerosis-linked mutations accelerate aggregation and increase toxicity. *J Biol Chem*, Vol.284, No.30, pp. 20329-20339, ISSN 0021-9258

Kabashi, E.; Valdmanis, P.N.; Dion, P.; Spiegelman, D.; McConkey, B.J.; Vande Velde, C.; Bouchard, J.P.; Lacomblez, L.; Pochigaeva, K.; Salachas, F.; Pradat, P.F.; Camu, W.; Meininger, V.; Dupre, N. & Rouleau, G.A. (2008). TARDBP mutations in individuals with sporadic and familial amyotrophic lateral sclerosis. *Nat Genet*, Vol.40, No.5, pp. 572-4, ISSN 1546-1718

Karch, C.M.; Prudencio, M.; Winkler, D.D.; Hart, P.J. & Borchelt, D.R. (2009). Role of mutant SOD1 disulfide oxidation and aggregation in the pathogenesis of familial ALS. *Proc Natl Acad Sci U S A*, Vol.106, No.19, pp. 7774-7779, ISSN 1091-6490

Kato, S.; Takikawa, M.; Nakashima, K.; Hirano, A.; Cleveland, D.W.; Kusaka, H.; Shibata, N.; Kato, M.; Nakano, I. & Ohama, E. (2000). New consensus research on neuropathological aspects of familial amyotrophic lateral sclerosis with superoxide dismutase 1 (SOD1) gene mutations: inclusions containing SOD1 in neurons and astrocytes. *Amyotroph Lateral Scler Other Motor Neuron Disord*, Vol.1, No.3, pp. 163-184, ISSN 1466-0822

Kawamata, H. & Manfredi, G. (2008). Different regulation of wild-type and mutant Cu,Zn superoxide dismutase localization in mammalian mitochondria. *Hum Mol Genet*, Vol.17, No.21, pp. 3303-3317, ISSN 1460-2083

Kerman, A.; Liu, H.N.; Croul, S.; Bilbao, J.; Rogaeva, E.; Zinman, L.; Robertson, J. & Chakrabartty, A. (2010). Amyotrophic lateral sclerosis is a non-amyloid disease in which extensive misfolding of SOD1 is unique to the familial form. *Acta Neuropathol*, Vol.119, No.3, pp. 335-344, ISSN 1432-0533

Klunk, W.E.; Jacob, R.F. & Mason, R.P. (1999). Quantifying amyloid by congo red spectral shift assay. *Methods Enzymol*, Vol.309, pp. 285-305, ISSN 0076-6879

Kraemer, B.C.; Schuck, T.; Wheeler, J.M.; Robinson, L.C.; Trojanowski, J.Q.; Lee, V.M. & Schellenberg, G.D. (2010). Loss of murine TDP-43 disrupts motor function and plays an essential role in embryogenesis. *Acta Neuropathol*, Vol.119, No.4, pp. 409-419, ISSN 1432-0533

Kwiatkowski, T.J., Jr.; Bosco, D.A.; Leclerc, A.L.; Tamrazian, E.; Vanderburg, C.R.; Russ, C.; Davis, A.; Gilchrist, J.; Kasarskis, E.J.; Munsat, T.; Valdmanis, P.; Rouleau, G.A.; Hosler, B.A.; Cortelli, P.; de Jong, P.J.; Yoshinaga, Y.; Haines, J.L.; Pericak-Vance, M.A.; Yan, J.; Ticozzi, N.; Siddique, T.; McKenna-Yasek, D.; Sapp, P.C.; Horvitz, H.R.; Landers, J.E. & Brown, R.H., Jr. (2009). Mutations in the FUS/TLS gene on chromosome 16 cause familial amyotrophic lateral sclerosis. *Science*, Vol.323, No.5918, pp. 1205-1208, ISSN 1095-9203

Lagier-Tourenne, C.; Polymenidou, M. & Cleveland, D.W. (2010). TDP-43 and FUS/TLS: emerging roles in RNA processing and neurodegeneration. *Hum Mol Genet*, Vol.19, pp. R46-R64, ISSN 1460-2083

Leitch, J.M.; Jensen, L.T.; Bouldin, S.D.; Outten, C.E.; Hart, P.J. & Culotta, V.C. (2009). Activation of Cu,Zn-superoxide dismutase in the absence of oxygen and the copper chaperone CCS. *J Biol Chem*, Vol.284, No.33, pp. 21863-21871, 0021-9258

Lelie, H.L.; Liba, A.; Bourassa, M.W.; Chattopadhyay, M.; Chan, P.K.; Gralla, E.B.; Miller, L.M.; Borchelt, D.R.; Valentine, J.S. & Whitelegge, J.P. (2011). Copper and zinc metallation status of copper-zinc superoxide dismutase from amyotrophic lateral sclerosis transgenic mice. *J Biol Chem*, Vol.286, No.4, pp. 2795-2806, ISSN 1083-351X

LeVine, H., 3rd (1999). Quantification of beta-sheet amyloid fibril structures with thioflavin T. *Methods Enzymol*, Vol.309, pp. 274-284, ISSN 0076-6879

Lin, W.L. & Dickson, D.W. (2008). Ultrastructural localization of TDP-43 in filamentous neuronal inclusions in various neurodegenerative diseases. *Acta Neuropathol*, Vol.116, No.2, pp. 205-213, ISSN 0001-6322

Liu, H.N.; Sanelli, T.; Horne, P.; Pioro, E.P.; Strong, M.J.; Rogaeva, E.; Bilbao, J.; Zinman, L. & Robertson, J. (2009). Lack of evidence of monomer/misfolded superoxide dismutase-1 in sporadic amyotrophic lateral sclerosis. *Ann Neurol*, Vol.66, No.1, pp. 75-80, ISSN 1531-8249

Luk, K.C.; Song, C.; O'Brien, P.; Stieber, A.; Branch, J.R.; Brunden, K.R.; Trojanowski, J.Q. & Lee, V.M. (2009). Exogenous alpha-synuclein fibrils seed the formation of Lewy body-like intracellular inclusions in cultured cells. *Proc Natl Acad Sci U S A*, Vol.106, No.47, pp. 20051-20056, ISSN 1091-6490

Mackenzie, I.R.; Bigio, E.H.; Ince, P.G.; Geser, F.; Neumann, M.; Cairns, N.J.; Kwong, L.K.; Forman, M.S.; Ravits, J.; Stewart, H.; Eisen, A.; McClusky, L.; Kretzschmar, H.A.; Monoranu, C.M.; Highley, J.R.; Kirby, J.; Siddique, T.; Shaw, P.J.; Lee, V.M. & Trojanowski, J.Q. (2007). Pathological TDP-43 distinguishes sporadic amyotrophic lateral sclerosis from amyotrophic lateral sclerosis with SOD1 mutations. *Ann Neurol*, Vol.61, No.5, pp. 427-434, ISSN 0364-5134

Mackenzie, I.R.; Ansorge, O.; Strong, M.; Bilbao, J.; Zinman, L.; Ang, L.C.; Baker, M.; Stewart, H.; Eisen, A.; Rademakers, R. & Neumann, M. (2011). Pathological heterogeneity in amyotrophic lateral sclerosis with FUS mutations: two distinct patterns correlating with disease severity and mutation. *Acta Neuropathol*, Vol.122, No.1, pp. 87-98, ISSN 1432-0533

Maruyama, H.; Morino, H.; Ito, H.; Izumi, Y.; Kato, H.; Watanabe, Y.; Kinoshita, Y.; Kamada, M.; Nodera, H.; Suzuki, H.; Komure, O.; Matsuura, S.; Kobatake, K.; Morimoto, N.; Abe, K.; Suzuki, N.; Aoki, M.; Kawata, A.; Hirai, T.; Kato, T.; Ogasawara, K.; Hirano, A.; Takumi, T.; Kusaka, H.; Hagiwara, K.; Kaji, R. & Kawakami, H. (2010). Mutations of optineurin in amyotrophic lateral sclerosis. *Nature*, Vol.465, No.7295, pp. 223-226, ISSN 1476-4687

McCord, J.M. & Fridovich, I. (1969). Superoxide dismutase. An enzymic function for erythrocuprein (hemocuprein). *J Biol Chem*, Vol.244, No.22, pp. 6049-6055,

Millecamps, S.; Salachas, F.; Cazeneuve, C.; Gordon, P.; Bricka, B.; Camuzat, A.; Guillot-Noel, L.; Russaouen, O.; Bruneteau, G.; Pradat, P.F.; Le Forestier, N.; Vandenberghe, N.; Danel-Brunaud, V.; Guy, N.; Thauvin-Robinet, C.; Lacomblez, L.; Couratier, P.; Hannequin, D.; Seilhean, D.; Le Ber, I.; Corcia, P.; Camu, W.; Brice, A.; Rouleau, G.; LeGuern, E. & Meininger, V. (2010). SOD1, ANG, VAPB, TARDBP, and FUS mutations in familial amyotrophic lateral sclerosis: genotype-phenotype correlations. *J Med Genet*, Vol.47, No.8, pp. 554-560, ISSN 1468-6244

Munch, C.; O'Brien, J. & Bertolotti, A. (2011). Prion-like propagation of mutant superoxide dismutase-1 misfolding in neuronal cells. *Proc Natl Acad Sci U S A*, Vol.108, No.9, pp. 3548-3553, ISSN 1091-6490

Neumann, M.; Sampathu, D.M.; Kwong, L.K.; Truax, A.C.; Micsenyi, M.C.; Chou, T.T.; Bruce, J.; Schuck, T.; Grossman, M.; Clark, C.M.; McCluskey, L.F.; Miller, B.L.; Masliah, E.; Mackenzie, I.R.; Feldman, H.; Feiden, W.; Kretzschmar, H.A.; Trojanowski, J.Q. & Lee, V.M. (2006). Ubiquitinated TDP-43 in frontotemporal lobar degeneration and amyotrophic lateral sclerosis. *Science*, Vol.314, No.5796, pp. 130-133, ISSN 1095-9203

Okamoto, K.; Mizuno, Y. & Fujita, Y. (2008). Bunina bodies in amyotrophic lateral sclerosis. *Neuropathology*, Vol.28, No.2, pp. 109-115, ISSN 0919-6544

Oztug Durer, Z.A.; Cohlberg, J.A.; Dinh, P.; Padua, S.; Ehrenclou, K.; Downes, S.; Tan, J.K.; Nakano, Y.; Bowman, C.J.; Hoskins, J.L.; Kwon, C.; Mason, A.Z.; Rodriguez, J.A.; Doucette, P.A.; Shaw, B.F. & Selverstone Valentine, J. (2009). Loss of metal ions, disulfide reduction and mutations related to familial ALS promote formation of amyloid-like aggregates from superoxide dismutase. *PLoS One*, Vol.4, No.3, pp. e5004, ISSN 1932-6203

Piao, Y.S.; Wakabayashi, K.; Kakita, A.; Yamada, M.; Hayashi, S.; Morita, T.; Ikuta, F.; Oyanagi, K. & Takahashi, H. (2003). Neuropathology with clinical correlations of sporadic amyotrophic lateral sclerosis: 102 autopsy cases examined between 1962 and 2000. *Brain Pathol*, Vol.13, No.1, pp. 10-22, ISSN 1015-6305

Rae, T.D.; Schmidt, P.J.; Pufahl, R.A.; Culotta, V.C. & O'Halloran, T.V. (1999). Undetectable intracellular free copper: The requirement of a copper chaperone for superoxide dismutase. *Science*, Vol.284, No.5415, pp. 805-808,

Rakhit, R.; Cunningham, P.; Furtos-Matei, A.; Dahan, S.; Qi, X.F.; Crow, J.P.; Cashman, N.R.; Kondejewski, L.H. & Chakrabartty, A. (2002). Oxidation-induced misfolding and aggregation of superoxide dismutase and its implications for amyotrophic lateral sclerosis. *J Biol Chem*, Vol.277, No.49, pp. 47551-47556,

Rakhit, R.; Crow, J.P.; Lepock, J.R.; Kondejewski, L.H.; Cashman, N.R. & Chakrabartty, A. (2004). Monomeric Cu,Zn-superoxide dismutase is a common misfolding intermediate in the oxidation models of sporadic and familial amyotrophic lateral sclerosis. *J. Biol. Chem.*, Vol.279, No.15, pp. 15499-15504,

Reaume, A.G.; Elliott, J.L.; Hoffman, E.K.; Kowall, N.W.; Ferrante, R.J.; Siwek, D.F.; Wilcox, H.M.; Flood, D.G.; Beal, M.F.; Brown, R.H., Jr.; Scott, R.W. & Snider, W.D. (1996). Motor neurons in Cu/Zn superoxide dismutase-deficient mice develop normally but exhibit enhanced cell death after axonal injury. *Nat Genet*, Vol.13, No.1, pp. 43-47,

Ren, P.H.; Lauckner, J.E.; Kachirskaia, I.; Heuser, J.E.; Melki, R. & Kopito, R.R. (2009). Cytoplasmic penetration and persistent infection of mammalian cells by polyglutamine aggregates. *Nat Cell Biol*, Vol.11, No.2, pp. 219-225, ISSN 1476-4679

Rodriguez, J.A.; Valentine, J.S.; Eggers, D.K.; Roe, J.A.; Tiwari, A.; Brown, R.H. & Hayward, L.J. (2002). Familial amyotrophic lateral sclerosis-associated mutations decrease the thermal stability of distinctly metallated species of human copper/zinc superoxide dismutase. *J Biol Chem*, Vol.277, No.18, pp. 15932-15937,

Rodriguez, J.A.; Shaw, B.F.; Durazo, A.; Sohn, S.H.; Doucette, P.A.; Nersissian, A.M.; Faull, K.F.; Eggers, D.K.; Tiwari, A.; Hayward, L.J. & Valentine, J.S. (2005). Destabilization of apoprotein is insufficient to explain Cu,Zn-superoxide dismutase-linked ALS pathogenesis. *Proc Natl Acad Sci U S A*, Vol.102, No.30, pp. 10516-10521,

Rosen, D.R.; Siddique, T.; Patterson, D.; Figlewicz, D.A.; Sapp, P.; Hentati, A.; Donaldson, D.; Goto, J.; O'Regan, J.P.; Deng, H.X. & et al. (1993). Mutations in Cu/Zn superoxide dismutase gene are associated with familial amyotrophic lateral sclerosis. *Nature*, Vol.362, No.6415, pp. 59-62,

Ross, C.A. & Poirier, M.A. (2004). Protein aggregation and neurodegenerative disease. *Nat Med*, Vol.10 Suppl, pp. S10-S17, ISSN 1078-8956

Serpell, L.C. & Smith, J.M. (2000). Direct visualisation of the beta-sheet structure of synthetic Alzheimer's amyloid. *J Mol Biol*, Vol.299, No.1, pp. 225-231, ISSN 0022-2836

Shaw, B.F.; Lelie, H.L.; Durazo, A.; Nersissian, A.M.; Xu, G.; Chan, P.K.; Gralla, E.B.; Tiwari, A.; Hayward, L.J.; Borchelt, D.R.; Valentine, J.S. & Whitelegge, J.P. (2008). Detergent-insoluble aggregates associated with amyotrophic lateral sclerosis in transgenic mice contain primarily full-length, unmodified superoxide dismutase-1. *J Biol Chem*, Vol.283, No.13, pp. 8340-8350, ISSN 0021-9258

Shibata, N.; Hirano, A.; Kobayashi, M.; Sasaki, S.; Kato, T.; Matsumoto, S.; Shiozawa, Z.; Komori, T.; Ikemoto, A.; Umahara, T. & et al. (1994). Cu/Zn superoxide dismutase-like immunoreactivity in Lewy body-like inclusions of sporadic amyotrophic lateral sclerosis. *Neurosci Lett*, Vol.179, No.1-2, pp. 149-152,

Shibata, N.; Asayama, K.; Hirano, A. & Kobayashi, M. (1996a). Immunohistochemical study on superoxide dismutases in spinal cords from autopsied patients with amyotrophic lateral sclerosis. *Dev Neurosci*, Vol.18, No.5-6, pp. 492-498, ISSN 0378-5866

Shibata, N.; Hirano, A.; Kobayashi, M.; Siddique, T.; Deng, H.X.; Hung, W.Y.; Kato, T. & Asayama, K. (1996b). Intense superoxide dismutase-1 immunoreactivity in intracytoplasmic hyaline inclusions of familial amyotrophic lateral sclerosis with posterior column involvement. *J Neuropathol Exp Neurol*, Vol.55, No.4, pp. 481-490, ISSN 0022-3069

Siddique, T.; Figlewicz, D.A.; Pericak-Vance, M.A.; Haines, J.L.; Rouleau, G.; Jeffers, A.J.; Sapp, P.; Hung, W.Y.; Bebout, J.; McKenna-Yasek, D. & et al. (1991). Linkage of a gene causing familial amyotrophic lateral sclerosis to chromosome 21 and evidence of genetic-locus heterogeneity. *N Engl J Med*, Vol.324, No.20, pp. 1381-1384, ISSN 0028-4793

Son, M.; Puttaparthi, K.; Kawamata, H.; Rajendran, B.; Boyer, P.J.; Manfredi, G. & Elliott, J.L. (2007). Overexpression of CCS in G93A-SOD1 mice leads to accelerated neurological deficits with severe mitochondrial pathology. *Proc Natl Acad Sci U S A*, Vol.104, No.14, pp. 6072-6077, ISSN 0027-8424

Soto, C. (2003). Unfolding the role of protein misfolding in neurodegenerative diseases. *Nat Rev Neurosci*, Vol.4, No.1, pp. 49-60, ISSN 1471-003X

Sreedharan, J.; Blair, I.P.; Tripathi, V.B.; Hu, X.; Vance, C.; Rogelj, B.; Ackerley, S.; Durnall, J.C.; Williams, K.L.; Buratti, E.; Baralle, F.; de Belleroche, J.; Mitchell, J.D.; Leigh, P.N.; Al-Chalabi, A.; Miller, C.C.; Nicholson, G. & Shaw, C.E. (2008). TDP-43 mutations in familial and sporadic amyotrophic lateral sclerosis. *Science*, Vol.319, No.5870, pp. 1668-1672, ISSN 1095-9203

Stathopulos, P.B.; Rumfeldt, J.A.; Scholz, G.A.; Irani, R.A.; Frey, H.E.; Hallewell, R.A.; Lepock, J.R. & Meiering, E.M. (2003). Cu/Zn superoxide dismutase mutants associated with amyotrophic lateral sclerosis show enhanced formation of aggregates in vitro. *Proc Natl Acad Sci USA*, Vol.100, No.12, pp. 7021-7026,

Subramaniam, J.R.; Lyons, W.E.; Liu, J.; Bartnikas, T.B.; Rothstein, J.; Price, D.L.; Cleveland, D.W.; Gitlin, J.D. & Wong, P.C. (2002). Mutant SOD1 causes motor neuron disease independent of copper chaperone-mediated copper loading. *Nat Neurosci*, Vol.5, No.4, pp. 301-307,

Sun, Z.; Diaz, Z.; Fang, X.; Hart, M.P.; Chesi, A.; Shorter, J. & Gitler, A.D. (2011). Molecular determinants and genetic modifiers of aggregation and toxicity for the ALS disease protein FUS/TLS. *PLoS Biol*, Vol.9, No.4, pp. e1000614, ISSN 1545-7885

Tiwari, A. & Hayward, L.J. (2003). Familial amyotrophic lateral sclerosis mutants of copper/zinc superoxide dismutase are susceptible to disulfide reduction. *J Biol Chem*, Vol.278, No.8, pp. 5984-5992, ISSN 0021-9258

Turner, B.J. & Talbot, K. (2008). Transgenics, toxicity and therapeutics in rodent models of mutant SOD1-mediated familial ALS. *Prog Neurobiol*, Vol.85, No.1, pp. 94-134, ISSN 0301-0082

Uranishi, H.; Tetsuka, T.; Yamashita, M.; Asamitsu, K.; Shimizu, M.; Itoh, M. & Okamoto, T. (2001). Involvement of the pro-oncoprotein TLS (translocated in liposarcoma) in nuclear factor-kappa B p65-mediated transcription as a coactivator. *J Biol Chem*, Vol.276, No.16, pp. 13395-13401, ISSN 0021-9258

Van Deerlin, V.M.; Leverenz, J.B.; Bekris, L.M.; Bird, T.D.; Yuan, W.; Elman, L.B.; Clay, D.; Wood, E.M.; Chen-Plotkin, A.S.; Martinez-Lage, M.; Steinbart, E.; McCluskey, L.; Grossman, M.; Neumann, M.; Wu, I.L.; Yang, W.S.; Kalb, R.; Galasko, D.R.; Montine, T.J.; Trojanowski, J.Q.; Lee, V.M.; Schellenberg, G.D. & Yu, C.E. (2008). TARDBP mutations in amyotrophic lateral sclerosis with TDP-43 neuropathology: a genetic and histopathological analysis. *Lancet Neurol*, Vol.7, No.5, pp. 409-416, ISSN 1474-4422

Vance, C.; Rogelj, B.; Hortobagyi, T.; De Vos, K.J.; Nishimura, A.L.; Sreedharan, J.; Hu, X.; Smith, B.; Ruddy, D.; Wright, P.; Ganesalingam, J.; Williams, K.L.; Tripathi, V.; Al-Saraj, S.; Al-Chalabi, A.; Leigh, P.N.; Blair, I.P.; Nicholson, G.; de Belleroche, J.; Gallo, J.M.; Miller, C.C. & Shaw, C.E. (2009). Mutations in FUS, an RNA processing protein, cause familial amyotrophic lateral sclerosis type 6. *Science*, Vol.323, No.5918, pp. 1208-1211, ISSN 1095-9203

Wang, J.; Xu, G.; Gonzales, V.; Coonfield, M.; Fromholt, D.; Copeland, N.G.; Jenkins, N.A. & Borchelt, D.R. (2002). Fibrillar inclusions and motor neuron degeneration in transgenic mice expressing superoxide dismutase 1 with a disrupted copper-binding site. *Neurobiol Dis*, Vol.10, No.2, pp. 128-38, 0969-9961 (Print)

Wang, J.; Xu, G.; Li, H.; Gonzales, V.; Fromholt, D.; Karch, C.; Copeland, N.G.; Jenkins, N.A. & Borchelt, D.R. (2005). Somatodendritic accumulation of misfolded SOD1-L126Z in motor neurons mediates degeneration: alphaB-crystallin modulates aggregation. *Hum Mol Genet*, Vol.14, No.16, pp. 2335-2347, 0964-6906 (Print)

Wang, Q.; Johnson, J.L.; Agar, N.Y. & Agar, J.N. (2008). Protein aggregation and protein instability govern familial amyotrophic lateral sclerosis patient survival. *PLoS Biol*, Vol.6, No.7, pp. e170, ISSN 1545-7885

Watanabe, M.; Dykes-Hoberg, M.; Culotta, V.C.; Price, D.L.; Wong, P.C. & Rothstein, J.D. (2001). Histological evidence of protein aggregation in mutant SOD1 transgenic mice and in amyotrophic lateral sclerosis neural tissues. *Neurobiol Dis*, Vol.8, No.6, pp. 933-941,

Wegorzewska, I.; Bell, S.; Cairns, N.J.; Miller, T.M. & Baloh, R.H. (2009). TDP-43 mutant transgenic mice develop features of ALS and frontotemporal lobar degeneration. *Proc Natl Acad Sci U S A*, Vol.106, No.44, pp. 18809-18814, ISSN 1091-6490

Wils, H.; Kleinberger, G.; Janssens, J.; Pereson, S.; Joris, G.; Cuijt, I.; Smits, V.; Ceuterick-de Groote, C.; Van Broeckhoven, C. & Kumar-Singh, S. (2010). TDP-43 transgenic mice develop spastic paralysis and neuronal inclusions characteristic of ALS and frontotemporal lobar degeneration. *Proc Natl Acad Sci U S A*, Vol.107, No.8, pp. 3858-3863, ISSN 1091-6490

Yang, L.; Embree, L.J.; Tsai, S. & Hickstein, D.D. (1998). Oncoprotein TLS interacts with serine-arginine proteins involved in RNA splicing. *J Biol Chem*, Vol.273, No.43, pp. 27761-27764, ISSN 0021-9258

Yang, Y.; Hentati, A.; Deng, H.X.; Dabbagh, O.; Sasaki, T.; Hirano, M.; Hung, W.Y.; Ouahchi, K.; Yan, J.; Azim, A.C.; Cole, N.; Gascon, G.; Yagmour, A.; Ben-Hamida, M.; Pericak-Vance, M.; Hentati, F. & Siddique, T. (2001). The gene encoding alsin, a protein with three guanine-nucleotide exchange factor domains, is mutated in a form of recessive amyotrophic lateral sclerosis. *Nat Genet*, Vol.29, No.2, pp. 160-165, ISSN 1061-4036

Zhou, H.; Huang, C.; Chen, H.; Wang, D.; Landel, C.P.; Xia, P.Y.; Bowser, R.; Liu, Y.J. & Xia, X.G. (2010). Transgenic rat model of neurodegeneration caused by mutation in the TDP gene. *PLoS Genet*, Vol.6, No.3, pp. e1000887, ISSN 1553-7404

Zinszner, H.; Sok, J.; Immanuel, D.; Yin, Y. & Ron, D. (1997). TLS (FUS) binds RNA in vivo and engages in nucleo-cytoplasmic shuttling. *J Cell Sci*, Vol.110 (Pt 15), pp. 1741-1750, ISSN 0021-9533

Zoghbi, H.Y. & Orr, H.T. (2000). Glutamine repeats and neurodegeneration. *Annu Rev Neurosci*, Vol.23, pp. 217-247, ISSN 0147-006X

15

The Kynurenine Pathway

Yiquan Chen[1] and Gilles Guillemin[1,2]
[1]*Department of Pharmacology, School of Medical Sciences, University of New South Wales, Sydney,*
[2]*St Vincent's Centre for Applied Medical Research, St Vincent's Hospital, Sydney, Australia*

1. Introduction

The kynurenine pathway represents a major route for the catabolism of tryptophan (TRP). In the body, TRP is transported around the periphery either bound to albumin (90%) or in free form (10%), the two states existing in equilibrium (McMenamy 1965). However, only free form TRP can be transported across the blood-brain barrier (BBB) by the competitive and non-specific L-type amino acid transporter (Hargreaves and Pardridge 1988). Once in the central nervous system (CNS), TRP acts as a precursor to several metabolic pathways, such as for the synthesis of kynurenine (KYN), serotonin, melatonin and protein (Fig. 1) (Ruddick *et al.* 2006).

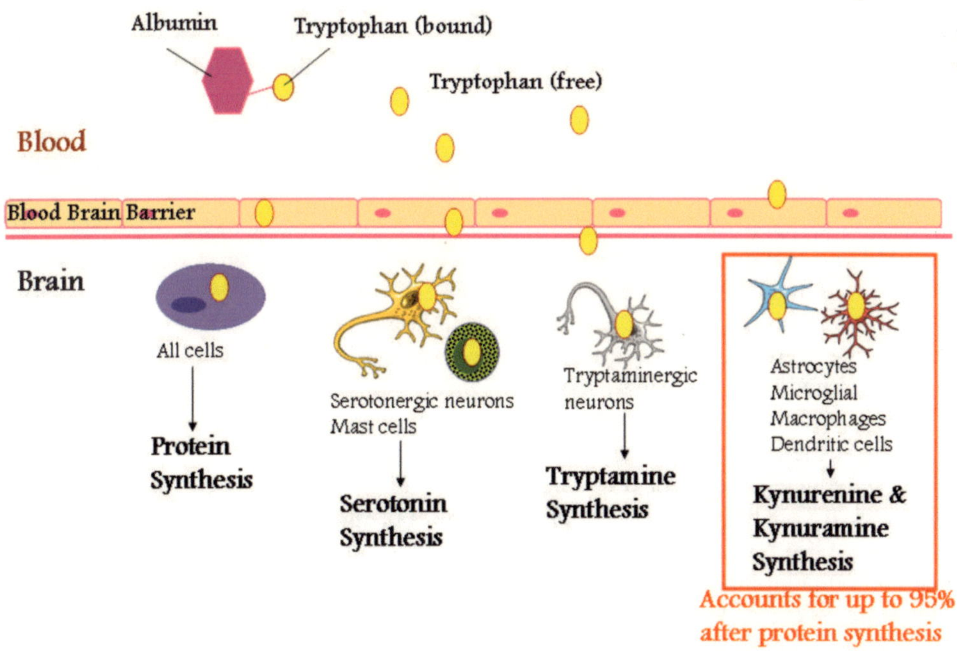

Fig. 1. TRP in the CNS. Only free TRP can cross the BBB and act as precursor for protein, serotonin, tryptamine, and kynurenine and kynuramine synthesis. The kynurenine pathway is a major pathway for TRP catabolism. Adapted from (Ruddick *et al.* 2006).

In the CNS, the kynurenine pathway is present to varying extents in most cell types, including astrocytes (Guillemin *et al.* 2000), neurons (Guillemin *et al.* 2007), infiltrating macrophages and microglia (Guillemin *et al.* 2003), oligodendrocytes (Lim *et al.* 2007), and endothelial cells (Owe-Young *et al.* 2008). Infiltrating macrophages, activated microglia and neurons have the complete repertoire of kynurenine pathway enzymes. On the other hand, neuroprotective astrocytes and oligodendrocytes lack the enzyme, kynurenine 3-monooxygenase (KMO) and indoleamine 2,3-dioxygenase 1 (IDO-1) respectively, and are incapable of synthesizing the excitotoxin, quinolinic acid (QUIN) (Guillemin *et al.* 2000; Lim *et al.* 2007).

The oxidation of TRP, initiating the kynurenine pathway (Fig. 2), may be catalyzed by one of three enzymes - TRP 2,3-dioxygenase (TDO), IDO-1 or IDO-2, a newly discovered IDO related enzyme (Salter and Pogson 1985; Takikawa *et al.* 1986; Ball *et al.* 2007; Metz *et al.* 2007). TDO resides primarily in the liver, although it is also expressed in low quantities in the brain, and is induced by TRP or corticosteroids (Salter and Pogson 1985; Miller *et al.* 2004). In contrast, IDO-1 is the predominant enzyme extra-hepatically and is found in numerous cells, including macrophages, microglia, neurons and astrocytes (Guillemin *et al.* 2001; Guillemin *et al.* 2003; Guillemin *et al.* 2005; Guillemin *et al.* 2007). IDO-1 is up regulated by certain cytokines and inflammatory molecules, such as lipopolysaccharides, amyloid peptides and human immunodeficiency virus (HIV) proteins (Fujigaki *et al.* 1998; Guillemin *et al.* 2003; Takikawa 2005), and its most potent stimulant is interferon gamma (IFN-γ) (Hayaishi and Yoshida 1978; Werner-Felmayer *et al.* 1989). IFN-γ induces both the gene expression and enzymatic activity of IDO-1 (Yasui *et al.* 1986; Dai and Gupta 1990). IDO-2 possesses similar structural and enzymatic activities as IDO-1. However, the two enzymes differ in their expression pattern and signalling pathway, and IDO-2 is preferentially inhibited by D-1-methyl-tryptophan (D-1-MT) (Ball *et al.* 2007; Metz *et al.* 2007).

The first stable intermediate from the kynurenine pathway is KYN. Subsequently, several neuroactive intermediates are generated. They include the free-radical generator, 3-hydroxyanthranilic acid (3HAA) (Goldstein *et al.* 2000), the excitotoxin and *N*-methyl *D*-aspartate (NMDA) receptor agonist, QUIN (Stone and Perkins 1981), the NMDA antagonist, kynurenic acid (KYNA) (Perkins and Stone 1982), and the neuroprotectant, picolinic acid (PIC) (Jhamandas *et al.* 1990).

The kynurenine pathway first aroused great interest when it was observed that an accelerated and sustained degradation of TRP occurred when activated T cells released IFN-γ during an immune response (Pfefferkorn 1984). The significance was speculated to be a defence mechanism that starved tumour cells, pathogens and parasites of TRP (Pfefferkorn 1984; Brown *et al.* 1991). Further research soon discovered that IDO-1 activity was necessary for the preservation of allogeneic foetuses in mice, and that TRP depletion had an anti-proliferative and apoptotic effect on T cells (Munn *et al.* 1998; Munn *et al.* 1999; Lee *et al.* 2002). Hence, the kynurenine pathway appeared to exert an immuno-regulatory effect. In particular, the general control non-derepressible-2 kinase (GCN2) was identified as a key mediator in IDO-1 induced TRP depletion immunosuppression (Munn *et al.* 2005). The activation of GCN2 triggered a stress-response program that resulted in cell-cycle arrest, differentiation, adaptation or apoptosis (de Haro *et al.* 1996; Rao *et al.* 2004; Bi *et al.* 2005). Furthermore, some of the kynurenines, such as QUIN and 3HAA, can selectively target immune cells undergoing activation, thus suppressing T cell proliferation (Frumento *et al.* 2002; Fallarino *et al.* 2003). They can also act in concert to produce an additive effect (Terness *et al.* 2002). Lastly, the production of the excitotoxic QUIN was often significantly increased following inflammation and resulting immune activation (Moffett *et al.* 1997).

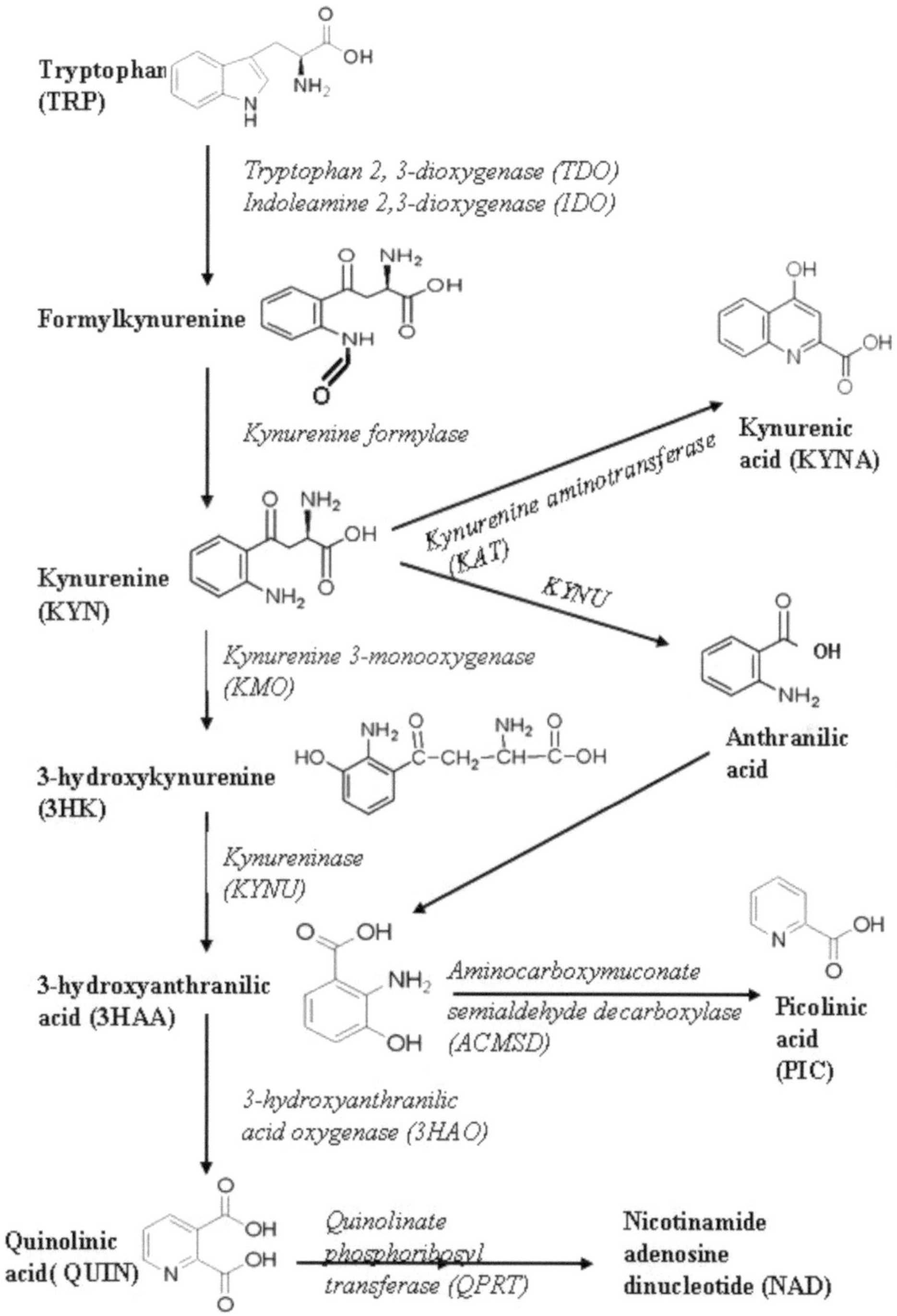

Fig. 2. The kynurenine pathway. Via the kynurenine pathway, TRP is converted to nicotinamide adenine dinucleotide (NAD) in a series of biochemical steps. In the process, neuroactive intermediates are produced. The neuroprotectants include kynurenic acid and picolinic, and the neurotoxin, QUIN.

To date, the kynurenine pathway has been implicated in a wide range of diseases and disorders, including infectious diseases (e.g. HIV), neurological disorders (e.g. Alzheimer's disease (AD), Huntington's disease (HD) and ALS), affective disorders (e.g. schizophrenia, depression and anxiety), autoimmune diseases (e.g. multiple sclerosis and rheumatoid arthritis), peripheral conditions (e.g. cardiovascular disease) and malignancy, and a key indicator is often the up-regulation in IDO-1 resulting in an accelerated and sustained degradation in TRP.

2. The kynurenine pathway and QUIN in ALS

The interest in the kynurenine pathway in the pathogenesis of ALS is relatively new. However, a number of studies have provided relevant results demonstrating the involvement of the kynurenine pathway in ALS.

For the kynurenine pathway to be involved in the pathogenesis and progression of ALS, a key prerequisite has to be met - the activation of the immune response, particularly the presence of: (1) IFN-γ, which is the most potent stimulator of IDO-1 (Takikawa *et al.* 1999); and (2) activated microglia and/or infiltrating macrophages, which are the main producers of QUIN in the CNS (Brew *et al.* 1995; Heyes *et al.* 1996). Figure 3 summarizes the main adverse events exerted by QUIN leading to motor neuron injury and death.

A few studies have provided direct evidence between TRP metabolism and ALS. Patients with severe clinical status had significantly higher cerebrospinal fluid (CSF) KYNA levels compared to controls; however, serum KYNA levels were significantly lower in patients with severe clinical status compared to either controls or patients with mild clinical status (Ilzecka *et al.* 2003). This increase in CSF KYNA in patients was conjectured to be associated with the neuroprotective effect of KYNA, produced mainly by activated astrocytes (Guillemin *et al.* 2001). ALS samples have also been found to have significantly higher levels of CSF and serum KYN and QUIN and decreased levels of serum PIC (Chen *et al.* 2010).

Another study looked at Trp-32 in superoxide dismutase 1 (SOD1) protein. The aggregation of SOD1 is one of the hallmarks of familial ALS. Trp-32 is the only aromatic residue in SOD1 protein and is found on the SOD1 protein surface (Zhang *et al.* 2003). The oxidation of Trp-32 to KYN is responsible for bicarbonate mediated peroxidase activity induced SOD1 aggregation (Zhang *et al.* 2003). By substituting Trp-32 with phenylalanine, which oxidizes more slowly, mutant SOD-1 motor neurons survived longer and were less likely to form cytoplasmic inclusions (Taylor *et al.* 2007).

3. Indirect evidence for the role of QUIN in ALS

In addition to the direct evidence demonstrating the link between the kynurenine pathway and ALS, numerous other studies have provided indirect evidence supporting the role of QUIN, in particular, in ALS.

3.1 QUIN and SOD1 expression

Mutations in SOD1 constitute about 20% of familial ALS cases. In rat brain, intracerebral injection of QUIN resulted in significant neuronal loss and a markedly increased level of SOD1 expression in a time-dependent manner (Noack *et al.* 1998). This increase in SOD1 expression was thought to be a neuroprotective response to limit the oxidative damage caused by QUIN. Presumably, QUIN could have a similar effect on mutant SOD1, which would amplify the deleterious effects associated with mutant SOD1 pathology in ALS.

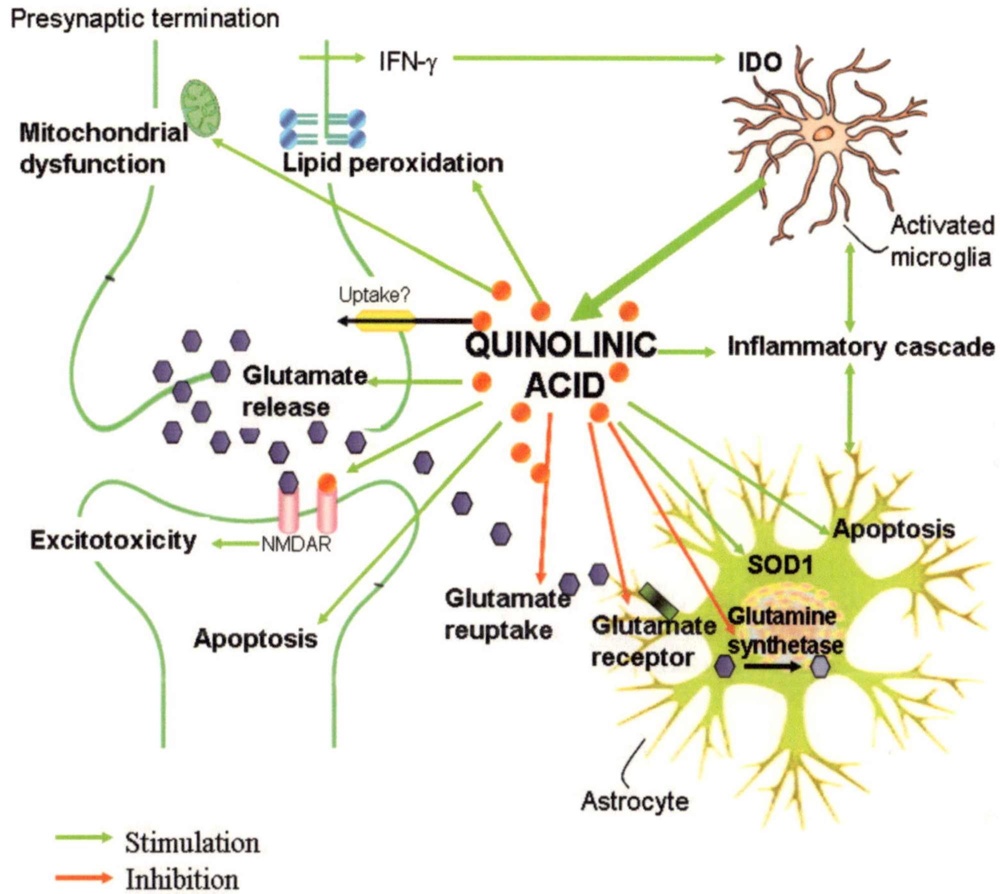

Fig. 3. Hypothetical model of the involvement of QUIN in the pathogenesis of ALS. QUIN, released from activated microglia, can induce various effects in astrocytes and motor neurons, including excitotoxicity, oxidative stress, apoptosis, mitochondrial dysfunction and the inflammatory cascade, all putatively thought to contribute to ALS disease pathogenesis and progression. Adapted from (Guillemin *et al.* 2005).

3.2 QUIN and excitotoxicity

QUIN is an excitotoxin and can be linked to excitotoxicity in ALS in two ways: (1) through the activation of the NMDA receptor; and (2) its effect on glutamate levels. The heteromeric NMDA receptor (NR) has three families of subunits: NR1 (A and B), NR2 (A to D) and NR3 (A and B). In the ventral and dorsal horns of ALS spinal cord, up to 78% loss of NR2A has been detected (Samarasinghe *et al.* 1996). Interestingly, QUIN acts on the NR subtypes, NR1+NR2A and NR1+NR2B (Priestley *et al.* 1995), and the loss of NR2A in ALS patients may possibly reflect an excitotoxic mechanism involving QUIN.

Glutamate induced toxicity has been implicated in the selective neuronal damage seen in ALS and counteracting glutamatergic toxicity, thus far, is the only treatment available for ALS. QUIN can potentiate its own toxicity and that of other excitatory amino acids, such as glutamate, under energy deprived conditions (Schurr and Rigor 1993). Moreover, QUIN contributes to excessive microenvironment glutamate concentrations and neurotoxicity via at least three mechanisms: (1) stimulation of synaptosomal glutamate release by neurons (Tavares *et al.* 2002); (2) inhibition of glutamate uptake into synaptic vesicle by astrocytes (Tavares *et al.* 2000); and (3) limiting glutamate to glutamine recycling in astrocytes by decreasing glutamine synthetase activity (Baverel *et al.* 1990).

3.3 QUIN and oxidative stress

One of the putative causes of ALS is the increased production and accumulation of reactive oxygen species (ROS) leading to oxidative stress and lipid peroxidation. Toxicity induced by QUIN has been related to increase ROS and oxidative stress. Intracerebral injection of QUIN shows neuronal damage and increase in ROS content occurring as early as 4 hrs after administration (Ganzella *et al.* 2006).

The lipid peroxidative effect of QUIN has also been demonstrated *in vivo* in adult rat brain (Rios and Santamaria 1991), and in rat brain synaptosomes *in vitro* (Santamaria *et al.* 2001). Similarly, in sheep foetal brain infused with QUIN, 4-hydroxynonenal (4-HNE), a toxic product of lipid peroxidation, immunoreactivity was observed in Purkinje cells and in the cytoplasm of cell bodies and dendrites, reaching into the molecular layer of the cerebellum (Yan *et al.* 2005). A sub-lethal dose of 4-HNE will also lead to the loss of spinal motor neurons in mice (Vigh *et al.* 2005). This may be a consequence of microglia activation, as 4-HNE is a potent activator of microglia, which will further contribute to neuroinflammation and oxidative stress in ALS (Hall *et al.* 1998).

In sporadic ALS patients, 4-HNE was enhanced in motor neurons and glia cells in the spinal cord (Shibata *et al.* 2001), and significantly elevated in the serum and CSF, correlating positively with the stage of disease (Simpson *et al.* 2004). CSF 4-HNE levels from sporadic ALS patients were also sufficient to cause the demise of motor neurons *in vitro* (Smith *et al.* 1998).

3.4 QUIN and mitochondrial dysfunction

Mitochondrial dysfunction is a prominent feature of ALS and predisposes motor neurons to ionotropic glutamate receptor-mediated excitotoxicity (Kanki *et al.* 2004). Excitotoxicity may lead to the activation of mitochondrial permeability transition pore, resulting in mitochondrial swelling and progressive motor neuron death (Bendotti *et al.* 2001). Intracerebral injection of QUIN, in addition to being excitotoxic, also produces progressive mitochondrial dysfunction leading to time-dependent energetic dysfunction, which may be a common and critical event in the cell death cascade seen in ALS (Bordelon *et al.* 1997).

3.5 QUIN and the inflammatory cascade

The presence of neuroinflammation is a pathological hallmark of ALS. Activated astrocytes and microglia are often seen in the degenerating areas surrounding injured motor neurons (McGeer and McGeer 2002). Elevated levels of chemokines and cytokines, such as monocyte chemoattractant protein 1 (MCP-1), macrophage inflammatory protein (MIP)1-α, chemokine ligand 5, interleukin (IL)-1 to IL-12, TNF-α and IFN-γ, have been detected in both G93A SOD1 mice and ALS patients (Hensley *et al.* 2003; Wilms *et al.* 2003; Henkel *et al.* 2004). It has been demonstrated that QUIN can induce astrocyte proliferation and the production of chemokines, particularly MCP-1 (Croitoru-Lamoury *et al.* 2003; Guillemin *et al.* 2003; Ting 2008), and IL-1β messenger ribonucleic acid (mRNA) expression (Guillemin *et al.* 2003) in human astrocytes and macrophages.

3.6 QUIN and apoptosis

In ALS, apoptosis is evident from the increased expression of pro-apoptotic proto-oncogenes, BCl-2 and c-jun, and caspases 1 and 3 in tissue, and from the morphological features of apoptosis displayed by dying motor neurons. QUIN has been demonstrated to induce neuronal and astrocytic apoptosis involving the activation of caspase 3 (Macaya *et al.* 1994; Jeon *et al.* 1999; Guillemin *et al.* 2005). Astrocytes are essential for the homeostasis of the CNS and so, the well-being of neurons. Hence, the loss of normal astrocytes in ALS would be detrimental to motor neurons and could exacerbate disease progression in ALS (Yamanaka *et al.* 2008).

4. Potential therapeutics targeted at the kynurenine pawthay for ALS

In 1995, riluzole became the first drug, and remains the only drug, approved by the FDA (USA) for treatment of ALS. The approval was based on two large placebo controlled clinical studies where riluzole decreased the rate of muscle deterioration and modestly improved the survival rate of ALS patients (Bensimon *et al.* 1994; Lacomblez *et al.* 1996). Though the precise mechanism of riluzole remains unclear, it appears to interfere with excitatory amino acid signalling, perhaps through the inhibition of glutamate release (Mizoule *et al.* 1985; Cheramy *et al.* 1992; Martin *et al.* 1993), blockade of inactivated sodium channels (Benoit and Escande 1991) and interaction with guanosine triphosphate (GTP)-binding proteins (Doble *et al.* 1992). 16 years on, there is still a lack of effective treatment available and an intense search is on going to discover better treatments for ALS.

In developing therapeutic agents aimed at modulating the kynurenine pathway, two approaches may be taken: (1) to develop analogues of the neuroprotective kynurenines; (2) to inhibit the synthesis of the neurotoxic QUIN. Figure 4 summarizes the drugs targeting the kynurenine pathway that could be potential candidates for ALS.

4.1 IDO inhibitors

As the first enzyme in the kynurenine pathway, suppression of IDO would lead to decrease QUIN production. Although it has not been specifically tested in neurodegenerative disorders, it is a novel therapeutic target in cancer research and the results have been positive. Using transgenic mouse model of breast cancer, IDO-1 inhibitors, 1-MT and methyl-thiohydantoin-tryptophan, were able to potentiate the efficacy of chemotherapy drugs, promoting tumour regression without increasing the side effects (Muller *et al.* 2005).

4.2 4-chlorokynurenine

QUIN neurotoxicity can be prevented by blocking the glycine modulatory site of the NMDA receptor (Foster *et al.* 1990; Hartley *et al.* 1990). 7-chlorokynurenate, a synthetic derivative of KYNA, is such an NMDA receptor antagonist (Kemp *et al.* 1988) but has difficulty crossing the BBB (Rao *et al.* 1993). On the other hand, its precursor, 4-chlorokynurenine, is rapidly transported across the BBB (Hokari *et al.* 1996). Intracerebral and intraperitoneal administration of 4-chlorokynurenine with QUIN showed successful enzymatic transamination of 4-chlorokynurenine into the neuroprotective 7-chlorokynurenate (Wu *et al.* 1997; Wu *et al.* 2000).

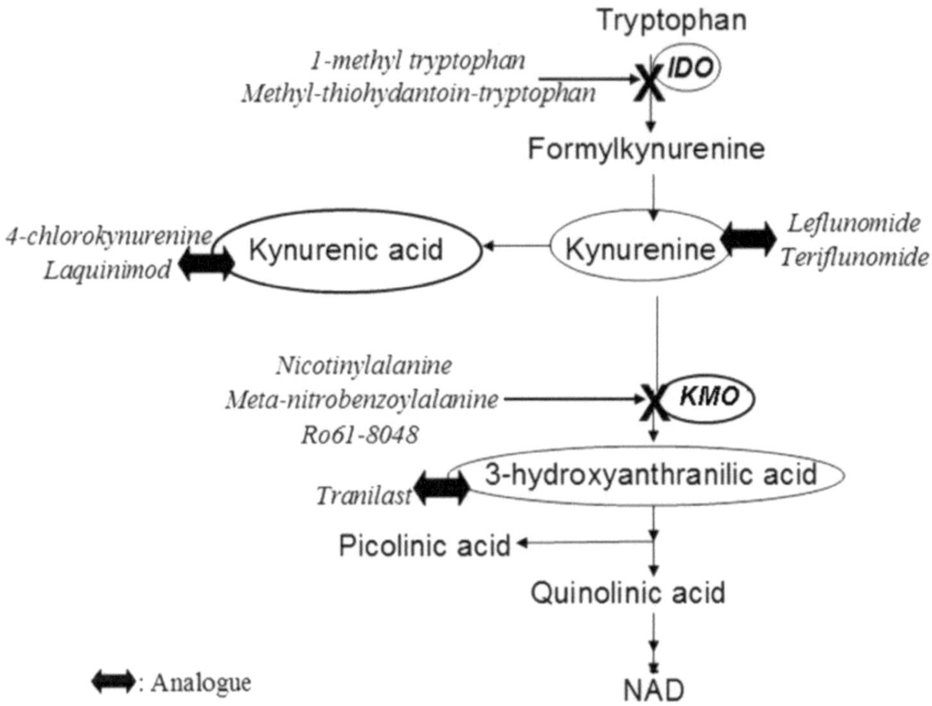

Fig. 4. Potential drug candidates targeting the kynurenine pathway for ALS. 1-MT, methyl-thiohydantoin-tryptophan, nicotinylalanine, meta-nitrobenzoylalanine and Ro61-8048 are kynurenine pathway inhibitors, while 4-chlorokynurenine, laquinimod, leflunomide, teriflunomide and tranilast are analogues of kynurenines.

4.3 Laquinimod

Laquinimod (ABR-215062) is a novel synthetic quinoline with high oral bioavailability. In preclinical trials, the compound exhibited immunomodulatory properties without immunosuppression (Brunmark *et al.* 2002; Zou *et al.* 2002; Yang *et al.* 2004). In rats with experimental autoimmune encephalomyelitis (EAE), a widely used animal model for MS, laquinimod inhibited disease progression and infiltration of CD4+ T cells and macrophages into the CNS (Yang *et al.* 2004). It also shifted the cytokine profile towards Th2/Th3 cytokines IL-4, IL-10 and transforming growth factor β (TGF-β) (Yang *et al.* 2004). Furthermore, laquinimod is able to act synergistically with IFN-β, though the mechanism of action is currently unknown but is independent of IFN-β (Runstrom *et al.* 2006). In addition, laquinimod has also successfully reduced the development of active lesions in patients with relapsing MS (Polman *et al.* 2005).

4.4 Leflunomide

Leflunomide (Avara®) is an immunosuppressive and anti-inflammatory pro-drug, which is converted *in vivo* to its active open-ring metabolite, teriflunomide (A771726), an inhibitor of mitochondrial dihydroorotate dehydrogenase, an essential enzyme for *de novo* pyrimidine synthesis (Williamson *et al.* 1995). Leflunomide is a potent inhibitor of the nuclear factor *kappa*-light-chain-enhancer of activated B cells (NF-κB) activation (Manna and Aggarwal

1999) and prevents Th1 cell activation while promoting Th2 cell differentiation (Dimitrova *et al.* 2002). The exact mechanism of action is still unclear though it has been shown to attenuate EAE independent of pyrimidine depletion (Korn *et al.* 2004).

In 1998, leflunomide was approved by the FDA (USA) for the treatment of rheumatoid arthritis. Leflunomide has also been successful in inhibiting disease progression in animal models of autoimmune diseases, such as experimental autoimmune neuritis (Ogawa *et al.* 1990), EAE (Bartlett *et al.* 1993) and experimental myasthenia gravis (Vidic-Dankovic *et al.* 1995). In a phase II trial recently, teriflunomide proved to be well tolerated and effective in reducing active lesions in patients with relapsing MS (O'Connor *et al.* 2006).

4.5 Tranilast

Tranilast (Rizaben®) is a synthetic anthranilic acid derivative drug with several inhibitory actions. It has the ability to inhibit the release of chemical mediators, such as histamine, during hypersensitivity reactions and from mast cells and also suppresses the release of TGF-β and inhibits angiogenesis (Suzawa *et al.* 1992; Isaji *et al.* 1997). Thus, it is effective against many diseases, including allergic rhinitis, atopic dermatitis, bronchial asthma, hypertrophic scar formation and keloid. Recently, tranilast showed promising results against EAE, shifting the cytokine profile towards favouring Th2 cells, inhibiting the actions of Th1 cells and promoting the generation of IL-10 producing Th2 cells, an effect similar to that of natural TRP catabolites (Platten *et al.* 2005).

4.6 Alanine derivatives

The synthesis of QUIN can also be blocked by inhibiting either KYNU or KMO activity, thus diverting the kynurenine pathway towards the synthesis of KYNA. Nicotinylalanine is one such agent (Decker *et al.* 1963). When administered together with probenecid (to allow for the accumulation of KYNA by inhibiting the organic acid transport system), nicotinylalanine increased the amount of KYNA produced in the brain and protected the brain from induced seizures (Connick *et al.* 1992; Russi *et al.* 1992) and QUIN induced striatal damage (Harris *et al.* 1998).

Another alanine derivative capable of inhibiting KMO is meta-nitrobenzoylalanine (Pellicciari *et al.* 1994). The inhibition of KMO results in an increase in brain KYN and KYNA, which is associated with sedation and anticonvulsant effects (Chiarugi and Moroni 1999) and reduction in neuronal loss from brain ischemia (Cozzi *et al.* 1999). In immune activated mice, meta-nitrobenzoylalanine also significantly reduced the formation of QUIN in the periphery and CNS (Chiarugi and Moroni 1999).

4.7 Ro61-8048

Ro61-8048 (3,4-dimethoxy-N-[4-(3-nitrophenyl)thiazol-2-yl] benzenesulfon-amide) is another potent KMO inhibitor (Rover *et al.* 1997). In addition to raising brain KYNA level, Ro61-8048 also reduces glutamate concentration in the extracellular spaces of the basal ganglia in rats without impairing the learning or memory process typically associated with glutamate receptor antagonists (Moroni *et al.* 2005). In rats with EAE, administration of Ro61-8048 significantly reduces the neurotoxic levels of 3-hydroxykynurenine and QUIN in the CNS (Chiarugi *et al.* 2001). Like meta-nitrobenzoylalanine, Ro61-8048 also decreases neuronal loss due to brain ischemia (Cozzi *et al.* 1999).

4.8 Clioquinol

Clioquinol (5-chloro-7-iodo-8-hydroxyquinoline) is a quinoline metal chelator that binds selectively to zinc and copper ions (Cherny *et al.* 2001). Having a hydrophobic nature, it crosses the BBB easily. Recent research with clioquinol in neurological disorders contributed by an imbalance in metal ions has led to promising results, presenting the possibility of a new therapeutic strategy. In AD transgenic mice, treatment with clioquinol resulted in the dissolution of aberrant neocortex beta amyloid (Aβ) aggregates, which are enriched with copper and zinc ions (Cherny *et al.* 2001). In a pilot phase II clinical trial, the drug was well tolerated and led to a significant decrease in Aβ plasma levels in AD patients, providing support for future trials (Ritchie *et al.* 2003). In PD, elevated levels of iron in the substantia nigra, the brain region affected in PD, has been reported. In mice, oral administration of clioquinol antagonized the action of the Parkinson's inducing agent 1-methyl-4-phenyl-1,2,3,6-tetra-pyridine (MPTP) (Kaur *et al.* 2003). In HD, where iron, copper and zinc have been implicated, clioquinol improved the symptoms and lifespan of transgenic HD mice (Nguyen *et al.* 2005).

A second generation 8-hydroxyquinoline, PBT2, has been developed to improve the safety and efficacy of clioquinol and also its pharmaceutical properties, such as solubility and bioavailability. In preclinical *in vivo* and *in vitro* trials on transgenic AD mice, PBT2 was more effective in lowering plaque formation and reducing plaque toxicity. More importantly, it may also improve cognition.

5. Conclusion

The current consensus is that ALS is a multifactorial disease. However, an explanation for the initiation of the putative causative mechanism of ALS remains elusive, and there lacks a hypothesis that can link all the mechanisms together. In recent years, the implication of the kynurenine pathway in multiple diseases, particularly neurodegenerative diseases, has led to an increase in assessing the efficacy of drugs targeting the kynurenine pathway in ameliorating disease symptoms and/or retarding disease progression.

The kynurenine pathway has been demonstrated to be involved in ALS and this provides an important link that ties together some of the major hypotheses underlying the pathogenesis of ALS, namely glutamate excitotoxicity, oxidative stress, non-cell-autonomous mechanism and apoptosis, which are also the major mechanisms via which QUIN exerts its neurotoxicity effects. Due to the multiple pathways involved in the pathogenesis and progression of ALS, it may be speculated that a combination therapy could be more efficacious. Hence, by targeting the kynurenine pathway, it is hoped that more effective therapeutic agents, acting in synergy with other agents, may uncover a better treatment for ALS.

6. Appendix

3HAA3-hydroxyanthranilic acid
4-HNE4-hydroxynonenal
Aβ Beta amyloid
ADAlzheimer's disease
ALSAmyotrophic lateral sclerosis
BBBBlood-brain barrier

CNSCentral nervous system
CSFCerebrospinal fluid
D-1-MTD-1-methyl-tryptophan
EAEExperimental autoimmune encephalomyelitis
GCN2General control non-derepressible-2 kinase
GTPGuanosine triphosphate
HDHuntington's disease
HIVHuman immunodeficiency virus
IDOIndoleamine 2,3-dioxygenase
IFN-γInterferon gamma
ILInterleukin
KMOKynurenine 3-monooxygenase
KYNKynurenine
KYNAKynurenic acid
MCPMonocyte chemoattractant protein
MIPMacrophage inflammatory protein
MPTPMethyl-4-phenyl-1,2,3,6-tetra-pyridine
mRNAMessenger ribonucleic acid
NF-κBNuclear factor *kappa*-light-chain-enhancer of activated *B* cells
NMDA*N*-methyl *D*-aspartate
NRNMDA receptor
PICPicolinic acid
QUINQuinolinic acid
ROSReactive oxygen species
SOD1Superoxide dismutase 1
TDOTryptophan 2,3-dioxygenase
TGF-βtransforming growth factor β
TRPTryptophan

7. References

Ball, H. J., A. Sanchez-Perez, *et al.* (2007). Characterization of an indoleamine 2,3-dioxygenase-like protein found in humans and mice. *Gene* 396(1): 203-13.

Bartlett, R. R., H. Anagnostopulos, *et al.* (1993). Effects of leflunomide on immune responses and models of inflammation. *Springer Semin Immunopathol* 14(4): 381-94.

Baverel, G., G. Martin, *et al.* (1990). Glutamine synthesis from aspartate in guinea-pig renal cortex. *Biochem J* 268(2): 437-42.

Bendotti, C., N. Calvaresi, *et al.* (2001). Early vacuolization and mitochondrial damage in motor neurons of FALS mice are not associated with apoptosis or with changes in cytochrome oxidase histochemical reactivity. *J Neurol Sci* 191(1-2): 25-33.

Benoit, E. and D. Escande (1991). Riluzole specifically blocks inactivated Na channels in myelinated nerve fibre. *Pflugers Arch* 419(6): 603-9.

Bensimon, G., L. Lacomblez, *et al.* (1994). A controlled trial of riluzole in amyotrophic lateral sclerosis. ALS/Riluzole Study Group. *N Engl J Med* 330(9): 585-91.

Bi, M., C. Naczki, *et al.* (2005). ER stress-regulated translation increases tolerance to extreme hypoxia and promotes tumor growth. *Embo J* 24(19): 3470-81.

Bordelon, Y. M., M. F. Chesselet, *et al.* (1997). Energetic dysfunction in quinolinic acid-lesioned rat striatum. *J Neurochem* 69(4): 1629-39.

Brew, B. J., J. Corbeil, *et al.* (1995). Quinolinic acid production is related to macrophage tropic isolates of HIV-1. *J Neurovirol* 1(5-6): 369-74.

Brown, R. R., Y. Ozaki, *et al.* (1991). Implications of interferon-induced tryptophan catabolism in cancer, auto-immune diseases and AIDS. *Adv Exp Med Biol* 294: 425-35.

Brunmark, C., A. Runstrom, *et al.* (2002). The new orally active immunoregulator laquinimod (ABR-215062) effectively inhibits development and relapses of experimental autoimmune encephalomyelitis. *J Neuroimmunol* 130(1-2): 163-72.

Chen, Y. and G. J. Guillemin (2009). Kynurenine pathway metabolites in humans: disease and healthy states. *International Journal of Tryptophan Research* 2: 1-19.

Cheramy, A., L. Barbeito, *et al.* (1992). Riluzole inhibits the release of glutamate in the caudate nucleus of the cat in vivo. *Neurosci Lett* 147(2): 209-12.

Cherny, R. A., C. S. Atwood, *et al.* (2001). Treatment with a copper-zinc chelator markedly and rapidly inhibits beta-amyloid accumulation in Alzheimer's disease transgenic mice. *Neuron* 30(3): 665-76.

Chiarugi, A., A. Cozzi, *et al.* (2001). Kynurenine 3-mono-oxygenase activity and neurotoxic kynurenine metabolites increase in the spinal cord of rats with experimental allergic encephalomyelitis. *Neuroscience* 102(3): 687-95.

Chiarugi, A. and F. Moroni (1999). Quinolinic acid formation in immune-activated mice: studies with (m-nitrobenzoyl)-alanine (mNBA) and 3,4-dimethoxy-[-N-4-(-3-nitrophenyl)thiazol-2yl]-benzenesul fonamide (Ro 61-8048), two potent and selective inhibitors of kynurenine hydroxylase. *Neuropharmacology* 38(8): 1225-33.

Connick, J. H., G. C. Heywood, *et al.* (1992). Nicotinylalanine increases cerebral kynurenic acid content and has anticonvulsant activity. *Gen Pharmacol* 23(2): 235-9.

Cozzi, A., R. Carpenedo, *et al.* (1999). Kynurenine hydroxylase inhibitors reduce ischemic brain damage: studies with (m-nitrobenzoyl)-alanine (mNBA) and 3,4-dimethoxy-[-N-4-(nitrophenyl)thiazol-2yl]-benzenesulfonamide (Ro 61-8048) in models of focal or global brain ischemia. *J Cereb Blood Flow Metab* 19(7): 771-7.

Croitoru-Lamoury, J., G. J. Guillemin, *et al.* (2003). Expression of chemokines and their receptors in human and simian astrocytes: evidence for a central role of TNF alpha and IFN gamma in CXCR4 and CCR5 modulation. *Glia* 41(4): 354-70.

Dai, W. and S. L. Gupta (1990). Regulation of indoleamine 2,3-dioxygenase gene expression in human fibroblasts by interferon-gamma. Upstream control

Decker, R. H., R. R. Brown, *et al.* (1963). Studies on the biological activity of nicotinylalanine, an analogue of kynurenine. *J Biol Chem* 238: 1049-53.

region discriminates between interferon-gamma and interferon-alpha. *J Biol Chem* 265(32): 19871-7.

de Haro, C., R. Mendez, *et al.* (1996). The eIF-2alpha kinases and the control of protein synthesis. *Faseb J* 10(12): 1378-87.

Dimitrova, P., A. Skapenko, *et al.* (2002). Restriction of de novo pyrimidine biosynthesis inhibits Th1 cell activation and promotes Th2 cell differentiation. *J Immunol* 169(6): 3392-9.

Doble, A., J. P. Hubert, *et al.* (1992). Pertussis toxin pretreatment abolishes the inhibitory effect of riluzole and carbachol on D-[3H]aspartate release from cultured cerebellar granule cells. *Neurosci Lett* 140(2): 251-4.

Fallarino, F., U. Grohmann, *et al.* (2003). T cell apoptosis by kynurenines. *Adv Exp Med Biol* 527: 183-90.

Foster, A. C., C. L. Willis, *et al.* (1990). Protection Against N-methyl-D-aspartate Receptor-Mediated Neuronal Degeneration In Rat Brain by 7-chlorokynurenate and 3-amino-1-hydroxypyrrolid-2-one, Antagonists at The Allosteric Site for Glycine. *Eur J Neurosci* 2(3): 270-277.

Frumento, G., R. Rotondo, *et al.* (2002). Tryptophan-derived catabolites are responsible for inhibition of T and natural killer cell proliferation induced by indoleamine 2,3-dioxygenase. *J Exp Med* 196(4): 459-68.

Fujigaki, S., K. Saito, *et al.* (1998). Species differences in L-tryptophan-kynurenine pathway metabolism: quantification of anthranilic acid and its related enzymes. *Arch Biochem Biophys* 358(2): 329-35.

Ganzella, M., F. M. Jardim, *et al.* (2006). Time course of oxidative events in the hippocampus following intracerebroventricular infusion of quinolinic acid in mice. *Neurosci Res* 55(4): 397-402.

Goldstein, L. E., M. C. Leopold, *et al.* (2000). 3-Hydroxykynurenine and 3-hydroxyanthranilic acid generate hydrogen peroxide and promote alpha-crystallin cross-linking by metal ion reduction. *Biochemistry* 39(24): 7266-75.

Guillemin, G. J., B. J. Brew, *et al.* (2005). Indoleamine 2,3 dioxygenase and quinolinic acid immunoreactivity in Alzheimer's disease hippocampus. *Neuropathol Appl Neurobiol* 31: 395-404.

Guillemin, G. J., J. Croitoru-Lamoury, *et al.* (2003). Quinolinic acid upregulates chemokine production and chemokine receptor expression in astrocytes. *Glia* 41: 371-381.

Guillemin, G. J., K. M. Cullen, *et al.* (2007). Characterization of the kynurenine pathway in human neurons. *J Neurosci* 27(47): 12884-12892.

Guillemin, G. J., S. J. Kerr, *et al.* (2004). Involvement of quinolinic acid in AIDS dementia complex. *Neurotox Res* 7: 103-124.

Guillemin, G. J., S. J. Kerr, *et al.* (2001). IFN-beta 1b induces kynurenine pathway metabolism in human macrophages: potential implications for multiple sclerosis treatment. *J Intereron Cytokine Res* 21(12): 1097-101.

Guillemin, G. J., S. J. Kerr, *et al.* (2001). Kynurenine pathway metabolism in human astrocytes: a paradox for neuronal protection. *Journal of Neurochemistry* 78: 842-853.

Guillemin, G. J., V. Meininger, *et al.* (2005). Implications for the kynurenine pathway and quinolinic acid in amyotrophic lateral sclerosis. *Neurodegener Dis.* 2(3-4): 166-76.

Guillemin, G. J., D. G. Smith, *et al.* (2000). Characterisation of kynurenine pathway metabolism in human astrocytes and implications in neuropathogenesis. *Redox Report* 5(2/3): 108-111.

Guillemin, G. J., D. G. Smith, *et al.* (2003). Expression of the kynurenine pathway enzymes in human microglia and macrophages. *Adv Exp Med Biol* 527: 105-12.

Guillemin, G. J., G. Smythe, *et al.* (2004). Expression of indoleamine 2,3-dioxygenase and production of quinolinic acid by human microglia, astrocytes, and neurons. *Glia* 49(1): 15-23.

Guillemin, G. J., G. A. Smythe, *et al.* (2003). A beta 1-42 induces production of quinolinic acid by human macrophages and microglia. *Neuroreport* 14(18): 2311-5.

Guillemin, G. J., L. Wang, *et al.* (2005). Quinolinic acid selectively induces apoptosis of human astrocytes: potential role in AIDS dementia complex. *J Neuroinflammation* 2: 16.

Guillemin, G. J., K. R. Williams, *et al.* (2003). Quinolinic acid in the pathogenesis of Alzheimer's disease. *Adv Exp Med Biol* 527: 167-76.

Hall, E. D., P. K. Andrus, *et al.* (1998). Relationship of oxygen radical-induced lipid peroxidative damage to disease onset and progression in a transgenic model of familial ALS. *J Neurosci Res* 53(1): 66-77.

Hargreaves, K. M. and W. M. Pardridge (1988). Neutral amino acid transport at the human blood-brain barrier. *J Biol Chem* 263(36): 19392-7.

Harris, C. A., A. F. Miranda, *et al.* (1998). Modulation of striatal quinolinate neurotoxicity by elevation of endogenous brain kynurenic acid. *Br J Pharmacol* 124(2): 391-9.

Hartley, D. M., H. Monyer, *et al.* (1990). 7-Chlorokynurenate Blocks NMDA Receptor-Mediated Neurotoxicity in Murine Cortical Culture. *Eur J Neurosci* 2(4): 291-295.

Hayaishi, O. and R. Yoshida (1978). Specific induction of pulmonary indoleamine 2,3-dioxygenase by bacterial lipopolysaccharide. *Ciba Found Symp*(65): 199-203.

Henkel, J. S., J. I. Engelhardt, *et al.* (2004). Presence of dendritic cells, MCP-1, and activated microglia/macrophages in amyotrophic lateral sclerosis spinal cord tissue. *Ann Neurol* 55(2): 221-35.

Hensley, K., J. Fedynyshyn, *et al.* (2003). Message and protein-level elevation of tumor necrosis factor alpha (TNF alpha) and TNF alpha-modulating cytokines in spinal cords of the G93A-SOD1 mouse model for amyotrophic lateral sclerosis. *Neurobiol Dis* 14(1): 74-80.

Heyes, M. P., C. L. Achim, *et al.* (1996). Human microglia convert l-tryptophan into the neurotoxin quinolinic acid. *Biochem J* 320 (Pt 2): 595-7.

Hokari, M., H. Q. Wu, *et al.* (1996). Facilitated brain uptake of 4-chlorokynurenine and conversion to 7-chlorokynurenic acid. *Neuroreport* 8(1): 15-8.

Ilzecka, J., T. Kocki, *et al.* (2003). Endogenous protectant kynurenic acid in amyotrophic lateral sclerosis. *Acta Neurol Scand* 107(6): 412-8.

Isaji, M., H. Miyata, *et al.* (1997). Tranilast inhibits the proliferation, chemotaxis and tube formation of human microvascular endothelial cells in vitro and angiogenesis in vivo. *Br J Pharmacol* 122(6): 1061-6.

Jeon, B. S., N. G. Kholodilov, *et al.* (1999). Activation of caspase-3 in developmental models of programmed cell death in neurons of the substantia nigra. *J Neurochem* 73(1): 322-33.

Jhamandas, K., R. J. Boegman, *et al.* (1990). Quinolinate-induced cortical cholinergic damage: modulation by tryptophan metabolites. *Brain Res* 529(1-2): 185-91.

Kanki, R., T. Nakamizo, *et al.* (2004). Effects of mitochondrial dysfunction on glutamate receptor-mediated neurotoxicity in cultured rat spinal motor neurons. *Brain Res* 1015(1-2): 73-81.

Kaur, D., F. Yantiri, *et al.* (2003). Genetic or pharmacological iron chelation prevents MPTP-induced neurotoxicity in vivo: a novel therapy for Parkinson's disease. *Neuron* 37(6): 899-909.

Kemp, J. A., A. C. Foster, *et al.* (1988). 7-Chlorokynurenic acid is a selective antagonist at the glycine modulatory site of the N-methyl-D-aspartate receptor complex. *Proc Natl Acad Sci U S A* 85(17): 6547-50.

Korn, T., T. Magnus, *et al.* (2004). Modulation of effector cell functions in experimental autoimmune encephalomyelitis by leflunomide--mechanisms independent of pyrimidine depletion. *J Leukoc Biol* 76(5): 950-60.

Lacomblez, L., G. Bensimon, *et al.* (1996). Dose-ranging study of riluzole in amyotrophic lateral sclerosis. Amyotrophic Lateral Sclerosis/Riluzole Study Group II. *Lancet* 347(9013): 1425-31.

Lee, G. K., H. J. Park, *et al.* (2002). Tryptophan deprivation sensitizes activated T cells to apoptosis prior to cell division. *Immunology* 107(4): 452-60.

Lim, C. K., G. A. Symthe, *et al.* (2007). Characterization of the kynurenine pathway in human oligodendrocytes. *International Congress Series* 1304: 213-217.

Ogawa, T., M. Inazu, *et al.* (1990). Effects of leflunomide on glomerulonephritis induced by antibasement membrane antibody in rats. *Agents Actions* 31(3-4): 321-8.

Macaya, A., F. Munell, *et al.* (1994). Apoptosis in substantia nigra following developmental striatal excitotoxic injury. *Proc Natl Acad Sci U S A* 91(17): 8117-21.

Manna, S. K. and B. B. Aggarwal (1999). Immunosuppressive leflunomide metabolite (A77 1726) blocks TNF-dependent nuclear factor-kappa B activation and gene expression. *J Immunol* 162(4): 2095-102.

Martin, D., M. A. Thompson, *et al.* (1993). The neuroprotective agent riluzole inhibits release of glutamate and aspartate from slices of hippocampal area CA1. *Eur J Pharmacol* 250(3): 473-6.

McGeer, P. L. and E. G. McGeer (2002). Inflammatory processes in amyotrophic lateral sclerosis. *Muscle Nerve* 26(4): 459-70.

McMenamy, R. H. (1965). Binding of indole analogues to human serum albumin. Effects of fatty acids. *J Biol Chem* 240(11): 4235-43.

Metz, R., J. B. Duhadaway, *et al.* (2007). Novel tryptophan catabolic enzyme IDO2 is the preferred biochemical target of the antitumor indoleamine 2,3-dioxygenase inhibitory compound D-1-methyl-tryptophan. *Cancer Res* 67(15): 7082-7.

Miller, C. L., I. C. Llenos, *et al.* (2004). Expression of the kynurenine pathway enzyme tryptophan 2,3-dioxygenase is increased in the frontal cortex of individuals with schizophrenia. *Neurobiol Dis* 15(3): 618-29.

Mizoule, J., B. Meldrum, *et al.* (1985). 2-Amino-6-trifluoromethoxy benzothiazole, a possible antagonist of excitatory amino acid neurotransmission--I. Anticonvulsant properties. *Neuropharmacology* 24(8): 767-73.

Moffett, J. R., T. Els, *et al.* (1997). Quinolinate immunoreactivity in experimental rat brain tumors is present in macrophages but not in astrocytes. *Exp Neurol* 144(2): 287-301.

Moroni, F., A. Cozzi, *et al.* (2005). Kynurenine 3-mono-oxygenase inhibitors reduce glutamate concentration in the extracellular spaces of the basal ganglia but not in those of the cortex or hippocampus. *Neuropharmacology* 48(6): 788-95.

Muller, A. J., J. B. DuHadaway, *et al.* (2005). Inhibition of indoleamine 2,3-dioxygenase, an immunoregulatory target of the cancer suppression gene Bin1, potentiates cancer chemotherapy. *Nat Med* 11(3): 312-9.

Munn, D. H., E. Shafizadeh, *et al.* (1999). Inhibition of T cell proliferation by macrophage tryptophan catabolism. *J Exp Med* 189(9): 1363-72.

Munn, D. H., M. D. Sharma, *et al.* (2005). GCN2 kinase in T cells mediates proliferative arrest and anergy induction in response to indoleamine 2,3-dioxygenase. *Immunity* 22(5): 633-42.

Munn, D. H., M. Zhou, *et al.* (1998). Prevention of allogeneic fetal rejection by tryptophan catabolism. *Science* 281(5380): 1191-3.

Nguyen, T., A. Hamby, *et al.* (2005). Clioquinol down-regulates mutant huntingtin expression in vitro and mitigates pathology in a Huntington's disease mouse model. *Proc Natl Acad Sci U S A* 102(33): 11840-5.

Noack, H., J. Lindenau, *et al.* (1998). Differential expression of superoxide dismutase isoforms in neuronal and glial compartments in the course of excitotoxically mediated neurodegeneration: relation to oxidative and nitrergic stress. *Glia* 23(4): 285-97.

O'Connor, P. W., D. Li, *et al.* (2006). A Phase II study of the safety and efficacy of teriflunomide in multiple sclerosis with relapses. *Neurology* 66(6): 894-900.

Owe-Young, R., N. L. Webster, *et al.* (2008). Kynurenine Pathway Metabolism in Human Blood-Brain Barrier Cells: Implications for Immune Tolerance & Neurotoxicity. *J Neurochem*.

Pellicciari, R., B. Natalini, *et al.* (1994). Modulation of the kynurenine pathway in search for new neuroprotective agents. Synthesis and preliminary evaluation of (m-nitrobenzoyl)alanine, a potent inhibitor of kynurenine-3-hydroxylase. *J Med Chem* 37(5): 647-55.

Perkins, M. N. and T. W. Stone (1982). An iontophoretic investigation of the actions of convulsant kynurenines and their interaction with the endogenous excitant quinolinic acid. *Brain Res* 247(1): 184-7.

Pfefferkorn, E. R. (1984). Interferon gamma blocks the growth of Toxoplasma gondii in human fibroblasts by inducing the host cells to degrade tryptophan. *Proc Natl Acad Sci U S A* 81(3): 908-12.

Platten, M., P. P. Ho, *et al.* (2005). Treatment of autoimmune neuroinflammation with a synthetic tryptophan metabolite. *Science* 310(5749): 850-5.

Polman, C., F. Barkhof, *et al.* (2005). Treatment with laquinimod reduces development of active MRI lesions in relapsing MS. *Neurology* 64(6): 987-91.

Priestley, T., P. Laughton, *et al.* (1995). Pharmacological properties of recombinant human N-methyl-D-aspartate receptors comprising NR1a/NR2A and NR1a/NR2B subunit assemblies expressed in permanently transfected mouse fibroblast cells. *Mol Pharmacol* 48(5): 841-8.

Rao, R. V., H. M. Ellerby, *et al.* (2004). Coupling endoplasmic reticulum stress to the cell death program. *Cell Death Differ* 11(4): 372-80.

Rao, T. S., N. M. Gray, *et al.* (1993). Indole-2-carboxylates, novel antagonists of the N-methyl-D-aspartate (NMDA)-associated glycine recognition sites: in vivo characterization. *Neuropharmacology* 32(2): 139-47.

Ritchie, C. W., A. I. Bush, *et al.* (2003). Metal-protein attenuation with iodochlorhydroxyquin (clioquinol) targeting Abeta amyloid deposition and toxicity in Alzheimer disease: a pilot phase 2 clinical trial. *Arch Neurol* 60(12): 1685-91.

Rover, S., A. M. Cesura, *et al.* (1997). Synthesis and biochemical evaluation of N-(4-phenylthiazol-2-yl)benzenesulfonamides as high-affinity inhibitors of kynurenine 3-hydroxylase. *J Med Chem* 40(26): 4378-85.

Ruddick, J. P., A. K. Evans, *et al.* (2006). Tryptophan metabolism in the central nervous system: medical implications. *Expert Rev Mol Med* 8(20): 1-27.

Runstrom, A., T. Leanderson, *et al.* (2006). Inhibition of the development of chronic experimental autoimmune encephalomyelitis by laquinimod (ABR-215062) in IFN-beta k.o. and wild type mice. *J Neuroimmunol* 173(1-2): 69-78.

Russi, P., M. Alesiani, *et al.* (1992). Nicotinylalanine increases the formation of kynurenic acid in the brain and antagonizes convulsions. *J Neurochem* 59(6): 2076-80.

Salter, M. and C. I. Pogson (1985). The role of tryptophan 2,3-dioxygenase in the hormonal control of tryptophan metabolism in isolated rat liver cells. Effects of glucocorticoids and experimental diabetes. *Biochem J* 229(2): 499-504.

Samarasinghe, S., L. Virgo, *et al.* (1996). Distribution of the N-methyl-D-aspartate glutamate receptor subunit NR2A in control and amyotrophic lateral sclerosis spinal cord. *Brain Res* 727(1-2): 233-7.

Santamaria, A., S. Galvan-Arzate, *et al.* (2001). Quinolinic acid induces oxidative stress in rat brain synaptosomes. *Neuroreport* 12(4): 871-4.

Schurr, A. and B. M. Rigor (1993). Quinolinate potentiates the neurotoxicity of excitatory amino acids in hypoxic neuronal tissue in vitro. *Brain Res* 617(1): 76-80.

Shibata, N., R. Nagai, *et al.* (2001). Morphological evidence for lipid peroxidation and protein glycoxidation in spinal cords from sporadic amyotrophic lateral sclerosis patients. *Brain Res* 917(1): 97-104.

Simpson, E. P., Y. K. Henry, *et al.* (2004). Increased lipid peroxidation in sera of ALS patients: a potential biomarker of disease burden. *Neurology* 62(10): 1758-65.

Smith, R. G., Y. K. Henry, *et al.* (1998). Presence of 4-hydroxynonenal in cerebrospinal fluid of patients with sporadic amyotrophic lateral sclerosis. *Ann Neurol* 44(4): 696-9.

Stone, T. W. and M. N. Perkins (1981). Quinolinic acid: a potent endogenous excitant at amino acid receptors in CNS. *Eur J Pharmacol* 72(4): 411-2.

Suzawa, H., S. Kikuchi, *et al.* (1992). The mechanism involved in the inhibitory action of tranilast on collagen biosynthesis of keloid fibroblasts. *Jpn J Pharmacol* 60(2): 91-6.

Takikawa, O. (2005). Biochemical and medical aspects of the indoleamine 2,3-dioxygenase-initiated L-tryptophan metabolism. *Biochem Biophys Res Commun* 338(1): 12-9.

Takikawa, O., Y. Tagawa, *et al.* (1999). Interferon-gamma-dependent/independent expression of indoleamine 2,3-dioxygenase. Studies with interferon-gamma-knockout mice. *Adv Exp Med Biol* 467: 553-7.

Takikawa, O., R. Yoshida, *et al.* (1986). Tryptophan degradation in mice initiated by indoleamine 2,3-dioxygenase. *J Biol Chem* 261(8): 3648-53.

Tavares, R. G., C. I. Tasca, *et al.* (2002). Quinolinic acid stimulates synaptosomal glutamate release and inhibits glutamate uptake into astrocytes. *Neurochem Int* 40(7): 621-7.

Tavares, R. G., C. I. Tasca, *et al.* (2000). Quinolinic acid inhibits glutamate uptake into synaptic vesicles from rat brain. *Neuroreport* 11(2): 249-53.

Taylor, D. M., B. F. Gibbs, *et al.* (2007). Tryptophan 32 potentiates aggregation and cytotoxicity of a copper/zinc superoxide dismutase mutant associated with familial amyotrophic lateral sclerosis. *J Biol Chem* 282(22): 16329-35.

Terness, P., T. M. Bauer, *et al.* (2002). Inhibition of allogeneic T cell proliferation by indoleamine 2,3-dioxygenase-expressing dendritic cells: mediation of suppression by tryptophan metabolites. *J Exp Med* 196(4): 447-57.

Ting, K. K. (2008). Quinolinic acid and its effect on the astrocyte with relevance to the pathogenesis of Alzheimer's disease [Thesis].

Vidic-Dankovic, B., D. Kosec, *et al.* (1995). Leflunomide prevents the development of experimentally induced myasthenia gravis. *Int J Immunopharmacol* 17(4): 273-81.

Vigh, L., R. G. Smith, *et al.* (2005). Sublethal dose of 4-hydroxynonenal reduces intracellular calcium in surviving motor neurons in vivo. *Acta Neuropathol* 109(6): 567-75.

Werner-Felmayer, G., E. R. Werner, *et al.* (1989). Characteristics of interferon induced tryptophan metabolism in human cells in vitro. *Biochim Biophys Acta* 1012(2): 140-7.

Williamson, R. A., C. M. Yea, *et al.* (1995). Dihydroorotate dehydrogenase is a high affinity binding protein for A77 1726 and mediator of a range of biological effects of the immunomodulatory compound. *J Biol Chem* 270(38): 22467-72.

Wilms, H., J. Sievers, *et al.* (2003). Intrathecal synthesis of monocyte chemoattractant protein-1 (MCP-1) in amyotrophic lateral sclerosis: further evidence for microglial activation in neurodegeneration. *J Neuroimmunol* 144(1-2): 139-42.

Wu, H. Q., S. C. Lee, *et al.* (2000). Systemic administration of 4-chlorokynurenine prevents quinolinate neurotoxicity in the rat hippocampus. *Eur J Pharmacol* 390(3): 267-74.

Wu, H. Q., F. G. Salituro, *et al.* (1997). Enzyme-catalyzed production of the neuroprotective NMDA receptor antagonist 7-chlorokynurenic acid in the rat brain in vivo. *Eur J Pharmacol* 319(1): 13-20.

Yamanaka, K., S. J. Chun, *et al.* (2008). Astrocytes as determinants of disease progression in inherited amyotrophic lateral sclerosis. *Nat Neurosci* 11(3): 251-3.

Yan, E., M. Castillo-Melendez, *et al.* (2005). Quinolinic acid promotes albumin deposition in Purkinje cell, astrocytic activation and lipid peroxidation in fetal brain. *Neuroscience* 134(3): 867-75.

Yang, J. S., L. Y. Xu, *et al.* (2004). Laquinimod (ABR-215062) suppresses the development of experimental autoimmune encephalomyelitis, modulates the Th1/Th2 balance and induces the Th3 cytokine TGF-beta in Lewis rats. *J Neuroimmunol* 156(1-2): 3-9.

Yasui, H., K. Takai, *et al.* (1986). Interferon enhances tryptophan metabolism by inducing pulmonary indoleamine 2,3-dioxygenase: its possible occurrence in cancer patients. *Proc Natl Acad Sci U S A* 83(17): 6622-6.

Zhang, H., C. Andrekopoulos, *et al.* (2003). Bicarbonate-dependent peroxidase activity of human Cu,Zn-superoxide dismutase induces covalent aggregation of protein: intermediacy of tryptophan-derived oxidation products. *J Biol Chem* 278(26): 24078-89.

Zou, L. P., N. Abbas, *et al.* (2002). Suppression of experimental autoimmune neuritis by ABR-215062 is associated with altered Th1/Th2 balance and inhibited migration of inflammatory cells into the peripheral nerve tissue. *Neuropharmacology* 42(5): 731-9.

Part 3

Cellular Pathophysiology, the Immune System and Stem Cell Strategies

16

The Astrocytic Contribution in ALS: Inflammation and Excitotoxicity

Kim Staats[1,2] and Ludo Van Den Bosch[1,2]
[1]*University of Leuven,*
[2]*VIB Vesalius Research Center,*
Belgium

1. Introduction

Amyotrophic Lateral Sclerosis (ALS) is a devastating progressive neurodegenerative disease, due to the loss of motor neurons and denervation of muscle fibres, resulting in increasing muscle weakness and paralysis. The disease has an incidence of 2.7 cases per 100,000 people in Europe (Longroscino et al., 2010). It is diagnosed from teen years onward, but is more prevalent in the later years of life. In lack of a medical cure, average life expectancy post diagnosis is between 2 and 5 years, though 10% of all patients live longer than 10 years. Patients mainly succumb to the disease by respiratory insufficiency or may opt for euthanasia where legislature permits (Maessen et al., 2010). Although ALS is characterised by degeneration of central nervous system tissue, mental functions remain largely unaffected resulting in a locked-in state (Kotchoubey et al., 2003). At current, there is but one medicine to treat the disease, riluzole, slowing disease progression moderately (Miller et al., 2007).

1.1 Basic genetics of ALS

Mutations in the ubiquitously expressed Cu/Zn superoxide dismutase 1 (SOD1) gene can cause ALS. SOD1 detoxifies cell damaging free radicals and its mutations account for 20% of the ALS patients suffering from the disease by familial origin (fALS) worldwide. The remaining 90% of ALS patients suffer from the disease by unknown sporadic causes (sALS), though a common mechanism is predicted as fALS and sALS patients display indistinguishable clinical phenotypes. Overexpression of mutant forms of human SOD1 causes the ALS phenotype of transgenic SOD1 mice, accounting for an invaluable contribution to ALS research (Gurney et al., 1994). Many hallmarks of the disease are shared between patients and this rodent model, including specific motor neuron loss, aggregate formation, astrogliosis, microgliosis and progressive paralysis. As the genetic ablation of SOD1 does not produce an ALS-like phenotype in mice (Reaume et al., 1996; Shefner et al., 1999) the pathogenic mechanism of mutant SOD1 is a toxic gain of function. This gain of function may be exerted by protein misfolding, aggregation, impaired proteasome functioning, impaired retrograde transport, excitotoxic cell death or other mechanisms (reviewed in Bruijn et al., 2004). Mutations in other genes also cause familial ALS, including mutations in vesicle-associated membrane protein-associated protein B (VAPB), TAR DNA binding protein (TDP-43), fused in sarcoma/translocated in liposarcoma (FUS/TLS), optineurin and valsolin containing protein (VCP) (Johnson et al.; Maruyama et al.; Rutherford et al., 2008; Van Deerlin et al., 2008; Del Bo et al., 2009; Kwiatkowski et al., 2009; Vance et al., 2009). Unfortunately, the discovery of these mutant genes has not yet progressed into useful ALS model organisms, so most of the work described below was conducted with mutant SOD1-based ALS models.

1.2 Non-cell autonomous ALS

Multiple cell types contribute to the pathology making ALS a non-cell autonomous disease (Boillee et al., 2006a). By addition or deletion of mutant SOD1 in specific cell types, it is known that mutant SOD1 influences the disease depending on the cell type, including astrocytes (Yamanaka et al., 2008; Wang et al., 2011a), microglia (Boillee et al., 2006b), Schwann cells (Lobsiger et al., 2009) and motor neurons (Jaarsma et al., 2008). Additionally, ablation of T-cells (Beers et al., 2008; Chiu et al., 2008), B-cells (Naor et al., 2009), CD4+ and CD8+ cells (Beers et al., 2008) decrease survival of ALS mice, demonstrating the role of immune cells in disease progression. Although ALS is a non-cell autonomous disease, mutant SOD1 expressed solely in motor neurons is sufficient to initiate the disease, albeit with a slower disease progression (Jaarsma et al., 2008). Motor neurons in the motor cortex, brainstem and spinal cord undergo cell death selectively in patients. A number of hypotheses attempt to explain this cell type selectivity, including the long axons of the motor neurons (Fischer and Glass, 2007), their poor intracellular calcium buffering capacity (Grosskreutz et al., 2010) and motor neuron specific cell death pathways (Raoul et al., 2002; Raoul et al., 2006; Genestine et al., 2011).

The contribution of mutant SOD1 expressing astrocytes in the non-cell autonomous character of ALS has been studied by excising mutant SOD1 from astrocytes which increases survival in two different mutant SOD1 mouse models (Yamanaka et al., 2008; Wang et al., 2011a). These results denote the toxic character of mutant SOD1 in astrocytes that accelerate disease progression significantly by mechanisms such as, but not exclusively, the below described mechanisms of neuroinflammation and excitotoxicity. This is schematically presented in figure 1.

1.3 Neuroinflammation observed in ALS

Neuroinflammation occurs in a number of neurodegenative diseases, including ALS (reviewed in Papadimitriou et al., 2010 and Philips and Robberecht, 2011), and entails the reactive state of astrocytes (astrogliosis) and microglia (microgliosis) and the infiltration of lymphocytes. Initially perceived as a bystander effect, neuroinflammation is currently seen as beneficial at first, removing damaged cells and secreting supportive factors, and potentially detrimental thereafter by excessive release of cytokines (Beers et al., 2011a). Evidence of inflammation is detected in post mortem tissue (Schiffer et al., 1996; Anneser et al., 2004; Casula et al., 2011; Sta et al., 2011; Wang et al., 2011b), in cerebrospinal fluid (CSF) (Baron et al., 2005; Tateishi et al., 2010) and in blood samples of ALS patients (Poloni et al., 2000). In accordance, similar parameters of neuroinflammation are detected in ALS rodent models (among many others in Kiaei et al., 2006; Keller et al., 2009; Beers et al., 2011b). Inflammation is generally perceived as hazardous in ALS, as increasing inflammation in ALS models exacerbates disease progression and diminishes survival (Nguyen et al., 2004; Gowing et al., 2009). Fittingly, therapeutic strategies targeting inflammation are often advantageous in ALS rodent models (see below).

1.4 Excitotoxicity in ALS

An additional detrimental mechanism in ALS is excitotoxicity; an overstimulation of neurons causing neurodegeneration. Glutamate binds to the N-methyl D-aspartate (NMDA) or α-amino-3-hydroxy-5-methyl-4-isoxazole proprionic acid (AMPA) receptors, allowing extracellular sodium and calcium to enter motor neurons. Increased levels of intracellular calcium consequently cause neuronal cell death. The importance of excitotoxicity in ALS is demonstrated by the beneficial effects obtained by treating patients with riluzole. Although the precise mechanism of this drug is not yet known, it blocks NMDA receptors, enhances re-uptake of glutamate from the synaptic cleft and inhibits glutamate release by blocking voltage-gated sodium channels (Siniscalhi et al., 1999), thus preventing motor neuron cell death. Riluzole treatment increases predicted lifespan with a significant 12% in ALS mice (Bensimon et al., 1994; Lacomblez et al., 1996) and increases the probability of one year survival in patients by 9% (Miller et al., 2007). Unfortunately, it does not halt disease progression.

An overview of the current knowledge of the astrocytic contribution in ALS will be addressed in this chapter separately for the mechanisms inflammation and excitotoxicity.

2. Astrocytes in inflammation

Despite that microglia are the main immune cells of the central nervous system (reviewed in Ransohoff, 2010), astrocytes can also become reactive and contribute to neuroinflammation and are the focus of this chapter, with microglial inflammatory effects residing beyond the scope of this chapter. During neuroinjury or neurodegeneration the production of cytokines induce astrogliosis in which astrocytes increase glial fibrillary acidic protein (GFAP) and vimentin expression as well as an array of other genes. This response increases neuronal survival and includes both supportive factors (e.g. growth factors and glutamate transporters) and cytokines to sustain/promote neuroinflammation. Interestingly, during neuroinflammation the number of astrocytes increases by the differentiation of chondroitin sulfate proteoglycan, NG2, positive cells to astrocytes and not by astrocytic proliferation (Gowing et al., 2008).

2.1 Increasing inflammation in ALS

To assess the effect of inflammation in ALS and thus to discover whether boosting the inherent inflammation would be beneficial, lipopolysaccharide (LPS) was daily administered to ALS mice (Nguyen et al., 2004). The effect of this treatment was a clear decrease in lifespan, implying that an increase of inflammation is detrimental in ALS (Nguyen et al., 2004). Another study, initially intended to decrease inflammation, administered macrophage colony stimulating factor (M-CSF) to ALS mice and observed an unexpected increase of microgliosis also leading to a decreased survival (Gowing et al., 2009). Although not directed specifically at astrocytes, this work has led to the understanding of the hazardous character of neuroinflammation in ALS.

2.2 Astrogliosis in ALS

Reactive astrocytes alter gene expression including an upregulation of the intermediate filaments GFAP and vimentin that allow for visualisation of astrogliosis by increased immunoreactivity of these filaments in patient and ALS model tissue. Post mortem spinal cord tissue from fALS and sALS patients display astrogliosis (Schiffer et al., 1996), implying that reactivity of astrocytes is not limited to the familial form of ALS. Interestingly, astrogliosis levels are similar between long surviving and short surviving ALS patients, although this is not the case for microglial activation and the amount of dendritic cells (Sta et al., 2011). An extra facet of astrogliosis in ALS is an increased immunoreactivity of toll-like receptor 4 in astrocytes of sALS patients (Casula et al., 2011). Astrogliosis in ALS mice is present at symptomatic stages preceeding microgliosis (Kiaei et al., 2006; Keller et al., 2009; Yang et al., 2011). Interestingly, GFAP is not necessary for astrogliosis as GFAP deficient astrocytes can still become reactive and do not affect survival of ALS mice (Yoshii et al., 2011).

2.3 Mutant SOD1 affects astrocytic inflammatory behaviour

The expression of mutant SOD1 in astrocytes alters their function in vivo and in vitro. To begin, deletion of mutant SOD1 in astrocytes in two distinct ALS models demonstrates the detrimental effect of mutant SOD1 in astrocytes mainly post onset, as deletion increased lifespan of ALS mice (Yamanaka et al., 2008; Wang et al., 2011a). Intriguingly, astrogliosis was unaltered, implying that the negative effect of mutant SOD1 in astrocytes is not due to altered levels of astrogliosis (Yamanaka et al., 2008), but potentially by astrocytes inducing microgliosis (Yamanaka et al., 2008; Wang et al., 2011a). An alternative approach arrives from the field of transplantation in which non-transgenic mesenchymal stem cells are transplanted into the spinal cord of ALS rats and differentiate into astrocytes, thus diluting the mutant SOD1 positive astrocytes in the spinal cord (Boucherie et al., 2009). This approach also shows unaltered astrogliosis, but also decreased microgliosis and cyclooxygenase 2 (COX2) expression, and extends murine ALS life span (Boucherie et al., 2009). The processes explaining this hazardous effect of mutant SOD1 in astrocytes has been investigated in vitro. To begin, an interesting approach of transducing human astrocytes with wild-type SOD1 or mutant SOD1 increases inflammation in mutant SOD1 cultures (Marchetto et al., 2008). In addition, the mutant SOD1 transduced astrocytes provide a less viable environment for human embryonic stem cell derived motor neurons (Marchetto et al., 2008). The latter was rescued by using a NADPH oxidase 2 (NOX2) inhibitor, apocynin (Marchetto et al., 2008). Other studies concur that mutant SOD1 primary astrocytes exhibit a higher gene expression of cytokines on baseline and when stimulated by interferon γ (IFNγ) or tumor necrosis factor α (TNFα) (Hensley et al., 2006), implying once again that mutant SOD1 expression may affect the threshold of astrocytes to produce proinflammatory cytokines. Accordingly, the expression of interferon simulated genes is detected in astrocytes of presymptomatic ALS mice (Wang et al., 2011b) and genetic ablation and knockdown of the interferon alpha receptor type 1 (IFNAR1) increase ALS mouse survival by 5% and 10%, respectively (Wang et al., 2011b). Intriguingly, Aebischer et al. stress the importance of interferon signalling in mutant SOD1 astrocytes by demonstrating that mutant SOD1 astrocytes trigger the selective death of motor neurons mediated by IFNγ (Aebischer et al., 2011). This mechanism is dependent on the activation of the lymphotoxin-β receptor by LIGHT (TNFSF14) and genetic ablation of LIGHT extends survival of ALS mice by 13%, but does not postpone disease onset (Aebischer et al., 2011). Although this is a large increase in disease survival, clearly other mechanisms remain to play a role.

The above described altered functioning of mutant SOD1 expressing astrocytes is induced by an overexpression of multiple copies of mutant SOD1. It is unclear whether these effects also play a role in fALS patients with only 1 allele of mutant SOD1 or in fALS/sALS patients without disease causing SOD1 mutations. Remarkable work by Haidet-Phillips et al., (2011) shows that astrocytes collected post mortem from fALS and sALS are both able to induced motor neuron selective death which is not observed with astrocytes obtained from controls (Haidet-Phillips et al., 2011). Gene expression analysis of the the fALS and sALS astrocytes demonstrated increased expression chemokines, proinflammatory cytokines and components of the complement pathway (Haidet-Phillips et al., 2011). This study confirms that the astrocytic inflammatory effects found in vitro and in vivo in ALS mice may also contribute to disease pathology in humans.

2.4 Genetic tools to minimise astrogliosis

Attempts to minimise the inflammatory effect of astrocytes in ALS include genetic strategies targeting astrocytic knockdown of certain cytokines. Targeting of nuclear factor κB (NF-κB) activation specifically in astrocytes does not alter disease onset nor life span in ALS mice (Crosio et al., 2011). Which may be in part due to the mere decreased astrogliosis at presymtomatic stage (Crosio et al., 2011). Additionally, complete ablation of TNFα does not affect disease parameters (Gowing et al., 2006), also implying deletion of a single cytokine may not be sufficient to affect disease progression, as a general decrease in inflammation can be beneficial (see below). Instead of targeting cytokine production, ablating proliferating astrocytes was attempted in ALS, showing no effect on survival (Lepore et al., 2008a). This may be explained by the inability of astrocytes to proliferate in ALS (Gowing et al., 2008).

2.5 Therapeutic strategies targeting inflammation in ALS

A number of strategies have been utilized to diminish inflammation in ALS mice, though often not specifically targeting astrocytes. It is worthwhile to note that it is commonly unclear whether anti-inflammatory strategies truly exert an anti-inflammatory function due to the age-matched analysis of astrogliosis instead of disease stage-matched analysis with drugs that successfully extend lifespan. Among these therapeutic strategies are those intended to pharmacologically block the cyclooxygenase (COX) pathway by administration of celecoxib, a selective COX-2 inhibitor, and deletion of the prostaglandin E2 receptor. Both strategies diminish inflammation, postpone disease onset and prolong survival in ALS mice (Drachman et al., 2002; Liang et al., 2008). Similarly, celastrol administration also postponed disease onset extended lifespan, while decreasing TNFα, nitric oxide synthases (iNOS), cluster of differentiation 40 (CD40) immunoreactivity and astrogliosis when assessing age-matched spinal cord tissue (Kiaei et al., 2005). Similar effects are obtained when providing ALS mice with folic acid (Zhang et al., 2008) or bee venom (Yang et al., 2010). Thalidomide extends survival in ALS mice by destabilising cytokine mRNA including TNFα (Kiaei et al., 2006). Additionally, its analog lenalidomide also prolongs survival (Kiaei et al., 2006), even when administered after symptom onset (Neymotin et al., 2009). To conclude, minocycline has shown a dramatic increase in survival of ALS mice and postpones symptom onset (Kriz et al., 2002; Van Den Bosch et al., 2002; Zhu et al., 2002). Interestingly, this effect is moment of administration dependent, as administration of minocycline post disease onset increases the astrocytic and microglial response in ALS mice, decreasing survival (Keller et al., 2011).

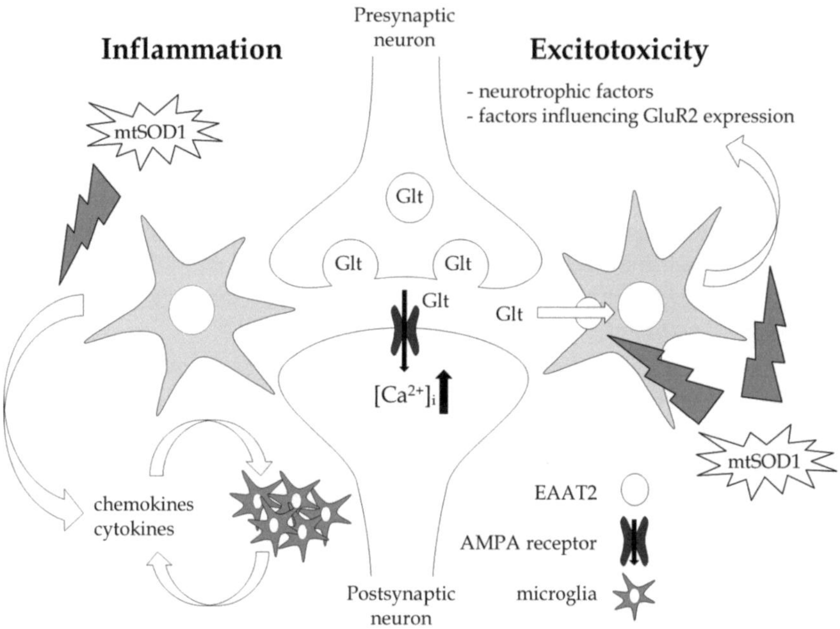

Fig. 1. Mutant SOD1 in astrocytes affecting (motor) neuron survival.

3. Astrocytes in excitotoxicity

In addition to the clear inflammatory role that astrocytes play in ALS, they also contribute to the mechanism of excitotoxicity. Their effect in the latter mechanism is two-fold: firstly, astrocytes facilitate the removal of excessive glutamate at the synaptic cleft and secondly, they affect the calcium permeability of AMPA receptors of motor neurons.

3.1 Excitotoxicity in ALS explained

Glutamate is the initiator of excitotoxicity in ALS. This neurotransmitter is the most abundant excitatory neurotransmitter in the brain and binds to NMDA, AMPA, and kainate (ionotropic) and metabotropic glutamate receptors (mGluR). Packaged into vesicles by the pre-synaptic neuron, glutamate is released into the synaptic cleft by the fusion of vesicles to the membrane of the neuron to excite the post synaptic neuron. This process is inhibited by riluzole (Siniscalhi et al., 1999). Increased levels of glutamate are detected in fALS, sALS (Fiszman et al., 2010; Spreux-Varoquaux et al., 2002) and is confirmed in spinal cords of ALS mice and rats. The detrimental role of glumate in the disease is demonstrated by the pronounced cell death that occurs to neurons in vitro when exposed to low levels of glutamate, even as low as physiologically detected in CSF (Cid et al., 2003). To further illustrate the detrimental role of glutamate in ALS, administration of compounds that block the formation of glutamate increase cell survival, both in vivo and in vitro (Cid et al., 2003).

3.2 Astrocytes in excitotoxicity in ALS: EAAT2/GLT-1

After glutamate release from the pre-synaptic neuron and binding of glutamate to ionotropic or metabotropic receptors on the post-synapse (increasing the concentration of intracellular calcium), glutamate is recycled for further use by the glial and endothelial cells, including astrocytes. Astrocytic glutamate re-uptake occurs by the glutamate transporters excitatory amino acid transporter 1 (EAAT1) and excitatory amino acid transporter 2 (EAAT2; also known as glutamate aspartate transporter (GLAST1) and glutamate transporter 1 (GLT-1), respectively). These transporters internalise glutamate, eg. into the astrocyte, for conversion to glutamine that is returned to the pre-synaptic neuron to be release again as glutamate (Laake et al., 1995).

Decreased glutamate uptake and EAAT2 protein levels are a common feature in both fALS and sALS and both in vitro and in vivo model systems (Staats and Van Den Bosch, 2009). In vitro transfection of primary cultured astrocytes with either mutant SOD1 or wild type human SOD1 down-regulates EAAT2 post transcriptionally (Tortarolo et al., 2004) and decreases EAAT2 transcription (Yang et al., 2009). Accordingly, glutamate transport is decreased in a neuronal cell line by mutant SOD1 transfection (Sala et al., 2005). Interestingly, this down-regulation also occurs in ALS model rats at pre-symptomatic stages through to end stage (Howland et al., 2002), at end stage only (Warita et al., 2002), in ALS model mice at end stage (Bendotti et al., 2001; Guo et al., 2010) and in post mortem patient spinal cords (Sasaki et al., 2001). In addition, in patient material the loss of EAAT2 and decreased tissue glutamate transport does not coincide with decreased levels of gene expression (Bristol and Rothstein, 1996), indicating that the loss is induced post transcriptionally, also in humans. Interestingly, a decrease of EAAT2 protein levels is not only in mutant SOD1 ALS models, but also a model of ALS/PDC (Wilson et al., 2003). In this model wild-type mice are fed with washed cycad flour containing β-methylamino-alanine (BMAA), which causes an ALS-like phenotype (Wilson et al., 2002). Although the loss of EAAT2 in ALS is apparent, it remains unclear whether this post transcriptional loss of EAAT2 proceeds or follows the loss of motor neurons.

3.3 Targeting (astrocytic) EAAT2

To assess whether the loss of glutamate transport or the loss of EAAT2 specifically results in motor neuron loss, pharmacological and genetic tools have been used. To begin, research conducted by pharmacologically inhibiting glutamate transport in the rat spinal cord, failed to show any motor neuron loss despite the increased levels of glutamate (Tovar et al., 2009). In contrast, a similar experiment has been performed to address whether EAAT2 loss specifically induces motor neuron loss. EAAT2 null mice live for approximately 6 weeks before they succumb to epileptic seizures and are vulnerability to acute brain injury (Tanaka et al., 1997). To this end, heterozygous mice demonstrated the effect of approximately 40% knockdown of EAAT2 in the spinal cord in ALS mice (Pardo et al., 2006). This knockdown resulted in a non-significant decrease of symptom onset and significant, but moderate, decrease of lifespan in ALS mice (Pardo et al., 2006).

To assess the expected beneficial role of EAAT2 in ALS, transgenic mice overexpressing human EAAT2 in specifically astrocytes were crossbred with mutant SOD1 mice. Although glutamate uptake is increased in vivo and an overexpression of human EAAT2 is protective on cortical neurons in vitro, an effect on symptom onset or lifespan was absent (Guo et al., 2003). Possibly, the expression levels were insufficient to induce an effect or human EAAT2 is not as efficient as murine EAAT2 in mouse, as administration of ceftriaxone (a β-lactam antibiotic) and GPI-1046 (a synthetic, non-immunosuppressive derivative of FK506) increase EAAT2 protein levels and extend lifespan of ALS mice (Rothstein et al., 2005; Ganel et al.,

2006) by enhancing EAAT2 transcription (Lee et al., 2008). In addition, EAAT2 is also expressed by other cells types than astrocytes alone (Anderson and Swanson, 2000), which are not targeted in this genetic experimental design. Interestingly, removal of mutant SOD1 from astrocytes leads to prolonged survival without affecting astrogliosis, but does preserve EAAT2 levels potentially explaining the extended lifespan (Wang et al., 2011a).

3.4 Astrocytic replacement therapy in ALS mice

The beneficial effect of EAAT2 is often used as an explanation of positive effects found by cell transfers in ALS model rodents. For instance, the systemic transplantation of c-kit positive cell from bone marrow in mutant SOD1 mice significantly increased the lifespan, which is, at least in part, attributed to increased EAAT2 expression induced by the transferred cells (Corti et al., 2010). The same holds true for the prolonged survival of ALS rats when treated with focal transplantation-based astrocyte replacement with wild type glial-restricted precursors (GRPs) (Lepore et al., 2008b). This study also focussed on EAAT2 by also transplanting EAAT2 overexpressing GRPs and EAAT2 null GRPs. The ALS mice treated with the EAAT2 overexpressing GRPs showed no additional increase of lifespan compared to wild type GRP treated ALS mice (already increased compared to controls). Intriguingly, this positive effect of transplantation of the wild type GRPs is diminished in mice transplanted with EAAT2 null GRPs (Lepore et al., 2008b). In addition, co-cultures of human adipose-derived stem cells with astrocytes induce higher levels of EAAT2 in astrocytes (Gu et al., 2010), though this treatment has not (yet) been shown to affect motor neuron survival in vitro or in vivo.

3.5 Astrocytes in excitotoxicity in ALS: AMPA receptor permeability

After the release of glutamate from the pre-synaptic neuron into the synaptic cleft, glutamate binds to NMDA, AMPA receptors or the metabotropic receptors. High levels of calcium entering through AMPA receptors into the post-synaptic neuron can cause neuronal death. The AMPA receptor is formed as a tetramer combining, usually pairwise, a combination of its four different subunits (glutamate receptor unit 1-4 (GluR1-4)) (Shi et al., 1999). Each subunit can bind glutamate and the channel opens after occupation of at least 2 binding locations (Mayer, 2005). The importance of this receptor in ALS is demonstrated by the ablation of glutamate induced apoptosis in cortical neurons in vitro (Cid et al., 2003) and in vivo when administering an AMPA receptor antagonist (Van Damme et al., 2003; Tortarolo et al., 2006).

The AMPA receptor plays an imperative role in excitotoxicity by its calcium permeability that is determined by the incorporation of the GluR2 subunit in the receptor complex. In most conditions, the AMPA receptor complex contains at least one GluR2 subunit and it prevents the influx of extracellular calcium into the neuron (Seeburg et al., 2001). In contrast, receptors lacking the GluR2 subunit are highly calcium permeable (Seeburg et al., 2001). A general decrease of GluR2 is found in ALS model mice, portraying an increased vulnerability of these mice to excitotoxic insults (Tortarolo et al., 2006; Zhao et al., 2008). The role of GluR2 in ALS is investigated by genetically ablating GluR2 in ALS mice, which decreases survival in vivo and decreases cell survival in vitro (Van Damme et al., 2005). The opposite has been shown by up-regulating GluR2 expression in motor neurons of ALS mice, as hereby survival is increased (Tateno et al., 2002). In addition, pharmacological inhibition of the AMPA receptor prolonged survival in ALS model mice (Van Damme et al., 2003; Tortarolo et al., 2006).

Interestingly, the surrounding astrocytes influence the expression level of the GluR2 subunit in motor neurons, as soluble factor(s) released from astrocytes effect GluR2 gene expression and neuronal vulnerability to excitotoxic insults, both in vitro and in vivo (Van Damme et al., 2007). Moreover, the presence of mutant SOD1 interferes with the production and/or secretion of this factor(s) to increase GluR2 expression and thus decreases motor neuronal resistance to excitotoxicity (Van Damme et al., 2007).

4. Conclusions and future directions

Astrocytes clearly contribute to ALS decrease progression in both neuroinflammation and excitotoxicity. An intriguing aspect of astrocytes in ALS disease pathology is whether the mutant SOD1 astrocytic properties, of LIGHT dependent cell death and diminished GluR2 editing for example, are also important in other ALS causing mutations and in sporadic cases of ALS. Initial work performed implies that these characteristics are not solely dependent on mutant SOD1 in patients. In addition, both mechanisms in which astrocytes function seem successfully targetable in mice. Future research may benefit from further assessing the role of also non-SOD1 ALS causing mutations in astrocytes on ALS and optimizing therapeutic strategies against neuroinflammation and excitotoxicity.

5. References

Aebischer, J., Cassina, P., Otsmane, B., Moumen, A., Seilhean, D., Meininger, V., Barbeito, L., Pettmann, B., and Raoul, C. (2011). IFNgamma triggers a LIGHT-dependent selective death of motoneurons contributing to the non-cell-autonomous effects of mutant SOD1. *Cell Death Differ* 18, 754-768.

Anderson, C.M., and Swanson, R.A. (2000). Astrocyte glutamate transport: review of properties, regulation, and physiological functions. *Glia* 32, 1-14.

Anneser, J.M., Chahli, C., Ince, P.G., Borasio, G.D., and Shaw, P.J. (2004). Glial proliferation and metabotropic glutamate receptor expression in amyotrophic lateral sclerosis. *J Neuropathol Exp Neurol* 63, 831-840.

Baron, P., Bussini, S., Cardin, V., Corbo, M., Conti, G., Galimberti, D., Scarpini, E., Bresolin, N., Wharton, S.B., Shaw, P.J., *et al.* (2005). Production of monocyte chemoattractant protein-1 in amyotrophic lateral sclerosis. *Muscle Nerve* 32, 541-544.

Beers, D.R., Henkel, J.S., Zhao, W., Wang, J., and Appel, S.H. (2008). CD4+ T cells support glial neuroprotection, slow disease progression, and modify glial morphology in an animal model of inherited ALS. *Proc Natl Acad Sci U S A* 105, 15558-15563.

Beers, D.R., Henkel, J.S., Zhao, W., Wang, J., Huang, A., Wen, S., Liao, B., and Appel, S.H. (2011a). Endogenous regulatory T lymphocytes ameliorate amyotrophic lateral sclerosis in mice and correlate with disease progression in patients with amyotrophic lateral sclerosis. *Brain* 134, 1293-1314.

Beers, D.R., Zhao, W., Liao, B., Kano, O., Wang, J., Huang, A., Appel, S.H., and Henkel, J.S. (2011b). Neuroinflammation modulates distinct regional and temporal clinical responses in ALS mice. *Brain Behav Immun* 25, 1025-1035.

Bendotti, C., Tortarolo, M., Suchak, S.K., Calvaresi, N., Carvelli, L., Bastone, A., Rizzi, M., Rattray, M., and Mennini, T. (2001). Transgenic SOD1 G93A mice develop reduced

GLT-1 in spinal cord without alterations in cerebrospinal fluid glutamate levels. *J Neurochem* 79, 737-746.

Bensimon, G., Lacomblez, L., and Meininger, V. (1994). A controlled trial of riluzole in amyotrophic lateral sclerosis. ALS/Riluzole Study Group. *N Engl J Med* 330, 585-591.

Boillee, S., Vande Velde, C., and Cleveland, D.W. (2006a). ALS: a disease of motor neurons and their nonneuronal neighbors. *Neuron* 52, 39-59.

Boillee, S., Yamanaka, K., Lobsiger, C.S., Copeland, N.G., Jenkins, N.A., Kassiotis, G., Kollias, G., and Cleveland, D.W. (2006b). Onset and progression in inherited ALS determined by motor neurons and microglia. *Science* 312, 1389-1392.

Boucherie, C., Schafer, S., Lavand'homme, P., Maloteaux, J.M., and Hermans, E. (2009). Chimerization of astroglial population in the lumbar spinal cord after mesenchymal stem cell transplantation prolongs survival in a rat model of amyotrophic lateral sclerosis. *J Neurosci Res* 87, 2034-2046.

Bristol, L.A., and Rothstein, J.D. (1996). Glutamate transporter gene expression in amyotrophic lateral sclerosis motor cortex. *Ann Neurol* 39, 676-679.

Bruijn, L.I., Miller, T.M., and Cleveland, D.W. (2004). Unraveling the mechanisms involved in motor neuron degeneration in ALS. *Annu Rev Neurosci* 27, 723-749.

Casula, M., Iyer, A.M., Spliet, W.G., Anink, J.J., Steentjes, K., Sta, M., Troost, D., and Aronica, E. (2011). Toll-like receptor signaling in amyotrophic lateral sclerosis spinal cord tissue. *Neuroscience* 179, 233-243.

Chiu, I.M., Chen, A., Zheng, Y., Kosaras, B., Tsiftsoglou, S.A., Vartanian, T.K., Brown, R.H., Jr., and Carroll, M.C. (2008). T lymphocytes potentiate endogenous neuroprotective inflammation in a mouse model of ALS. *Proc Natl Acad Sci U S A* 105, 17913-17918.

Cid, C., Alvarez-Cermeno, J.C., Regidor, I., Salinas, M., and Alcazar, A. (2003). Low concentrations of glutamate induce apoptosis in cultured neurons: implications for amyotrophic lateral sclerosis. *J Neurol Sci* 206, 91-95.

Corti, S., Nizzardo, M., Nardini, M., Donadoni, C., Salani, S., Simone, C., Falcone, M., Riboldi, G., Govoni, A., Bresolin, N., *et al.* (2010). Systemic transplantation of c-kit+ cells exerts a therapeutic effect in a model of amyotrophic lateral sclerosis. *Hum Mol Genet* 19, 3782-3796.

Crosio, C., Valle, C., Casciati, A., Iaccarino, C., and Carri, M.T. (2011). Astroglial inhibition of NF-kappaB does not ameliorate disease onset and progression in a mouse model for amyotrophic lateral sclerosis (ALS). *PLoS One* 6(3): e17187. doi:10.1371/journal.pone.0017187.

Del Bo, R., Ghezzi, S., Corti, S., Pandolfo, M., Ranieri, M., Santoro, D., Ghione, I., Prelle, A., Orsetti, V., Mancuso, M., *et al.* (2009). TARDBP (TDP-43) sequence analysis in patients with familial and sporadic ALS: identification of two novel mutations. *Eur J Neurol* 16, 727-732.

Drachman, D.B., Frank, K., Dykes-Hoberg, M., Teismann, P., Almer, G., Przedborski, S., and Rothstein, J.D. (2002). Cyclooxygenase 2 inhibition protects motor neurons and prolongs survival in a transgenic mouse model of ALS. *Ann Neurol* 52, 771-778.

Fischer, L.R., and Glass, J.D. (2007). Axonal degeneration in motor neuron disease. *Neurodegener Dis* 4, 431-442.

Fiszman, M.L., Ricart, K.C., Latini, A., Rodriguez, G., and Sica, R.E. (2010). In vitro neurotoxic properties and excitatory aminoacids concentration in the cerebrospinal fluid of amyotrophic lateral sclerosis patients. Relationship with the degree of certainty of disease diagnoses. *Acta Neurol Scand* 121, 120-126.

Ganel, R., Ho, T., Maragakis, N.J., Jackson, M., Steiner, J.P., and Rothstein, J.D. (2006). Selective up-regulation of the glial Na+-dependent glutamate transporter GLT1 by a neuroimmunophilin ligand results in neuroprotection. *Neurobiol Dis* 21, 556-567.

Genestine, M., Caricati, E., Fico, A., Richelme, S., Hassani, H., Sunyach, C., Lamballe, F., Panzica, G.C., Pettmann, B., Helmbacher, F., *et al.* (2011). Enhanced neuronal Met signalling levels in ALS mice delay disease onset. *Cell Death Dis* 2, e130; doi:10.1038/cddis.2011.11.

Gowing, G., Dequen, F., Soucy, G., and Julien, J.P. (2006). Absence of tumor necrosis factor-alpha does not affect motor neuron disease caused by superoxide dismutase 1 mutations. *J Neurosci* 26, 11397-11402.

Gowing, G., Lalancette-Hebert, M., Audet, J.N., Dequen, F., and Julien, J.P. (2009). Macrophage colony stimulating factor (M-CSF) exacerbates ALS disease in a mouse model through altered responses of microglia expressing mutant superoxide dismutase. *Exp Neurol* 220, 267-275.

Gowing, G., Philips, T., Van Wijmeersch, B., Audet, J.N., Dewil, M., Van Den Bosch, L., Billiau, A.D., Robberecht, W., and Julien, J.P. (2008). Ablation of proliferating microglia does not affect motor neuron degeneration in amyotrophic lateral sclerosis caused by mutant superoxide dismutase. *J Neurosci* 28, 10234-10244.

Grosskreutz, J., Van Den Bosch, L., and Keller, B.U. (2010). Calcium dysregulation in amyotrophic lateral sclerosis. *Cell Calcium* 47, 165-174.

Gu, R., Hou, X., Pang, R., Li, L., Chen, F., Geng, J., Xu, Y., and Zhang, C. (2010). Human adipose-derived stem cells enhance the glutamate uptake function of GLT1 in SOD1(G93A)-bearing astrocytes. *Biochem Biophys Res Commun* 393, 481-486.

Guo, H., Lai, L., Butchbach, M.E., Stockinger, M.P., Shan, X., Bishop, G.A., and Lin, C.L. (2003). Increased expression of the glial glutamate transporter EAAT2 modulates excitotoxicity and delays the onset but not the outcome of ALS in mice. *Hum Mol Genet* 12, 2519-2532.

Guo, Y., Duan, W., Li, Z., Huang, J., Yin, Y., Zhang, K., Wang, Q., Zhang, Z., and Li, C. (2010). Decreased GLT-1 and increased SOD1 and HO-1 expression in astrocytes contribute to lumbar spinal cord vulnerability of SOD1-G93A transgenic mice. *FEBS Lett* 584, 1615-1622.

Gurney, M.E., Pu, H., Chiu, A.Y., Dal Canto, M.C., Polchow, C.Y., Alexander, D.D., Caliendo, J., Hentati, A., Kwon, Y.W., Deng, H.X., *et al.* (1994). Motor neuron degeneration in mice that express a human Cu,Zn superoxide dismutase mutation. *Science* 264, 1772-1775.

Haidet-Phillips, A.M., Hester, M.E., Miranda, C.J., Meyer, K., Braun, L., Frakes, A., Song, S., Likhite, S., Murtha, M.J., Foust, K.D., *et al.* (2011). Astrocytes from familial and sporadic ALS patients are toxic to motor neurons. *Nat Biotechnol* doi: 10.1038/ nbt.1957

Hensley, K., Abdel-Moaty, H., Hunter, J., Mhatre, M., Mou, S., Nguyen, K., Potapova, T., Pye, Q.N., Qi, M., Rice, H., *et al.* (2006). Primary glia expressing the G93A-SOD1 mutation present a neuroinflammatory phenotype and provide a cellular system for studies of glial inflammation. *J Neuroinflammation* 3, 2.

Howland, D.S., Liu, J., She, Y., Goad, B., Maragakis, N.J., Kim, B., Erickson, J., Kulik, J., DeVito, L., Psaltis, G., *et al.* (2002). Focal loss of the glutamate transporter EAAT2 in a transgenic rat model of SOD1 mutant-mediated amyotrophic lateral sclerosis (ALS). *Proc Natl Acad Sci U S A* 99, 1604-1609.

Jaarsma, D., Teuling, E., Haasdijk, E.D., De Zeeuw, C.I., and Hoogenraad, C.C. (2008). Neuron-specific expression of mutant superoxide dismutase is sufficient to induce amyotrophic lateral sclerosis in transgenic mice. *J Neurosci* 28, 2075-2088.

Johnson, J.O., Mandrioli, J., Benatar, M., Abramzon, Y., Van Deerlin, V.M., Trojanowski, J.Q., Gibbs, J.R., Brunetti, M., Gronka, S., Wuu, J., *et al.* Exome sequencing reveals VCP mutations as a cause of familial ALS. *Neuron* 68, 857-864.

Keller, A.F., Gravel, M., and Kriz, J. (2009). Live imaging of amyotrophic lateral sclerosis pathogenesis: disease onset is characterized by marked induction of GFAP in Schwann cells. *Glia* 57, 1130-1142.

Keller, A.F., Gravel, M., and Kriz, J. (2011). Treatment with minocycline after disease onset alters astrocyte reactivity and increases microgliosis in SOD1 mutant mice. *Exp Neurol* 228, 69-79.

Kiaei, M., Kipiani, K., Petri, S., Chen, J., Calingasan, N.Y., and Beal, M.F. (2005). Celastrol blocks neuronal cell death and extends life in transgenic mouse model of amyotrophic lateral sclerosis. *Neurodegener Dis* 2, 246-254.

Kiaei, M., Petri, S., Kipiani, K., Gardian, G., Choi, D.K., Chen, J., Calingasan, N.Y., Schafer, P., Muller, G.W., Stewart, C., *et al.* (2006). Thalidomide and lenalidomide extend survival in a transgenic mouse model of amyotrophic lateral sclerosis. *J Neurosci* 26, 2467-2473.

Kriz, J., Nguyen, M.D., and Julien, J.P. (2002). Minocycline slows disease progression in a mouse model of amyotrophic lateral sclerosis. *Neurobiol Dis* 10, 268-278.

Kotchoubey, B., Lang, S., Winter, S., and Birbaumer, N. (2003). Cognitive processing in completely paralyzed patients with amyotrophic lateral sclerosis. *Eur J Neurol* 10, 551-558.

Kwiatkowski, T.J., Jr., Bosco, D.A., Leclerc, A.L., Tamrazian, E., Vanderburg, C.R., Russ, C., Davis, A., Gilchrist, J., Kasarskis, E.J., Munsat, T., *et al.* (2009). Mutations in the FUS/TLS gene on chromosome 16 cause familial amyotrophic lateral sclerosis. *Science* 323, 1205-1208.

Laake, J.H., Slyngstad, T.A., Haug, F.M., and Ottersen, O.P. (1995). Glutamine from glial cells is essential for the maintenance of the nerve terminal pool of glutamate: immunogold evidence from hippocampal slice cultures. *J Neurochem* 65, 871-881.

Lacomblez, L., Bensimon, G., Leigh, P.N., Guillet, P., and Meininger, V. (1996). Dose-ranging study of riluzole in amyotrophic lateral sclerosis. Amyotrophic Lateral Sclerosis/Riluzole Study Group II. *Lancet* 347, 1425-1431.

Lee, S.G., Su, Z.Z., Emdad, L., Gupta, P., Sarkar, D., Borjabad, A., Volsky, D.J., and Fisher, P.B. (2008). Mechanism of ceftriaxone induction of excitatory amino acid transporter-2 expression and glutamate uptake in primary human astrocytes. *J Biol Chem* 283, 13116-13123.

Lepore, A.C., Dejea, C., Carmen, J., Rauck, B., Kerr, D.A., Sofroniew, M.V., and Maragakis, N.J. (2008a). Selective ablation of proliferating astrocytes does not affect disease outcome in either acute or chronic models of motor neuron degeneration. *Exp Neurol* 211, 423-432.

Lepore, A.C., Rauck, B., Dejea, C., Pardo, A.C., Rao, M.S., Rothstein, J.D., and Maragakis, N.J. (2008b). Focal transplantation-based astrocyte replacement is neuroprotective in a model of motor neuron disease. *Nat Neurosci* 11, 1294-1301.

Liang, X., Wang, Q., Shi, J., Lokteva, L., Breyer, R.M., Montine, T.J., and Andreasson, K. (2008). The prostaglandin E2 EP2 receptor accelerates disease progression and inflammation in a model of amyotrophic lateral sclerosis. *Ann Neurol* 64, 304-314.

Lobsiger, C.S., Boillee, S., McAlonis-Downes, M., Khan, A.M., Feltri, M.L., Yamanaka, K., and Cleveland, D.W. (2009). Schwann cells expressing dismutase active mutant SOD1 unexpectedly slow disease progression in ALS mice. *Proc Natl Acad Sci U S A* 106, 4465-4470.

Logroscino, G., Traynor, B.J., Hardiman, O., Chio, A., Mitchell, D., Swingler, R.J., Millul, A., Benn, E., and Beghi, E. (2010). Incidence of amyotrophic lateral sclerosis in Europe. *J Neurol Neurosurg Psychiatry* 81(4):385-90

Maessen, M., Veldink, J.H., van den Berg, L.H., Schouten, H.J., van der Wal, G., and Onwuteaka-Philipsen, B.D. (2010). Requests for euthanasia: origin of suffering in ALS, heart failure, and cancer patients. *J Neurol* 257, 1192-1198.

Marchetto, M.C., Muotri, A.R., Mu, Y., Smith, A.M., Cezar, G.G., and Gage, F.H. (2008). Non-cell-autonomous effect of human SOD1 G37R astrocytes on motor neurons derived from human embryonic stem cells. *Cell Stem Cell* 3, 649-657.

Maruyama, H., Morino, H., Ito, H., Izumi, Y., Kato, H., Watanabe, Y., Kinoshita, Y., Kamada, M., Nodera, H., Suzuki, H., *et al.* Mutations of optineurin in amyotrophic lateral sclerosis. *Nature* 465, 223-226.

Mayer, M.L. (2005). Glutamate receptor ion channels. *Curr Opin Neurobiol* 15, 282-288.

Miller, R.G., Mitchell, J.D., Lyon, M., and Moore, D.H. (2007). Riluzole for amyotrophic lateral sclerosis (ALS)/motor neuron disease (MND). *Cochrane Database Syst Rev*, CD001447.

Naor, S., Keren, Z., Bronshtein, T., Goren, E., Machluf, M., and Melamed, D. (2009). Development of ALS-like disease in SOD-1 mice deficient of B lymphocytes. *J Neurol* 256, 1228-1235.

Neymotin, A., Petri, S., Calingasan, N.Y., Wille, E., Schafer, P., Stewart, C., Hensley, K., Beal, M.F., and Kiaei, M. (2009). Lenalidomide (Revlimid) administration at symptom onset is neuroprotective in a mouse model of amyotrophic lateral sclerosis. *Exp Neurol* 220, 191-197.

Nguyen, M.D., D'Aigle, T., Gowing, G., Julien, J.P., and Rivest, S. (2004). Exacerbation of motor neuron disease by chronic stimulation of innate immunity in a mouse model of amyotrophic lateral sclerosis. *J Neurosci* 24, 1340-1349.

Papadimitriou, D., Le Verche, V., Jacquier, A., Ikiz, B., Przedborski, S., and Re, D.B. (2010). Inflammation in ALS and SMA: sorting out the good from the evil. *Neurobiol Dis* 37, 493-502.

Pardo, A.C., Wong, V., Benson, L.M., Dykes, M., Tanaka, K., Rothstein, J.D., and Maragakis, N.J. (2006). Loss of the astrocyte glutamate transporter GLT1 modifies disease in SOD1(G93A) mice. *Exp Neurol* 201, 120-130.

Philips, T., and Robberecht, W. (2011). Neuroinflammation in amyotrophic lateral sclerosis: role of glial activation in motor neuron disease. *Lancet Neurol* 10, 253-263.

Poloni, M., Facchetti, D., Mai, R., Micheli, A., Agnoletti, L., Francolini, G., Mora, G., Camana, C., Mazzini, L., and Bachetti, T. (2000). Circulating levels of tumour necrosis factor-alpha and its soluble receptors are increased in the blood of patients with amyotrophic lateral sclerosis. *Neurosci Lett* 287, 211-214.

Ransohoff, R.M., and Cardona, A.E. (2010). The myeloid cells of the central nervous system parenchyma. *Nature* 468, 253-262.

Raoul, C., Buhler, E., Sadeghi, C., Jacquier, A., Aebischer, P., Pettmann, B., Henderson, C.E., and Haase, G. (2006). Chronic activation in presymptomatic amyotrophic lateral sclerosis (ALS) mice of a feedback loop involving Fas, Daxx, and FasL. *Proc Natl Acad Sci U S A* 103, 6007-6012.

Raoul, C., Estevez, A.G., Nishimune, H., Cleveland, D.W., deLapeyriere, O., Henderson, C.E., Haase, G., and Pettmann, B. (2002). Motoneuron death triggered by a specific pathway downstream of Fas. potentiation by ALS-linked SOD1 mutations. *Neuron* 35, 1067-1083.

Reaume, A.G., Elliott, J.L., Hoffman, E.K., Kowall, N.W., Ferrante, R.J., Siwek, D.F., Wilcox, H.M., Flood, D.G., Beal, M.F., Brown, R.H., Jr., *et al.* (1996). Motor neurons in Cu/Zn superoxide dismutase-deficient mice develop normally but exhibit enhanced cell death after axonal injury. *Nat Genet* 13, 43-47.

Rothstein, J.D., Patel, S., Regan, M.R., Haenggeli, C., Huang, Y.H., Bergles, D.E., Jin, L., Dykes Hoberg, M., Vidensky, S., Chung, D.S., *et al.* (2005). Beta-lactam antibiotics offer neuroprotection by increasing glutamate transporter expression. *Nature* 433, 73-77.

Rutherford, N.J., Zhang, Y.J., Baker, M., Gass, J.M., Finch, N.A., Xu, Y.F., Stewart, H., Kelley, B.J., Kuntz, K., Crook, R.J., *et al.* (2008). Novel mutations in TARDBP (TDP-43) in patients with familial amyotrophic lateral sclerosis. *PLoS Genet* 4, e1000193.

Sala, G., Beretta, S., Ceresa, C., Mattavelli, L., Zoia, C., Tremolizzo, L., Ferri, A., Carri, M.T., and Ferrarese, C. (2005). Impairment of glutamate transport and increased vulnerability to oxidative stress in neuroblastoma SH-SY5Y cells expressing a Cu,Zn superoxide dismutase typical of familial amyotrophic lateral sclerosis. *Neurochem Int* 46, 227-234.

Sasaki, S., Warita, H., Abe, K., Komori, T., and Iwata, M. (2001). EAAT1 and EAAT2 immunoreactivity in transgenic mice with a G93A mutant SOD1 gene. *Neuroreport* 12, 1359-1362.

Schiffer, D., Cordera, S., Cavalla, P., and Migheli, A. (1996). Reactive astrogliosis of the spinal cord in amyotrophic lateral sclerosis. *J Neurol Sci* 139 Suppl, 27-33.

Seeburg, P.H., Single, F., Kuner, T., Higuchi, M., and Sprengel, R. (2001). Genetic manipulation of key determinants of ion flow in glutamate receptor channels in the mouse. *Brain Res* 907, 233-243.

Shefner, J.M., Reaume, A.G., Flood, D.G., Scott, R.W., Kowall, N.W., Ferrante, R.J., Siwek, D.F., Upton-Rice, M., and Brown, R.H., Jr. (1999). Mice lacking cytosolic copper/zinc superoxide dismutase display a distinctive motor axonopathy. *Neurology* 53, 1239-1246.

Shi, S.H., Hayashi, Y., Petralia, R.S., Zaman, S.H., Wenthold, R.J., Svoboda, K., and Malinow, R. (1999). Rapid spine delivery and redistribution of AMPA receptors after synaptic NMDA receptor activation. *Science* 284, 1811-1816.

Siniscalchi, A., Zona, C., Sancesario, G., D'Angelo, E., Zeng, Y.C., Mercuri, N.B., and Bernardi, G. (1999). Neuroprotective effects of riluzole: an electrophysiological and histological analysis in an in vitro model of ischemia. *Synapse* 32, 147-152.

Spreux-Varoquaux, O., Bensimon, G., Lacomblez, L., Salachas, F., Pradat, P.F., Le Forestier, N., Marouan, A., Dib, M., and Meininger, V. (2002). Glutamate levels in cerebrospinal fluid in amyotrophic lateral sclerosis: a reappraisal using a new HPLC method with coulometric detection in a large cohort of patients. *J Neurol Sci* 193, 73-78.

Sta, M., Sylva-Steenland, R.M., Casula, M., de Jong, J.M., Troost, D., Aronica, E., and Baas, F. (2011). Innate and adaptive immunity in amyotrophic lateral sclerosis: evidence of complement activation. *Neurobiol Dis* 42, 211-220.

Staats, K.A., and Van Den Bosch, L. (2009). Astrocytes in amyotrophic lateral sclerosis: direct effects on motor neuron survival. *J Biol Phys* 35(4): p. 337-46.

Tanaka, K., Watase, K., Manabe, T., Yamada, K., Watanabe, M., Takahashi, K., Iwama, H., Nishikawa, T., Ichihara, N., Kikuchi, T., *et al.* (1997). Epilepsy and exacerbation of brain injury in mice lacking the glutamate transporter GLT-1. *Science* 276, 1699-1702.

Tateishi, T., Yamasaki, R., Tanaka, M., Matsushita, T., Kikuchi, H., Isobe, N., Ohyagi, Y., and Kira, J. (2010). CSF chemokine alterations related to the clinical course of amyotrophic lateral sclerosis. *J Neuroimmunol* 222, 76-81.

Tateno, M., Sugimoto, H., Tanaka, S., Itohara, H., Hama, A., Miyawaki, R.M., Shin, M.M., Masumada, T., Aosaki, H., Misawa, R., *et al.* (2002). GluR2 overexpression in motor neurons renders AMPA receptors impermeable to calcium and delays disease onset in an ALS transgenic mouse model. *Soc for Neurosci Abstr* 789.21

Tortarolo, M., Crossthwaite, A.J., Conforti, L., Spencer, J.P., Williams, R.J., Bendotti, C., and Rattray, M. (2004). Expression of SOD1 G93A or wild-type SOD1 in primary cultures of astrocytes down-regulates the glutamate transporter GLT-1: lack of involvement of oxidative stress. *J Neurochem* 88, 481-493.

Tortarolo, M., Grignaschi, G., Calvaresi, N., Zennaro, E., Spaltro, G., Colovic, M., Fracasso, C., Guiso, G., Elger, B., Schneider, H., *et al.* (2006). Glutamate AMPA receptors change in motor neurons of SOD1(G93A) transgenic mice and their inhibition by a noncompetitive antagonist ameliorates the progression of amytrophic lateral sclerosis-like disease. *J Neurosci Res* 83, 134-146.

Tovar, Y.R.L.B., Santa-Cruz, L.D., Zepeda, A., and Tapia, R. (2009). Chronic elevation of extracellular glutamate due to transport blockade is innocuous for spinal motoneurons in vivo. *Neurochem Int* 54, 186-191.

Van Damme, P., Bogaert, E., Dewil, M., Hersmus, N., Kiraly, D., Scheveneels, W., Bockx, I., Braeken, D., Verpoorten, N., Verhoeven, K., *et al.* (2007). Astrocytes regulate GluR2 expression in motor neurons and their vulnerability to excitotoxicity. *Proc Natl Acad Sci U S A* 104, 14825-14830.

Van Damme, P., Braeken, D., Callewaert, G., Robberecht, W., and Van Den Bosch, L. (2005). GluR2 deficiency accelerates motor neuron degeneration in a mouse model of amyotrophic lateral sclerosis. *J Neuropathol Exp Neurol* 64, 605-612.

Van Damme, P., Leyssen, M., Callewaert, G., Robberecht, W., and Van Den Bosch, L. (2003). The AMPA receptor antagonist NBQX prolongs survival in a transgenic mouse model of amyotrophic lateral sclerosis. *Neurosci Lett* 343, 81-84.

Van Deerlin, V.M., Leverenz, J.B., Bekris, L.M., Bird, T.D., Yuan, W., Elman, L.B., Clay, D., Wood, E.M., Chen-Plotkin, A.S., Martinez-Lage, M., *et al.* (2008). TARDBP mutations in amyotrophic lateral sclerosis with TDP-43 neuropathology: a genetic and histopathological analysis. *Lancet Neurol* 7, 409-416.

Van Den Bosch, L., Tilkin, P., Lemmens, G., and Robberecht, W. (2002). Minocycline delays disease onset and mortality in a transgenic model of ALS. *Neuroreport* 13, 1067-1070.

Vance, C., Rogelj, B., Hortobagyi, T., De Vos, K.J., Nishimura, A.L., Sreedharan, J., Hu, X., Smith, B., Ruddy, D., Wright, P., *et al.* (2009). Mutations in FUS, an RNA processing protein, cause familial amyotrophic lateral sclerosis type 6. *Science* 323, 1208-1211.

Wang, L., Gutmann, D.H., and Roos, R.P. (2011a). Astrocyte loss of mutant SOD1 delays ALS disease onset and progression in G85R transgenic mice. *Hum Mol Genet* 20, 286-293.

Wang, R., Yang, B., and Zhang, D. (2011b). Activation of interferon signaling pathways in spinal cord astrocytes from an ALS mouse model. *Glia* 59, 946-958.

Warita, H., Manabe, Y., Murakami, T., Shiote, M., Shiro, Y., Hayashi, T., Nagano, I., Shoji, M., and Abe, K. (2002). Tardive decrease of astrocytic glutamate transporter protein in transgenic mice with ALS-linked mutant SOD1. *Neurol Res* 24, 577-581.

Wilson, J.M., Khabazian, I., Pow, D.V., Craig, U.K., and Shaw, C.A. (2003). Decrease in glial glutamate transporter variants and excitatory amino acid receptor down-regulation in a murine model of ALS-PDC. *Neuromolecular Med* 3, 105-118.

Wilson, J.M., Khabazian, I., Wong, M.C., Seyedalikhani, A., Bains, J.S., Pasqualotto, B.A., Williams, D.E., Andersen, R.J., Simpson, R.J., Smith, R., *et al.* (2002). Behavioral and neurological correlates of ALS-parkinsonism dementia complex in adult mice fed washed cycad flour. *Neuromolecular Med* 1, 207-221.

Yamanaka, K., Chun, S.J., Boillee, S., Fujimori-Tonou, N., Yamashita, H., Gutmann, D.H., Takahashi, R., Misawa, H., and Cleveland, D.W. (2008). Astrocytes as determinants of disease progression in inherited amyotrophic lateral sclerosis. *Nat Neurosci* 11, 251-253.

Yang, E.J., Jiang, J.H., Lee, S.M., Yang, S.C., Hwang, H.S., Lee, M.S., and Choi, S.M. (2010). Bee venom attenuates neuroinflammatory events and extends survival in amyotrophic lateral sclerosis models. *J Neuroinflammation* 7, 69.

Yang, W.W., Sidman, R.L., Taksir, T.V., Treleaven, C.M., Fidler, J.A., Cheng, S.H., Dodge, J.C., and Shihabuddin, L.S. (2011). Relationship between neuropathology and disease progression in the SOD1(G93A) ALS mouse. *Exp Neurol* 227, 287-295.

Yang, Y., Gozen, O., Watkins, A., Lorenzini, I., Lepore, A., Gao, Y., Vidensky, S., Brennan, J., Poulsen, D., Won Park, J., *et al.* (2009). Presynaptic regulation of astroglial excitatory neurotransmitter transporter GLT1. *Neuron* 61, 880-894.

Yoshii, Y., Otomo, A., Pan, L., Ohtsuka, M., and Hadano, S. (2011). Loss of glial fibrillary acidic protein marginally accelerates disease progression in a SOD1(H46R) transgenic mouse model of ALS. *Neurosci Res* 70, 321-329.

Zhang, X., Chen, S., Li, L., Wang, Q., and Le, W. (2008). Folic acid protects motor neurons against the increased homocysteine, inflammation and apoptosis in SOD1 G93A transgenic mice. *Neuropharmacology* 54, 1112-1119.

Zhao, P., Ignacio, S., Beattie, E.C., and Abood, M.E. (2008). Altered presymptomatic AMPA and cannabinoid receptor trafficking in motor neurons of ALS model mice: implications for excitotoxicity. *Eur J Neurosci* 27, 572-579.

Zhu, S., Stavrovskaya, I.G., Drozda, M., Kim, B.Y., Ona, V., Li, M., Sarang, S., Liu, A.S., Hartley, D.M., Wu du, C., *et al.* (2002). Minocycline inhibits cytochrome c release and delays progression of amyotrophic lateral sclerosis in mice. *Nature* 417, 74-78.

17

Innate Immunity in ALS

John D. Lee[1], Jia Y. Lee[1], Stephen M. Taylor[1],
Peter G. Noakes[1, 2] and Trent M. Woodruff[1]
[1]*School of Biomedical Sciences,*
[2]*Queensland Brain Institute, University of Queensland,*
Australia

1. Introduction

Amyotrophic Lateral Sclerosis (ALS), also known as Lou Gehrig's disease, is the most common form of motor neuron disease. It is a debilitating, late onset neurodegenerative disorder that is characterized by the progressive death of upper and α-motor neurons within the central nervous system (CNS) (Bruijn and Cleveland, 1996). This results in symptoms of muscle weakness and atrophy of skeletal muscles, leading to paralysis and eventual death due to failure of respiratory muscles (Cozzolino et al., 2008). ALS has a prevalence of approximately 1~2 per 100,000 worldwide with males being more susceptible than females (1.3 ~ 1.6: 1) (Strong, 2003, Woodruff et al., 2008b, Worms, 2001). The majority of ALS cases (~90%) are thought to be sporadic with unknown aetiology and no robust environmental risk factors, with the remaining 10% being familial ALS. Of this 10%, approximately 20% have been linked to dominant mis-sense point mutations in the Copper/Zinc superoxide dismutase 1 (SOD1) gene which results in a gain of unidentified deleterious properties (Rosen et al., 1993). The two aetiologies of ALS (i.e. sporadic and familial) are indistinguishable on the basis of their clinical and pathological features, including progressive muscle weakness, atrophy and spasticity, each of which reflects the degeneration and death of upper and α-motor neurons (Boillee et al., 2006). The mechanisms leading to ALS are still unclear but theories have suggested that glutamate excitoxicity, oxidative stress, protein aggregation, mitochondrial dysfunction, cytoskeletal abnormalities and neuro-inflammation may all play a role (Bruijn et al., 2004). The present chapter will review the role of innate immune system, in particular the complement system, during the disease progression of ALS. It will review evidence for an involvement of the innate immune Toll-like receptor (TLR) system and receptor for advanced glycosylation end products (RAGE) in ALS patients and animal models of ALS. It will also comprehensively evaluate the role of the innate immune complement cascade in this disease. Finally, the future therapeutic possibilities for ALS, aimed at targeting components of the innate immune system will be discussed. We provide compelling evidence for specific inhibitors of complement C5a receptors as novel treatment strategies for ALS.

2. Innate immunity in neurodegenerative disease

Innate immunity is an evolutionary ancient system that provides the host with immediately available defence mechanisms. It is a rapid and coordinated cascade of reactions by host cells to protect them against foreign pathogens and insults (Akira et al., 2001, Nguyen et al., 2004). Until recently, the CNS was considered to be immunologically privileged because of its inability to mount an immune response and process antigens. Recent studies have revealed that immune surveillance and differentiation between self and non-self does take place in the CNS, where glial cells, including microglia, astrocytes and oligodendrocytes, act as CNS immune effector cells (Hanisch et al., 2008, Lehnardt, 2010, Ricklin et al., 2010).

The role of innate immune system in the CNS is mainly to provide protection to the neurons from foreign pathogens and injurious stimuli, and to maintain CNS homeostasis. It is also required for tissue modelling during development and following injury (Benard et al., 2008, Mastellos et al., 2005, Rahpeymai et al., 2006, Stevens et al., 2007). However sustained chronic inflammation might be harmful for neuronal integrity and may result in cellular dysfunction which triggers neurodegeneration. There is increasing evidence that suggests an involvement of the innate immune system in the development of neuro-inflammation which may drive the progression of many neurodegenerative diseases including ALS. Two major constituents of innate immune system are the TLRs and the complement cascade, each of which are described below.

3. Toll-like receptors (TLRs) and receptor for advanced glycosylation end products (RAGE) in ALS

TLRs are a large family of evolutionarily conserved transmembrane glycoproteins that initiate immune responses for host defence upon activation. These receptors are pattern recognition receptors that recognise pathogen-associated molecular patterns (PAMPs) from diverse organisms including bacteria, viruses, fungi and parasites (Liew et al., 2005). TLRs are expressed in various cell types in the CNS including microglia, astrocytes, oligodendrocytes and neurons (Aravalli et al., 2007, Bowman et al., 2003, Olson and Miller, 2004, Tang et al., 2007). This pathway has recently been implicated in the pathogenesis of ALS. Increased levels of TLRs (TLR1, TLR2, TLR5, TLR7 and TLR9) have been observed in mutant SOD1 mice as compared to controls (Letiembre et al., 2009) and mutant SOD1 expression in ALS has been suggested to facilitate microglial neurotoxic inflammatory responses via TLR2 (Liu et al., 2009). In addition, it has recently been shown that mutant SOD1 binds to CD14, which is a co-receptor of TLR2 and TLR4, and that microglial activation mediated by mutant SOD1 (G93A) can be attenuated using TLR2, TLR4 and CD14 blocking antibodies (Zhao et al., 2010). The involvement of TLR signalling in the pathogenesis of ALS is also supported by up-regulation of TLR2 and TLR4 mRNA and protein in the ALS patients, compared to control spinal cords. The increased expression level of TLR2 and TLR4 was shown on microglia and reactive astrocytes respectively (Casula et al., 2011). This suggests that TLRs could play a role in the progressive degeneration of motor neurons in ALS and indicates that the innate immune system is important in sensing neuronal injury and driving the progression of this disease.

In absence of pathogens, TLR signalling can also be activated via molecules called damage associated molecular patterns (DAMPs) including the high mobility group box 1 (HMGB1) protein released by injured tissues (Bianchi and Manfredi, 2009). HMGB1 is a nearly ubiquitous chromatin component that can regulate transcription of different sets of genes, including pro-inflammatory genes (Bianchi and Manfredi, 2009, Mouri et al., 2008). It can also be released passively by necrotic cells and actively secreted by stimulated monocytes/macrophages and astrocytes, which then bind to RAGE, TLR2 and TLR4. (Andersson et al., 2008, Hreggvidsdottir et al., 2009, Parker et al., 2004, Scaffidi et al., 2002). Therefore, HMGB1 can act as a potent pro-inflammatory cytokine-like mediator, thus contributing to amplification of the inflammatory response (Bianchi and Manfredi, 2007, Hreggvidsdottir et al., 2009). HMGB1-RAGE signalling has also been implicated in the progression of ALS where there was a significant increase in HMGB1 mRNA expression in ALS patient spinal cords when compared to normal individuals (Casula et al., 2011). The increased expression of HMGB1 was expressed by activated microglia and astrocytes in the spinal cord (Casula et al., 2011). Interestingly, there were no significant changes in RAGE mRNA expression in 12 ALS patients when compared to 6 controls. This observation could be due to the loss of motor neurons expressing RAGE in ALS patients, thus reducing the endogenous pool of RAGE mRNA. This same study also demonstrated that there is an increased expression of RAGE on astrocytes and microglia when compared to controls (Casula et al., 2011). Furthermore, serum soluble RAGE (sRAGE) levels were decreased in the serum of ALS patients when compared to normal individuals, where sRAGE is known to be a possible modulator of inflammation in several diseases (Ilzecka, 2009). Hence it is possible that low sRAGE levels may accelerate the neurodegeneration and could be a risk factor in ALS. This suggests that TLR/RAGE signalling may play a role in the disease progression of ALS, by activating microglia and astrocytes in the vicinity of motor neuron death. Targeting TLRs and RAGE may therefore be a novel therapeutic strategy to treat degenerative neuronal loss occurring in ALS.

4. The complement system in the CNS

The complement system is a key component of the innate immune system, which participates in the recognition, trafficking and elimination of pathogens and unwanted host materials. The complement system is an enzymatic cascade consisting of more than 30 plasma proteins and glycoproteins, and either soluble or membrane-bound receptors (Guo and Ward, 2005). Complement activation participates in host defence against pathogens primarily by cytotoxic and cytolytic activity through triggering formation of the membrane attack complex (MAC or C5b-9) on the target cell membrane (van Beek et al., 2003). It is activated via three major pathways: the classical, alternative, and lectin pathways; it is also activated by a recently identified fourth, extrinsic protease pathway (Huber-Lang et al., 2006, Thoman et al., 1984) (Figure 1).

The classical pathway is primarily activated in response to the recognition molecule C1q binding to antigen-antibody complexes such as immunoglobins (IgG and IgM) and pentraxins (such as C-reactive protein) bound to their targets (Ricklin et al., 2010, Woodruff et al., 2010). C1q may also bind directly to pathogen surfaces and to non-pathogen surfaces such as beta-amyloid and liposomes (Jiang et al., 1994, Marjan et al., 1994). The alternative pathway is activated by foreign surfaces which amplifies the slow spontaneous hydrolysis of C3 which leads to the formation of C3 convertases (Pangburn et al., 1981, Ricklin et al., 2010), whereas lectin pathway is initiated following the binding of mannose-binding lectin to carbohydrate groups on the surfaces of some pathogens (Woodruff et al., 2010). The activation of each of these pathways results in assembly of C3 and C5 convertase enzymes which cleave their respective inactive complement factors C3 and C5 into their active fragments C3a, C3b, C5a and C5b. This leads to the formation of MAC through the non-enzymatic assembly of C5b with complement factors C6-C9, forming C5b-9 on the cell membrane, which creates a transmembrane pore, ultimately leading to cell lysis (Podack et al., 1982). A recently identified fourth extrinsic pathway involves direct cleavage of complement 3 (C3) and complement 5 (C5) into C3a/C3b and C5a/C5b by proteolytic enzymes (serine proteases) such as kallikrein, thrombin and cell-derived proteases (Huber-Lang et al., 2002, Huber-Lang et al., 2006). As a result, synthesis of C5 by local inflammatory cells can produce C5a via cleavage of C5 with cell derived proteases, even when devoid of the complement cascade precursor, C3 (Huber-Lang et al., 2006). This pathway may provide a source of complement activation factors in the absence of upstream complement activation, and in a local tissue environment such as the CNS (Woodruff et al., 2010).

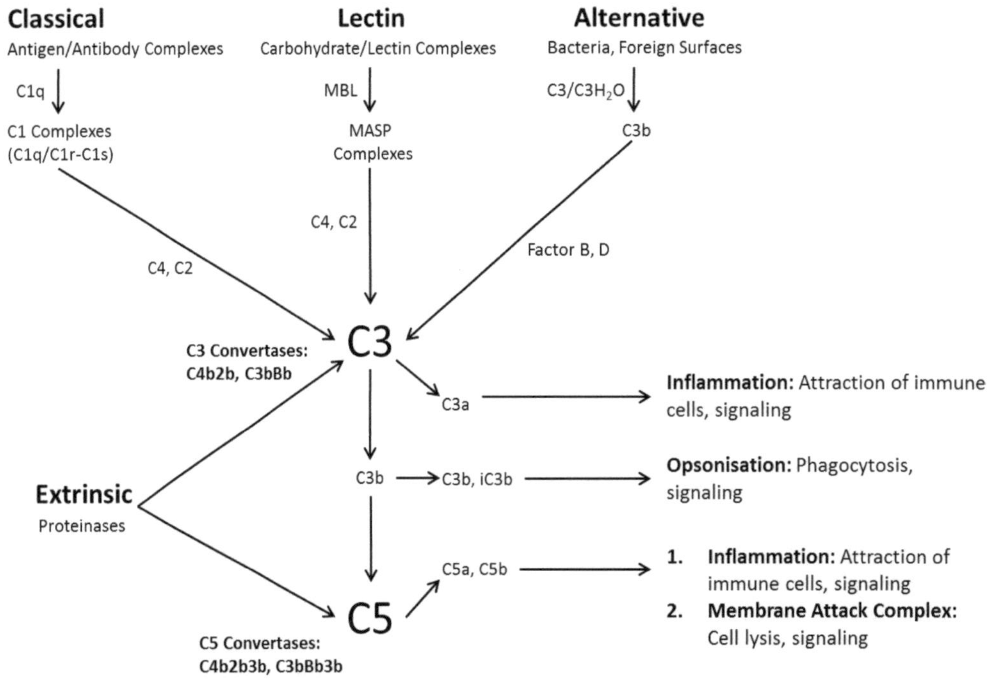

Fig. 1. Complement Cascade: Complement is part of the innate immune system and can be activated via four different pathways: the classical pathway, an antigen-antibody complex; the alternative pathway, activated by bacteria and foreign surfaces; the lectin pathway activated by mannose binding lectin; and recently discovered extrinsic protease pathway involving direct cleavage of C3 and C5. Each pathway converges at C3 and leads to a common terminal point which involves the formation of the cytolytic membrane attack complex (MAC) leading to cell lysis. Formation of pro-inflammatory anaphylatoxins C3a and C5a induces glial chemotaxis, generation of superoxide radicals and release of inflammatory mediators. C3b and iC3b facilitates phagocytosis by opsonising foreign pathogens.

The primary function of complement activation is to provide a rapid response to infection and injury by initiating the production of opsonins C1q and C3b to opsonise pathogens, the production of the pro-inflammatory anaphylatoxins C3a and C5a to recruit immune and inflammatory cells through ligand-receptor interactions with their corresponding receptors, C3aR and CD88, and the formation of cytolytic MAC, which ultimately leads to the destruction of invading organisms by cell apoptosis/necrosis (Liszewski et al., 1996).

C5a is considered to be the most potent inflammatory molecule generated upon complement activation and exhibits a broad range of functions. C5a exerts its effect through two high affinity receptors, the classical C5aR (CD88), and the C5a-like receptor 2 (C5L2/GPR77). The main C5a receptor, CD88 is a member of the rhodopsin family of seven transmembrane domain receptors coupled to the hetero-metric G proteins of the Gi subtype: pertussis toxin-sensitive $G_{\alpha i2}$, $G_{\alpha i3}$ or pertussis toxin-insensitive $G_{\alpha 16}$ (Amatruda et al., 1993, Johswich and Klos, 2007, Rollins et al., 1991). Cellular activation of CD88 involves intracellular calcium mobilization and activation of different signaling pathways including phosphatidylinositol-3-kinase/Akt (PI3Kγ; Perianayagam et al., 2002), Ras/B-Raf/mitogen-activated protein kinase (MAPK)/extracellular signal-related kinase (ERK) (Buhl et al., 1994), phospholipase A_2, phospholipase D (Cockcroft, 1992, Mullmann et al., 1990), protein kinase C (PKC; Buhl et al., 1994), p21-activated kinases, Rac GTPases (Huang et al., 1998), signal transducers and activators of transcription, sphingosine kinase (Melendez and Ibrahim, 2004) and NF-κB (Kastl et al., 2006). It is widely expressed on variety of cells and tissues, and its activation is known to have pro-inflammatory functions such as chemotaxis, degranulation, superoxide production, and release of proteases, eicosanoids, cytokines and chemokines from inflammatory cells (Gomez-Cambronero et al., 2007, Melendez and Ibrahim, 2004, Torres and Forman, 1999, Tsai et al., 2004).

The recently discovered C5a receptor, C5L2 has the conventional G-protein coupled receptor structure but it is not coupled to intracellular G-protein activated signaling pathways (Bamberg et al., 2010, Okinaga et al., 2003). Binding of C5a to C5L2 failed to induce intracellular calcium mobilization, extracellular signal-related kinase phosphorylation or receptor internalization, by contrast to CD88 (Cain and Monk, 2002, Okinaga et al., 2003). This has led to the proposal that C5L2 may act as a decoy anaphylatoxin receptor by regulating the availability of C5a to CD88, or by forming oligomers with CD88 to interrupt C5a-CD88 signaling (Rabiet et al., 2007). Although the mechanisms underlying C5L2 activation are still unknown, several recent studies in C5L2 knockout mice have showed greater response to C5a, a greater influx of inflammatory cells and a greater release of IL-6 and TNF-α compared to the wild-type mice (Rabiet et al., 2007). This suggests that C5a signaling via C5L2 may exert anti- inflammatory functions which buffer the effects of the inflammatory C5a-CD88 signaling pathway (Rabiet et al., 2007). Furthermore, studies have shown that C5L2 may function as an intracellular receptor, which becomes activated only after ligand binds to CD88. It was suggested that C5L2 negatively modulates C5a-CD88 signaling and limits the signaling capacity of C5a via its interaction with CD88 and β-arrestins (Bamberg et al., 2010, Van Lith et al., 2009). Any role for C5L2 in neurodegenerative diseases has yet to be properly elucidated.

Although the CNS does not receive the same composition of circulating complement factors synthesised in the liver by hepatocytes, due to the blood brain barrier (BBB), many studies have revealed that the CNS contains components of complement cascade, where they are expressed by astrocytes, microglia, oligodendrocytes and neurons (Barnum, 1995, Gasque et al., 1997, Nataf et al., 2001, O'Barr et al., 2001). Similar to the peripheral system, the role of complement activation within the CNS is thought to primarily protect the neurons from foreign pathogens through activation of inflammatory and immune cascades by surrounding glial cells. In addition to their immune surveillance functions, recent studies have shown that complement molecules also have a role in adaptive immune response, nervous system development, regeneration and regulating CNS homeostasis by clearing cellular debris and also eliminating excess synapses (i.e. synaptic pruning) (Stevens et al., 2007). Intriguingly, synaptic loss is not only a feature of neural development but is also a key pathological feature of neurodegenerative diseases (Schafer and Stevens, 2010, Woodruff et al., 2010). Hence it has been proposed that complement has multiple central roles in the CNS other than its canonical functions associated with host defence (Benard et al., 2008, Rahpeymai et al., 2006, Stevens et al., 2007). Therefore dysregulation or imbalance of the complement system in the CNS can be harmful to the neurons and may lead to, or contribute to, neurodegenerative diseases including ALS.

5. Clinical evidence of complement involvement in ALS

Several studies have been conducted on ALS patients in an attempt to identify whether complement components are up-regulated in disease progression (Table 1). It has been proposed that the classical complement system is involved in the pathophysiology of ALS, as studies have shown that activation fragments of complement components C3 and C4 are increased in the serum, cerebrospinal fluid (CSF), and neurological tissue (including spinal cord and motor cortex) of ALS patients (Annunziata and Volpi, 1985, Apostolski et al., 1991, Goldknopf et al., 2006, Kawamata et al., 1992, Trbojevic-Cepe et al., 1998). The first of these studies examined C3 immunofluorescence in spinal cord and motor cortex of 16 ALS patients and demonstrated significant C3 deposition, which appeared to be on astrocyte-like cells with no apparent neuronal staining (Donnenfeld et al., 1984). Subsequent studies measured C3c, C4, C1 inactivator and C3 activator fractions in the serum and CSF of 13 ALS patients but only detected increased levels of C3c in the CSF of ALS patients compared to normal individuals (Annunziata and Volpi, 1985). Furthermore Apopstolski and colleagues (1991) measured serum C4, C3 and Factor B levels in 33 ALS patients and found an increase in C4 levels when compared to normal individuals. Increased clusters of C3d and C4d coated fibers on oligodendroglia and degenerating neurites in spinal cord and motor cortex was also found in 8 ALS patients compared to 5 normal individuals (Kawamata et al., 1992). Two separate studies also investigated C1q, C4d and C4 levels in the serum and CSF of ALS patients and found C4d levels significantly increased in 15 ALS patients which also correlated with disease severity (Tsuboi and Yamada, 1994); another study also detected upregulation of C4 in ALS patients (Trbojevic-Cepe et al., 1998). Studies by Grewal and colleagues (Grewal et al., 1999) and Jiang and colleagues (Jiang et al., 2005) have identified increased mRNA of upstream complement components (C1q and C2) in the spinal cord of ALS patients. Recently, Sta and colleagues have found increased levels of C1q, C3c, C3d and C5b-9 in the spinal cord and motor cortex of ALS patients compared to normal individuals (Sta et al., 2011). The expression of these complement components was observed in glial cells rather than neurons (Sta et al., 2011). Lastly, complement component C3 was also found to be upregulated in the CSF of 71 ALS patients when compared to 40 normal individuals (Ganesalingam et al., 2011).

These findings of upregulated complement components and activation fragments, predominantly composing the classical pathway, in the serum, CSF, and neurological tissue in ALS patients strongly suggest that the classical complement pathway is involved in the progression of disease in ALS. However it is currently unknown where these complement factors originate, and what initiates their activation. Complement factors can be produced by various cells of the CNS and thus these complement factors could be produced locally in response to disturbance in CNS homeostasis due to immunoglobulin deposits and auto-antibodies in the CNS of ALS patients (Donnenfeld et al., 1984, Niebroj-Dobosz et al., 2006). Also the circulation could be a source of these complement factors as there is BBB breakdown in the end stages of ALS (Apostolski et al., 1991). Overall, evidence from these clinical studies helps us to propose that complement system activation occurs in ALS patients, and may play a role in the disease pathology. This is also supported by evidence of studies showing involvement of complement factors in animal models of ALS.

Complement factors	mRNA/Protein	Sample	Methods
C3	Protein	Spinal Cord, Motor cortex	Immunofluorescence
C3c	Protein	Serum, CSF	Single radial immuno-diffusion
C4	Protein	Serum	Single radial immuno-diffusion
C3d, C4d	Protein	Spinal Cord, Motor cortex	Immunohistochemistry
C4d	Protein	CSF	Sandwich ELISA
C4	Protein	CSF	Laser nephelometry
C1q	mRNA	Spinal Cord, Motor cortex	Northern blot, *In situ* hybridization
C2	mRNA	Spinal Cord	Microarray
C3c, C3dg, Factor H	Protein	Serum	2D gel electrophoresis
C1q, C3c, C3d, C5b-9	mRNA/Protein	Spinal Cord, Motor cortex	qPCR, immunohistochemistry
C3	Protein	CSF	Sandwich ELISA

Table 1. Clinical evidence of complement activation in ALS patients

6. Experimental evidence of complement involvement in ALS

Many studies in animal models of ALS have shown the involvement of the complement system during disease progression, supporting findings in ALS patients (Table 2). Although the SOD1 gene mutation only accounts for 2% of total ALS cases, mouse models carrying over-expression of mutant SOD1 enzyme are widely used, as it leads to progressive symptoms which are very similar to the human condition.

Complement factors	mRNA/Protein	Transgenic model	Reference
C1q	mRNA	Mouse SOD1 ^{G93A}	(Perrin et al., 2005)
C1q, DAF	mRNA	Mouse SOD1 ^{G37R} and SOD1 ^{G85R}	(Lobsiger et al., 2007)
C1q, C4	mRNA/Protein	Mouse SOD1 ^{G93A}	(Ferraiuolo et al., 2007)
C1q	mRNA	Mouse SOD1 ^{L126delTT}	(Fukada et al., 2007)
CD88	mRNA/Protein	Rat SOD1 ^{G93A}	(Woodruff et al., 2008a)
CD88	mRNA/Protein	Mouse NFL -/-	(Humayun et al., 2009)
C1q, C3	mRNA/Protein	Mouse SOD1 ^{G93A}	(Heurich et al., 2011)

Table 2. Experimental evidence of complement activation in animal models of ALS

The first study to demonstrate experimentally the involvement of complement factors in a SOD1 transgenic mouse model was performed by Perrin and colleagues in 2005. They isolated the ventral motor neurons from the lumbar spinal cord of SOD1^{G93A} transgenic mouse using laser-capture micro-dissection and then using microarray analysis they detected increased levels of all subcomponents of C1q in these mice at early symptomatic and end stage when compared to motor neurons from wild-type mice (~5 and ~8 fold respectively) (Perrin et al., 2005).

Subsequent studies in two distinct SOD1 transgenic mouse models also used laser-capture micro-dissection to isolate lumbar motor neurons from SOD1^{G37R} and SOD1^{G85R} transgenic mice which showed upregulation of genes for all three C1q subcomponents when compared to SOD1^{WT} mice 2 months prior to clinical onset (P105) (Lobsiger et al., 2007). In addition, this group demonstrated that the complement regulatory molecule, decay accelerating factor (DAF) also decreased at this time point (Lobsiger et al., 2007). Furthermore they showed that C1q protein was expressed by motor neurons using immunohistochemistry on spinal cord sections of both SOD1^{G37R} and SOD1^{G85R} transgenic mice but absent in the age-matched control mice (Lobsiger et al., 2007).

A separate group also used laser-capture microdissection to isolate the lumbar motor neurons from SOD1^{G93A} transgenic mice. Using microarray analysis and real time quantitative PCR, they showed there were increased levels of C1q (subcomponent B) and C4 mRNA at disease onset (P90) and late-stage disease (P120) (~7 and ~8 fold respectively) (Ferraiuolo et al., 2007). A similar study also used microarray analysis in a separate SOD1 transgenic mouse model using whole lumbar spinal cord homogenate (Fukada et al., 2007). This study used SOD1^{L126delTT} transgenic mice and showed elevated levels of C1q (subcomponent B) mRNA in post-symptomatic (P154) mice compared to wild-type mice. A very recent study has shown increased levels of C1q in the neuromuscular junction of SOD1^{G93A} transgenic mice compared to wild-type mice (Heurich et al., 2011).

By contrast to the above studies, which indicates a role for the classical complement pathway in the progression of pathology of the SOD1 transgenic mouse, a recent study has demonstrated that when SOD1^{G93A} transgenic mice were bred onto a background deficient in complement C4 (a necessary component of the classical complement pathway, downstream of C1q), there was a difference in the macrophage levels and activation in the peripheral nervous system but no difference in the onset of motor symptoms and survival when compared to wild-type mice (Chiu et al., 2009). This study indicates that other molecular pathways such as the alternative or extrinsic pathway may play compensatory roles in immune activation and macrophage recruitment in the absence of the classical pathway in these mice. To support this, recent studies in SOD1^{G93A} transgenic mouse showed increases in the C3 mRNA and protein levels in the spinal cord when compared to wild-type animals at symptomatic stage (P126) (Heurich et al., 2011). They also observed upregulation of C3 at the motor end plate and nerve terminals in the SOD1^{G93A} transgenic mice at pre-symptomatic stage (P47) when compared to wild-type animal (Heurich et al., 2011).

To further validate the involvement of downstream components of the complement cascade in the disease progression of ALS, upregulation of C5a receptor CD88 mRNA and protein was observed in mice deficient in the low molecular weight neurofilament (NFL) subunit protein, a mouse model of motor neuron degeneration in which neurofilament aggregates in a similar fashion to that in ALS patients (Humayun et al., 2009). This study showed there was a 4 and 3 fold increase in CD88 mRNA expression level at 2 and 3 months respectively, a time which is early in the disease process (Humayun et al., 2009). There was also an increased immunoreactivity of CD88 in motor neurons of NFL deficient mice when compared to wild-type mice at 3, 4 and 5 months. Our own findings also support a pathogenic role for C5a in ALS (Woodruff et al., 2008a). Chronic administration of a specific C5a receptor antagonist, developed in our laboratories (Wong et al., 1998) in SOD1^{G93A} transgenic rats, markedly delayed the onset of motor symptoms and increased survival, compared to untreated animals (Woodruff et al., 2008a). We also showed upregulation of CD88 in the lumbar spinal cord of SOD1^{G93A} transgenic rats, which increased as disease progressed (Woodruff et al., 2008a).

These findings of upregulated complement components in different animal models of ALS suggest that the activation of complement system is critically linked with disease progression in ALS. Whilst inhibition of one component of the classical and lectin complement pathway, C4, failed to ameliorate disease in SOD1^{G93A} transgenic mice, inhibition of the classical receptor for C5a, CD88, reduced disease pathology in SOD1^{G93A} transgenic rats. It should be noted that C5a is expressed following activation of all complement pathways (Figure 1). Hence inhibiting central components of the complement system, at the C3 and C5 level, may have benefits in slowing disease progression in ALS, as opposed to inhibiting an individual activation pathway. Specifically, our studies suggest that inhibiting the pro-inflammatory C5 activation fragment, C5a, which is central to, and generated by, all complement pathways, may be a novel therapeutic strategy to treat ALS.

7. Future directions: Therapeutic applications

To date, riluzole (Rilutek, Aventis Pharmaceuticals Inc) is the only approved therapeutic to treat ALS; it is known to prevent the pre-synaptic release of glutamine (Bellingham, 2011, Miller et al., 2007). In clinical trials, it has been shown to extend survival by around 2 ~ 3 months and delay the onset of ventilator dependence or tracheostomy (Bellingham, 2011, Miller et al., 2007). It is not clear that the drug improves the quality of life, however. Given this modest extension of ~2-3 months in survival there is an urgent need to develop new therapeutics which will significantly extend survival and also decrease morbidity in ALS.

Recent studies have suggested that the innate immune system is important in sensing ALS progression and its subsequent upregulation may drive the progression of this disease (Woodruff et al., 2008b). The complement system would be a logical and viable pathway to target, given the steadily accumulating clinical evidence of complement involvement in this disease. This is also supported by our findings where using specific C5a receptor antagonist improved motor symptoms and extended survival in the $SOD1^{G93A}$ transgenic rat (Woodruff et al., 2008a).

Our laboratories have developed a series of cyclic peptide C5a receptor antagonists which are potent inhibitors of C5a receptors on human inflammatory cells (Woodruff et al., 2011). PMX53 (AcF-[OPdChaWR] and PMX205 (hydrocinnamate-[OPdChaWR]) are orally active cyclic hexapeptides, which were derived from the linear CD88 antagonist, Me-FKPdChaWR (Konteatis et al., 1994) that were cyclised to induce structural and metabolic stability(Finch et al., 1999, March et al., 2004). These drugs have been shown to display therapeutic efficacy in numerous rodent models of inflammatory disease including rheumatoid arthritis (Woodruff et al., 2002), ischemic reperfusion injuries (Arumugam et al., 2004) and inflammatory bowel disease (Woodruff et al., 2003), as well as acute neurodegeneration (Woodruff et al., 2006). PMX205 is more lipophilic than the original CD88 antagonist PMX53, which results in increased potency in certain inflammatory models (Woodruff et al., 2005) and increased CNS penetrance (Woodruff et al., 2006). Hence, it has been used to reduce disease severity and prolong survival in animal models of neural degeneration including Huntington's disease, Alzheimer's disease and ALS (Ager et al., 2010, Fonseca et al., 2009, Woodruff et al., 2006, Woodruff et al., 2008a). As a result of this work, PMX205 would be the particular PMX series compound we would promote for any future clinical trialling in ALS.

In addition to inhibiting C5a receptors, targeting other factors of the complement system may provide viable therapeutic options to treat ALS. Several complement inhibitors have been developed over the years and compounds such as sCR1, C5 antibodies, compstatin or others could be used as potential therapies for ALS. However, due to the need to chronically administer a drug in ALS, a small, orally active and BBB permeable complement inhibitor, such as PMX205, would be required. The selectivity of PMX205 towards the classical C5a receptor leaves other components of the complement system intact, allowing for the production of complement factors including the MAC, thus reducing immune suppression -

a likely side effect of other inhibitors of complement which act more upstream in the system, were they are to be used chronically. Finally, PMX53, an analogue to PMX205 has already been shown to be safe when administered to humans, successfully completing three Phase I/IIa clinical trials, thus promoting the safety of these classes of drugs in humans (Woodruff et al., 2011).

In addition to anti-complement agents, combined therapies targeting multiple and disparate pathways will most likely be needed to effectively treat ALS. Extensive controlled clinical trials will need to be conducted in order to ascertain any potential therapeutic benefit of a complement inhibitor to treat the devastating and intractable nature of ALS.

8. Conclusion

There is increasing evidence that implicates the involvement of the innate immune system in the progression of ALS. In particular, the inappropriate activation or dysregulation of the complement system may play a role in ALS pathology. Evidence for this includes elevated levels of complement activation fragments in the serum, CSF, spinal cord and motor cortex of ALS patients. This has also been supported with elevated levels of complement activation fragments in various animal models of ALS. Moreover, inhibition of the C5a receptor using a specific C5a receptor antagonist ameliorated disease symptoms in a rat model of ALS. Collectively, these studies suggest that complement activation may play a crucial role in the progression of ALS. Hence reducing complement-induced inflammation using inhibitors to target complement factors could be an important therapeutic strategy to treat ALS.

9. Acknowledgments

We acknowledge the funding support of the Motor Neuron Disease Research Institute of Australia (Charles & Shirley Graham MND Research Grant 2010), and the National Health and Medical Research Council of Australia (Project Grants 455856 and APP1004455).

10. References

Ager, R. R., Fonseca, M. I., Chu, S. H., Sanderson, S. D., Taylor, S. M., Woodruff, T. M. & Tenner, A. J. (2010). Microglial C5aR (CD88) expression correlates with amyloid-beta deposition in murine models of Alzheimer's disease. *J Neurochem*, Vol.113, No.2, (April 2010), pp.389-401, ISSN 1471-4159.

Akira, S., Takeda, K. & Kaisho, T. (2001). Toll-like receptors: critical proteins linking innate and acquired immunity. *Nature immunology*, Vol.2, No.8, (August 2001), pp.675-680, ISSN 1529-2908.

Amatruda, T. T., 3RD, Gerard, N. P., Gerard, C. & Simon, M. I. (1993). Specific interactions of chemoattractant factor receptors with G-proteins. *The Journal of biological chemistry*, Vol.268, No.14, (May 1993), pp.10139-10144, ISSN 0021-9258.

Andersson, A., Covacu, R., Sunnemark, D., Danilov, A. I., Dal Bianco, A., Khademi, M., Wallstrom, E., Lobell, A., Brundin, L., Lassmann, H. & Harris, R. A. (2008). Pivotal advance: HMGB1 expression in active lesions of human and experimental multiple sclerosis. *Journal of leukocyte biology*, Vol.84, No.5, (November 2008), pp.1248-1255, ISSN 0741-5400.

Annunziata, P. & Volpi, N. (1985). High levels of C3c in the cerebrospinal fluid from amyotrophic lateral sclerosis patients. *Acta neurologica Scandinavica,* Vol.72, No.1, (July 1985), pp.61-64, ISSN 0001-6314.

Apostolski, S., Nikolic, J., Bugarski-Prokopljevic, C., Miletic, V., Pavlovic, S. & Filipovic, S. (1991). Serum and CSF immunological findings in ALS. *Acta neurologica Scandinavica,* Vol.83, No.2, (February 1991), pp.96-98, ISSN 0001-6314.

Aravalli, R. N., Peterson, P. K. & Lokensgard, J. R. (2007). Toll-like receptors in defense and damage of the central nervous system. *Journal of neuroimmune pharmacology : the official journal of the Society on NeuroImmune Pharmacology,* Vol.2, No.4, (December 2007), pp.297-312, ISSN 1557-1904.

Arumugam, T. V., Shiels, I. A., Woodruff, T. M., Granger, D. N. & Taylor, S. M. (2004). The role of the complement system in ischemia-reperfusion injury. *Shock,* Vol.21, No.5, (May 2004), pp.401-409, ISSN 1073-2322.

Bamberg, C. E., Mackay, C. R., Lee, H., Zahra, D., Jackson, J., Lim, Y. S., Whitfeld, P. L., Craig, S., Corsini, E., Lu, B., Gerard, C. & Gerard, N. P. (2010). The C5a receptor (C5aR) C5L2 is a modulator of C5aR-mediated signal transduction. *Journal of Biological Chemistry,* Vol.285, No.10, (March 2010), pp.7633-7644, ISSN 1083-351X.

Barnum, S. R. (1995). Complement biosynthesis in the central nervous system. *Crit Rev Oral Biol Med,* Vol.6, No.2, (January 1995), pp.132-146, ISSN 1045-4411.

Bellingham, M. C. (2011). A review of the neural mechanisms of action and clinical efficiency of riluzole in treating amyotrophic lateral sclerosis: what have we learned in the last decade? *CNS neuroscience & therapeutics,* Vol.17, No.1, (February 2011), pp.4-31, ISSN 1755-5949.

Benard, M., Raoult, E., Vaudry, D., Leprince, J., Falluel-Morel, A., Gonzalez, B. J., Galas, L., Vaudry, H. & Fontaine, M. (2008). Role of complement anaphylatoxin receptors (C3aR, C5aR) in the development of the rat cerebellum. *Molecular immunology,* Vol.45, No.14, (August 2008), pp.3767-3774, ISSN 0161-5890.

Bianchi, M. E. & Manfredi, A. A. (2007). High-mobility group box 1 (HMGB1) protein at the crossroads between innate and adaptive immunity. *Immunological reviews,* Vol.220, (December 2007), pp.35-46, ISSN 0105-2896.

Bianchi, M. E. & Manfredi, A. A. (2009). Immunology. Dangers in and out. *Science,* Vol.323, No.5922, (March 2009), pp.1683-1684, ISSN 1095-9203.

Boillee, S., Vande Velde, C. & Cleveland, D. W. (2006). ALS: a disease of motor neurons and their nonneuronal neighbors. *Neuron,* Vol.52, No.1, (October 2006), pp.39-59, ISSN 0896-6273.

Bowman, C. C., Rasley, A., Tranguch, S. L. & Marriott, I. (2003). Cultured astrocytes express toll-like receptors for bacterial products. *Glia,* Vol.43, No.3, (September 2003), pp.281-291, ISSN 0894-1491.

Bruijn, L. I. & Cleveland, D. W. (1996). Mechanisms of selective motor neuron death in ALS: insights from transgenic mouse models of motor neuron disease. *Neuropathol Appl Neurobiol,* Vol.22, No.5, (October 1996), pp.373-387, ISSN 0305-1846.

Bruijn, L. I., Miller, T. M. & Cleveland, D. W. (2004). Unraveling the mechanisms involved in motor neuron degeneration in ALS. *Annu Rev Neurosci,* Vol.27, (June 2004), pp.723-749, ISSN 0147-006X.

Buhl, A. M., Avdi, N., Worthen, G. S. & Johnson, G. L. (1994). Mapping of the C5a receptor signal transduction network in human neutrophils. *Proc Natl Acad Sci U S A,* Vol.91, No.19, (September 1994), pp.9190-9194, ISSN 0027-8424.

Cain, S. A. & Monk, P. N. (2002). The orphan receptor C5L2 has high affinity binding sites for complement fragments C5a and C5a des-Arg(74). *Journal of Biological Chemistry,* Vol.277, No.9, (March 2002), pp.7165-7169, ISSN 0021-9258.

Casula, M., Iyer, A. M., Spliet, W. G., Anink, J. J., Steentjes, K., Sta, M., Troost, D. & Aronica, E. (2011). Toll-like receptor signaling in amyotrophic lateral sclerosis spinal cord tissue. *Neuroscience,* Vol.179, (April 2011), pp.233-243, ISSN 1873-7544.

Chiu, I. M., Phatnani, H., Kuligowski, M., Tapia, J. C., Carrasco, M. A., Zhang, M., Maniatis, T. & Carroll, M. C. (2009). Activation of innate and humoral immunity in the peripheral nervous system of ALS transgenic mice. *Proceedings of the National Academy of Sciences of the United States of America,* Vol.106, No.49, (December 2009), pp.20960-20965, ISSN 1091-6490.

Cockcroft, S. (1992). G-protein-regulated phospholipases C, D and A2-mediated signalling in neutrophils. *Biochim Biophys Acta,* Vol.1113, No.2, (August 1992), pp.135-160, ISSN 0006-3002.

Cozzolino, M., Ferri, A. & Carri, M. T. (2008). Amyotrophic lateral sclerosis: from current developments in the laboratory to clinical implications. *Antioxid Redox Signal,* Vol.10, No.3, (March 2008), pp.405-443, ISSN 1523-0864.

Donnenfeld, H., Kascsak, R. J. & Bartfeld, H. (1984). Deposits of IgG and C3 in the spinal cord and motor cortex of ALS patients. *Journal of neuroimmunology,* Vol.6, No.1, (February 1984), pp.51-57, ISSN 0165-5728.

Ferraiuolo, L., Heath, P. R., Holden, H., Kasher, P., Kirby, J. & Shaw, P. J. (2007). Microarray analysis of the cellular pathways involved in the adaptation to and progression of motor neuron injury in the SOD1 G93A mouse model of familial ALS. *The Journal of neuroscience : the official journal of the Society for Neuroscience,* Vol.27, No.34, (August 2007), pp.9201-9219, ISSN 1529-2401.

Finch, A. M., Wong, A. K., Paczkowski, N. J., Wadi, S. K., Craik, D. J., Fairlie, D. P. & Taylor, S. M. (1999). Low-molecular-weight peptidic and cyclic antagonists of the receptor for the complement factor C5a. *Journal of medicinal chemistry,* Vol.42, No.11, (June 1999), pp.1965-1974, ISSN 0022-2623.

Fonseca, M. I., Ager, R. R., Chu, S. H., Yazan, O., Sanderson, S. D., Laferla, F. M., Taylor, S. M., Woodruff, T. M. & Tenner, A. J. (2009). Treatment with a C5aR antagonist decreases pathology and enhances behavioral performance in murine models of Alzheimer's disease. *J Immunol,* Vol.183, No.2, (July 2009), pp.1375-1383, ISSN 1550-6606.

Fukada, Y., Yasui, K., Kitayama, M., Doi, K., Nakano, T., Watanabe, Y. & Nakashima, K. (2007). Gene expression analysis of the murine model of amyotrophic lateral sclerosis: studies of the Leu126delTT mutation in SOD1. *Brain research,* Vol.1160, (July 2007), pp.1-10, ISSN 0006-8993.

Ganesalingam, J., An, J., Shaw, C. E., Shaw, G., Lacomis, D. & Bowser, R. (2011). Combination of neurofilament heavy chain and complement C3 as CSF biomarkers for ALS. *Journal of neurochemistry,* Vol.117, No.3, (May 2011), pp.528-537, ISSN 1471 4159.

Gasque, P., Singhrao, S. K., Neal, J. W., Gotze, O. & Morgan, B. P. (1997). Expression of the receptor for complement C5a (CD88) is up-regulated on reactive astrocytes, microglia, and endothelial cells in the inflamed human central nervous system. *Am J Pathol,* Vol.150, No.1, (January 1997), pp.31-41, ISSN 0002-9440.

Goldknopf, I. L., Sheta, E. A., Bryson, J., Folsom, B., Wilson, C., Duty, J., Yen, A. A. & Appel, S. H. (2006). Complement C3c and related protein biomarkers in amyotrophic lateral sclerosis and Parkinson's disease. *Biochem Biophys Res Commun,* Vol.342, No.4, (April 2006), pp.1034-1039, ISSN 0006-291X.

Gomez-Cambronero, J., Di Fulvio, M. & Knapek, K. (2007). Understanding phospholipase D (PLD) using leukocytes: PLD involvement in cell adhesion and chemotaxis. *J Leukoc Biol,* Vol.82, No.2, (August 2007), pp.272-281, ISSN 0741-5400.

Grewal, R. P., Morgan, T. E. & Finch, C. E. (1999). C1qB and clusterin mRNA increase in association with neurodegeneration in sporadic amyotrophic lateral sclerosis. *Neurosci Lett,* Vol.271, No.1, (August 1999), pp.65-67, ISSN 0304-3940.

Guo, R. F. & Ward, P. A. (2005). Role of C5a in inflammatory responses. *Annu Rev Immunol,* Vol.23, (March 2005), pp.821-852, ISSN 0732-0582.

Hanisch, U. K., Johnson, T. V. & Kipnis, J. (2008). Toll-like receptors: roles in neuroprotection? *Trends in neurosciences,* Vol.31, No.4, (April 2008), pp.176-182, ISSN 0166-2236.

Heurich, B., El Idrissi, N. B., Donev, R. M., Petri, S., Claus, P., Neal, J., Morgan, B. P. & Ramaglia, V. (2011). Complement upregulation and activation on motor neurons and neuromuscular junction in the SOD1 G93A mouse model of familial amyotrophic lateral sclerosis. *Journal of neuroimmunology,* Vol.235, No.1-2, (June 2011), pp.104-109, ISSN 1872-8421.

Hreggvidsdottir, H. S., Ostberg, T., Wahamaa, H., Schierbeck, H., Aveberger, A. C., Klevenvall, L., Palmblad, K., Ottosson, L., Andersson, U. & Harris, H. E. (2009). The alarmin HMGB1 acts in synergy with endogenous and exogenous danger signals to promote inflammation. *Journal of leukocyte biology,* Vol.86, No.3, (September 2009), pp.655-662, ISSN 1938-3673.

Huang, R., Lian, J. P., Robinson, D. & Badwey, J. A. (1998). Neutrophils stimulated with a variety of chemoattractants exhibit rapid activation of p21-activated kinases (Paks): separate signals are required for activation and inactivation of paks. *Mol Cell Biol,* Vol.18, No.12, (December 1998), pp.7130-7138, ISSN 0270-7306.

Huber-Lang, M., Sarma, J. V., Zetoune, F. S., Rittirsch, D., Neff, T. A., Mcguire, S. R., Lambris, J. D., Warner, R. L., Flierl, M. A., Hoesel, L. M., Gebhard, F., Younger, J. G., Drouin, S. M., Wetsel, R. A. & Ward, P. A. (2006). Generation of C5a in the absence of C3: a new complement activation pathway. *Nat Med,* Vol.12, No.6, (June 2006), pp.682-687, ISSN 1078-8956.

Huber-Lang, M., Younkin, E. M., Sarma, J. V., Riedemann, N., Mcguire, S. R., Lu, K. T., Kunkel, R., Younger, J. G., Zetoune, F. S. & Ward, P. A. (2002). Generation of C5a by phagocytic cells. *Am J Pathol,* Vol.161, No.5, (November 2002), pp.1849-1859, ISSN 0002-9440.

Humayun, S., Gohar, M., Volkening, K., Moisse, K., Leystra-Lantz, C., Mepham, J., Mclean, J. & Strong, M. J. (2009). The complement factor C5a receptor is upregulated in

NFL-/- mouse motor neurons. *J Neuroimmunol,* Vol.210, No.1-2, (May 2009), pp.52-62, ISSN 1872-8421.

Ilzecka, J. (2009). Serum-soluble receptor for advanced glycation end product levels in patients with amyotrophic lateral sclerosis. *Acta neurologica Scandinavica,* Vol.120, No.2, (August 2009), pp.119-122, ISSN 1600-0404.

Jiang, H., Burdick, D., Glabe, C. G., Cotman, C. W. & Tenner, A. J. (1994). beta-Amyloid activates complement by binding to a specific region of the collagen-like domain of the C1q A chain. *Journal of immunology,* Vol.152, No.10, (May 1994), pp.5050-5059, ISSN 0022-1767.

Jiang, Y. M., Yamamoto, M., Kobayashi, Y., Yoshihara, T., Liang, Y., Terao, S., Takeuchi, H., Ishigaki, S., Katsuno, M., Adachi, H., Niwa, J., Tanaka, F., Doyu, M., Yoshida, M., Hashizume, Y. & Sobue, G. (2005). Gene expression profile of spinal motor neurons in sporadic amyotrophic lateral sclerosis. *Ann Neurol,* Vol.57, No.2, (February 2005), pp.236-251, ISSN 0364-5134.

Johswich, K. & Klos, A. (2007). C5L2--an anti-inflammatory molecule or a receptor for acylation stimulating protein (C3a-desArg)? *Advances in experimental medicine and biology,* Vol.598, (September 2007), pp.159-180, ISSN 0065-2598.

Kastl, S. P., Speidl, W. S., Kaun, C., Rega, G., Assadian, A., Weiss, T. W., Valent, P., Hagmueller, G. W., Maurer, G., Huber, K. & Wojta, J. (2006). The complement component C5a induces the expression of plasminogen activator inhibitor-1 in human macrophages via NF-kappaB activation. *J Thromb Haemost,* Vol.4, No.8, (August 2006), pp.1790-1797, ISSN 1538-7933.

Kawamata, T., Akiyama, H., Yamada, T. & Mcgeer, P. L. (1992). Immunologic reactions in amyotrophic lateral sclerosis brain and spinal cord tissue. *The American journal of pathology,* Vol.140, No.3, (March 1992), pp.691-707, ISSN 0002-9440.

Konteatis, Z. D., Siciliano, S. J., Van Riper, G., Molineaux, C. J., Pandya, S., Fischer, P., Rosen, H., Mumford, R. A. & Springer, M. S. (1994). Development of C5a receptor antagonists. Differential loss of functional responses. *Journal of immunology,* Vol.153, No.9, (November 1994), pp.4200-4205, ISSN 0022-1767.

Lehnardt, S. (2010). Innate immunity and neuroinflammation in the CNS: the role of microglia in Toll-like receptor-mediated neuronal injury. *Glia,* Vol.58, No.3, (February 2010), pp.253-263, ISSN 1098-1136.

Letiembre, M., Liu, Y., Walter, S., Hao, W., Pfander, T., Wrede, A., Schulz-Schaeffer, W. & Fassbender, K. (2009). Screening of innate immune receptors in neurodegenerative diseases: a similar pattern. *Neurobiology of aging,* Vol.30, No.5, (May 2009), pp.759-768, ISSN 1558-1497.

Liew, F. Y., Xu, D., Brint, E. K. & O'neill, L. A. (2005). Negative regulation of toll-like receptor-mediated immune responses. *Nature reviews. Immunology,* Vol.5, No.6, (June 2005), pp.446-458, ISSN 1474-1733.

Liszewski, M. K., Farries, T. C., Lublin, D. M., Rooney, I. A. & Atkinson, J. P. (1996). Control of the complement system. *Advances in immunology,* Vol.61, (January 1996), pp.201-283, ISSN 0065-2776.

Liu, Y., Hao, W., Dawson, A., Liu, S. & Fassbender, K. (2009). Expression of amyotrophic lateral sclerosis-linked SOD1 mutant increases the neurotoxic potential of microglia via TLR2. *The Journal of biological chemistry,* Vol.284, No.6, (February 2009), pp.3691-3699, ISSN 0021-9258.

Lobsiger, C. S., Boillee, S. & Cleveland, D. W. (2007). Toxicity from different SOD1 mutants dysregulates the complement system and the neuronal regenerative response in ALS motor neurons. *Proc Natl Acad Sci U S A,* Vol.104, No.18, (May 2007), pp.7319-7326, ISSN 0027-8424.

March, D. R., Proctor, L. M., Stoermer, M. J., Sbaglia, R., Abbenante, G., Reid, R. C., Woodruff, T. M., Wadi, K., Paczkowski, N., Tyndall, J. D., Taylor, S. M. & Fairlie, D. P. (2004). Potent cyclic antagonists of the complement C5a receptor on human polymorphonuclear leukocytes. Relationships between structures and activity. *Mol Pharmacol,* Vol.65, No.4, (April 2004), pp.868-879, ISSN 0026-895X.

Marjan, J., Xie, Z. & Devine, D. V. (1994). Liposome-induced activation of the classical complement pathway does not require immunoglobulin. *Biochimica et biophysica acta,* Vol.1192, No.1, (June 1994), pp.35-44, ISSN 0006-3002.

Mastellos, D., Germenis, A. E. & Lambris, J. D. (2005). Complement: an inflammatory pathway fulfilling multiple roles at the interface of innate immunity and development. *Current drug targets. Inflammation and allergy,* Vol.4, No.1, (February 2005), pp.125-127, ISSN 1568-010X.

Melendez, A. J. & Ibrahim, F. B. (2004). Antisense knockdown of sphingosine kinase 1 in human macrophages inhibits C5a receptor-dependent signal transduction, Ca2+ signals, enzyme release, cytokine production, and chemotaxis. *J Immunol,* Vol.173, No.3, (August 2004), pp.1596-1603, ISSN 0022-1767.

Miller, R. G., Mitchell, J. D., Lyon, M. & Moore, D. H. (2007). Riluzole for amyotrophic lateral sclerosis (ALS)/motor neuron disease (MND). *Cochrane Database Syst Rev,* No.1, (January 2007), pp.CD001447, ISSN 1469-493X.

Mouri, F., Tsukada, J., Mizobe, T., Higashi, T., Yoshida, Y., Minami, Y., Izumi, H., Kominato, Y., Kohno, K. & Tanaka, Y. (2008). Intracellular HMGB1 transactivates the human IL1B gene promoter through association with an Ets transcription factor PU.1. *European journal of haematology,* Vol.80, No.1, (January 2008), pp.10-19, ISSN 1600-0609.

Mullmann, T. J., Siegel, M. I., Egan, R. W. & Billah, M. M. (1990). Complement C5a activation of phospholipase D in human neutrophils. A major route to the production of phosphatidates and diglycerides. *J Immunol,* Vol.144, No.5, (March 1990), pp.1901-1908, ISSN 0022-1767.

Nataf, S., Levison, S. W. & Barnum, S. R. (2001). Expression of the anaphylatoxin C5a receptor in the oligodendrocyte lineage. *Brain Res,* Vol.894, No.2, (March 2001), pp.321-326, ISSN 0006-8993.

Nguyen, M. D., D'aigle, T., Gowing, G., Julien, J. P. & Rivest, S. (2004). Exacerbation of motor neuron disease by chronic stimulation of innate immunity in a mouse model of amyotrophic lateral sclerosis. *The Journal of neuroscience : the official journal of the Society for Neuroscience,* Vol.24, No.6, (February 2004), pp.1340-1349, ISSN 1529-2401.

Niebroj-Dobosz, I., Dziewulska, D. & Janik, P. (2006). Auto-antibodies against proteins of spinal cord cells in cerebrospinal fluid of patients with amyotrophic lateral sclerosis (ALS). *Folia neuropathologica / Association of Polish Neuropathologists and Medical*

Research Centre, Polish Academy of Sciences, Vol.44, No.3, (October 2006), pp.191-196, ISSN 1641-4640.

O'barr, S. A., Caguioa, J., Gruol, D., Perkins, G., Ember, J. A., Hugli, T. & Cooper, N. R. (2001). Neuronal expression of a functional receptor for the C5a complement activation fragment. *J Immunol,* Vol.166, No.6, (March 2001), pp.4154-4162, ISSN 0022-1767.

Okinaga, S., Slattery, D., Humbles, A., Zsengeller, Z., Morteau, O., Kinrade, M. B., Brodbeck, R. M., Krause, J. E., Choe, H. R., Gerard, N. P. & Gerard, C. (2003). C5L2, a nonsignaling C5A binding protein. *Biochemistry,* Vol.42, No.31, (August 2003), pp.9406-9415, ISSN 0006-2960.

Olson, J. K. & Miller, S. D. (2004). Microglia initiate central nervous system innate and adaptive immune responses through multiple TLRs. *Journal of immunology,* Vol.173, No.6, (September 2004), pp.3916-3924, ISSN 0022-1767.

Pangburn, M. K., Schreiber, R. D. & Muller-Eberhard, H. J. (1981). Formation of the initial C3 convertase of the alternative complement pathway. Acquisition of C3b-like activities by spontaneous hydrolysis of the putative thioester in native C3. *The Journal of experimental medicine,* Vol.154, No.3, (September 1981), pp.856-867, ISSN 0022-1007.

Parker, L. C., Whyte, M. K., Vogel, S. N., Dower, S. K. & Sabroe, I. (2004). Toll-like receptor (TLR)2 and TLR4 agonists regulate CCR expression in human monocytic cells. *Journal of immunology,* Vol.172, No.8, (April 2004), pp.4977-4986, ISSN 0022-1767.

Perianayagam, M.C., Balakrishnan, V.S., King, A.J., Pereira, B.J., Jaber, B.L., (2002). C5a delays apoptosis of human neutrophils by a phosphatidylinositol 3-kinase signaling pathway. *Kidney Int,* Vol.61, No.2, (February 2002), pp.456-463, ISSN 0085-2538.

Perrin, F. E., Boisset, G., Docquier, M., Schaad, O., Descombes, P. & Kato, A. C. (2005). No widespread induction of cell death genes occurs in pure motoneurons in an amyotrophic lateral sclerosis mouse model. *Human molecular genetics,* Vol.14, No.21, (November 2005), pp.3309-3320, ISSN 0964-6906.

Podack, E. R., Tschoop, J. & Muller-Eberhard, H. J. (1982). Molecular organization of C9 within the membrane attack complex of complement. Induction of circular C9 polymerization by the C5b-8 assembly. *The Journal of experimental medicine,* Vol.156, No.1, (July 1982), pp.268-282, ISSN 0022-1007.

Rabiet, M. J., Huet, E. & Boulay, F. (2007). The N-formyl peptide receptors and the anaphylatoxin C5a receptors: an overview. *Biochimie,* Vol.89, No.9, (Septmeber 2007), pp.1089-1106, ISSN 0300-9084.

Rahpeymai, Y., Hietala, M. A., Wilhelmsson, U., Fotheringham, A., Davies, I., Nilsson, A. K., Zwirner, J., Wetsel, R. A., Gerard, C., Pekny, M. & Pekna, M. (2006). Complement: a novel factor in basal and ischemia-induced neurogenesis. *The EMBO journal,* Vol.25, No.6, (March 2006), pp.1364-1374, ISSN 0261-4189.

Ricklin, D., Hajishengallis, G., Yang, K. & Lambris, J. D. (2010). Complement: a key system for immune surveillance and homeostasis. *Nature immunology,* Vol.11, No.9, (September 2010), pp.785-797, ISSN 1529-2916.

Rollins, T. E., Siciliano, S., Kobayashi, S., Cianciarulo, D. N., Bonilla-Argudo, V., Collier, K. & Springer, M. S. (1991). Purification of the active C5a receptor from human polymorphonuclear leukocytes as a receptor-Gi complex. *Proceedings of the National Academy of Sciences of the United States of America,* Vol.88, No.3, (February 1991), pp.971-975, ISSN 0027-8424.

Rosen, D. R., Siddique, T., Patterson, D., Figlewicz, D. A., Sapp, P., Hentati, A., Donaldson, D., Goto, J., O'regan, J. P., Deng, H. X. & Et Al. (1993). Mutations in Cu/Zn superoxide dismutase gene are associated with familial amyotrophic lateral sclerosis. *Nature,* Vol.362, No.6415, (March 1993), pp.59-62, ISSN 0028-0836.

Scaffidi, P., Misteli, T. & Bianchi, M. E. (2002). Release of chromatin protein HMGB1 by necrotic cells triggers inflammation. *Nature,* Vol.418, No.6894, (July 2002), pp.191-195, ISSN 0028-0836.

Schafer, D. P. & Stevens, B. (2010). Synapse elimination during development and disease: immune molecules take centre stage. *Biochem Soc Trans,* Vol.38, No.2, (April 2010), pp.476-481, ISSN 1470-8752.

Sta, M., Sylva-Steenland, R. M., Casula, M., De Jong, J. M., Troost, D., Aronica, E. & Baas, F. (2011). Innate and adaptive immunity in amyotrophic lateral sclerosis: evidence of complement activation. *Neurobiology of disease,* Vol.42, No.3, (June 2011), pp.211-220, ISSN 1095-953X.

Stevens, B., Allen, N. J., Vazquez, L. E., Howell, G. R., Christopherson, K. S., Nouri, N., Micheva, K. D., Mehalow, A. K., Huberman, A. D., Stafford, B., Sher, A., Litke, A. M., Lambris, J. D., Smith, S. J., John, S. W. & Barres, B. A. (2007). The classical complement cascade mediates CNS synapse elimination. *Cell,* Vol.131, No.6, (December 2007), pp.1164-1178, ISSN 0092-8674.

Strong, M. J. (2003). The basic aspects of therapeutics in amyotrophic lateral sclerosis. *Pharmacology & Therapeutics,* Vol.98, No.3, (n.d.), pp.379-414, ISSN 01637258.

Tang, S. C., Arumugam, T. V., Xu, X., Cheng, A., Mughal, M. R., Jo, D. G., Lathia, J. D., Siler, D. A., Chigurupati, S., Ouyang, X., Magnus, T., Camandola, S. & Mattson, M. P. (2007). Pivotal role for neuronal Toll-like receptors in ischemic brain injury and functional deficits. *Proceedings of the National Academy of Sciences of the United States of America,* Vol.104, No.34, (August 2007), pp.13798-13803, ISSN 0027-8424.

Thoman, M. L., Meuth, J. L., Morgan, E. L., Weigle, W. O. & Hugli, T. E. (1984). C3d-K, a kallikrein cleavage fragment of iC3b is a potent inhibitor of cellular proliferation. *Journal of immunology,* Vol.133, No.5, (November 1984), pp.2629-2633, ISSN 0022-1767.

Torres, M. & Forman, H. J. (1999). Activation of several MAP kinases upon stimulation of rat alveolar macrophages: role of the NADPH oxidase. *Arch Biochem Biophys,* Vol.366, No.2, (June 1999), pp.231-239, ISSN 0003-9861.

Trbojevic-Cepe, M., Brinar, V., Pauro, M., Vogrinc, Z. & Stambuk, N. (1998). Cerebrospinal fluid complement activation in neurological diseases. *Journal of the neurological sciences,* Vol.154, No.2, (February 1998), pp.173-181, ISSN 0022-510X.

Tsai, H. R., Yang, L. M., Tsai, W. J. & Chiou, W. F. (2004). Andrographolide acts through inhibition of ERK1/2 and Akt phosphorylation to suppress chemotactic migration. *Eur J Pharmacol,* Vol.498, No.1-3, (September 2004), pp.45-52, ISSN 0014-2999.

Tsuboi, Y. & Yamada, T. (1994). Increased concentration of C4d complement protein in CSF in amyotrophic lateral sclerosis. *Journal of neurology, neurosurgery, and psychiatry,* Vol.57, No.7, (July 1994), pp.859-861, ISSN 0022-3050.

Van Beek, J., Elward, K. & Gasque, P. (2003). Activation of complement in the central nervous system: roles in neurodegeneration and neuroprotection. *Ann N Y Acad Sci,* Vol.992, (May 2003), pp.56-71, ISSN 0077-8923.

Van Lith, L. H., Oosterom, J., Van Elsas, A. & Zaman, G. J. (2009). C5a-stimulated recruitment of beta-arrestin2 to the nonsignaling 7-transmembrane decoy receptor C5L2. *J Biomol Screen,* Vol.14, No.9, (October 2009), pp.1067-1075, ISSN 1552-454X.

Wong, A. K., Finch, A. M., Pierens, G. K., Craik, D. J., Taylor, S. M. & Fairlie, D. P. (1998). Small molecular probes for G-protein-coupled C5a receptors: conformationally constrained antagonists derived from the C terminus of the human plasma protein C5a. *Journal of medicinal chemistry,* Vol.41, No.18, (August 1998), pp.3417-3425, ISSN 0022-2623.

Woodruff, T. M., Ager, R. R., Tenner, A. J., Noakes, P. G. & Taylor, S. M. (2010). The role of the complement system and the activation fragment C5a in the central nervous system. *Neuromolecular Med,* Vol.12, No.2, (June 2010), pp.179-192, ISSN 1559-1174.

Woodruff, T. M., Arumugam, T. V., Shiels, I. A., Reid, R. C., Fairlie, D. P. & Taylor, S. M. (2003). A potent human C5a receptor antagonist protects against disease pathology in a rat model of inflammatory bowel disease. *J Immunol,* Vol.171, No.10, (Nov ember 2003), pp.5514-5520, ISSN 0022-1767.

Woodruff, T. M., Costantini, K. J., Crane, J. W., Atkin, J. D., Monk, P. N., Taylor, S. M. & Noakes, P. G. (2008a). The complement factor C5a contributes to pathology in a rat model of amyotrophic lateral sclerosis. *J Immunol,* Vol.181, No.12, (Dec ember 2008), pp.8727-8734, ISSN 1550-6606.

Woodruff, T. M., Costantini, K. J., Taylor, S. M. & Noakes, P. G. (2008b). Role of complement in motor neuron disease: animal models and therapeutic potential of complement inhibitors. *Adv Exp Med Biol,* Vol.632, (November 2008), pp.143-158, ISSN 0065-2598.

Woodruff, T. M., Crane, J. W., Proctor, L. M., Buller, K. M., Shek, A. B., De Vos, K., Pollitt, S., Williams, H. M., Shiels, I. A., Monk, P. N. & Taylor, S. M. (2006). Therapeutic activity of C5a receptor antagonists in a rat model of neurodegeneration. *FASEB J,* Vol.20, No.9, (July 2006), pp.1407-1417, ISSN 1530-6860.

Woodruff, T. M., Nandakumar, K. S. & Tedesco, F. (2011). Inhibiting the C5-C5a receptor axis. *Molecular immunology,* Vol.48, No.14, (August 2011), pp.1631-1642, ISSN 1872-9142.

Woodruff, T. M., Pollitt, S., Proctor, L. M., Stocks, S. Z., Manthey, H. D., Williams, H. M., Mahadevan, I. B., Shiels, I. A. & Taylor, S. M. (2005). Increased potency of a novel complement factor 5a receptor antagonist in a rat model of inflammatory bowel disease. *J Pharmacol Exp Ther,* Vol.314, No.2, (August 2005), pp.811-817, ISSN 0022-3565.

Woodruff, T. M., Strachan, A. J., Dryburgh, N., Shiels, I. A., Reid, R. C., Fairlie, D. P. & Taylor, S. M. (2002). Antiarthritic activity of an orally active C5a receptor antagonist against antigen-induced monarticular arthritis in the rat. *Arthritis Rheum,* Vol.46, No.9, (September 2002), pp.2476-2485, ISSN 0004-3591.

Worms, P. M. (2001). The epidemiology of motor neuron diseases: a review of recent studies. *Journal of the neurological sciences,* Vol.191, No.1-2, (October 2001), pp.3-9, ISSN 0022-510X.

Zhao, W., Beers, D. R., Henkel, J. S., Zhang, W., Urushitani, M., Julien, J. P. & Appel, S. H. (2010). Extracellular mutant SOD1 induces microglial-mediated motoneuron injury. *Glia,* Vol.58, No.2, (January 2010), pp.231-243, ISSN 1098-1136.

18

The Role of TNF-Alpha in ALS: New Hypotheses for Future Therapeutic Approaches

Cristina Cereda[1*], Stella Gagliardi[1*],
Emanuela Cova[1], Luca Diamanti[2,3] and Mauro Ceroni[2,3]
[1]*Laboratory of Experimental Neurobiology, IRCCS,*
National Neurological Institute "C. Mondino", Pavia,
[2]*General Neurology Department, IRCCS,*
National Neurological Institute "C. Mondino", Pavia,
[3]*Department of Neurological Sciences, University of Pavia, Pavia,*
Italy

1. Introduction

The pathophysiological origins of neurodegenerative disorders are a complex combination of both environmental and genetic factors. However, in many of these disorders, processes such as inflammation and oxidative stress activate common and final pathways leading to toxicity and cellular death. High levels of oxidative damage within the brain and the activation of neuroinflammation factors are a prominent feature in patients with Alzheimer's disease (AD), Parkinson's disease (PD), Huntington's disease (HD), Amyotrophic Lateral Sclerosis (ALS) and inherited ataxias (Halliwell, 2006; Lin & Beal, 2006). Regarding the immunological point of view, the brain was considered an immune privileged organ because it was isolated from the systemic circulation by protective blood-brain barrier that controls the infiltration of pathogens, the transition of pro or anti inflammatory factors and peripheral blood cells (Itzhaki et al., 2004). Despite that, in recent years, the relationship between neuroinflammation and neurodegeneration has been described with particular attention to the lymphocytes activation and cytokines production (Appel, 2009; Tansey et al., 2007). Moreover, it is well known the implication of glial cells in the progression of neurodegeneration: they are involved in many types of damage, they migrate to the damaged cells and also they have a role in clearing the debris of the dead cells. Through such processes, microglia releases reactive oxygen species, proinflammatory cytokines, complement factors, and neurotoxic molecules, leading to further neuronal dysfunction and death (Heneka et al., 2011; Lasiene et al., 2011). In addition, the implication of the peripheral system and its participation in the cellular mechanisms that direct to neurodegeneration, as white blood cells, is well documented (Calvo et al., 2010; Ghezzi et al., 1998; Gowing et al., 2006).
Many data from autoptic spinal cord and blood examinations of the ALS patients, animal and cellular models support an immune system involvement in ALS pathogenesis. Since

---

*These authors contributed equally to this work.

1984 the presence of an autoimmunity component in ALS was proven when immunoglobulin depositories have been described in spinal cord (Donnenfeld et al., 1984). At present the implication of the neuronal and non-neuronal immunological cells and activation of the inflammatory processes have been extensively described in ALS (Engelhardt et al., 1995; Henkel et al., 2004; Troost et al., 1990).
Starting from literature data about implication of the innate and adaptive immunity in ALS, we would like to point out the role of the TNF alpha (TNF-α) system and its interactions in ALS pathway with particular attention to SOD1 protein, the most important player in the ALS pathogenesis. We will focus this book section on TNF-α cytokine because its involvement both in immunological pathways and in oxidative stress is known in ALS disease. Moreover we will try to define the immunological actors that exert a protective function and how they could be used in a possible therapy.

2. ALS and immunity

In the last decades, increasing numbers of experimental and clinical observations have reported inflammatory reactions in ALS tissues which indicate the involvement of both the innate and adaptive immune responses (Fig. 1) (McGeer & McGeer, 2006; Moisse & Strong, 2006; Sta et al., 2011; Weydt et al., 2002).
So far it is not clear how immune system is involved in ALS disease, whether the adaptive or innate immunity has a major role and whether immunity is part of damaging or neuroprotective response to the pathological process.

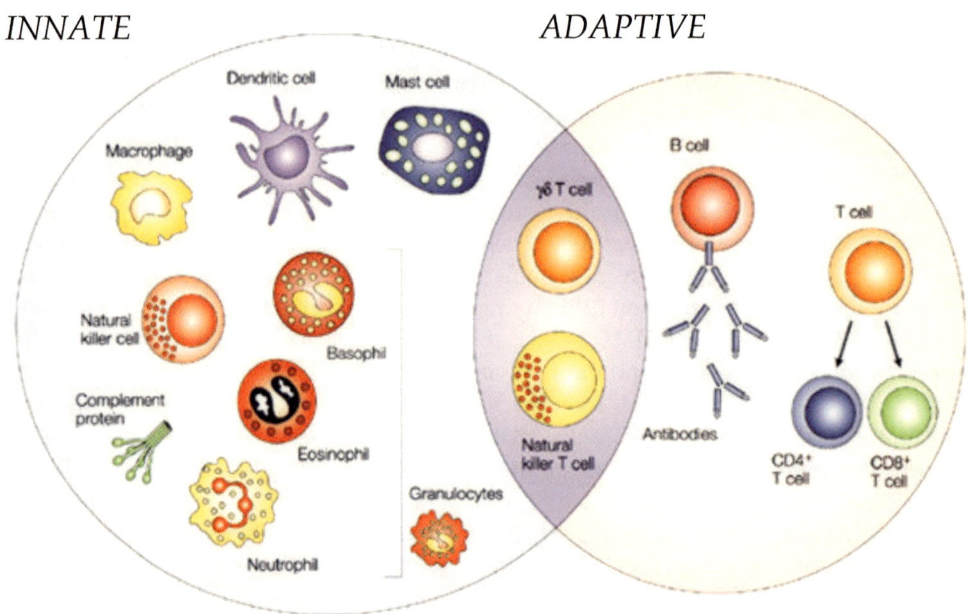

Fig. 1. Innate and adaptive immunity.

2.1 Innate immune system

Innate immunity is naturally present and is not stimulated by antigens or mediated by antibodies. It is therefore non-specific and is executed by a variety of cells: granulocytes, as eosinophils and basophils, white blood cells as natural killer and mast cells. Instead, microglia belongs to the central nervous system and is involved in the local innate immunity. Inflammation is one of the aspects of the innate immune response.

Interactions between innate immune system, brain and neurodegenerative diseases are known (Ghezzi et al., 1998; Gowing et al., 2006) and it has been reported that mast cells, macrophages, dendritic cells, microglia, complement and cytokines participate in limiting the damage (Calvo et al., 2010).

Innate system was found activated in central and in peripheral system of ALS patients (Chandels et al., 2001; Elliott et al., 2001; Sta et al., 2011).

Several studies regarding peripheral innate immune system changes in sporadic ALS reveal that there are increased levels of circulating monocytes and macrophages (Harman et al., 1991; Hemnani et al, 1998). The presence of T cells, IgG, activated microglia, macrophages, and reactive astrocytes, as well as other indications of inflammation are found in ALS spinal cord tissue (Henkel et al., 2004; Engelhardt et al., 1995; Troost et al., 1990).

In ALS there is morphological and neurochemical evidence for the proliferation and activation of microglia in areas of significant motor neuron loss, as spinal cord (Henkel et al., 2004; Kawamata et al., 1992; Moisse et al., 2006). This activation may be a consequence of stressed neurons that induced proliferation and activation of microglial cells activating complement system and pro-cytokine response involved in neuronal death (Fig. 2). Motor neuron loss and immune system activation may increase neuron stress leading to increase of neuroinflammation.

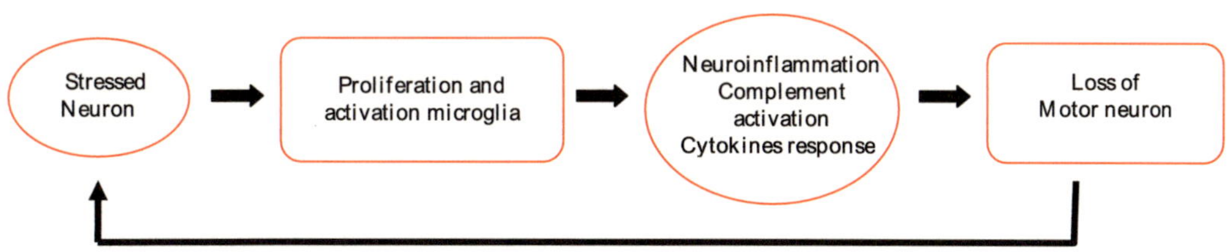

Fig. 2. Hypothesis of activation of innate immunity in ALS.

2.2 Adaptive immune system

As innate immunity, adaptive immunity has a role in ALS (Sta et al., 2011). Unlike innate immune responses, the adaptive responses are highly specific and they consist of antibodies, lymphocytes activation and cell mediated response. The cells of the adaptive immune system are B and T lymphocytes: B cells, which are derived from the bone marrow, become the cells that produce antibodies. T cells can cross-talk with neurons and microglia, and either damage or protect neurons from stressful stimuli (Alexaniu et al., 2001), also in spinal cord and brain (Chiu et al., 2008).

T-helper cells have been observed in proximity of degenerating corticospinal tracts; T-helper and T-suppressor cells, with a variable number of macrophages, have been found in ventral horns of the spinal cord (Troost et al., 1990).

Infiltration of T cells compatible with adaptive response have been found in the areas of motor neuron destruction in the CNS but no correlation was found between clinical

parameters and infiltrating T cells (Holmoy et al., 2008). The majority of T cells characterized in the infiltration were CD8+ cytotoxic T cells, but a substantial number of T CD4+ cells were also present (Beers et al., 2008).
Alterations of total lymphocyte count (Provinciali et al., 1988; Tavolato et al., 1975) and T subset distribution in peripheral system of ALS patients (Westall et al., 1983) have been reported. Low T cells numbers and decreased proliferative capacity in T cells are found in the blood of ALS patients (Holmoy et al., 2008).
As concerned CD8+ and natural killer T cells, they were found increased in ALS patients compared to control cohort (Rentzos et al., 2011).
Interestingly, ALS patients showed a reduction of CD4+/CD25+ regulatory T cells that are known to interact with the local microglia, reinforcing the hypothesis of the involvement of the adaptive immune system associated with neuroinflammatory process in ALS (Mantovani et al., 2009). Beers and colleagues (Beers et al., 2011) observed that regulatory T cells as CD4+/CD25+/FoxP3 correlated with disease progression; in fact, the number of T cells were found inversely correlated with disease progression rate.
Animal studies showed that in ALS model T cells deficiency decreases microglia reactivity and accelerates ALS disease progression; specific and progressive accumulation of monocytes/macrophages was observed along the length of degenerating nerve fibers and activated microglia was detected in spinal cord of ALS model mice (Chiu et al., 2009).
No infiltrating B-cells have been found even if a role of B lymphocytes in the pathogenesis of ALS has been hypothesized, as secreted autoantibodies by B cells identified in CSF and serum from ALS patients (Naor et al., 2009).
As concern antibodies, since the eighties the presence of IgG in serum or tissues of ALS patients has been documented (anti-ganglioside GM1, anti-sulfoglucuronyl paragloboside, anti-neurofilaments and anti-Fas) (Sengun & Appel, 2003; Yi et al., 2000). Indeed, IgG deposits have been demonstrated in motor cortex, spinal cord and in motor neurons from ALS patients (Donnenfeld et al., 1984; Engelhardt & Appel, 1990; Fishman & Drachman, 1995). Serum immunoglobulins from ALS patients showed enhanced binding to rat spinal cord cells *in vitro* (Digby et al., 1985), demonstrating cytotoxic effects when they were added to a motor neuron cell cultures (Alexianu et al., 1994; Demestre et al., 2005) and that the presence of an immune response to spinal cord cell membrane components in patients with motor neuron disease was a damaging event.
IgG from ALS patients reacts with the skeletal muscle DHP (bisognerebbe spiegare cosa è)-sensitive Ca^{2+} channels reducing the peak of the Ca^{2+} current and the charge movement in single cut fibres from the rat extensor muscle (Delbono et al., 1991). About 60% of ALS sera contained different monoclonal immunoglobulins: in particular IgG (72.7%) and IgM (27.3%) have been found (Duarte et al., 1991).

2.3 Cytokines

Different interactions have been found between innate and adaptive immunity in ALS, as concern cytokines involvement. Cytokines have an effect on the expression of other inflammatory factors and on each other, and these functional relationships are non-linear: the causal relationships of cytokines and disease are complex and difficult to prove (Marklund et al., 1992).
Several studies regarding immune system changes in sporadic ALS reveal that there are increased levels of circulating monocytes and macrophages, producing cytokines as IL-1

and IFN-γ, (Harman et al., 1991; Hemnani et al., 1998). Furthermore, high cytokine levels have been described in plasma, serum and cerebral fluid (CSF) from ALS patients and sometimes correlate with the clinical status (Kelly et al., 1994; Lee et al., 2005; Khule et al., 2009; Tateishi et al., 2010).

As concern inflammatory cytokines (IL-7, 9, 12, 17 and IL-1β) levels were found higher in CSF of sporadic ALS patients (Tateishi et al., 2010). IL-15 and IL-12 serum levels, they also have been found higher in patients with ALS (Rentzos et al., 2010). The same authors measured IL-17 and IL-23 levels in serum and CSF from ALS patients that were found increased compared to controls (Rentzos et al., 2010). TGF-β1 concentrations in the serum and CSF of ALS patients did not differ from controls, but TGF-β1 serum concentration was significantly higher in ALS patients at the terminal clinical status (Ilzecka et al., 2002). Higher amount of IL-6 has been found in sera and CSF from sporadic ALS patients and it has been related to hypoxemia severity rather than pathological condition (Moreau et al., 2005).

Plasma concentration of TNF-α, TNF-R1 and TNF-R2 and their time course during disease progression were studied in ALS patients in order to assess the TNF-α system implication in ALS pathogenesis. In all plasma patients soluble forms of the TNF-α and its receptors are found increased already at disease onset and remain over the normal range during the disease progression time (Cereda et al., 2008). In addition TNF-α amounts have been found higher in sera from sporadic ALS patients but no correlation was found with the clinical criteria (Poloni et al., 2000; Cereda et al., 2008). TNF-α role in neurodegeneration will be further highlight in the next paragraph.

3. Tumor necrosis factor-alpha (TNF-α)

The Tumour Necrosis Factor Alpha (TNF-α) is a pro-inflammatory cytokine produced by monocytes/macrophages and activated by mast cells, endothelial cells, fibroblasts, neurons and glial cells during acute inflammation and it is responsible for a wide range of cell signals about cell viability, gene expression, homeostasis control and synaptic integrity.

TNF-α was described for the first time by Carswell et al. in 1975 as a protein component of serum of mice stimulated with bacterial antigens, and was brought to light the ability to induce death in cancer cell lines in vitro and in vivo to destroy transplanted sarcomas. Characteristically, this cytokine was able to cause tumor cells death without compromising the viability of healthy cells. The subsequent isolation and molecular characterization of the gene have provided information on the structure and functioning of this molecule.

3.1 TNF-α gene

The gene coding for TNF-α is located on chromosome 6 within the region encoding the Major Histocompatibility Complex (MCH), HLA in human, between the HLA-DR class II and HLA-B class I genes (Fig. 3). Its location and strict linkage disequilibrium present between some alleles of class I and class II genes has permitted to hypothesize associations between TNF-α alleles and some diseases. The gene for TNF-α include about 3 Kb and contains four exons (almost 80% of the protein is codified by the exon four) and three introns.

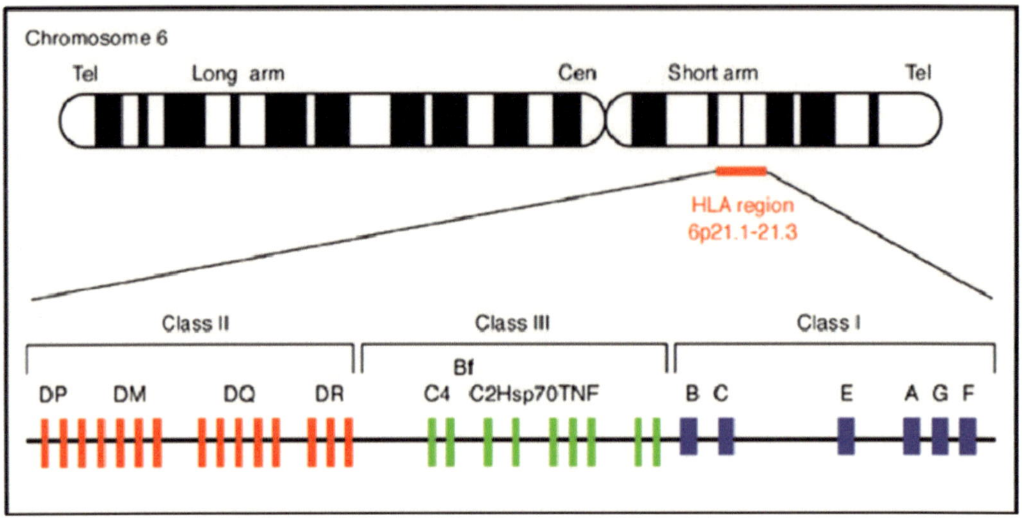

Fig. 3. Localization of TNF-α gene on chromosome 6 (6p21.3)

TNF-α gene codifies for a protein of 233 amino acids with a molecular weight of 25.6 kDa. TNF-α is, at the beginning, a transmembrane protein of 212 amino acids associated to homotrimers; the N-terminal portion loses 76 amino acid by cleavage of TNF-α converting enzyme (TACE or ADAM-17), producing a soluble monomeric TNF-α form (17 kD) and next, the trimetric form of 51 kD (Bazzoni & Beutler, 1996; Reddy et al., 2000).

The trimer is the biological active soluble form because of its ability to bind its receptors. However, the trimeric soluble form spontaneously tends to dissociate into a monomeric inactive form, that is a physiological process that allows to limit the deleterious effects of excessive concentration of TNF-α (Smith et al., 1987).

TNF-α response to a variety of extracellular signals is very rapid and transient and includes a transcriptional component as well as posttranscriptional events. Its transcriptional control occurs predominantly at the level of transcriptional initiation.

The approximately 1000 base pairs of the TNF-α gene's 5' flanking region contains a number of important regulatory elements that affect TNF-α transcription in response to various stimuli. The basic promoter region is defined by TATA box sequence, located about 20 bp upstream from the transcription site and about 200 bp form the translation start codon. Multiple potential regulatory sites, including consensus sequences for the AP-1 (Activator Protein-1) and AP-2 (Activator Protein-2) sites, the cAMP-responsive element, and sequences similar to the NF-kB, (Nuclear Factor kappa-light-chain-enhancer of activated B cells) sequences found in immunoglobulin and cytokine regulatory elements are present in 5' flanking region. This sequence has been demonstrated to be responsive to LPS (lipolysaccharide) and TNF-α stimulation. The 3' untranslated region contains a sequence element affecting posttranslational control of TNF-α through mRNA stability and translation efficiency.

Many polymorphisms have been described in TNF-α promoter region (-308, -857, -863, -238, -1031) defining its correlation with TNF-α mRNA amounts: wild-308G allele is responsible for a higher transcription gene (Helmig et al., 2011), as the A mutated allele at position -857 results in a high production of TNF-α (McCusker et al., 2001).

As concerned -238 polymorphism, has been described a direct effect on gene expression, although studies suggest that this region contains a strong repressor site (-280 to -172). -238 TNFG/A allele genotype may be in linkage disequilibrium with a functional polymorphism that impacts TNF production (Liu et al., 2008).

Several of these polymorphisms have been studied extensively in some diseases, mainly -308 and -857 SNPs.

The mutated allele -308A is a marker of susceptibility to several autoimmune and inflammatory diseases such as lupus erythematosus, celiac disease and Alzheimer's disease (Candor et al., 2002 and 2004), but so far it has been published in a very large number of works in order to reach the correct conclusions on the role of these polymorphisms.

Most SNPs (-863, -238, -1031) do not affect the levels of expression but their pathologic involvement is related to the variation of allelic or genotypic frequencies.

As concerned SNPs in coding region, some polymorphisms are described (http://www.ncbi.nlm.nih.gov/SNP) but they are not correlated with any diseases or functions.

3.2 TNF-α protein function

The functions of TNF-α are biologically dependent on the amount of cytokine produced. If it is present in small amounts, TNF-α acts locally as autocrine and paracrine mediator of inflammation in leukocytes and endothelial cells, determines the expression of surface receptors for leukocyte migration, acting as an angiogenic factor, such as fibroblast growth factor and induces apoptosis in certain cell types. If it is present in high amounts, however, is distributed in the systemic circulation where it stimulates the production of IL-1 and IL-6 by leukocytes and the synthesis of acute phase proteins in the liver (such as fibrinogen) and activates the intravascular thrombus formation.

TNF-α exerts many of its effects by binding, as a trimer, the cell membrane receptor TNF-R1 of 55 kDa (p55) or TNF-R2 of 75 kDa (p75) belonging to the superfamily of TNF receptors, which also includes FAS, CD40, CD27 and RANK.

TNF-R1 is expressed in almost all tissues and may be activated by trimeric soluble form and also by membrane-associated form of TNF-α; TNF-R2 is expressed only by cells of the immune system and it is activated only by trimeric soluble form of the TNF-α. Differently from TNF-R1, TNF-R2 do not own a death domain (DD), and its activation may only induce the survival pathway (Fig. 4).

Instead, the binding of TNF-α to the TNF-R1 may cause both cell death or survival depending on which pathway is activated and it also depends on the second signal involved (Hsu et al., 1996; Darnay et al.,1997). Following the binding of TNF-α, TNF-R1 produces a conformational change that determines the separation of the intracellular death domain (DD). This dissociation allows the adapter protein TRADD to bind the domain of death (DD) to induce apoptosis or form a platform for the subsequent binding proteins to make cell survival. If TRADD directly binds FADD, which in turn recruits caspase-8, the apoptosis way is activated. High concentrations of caspase-8 induce its proteolytic activation and subsequent cleavage of downstream caspases, leading to cell apoptosis. Cell death induced by TNF-α plays a minor role compared to the role of this cytokine in inflammation. Its ability to induce apoptosis is in fact modest when compared to that of other members of the family as Fas and often masked by the anti-apoptotic effects.

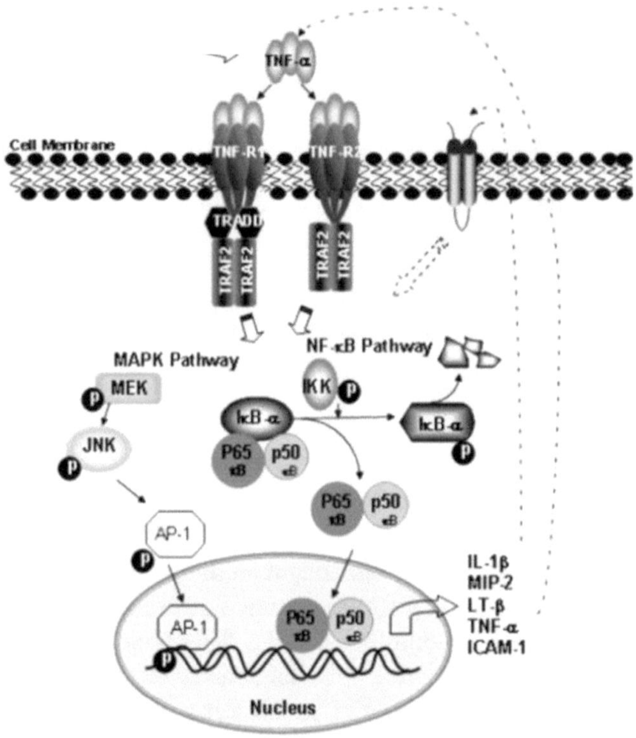

Fig. 4. TNF-α and TNFR pathway (Rosenquist M., 2003)

Both TNF-α receptors activate different survival intracellular signalling pathways, especially because of the IkB kinase (IKK) and the cascade of MAP kinases (MAPKs) that control the gene expression through NF-kB, and AP-1 respectively. In detail the term NF-kB refers to a family of five structurally-related transcription factors (p50, p52, RelA/ p65, c-Rel and RelB), all containing the Rel homology domain (RHD) within the N-terminus and acting as homo- and heterodimeric DNA binding complexes (O'Dea et al., 2010). Several studies showed that NF-kB activity is induced in most cell types in response to a broad variety of stimuli, ranging from cytokines, radiation and reactive oxygen species (ROS) (such as exposure to H_2O_2), with major roles in coordinating innate and adaptative immunity, cell activation and proliferation, survival, development and apoptosis (Ghosh et al., 2008; Vallabhapurapu et al., 2009).

TRADD recruits TRAF2 (TNF receptor-associated factor 2) and RIP (receptor interacting protein). TRAF2 in turn recruits the protein kinase IKK (inhibitor of nuclear factor kappa-B kinase), which is activated by RIP. The IKBα inhibitory protein that normally binds the NF-kB and inhibits its translocation, is phosphorylated by IKK and then is degraded, releasing NF-kB. The latter NF-kB is a transcription factor that translocates into the nucleus and mediates the transcription of a wide variety of genes and theirs products involved in survival and cell proliferation, in the inflammatory response and anti-apoptotic factors.

As concerns the activation of MAP kinase (MAPK), TNF-α induces a strong activation of JNK (c-Jun N-terminal Kinase), one of three major cascades of MAPK, evokes a moderate response of the p38-MAPK, and is responsible of a minimal activation of ERK. TRAF2 actives MEKK1 and ASK1 directly or indirectly, which phosphorylate MKK7, which in turn activates JNK. The latter AP-1 translocates into the nucleus and activates transcription factors such as c-Jun and AFT2. The way of JNK is involved in differentiation, cell proliferation and apoptosis.

3.3 TNF-α and nervous system

In the central nervous system TNF-α is produced by astrocytes, microglia and neurons in response to several stimuli both intra and extracellular, and seems to play a central role in the genesis and perpetuation of neuroinflammatory signal. An alteration in the regulatory mechanisms of TNF-α was found in a wide variety of disorders such as depression, carcinogenesis, and Alzheimer's disease. In the nervous system different TNF-α activities were defined, as inducer or inhibitor of neuronal apoptosis underlining how complex TNF-α pathway may be.

Moreover, electrophysiological experiments have shown a negative effect determined by TNF-α on neuronal function. Studies of hippocampal sections showed that the addition of pro-inflammatory cytokines decreased the long-term potentiation (Long-term potentiation, LTP), a correlate of learning and memory processes (Tancredi et al., 1992). The mechanism by which this occurs is still under investigation, but it has been suggested that activation of p38 plays a major role in reducing the early phase of LTP in response to TNF-α, while the protein expression changes would play a role in the late phase (Butler et al., 2004).

However, other studies have shown that TNF-α alone is not able to initiate apoptosis in the absence of a second signal and may actually prevent apoptosis in response to certain types of cell damage (Badiola et al., 2009). In fact, although apoptosis is primarily triggered by the TRADD, TNF-α may also be associated with cell survival signals, because it is also able to facilitate the binding of other molecules such as JNK and NF-kB, which were instead important in cells endurance, indicating how complex are the signalling pathways of TNF-α. In fact, TNF-α facilitates axonal regeneration, induces neuronal survival through the anti-apoptotic pathway mediated by NF-kB, limits the demyelination in experimental autoimmune encephalomyelitis, but these effects appear to be highly dose-dependent and related to the exposure time and interaction with other factors (Schwartz et al., 1991).

The protective effect of the cascade triggered by TNF-α has been documented experimentally: mice lacking the receptor for TNF-α were subjected to cerebral ischemia. This result was attributed to an increase of reactive oxygen species, suggesting that TNF-α could induce an antioxidant protection due to ischemic events (Bruce et al., 1996). Similarly, in a model of glutamatergic excitotoxicity, stimulation of TNF-R2 with TNF-α led to protection against this toxicity (Marchetti et al., 2004). In conclusion, these data suggest that TNF-α could affect neuronal viability in different ways depending on the receptor subtype involved and the presence/absence of secondary signals from endogenous or exogenous stimuli.

In neurodegenerative disease, as Parkinson's (PD) and Alzheimer's (AD), neuroinflammatory processes appear to play key roles in neuronal dysfunction and death (Hakansson et al., 2005). TNF-α was found increased in striatum and CSF from PD patients compared to controls (Nagatsu et al., 2000), and a large number of TNF-α immunoreactive glial cells were detected in CSN from PD patients (Imamura et al., 2003).

As concern AD, TNF-α was found upregulated in both CSF and serum, and its levels correlate with disease severity (Dickson, 1997; Fillit et al., 1991; Paganelli et al., 2002); examination of post-mortem AD brains reveals that TNF-α increased and co-localizes with Aβ plaques (Montgomery et al., 2011). AD patients showed elevated levels of TNF-α in the brain (Tarkowski et al., 2000) and in vitro studies have shown that TNF-α induces the production of Aβ peptides through the regulation of the gamma secretase complex (Blasko et al., 1999).

4. TNF-α system and ALS

Starting from TNF-α literature in ALS disease, the data often come from ALS animal model: TNF-α mRNA was found in the spinal cord of G93A mice in the early stages of the disease (4 months of age) in correlation with the astroglia activation (Hensley et al., 2003) . Moreover gene expression in mice increases with age up to a peak at the final stages of the disease (7-8 months). Although transcripts of both receptors, TNF-R1 and TNF-R2, have been identified in the spinal cord of the G93A rat (Elliot et al., 2001; Hensley et al., 2003). Yoshihara et al. (2002) have shown that the expression of TNF-α in the marrow of G93A mice overlaps with the activation of microglia already in a pre-symptomatic stage. Then, using immunohistochemistry approach authors found that TNF-α was located mainly at the level of motor neurons and microglia. Some genes involved in apoptosis showed the same pattern of TNF-α gene expression, suggesting a correlation between the inflammatory reaction and the apoptotic pathway (Yoshihara et al., 2002). To this regard, Hensley et al. (2003) have characterized the relationship between the inflammatory genes, oxidative stress and apoptotic events in the G93A mice. In the spinal cord of mice at the presymptomatic stadium expression of FADD and TNF-R1 and many members of the caspase apoptotic cascade were found increased; however, they were expressed at the highest level only in the early stage of the disease, during which an increased protein oxidation was also observed.

Kiaei et al. (2006) have seen an increase in immunoreactivity for TNF-α in sections of the spinal cord of G93A mice and familial or sporadic ALS patients; in G93A mice treatment with thalidomide and lenalidomide, drugs capable of inhibiting the expression of TNF-α, attenuates disease progression was. This result is a further confirmation of the hypothesis that TNF-α plays an important role in the pathogenesis of ALS, probably giving rise to an apoptotic pathway (Kiaei et al., 2006).

Veglianese et al. (2006), showed p38MAPK activation in the G93A mice in the presymptomatic stage at the level of motor neurons, and in later phase also in astrocytes and microglia. It has also been demonstrated to be involved in the activation of kinases upstream of MAPK pathway. An increased expression of both receptors of TNF-α is also observed in the presymptomatic stage, confirming the activation, mediated by TNF-α, of the signalling cascade that leads to MAPK. The MAPK seems to be implicated in the development and disease progression in G93A mice, as already said. Once activated it is able to phosphorylate neurofilaments, causing their accumulation within motor neurons, which is considered one of the pathogenetic features of ALS. In addition, p38MAPK is able to stimulate nitric oxide synthase in neurons and in glia, leading to the formation of peroxynitrite (Wengenack et al., 2004). The generation of SOD1 knock-out mice for TNF-α, however, has shown that the absence of TNF-α has no effect on axonal degeneration but influences onset, severity and progression of the disease in G93A mice; these data suggest that TNF-α, despite its high expression during disease, is not the only factor involved in the degeneration caused by mutations in SOD1 motor neurons in animal models (Gowing et al., 2006).

4.1 TNF-α level in peripheral blood of ALS patients

TNF-α and its soluble receptors, sTNFRs, were already found significantly higher in plasma of ALS patients than in those of healthy controls (Poloni et al., 2000). They found a significant correlation between levels of TNF-α and sTNF-R1 and sTNF-R2, confirming that a general activation of the TNF-α system occurred in ALS patients. Activation of the TNF-α system however did not correlate neither with the disease duration nor with the disease severity. Even after dividing the patients in two subgroups, with high and low TNF-α levels, they did not find any difference in terms of clinical parameters of the disease (Poloni et al., 2000).

Our research group analyzed the possible implication of TNF-α pathway in ALS pathogenesis (Cereda et al., 2008). We assayed both the levels of TNF-α and its soluble receptors in plasma from ALS patients overtime during disease progression. We assayed the concentrations of TNF-α and its soluble receptors in plasma of 88 patients with sporadic ALS and 40 healthy controls; blood sample from each patient was taken since two months after diagnosis up to death, or along 80 months. We found that circulating levels of TNF-α and its two soluble receptors were significantly increased in the plasma of patients with sporadic ALS. Our data show that TNF-α high plasma concentration is present already at disease onset in the majority of ALS patients and remains over the normal range during the whole disease progression time, even though it slightly decreases during disease progression.

We hypothesised that in the majority of ALS patients TNF-α plasma concentration has already reached its peak at disease onset, remains high during all disease duration and starts to decrease at the end of the disease. This finding suggests that TNF-α pathway could be activated in the first stage of the disease and it decreases its effect with the progression of the disease (Cereda et al., 2008).

4.2 Polymorphisms and TNF-α transcription gene

Preliminary genetic analysis are documented in ALS only about (-308, -857) TNF-α promoter polymorphisms and they do not show statistically significant differences in allelic and genotypic frequencies (Cereda et al., 2008). In 2008 over 100 sporadic ALS patients' DNA samples collected at the Neurological Institute "C. Mondino" (Pavia, Italy) and DNA sample from 228 healthy controls were used to study polymorphisms of TNF-α, TNF-R1 and TNF-R2 genes by RFLP.

In our work we studied -308 G/A and -857 A/G. Moreover, we investigated MspaI polymorphism in exon 1 TNF-R1 gene, a SNP at +36 A/G positions, and Nla III polymorphism in exon 6 TNF-R2 that identified a SNP (T/G) at 196 codon, which leads to an amino acid substitution (Met/Arg). We found no statistically significant differences in allele and genotype frequencies between patients and controls for polymorphisms considered. In our recent work, we performed a molecular study of polymorphisms of many cytokines (IL-1α, IL-1β, IL-1R, IL-1R, IL-4Rα, IL-12, IFN-γ, TGF-β1, IL-2, IL-4, IL-6, IL-10) including -238 TNF-α on 70 ALS patients (unpublished data). Although no difference was found in allele frequencies of this polymorphism, we observed a statistical significance in AA genotype of the TNF-α -238 SNPs comparing ALS patients respect to healthy control. The most common G allele of -238 polymorphism of TNF-α gene is associated with high production of TNF-α (Huizinga et al., 1991; Wilson et al., 1997) but no data is available on the relationship between the minor allele and transcriptional level. Indeed the results obtained from studies on multiple sclerosis, a chronic inflammatory disease, suggest a possible protective effect of A allele in -238 position.

Our study shows that mRNAs of TNF-α were expressed at higher level in lymphocytes of sporadic ALS patients than in controls but there was not relationship with site of disease onset (spinal or bulbar), disease duration at the time of blood sample withdrawal or disease severity. We suppose that mRNA level increase may be due to an ALS disease's point common, as oxidative stress involvement, in all patients analyzed (Carrì et al., 1997; Ciriolo et al., 2002). Interaction between TNF-α, oxidative stress and SOD1 will be better described in the next paragraph.

4.3 TNF-α and SOD1 pathways

Several data support the hypothesis that TNF-α and SOD1 may not only take part to a common cellular pathway but they may also regulate directly and indirectly their self. In fact, an inverse correlation between the expression of SOD1 and TNF-α has been described: cytotoxic effects of TNF-α can be reduced by increasing levels of SOD1 as inhibition of SOD1 mRNA and protein may result in a decrease in the protective effect of SOD1 against inflammation (Meier et al.,1989; Wong & Goeddel ,1988).

In 2006 Afonso and collaborators demonstrated that, in U937 cells, TNF-α down-regulated SOD1 protein expression in a time-dependent manner (Alfonso et al., 2006). Afonso and colleagues performed different experiments treating U937 cells with TNF-α (10 ng/ml) for 1, 4 , 24 hours and their data showed a decline of SOD1 mRNA at 1 hour (22%), maximal suppressor at 4 h (54%) and lesser at 24h (38%).

Although SOD1 activity is modified in some specific situations, the direct effect of the proinflammatory cytokine TNF-α on SOD1 promoter has not been reported. Variable results were reported regarding SOD1 regulation by TNF-α (Chovolou et al.,2003), confirmed by gene expression studies that show the same tendency of SOD1 and TNF-α and suggest that these two genes may have a common system, or, at least, they may take part to the same one.

As concern SOD1 and TNF-α, it is well documented that both TNF-α and SOD1 pathways are regulated by reactive oxygen species (ROS) concentration and we suppose that oxidative stress is a common regulation point thought NF-kB activation.

The important role of ROS is reported in TNF-α signalling although it is unclear whether the TNF-α action may be producer or reducer of ROS concentration. In fact, TNF-α has been reported to increase ROS production from electron transport in mitochondria, plasma membrane NADPH oxidase and cytosolic phospholipase A2-linked cascade through signal transduction pathways triggered by TNFR-related proteins (Chandel et al., 2001; Micheau et al., 2003; Woo et al., 2000). Multimerization of TNFRs may lead to recruitment of TRAFs (TNFR-associated factors) by the receptors resulting in activation of kinases and transcription factors, such as c-Jun and NF-kB (Chandel et al., 2001).

About the reducer role, in a mice model it was demonstrated that TNF-α stimulation in mice deficient in TNF receptor-associated factor 2 (TRAF2) or p65 NF-kB subunit did not induce ROS accumulation, indicating that TRAF-mediated NF-kB activation normally suppresses the TNF-induced ROS accumulation (Sakon et al., 2003). ROS in lower concentrations may function as second messengers in mediating TNF-α activated signal transduction pathways that regulate the NF-kB system (Grisham et al.,1998; Janssen-Heininger et al.,2000).

As concern ROS role, Scott and collaborators demonstrated that ROS may up-regulate TACE activity and consequently, this increased activity may change TNF-α cleavage by TACE (Scott et al., 2011).

In fact, hydrogen peroxide serves as a messenger mediating directly or indirectly the activation of transcription factors such as NF-kB that mediates the induction of various proinflammatory genes (Schreck et al.,1991).
Regarding NF-kB, its pathway is also involved in SOD1, NF-κB was one of the first transcription factor shown to be redox-regulated. Rojo and colleagues (Rojo et al., 2004) showed that cell treatment with H_2O_2 initiates the PI3K/Akt cascades, which participates in NF-κB activation and in subsequent SOD1 transcriptional induction. Indeed, NF-κB binding site was identified in the human SOD1 promoter (GGTAAGTCCC) demonstrating that Akt-activated NF-κB presents increased binding to this sequence, mediating the up-regulation of SOD1 expression.
About ALS disease, we have already underlined the importance of NF-kB role in SOD1 activity, which altered expression and mutations are implicated in ALS disease. Our laboratory studied SOD1 mRNA expression (Gagliardi et al., 2010), we demonstrated that SOD1 mRNA level were altered in ALS patients. In fact we found that the SOD1 gene expression was increased in ALS patients than in controls population. Our unpubblished data show that TNF-α mRNA level is higher in patients' lymphocytes than controls as mRNA SOD1 gene. Unfortunately only few data are available about NF-kB and ALS, that may help to understand the relationship between SOD1 and ALS, so far NF-kB have been studied in ALS mouse model but the inhibition of NF-kB pathway has not effect on the progression of the disease (Crosio et al., 2011).

5. Therapeutic strategies

5.1 Classic immunotherapy in ALS

Several trials both controlled and uncontrolled using immunomodulating agents have been conduced in patients with ALS. These have included plasma exchange, steroids, azathioprine, cyclophosphamide, recombinant human IFN, cyclosporine, immunoglobulin, glatiramer acetate, minocycline.
High-dose therapy with intravenous immunoglobulins was used in ALS, the rationale was strengthened by observations that Ig was effective in improving the muscle strength of patients with a paraproteinemic or conduction block polyneuropathy and also in other autoimmune neuromuscular disease. The authors (Meucci et al. 1996, Dalakas et al. 1994) concluded that IVIg had no apparent therapeutic role in improving the symptoms or arresting the progression in ALS patients (Meucci et al. 1996). Meucci et al included in the study seven patients with a diagnosis of definite or probable ALS according to El Escorial criteria. All patients were treated with intravenous infusions of IVIg 0,4 g/kg/die for 5 consecutive days, followed by monthly, two day infusions at the same daily dosage for 4 to 13 months. All patients were concomitantly treated with oral cyclophosphamide, 1-2 mg/kg/die, as this therapy is effective delaying the frequency of IVIg maintenance infusions in other diseases. The response to treatment was assessed by the Medical Research Council rating scale for muscle strength on ten muscles per limb, a clinical bulbar function scale, a modified Rankin disability scale. The effect of treatment on the progression of the disease was evaluated by comparing the monthly rate of progression of upper and lower limb muscle weakness before and during treatment. All patients continued to deteriorate during treatment, reflected by the worsening of scores after treatment compared with the scores before therapy. The monthly rate of progression of limb weakness during therapy

was not better and possibly worse than that estimated in the period before therapy. No major side effect was reported by the patients.

Dalakas and collaborators (Dalakas et al. 1994) used intravenous infusions of high-dose immunoglobulin administered once a month for 3 months (total dose 2g/kg, divided into two daily doses) in nine ALS patients (El Escorial criteria) with a rapidly progressive course of disease. The efficacy of treatment was assessed by objective measurement of maximum voluntary isometric contraction in all muscle groups of two limbs or with Medical Research Council sores, before and after therapy. All patients worsened during the study and, by the end of the third month, their mean total muscle scores had declined. The pace of progression did not change during the observation period. All patients tolerated the intravenous immunoglobulin infusions well and adverse effects were noted.

Another approach was designed by Drachman lab's group (Drachman et al., 1994), who assessed a more powerful and prolonged immunosuppression obtained by total lymphoid irradiation (TLI) in ALS patients. The discovery that TLI produces powerful immunosuppression in humans led to its use in the treatment of autoimmune diseases. The basic principles of TLI therapy involve the lymphoid organs while shielding non-lymphoid tissues and delivering the radiation in multiple small fractions. The study included thirty patients with ALS. The radiation field consisted of an extended mantle, a para-aortic field and an inverted-Y including the spleen. Patients received anterior and posterior irradiation 5 days/week at a rate of 1,8 Gy/day. Blood counts were obtained 1 to 3 times/week as needed to detect haematological toxicity. Four types of parameters of motor function were evaluated: quantitative dynamometry (4 pairs of muscles in the upper extremities and 5 pairs of muscles in the lower extremities), manual muscle testing, functional tests (swallowing, breathing), activity indexes. Tests of immune function were: leukocytes (absolute lymphocyte counts, decrease in CD4 cells, CD4/CD8 ratio), cell-mediated immunity (negative conversion of skin tests), humoral immunity (tetanus antibody response). To assess whether the effectiveness of immunosuppression had an influence on the course of ALS, they analysed the relationships between parameters of immunosuppression and the measures of progression of ALS. This analysis showed that evidence of more effective immunosuppression did not correlate with a more favourable disease course.

Another immunotherapy tried in ALS was liquorpheresis (Andrich et al. 1996; Finsterer et al., 1999) with no results both in sporadic and familial ALS.

IFNs alpha and beta cytokines can regulate the major histocompatibility complex and the presentation of antigens to T-cell receptors. They have been used in variable doses for up to 6 months in small trials in ALS patients with negative results, however the small sample size, the possibility inadequate dose and the short period of follow-up prevented definite conclusions about the efficacy of IFNs. For these reasons a study was undertaken in which recombinant IFNbeta-1a was used in a large patient population at a dose twice as large as that found to be effective in patient with MS. Beghi et al. (2000) recruited patients with 6 to 24 months history of confirmed ALS, that received 12 mIU of IFN subcutaneously three times a week for 6 months and were followed up for an additional 6 months. Medical Research Council scale, Norris scale, bulbar scores were used to assess disability; selected electrophysiologic measures were also used. There were no significant differences of disease progression and disability in patients treated with IFN. Common adverse events were flu-like syndrome, local erythema, gastrointestinal symptomps.

Glatiramer acetate (GA) is a synthetic copolymer composed of four amino acids, used in MS for reduction of the frequency of relapses. GA induces a wide variety of actions on T-cells and leads to generalized, antigen-non-specific alterations of various types of antigen presenting cells in such a way that they stimulate Th2-like responses. It blocks the release of TNF-α and interleukin in monocytes and dendritic cells. So GA has neuroprotective as well as immunomodulatory actions. Meininger and collaborators (Meininger et al., 2009) recruited patients with El Escorial definite, probable or laboratory probable ALS of less than three years duration. Patients were given 40 mg GA daily for a period of 52 weeks. The prospectively defined primary efficacy outcome was the slope of ALSFRS score, the secondary efficacy outcome was time to death, tracheostomy or positive pressure ventilation more than 23 h per day. Additional functional endpoints included mean change from baseline and across visits in ALSFRS score, manuasl muscle testing score and slow vital capacity. GA was shown to be safe and well tolerated, the most significant adverse event was the injection site reaction. This study suggested that glatiramer acetate didn't show any beneficial effect in ALS patients either for course or survival.

Minocycline has anti-apoptotic and anti-inflammatory effects in vitro in CNS, so several trials are planned or are in progress to assess whether minocycline slows human neurodegeneration. Gordon (Gordon et al., 2007) did a multicentre trial in which patients with diagnosis of ALS (according to El Escorial criteria) received minocycline escalating doses of up to 400 mg/day for 9 months (started at 100 mg twice per day and increased every week by 50 mg twice per day to the highest dose of 400 mg). The primary outcome measures was the changes in ALSFRS-r, the secondary outcome measures were forced vital capacity, manual muscle testing, quality of life, time of tracheostomy, chronic assisted ventilation, survival and safety. ALSFRS-r score deterioration was faster in the minocycline group of patients and greater mortality during the 9-months treatment phase was registered in the same group.

Adverse events were most commonly reported in the respiratory system, gastrointestinal system (nausea, diarrhoea, costipation), neurological system (dizziness, fatigue).

5.2 TNF-α and new approaches in immunotherapy

The discovery, in 1988, of a naturally occurring TNF-α inhibitor in human urine (Seckinger et al., 1990), which was identified as a soluble form of the TNF-receptor that acted by neutralizing the cytokine, opened the way to immunotherapy. Subsequently two TNF-binding proteins were purified that were capable of inhibiting the binding of TNF-α to cells (Engelmann et al., 1990). The identification of soluble TNF-α receptors paved the way for the development of soluble TNF-α receptors antibodies currently used for the treatment of several systemic inflammatory diseases, including rheumatoid arthritis, juvenile polyarticular rheumatoid arthritis, inflammatory bowel diseases, psoriatic arthritis and ankylosing spondylitis (Sfikakis et al., 2010).

There are three anti-TNF-α agents approved for clinical use: Etancercept, Infliximab, Adalimumab. The latter two are full-length bivalent IgG monoclonal antibodies specific for sTNF and tmTNF, whereas Etanercept is a genetically engineered Fc fusion protein generated from the extracellular domain of human TNF-R2 and functions as a decoy receptor to block sTNF, tmTNF and distinct ligands of lymphotoxin, a TNF-related protein (Tracey et al., 2005).

The important side effects that have been most extensively related to TNF-α inhibitors include: lymphoma (hepatosplenic T-cell lymphoma in young patients being treated for

Chron disease and ulcerative colitis), infections (fungal infections such as histoplasmosis, coccidioidomycosis, blastomycosis and tuberculosis), congestive heart failure, demyelinating disease, a lupus-like syndrome, induction of auto-antibodies, injection site reactions and systemic side effects (Scheinfeld et al., 2006).

Clinical trials examining the effects of TNF-α inhibition have been conducted on patients with Multiple Sclerosis (MS) and Alzheimer disease (AD).

Strategies to inhibit TNF-α in MS seemed promising in preclinical applications but have widely failed in human clinical trials due to the lack of therapeutic selectivity. During an open-label phase I trial, a monoclonal TNF-α antibody was infused into two human patients exhibiting rapidly progressing disease. Subsequently, in a double-blinded, placebo controlled, multicentered phase II study, 168 relapsing-remitting MS patients were administered Lenercept, a sTNF-R1 fusion protein that neutralizes TNF-α. Lenercept-treated individuals experienced higher occurrence of relapse and increased neurological deficits (Van oosten et al., 1996). The ineffectiveness of anti-TNF-α therapy in MS may be a consequence of divergent roles for the TNF receptors, considering that blocking TNF-R1 in mouse models dampens disease severity, while suppressing TNF-R2, the receptor that induces remyelination and harbors immunosuppressive properties, results in exacerbated disease (Arnett et al., 2001; Kassiotis et al., 2011). Recently, pharmacological agents selectively targeting TNF-R1 have been investigated. Using phage display technology, a TNF-R1 antagonist was developed and upon evaluation in mice it was found that administration of this selective antagonist improved clinical scores, reduced cerebral demyelination and suppressed the number of infiltrating inflammatory cells (Nomura et al., 2011).

TNF-α intervention in AD has been evaluated in open-labeled phase I clinical trials where perispinal extrathecal administration of Etanercept was administered weekly to a small number of patients ranging from mild to severe AD for a short duration of 6 months that claimed substantial cognitive and behavioural improvements, including verbal fluency and aphasia (Tobinick et al., 2006; Tobinick et al., 2008). Currently a phase II study is recruiting to evaluate the safety and tolerability of Etanercept in AD. These results seem promising but conclusions regarding the promise of such a therapeutic strategy should be reserved until after extensive chronic suppression of TNF-α activity is performed in preclinical models and double-blind human clinical trials have been conducted and results critically reviewed by the research community.

Trails on the immunological hypothesis in ALS are not yet established although TNF-α system implications have been described for a long time. This therapeutic approach was not considered using neither synthetic TNF-α-receptor inhibitors nor monoclonal anti-TNF-α antibody.

6. Conclusions

There is no doubt that TNF-α play key roles in degenerative conditions afflicting CNS, also in ALS. The precise role TNF-α plays remain highly controversial due to the complexity and pleiotropic nature of this cytokine and its activities during critical developmental and homeostatic cellular processes. Multiple factors determine whether TNF-α will exert deleterious or beneficial effects for neuronal survival and some of these differential actions relate to its duration of expression, concentration, receptor conformation. Despite the

elaborate and promising data collected thus far to assign function to TNF-α in neurodegeneration, surprisingly little is still known about the cellular and stage-specific roles of this cytokine.
The data reported in this chapter also underline the importance of TNF-α pathways in ALS pathology due to the interaction with SOD1 gene.
In fact, the data that demonstrated the down-regulation of SOD1 after treatment with TNF-α (Afonso et al., 2006), related to the up-regulation of SOD1 mRNA expression in ALS patients suggest to carry on the studies about TNF-α in ALS disease to better define the TNF-α function in neurodegeneration. A better understanding of SOD1 regulation related to TNF-α function may permit to develop novel immunotherapy application in ALS disease.

7. Acknowledgement

We are grateful to "our" ALS patients and their families that trust our work. Moreover we would like to thank National and International Research Agencies and Italian Health Minister that found our research projects.

8. References

Aisen P.S., J. Schmeidler, G.M. Pasinetti. (2002). Randomized pilot study of nimesulide treatment in Alzheimer disease. Neurology, 58, 1050-1054.

Aisen P.S., K.A. Schafer, M Grundman, E. Pfeiffer, M. Sano, K.L. Davis, M.R. Farlow, S. Jin, R.G. Thomas, L.J. Thal. (2003). Effects of rofecoxib or naproxen vs placebo on Alzheimer disease progression: a randomized controlled trial. JAMA, 289, 2819-2826.

Aisen P.S., K.L. Davis, J.D. Berg, K. Schafer, K. Campbell, R.G. Thomas, M.F. Weiner, M.R. Farlow, M. Sano, M. Grundman, L.J. Thal. (2000). A randomized controlled trial of prednisone in Alzheimer disease. Neurology, 54, 588-593. Alexianu ME, Kozovska M, Appel SH. (2001) Immune reactivity in a mouse model of familial ALS correlates with disease progression. Neurology.57:1282–1289.

Arnett H.A., J. Mason, M. Marino, K. Suzuki, G.K. Matsushima, J.P. Ting. (2001). TNF-alpha promotes proligeration of oligdendrocyte progenitors and remyelination. Nat Neurosci, 4, 1116-1122.

Badiola N, Malagelada C, Llecha N, Hidalgo J, Comella JX, Sabriá J, Rodríguez-Alvarez J. (Sep 2009). Activation of caspase-8 by tumour necrosis factor receptor 1 is necessary for caspase-3 activation and apoptosis in oxygen-glucose deprived cultured cortical cells. Neurobiol Dis.;35(3):438-47. Epub 2009 Jun 23.

Baker SJ, Reddy EP.Modulation of life and death by the TNF receptor superfamily. Oncogene. (Dec 1998). 24;17(25):3261-70.

Bazzoni F, Beutler B. The tumor necrosis factor ligand and receptor families. N Engl J Med. (Jun 1996) 27;334(26):1717-25.

Beers DR, Henkel JS, Zhao W, Wang J, Appel. (Oct 2008). SH.CD4+ T cells support glial neuroprotection, slow disease progression, and modify glial morphology in an animal model of inherited ALS.Proc Natl Acad Sci U S A. 7;105(40):15558-63. Epub 2008 Sep 22.

Beghi E, A. Chiò, M. Inghilleri, L. Mazzini, A. Micheli, G. Mora, M. Poloni, R. Riva, L. Serlenga, D. Testa, P. Tonali; A randomized controlled trial of recombinant interferon beta-1a in ALS. Neurology,. (2000). 54, 469-474.

Blasko I, Marx F, Steiner E, Hartmann T, Grubeck-Loebenstein B. (Jan 1999). TNFalpha plus IFNgamma induce the production of Alzheimer beta-amyloid peptides and decrease the secretion of APPs.FASEB J.13(1):63-8.

Bruce AJ, Boling W, Kindy MS, Peschon J, Kraemer PJ, Carpenter MK, Holtsberg FW, Mattson MP. (Jul 1996). Altered neuronal and microglial responses to excitotoxic and ischemic brain injury in mice lacking TNF receptors.Nat Med.2(7):788-94.

Bruijn LI, Houseweart MK, Kato S, Anderson KL, Anderson SD, Ohama E, Reaume AG, Scott RW, Cleveland DW. (Sep 1998). Aggregation and motor neuron toxicity of an ALS-linked SOD1 mutant independent from wild-type SOD1. Science. 281(5384):1851-4.

Butler MP, O'Connor JJ, Moynagh PN. (2004). Dissection of tumor-necrosis factor-alpha inhibition of long-term potentiation (LTP) reveals a p38 mitogen-activated protein kinase-dependent mechanism which maps to early-but not late-phase LTP. Neuroscience.124(2):319-26.

Calvo A., C. Moglia, M. Balma, A. Chiò. (2010). Involvement of immune response in the pathogenesis of Amyotrofic Lateral Sclerosis: a therapeutic opportunity? CNS & neurological disorders - Drugs Targets, , 9, 325-330.

Carlo-Stella N, Badulli C, De Silvestri A, Bazzichi L, Martinetti M, Lorusso L, Bombardieri S, Salvaneschi L, Cuccia M. (2006). A first study of cytokine genomic polymorphisms in CFS: Positive association of TNF-857 and IFNgamma 874 rare alleles. Clin Exp Rheumatol.24:179 182.

Carswell EA, Old LJ, Kassel RL, Green S, Fiore N, Williamson B. (Sep 1975). An endotoxin-induced serum factor that causes necrosis of tumors. Proc Natl Acad Sci U S A.72(9):3666-70.

Cereda C, Boiocchi C, Bongioanni P, Cova E, Guareschi S, Metelli MR, Rossi B, Sbalsi I, Cuccia MC, Ceroni M. (2008). TNF and sTNFR1/2 plasma levels in ALS patients. J Neuroimmunol. 194:123-131,.

Chandel NS, Schumacker PT, Arch RH. (2001). Reactive oxygen species are downstream products of TRAF-mediated signal transduction. J. Biol. Chem. 276: 42728-42736,.

Chiu IM, (2008). T lymphocytes potentiate endogenous neuroprotective inflammation in a mouse model of ALS. Proc Natl Acad Sci USA.;105:17913–17918

Chovolou Y, Watjen W, Kampkotter A, Kahl R. (Aug 2003). Resistance to tumor necrosis factor-alpha (TNF-alpha)-induced apoptosis in rat hepatoma cells expressing TNF-alpha is linked to low antioxidant enzyme expression. J Biol Chem. 8;278(32):29626-32. Epub 2003 May 29.

Crosio C, Valle C, Casciati A, Iaccarino C, Carrì MT. (Mar 2011). Astroglial inhibition of NF-κB does not ameliorate disease onset and progression in a mouse model for amyotrophic lateral sclerosis (ALS). PLoS One. 6(3):e17187.

Cudkowicz ME, Katz J, Moore DH, O'Neill G, Glass JD, Mitsumoto H, Appel S, Ravina B, Kieburtz K, Shoulson I, Kaufmann P, Khan J, Simpson E, Shefner J, Levin B, Cwik V, Schoenfeld D, Aggarwal S, McDermott MP, Miller RG. (May 2010). Toward more efficient clinical trials for amyotrophic lateral sclerosis. Amyotroph Lateral Scler. 11(3):259-65. Review.

Dal Canto MC, Gurney ME. (1994). Development of central nervous system pathology in a murine transgenic model of human amyotrophic lateral sclerosis. Am J Clin Pathol.;145:1271–9.

Dalakas M.C., D.P. Stein, C. Otero, E. Sekul, E.J. Cupler, S. McCrosky. (1994). Effect of high-dose intravenous immunoglobulin on ALS and multifocal motor neuropathy. Arch. Neurol., , 51, 861-864

Darnay BG. and Aggarwal B.B., (1997). Early events in TNF signaling : a story of associations and dissociations. Journal of Leukocyte Biology 61:559-566

Dickson DW (1997) The pathogenesis of senile plaques. J Neuropathol Exp Neurol 56:321–339

Drachman D.B, V. Chaudhry, D. Cornblath, R.W. Kuncl, A. Pestronk, L. Clawson, E.D Mellits, S. Quaskey, T. Quinn, A. Calkins, S. Order. (1994). Trial of immunosuppression in ALS using total lymphoid irradiation. Ann. Neurol., 35, 142-150

Elliott J.L., (2001). Cytokine upregulation in a murine model of familial amyotrophic lateral sclerosis. Brain Res. Mol. Brain Res. 95:172-178

Engelhardt JI, Tajti J, Appel SH. Lymphocytic infiltrates in the spinal cord in amyotrophic lateral sclerosis. Arch Neurol 1993;50:30 -36.

Engelmann H., D. Novick, D. Wallach. (1990). Two TNF-binding proteins purified from human urine, evidence for immunological cross-reactivity with cell surface TNF-receptors. J. Biol. Chem., , 265, 1531-1536.-Estevez AY, O'Regan MH, Song D, Phillis JW. (1999). Hyposmotically induced amino acid release from the rat cerebral cortex: role of phospholipases and protein kinases. Brain Res. Oct 9;844(1-2):1-9.

Fillit H, Ding WH, Buee L, Kalman J, Altstiel L, Lawlor B, Wolf- Klein G (1991) Elevated circulating tumor necrosis factor levels

Finsterer, B. Mamoli. (1999). Liquorpheresis in familial ALS. Spinal Cord., , 37, 592-593

Ghosh S, Hayden MS. (2008). New regulators of NF-κB in inflammation. Nat Rev Immunol 8: 837–848.

Glezer I, Simard AR, Rivest S. (Jul 2007). Neuroprotective role of the innate immune system by microglia. Neuroscience. 147(4):867-83. Apr 24. Review.

Gordon P.H., D.H. Moore, R.G. Miller, J.M. Florence, J.L. Verheijde, C. Doorish, J.F. Hilton, G.M. Spitalny, R.B. MacArthur, H. Mitsumoto, H.E. Neville, K. Boylan, T. Mozaffar, J.M. Belsh, J. Ravits, R.S. Bedlack, M.C. Graves, L.F. Mccluskey, R.J. Barohn, R. Tundan. (2007), Efficacy of minocycline in patients with ALS: a phase III randomized trial. Lancet Neurol., 6, 1045-1053

Gowing G, Dequen F, Soucy G, Julien JP. (2006). Absence of tumor necrosis factor-alpha does not affect motor neuron disease caused by superoxide dismutase 1 mutations. J Neurosci. 26(44):11397-402

Grisham MB, Granger DN, Lefer DJ. (1998). Modulation of leukocyte-endothelial interactions by reactive metabolites of oxygen and nitrogen: relevance to ischemicheart disease. Free Radic. Biol. Med. 25: 404-433.

Halliwell B. (Jun 2006). Oxidative stress and neurodegeneration: where are we now? J Neurochem.97(6):1634-58. Review.

Hemnani T and Parihar MS. (1998). Reactive oxygen species and oxidative DNA damage. Ind. J. Physiol. Pharmacol. 42: 440-452.

Heneka M. T., J. J. Rodr´ıguez, and A. Verkhratsky. (2010). Neuroglia in neurodegeneration, Brain Research Reviews, vol. 63, no. 1- 2, pp. 189–211.

Hensley K., Fedynyshyn J., Ferrell S., Floyd R.A., Gordon B., Grammas P., Hamdheydari L., Mhatre M., Mou S., Pye Q.N., Stewart C., West M., West S., Williamson K.S. (2003). Message and protein-level elevation of tumor necrosis factor alpha (TNF alpha) and TNF alphamodulating cytokines in spinal cords of the G93A-SOD1 mouse model for amyotrophiclateral sclerosis. Neurobiol. Dis. 14:74-80

Holmøy T. (Apr 2008). T cells in amyotrophic lateral sclerosis. Eur J Neurol.15(4):360-6. Epub 2008 Feb 11. Review.

Hsu H., Shu H.B., Pan M.G., Goeddel D.V., (1996). TRADD-TRAF2 and TRADD-FADD interactions define two distinct TNF receptor 1 signal transduction pathways. Cell 84:299-308

Huizinga TW, Westendorp RG, Bollen EL, Keijsers V, Brinkman BM, Langermans JA, et al. (1997). TNF-alpha promoter polymorphisms, production and susceptibility to multiple sclerosis in different groups of patients. J Neuroimmunol.;72:149 153.

Håkansson A, Westberg L, Nilsson S, Buervenich S, Carmine A, Holmberg B, Sydow O, Olson L, Johnels B, Eriksson E, Nissbrandt H. (2005). Investigation of genes coding for inflammatory components in Parkinson's disease. Mov Disord. May;20(5):569-73.

Iłzecka J, Stelmasiak Z, Dobosz B. (Dec 2002). Transforming growth factor-Beta 1 (tgf-Beta 1) in patients with amyotrophic lateral sclerosis. Cytokine. 7;20(5):239-43.

Ilzecka J, Stelmasiak, Z, Dobosz B. (2002). Transforming growth factor-Beta 1 (tgf-Beta 1) in patients with amyotrophic lateral sclerosis. Cytokine;20:239 243.

Imamura K, Hishikawa N, Sawada M, Nagatsu T, Yoshida M, Hashizume Y. (1988). Distribution of major histocompatibility complex class II-positive microglia and cytokine profile of Parkinson's disease brains.Immunity assessment in the early stages of amyotrophic lateral sclerosis: a study of virus antibodies and lymphocyte subsets. Acta Neurol Scand. Dec;78(6):449-54.

Itzhaki RF, Wozniak MA, Appelt DM, Balin BJ. (2004). Infiltration of the brain by pathogens causes Alzheimer's disease.Neurobiol Aging. May-Jun;25(5):619-27. Review.

Janssen-Heininger YMW, Poynter ME, Baeuerle PA. (2000). Recent advances towards understanding redox mechanisms in the activation of nuclear factor kappaB. Radic. Biol. Med. 28: 1317-1327,

Kassiotis G., G. Kollias. (2001). Uncoupling the proinflammatory from the immunosuppressive properties of TNF at the p55 TNF receptor level: implications for pathogenesis and therapy of autoimmune demyelination. J Exp Med, , 193, 427-434.

Kawamata T, Akiyama H, Yamada T, McGeer PL. (Mar 1992). Immunologic reactions in amyotrophic lateral sclerosis brain and spinal cord tissue.Am J Pathol.140(3):691-707.

Kelly KA, Hill MR, Youkhana K, Wanker F, Gimble JM. (1994). Dimethyl sulfoxide modulates NF-kappa B and cytokine activation in lipopolysaccharide-treated murine macrophages. Infect. Immun. 62: 3122-3128,.

Kiaiei M. et al., (2006). Thalidomide and Lenalidomide extend survival in a transgenic mouse model of amyotrophic lateral sclerosis. The Journal of Neuroscience, 26(9):2467-2473

Kuhle, R. L. P. Lindberg, A. Regeniter, M. Mehling, A. J. Steck, L. Kappos and A. Czaplinski (2009). Increased levels of inflammatory chemokines in amyotrophic lateral sclerosis. European Journal of Neurology, 16: 771–774

Lasiene J, Yamanaka K. Glial cells in amyotrophic lateral sclerosis (2011). Neurol Res Int. 2011;2011:718987. Epub Jun 7.

Lee ,Choi EM. Biochanin A. (2005) stimulates osteoblastic differentiation and inhibits hydrogen peroxide-induced production of inflammatory mediators in MC3T3-E1 cells. Biol. Pharm. Bull. 28:1948-1953

Li N, Karin M. (1999). Is NF-kappaB the sensor of oxidative stress? FASEB J. 13(10):1137-43.

Lin MT, Beal MF. Mitochondrial dysfunction and oxidative stress in neurodegenerative diseases. Nature. 2006 Oct 19;443(7113):787-95. Review.

Liu C, Wang J, Zhou S, Wang B, Ma X. (Sep 2010). Association between -238 but not -308 polymorphism of Tumor necrosis factor alpha (TNF-alpha)v and unexplained recurrent spontaneous abortion (URSA) in Chinese population. Reprod Biol Endocrinol.8:114.

Manna SK, Mukhopadhyay A, Aggarwal BB. (2000). Resveratrol suppresses TNF-induced activation of nuclear transcription factors NF-kappa B, activator protein-1, and apoptosis: potential role of reactive oxygen intermediates and lipid peroxidation. J. Immunol. 164: 6509-6519,.

Mantovani S, Garbelli S, Pasini A, Alimonti D, Perotti C, Melazzini M, Bendotti C, Mora G. (May 2009). Immune system alterations in sporadic amyotrophic lateral sclerosis patients suggest an ongoing neuroinflammatory process. J Neuroimmunol. 210(1-2):73-9.

Marchetti L, Klein M, Schlett K, Pfizenmaier K, Eisel UL. (2004). Tumor necrosis factor (TNF)-mediated neuroprotection against glutamate-induced excitotoxicity is enhanced by N-methyl-D-aspartate receptor activation. Essential role of a TNF receptor 2-mediated phosphatidylinositol 3-kinase-dependent NF-kappa B pathway. J Biol Chem. Jul 30;279(31):32869-81.

McGeer, P.L., McGeer, E.G., (2006). Inflammatory processes in amyotrophic lateral sclerosis. Muscle Nerve 26, 459–470.

Meier B, Radeke HH, Selle S, Younes M, Sies H, Resch K, Habermehl GG. (1989). Human fibroblasts release reactive oxygen species in response to interleukin-1 or tumour necrosis factor-alpha. Biochem. J. 269:539-545,.

Meininger V, V.E. Drory, P.N. Leigh, A. Ludolph, W. Robberecht, V. Silani (2009). Glatiramer acetate has no impact on disease progression in ALS at 40 mg/day: a double-blind, randomized, multicentre, placebo-controlled trial. Amyotrofic Lat. Scler., 10, 378-383

Meucci N, E. Nobile-Orazio, G. Scarlato. (1996). Intravenous immunoglobulin therapy in ALS. J. Neurol., 243, 117-120

Micheau O., J. Tschopp. (2003). Induction of TNF receptor I-mediated apoptosis via two sequential signaling complexes, Cell 114 181–190.

Moisse, K., Strong, M.J. (2006). Innate immunity in amytrophic lateral sclerosis. Biochim. Biophys. Acta 1762, 1083–1093.

-Montgomery S.L., W.J. Bowers. (2011). Tumor necrosis factor-alpha and the roles it plays in homeostatic and degenerative processes within the central nervous system. J Neuroimmune Pharmacol,.

Moodie FM, Marwick JA, Anderson CS, Szulakowski P, Biswas SK, Bauter MR, Kilty I, Rahman I. (2004). Oxidative stress and cigarette smoke alter chromatin remodeling but differentially regulate NF-kappaB activation and proinflammatory cytokine release in alveolar epithelial cells. FASEB J. 18: 1897-1899,.

Moon DO, Kim MO, Lee JD, Choi YH, Kim GY. (2009). Rosmarinic acid sensitizes cell death through suppression of TNF-alpha-induced NF-kappaB activation and ROS generation in human leukemia U937 cells. Cancer Lett. 2010 Feb 28;288(2):183-91. Jul 19.

Moreau C, Devos D, Brunaud-Danel V, Defebvre L, Perez T, Destée A, Tonnel AB, Lassalle P, Just N. (Dec 2005). Elevated IL-6 and TNF-alpha levels in patients with ALS: inflammation or hypoxia? Neurology. 27;65(12):1958-60.

Nagatsu T, Mogi M, Ichinose H, Togari A. (Dec 2003). Changes in cytokines and neurotrophins in Parkinson's disease. J Neural Transm Suppl. 2000;(60):277-90. Review. Acta Neuropathol.;106(6):518-26.

Naor S, Keren Z, Bronshtein T, Goren E, Machluf M, Melamed D. (Aug 2009). Development of ALS-like disease in SOD-1 mice deficient of B lymphocytes.J Neurol.256(8):1228-35. Epub 2009 Mar 12.

Nomura et al. T. (2011). Therapeutic effect of PEGylated TNF-R1 selective antagonistic mutant TNF in experimental autoimmune encephalomyelitis mice. J Control Release, 149, 8-14.

O'Dea E, Hoffmann A. (2010) The regulatory logic of the NF-kappaB signaling system. Cold Spring Harb Perspect Biol. Jan;2(1):a000216.

Oppenheim RW. (1996). Neurotrophic survival molecules for motoneurons: an embarrassment of riches. Neuron 17:195–197,

Paganelli R, Di Iorio A, Patricelli L, Ripani F, Sparvieri E, Faricelli R, Iarlori C, Porreca E, Di Gioacchino M, Abate G (2002) Proinflammatory cytokines in sera of elderly patients with dementia: levels in vascular injury are higher than those of mild-moderate Alzheimers disease patients. Exp Gerontol 37:257–263

Pettmann B, Henderson CE (Feb 1998) Neuronal cell death. Neuron 20:633–647. Presence of dendritic cells, MCP-1, and activated microglia/macrophages in amyotrophic lateral sclerosis spinal cord tissue. Ann Neurol. 2004;55(2):221-35.

Provinciali L, Laurenzi MA, Vesprini L, Giovagnoli AR, Bartocci C, Montroni M, Bagnarelli P, Clementi M, Varaldo PE. Reaume AG, Elliott JL, Hoffman EK, Kowall NW, Ferrante RJ, Siwek DF, Wilcox HM, Flood DG, Beal MF, Brown RH Jr, Scott RW, Snider WD. (May 1996) Motor neurons in Cu/Zn superoxide dismutase-deficient mice develop normally but exhibit enhanced cell death after axonal injury.Nat Genet.13(1):43-7.

Reddy P, Slack JL, Davis R, Cerretti DP, Kozlosky CJ, Blanton RA, Shows D, Peschon JJ, Black RA. (2000) Functional analysis of the domain structure of tumor necrosis factor-alpha converting enzyme. J Biol Chem. May 12;275(19):14608-14.

Rentzos M, Evangelopoulos E, Sereti E, Zouvelou V, Marmara S, Alexakis T, Evdokimidis I. (2011). Alterations of T cell subsets in ALS: a systemic immune activation? Acta Neurol Scand. Jun 9. doi: 10.1111/j.1600-0404.2011.01528.x. [Epub ahead of print]

Rentzos M, Rombos A, Nikolaou C, Zoga M, Zouvelou V, Dimitrakopoulos A, Alexakis T, Tsoutsou A, Samakovli A, Michalopoulou M, Evdokimidis I. (2010). Interleukin-15 and interleukin-12 are elevated in serum and cerebrospinal fluid of patients with amyotrophic lateral sclerosis. Eur Neurol.;63(5):285-90. Epub 2010 Apr 14.

Rentzos M, Rombos A, Nikolaou C, Zoga M, Zouvelou V, Dimitrakopoulos A, Alexakis T, Tsoutsou A, Samakovli A, Michalopoulou M, Evdokimidis J. (2010). Interleukin-17 and interleukin-23 are elevated in serum and cerebrospinal fluid of patients with ALS: a reflection of Th17 cells activation? Acta Neurol Scand. Dec;122(6):425-9.

Rojo AI, Salinas M, Martín D, Perona R, Cuadrado A. (2004). Regulation of Cu/Zn-superoxide dismutase expression via the phosphatidylinositol 3 kinase/Akt pathway and nuclear factor-kappaB. J Neurosci. Aug 18;24(33):7324-34.

Rosenquist M. 14-3-3 proteins in apoptosis. Braz J Med Biol Res. (Apr 2003).;36(4):403-8. Epub 2003 Apr 8. Review.

Sakon S, Xue X, Takekawa M, Sasazuki T, Okazaki T, Kojima Y, Piao JH, Yagita H, Okumura K, Doi T, Nakano H. (2003). NF-kappaB inhibits TNF-induced accumulation of ROS that mediate prolonged MAPK activation and necrotic cell death. EMBO J. 22: 3898-3909.

Scharf S., A. Mander, A. Ugoni, F. Vajda, N. Christophidis. (2003) A double-blind, placebo-controlled trial of diclofenac/misoprostol in Alzheimer disease. Neurology, 53, 197-201.

Scheinfeld N. (2004) A comprehensive review and evaluation of the side effects of the TNF blockers etanercept, infliximab and adalimumab. J Dermatolog Treat, 15, 280-294.

Schreck R, Rieber P, Baeuerle PA. (Aug 1991). Reactive oxygen intermediates as apparently widely used messengers in the activation of the NF-kappa B transcription factor and HIV-1. EMBO J.10(8):2247-58.

Schwartz M, Solomon A, Lavie V, Ben-Bassat S, Belkin M, Cohen A. (1991). Tumor necrosis factor facilitates regeneration of injured central nervous system axons. Brain Res. Apr 5;545(1-2):334-8.

Scott AJ, O'Dea KP, O'Callaghan D, Williams L, Dokpesi JO, Tatton L, Handy JM, Hogg PJ, Takata M. (2011). Reactive oxygen species and p38 MAPK mediate TNF-alpha converting enzyme (TACE/ADAM17) activation in primary human monocytes. J Biol Chem. Aug 24. [Epub ahead of print]

Seckinger P., J.H. Zhang, B. Hauptmann, J.M. Dayer. (1990). Characterization of a TNF-alpha inhibitor: evidence of immunological cross-reactivity with the TNF receptor. Proc. Natl. Acad. Sci., 87, 5188-5192.

Sfikakis P.P. (2010). The first decade of biologic TNF antagonists in clinical practice: lessons learned, unresolved issues and future directions. Curr. Dir. Autoimmun, , 11, 180-210.

Smith RA, Baglioni C.The active form of tumor necrosis factor is a trimer.J Biol Chem. (1987) May 25;262(15):6951-4.

Sta M, Sylva-Steenland RM, Casula M, de Jong JM, Troost D, Aronica E, Baas F. (2011). Innate and adaptive immunity in amyotrophic lateral sclerosis: Evidence of complement activation. Neurobiol Dis. [Epub ahead of print]

Stewart W.F., C. Kawas, M. Corrada, E.J. Metter. (1997) Risk of Alzheimer disease and duration of NSAID use. Neurology, 48, 626-632.

Tancredi V, D'Arcangelo G, Grassi F, Tarroni P, Palmieri G, Santoni A, Eusebi F. (1992). Tumor necrosis factor alters synaptic transmission in rat hippocampal slices. Neurosci Lett. Nov 9;146(2):176-8.

Tansey MG, Frank-Cannon TC, McCoy MK, Lee JK, Martinez TN, McAlpine FE, Ruhn KA, Tran TA. (2008). Neuroinflammation in Parkinson's disease: is there sufficient evidence for mechanism-based interventional therapy? Front Biosci. Jan 1;13:709-17. Review.

Tarkowski E, Ringqvist A, Blennow K, Wallin A, Wennmalm A. (2000). Intrathecal release of nitric oxide in Alzheimer's disease and vascular dementia.Dement Geriatr Cogn Disord. Nov-Dec;11(6):322-6.

Tateishi T, Yamasaki R, Tanaka M, Matsushita T, Kikuchi H, Isobe N, Ohyagi Y, Kira JI. (2010). CSF chemokine alterations related to the clinical course of amyotrophic lateral sclerosis. J Neuroimmunol. Apr 8. [Epub ahead of print]

Tavolato BF. (1975). Immunoglobulin G distribution in multiple sclerosis brain. An immunofluorescence study. J Neurol Sci. Jan;24(1):1-11.

Tobinick E., H. Gross, A. Weinberger, H. Cohen. (2006). TNF-alpha modulation for treatment of Alzheimer disease: a 6-month pilot study. MedGenMed, 8, 25.

Tobinick E., H. Gross. (2008). Rapid improvement in verbal fluency and aplasia following perispinal etanercept in Alzheimer disease. BMC Neurol, 8, 27.

Tracey D., L. Klareskog, E.H. Sasso, J.G. Salfeld, P.P. Tak. (2008). TNF antagonist mechanisms of action : a comprehensive review. Pharmacol Ther, 117, 244-279.

Troost D, Van den Oord JJ, Vianney de Jong JM. (1990). Immunohistochemical characterization of the inflammatory infiltrate in amyotrophic lateral sclerosis. Neuropathol Appl Neurobiol. Oct;16(5):401-10.

Van oosten B.W., F. Barkhof, L. Truyen, J.B. Boringa, F.W. Bertelsmann, B.M. Von Blomberg, J.N. Woody, H.P. Hartung, C.H. Polman (1996). Increased MRI activity and immune activation in two multiple sclerosis patients treated with the monoclonal anti-TNF antibody cA2. Neurology, 47, 1531-1534.

Veglianese P, Lo Coco D, Bao Cutrona M, Magnoni R, Pennacchini D, Pozzi B, Gowing G, Julien JP, Tortarolo M, Bendotti C. (2006). Activation of the p38MAPK cascade is associated with upregulation of TNF alpha receptors in the spinal motor neurons of mouse models of familial ALS. Mol Cell Neurosci. 31(2):218-31

Wengenack TM. (2004). Activation of programmed cell death markers in ventral horn motor neurons during early presyntomatic stages of amyotrophic lateral sclerosis in a transgenic mouse model. Brain Res. 1027:73-86

Westall FC, Rubin R, Gospodarowicz D. (1983). Brain-derived fibroblast growth factor: a study of its inactivation. Life Sci. Dec 12;33(24):2425-9.

Weydt, P., Weiss, M.D., Möller, T., Carter, G.T. (2002). Neuro-inflammation as a therapeutic target amyotrophic lateral sclerosis. Curr. Opin. Investig. Drugs 12, 1720–1724.

Wilson AG, Symons JA, McDowell TL, McDevitt HO, Duff GW. (1997). Effects of a polymorphism in the human tumor necrosis factor alpha pronoter on transcriptional activation. Proc Natl Acad Sci USA; 94:3195-3199.

Vlahopoulos S, Boldogh I, Casola A, Brasier AR. (1999). Nuclear factor-kappaB-dependent induction of interleukin-8 gene expression by tumor necrosis factor alpha: evidence for an antioxidant sensitive activating pathway distinct from nuclear translocation. Blood 94: 1878-1889.

Wong GHW and Goeddel DV. (1988). Induction of manganous superoxide dismutase by tumor necrosis factor: possible protective mechanism. Science 242: 941-944.

Woo CH, Eom YW, Yoo MH, You HJ, Han HJ, Song WK, Yoo YJ, Chun JS, Kim JH. (2000). Tumor necrosis factor-alpha generates reactive oxygen species via acytosolic phospholipase A2-linked cascade. J. Biol. Chem. 275: 32357-32362.

Yoshihara T., Ishigaki S., Yamamoto M., Liang Y., Niwa J., Takeuchi H., Doyu M., Sobue G. (2002). Differential expression of inflammation- and apoptosis-related genes in spinal cords of a mutant SOD1 transgenic mouse model of familial amyotrophic lateral sclerosis. J.Neurochem. 80:158-167

Zhao X, Bausano B, Pike BR, Newcomb-Fernandez JK, Wang KK, Shohami E, Ringger NC, DeFord SM, Anderson DK, Hayes RL. (2001). TNF-alpha stimulates caspase-3 activation and apoptotic cell death in primary septo-hippocampal cultures. J Neurosci Res 64:121–131

19

Stem Cell Application for Amyotrophic Lateral Sclerosis: Growth Factor Delivery and Cell Therapy

Masatoshi Suzuki, Chak Foon Tso and Michael G. Meyer
University of Wisconsin-Madison
U. S. A.

1. Introduction

1.1 ALS and the SOD1 rodent models

Amyotrophic lateral sclerosis (ALS) is a progressive disorder that leads to degeneration of upper and lower motor neurons, muscular atrophy, and (ultimately) death. A clinical diagnosis of ALS requires signs of progressive degeneration in both upper and lower motor neurons, with no evidence that suggest that the signs can be explained by other disease processes (Brooks et al., 1994, 2000). The incidence rate of the disease is around 2 in 100,000 people (Hirtz et al., 2007). The onset age of sporadic and most familial form of ALS is between 50-60 years, and is generally fatal within 1-5 years of onset (Cleveland & Rothstein, 2001). Riluzile is the only drug that demonstrates a beneficial effect on ALS patients, but only increases survival by a matter of months (Zoccolella et al., 2009).

Motor neuron cell death in ALS probably involves multiple pathways. Most ALS cases are sporadic in nature, while ~10% arise from a dominantly inherited trait (familial ALS or FALS) (Brown, 1995). The cause for sporadic ALS remains unclear, while 20% of FALS patients have a point mutation in the cytosolic Cu^{2+}/Zn^{2+} superoxide dismutase 1 (SOD1) gene (Rosen et al., 1993). Recent reports suggested that other causes of FALS also include mutations in TDP-43 (the 43-KDa TAR DNA binding protein) and FUS (Fused in sarcoma/translocated in liposarcoma) genes (Ticozzi et al, 2011). From various lines of transgenic mice, we can observe that motor neuron disease is developed in mutants with elevated SOD1 levels (ex. hSOD1-G93A line), while no symptoms are observed in SOD1 knockout mice. The combined effect shows that SOD1 acts through a toxic gain of function rather than loss of dismutase activity (Julien et al., 2001). Both mouse and rat models over-expressing SOD1 genes show similar disease phenotypes and disease progression to those observed in human ALS patients (Gurney, 1994; Nagai et al., 2001; Howland et al., 2002).

The mechanism underlying motor neuron death in ALS is still unknown. However, SOD1 mutant induces non-cell-autonomous motor neuron killing by an unknown gain of toxicity, which means the gain of toxicity arises from damage to cells other than motor neurons (Boillée et al., 2006a). Multiple mechanisms account for the selective vulnerability of motor neurons including protein misfolding, mitochondrial dysfunction, oxidative damage, defective axonal transport, excitoxicity, insufficient growth factor signaling, and inflammation (Boillée et al., 2006a). Of course there are a lot of shortcomings for using

G93A and other SOD1 transgenic rodent models as SOD1 mutation is only found in a small proportion of human ALS patients. However, it is still an excellent tool for ALS researchers as transgenic mice have proven to be one of the most useful tools to understand the complexity of neurodegenerative diseases because of their usefulness to unveil underlying mechanisms of the disease and evaluating potential treatments (Rothstein, 2004). In this review we will overview the extensive use of SOD1 transgenic rodent models in ALS research and how those findings can be transferred to treat human ALS patients.

1.2 Chapter overview

Topics covered in this chapter include growth factor therapy and stem cell therapy for ALS. For growth factor therapy, we will introduce different delivery methods and injection sites. As for stem cell transplantation therapy, we will look into strategies that aim to replace or protect motor neurons. After that, we will summarize studies that utilize stem cells as a tool to deliver growth factors. We will conclude the chapter by looking forward to future development in the field.

2. Growth factors and gene therapy in ALS

2.1 Growth factors and the nervous system

Growth factors are a class of naturally occurring proteins that are capable of stimulating cell growth, proliferation, and differentiation. In development of the nervous system, they are crucial because they are essential for neuronal survival and differentiation. For adults, they are also required in some cases to maintain normal function of the nervous system, but only at very low levels. However, the presence of low levels of growth factors in adult tissues is critical because motor neurons rely on them for survival and repair upon stress and injury. Experiments have been performed to investigate the effect of growth factors on alleviating the symptoms of ALS. Those growth factors includes glial cell line-derived neurotrophic factor (GDNF), insulin growth factor 1 (IGF-1), vascular endothelial growth factor (VEGF), and brain derived neurotrophic factor (BDNF). For each of the growth factors listed above, there are studies on hSOD1-G93A transgenic rodent models that show some degree of improvement, which includes some or all of the following: delay onset, slow disease progression, decrease motor neuron loss, preserve neuromuscular junction and prolong survival.

2.2 Strategies of growth factor delivery

2.2.1 Methods of delivery

Currently, three different methods of have been used to deliver the growth factor into the motor nervous system to ALS patients or rodent models. The first is subcutaneous injection of the growth factor protein. The obvious advantage of this method is the ease and simplicity to administrate. Some growth factors are pharmaceutically available to treat other neurodevelopmental diseases, such as IGF-1 to treat IGF deficiency in children. This is the reason why it is the only method of delivery that has been tested on human ALS patients. However, a statistically significant result has not been observed in this method of delivery. The only successful case is the North American study on IGF-1 in 1997 (Lai et al., 1997), but was immediately challenged by an almost identical study in Europe in 1998 (Borasio et al., 1998) and other later studies. The failure of this classical method of delivery to alleviate ALS symptoms includes (i) inability of some of the chemical of interest to pass the blood-brain barrier; (ii) unwanted side effects in non-targeted sites, and (iii) a relative short half-life of the protein. The significance of these issues is amplified in the human nervous system because of greater cross-sectional area when compared to rodents. Further penetration is needed for the injected growth factor to reach the deep structure in the brain or spinal cord to give its desired effect. Similar issues are found in clinical trials for patients with Parkinson's disease using the same strategy to deliver growth factors.

The second method is to deliver the chemical of interest by implanting a catheter directly into the site of the brain that needs the growth factor, as seen in a couple Parkinson's disease studies (Gill et al., 2003; Slevin et al., 2005). It is better than the previous method as it overcomes the distance problem seen in large animals. However, there are a couple of drawbacks if this is applied to ALS patients to deliver the growth factor into the spinal cord instead of the brain for Parkinson's disease. The implanted catheter might interrupt the ascending and/or descending white matter track, and the natural movement of the spinal cord in patients increase the shearing forces may cause further damage. Therefore catheter delivery would not be a desirable method of ALS growth factor delivery.

The last approach uses viral vectors to circumvent all those issues. Those viruses include lentivirus (Cisterni et al., 2000; Hottinger et al., 2000; Azzouz et al., 2004), adenovirus (Acsadi et al., 2002; Hasse et al., 2007), and adeno-associated virus (AAV) (Kasper et al., 2003; Wang et al., 2002). They are used because of the ability to deliver genes to non-dividing cells, which includes mature neurons. Thus they are ready to be engineered to encode the therapeutic protein. Extensive studies of AAV delivery of potential drugs to specific brain regions have been published, suggesting viral vector delivery is a practical method.

2.2.2 Sites of delivery

Studies have been done to inject vectors encoding the growth factor of interest into two distinctive types of tissues: (i) limb/respiratory muscles and (ii) the connecting motor neurons. In most ALS studies the vectors are injected in the muscle. Although positive results are shown in studies with GDNF and IGF-1, researchers believes that motor neurons may detach from the muscle at early stages of the disease (Fischer et al., 2004), or the cellular transport mechanism is heavily impaired (Williamson & Cleveland, 1999; De Vos et al., 2007). Again due to their large cross-sectional area, retrograde transport is more severely affected in larger mammals when compared to mice, and thus requires a longer distance of transport. This factor may slow the translation of this successful strategy to clinical trials.

To overcome the potential problems of retrograde transport that may be encountered in muscle injections in humans, studies that inject vectors directly to motor neurons within spinal cord has been performed. Surprisingly, only a few studies have been published on this approach and the effect is less significant than the muscle injection studies. In a GDNF study on ALS mice, neuroprotection is only seen on facial but not lumbar motor neurons (Guillot, 2004). Another study supports the above idea by showing that GDNF is neuroprotective when it is overexpressed in skeletal muscles, but has no effect when the growth factor is overexpressed in motor neurons (Li et al., 2007). Disease progression is only slowed when GDNF is expressed in skeletal muscles, but not when it is expressed in the motor neurons.

2.3 Insights from growth factor studies to understand ALS disease progression

Although the ultimate goal of growth factor therapy for ALS is to alleviate symptoms, prolong survival, delay onset, and slow disease progression, during the course of investigation several interesting findings have been observed and may provide insights to better understand the underlying mechanism of the disease. For example, finding growth factors' targets may help us find how the disease is initiated. Currently, the growth factors' targets are not fully known. It could be the degenerating motor neuron itself, the neighboring neuron, or surrounding glial cells. But a recent report about wild type non-neuronal cells extending survival of SOD1 mutant motor neurons in chimeric ALS mice (Clement et al., 2003) may provide adequate evidence showing that the growth factor's target is the supporting glia instead of neurons.

Another point of interest is the similarity of the growth factors that have been used. All GDNF, IGF-1, VEGF, and BDNF interact with receptor tyrosine kinases to produce downstream effects. Experiments have shown that those growth factors indeed work in a similar pathway and mechanism as there is no additional improvement observed when they work in combination (IGF-1 and VEGF) as compared to working individually (Dodge et al. 2010). Another article reports that VEGF promotes motor neuron survival by blocking Caspase through Phosphoinositide 3-kinase/ protein kinase B (PI3K/Akt) pathway (Lunn et al., 2009). Further investigation on the PI3K/Akt pathway may provide clues on how motor neuron death is triggered in ALS.

3. Stem cell therapy for ALS

3.1 The motor neuron replacement strategy

As motor neuron loss is the key diagnostic feature of ALS, the most straightforward strategy is to derive motor neurons from various types of stem cells and try to use them to replace the dead motor neurons in patients. For adult stem cells, cells expressing neuron and glial lineage markers were successfully derived from trans-differentiation of human umbilical cord blood cells (McGuckin et al., 2004) and mouse bone marrow stem cells (Croft et al. 2006). However, those cells' electrophysiological properties, survival, differentiation, and efficacy of integration to functional neurons and glial cells either *in vitro* or *in vivo* were not tested. Neural stem cells are the only type of adult stem cells which have successfully derived motor neurons that are functional *in vivo* (Gao et al., 2005). Human neural stem cells, which are scarce in the human body, are usually derived from embryonic stem cells or fetal brain tissues (Tai & Svendsen, 2004).

More promising results were shown in experiments using pluripotent stem cells. From mouse embryonic stem (ES) cells, motor neurons were successfully generated by induction of developmentally relevant signaling factors. The derived cells survive when transplanted into chick embryonic spinal cord, extend axons, and exhibit signs of presynaptic specialization when reaching targeted muscles (Wichterle et al., 2002). Another study shows that those cells possess immunohistochemical and electrophysiological features of normal motor neurons (Miles et al., 2004). Similar to mouse ES cells, human ES cells have been reported to form functional neurons (Li et al., 2005; Lee et al., 2007).

Functional motor neurons can also be derived from human induced pluripotent stem (iPS) cells, a possible alternative that may avoid the ethical concerns for the use of human ES cells (Karumbayaram et al., 2009). iPS cells are somatic cells that are reprogrammed into pluripotent stem cells (Yu et al., 2007; Takahashi, 2007), with great similarity to embryonic stem cells. They are capable of deriving patient-specific differentiated cells like neurons and glia, which allows them to potentially be used for autologous cell replacement in ALS patients. iPS cells have been generated from ALS patients and the cells are capable of differentiating into motor neurons

(Dimos, 2008). However, introduction of new genes during the production of iPS cells may give rise to additional technical concerns when translating to clinical studies.

Mouse ES-derived motor neurons reportedly grow around the ventral horn when transplanted into the spinal cord of rats with impaired motor neurons (Harper et al., 2004). In combination with chemicals that overcome myelin-mediated repulsion and GDNF that stimulates axon guidance towards skeletal muscles, further improvement in survival and engraftment of the transplanted cells was observed. Improvement in motor function of the paralyzed rats was also observed (Despande et al., 2006).

Despite the excitement that these transplantation studies brings to the field, the fact that these studies were performed on static models of motor neuron loss does not guarantee success in progressive motor neuron diseases like ALS. In addition, in order for the motor neuron replacement strategy to be successful, the transplanted motor neuron will first need to receive synaptic input from the presynaptic neurons and extend it's axon all the way to the targeted muscle at a rate of 1-3 mm/day, which takes months to years in humans, before innervation to the targeted muscle can be possible (Papadeas & Maragakis, 2009). Therefore motor neuron replacement may not be a legitimate treatment at this moment.

3.2 The neuroprotection strategy

3.2.1 Non-cell autonomous nature of motor neuron death in ALS

Previously, little attention has been paid to the function of glial cells in the nervous system. However, we now know that glial cells modulate neuronal functions such as glutamate uptake, synaptic plasticity, trophic factor support, and even neuronal transmission (Kirchhoff et al., 2001). Studies also show that motor neuron death in ALS is non-cell autonomous, or mediated by astrocytes and microglia (Hall et al., 1998; Barbeito et al., 2004). Researchers also hypothesize that astrocytes and/or microglia form a positive feedback loop with motor neurons that leads to further propagation of the disease (Rao & Weiss, 2004). Moreover, chimeric mice with increased proportion of healthy, wild type glial cells increase survival of nearby human SOD1 mutant neurons *in vivo* (Clement et al., 2003). Using a CRE-lox system, selective reduction of the mutant gene in microglia and astrocytes in SOD1 transgenic mice slows disease progression, but has no effect on disease onset (Boillée et al., 2006b; Yamanaka et al., 2008).

Additional evidence is provided by stem cell-derived motor neurons/astrocytes co-culture. A study in 2007 shows that primary and ES cell-derived motor neurons are complementary in an *in vitro* motor neuron/astrocytes study for ALS (Nagai et al., 2007). From then on, studies using the following combinations have been performed: hES cell derived motor neurons with primary hSOD1-G93A or wild type mouse primary astrocytes (Di Giorgio et al. 2008); hSOD1-G93A mouse ES derived motor neuron with hSOD1-G93A derived mouse primary astrocytes (Di Giorgio 2007); and hES cells derived motor neuron with primary human astrocytes transfected with hSOD1-G47R genes (Marchetto, 2008). The Marchetto paper also uses that approach to verify a potential drug that has been beneficial in ALS rodent models. The success in this approach provides an easily accessible *in vitro* testing platform for cell-cell interactions in ALS and underlying disease mechanisms. Drug discovery will also accelerate as high throughput drug screening can be performed on the cultures.

3.2.2 Astrocyte replacement

Based on non-cell autonomous nature of motor neuron death in ALS, astrocyte replacement is another feasible strategy for ALS stem cell therapy. Researchers transplant glial restricted precursor (GRP) cells (lineage-restricted as derived from developing spinal cord) focally to cervical spinal cord that controls respiratory function in SOD1 rats (Lepore et al., 2008). The effect of the GRP transplant is significant: GRP cells survive and differentiated into mature astrocytes *in vivo.* The treatment also reduces microgliosis, prolongs survival, ameliorates motor neuron loss, and slows motor function decline. The group also found that the ALS rats with grafted GRP cells maintain normal level of glutamate transporter (GLT-1), an astrocyte-specific protein that has reduced expression in both ALS model rats and human patients (Howland et al., 2002; Rothstein et al., 1995). This may provide further evidence that astrocyte replacement is a sound strategy for ALS cell therapy.

3.2.3 Immunomodulation

Other than replacement strategies, some stem cell therapies modulate the immunological environment around the degenerating motor neurons to prevent them from dying. Bone marrow cells provide a rich source of mesenchymal stem cells (MSCs) and hematopoietic stem cells (HSCs). HSCs can give rise to a great variety of blood cells and cells in the immune system, but will particularly differentiate into microglia when introduced to the nervous system (Vitry et al., 2003). MSCs do not have the ability to differentiate into cells in the nervous system, but contribute to improved locomotion by differentiating into cells in the skeletal muscle lineage (Corti et al., 2004). Bone marrow transplanted into irradiated $SOD1^{G93A}/PU1^{-/-}$ double mutants (born without microglia and peripheral immune cells) prolonged survival and slowed disease progression (Beers et al., 2006). Another similar experiment confirms the result (Corti et al., 2004). This led to clinical trials of MSC and HSC transplants to sporadic ALS patients (Appel et al., 2008; Mazzini et al., 2008). Some of these studies show promising results **(Table 1)**.

3.3 Protective effect of neural stem cell and other cells in the neural lineage

Although most transplantations involving cells in the neural lineage were aimed at replacement of motor neurons, researchers now find that neuro-protection was instead the main effect. Various cell transplantations have been performed on hSOD1-G93A rodent models. They include: i) human embryonic germ cell delivered to cerebral spinal fluid (Kerr et al., 2003); ii) human neural stem cells grafted into the spinal cord (Yan et al., 2006); iii) hNT neurons derived from a human teratocarcinoma cell line grafted into spinal cord (Garbuzova-Davis et al., 2002); mouse Sertoli cells into parenchyma (Hemendinger et al., 2005); and human umbilical cord blood cells transfused into the systemic circulation (Habisch et al., 2007). In each of the cases, there was some degree of positive effect on motor neuron survival and life span of the animals. In addition, in most cases the positive effect is related to growth factor release (Suzuki & Svendsen, 2008). However, these studies do not specify which cell types are eventually exerting the protective effect or releasing the growth factors, though they are expected to be astrocytes (See Section 3.2 of this chapter). However, one human neural stem cell (NSC) transplant study suggests that the neuroprotective effect of host motor neurons stems from the ability of NSCs to differentiate into neuronal subtypes other than motor neurons such as GABAergic neurons that forms synaptic connection between grafted and host motor neurons (Xu et al., 2009). These neurons may provide additional benefits other than that from glial cells.

Cell type	Subject	Injection Site	Effect	Paper
Mouse GRP	hSOD1-G93A rats	bilateral cervival spinal cord injection	cells survive and differentiated into mature astrocytes; reduces microgliosis; prolongs survival, ameliorates motor neuron loss and slows down motor function decline; normal GLT-1 level	Lepore et al. 2008
Mouse bone marrow cell	hSOD1-G93A /PU1-/- double mutant mice	i.p. injection	cells effectively differentiated into microglia cells; prolongs survival; suppressed cytotoxicity; restore glial activation	Beers et al. 2006
Mouse Bone marrow transplant	hSOD1-G93A mice	i.p. injection	delayed onset, increase life span	Corti et al. 2004
Human embryonic germ cell	rats with diffused motor neuron injury	i.c.v injection (CSF)	cells distributed extensively over the rostrocaudal length of the spinal cord and migrated into the spinal cord parenchymal partially recovered motor function 12 and 24 weeks after transplantation	Kerr et al. 2003
hNT cell	hSOD1-G93A mice	L4-L5 segments of the ventral horn spinal cord	delay onset, prolong survival,	Garbuzova-Davis et al. 2002
Mouse Sertoli cell	hSOD1-G93A	unilateral spinal injection into the L4-L5 ventral horn	significant increase in motor neuron survival; no effect on disease onset and progression	Hemendiner et al. 2005
Neuroectodermal derivatives of hUBS (hUBS-NSCs)	hSOD1-G93A	direct injection into the CSF (the cisterna magna).	No effect	Habisch et al. 2007

Cell type	Subject	Injection Site	Effect	Paper
hUBC	hSOD1-G93A mice	i.v. injection	reduce microgliosis; increased lifespan; delayed disease progrssion	Garbuzova-Davis et al. 2008
hNPC-GDNF	hSOD1-G93A rats	Unilateral lumbar spinal cord injection	Robust migration of the transplanted cells into the degenerating region; efficient delivery of GDNF as well as preservation of a large proportion of motor neurons; no continued innervations of motor neuron to the skeletal muscle end plates, no effect on ipsilateral hind limb function.	Suzuki et al. 2007
hMSC-GDNF	hSOD1-G93A rats	Skeletal muscles	Transplanted cells survive within host skeletal muscles and release GDNF; significant increase in neuromuscular junctions; improves motor neuron survival	Suzuki et al. 2008
CD34+ HSCs, HLA-matched sibling donors	ALS patients	i.v. injection	No clinical benefits	Appel et al. 2008
Autologous bone marrow derived MSCs	ALS patients	multiple thoracic spinal cord injection	Decelerated linear decline of the forced vital capacity and of the ALS-FRS score in some patients	Mazzini et al. 2010
Autologous CD133+ cells	ALS patients	bilateral injection into frontal motor cortex	lives 47 months more than the control group	Martinez et al. 2009

Table 1. Stem Cell Trials for ALS GRP. Glial restricted precursor; hUBC: human umbilical cord blood cells; NSCs: neural stem cells; hNPC: human neural progenitor cell; hMSC: human mesenchymal stem cell; HSCs: hematopoietic stem cells.

4. Working in combination: Genetically engineered stem cells as a tool of growth factor delivery for ALS

We have introduced two successful strategies for slowing ALS disease progression in the previous sections of this chapter. Although both of them in some degree involve the release of neuroprotective growth factors, both strategies have their shortcomings. In viral delivery of growth factors, the cells still carry the mutant SOD1 gene or has the disease phenotype. Therefore the cells that are delivering the treatment are indeed still doing harm on the surrounding cells at the same time. On the other hand, neuroprotective strategy of stem cell transplants, though increases the proportion of wild type (normal) cells around the injection site(s), the transplanted cells may not naturally produce the desired neuroprotective growth factors in a pharmaceutically adequate amount (Gonzalez, 2009). Therefore, it is reasonable for us to combine the two strategies and see if they can complement each other and produce a great synergic effect.

4.1 hNPC-GDNF injection to spinal cord

Based on the logic above, our group genetically engineered human neural progenitor cells (hNPC) that express and secrete GDNF through lentiviral infection (Klein et al., 2005; Suzuki et al., 2007). hNPC are comprised of multiple classes of neural stem cells and lineage-restricted precursors. They are isolated from fetal brain cortical tissue (Svendsen et al., 1996; Keyoung et al., 2001; Tamaki et al., 2006; Suslov, 2002) and can be maintained for over 50 weeks in the presence of mitogen while retaining the ability to differentiate into astrocytes (Wright et al, 2003). With their special properties, hNPC can thus serve as "mini-pumps" to provide glial replacement and deliver trophic factors through transplantation into specific sites in the brain and spinal cord of diseased animals and patients. hNPC-GDNF were transplanted to the lumbar region of the spinal cord of hSOD1-G93A rats. We observed robust migration of the transplanted cells into the degenerating region, efficient delivery of GDNF, as well as preservation of a large proportion of motor neurons at both early and late stages of the disease within chimeric regions (Suzuki et al. 2007). However, the preservation of motor neurons does not accompany with continued innervations of motor neuron to the skeletal muscle end plates, thus had no effect on ipsilateral hind limb function.

4.2 hMSC-GDNF injection to skeletal muscles

Skeletal muscles clearly play an important role in guiding and attracting the developing neurons; and provide trophic support to maintain motor neuron function (Dobrowolny et al., 2005). A previous study showed that transplants of genetically engineered myoblasts (a kind of skeletal muscle precursor which has the ability to fuse with mature myofibers) secreting GDNF ameliorates motor neuron loss in ALS mice (Mohajeri et al., 1999). Thus we genetically engineered human MSCs (hMSCs) that express and secrete GDNF and transplanted them to three muscle groups in hSOD1-G93A rats (Suzuki et al., 2008). MSCs can be easily obtained from bone marrow from donations and have the ability to differentiate into the skeletal muscle lineage (Caplan & Arnold, 2009). The transplanted cells survives in the host skeletal muscle and releases GDNF. Moreover, it significantly increases the number of functional neuromuscular junctions and improves motor neuron survival in spinal cord at the mid-stage of disease. Furthermore, intramuscular hMSC-GDNF transplantation remarkably prolongs disease progression, increasing overall life span up to 28 days, which is one of the greatest improvements ever observed in familial ALS model rats.

4.3 Future research directions

From the two sets of experiments described in this section, we can conclude that stem cell delivery of growth factors is an effective strategy for ALS treatment. We also know that different sets of delivery tools are needed for the motor neuron cell bodies in the spinal cord and their synaptic connections to the skeletal muscles. Our current knowledge leads us to an initial thought for future development of the field of ALS growth factor/stem cell therapy. Motor neuron cell body protection will be provided by stem cell derived wild type astrocytes and microglia (from hNPC for example); while synaptic/axonal protection will be provided by stem cell derived myoblasts (from hMSC for example). Those cells will be genetically modified to enhance delivery of neurotrophic factors. Lastly, GDNF is only one of the many neurotrophic factors that showed to have beneficial effect on ALS rodent models as mentioned in Section 2 of this chapter. We expect there will soon be tests on the other neurotrophic factors.

5. Clinical translation

Despite the exciting breakthroughs in stem cell research aiming to treat ALS, there is still a long way to go to translate those successes to the clinic and help patients. Since we are still uncertain about the fate of stem cells after transplantation, thorough safety tests are needed. Then, optimal cell dose, source of cells, stage of cells, route of delivery, injection sites, and immunosuppressive regimen (to ensure grafted cell survival in host) will need to be determined as well (Papadeas and Margaskis, 2009).

Clinical trials that involve stem cells on ALS patients are in the initial stage. In 2010 the phrase I clinical trial of hMSC transplantation performed in Italy was reported. (Mazzini et. al., 2010) Autologous MSC isolated from bone marrow derived cells were transplanted to the thoracic region of 9 ALS patients. Neither adverse effect nor significant improvement was found. However, it provides initial evidence that MSC injection is safe. Large volume (1 mL) of cells can be infused to the spinal cord without causing observable defects.

Neuralstem and Emory ALS center have begun the phase I trial of spinal cord derived stem cells for patients with ALS. The advantages of using neural stem cells derived from human fetal spinal cord are no tumor formation and minimal HLA (human leukocyte antigen) expression, thus, resulting in a low overall antigenicity of the cells. The first surgery of the trial took place a year ago, and the 9th surgery was performed earlier in 2011, without the need for patients to be on ventilators or to be taken to intensive care post-operation. The trial was staged, first enrolling non-ambulatory patients, and the first ambulatory patient was enrolled early 2011.

6. Conclusion

In this chapter, we introduced the current application of stem cells in ALS (summarized in Figure 1). There are three points we should keep in mind about this topic. First, stem cell therapy design should be aimed at neuroprotection rather than motor neuron replacement. Motor neuron replacement is technically difficult to achieve. Also, in theory it will not bring much improvement to the patients because the evidence shows that glial cells are the actual determinant of ALS disease progression. Secondly, combining stem cell transplantation and growth factor delivery provides the best result in slowing disease progression and prolonging survival, as the two greatly complement each other. Finally, we are now convinced that injections of stem cells in multiple sites are needed in order to alleviate symptoms of ALS. There should be at least one injection that focuses on protecting cell bodies of motor neurons and another that aims to maintain neuromuscular connections. To sum up, stem cell applications have made a lot of contributions to ALS research and have great potential to bring breakthroughs to the field in the near future.

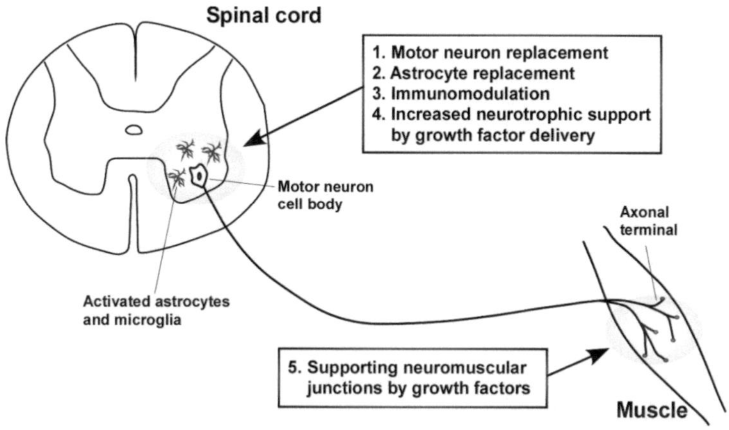

Fig. 1. Schematic illustration of possible stem cell interventions for ALS therapies. These could include: (1) Motor neuron replacement, differentiation of neural progenitor cells to motor neurons and projection to the periphery; (2) Differentiation and replacement of dysfunctional astrocytes; (3) Modulation of immunological environment around the degenerating motor neuron; (4) Trophic/growth factor delivery via stem cells to provide neuroprotective support for the endogenous populations; (5) Local delivery of growth factors to support neuromuscular junctions and axon integrity.

7. Acknowledgment

This work was support by grants from the ALS association, NIH/NINDS (R21NS06104), the University of Wisconsin Foundation, and the Les Turner ALS Foundation.

8. References

Acsadi G, Anguelov RA, Yang H, Toth G, Thomas R, Jani A, Wang Y, Ianakova E, Mohammad S, Lewis RA & Shy ME. (2002) Increased survival and function of SOD1 mice after glial cell-derived neurotrophic factor gene therapy. *Hum Gene Ther.* 2002 Jun 10; Volume 13(9); Pages 1047-59.

Appel SH, Engelhardt JI, Henkel JS, Siklos L, Beers DR, Yen AA, Simpson EP, Luo Y, Carrum G, Heslop HE, Brenner MK & Popat U. (2008) Hematopoietic stem cell transplantation in patients with sporadic amyotrophic lateral sclerosis. *Neurology.* 2008 Oct 21; Volume 71(17); Pages 1326-34.

Azzouz M, Ralph GS, Storkebaum E, Walmsley LE, Mitrophanous KA, Kingsman SM, Carmeliet P & Mazarakis ND. (2004) VEGF delivery with retrogradely transported lentivector prolongs survival in a mouse ALS model. *Nature.* 2004 May 27; Volume 429(6990); Pages 413-7.

Barbeito LH, Pehar M, Cassina P, Vargas MR, Peluffo H, Viera L, Estévez AG & Beckman JS. (2004) A role for astrocytes in motor neuron loss in amyotrophic lateral sclerosis. *Brain Res Brain Res Rev.* 2004 Dec; Volume 47(1-3): Pages 263-74.

Beers DR, Henkel JS, Xiao Q, Zhao W, Wang J, Yen AA, Siklos L, McKercher SR & Appel SH. (2006) Wild-type microglia extend survival in PU.1 knockout mice with familial amyotrophic lateral sclerosis. *Proc Natl Acad Sci U S A.* 2006 Oct 24; Volume 103(43); Pages 16021-6.

Boillée S, Vande Velde C & Cleveland DW. (2006a) ALS: a disease of motor neurons and their nonneuronal neighbors. *Neuron.* 2006 Oct 5; Volume 52(1): Pages 39-59.

Boillée S, Yamanaka K, Lobsiger CS, Copeland NG, Jenkins NA, Kassiotis G, Kollias G & Cleveland DW. (2006b) Onset and progression in inherited ALS determined by motor neurons and microglia. *Science.* 2006 Jun 2; Volume 312(5778); Pages 1389-92.

Borasio GD, Robberecht W, Leigh PN, Emile J, Guiloff RJ, Jerusalem F, Silani V, Vos PE, Wokke JH & Dobbins T. (1998) A placebo-controlled trial of insulin-like growth factor-I in amyotrophic lateral sclerosis. European ALS/IGF-I Study Group. *Neurology.* 1998 Aug; Volume 51(2); Pages 583-6.

Brooks BR (1994) El escorial World Federation of Neurology criteria for the diagnosis of amyotrophic lateral sclerosis. *Journal of the Neurological Sciences.* Volume 124 (Supplement 1), 1994 July, Pages 96-107, ISSN 0022-510X

Brooks BR, Miller RG, Swash M & Munsat TL. (2000) World Federation of Neurology Research Group on Motor Neuron Diseases. El Escorial revisited: revised criteria for the diagnosis of amyotrophic lateral sclerosis. *Amyotroph Lateral Scler Other Motor Neuron Disord.* 2000 Dec; Volume 1(5); Pages 293-9.

Brown RH Jr. (1995) Superoxide dismutase in familial amyotrophic lateral sclerosis: models for gain of function. *Curr Opin Neurobiol.* 1995 Dec; Volume 5(6); Pages 841-6.

Caplan, Arnold I. (2009) Mesenchymal Stem Cell, In: *Essentials of Stem Cell Biology*, Robert Lanza, pp 485-496, Academic Press, ISBN 9780123747297, U. S. A.

Cisterni C, Henderson CE, Aebischer P, Pettmann B & Déglon N. (2000) Efficient gene transfer and expression of biologically active glial cell line-derived neurotrophic factor in rat motoneurons transduced wit lentiviral vectors. *J Neurochem.* 2000 May; Volume 74(5); Pages 1820-8.

Clement AM, Nguyen MD, Roberts EA, Garcia ML, Boillée S, Rule M, McMahon AP, Doucette W, Siwek D, Ferrante RJ, Brown RH Jr, Julien JP, Goldstein LS & Cleveland DW. (2003) Wild-type nonneuronal cells extend survival of SOD1 mutant motor neurons in ALS mice. *Science.* 2003 Oct 3; Volume 302(5642); Pages 113-7. Erratum in: *Science.* 2003 Oct 24; Volume 302(5645): Page 568.

Cleveland DW & Rothstein JD. (2001) From Charcot to Lou Gehrig: deciphering selective motor neuron death in ALS. *Nat Rev Neurosci.* 2001 Nov; Volume 2(11); Pages 806-19.

Croft AP & Przyborski SA. (2006) Formation of neurons by non-neural adult stem cells: potential mechanism implicates an artifact of growth in culture. *Stem Cells.* 2006 Aug; Volume 24(8); Pages 1841-51.

Corti S, Locatelli F, Donadoni C, Guglieri M, Papadimitriou D, Strazzer S, Del Bo R & Comi GP. (2004) Wild-type bone marrow cells ameliorate the phenotype of SOD1-G93A

ALS mice and contribute to CNS, heart and skeletal muscle tissues. *Brain.* 2004 Nov; Volume 127(Pt 11); Pages 2518-32..

Deshpande DM, Kim YS, Martinez T, Carmen J, Dike S, Shats I, Rubin LL, Drummond J, Krishnan C, Hoke A, Maragakis N, Shefner J, Rothstein JD & Kerr DA. (2006) Recovery from paralysis in adult rats using embryonic stem cells. *Ann Neurol.* 2006 Jul; Volume 60(1); Pages 32-44.

De Vos KJ, Chapman AL, Tennant ME, Manser C, Tudor EL, Lau KF, Brownlees J, Ackerley S, Shaw PJ, McLoughlin DM, Shaw CE, Leigh PN, Miller CC & Grierson AJ. (2007) Familial amyotrophic lateral sclerosis-linked SOD1 mutants perturb fast axonal transport to reduce axonal mitochondria content. *Hum Mol Genet.* 2007 Nov 15; Volume 16(22); Pages 2720-8.

Dimos JT, Rodolfa KT, Niakan KK, Weisenthal LM, Mitsumoto H, Chung W, Croft GF, Saphier G, Leibel R, Goland R, Wichterle H, Henderson CE & Eggan K. (2008) Induced pluripotent stem cells generated from patients with ALS can be differentiated into motor neurons. *Science.* 2008 Aug 29; Volume 321(5893); Pages 1218-21..

Di Giorgio FP, Carrasco MA, Siao MC, Maniatis T & Eggan K. (2007) Non-cell autonomous effect of glia on motor neurons in an embryonic stem cell-based ALS model. *Nat Neurosci.* 2007 May; Volume 10(5); Pages 608-14.

Di Giorgio FP, Boulting GL, Bobrowicz S & Eggan KC. (2008) Human embryonic stem cell-derived motor neurons are sensitive to the toxic effect of glial cells carrying an ALS-causing mutation. *Cell Stem Cell.* 2008 Dec 4; Volume 3(6): Pages 637-48.

Dobrowolny G, Giacinti C, Pelosi L, Nicoletti C, Winn N, Barberi L, Molinaro M, Rosenthal N & Musarò A. (2005) Muscle expression of a local Igf-1 isoform protects motor neurons in an ALS mouse model. *J Cell Biol.* 2005 Jan 17; Volume 168(2): Pages 193-9.

Dodge JC, Treleaven CM, Fidler JA, Hester M, Haidet A, Handy C, Rao M, Eagle A, Matthews JC, Taksir TV, Cheng SH, Shihabuddin LS & Kaspar BK. (2010) AAV4-mediated expression of IGF-1 and VEGF within cellular components of the ventricular system improves survival outcome in familial ALS mice. *Mol Ther.* 2010 Dec; Volume 18(12): Pages 2075-84.

Fischer LR, Culver DG, Tennant P, Davis AA, Wang M, Castellano-Sanchez A, Khan J, Polak MA & Glass JD. (2004) Amyotrophic lateral sclerosis is a distal axonopathy: evidence in mice and man. *Exp Neurol.* 2004 Feb; Volume 185(2) Pages 232-40.

Gao J, Coggeshall RE, Tarasenko YI, Wu P. (2005) Human neural stem cell-derived cholinergic neurons innervate muscle in motoneuron deficient adult rats. *Neuroscience.* 2005; Volume 131(2); Pages 257-62.

Garbuzova-Davis S, Willing AE, Milliken M, Saporta S, Zigova T, Cahill DW & Sanberg PR. (2002) Positive effect of transplantation of hNT neurons (NTera 2/D1 cell-line) in a model of familial amyotrophic lateral sclerosis. *Exp Neurol.* 2002 Apr; Volume 174(2): Pages 169-80. Erratum in: *Exp Neurol* 2002 Jun; Volume 175(2); Pages 451.

Garbuzova-Davis S, Sanberg CD, Kuzmin-Nichols N, Willing AE, Gemma C, Bickford PC, Rossi R, & Sanberg PR. (2008) Human umbilical cord blood treatment in a mouse model of ALS: optimization of cell dose. *PLoS One.* 2008 Jun; Volume 3(6); Page e2494.

Gill SS, Patel NK, Hotton GR, O'Sullivan K, McCarter R, Bunnage M, Brooks DJ, Svendsen CN & Heywood P. (2003) Direct brain infusion of glial cell line-derived neurotrophic factor in Parkinson disease. *Nat Med.* 2003 May; Volume 9(5); Pages 589-95.

Gonzalez, Rodolfo. (2009) Neural Stem Cells for Central Nervous System Repair, In: *Essentials of Stem Cell Biology*, Robert Lanza, pp 485-496, Academic Press, ISBN 9780123747297, U. S. A.

Guillot S, Azzouz M, Déglon N, Zurn A & Aebischer P. (2004) Local GDNF expression mediated by lentiviral vector protects facial nerve motoneurons but not spinal motoneurons in SOD1(G93A) transgenic mice. *Neurobiol Dis.* 2004 Jun; Volume 16(1); Pages 139-49.

Gurney ME. (1994) Transgenic-mouse model of amyotrophic lateral sclerosis. *N Engl J Med.* 1994 Dec 22; Volume 331(25); Pages 1721-2.

Haase G, Kennel P, Pettmann B, Vigne E, Akli S, Revah F, Schmalbruch H & Kahn A. (1997) Gene therapy of murine motor neuron disease using adenoviral vectors for neurotrophic factors. *Nat Med.* 1997 Apr; Volume 3(4); Pages 429-36.

Habisch HJ, Janowski M, Binder D, Kuzma-Kozakiewicz M, Widmann A, Habich A, Schwalenstöcker B, Hermann A, Brenner R, Lukomska B, Domanska-Janik K, Ludolph AC & Storch A. (2007) Intrathecal application of neuroectodermally converted stem cells into a mouse model of ALS: limited intraparenchymal migration and survival narrows therapeutic effects. *J Neural Transm.* 2007; Volume 114(11); Pages 1395-406.

Hall ED, Oostveen JA & Gurney ME. (1998) Relationship of microglial and astrocytic activation to disease onset and progression in a transgenic model of familial ALS. *Glia.* 1998 Jul; Volume 23(3); Pages 249-56.

Harper JM, Krishnan C, Darman JS, Deshpande DM, Peck S, Shats I, Backovic S, Rothstein JD & Kerr DA. (2004) Axonal growth of embryonic stem cell-derived motoneurons in vitro and in motoneuron-injured adult rats. *Proc Natl Acad Sci U S A.* 2004 May 4; Volume 101(18):Pages 7123-8.

Hemendinger R, Wang J, Malik S, Persinski R, Copeland J, Emerich D, Gores P, Halberstadt C & Rosenfeld J. (2005) Sertoli cells improve survival of motor neurons in SOD1 transgenic mice, a model of amyotrophic lateral sclerosis. *Exp Neurol.* 2005 Dec; Volume 196(2); Pages 235-43.

Hirtz D, Thurman DJ, Gwinn-Hardy K, Mohamed M, Chaudhuri AR & Zalutsky R. (2007) How common are the "common" neurologic disorders? *Neurology.* 2007 Jan 30; Volume 68(5); Pages 326-37.

Hottinger AF, Azzouz M, Déglon N, Aebischer P & Zurn AD. (2000) Complete and long-term rescue of lesioned adult motoneurons by lentiviral-mediated expression of glial cell line-derived neurotrophic factor in the facial nucleus. *J Neurosci.* 2000 Aug 1; Volume 20(15); Pages 5587-93.

Howland DS, Liu J, She Y, Goad B, Maragakis NJ, Kim B, Erickson J, Kulik J, DeVito L, Psaltis G, DeGennaro LJ, Cleveland DW & Rothstein JD. (2002) Focal loss of the glutamate transporter EAAT2 in a transgenic rat model of SOD1 mutant-mediated amyotrophic lateral sclerosis (ALS). *Proc Natl Acad Sci U S A.* 2002 Feb 5; Volume 99(3): Pages 1604-9.

Julien JP. (2001) Amyotrophic lateral sclerosis. unfolding the toxicity of the misfolded. *Cell.* 2001 Feb 23; Volume 104(4) Pages 581-91..

Karumbayaram S, Novitch BG, Patterson M, Umbach JA, Richter L, Lindgren A, Conway AE, Clark AT, Goldman SA, Plath K, Wiedau-Pazos M, Kornblum HL & Lowry WE. (2009) Directed differentiation of human-induced pluripotent stem cells generates active motor neurons. *Stem Cells.* 2009 Apr; Volume 27(4); Pages 806-11.

Kaspar BK, Lladó J, Sherkat N, Rothstein JD & Gage FH. (2003) Retrograde viral delivery of IGF-1 prolongs survival in a mouse ALS model. *Science.* 2003 Aug 8; Volume 301(5634); Pages 839-42.

Kerr DA, Lladó J, Shamblott MJ, Maragakis NJ, Irani DN, Crawford TO, Krishnan C, Dike S, Gearhart JD & Rothstein JD. (2003) Human embryonic germ cell derivatives facilitate motor recovery of rats with diffuse motor neuron injury. *J Neurosci.* 2003 Jun 15; Voluem 23(12); Pages 5131-40.

Keyoung HM, Roy NS, Benraiss A, Louissaint A Jr, Suzuki A, Hashimoto M, Rashbaum WK, Okano H & Goldman SA. (2001) High-yield selection and extraction of two promoter-defined phenotypes of neural stem cells from the fetal human brain. *Nat Biotechnol.* 2001 Sep; Volume 19(9); Pages 843-50.

Kirchhoff F, Dringen R & Giaume C. (2001) Pathways of neuron-astrocyte interactions and their possible role in neuroprotection. *Eur Arch Psychiatry Clin Neurosci.* 2001 Aug; Volume 251(4); Pages 159-69..

Klein SM, Behrstock S, McHugh J, Hoffmann K, Wallace K, Suzuki M, Aebischer P & Svendsen CN. (2005) GDNF delivery using human neural progenitor cells in a rat model of ALS. *Hum Gene Ther.* 2005 Apr; Volume 16(4); Pages 509-21.

Lai EC, Felice KJ, Festoff BW, Gawel MJ, Gelinas DF, Kratz R, Murphy MF, Natter HM, Norris FH & Rudnicki SA. (1997) Effect of recombinant human insulin-like growth factor-I on progression of ALS. A placebo-controlled study. The North America ALS/IGF-I Study Group. *Neurology.* 1997 Dec;Volume 49(6); Pages 1621-30.

Lee H, Shamy GA, Elkabetz Y, Schofield CM, Harrsion NL, Panagiotakos G, Socci ND, Tabar V & Studer L. (2007) Directed differentiation and transplantation of human embryonic stem cell-derived motoneurons. *Stem Cells.* 2007 Aug; Voluem 25(8); Pages 1931-9.

Lepore AC, Rauck B, Dejea C, Pardo AC, Rao MS, Rothstein JD & Maragakis NJ. (2008) Focal transplantation-based astrocyte replacement is neuroprotective in a model of motor neuron disease. *Nat Neurosci.* 2008 Nov; Volume 11(11): Pages 1294-301.

Li W, Brakefield D, Pan Y, Hunter D, Myckatyn TM & Parsadanian A. (2007) Muscle-derived but not centrally derived transgene GDNF is neuroprotective in G93A-SOD1 mouse model of ALS. *Exp Neurol.* 2007 Feb; Volume 203(2); Pages 457-71.

Li XJ, Du ZW, Zarnowska ED, Pankratz M, Hansen LO, Pearce RA & Zhang SC. (2005) Specification of motoneurons from human embryonic stem cells. *Nat Biotechnol.* 2005 Feb; Volume 23(2); Pages 215-21..

Lunn JS, Sakowski SA, Kim B, Rosenberg AA & Feldman EL. (2009) Vascular endothelial growth factor prevents G93A-SOD1-induced motor neuron degeneration. *Dev Neurobiol.* 2009 Nov; Volume 69(13); Pages 871-84.

Marchetto MC, Muotri AR, Mu Y, Smith AM, Cezar GG & Gage FH. (2008) Non-cell-autonomous effect of human SOD1 G37R astrocytes on motor neurons derived from human embryonic stem cells. *Cell Stem Cell.* 2008 Dec 4; Volume 3(6); Pages 649-57.

Martinez HR, Gonzalez-Garza MT, Moreno-Cuevas JE, Caro E, Gutierrez-Jimenez E & Segura JJ. (2009) Stem-cell transplantation into the frontal motor cortex in amyotrophic lateral sclerosis patients. *Cytotherapy.* 2009; Volume 11(1); Pages 26-34.

Mazzini L, Mareschi K, Ferrero I, Vassallo E, Oliveri G, Nasuelli N, Oggioni GD, Testa L & Fagioli F. (2008) Stem cell treatment in Amyotrophic Lateral Sclerosis. *J Neurol Sci.* 2008 Feb 15; Volume 265(1-2); Pages 78-83.

Mazzini L, Ferrero I, Luparello V, Rustichelli D, Gunetti M, Mareschi K, Testa L, Stecco A, Tarletti R, Miglioretti M, Fava E, Nasuelli N, Cisari C, Massara M, Vercelli R, Oggioni GD, Carriero A, Cantello R, Monaco F & Fagioli F. (2010) Mesenchymal stem cell transplantation in amyotrophic lateral sclerosis: A Phase I clinical trial. *Exp Neurol.* 2010 May; Volume 223(1); Pages 229-37.

McGuckin CP, Forraz N, Allouard Q & Pettengell R. (2004) Umbilical cord blood stem cells can expand hematopoietic and neuroglial progenitors in vitro. *Exp Cell Res.* 2004 May 1; Volume 295(2); Pages 350-9.

Miles GB, Yohn DC, Wichterle H, Jessell TM, Rafuse VF & Brownstone RM. (2004) Functional properties of motoneurons derived from mouse embryonic stem cells. *J Neurosci.* 2004 Sep 8; Volume 24(36); Pages 7848-58.

Mohajeri MH, Figlewicz DA & Bohn MC. (1999) Intramuscular grafts of myoblasts genetically modified to secrete glial cell line-derived neurotrophic factor prevent motoneuron loss and disease progression in a mouse model of familial amyotrophic lateral sclerosis. *Hum Gene Ther.* 1999 Jul 20; Volume 10(11): Pages1853-66.

Nagai M, Aoki M, Miyoshi I, Kato M, Pasinelli P, Kasai N, Brown RH Jr & Itoyama Y. (2001) Rats expressing human cytosolic copper-zinc superoxide dismutase transgenes with amyotrophic lateral sclerosis: associated mutations develop motor neuron disease. *J Neurosci.* 2001 Dec 1; Volume 21(23); Pages 9246-54.

Nagai M, Re DB, Nagata T, Chalazonitis A, Jessell TM, Wichterle H & Przedborski S. (2007) Astrocytes expressing ALS-linked mutated SOD1 release factors selectively toxic to motor neurons. *Nat Neurosci.* 2007 May; Volume 10(5); Pages 615-22.

Papadeas ST & Maragakis NJ. (2009) Advances in stem cell research for Amyotrophic Lateral Sclerosis. *Curr Opin Biotechnol.* 2009 Oct; Volume 20(5); Pages 545-51.

Rao SD & Weiss JH. (2004) Excitotoxic and oxidative cross-talk between motor neurons and glia in ALS pathogenesis. *Trends Neurosci.* 2004 Jan; Volume 27(1); Pages 17-23.

Rosen DR, Siddique T, Patterson D, Figlewicz DA, Sapp P, Hentati A, Donaldson D, Goto J, O'Regan JP, Deng HX, et al. (1993) Mutations in Cu/Zn superoxide dismutase gene are associated with familial amyotrophic lateral sclerosis. *Nature.* 1993 Mar 4; Volume 362(6415); Pages 59-62. Erratum in: *Nature.* 1993 Jul 22; Volume 364(6435); Page 362.

Rothstein JD, Van Kammen M, Levey AI, Martin LJ & Kuncl RW. (1995) Selective loss of glial glutamate transporter GLT-1 in amyotrophic lateral sclerosis. *Ann Neurol.* 1995 Jul; Volume 38(1): Pages 73-84.

Rothstein J. (2004) Preclinical studies: how much can we rely on?. *Amyotrophic Lateral Sclerosis & Other Motor Neuron Disorders* . September 2, 2004; Volume 5; Pages 22-25.

Slevin JT, Gerhardt GA, Smith CD, Gash DM, Kryscio R & Young B. (2005) Improvement of bilateral motor functions in patients with Parkinson disease through the unilateral intraputaminal infusion of glial cell line-derived neurotrophic factor. *J Neurosurg.* 2005 Feb; Volume 102(2); Pagees 216-22.

Suslov ON, Kukekov VG, Ignatova TN & Steindler DA. (2002) Neural stem cell heterogeneity demonstrated by molecular phenotyping of clonal neurospheres. *Proc Natl Acad Sci U S A.* 2002 Oct 29; Volume 99(22); Pages 14506-11.

Suzuki M, McHugh J, Tork C, Shelley B, Klein SM, Aebischer P, Svendsen CN. (2007) GDNF secreting human neural progenitor cells protect dying motor neurons, but not their projection to muscle, in a rat model of familial ALS. *PLoS One.* 2007 Aug 1; Volume 2(8).

Suzuki M & Svendsen CN. (2008) Combining growth factor and stem cell therapy for amyotrophic lateral sclerosis. *Trends Neurosci.* 2008 Apr; Volume 31(4): Pages 192-8.

Suzuki M, McHugh J, Tork C, Shelley B, Hayes A, Bellantuono I, Aebischer P & Svendsen CN. (2008) Direct muscle delivery of GDNF with human mesenchymal stem cells improves motor neuron survival and function in a rat model of familial ALS. *Mol Ther.* 2008 Dec; Volume 16(12); Pages 2002-10.

Svendsen CN, Clarke DJ, Rosser AE, Dunnett SB. (1996) Survival and differentiation of rat and human epidermal growth factor-responsive precursor cells following grafting into the lesioned adult central nervous system. *Exp Neurol.* 1996 Feb; Volume 137(2); Pages 376-88.

Tai YT & Svendsen CN. (2004) Stem cells as a potential treatment of neurological disorders. *Curr Opin Pharmacol.* 2004 Feb; Volume 4(1); Pages 98-104.

Tamaki S, Eckert K, He D, Sutton R, Doshe M, Jain G, Tushinski R, Reitsma M, Harris B, Tsukamoto A, Gage F, Weissman I & Uchida N. (2002) Engraftment of sorted/expanded human central nervous system stem cells from fetal brain. *J Neurosci Res.* 2002 Sep 15; Volume 69(6); Pages 976-86.

Takahashi K, Tanabe K, Ohnuki M, Narita M, Ichisaka T, Tomoda K & Yamanaka S. (2007) Induction of pluripotent stem cells from adult human fibroblasts by defined factors. *Cell.* 2007 Nov 30; Volume 131(5); Pages 861-72.

Ticozzi N, Tiloca C, Morelli C, Colombrita C, Poletti B, Doretti A, Maderna L, Messina S, Ratti A & Silani V. (2011) Genetics of familial Amyotrophic lateral sclerosis. *Arch Ital Biol.* 2011 Mar; Volume 149(1); Pages 65-82.

Vitry S, Bertrand JY, Cumano A & Dubois-Dalcq M. (2003) Primordial hematopoietic stem cells generate microglia but not myelin-forming cells in a neural environment. *J Neurosci.* 2003 Nov 19; Volume 23(33); Pages 10724-31.

Wang LJ, Lu YY, Muramatsu S, Ikeguchi K, Fujimoto K, Okada T, Mizukami H, Matsushita T, Hanazono Y, Kume A, Nagatsu T, Ozawa K & Nakano I. (2002) Neuroprotective effects of glial cell line-derived neurotrophic factor mediated by an adeno-associated virus vector in a transgenic animal model of amyotrophic lateral sclerosis. *J Neurosci.* 2002 Aug 15; Volume 22(16); Pages 6920-8.

Wichterle H, Lieberam I, Porter JA, Jessell TM. (2002) Directed differentiation of embryonic stem cells into motor neurons. *Cell.* 2002 Aug 9; Volume 110(3); Pages 385-97.

Williamson TL & Cleveland DW. (1999) Slowing of axonal transport is a very early event in the toxicity of ALS-linked SOD1 mutants to motor neurons. *Nat Neurosci.* 1999 Jan; Volume 2(1); Pages 50-6.

Wright LS, Li J, Caldwell MA, Wallace K, Johnson JA & Svendsen CN. (2003) Gene expression in human neural stem cells: effects of leukemia inhibitory factor. *J Neurochem.* 2003 Jul; Volume 86(1): Pages 179-95.

Xu L, Ryugo DK, Pongstaporn T, Johe K & Koliatsos VE. (2009) Human neural stem cell grafts in the spinal cord of SOD1 transgenic rats: differentiation and structural integration into the segmental motor circuitry. *J Comp Neurol.* 2009 Jun 1; Volume 514(4); Pages 297-309.

Yamanaka K, Chun SJ, Boillee S, Fujimori-Tonou N, Yamashita H, Gutmann DH, Takahashi R, Misawa H & Cleveland DW. (2008) Astrocytes as determinants of disease progression in inherited amyotrophic lateral sclerosis. *Nat Neurosci.* 2008 Mar; Volume 11(3); Pages 251-3.

Yan J, Xu L, Welsh AM, Chen D, Hazel T, Johe K & Koliatsos VE. (2006) Combined immunosuppressive agents or CD4 antibodies prolong survival of human neural stem cell grafts and improve disease outcomes in amyotrophic lateral sclerosis transgenic mice. *Stem Cells.* 2006 Aug; Volume 24(8); Pages 1976-85.

Yu J, Vodyanik MA, Smuga-Otto K, Antosiewicz-Bourget J, Frane JL, Tian S, Nie J, Jonsdottir GA, Ruotti V, Stewart R, Slukvin II & Thomson JA. (2007) Induced pluripotent stem cell lines derived from human somatic cells. *Science.* 2007 Dec 21; Volume 318(5858); Pages 1917-20.

Zoccolella S, Santamato A & Lamberti P. (2009) Current and emerging treatments for amyotrophic lateral sclerosis. *Neuropsychiatr Dis Treat.* 2009 May Pages 577-95. Epub 2009 Nov 16.

20

Glial Cells as Therapeutic Targets for ALS

Amanda M. Haidet-Phillips and Nicholas J. Maragakis
Department of Neurology, Johns Hopkins University, Baltimore, Maryland, USA

1. Introduction

Although Amyotrophic Lateral Sclerosis (ALS) is a neurodegenerative disease characterized by motor neuron death, recent studies now implicate the non-neuronal environment as a major contributor to motor neuron loss. This body of evidence has been amassed over the past 10-15 years and highlights glial cells as new therapeutic targets for ALS. Glial cells, once thought to be simply the "glue" of the central nervous system (CNS), are now realized to actively participate in neural transmission and serve complex roles in regulation of the CNS environment.

Several glial cell types including astrocytes, microglia, and oligodendrocytes exist in the CNS; each serves a distinct function. Astrocytes comprise the majority of the CNS cellular space and act to regulate neurotransmitter concentrations at synapses, provide trophic support for neurons, and maintain metabolic and ionic homeostasis. Astrocytes can participate in the immune response, however, microglia serve as the resident immune cell of the CNS. Microglia are mobile, phagocytic, and constantly screening the CNS for possible infection or injury. Upon activation, microglia can secrete pro-inflammatory cytokines and chemokines to promote the clearance of any infectious agents and recruit other immune cells to the site of injury. Depending on the stimuli, microglia also are known to release neurotrophic growth factors and anti-inflammatory molecules to aid in repair and resolution of neural damage. Oligodendrocytes are the myelinating glia of the CNS which intimately interact with, and provide metabolic support to neurons. Oligodendrocytes are capable of producing myelin sheaths which insulate axons and aid in the conduction of action potentials.

Ongoing research strives to define exactly how glial cells affect motor neuron survival in ALS. Furthermore, translation of these studies to the clinical setting begs for novel approaches to treat this new target for ALS.

2. Non-neuronal cells contribute to motor neuron death in ALS

The bulk of work on glial cells in ALS is derived from studies in rodent ALS models. The most widely used ALS models are rodents that ubiquitously express the human mutant superoxide dismutase 1 (SOD1) protein associated with dominantly-inherited familial ALS (fALS) (Gurney et al., 1994). Currently, 12 different SOD1 mutations have been expressed in lines of transgenic mice leading to development of motor neuron disease. By far, the most commonly used model is the SOD1 G93A mutant mouse which contains 25 copies of the

human SOD1 G93A transgene corresponding to a 10-15 fold increase in SOD1 protein (Chiu et al., 1995; Gurney et al., 1994). These mice develop a severe motor neuron disease which resembles many of the clinical and pathological features of human ALS. One of the first indications that non-neuronal cells were involved in disease came from studies where the mutant SOD1 gene was expressed only in neurons instead of ubiquitously. Lines of transgenic mice were generated where mutant SOD1 expression was driven by either the Thy1 promoter or neurofilament light chain promoter (Jaarsma et al., 2008; Lino et al., 2002; Pramatarova et al., 2001). In two of these three studies (Lino et al., 2002; Pramatarova et al., 2001), the mice did not develop any neurological disease phenotype leading to the hypothesis that mutant SOD1 must be expressed in multiple cell types to trigger ALS. A subsequent study did report motor neuron disease with neuronal mutant SOD1 expression, however, the disease onset was very late (~500 days of age) and highly variable, suggesting a possible contribution of mutant non-neuronal cells in disease (Jaarsma et al., 2008).
Further studies combining various approaches continue to support this hypothesis (Clement et al., 2003; Miller et al., 2005). To evaluate the contribution of mutant SOD1 expression in different cell populations, chimeric mice were generated from a mixture of wild-type cells and cells that expressed mutant SOD1 (Clement et al., 2003). It was observed that mice with a greater proportion of wild-type cells to mutant SOD1 cells had extended survival. In addition, motor neurons expressing mutant SOD1 that were surrounded by wild-type non-neuronal cells had less severe pathology. Likewise, wild-type motor neurons surrounded by non-neuronal cells expressing mutant SOD1 appeared to be degenerating, suggesting that neighboring non-neuronal cells may play a direct role in the death of MNs. To more directly discern the contribution of mutant SOD1 in motor neurons, transgenic mice were created where mutant SOD1 was removed by Hb9-driven cre recombinase solely in motor neurons. Although these mice have greatly reduced mutant SOD1 expression in motor neurons, they still develop motor neuron disease albeit a significant delay in disease onset (Boillee et al., 2006a). Furthermore, targeting only the motor neurons with an siRNA to reduce mutant SOD1 levels showed only a transient effect of motor neuron protection, suggesting that other cell types were contributing to the ultimate demise of motor neurons (Miller et al., 2005). Collectively, these studies suggest that ALS is a non-cell autonomous disease; non-neuronal mutant SOD1-expressing cells can directly cause wild-type motor neurons to exhibit a disease phenotype.

2.1 Astrocytes influence the course of disease in ALS

Specific populations of glial cells have been analyzed to determine their precise role in motor neuron death in ALS. Astrocytes are glial cells with diverse roles including regulation of the extracellular CNS environment, maintenance of cell-cell communication, CNS vascular control, growth factor production, and neurotransmitter metabolism (Maragakis & Rothstein, 2006). Astrocytes can also become reactive and proliferative in response to neuronal death or CNS injury. Indeed, reactive astrocytosis and inflammation are prominent features in both the human ALS spinal cord as well as in rodent ALS models. Moreover, astrocytes have long been suspected to exacerbate motor neuron death due to their reported loss of glial glutamate transporter 1 (GLT1) [excitatory amino acid transporter 2 (EAAT2) in humans](Bendotti et al., 2001; Bristol & Rothstein, 1996; Bruijn et al., 1997; Rothstein et al., 1995). GLT1 is a glutamate transporter responsible for removing 90% of the extrasynaptic glutamate to prevent continued neuronal firing. Increased levels of glutamate have been found in the cerebrospinal fluid of ALS patients (Rothstein et al., 1990; Shaw et al., 1995). Chronic reduction in glutamate uptake results in a buildup of extracellular glutamate, leading to increased neuronal synaptic transmission and excitotoxic neuronal death. The ALS-linked GLT1 loss is found in both human ALS and in several rodent models and signifies astrocyte pathology as consistent theme in ALS pathobiology. However, it is difficult to discern whether astrocytes become dysfunctional due to motor neuron degeneration or whether dysfunction is a secondary event in the disease course.

Recent studies aim to answer these questions by evaluating how mutant SOD1 expression in astrocytes affects disease course in the mutant SOD1 mouse model. In these sets of experiments, cre recombinase was driven using the GFAP promoter to excise the floxed mutant SOD1 gene solely in astrocytes. Depending on which SOD1 mutation was present, the reduction of mutant SOD1 in astrocytes either slows disease progression (SOD1 G37R)(Yamanaka et al., 2008b) or slows disease onset and progression (SOD1 G85R)(Wang et al., 2011). Microgliosis was reduced and astrocytic GLT1 expression was maintained in one study (Wang et al., 2011), however, the exact mechanism for prolonged survival in these mice is still undefined. Nevertheless, it seems that the mutant SOD1 protein directly causes astrocytes to become aberrant in the SOD1 mouse model and rescue of diseased astrocytes can significantly influence disease course. It is also interesting to note that complete ablation of proliferating mutant SOD1 astrocytes in the SOD1 mouse model does not affect any measure of motor neuron disease in these mice. Therefore, astrocyte proliferation itself or the presence of mutant SOD1 in the proliferating astrocyte population does not seem to contribute to motor neuron degeneration (Lepore et al., 2008a).

2.2 Microglia direct disease progression in ALS mouse models

In addition to astrocytes, microglia are another important glial cell type in ALS pathogenesis due to their phagocytic properties and capacity to produce a wide array of cytokines and chemokines, attracting other cells to the site of injury. Indeed, extensive microglial activation and proliferation characterizes sites of motor neuron injury in human ALS and rodent models and this microgliosis increases as disease worsens (Henkel et al., 2009). Interestingly, investigations are ongoing as to whether microglia are neuroprotective, neurotoxic, or situationally both in ALS.

To directly assess the role of mutant SOD1 in microglia of the SOD1 mouse model, two parallel studies sought to remove the mutant SOD1 G37R specifically from microglia in these transgenic mice. In one study, the floxed mutant SOD1 gene was excised from microglia using cre recombinase driven by the Cd11b promoter, removing the gene from microglia and peripheral macrophages only (Boillee et al., 2006b). In the other parallel study, microglia were genetically ablated in the mutant SOD1 mouse followed by reconstitution with wild-type microglia through a bone-marrow transplant (Beers et al., 2006). The result from both studies was a slowed disease progression resulting in a dramatic extension in life in these mice. More recently, an additional study also showed slowed disease progression when a different SOD1 mutant, SOD1 G85R, was excised by cre recombinase solely in microglia (Wang et al., 2009). Collectively, these studies suggest the presence of mutant SOD1 in microglia causes these cells to adopt a more neurotoxic phenotype and directly affects motor neuron survival in the mutant SOD1 mouse model.

Other studies suggest that microglia may actually play a neuroprotective role in motor neuron disease. Evidence from other disease and injury models indicates that as microglia become activated, they can adopt either an "M1" proinflammatory phenotype or an "M2" alternatively activated phenotype leading to secretion of anti-inflammatory cytokines and neurotrophic factors (Henkel et al., 2009). Although mutant SOD1 expression seems to cause microglia to lean toward proinflammatory M1 activation, microglia have also been shown to produce anti-inflammatory cytokines and neuroprotective growth factors during the early phase of disease in the ALS mice (Chiu et al., 2008). Interestingly, several studies have indicated that T cells directly influence microglial activation and their differentiation toward a neuroprotective or proinflammatory phenotype. When SOD1 G93A mice were bred with a strain of mice lacking T cells, disease course was accelerated and this worsening of disease was accompanied by a decrease in alternative M2 microglial activation, although astrocytosis remained unchanged (Chiu et al., 2008). In addition, increased numbers of regulatory T cells are associated with the stable phase of disease in both mice and ALS patients and these regulatory T cells can promote microglia to adopt an anti-inflammatory M2 phenotype (Beers et al., 2011). Over the course of disease, these regulatory T cells decrease in number accompanied by a shift in microglia from protective M2 to the proinflammatory M1 phenotype. Therefore, this evidence suggests microglia adopt an activated neuroprotective M2 phenotype during early disease, but then develop into proinflammatory M1 microglia as disease progresses. Therapeutic approaches that promote M2 microglial differentiation or maintenance may prove to be an alternative to the limitation of microglial activation.

2.3 The undefined role of oligodendrocytes and their progenitors in ALS

While focus has been on the involvement of neurons, astrocytes and microglia in ALS pathogenesis, a few studies have investigated other glial cell lineages as well. In particular, myelinating oligodendrocytes of the central nervous system and Schwann cells of the peripheral nervous system form intimate connections with motor neurons and their axons, promote neuronal health through production of neurotrophic factors, and aid in regeneration after neuronal injury. Surprisingly little is known about the role of Schwann cells and oligodendrocytes in ALS, although pathological aberrations in myelin have been reported along peripheral nerves in human patients (Perrie et al., 1993). As with glial inflammation, these myelin abnormalities may be primary or secondary to motor neuron degeneration. To specifically investigate whether mutant SOD1 alters Schwann cells, transgenic mice were created with SOD1 G93A expression restricted to myelinating Schwann cells using the myelin protein zero (P0) promoter (Turner et al., 2010). No evidence of motor neuron disease was observed in these mice, suggesting the mutant SOD1 protein is not detrimental to this Schwann cell population. In contrast, the specific removal of floxed mutant SOD1 in Schwann cells by P0-driven cre recombinase seems to modestly accelerate disease progression in the SOD1 G37R mice (Lobsiger et al., 2009). This curious disease acceleration is hypothesized to be a result of reducing SOD1's normal dismutase activity in Schwann cells, which may serve an unrealized neuroprotective function during the nerve regeneration process. Thus, a clear role of mutant SOD1-expressing Schwann cells has not been determined in rodent ALS models.

Another open question in the field is whether oligodendrocytes and their NG2+ progenitor cells directly affect motor neuron loss in ALS. To date, only one study has investigated how mutant SOD1 in oligodendrocytes influences motor neuron loss and the experimental design causes the results to be difficult to interpret. In this study, chimeric mice were created by mixing embryonic cells expressing SOD1 G37R with wild-type cells lacking the Olig1 transcription factor (Yamanaka et al., 2008a). The Olig1 -/- mice are unable to form motor neurons or oligodendrocytes. Therefore, the motor neurons and oligodendrocytes in the chimeric mice were generated from the mutant SOD1 G37R cells which have normal Olig1 levels. The result is a chimeric mouse with mutant motor neurons and oligodendrocytes, but with all other cells being a mixture of mutant and wild-type cells. These mice did not develop the motor neuron disease typical in the SOD1 G37R mouse model and the authors suggest that mutant SOD1 expression in oligodendrocytes is not a significant contributor to motor neuron degeneration. However, technical limitations prohibited verifying that all oligodendrocytes expressed the mutant SOD1 so it is difficult to draw a strong conclusion from these studies.

Interest in the oligodendrocyte progenitor cells, also called NG2+ cells, has risen in the ALS field due to recent reports of their aberrant proliferation in rodent models. These NG2+ cells are found widely throughout the CNS and are mitotically active, especially in areas of injury or neuronal degeneration. Although the specific functions of these cells is still under investigation, these NG2+ cells can divide and differentiate into myelinating oligodendrocytes, but not into astrocytes or neurons *in vivo* (Kang et al., 2010). Several studies have reported a dramatic (20-fold) increase in proliferation of NG2+ cells over the course of disease in ALS mouse models, with NG2+ cells contributing to over half of the total dividing cell population in the spinal cord of symptomatic mice (Kang et al., 2010; Lepore et al., 2008a; Magnus et al., 2008). Differentiation of these NG2+ cells into oligodendrocytes is also enhanced in mutant SOD1 mice compared to wild-type mice for reasons still unknown (Kang et al., 2010). It has been proposed that oligodendrocytes undergo degeneration in response to motor neuron loss and the NG2+ cell proliferation and differentiation is an attempt to restore these lost oligodendrocytes. However, it will be crucial to dissect what effects are primary and secondary to motor neuron loss and what role, if any, NG2+ cells play in disease course. Studies investigating how mutant SOD1 influences normal NG2+ cell behavior are warranted, including analysis of whether mutant SOD1 NG2+ cells share a similar non-cell autonomous toxicity as astrocytes and microglia.

2.4 Glial cell involvement in TDP43/FUS ALS?

A defining pathological feature in post-mortem ALS tissue is ubiquitin-positive inclusions within neurons and glia in the spinal cord, brainstem, and motor cortex. In patients with SOD1 mutations, these inclusions contain misfolded SOD1 protein (Bruijn et al., 1998). However, in ALS patients lacking SOD1 mutations, these inclusions contain one of two RNA/DNA binding proteins: TAR DNA-binding protein 43 (TDP43) or fused in sarcoma protein (FUS) (Kwiatkowski et al., 2009; Mackenzie et al., 2007; Neumann et al., 2006; Vance et al., 2009). Genetic analyses have also revealed disease-linked mutations in both TDP43 and FUS in subsets of familial and few sporadic ALS patients, adding to evidence that these proteins are involved in ALS pathogenesis (Kabashi et al., 2008; Kwiatkowski et al., 2009; Sreedharan et al., 2008; Vance et al., 2009). However, a major question that remains is whether glial cells play an active role in ALS disease caused by TDP43 or FUS mutations.

Animal models are in development to better understand pathological disease mechanisms in TDP43 and FUS ALS. Thus far, a number of rodent models have been described for TDP43 ALS and these models vary in the TDP43 mutations expressed and the promoter used to drive expression (Cohen et al., 2011). The phenotypes observed in these models have been somewhat perplexing due to the difficulties in dissecting the effects of human TDP43 protein overexpression from mutant-specific effects. Nonetheless, a common theme in these animals is neurodegeneration accompanied by neuronal cytoplasmic aggregates in affected regions. None of the models to this point have reported glial pathology other than an increase in gliosis at sites of neuronal injury which may be secondary to neuronal death. Likewise, in the first reported rodent model for FUS ALS, astrogliosis and microgliosis were the only noted glial-specific pathologies (Huang et al., 2011). In contrast, TDP43- and FUS-positive inclusions are found in glial cells in post-mortem ALS spinal cord and it is difficult to know whether these inclusions were overlooked in the early animal models or whether they represent a discrepancy between human ALS and rodent models (Mackenzie et al., 2010). Careful dissection of the effects of mutant TDP43 and FUS in astrocytes, microglia, and oligodendrocytes (as well as NG2+ progenitors) will be essential to determine whether the non-cell autonomous disease nature extensively noted in SOD1 ALS is also recapitulated in TDP43- and FUS-mediated ALS.

3. ALS disease modeling using glial cells

Transgenic mouse models have played a key role in elucidating how glial cells affect the disease course of ALS. There are obvious advantages to *in vivo* models; however, it is often difficult to dissect the specific contributions of various cell populations from other influences in the CNS milieu. In parallel with these *in vivo* studies, several groups have established novel *in vitro* ALS models that recapitulate the glial-mediated motor neuron toxicity observed in transgenic ALS mouse models. Most of these *in vitro* models involve a co-culture where wildtype motor neurons are co-cultured with mutant SOD1 glia or wild-type glia. The goal is to determine the direct effects of diseased glia on motor neurons. Furthermore, *in vitro* models allow for the study of human cells derived from ALS patients. Most studies striving to correlate work from the ALS rodent model with human ALS rely on post-mortem tissue analysis, which makes it difficult to sort out primary contributors to motor neuron loss from secondary effects caused by neurodegeneration and the inflammatory response in the endstage spinal cord. These *in vitro* models provide a unique avenue to study human ALS in real-time and evaluate therapeutics and disease mechanisms.

3.1 Motor neuron-glial cell co-cultures recapitulate glial-derived motor neuron damage

Transgenic models have shown that removing the mutant SOD1 gene in microglia reduces motor neuron loss in the mutant SOD1 mouse model (Beers et al., 2006; Boillee et al., 2006b). Similar work has recapitulated this motor neuron loss using primary microglia isolated from mutant SOD1 mice in a co-culture with motor neurons. These studies have demonstrated that mutant SOD1-expressing microglia are more neurotoxic compared to wild-type microglia (Beers et al., 2006; Weydt et al., 2004; Xiao et al., 2007) which is not surprising given that mutant SOD1 microglia release an array of toxic inflammatory factors including nitric oxide, reactive oxygen species, TNF-α, and IL-1 (Almer et al., 1999; Henkel et al., 2009; Hensley et al., 2003; Nguyen et al., 2001; Sasaki et al., 2000; Weydt et al., 2004; Xiao et al., 2007). Motor neurons co-cultured with mutant SOD1-expressing microglia show a reduction in the number and length of neurites and reduced survival in the co-culture paradigm (Xiao et al., 2007). In addition, microglia treated with extracellular mutant SOD1 protein become inflamed and damaging to motor neurons in co-culture (Urushitani et al., 2006; Zhao et al., 2010). The extracellular mutant SOD1 only caused motor neuron death when microglia were added into the culture, indicating the motor neuron damage was directly initiated by microglia (Zhao et al., 2010). These *in vitro* systems could provide a platform for testing therapeutics that could potentially block neurotoxic microglia. For example, *in vitro* treatment with IL-4 caused mutant SOD1-expressing microglia to differentiate from an "M1" proinflammatory phenotype to an "M2" neuroprotective phenotype and improved motor neuron survival in co-culture (Zhao et al., 2006). It remains to be determined whether IL-4 will have the same effect when delivered to microglia *in vivo*. More efforts have focused on studying aberrant astrocyte function in mutant SOD1-based *in vitro* ALS models. Several studies have demonstrated that astrocytes isolated from mutant SOD1 mice (Di Giorgio et al., 2007; Nagai et al., 2007) as well as astrocytes derived from neural stem cells from these mice (Dodge et al., 2008) are toxic to wild-type motor neurons in co-culture. In these studies, primary motor neurons as well as motor neurons derived from mouse embryonic stem cells were shown to die more quickly *in vitro* when cultured on top of SOD1 G93A astrocytes compared to wild-type astrocytes. It has also been recently shown that human motor neurons differentiated from embryonic stem cells are susceptible to the same astrocytes isolated from the SOD1 G93A mouse model (Di Giorgio et al., 2008). Furthermore, human motor neurons derived from embryonic stem cells die in the presence of human fetal primary astrocytes overexpressing mutant SOD1 by lentivirus (Marchetto et al., 2008). These *in vitro* models support that mutant SOD1-expressing astrocytes are toxic to motor neurons regardless of the species and provide a way to study familial ALS utilizing human cells. While these results have been exciting, no consistent pathway has been implicated in these *in vitro* studies for causing motor neuron death; however, one common finding is that the toxicity is transferred through the media, suggesting a secreted factor may be responsible. Future studies will hopefully identify the specific factor(s) involved in this toxicity.

3.2 ALS disease modeling using human-derived cells

Development of *in vitro* ALS models provides another tool to investigate disease mechanisms and test therapeutics for ALS. Unfortunately, there has been a disconnect in the translation of drugs from rodent models of ALS to human clinical trials. While various drugs have shown promise in rodent models, there continues to be disappointment in clinical trials which may be a result of various factors including poor preclinical testing regimen, ineffective clinical design and delivery, or use of an animal model that does not accurately reflect human disease (Benatar, 2007). Indeed, most ALS models currently used for therapeutic testing are based on fALS caused by SOD1 mutations. Since fALS only accounts for 5-10% of ALS cases and SOD1 mutations are only present in 20% of these fALS patients, rodent ALS models may only represent 2% of all ALS cases. Thus, efforts have been focused on developing *in vitro* cell based models for sALS, representing the majority of the patient population. Human ALS-based *in vitro* models could be a helpful tool to identify drugs which modulate glial activity and be utilized as a complement to the mutant SOD1 mouse model to select more effective drugs for further clinical development.

Several methods can be employed to derive patient-specific glia for *in vitro* study. While it is difficult to isolate primary astrocytes or microglia from post-mortem tissue in large enough quantities, neural progenitor cells can be harvested from post-mortem brain and spinal cord tissue (Palmer et al., 2001). These human neural progenitor cells can be continuously expanded *in vitro* and differentiated into neurons, astrocytes, or oligodendrocytes for study. Recently, it has been shown that isolation of neural progenitor cells from post-mortem ALS spinal cord is feasible and astrocytes can be generated from these progenitors (Haidet-Phillips et al., 2011). Astrocytes derived from a fALS patient harboring a SOD1 mutation were co-cultured with wild-type motor neurons and a 50% increase in neuronal cell death was observed compared to co-culture with astrocytes from non-ALS controls, recapitulating evidence from the mutant SOD1 mouse model. However, it was also shown for the first time that astrocytes derived from sALS patients, which represent the majority of ALS patients, were similarly toxic to motor neurons in co-culture. The motor neuron death was shown to be triggered by conditioned astrocyte media, suggesting toxic secreted factors are responsible for motor neuron damage as seen in the mouse astrocyte co-culture studies. These results indicate a shared mechanism leading to motor neuron death between fALS and sALS through astrocyte-mediated toxicity and suggest therapies directed at astrocytes may be beneficial for both ALS populations.

In addition to neural progenitor cells, there are other stem cell sources which can be potentially used to derive patient-specific glial cells or motor neurons *in vitro*. With the development of induced pluripotent stem cell (iPSC) technology, many groups are also striving to create populations of neurons and astrocytes from iPSCs for disease modeling. iPSCs are pluripotent stem cells generated by reprogramming somatic cells through forced expression of specific pluripotency transcription factors. Like embryonic stem cells, iPSCs are characterized by an immense proliferative capacity and the ability to differentiate into all three germ lineages (endoderm, ectoderm, and mesoderm) which can eventually give rise to all tissues of the body (Yamanaka & Blau, 2010). A variety of different cell types have now been reprogrammed into iPSCs including both mouse and human somatic cells (Okita et al., 2007; Park et al., 2008; Takahashi et al., 2007; Takahashi & Yamanaka, 2006; Wernig et al., 2007; Yu et al., 2007). Importantly, protocols have also been developed for the differentiation of motor neurons, astrocytes, and oligodendrocytes from human iPSCs, which allow for *in vitro* ALS disease modeling (Czepiel et al., 2011; Dimos et al., 2008; Krencik et al., 2011; Liu et al., 2011).

Several groups have reprogrammed human fibroblasts from ALS patients into iPSCs and successfully differentiated motor neurons from these iPSCs (Boulting et al., 2011; Dimos et al., 2008). However, the major hurdle thus far has been demonstration of a disease-related phenotype in the iPSC-derived motor neurons. It may be necessary to either stress the iPSC-derived motor neurons or co-culture with astrocytes also generated from ALS patient iPSCs in order to observe motor neuron damage. Still, it may be difficult to reproduce a relevant *in vitro* phenotype when working with diseases that are complex and likely multifactorial such as sALS. Another question posed by these experiments is whether or not reprogramming a cell and concordant epigenetic remodeling causes the loss of the ALS "signature". If sporadic ALS is triggered in part by epigenetic modifications, reprogramming may eliminate this epigenetic profile leaving essentially a "wild-type" cell. Therefore,

comparisons between cells derived from ALS post-mortem tissues (not reprogrammed) and ALS-derived iPSCs may be crucial for dissecting these issues.
Although still in development, these *in vitro*-based ALS models provide a valuable platform for further mechanistic and therapeutic studies. Many of these models employ the use of Hb9-GFP reporter cell lines to generate motor neurons allowing for easy visualization of motor neuron survival over time in co-culture. With the reported ability to track motor neuron survival in real-time in a 96 well plate format (Haidet-Phillips et al., 2011), the development of high-throughput screens is foreseeable. Therapeutic compounds could be quickly screened for motor neuron protection against glial-cell mediated toxicity in this format. Additionally, one could envision genetic screens for modifiers of glial-cell derived motor neuron damage, leading to new therapeutic approaches or insights into disease mechanisms. Since there are currently no models for sALS, these *in vitro*-based systems utilizing either post-mortem neural progenitor or iPS-derived cells could provide a much needed novel platform for drug discovery. Although promising, some limitations do exist for *in vitro* modeling systems. For example, the time course for modeling motor neuron disease *in vitro* is short (days to weeks) whereas ALS is a late onset disorder which usually does not develop until 40-60 years of age. Additionally, the heterogeneity of ALS cases may pose another challenge, requiring a large number of both disease and control samples in order to identify relevant disease-related changes *in vitro*. Lastly, although *in vitro* modeling allows for dissection of cell-specific phenotypes, it will be important to evaluate any noticed changes in an *in vivo* context where many cell types interact and can influence disease.

4. Therapeutic advances to target glial cells in ALS

In recent years, much emphasis has been placed on the role of glial cells in mutant SOD1 mouse models and some of these findings have been recapitulated *in vitro* using human ALS patient-derived cells. Thus, many groups are devoting significant efforts to development of therapies directed at modulating glial cell activity. Indeed, glial cells have been suggested to affect both disease onset and progression in ALS mouse models. Since the majority of ALS patients are only diagnosed well after the onset of disease, therapies targeting disease progression by modification of glial cells may be beneficial in slowing symptomatic disease processes.

4.1 Therapeutic agents to target astrocytes and microglia

Currently, there is only one US Food and Drug Administration (FDA)-approved drug for the treatment of ALS and its therapeutic effects are hypothesized to derive from counteracting aberrant glutamate metabolism. Riluzole is an inhibitor of presynaptic glutamate release which may offset excitotoxicity seen in ALS. Riluzole has been confirmed to alter ALS disease survival in four independent clinical trials providing strong support for its therapeutic benefits (Miller et al., 2007). Unfortunately, riluzole only extends lifespan in ALS patients by an average of 3 months so efforts have focused on identifying other compounds which can counteract glutamate excitotoxicity. A variety of other drugs targeting glutamatergic pathways (talampanel, memantine, topiramate, lamotrigine, gabapentin, ONO-2506) have been evaluated in ALS patients, but the results have not suggested a benefit on disease course (Cudkowicz et al., 2003; de Carvalho et al., 2010; Miller et al., 2001; Ryberg et al., 2003; Zinman & Cudkowicz, 2011).

To identify new medications which may modulate glutamatergic pathways, an *in vitro* screening of over 1000 compounds already approved by the US Food and Drug Administration was completed (Rothstein et al., 2005). From this screen, β-lactam antibiotics were found to upregulate expression of the glutamate transporter, GLT1, and one of these antibiotics, ceftriaxone, was shown to significantly delay disease progression in the SOD1 G93A mouse model. Clinical trials testing intravenous ceftriaxone administration in ALS patients have already passed safety and tolerability stages and are currently in the final phase III of evaluation (Zinman & Cudkowicz, 2011).

In contrast to specific targeting of glutamatergic pathways, a variety of anti-inflammatory agents have been tested with hopes to combat the extensive glial reaction observed in ALS patient brain and spinal cord. Prostaglandins are mediators of the inflammatory response that can be released in response to immune stimuli and production of prostaglandins is increased in the spinal cord of ALS patients (Kondo et al., 2002). Prostaglandin stimulation can be reduced by inhibiting cyclooxygenase 2 (COX2), an inducible enzyme involved in the synthesis of prostaglandins. Treatment of SOD1 G93A mice with COX2 inhibitors lowers prostaglandin levels and prolongs survival in these mice (Drachman et al., 2002; Klivenyi et al., 2004; Pompl et al., 2003). Unfortunately, the COX2 inhibitor, celecoxib, was ineffective at increasing survival in a clinical trial of ALS patients (Cudkowicz et al., 2006). However, prostaglandin E2 levels in the CSF of these patients was unaltered by celecoxib therapy indicating the dose may have been too low to reach therapeutic levels in the CNS (Aggarwal & Cudkowicz, 2008).

Additional efforts to modulate the immune response in ALS have also been unsuccessful. The anti-microbial drug, minocycline, was shown to inhibit microglial activation and lengthen survival in mouse models of ALS (Kriz et al., 2002; Van Den Bosch et al., 2002; Zhu et al., 2002). Nonetheless, in a multicenter, randomized, phase III clinical trial of over 400 ALS patients, minocycline did not increase survival and in fact, was shown to worsen disease course in these patients (Gordon et al., 2007). The apparent divergence in results between preclinical animal studies and the clinical trial may have been due to the timing of minocycline treatment. When tested in animal models, minocycline was administered prior to symptomatic disease onset, whereas patients received the drug only after clinical onset of ALS. Indeed, a recent study showed that treatment of SOD1 G93A mice with minocycline administered after disease onset conferred no survival benefit and highlights the importance of a clinically-relevant testing regimen in ALS mouse studies (Keller et al., 2011). Compounds which modify neuroinflammation already present in the spinal cord, in contrast to preventing inflammation, may be more successful in the clinical setting.

4.2 Stem cell therapies for ALS

Because mounting data indicate that pathogenic glial cells actively contribute to motor neuron loss in ALS, one developing strategy is to replace the diseased glia with healthy cells which may alter the endogenous spinal cord environment and promote motor neuron survival. Transplantation of terminally differentiated glia to the CNS may pose technical difficulties since these cells are typically mature with limited proliferative and migratory capacity. Therefore, exploration of stem cells as a source for glial replacement has been sought after by many groups.

Mutant SOD1-expressing microglia are key drivers of disease progression in mouse models of fALS. Since microglia are derived from the hematopoietic lineage, hematopoietic stem cells are one possible source for microglial cell replacement. When SOD1 mice lacking microglia are given bone marrow transplants from wild-type mice, the microglial cell population is reconstituted with healthy microglia and survival is prolonged (Beers et al., 2006). In translating this line of investigation to ALS patients, allogeneic peripheral blood hematopoietic stem cells were transplanted into ALS patients following full body irradiation (Appel et al., 2008). Although transplanted cells remarkably migrated to sites of motor neuron injury, no clinical change in disease was observed. It is possible that either the transplanted cells did not differentiate into microglia or that a large proportion of endogenous microglia survived post-irradiation which outnumbered healthy, transplanted stem cells. Trials are ongoing to similarly test intraparenchymal transplantation of hematopoietic stem cells to ALS patients (Deda et al., 2009), but results may be difficult to interpret based on the use of autologous (and potentially diseased) stem cells as a source instead of allogeneic (from a matched donor) derived stem cells. Further studies are needed in ALS rodent models to determine the optimal cell type, number, and delivery method for transplantation to establish a critical proof-of-principle for these paradigms.

Further efforts have focused on replacement of diseased astrocytes using various cell sources and delivery approaches. In contrast to microglia, astrocytes are derived from the neural lineage and can be differentiated from several stem cell sources including both glial-restricted precursors as well as neural stem and progenitor cells. Thus far, transplantation of neural progenitor cells to rodent ALS models has resulted in either a lack of differentiation *in vivo* (Klein et al., 2005; Suzuki et al., 2007) or differentiation to mostly neurons after neural stem cell transplantation, but not to astrocytes (Xu et al., 2009; Xu et al., 2011).

In contrast, glial-restricted precursors are lineage-restricted and can only become astrocytes or oligodendrocytes. Transplantation of glial-restricted precursors to the cervical spinal cord of SOD1 G93A rats led to extensive differentiation of grafted cells into astrocytes (>85% of transplanted cells) which reduced significant motor neuron loss (Lepore et al., 2008b). The graft-derived astrocytes expressed increased levels of GLT1 in comparison to endogenous diseased astrocytes, which likely played a major role in protecting motor neurons. Importantly, rats receiving transplants also survived longer and showed preserved forelimb grip strength and respiratory function, attributable to the focal delivery of glial-restricted precursor cells to the cervical region of the spinal cord. This work provides a proof-of-principle for astrocyte replacement in ALS and sets the stage for future clinical trials testing transplantation of human glial-restricted precursors in ALS patients. Questions still remain as to whether human glial-restricted precursors will survive and differentiate after transplantation into humans and which spinal cord regions are most practical for targeting in ALS patients.

With the advancement of stem cell technology, astrocytes as well as neural progenitors (and possibly glial-restricted precursors) can now be derived from human iPS cells. This novel stem cell source provides another option for glial-cell replacement therapies since iPS cells have immense expansive abilities *in vitro*. A major potential advantage to iPS cells is that these cells can be derived directly from a living patient. In theory, use of autologous iPS cells for transplantation therapies may lessen worries of graft rejection and obviate the need for continued immunosuppressive therapy. However, one study testing this paradigm documented rejection of mouse iPS cells after transplantation to an autologous recipient, cautioning that transplantation of these cells may be more complex than originally thought (Zhao et al., 2011). Another issue is whether stem cells derived from ALS patients carry the disease phenotype. If so, any cells differentiated from the patient iPS cells may not provide the desired therapeutic benefit. In cases where there exists a disease-associated mutation such as SOD1, ex-vivo genetic correction of the mutation through homologous recombination, viral vectors, or zinc finger technology may be possible (Amabile & Meissner, 2009). However, most ALS patients have no identified genetic mutation responsible for the disease. Additionally, there remain many unresolved challenges with iPS cell therapy such as obtaining efficient differentiation of the iPS cells to the desired cell population, purifying a safe and non-tumorgenic population for transplantation, and optimizing delivery methods for transplantation of the iPS-derived cells back to the patient.

In addition to benefits derived from replacing diseased glia, transplanted populations of stem cells may also be used to deliver therapeutics to the brain and spinal cord. Stem cells can be genetically modified *in vitro* by transduction with viral vectors which can integrate into the genome and stably express therapeutic genes long-term. Since many therapeutic proteins have short half-lives after direct injection, genetically modified stem cells transplanted to the brain or spinal cord would allow for continuous production of the desired protein at the site of neurodegeneration, serving as "therapeutic pumps" *in vivo*. For example, human neural progenitor cells transduced with a lentivirus expressing glial-derived neurotrophic factor (GDNF) and transplanted to the ALS rat spinal cord can produce GDNF *in vivo* and protect motor neurons (Klein et al., 2005; Suzuki et al., 2007). One could envision using stem cells to deliver not only neuroprotective factors, but also therapies to modulate the glial environment such as anti-inflammatory proteins or anti-glutamatergic agents.

4.3 Gene-targeted therapies for ALS

The mechanisms leading to motor neuron death in ALS are still unclear; however, it is generally agreed in the field that in cases of SOD1 fALS, the mutant SOD1 protein harbors a toxic gain-of-function and reduction of mutant SOD1 is likely to be beneficial in these patients. Additionally, several studies have implicated a pathogenic role for wild-type SOD1 in cases of sALS (Bosco et al., 2010; Gruzman et al., 2007), including a potential role in glial cells (Haidet-Phillips et al., 2011). Therefore, therapies aimed at reducing SOD1 levels may potentially be applicable for not only SOD1 fALS patients, but for other ALS patient populations as well.

A variety of approaches have been attempted to reduce SOD1 levels in rodent models of ALS. RNA interference (RNAi) is a post-transcriptional gene-silencing mechanism initiated by small interfering RNAs (siRNA) which are double-stranded pieces of RNA 21-23 nucleotides in length (Sah & Aronin, 2011). Within the cytoplasm, the siRNA gets recognized and directed to the RNA-induced silencing complex. The silencing complex then uses the sequence-specific information on the siRNA to initiate degradation of endogenous complementary mRNA sequences, leading to subsequent gene silencing. Targeted siRNA can be exogenously delivered to a cell although naked siRNA is instable with a relatively short half life (Sah & Aronin, 2011). Alternatively, viral vectors can be used to continuously transcribe RNA containing short complementary sequences (Miller et al., 2008). These complementary sequences can bind, leading to duplex hairpin formation (short hairpin RNA or shRNA). Once transcribed, the shRNA gets recognized by the cellular machinery and cleaved by the Dicer enzyme to produce short, double-stranded siRNA sequences.

Sequences of siRNA targeted against SOD1 mRNA have been designed to reduce levels of the mutant SOD1 protein. Similar to many small molecule therapies, siRNA does not cross the blood-brain-barrier, creating challenges for delivery to the CNS (Sah & Aronin, 2011). Viral-mediated delivery of SOD1 shRNA has been attempted in rodent models of ALS with successful knockdown of SOD1 levels by both lentivirus and adeno-associated virus (AAV) (Miller et al., 2005; Ralph et al., 2005; Towne et al., 2011). However, these studies have targeted only motor neurons, transduced after retrograde transport from muscles injected with the virus. These strategies were unsuccessful in slowing disease progression, most likely due to the fact that motor neurons were solely targeted, although glial cells play a significant role in the disease process.

Other approaches have strived to target both motor neurons and glial cells with SOD1 shRNA. Intraparenchymal injection to the lumbar spinal cord of a lentivirus encoding SOD1 shRNA was shown to reduce SOD1 levels and retard disease onset and progression in the SOD1 G93A mouse (Raoul et al., 2005). Yet, the vast anatomical distribution of diseased cells throughout the motor cortex, brain stem and spinal cord pose a hurdle for direct injection of viral therapy with limited diffusive capacity. A novel version of AAV, AAV serotype 9, has recently shown potential for extensive targeting of CNS tissues (Foust et al., 2009). In this study, AAV9 was able to cross the blood-brain-barrier after vascular delivery and transduce over 60% of astrocytes in the brain and spinal cord. Additional evaluation in non-human primates verified that AAV9 is capable of efficiently targeting both motor neurons and glia in the brain and spinal cord after vascular delivery to a large species (Bevan et al., 2011). Use of this virus to deliver SOD1 shRNA is conceivable, although steps may be needed to target viral expression away from peripheral organs and only to CNS tissues.

Instead of using a viral vector to deliver shRNA sequences, others have sought to create more stable siRNA for direct delivery through chemically modifying the siRNA (Wang et al., 2008). Intrathecal infusion of chemically-modified SOD1 siRNA using an osmotic pump generated a 15% knockdown in SOD1 protein levels and a modest therapeutic effect in the SOD1 G93A mice. One potential advantage to infusion of naked, stabilized siRNA over viral delivery is the ability to halt the treatment at any time following adverse effects. Therefore, this type of RNAi therapy seems promising at least for treatment of ALS patients with SOD1 mutations.

A similar approach to RNAi therapy involves the use of antisense oligonucleotides to enact post-transcriptional gene silencing (Sah & Aronin, 2011). Antisense oligonucleotides are short (15-25 nucleotides) single stranded pieces of synthetic DNA which can bind to complementary mRNA sequences in the cytoplasm. Once bound, these DNA-mRNA complexes are targeted for degradation by the enzyme RNase H. Additionally, translation of mRNA bound by antisense oligonucleotides can be physically blocked, leading to further gene silencing for targeted mRNA sequences. Antisense oligonucleotides are generally more stable than naked siRNA with a half life of 2-6 weeks after delivery to the mouse and monkey CNS (Sah & Aronin, 2011). Like siRNA, antisense oligonucleotides can be absorbed by both neurons and glia to execute gene silencing. Sequence specific targeting of antisense oligonucleotides to SOD1 mRNA has been attainable, with a 50% reduction in SOD1 protein levels in the brain and spinal cord of SOD1 G93A rats infused for 28 days with antisense oligonucleotides into the right ventricle (Smith et al., 2006). The rats treated with SOD1 antisense oligonucleotides showed a slowed disease progression and this same SOD1 antisense oligonucleotide was demonstrated to lower SOD1 levels in fibroblasts isolated from an ALS patient. A phase I clinical trial has been initiated in fALS patients with SOD1 mutations testing intrathecal infusion of this same antisense oligonucleotide against SOD1. This dose-escalation trial will evaluate safety, tolerability, and pharmacokinetics in patients treated with antisense oligonucleotide infusion for 12 hours. If proven safe, this strategy holds considerable promise to treat SOD1 fALS patients.

While a great deal of progress has been made in the development of anti-SOD1 therapies, additional work needs to be focused on advancing novel treatments for non-SOD1 ALS patient populations. As additional genetic mutations are linked to ALS, these genes might present new targets for gene-based therapeutic approaches. However, in the case of TDP43 and FUS mutations, a great deal of basic research is still required to evaluate whether a loss-of-function or gain-of-function mechanism is responsible for disease caused by these mutations and whether glial cells are also a target in these cases. Until these crucial questions are answered, it will be difficult to develop RNAi or gene therapy treatments for these patients. Efforts to reach a broad ALS patient population may benefit most from the design of therapies which interfere with downstream mechanisms prevalent in most patients, such as glial-mediated glutamate excitotoxicity or neuroinflammation. Many of the siRNA and antisense oligonucleotide approaches can be amenable to inhibit potentially damaging genes involved in these glial responses. Additionally, viral vectors have been developed that can deliver gene therapies to glial cells in the CNS, allowing for potential immune modulation. With increasingly innovative developments in RNAi and gene therapy, the door is open for novel gene-based therapies to alter the ALS disease process.

5. Conclusion

The field of ALS research has progressed significantly in recent years with the identification of glial cells as an active contributor to the disease process. Specifically, astrocytes and microglia have been recognized as glial cell types which undeniably influence survival in rodent models of ALS. Efforts are underway to test therapies aimed at modifying the glial cell population in hopes of slowing ALS disease progression and extending patient survival.

While rodent models of ALS have been key in revealing glial cells as a disease contributor in SOD1 fALS, it still remains to be determined to what extent glial cells are involved in disease processes in other patient populations. New genes have been recently linked ALS including TDP43 and FUS, suggesting a possible role for RNA metabolism in disease pathogenesis. Creation of both rodent and *in vitro* models mimicking these forms of ALS is underway and will hopefully reveal whether glial cells are also a target in patients harboring these mutations.

Although glial cell targets have been identified, much work remains to elucidate the mechanisms behind their neural toxicity. Several groups have been able to model the glial-motor neuron interface *in vitro* using unique stem-cell based models to study the effects of diseased glia on motor neurons. While these studies have yet to identify relevant mechanisms involved in glial-mediated toxicity, *in vitro* models present the opportunity to study human patient-derived glial cells from both fALS and sALS patients. With the development of iPSC technology, there exists potential to study patient-specific glial cells and evaluate therapies in a high-throughput fashion.

Discovery of mechanisms involved in glial pathogenicity will likely lead to the development of promising therapeutic interventions. Detection of additional pathways of importance will hopefully shed light on new compounds which may be capable of targeting glial-mediated motor neuron damage. Furthermore, stem cell and gene-based therapies have reached evaluation in clinical trials, creating excitement and optimism in the field. As new knowledge of disease mechanisms arises, there is great hope for novel interventions to target glial cells and significantly change the ALS disease course.

6. References

Aggarwal, S. & Cudkowicz, M., (2008). ALS drug development: reflections from the past and a way forward. *Neurotherapeutics*. Vol. 5, No. 4, pp. 516-27.

Almer, G., Vukosavic, S., Romero, N. & Przedborski, S., (1999). Inducible nitric oxide synthase up-regulation in a transgenic mouse model of familial amyotrophic lateral sclerosis. *J Neurochem*. Vol. 72, No. 6, pp. 2415-25.

Amabile, G. & Meissner, A., (2009). Induced pluripotent stem cells: current progress and potential for regenerative medicine. *Trends Mol Med*. Vol. 15, No. 2, pp. 59-68.

Appel, S.H., Engelhardt, J.I., Henkel, J.S., Siklos, L., Beers, D.R., Yen, A.A., Simpson, E.P., Luo, Y., Carrum, G., Heslop, H.E., Brenner, M.K. & Popat, U., (2008). Hematopoietic stem cell transplantation in patients with sporadic amyotrophic lateral sclerosis. *Neurology*. Vol. 71, No. 17, pp. 1326-34.

Beers, D.R., Henkel, J.S., Xiao, Q., Zhao, W., Wang, J., Yen, A.A., Siklos, L., McKercher, S.R. & Appel, S.H., (2006). Wild-type microglia extend survival in PU.1 knockout mice with familial amyotrophic lateral sclerosis. *Proc Natl Acad Sci U S A*. Vol. 103, No. 43, pp. 16021-6.

Beers, D.R., Henkel, J.S., Zhao, W., Wang, J., Huang, A., Wen, S., Liao, B. & Appel, S.H., (2011). Endogenous regulatory T lymphocytes ameliorate amyotrophic lateral sclerosis in mice and correlate with disease progression in patients with amyotrophic lateral sclerosis. *Brain*. Vol. 134, No. Pt 5, pp. 1293-314.

Benatar, M., (2007). Lost in translation: treatment trials in the SOD1 mouse and in human ALS. *Neurobiol Dis*. Vol. 26, No. 1, pp. 1-13.

Bendotti, C., Tortarolo, M., Suchak, S.K., Calvaresi, N., Carvelli, L., Bastone, A., Rizzi, M., Rattray, M. & Mennini, T., (2001). Transgenic SOD1 G93A mice develop reduced GLT-1 in spinal cord without alterations in cerebrospinal fluid glutamate levels. *J Neurochem*. Vol. 79, No. 4, pp. 737-46.

Bevan, A.K., Duque, S., Foust, K.D., Morales, P.R., Braun, L., Schmelzer, L., Chan, C.M., McCrate, M., Chicoine, L.G., Coley, B.D., Porensky, P.N., Kolb, S.J., Mendell, J.R., Burghes, A.H. & Kaspar, B.K., (2011). Systemic Gene Delivery in Large Species for Targeting Spinal Cord, Brain, and Peripheral Tissues for Pediatric Disorders. *Mol Ther*. Vol., No., pp.

Boillee, S., Vande Velde, C. & Cleveland, D.W., (2006a). ALS: a disease of motor neurons and their nonneuronal neighbors. *Neuron*. Vol. 52, No. 1, pp. 39-59.

Boillee, S., Yamanaka, K., Lobsiger, C.S., Copeland, N.G., Jenkins, N.A., Kassiotis, G., Kollias, G. & Cleveland, D.W., (2006b). Onset and Progression in Inherited ALS Determined by Motor Neurons and Microglia. *Science*. Vol. 312, No. 5778, pp. 1389-92.

Bosco, D.A., Morfini, G., Karabacak, N.M., Song, Y., Gros-Louis, F., Pasinelli, P., Goolsby, H., Fontaine, B.A., Lemay, N., McKenna-Yasek, D., Frosch, M.P., Agar, J.N., Julien, J.P., Brady, S.T. & Brown, R.H., Jr., (2010). Wild-type and mutant SOD1 share an aberrant conformation and a common pathogenic pathway in ALS. *Nat Neurosci*. Vol. 13, No. 11, pp. 1396-403.

Boulting, G.L., Kiskinis, E., Croft, G.F., Amoroso, M.W., Oakley, D.H., Wainger, B.J., Williams, D.J., Kahler, D.J., Yamaki, M., Davidow, L., Rodolfa, C.T., Dimos, J.T., Mikkilineni, S., MacDermott, A.B., Woolf, C.J., Henderson, C.E., Wichterle, H. & Eggan, K., (2011). A functionally characterized test set of human induced pluripotent stem cells. *Nat Biotechnol.* Vol. 29, No. 3, pp. 279-86.

Bristol, L.A. & Rothstein, J.D., (1996). Glutamate transporter gene expression in amyotrophic lateral sclerosis motor cortex. *Ann Neurol.* Vol. 39, No. 5, pp. 676-9.

Bruijn, L.I., Becher, M.W., Lee, M.K., Anderson, K.L., Jenkins, N.A., Copeland, N.G., Sisodia, S.S., Rothstein, J.D., Borchelt, D.R., Price, D.L. & Cleveland, D.W., (1997). ALS-linked SOD1 mutant G85R mediates damage to astrocytes and promotes rapidly progressive disease with SOD1-containing inclusions. *Neuron.* Vol. 18, No. 2, pp. 327-38.

Bruijn, L.I., Houseweart, M.K., Kato, S., Anderson, K.L., Anderson, S.D., Ohama, E., Reaume, A.G., Scott, R.W. & Cleveland, D.W., (1998). Aggregation and motor neuron toxicity of an ALS-linked SOD1 mutant independent from wild-type SOD1. *Science.* Vol. 281, No. 5384, pp. 1851-4.

Chiu, A.Y., Zhai, P., Dal Canto, M.C., Peters, T.M., Kwon, Y.W., Prattis, S.M. & Gurney, M.E., (1995). Age-dependent penetrance of disease in a transgenic mouse model of familial amyotrophic lateral sclerosis. *Mol Cell Neurosci.* Vol. 6, No. 4, pp. 349-62.

Chiu, I.M., Chen, A., Zheng, Y., Kosaras, B., Tsiftsoglou, S.A., Vartanian, T.K., Brown, R.H., Jr. & Carroll, M.C., (2008). T lymphocytes potentiate endogenous neuroprotective inflammation in a mouse model of ALS. *Proc Natl Acad Sci U S A.* Vol. 105, No. 46, pp. 17913-8.

Clement, A.M., Nguyen, M.D., Roberts, E.A., Garcia, M.L., Boillee, S., Rule, M., McMahon, A.P., Doucette, W., Siwek, D., Ferrante, R.J., Brown, R.H., Jr., Julien, J.P., Goldstein, L.S. & Cleveland, D.W., (2003). Wild-type nonneuronal cells extend survival of SOD1 mutant motor neurons in ALS mice. *Science.* Vol. 302, No. 5642, pp. 113-7.

Cohen, T.J., Lee, V.M. & Trojanowski, J.Q., (2011). TDP-43 functions and pathogenic mechanisms implicated in TDP-43 proteinopathies. *Trends Mol Med.* Vol., No., pp.

Cudkowicz, M.E., Shefner, J.M., Schoenfeld, D.A., Brown, R.H., Jr., Johnson, H., Qureshi, M., Jacobs, M., Rothstein, J.D., Appel, S.H., Pascuzzi, R.M., Heiman-Patterson, T.D., Donofrio, P.D., David, W.S., Russell, J.A., Tandan, R., Pioro, E.P., Felice, K.J., Rosenfeld, J., Mandler, R.N., Sachs, G.M., Bradley, W.G., Raynor, E.M., Baquis, G.D., Belsh, J.M., Novella, S., Goldstein, J. & Hulihan, J., (2003). A randomized, placebo-controlled trial of topiramate in amyotrophic lateral sclerosis. *Neurology.* Vol. 61, No. 4, pp. 456-64.

Cudkowicz, M.E., Shefner, J.M., Schoenfeld, D.A., Zhang, H., Andreasson, K.I., Rothstein, J.D. & Drachman, D.B., (2006). Trial of celecoxib in amyotrophic lateral sclerosis. *Ann Neurol.* Vol. 60, No. 1, pp. 22-31.

Czepiel, M., Balasubramaniyan, V., Schaafsma, W., Stancic, M., Mikkers, H., Huisman, C., Boddeke, E. & Copray, S., (2011). Differentiation of induced pluripotent stem cells into functional oligodendrocytes. *Glia.* Vol. 59, No. 6, pp. 882-92.

de Carvalho, M., Pinto, S., Costa, J., Evangelista, T., Ohana, B. & Pinto, A., (2010). A randomized, placebo-controlled trial of memantine for functional disability in amyotrophic lateral sclerosis. *Amyotroph Lateral Scler.* Vol. 11, No. 5, pp. 456-60.

Deda, H., Inci, M.C., Kurekci, A.E., Sav, A., Kayihan, K., Ozgun, E., Ustunsoy, G.E. & Kocabay, S., (2009). Treatment of amyotrophic lateral sclerosis patients by autologous bone marrow-derived hematopoietic stem cell transplantation: a 1-year follow-up. *Cytotherapy*. Vol. 11, No. 1, pp. 18-25.

Di Giorgio, F.P., Carrasco, M.A., Siao, M.C., Maniatis, T. & Eggan, K., (2007). Non-cell autonomous effect of glia on motor neurons in an embryonic stem cell-based ALS model. *Nat Neurosci*. Vol. 10, No. 5, pp. 608-614.

Di Giorgio, F.P., Boulting, G.L., Bobrowicz, S. & Eggan, K.C., (2008). Human embryonic stem cell-derived motor neurons are sensitive to the toxic effect of glial cells carrying an ALS-causing mutation. *Cell Stem Cell*. Vol. 3, No. 6, pp. 637-48.

Dimos, J.T., Rodolfa, K.T., Niakan, K.K., Weisenthal, L.M., Mitsumoto, H., Chung, W., Croft, G.F., Saphier, G., Leibel, R., Goland, R., Wichterle, H., Henderson, C.E. & Eggan, K., (2008). Induced pluripotent stem cells generated from patients with ALS can be differentiated into motor neurons. *Science*. Vol. 321, No. 5893, pp. 1218-21.

Dodge, J.C., Haidet, A.M., Yang, W., Passini, M.A., Hester, M., Clarke, J., Roskelley, E.M., Treleaven, C.M., Rizo, L., Martin, H., Kim, S.H., Kaspar, R., Taksir, T.V., Griffiths, D.A., Cheng, S.H., Shihabuddin, L.S. & Kaspar, B.K., (2008). Delivery of AAV-IGF-1 to the CNS extends survival in ALS mice through modification of aberrant glial cell activity. *Mol Ther*. Vol. 16, No. 6, pp. 1056-64.

Drachman, D.B., Frank, K., Dykes-Hoberg, M., Teismann, P., Almer, G., Przedborski, S. & Rothstein, J.D., (2002). Cyclooxygenase 2 inhibition protects motor neurons and prolongs survival in a transgenic mouse model of ALS. *Ann Neurol*. Vol. 52, No. 6, pp. 771-8.

Foust, K.D., Nurre, E., Montgomery, C.L., Hernandez, A., Chan, C.M. & Kaspar, B.K., (2009). Intravascular AAV9 preferentially targets neonatal neurons and adult astrocytes. *Nat Biotechnol*. Vol. 27, No. 1, pp. 59-65.

Gordon, P.H., Moore, D.H., Miller, R.G., Florence, J.M., Verheijde, J.L., Doorish, C., Hilton, J.F., Spitalny, G.M., MacArthur, R.B., Mitsumoto, H., Neville, H.E., Boylan, K., Mozaffar, T., Belsh, J.M., Ravits, J., Bedlack, R.S., Graves, M.C., McCluskey, L.F., Barohn, R.J. & Tandan, R., (2007). Efficacy of minocycline in patients with amyotrophic lateral sclerosis: a phase III randomised trial. *Lancet Neurol*. Vol. 6, No. 12, pp. 1045-53.

Gruzman, A., Wood, W.L., Alpert, E., Prasad, M.D., Miller, R.G., Rothstein, J.D., Bowser, R., Hamilton, R., Wood, T.D., Cleveland, D.W., Lingappa, V.R. & Liu, J., (2007). Common molecular signature in SOD1 for both sporadic and familial amyotrophic lateral sclerosis. *Proc Natl Acad Sci U S A*. Vol. 104, No. 30, pp. 12524-9.

Gurney, M.E., Pu, H., Chiu, A.Y., Dal Canto, M.C., Polchow, C.Y., Alexander, D.D., Caliendo, J., Hentati, A., Kwon, Y.W., Deng, H.X. & et al., (1994). Motor neuron degeneration in mice that express a human Cu,Zn superoxide dismutase mutation. *Science*. Vol. 264, No. 5166, pp. 1772-5.

Haidet-Phillips, A.M., Hester, M.E., Miranda, C.J., Meyer, K., Braun, L., Frakes, A., Song, S., Likhite, S., Murtha, M.J., Foust, K.D., Rao, M., Eagle, A., Kammesheidt, A., Christensen, A., Mendell, J.R., Burghes, A.H. & Kaspar, B.K., (2011). Astrocytes from familial and sporadic ALS patients are toxic to motor neurons. *Nat Biotechnol*. Vol., No., pp.

Henkel, J.S., Beers, D.R., Zhao, W. & Appel, S.H., (2009). Microglia in ALS: The Good, The Bad, and The Resting. *J Neuroimmune Pharmacol*. Vol., No., pp.

Hensley, K., Fedynyshyn, J., Ferrell, S., Floyd, R.A., Gordon, B., Grammas, P., Hamdheydari, L., Mhatre, M., Mou, S., Pye, Q.N., Stewart, C., West, M., West, S. & Williamson, K.S., (2003). Message and protein-level elevation of tumor necrosis factor alpha

(TNF alpha) and TNF alpha-modulating cytokines in spinal cords of the G93A-SOD1 mouse model for amyotrophic lateral sclerosis. *Neurobiol Dis.* Vol. 14, No. 1, pp. 74-80.

Huang, C., Zhou, H., Tong, J., Chen, H., Liu, Y.J., Wang, D., Wei, X. & Xia, X.G., (2011). FUS transgenic rats develop the phenotypes of amyotrophic lateral sclerosis and frontotemporal lobar degeneration. *PLoS Genet.* Vol. 7, No. 3, pp. e1002011.

Jaarsma, D., Teuling, E., Haasdijk, E.D., De Zeeuw, C.I. & Hoogenraad, C.C., (2008). Neuron-specific expression of mutant superoxide dismutase is sufficient to induce amyotrophic lateral sclerosis in transgenic mice. *J Neurosci.* Vol. 28, No. 9, pp. 2075-88.

Kabashi, E., Valdmanis, P.N., Dion, P., Spiegelman, D., McConkey, B.J., Vande Velde, C., Bouchard, J.P., Lacomblez, L., Pochigaeva, K., Salachas, F., Pradat, P.F., Camu, W., Meininger, V., Dupre, N. & Rouleau, G.A., (2008). TARDBP mutations in individuals with sporadic and familial amyotrophic lateral sclerosis. *Nat Genet.* Vol. 40, No. 5, pp. 572-4.

Kang, S.H., Fukaya, M., Yang, J.K., Rothstein, J.D. & Bergles, D.E., (2010). NG2+ CNS glial progenitors remain committed to the oligodendrocyte lineage in postnatal life and following neurodegeneration. *Neuron.* Vol. 68, No. 4, pp. 668-81.

Keller, A.F., Gravel, M. & Kriz, J., (2011). Treatment with minocycline after disease onset alters astrocyte reactivity and increases microgliosis in SOD1 mutant mice. *Exp Neurol.* Vol. 228, No. 1, pp. 69-79.

Klein, S.M., Behrstock, S., McHugh, J., Hoffmann, K., Wallace, K., Suzuki, M., Aebischer, P. & Svendsen, C.N., (2005). GDNF delivery using human neural progenitor cells in a rat model of ALS. *Hum Gene Ther.* Vol. 16, No. 4, pp. 509-21.

Klivenyi, P., Kiaei, M., Gardian, G., Calingasan, N.Y. & Beal, M.F., (2004). Additive neuroprotective effects of creatine and cyclooxygenase 2 inhibitors in a transgenic mouse model of amyotrophic lateral sclerosis. *J Neurochem.* Vol. 88, No. 3, pp. 576-82.

Kondo, M., Shibata, T., Kumagai, T., Osawa, T., Shibata, N., Kobayashi, M., Sasaki, S., Iwata, M., Noguchi, N. & Uchida, K., (2002). 15-Deoxy-Delta(12,14)-prostaglandin J(2): the endogenous electrophile that induces neuronal apoptosis. *Proc Natl Acad Sci U S A.* Vol. 99, No. 11, pp. 7367-72.

Krencik, R., Weick, J.P., Liu, Y., Zhang, Z.J. & Zhang, S.C., (2011). Specification of transplantable astroglial subtypes from human pluripotent stem cells. *Nat Biotechnol.* Vol. 29, No. 6, pp. 528-34.

Kriz, J., Nguyen, M.D. & Julien, J.P., (2002). Minocycline slows disease progression in a mouse model of amyotrophic lateral sclerosis. *Neurobiol Dis.* Vol. 10, No. 3, pp. 268-78.

Kwiatkowski, T.J., Jr., Bosco, D.A., Leclerc, A.L., Tamrazian, E., Vanderburg, C.R., Russ, C., Davis, A., Gilchrist, J., Kasarskis, E.J., Munsat, T., Valdmanis, P., Rouleau, G.A., Hosler, B.A., Cortelli, P., de Jong, P.J., Yoshinaga, Y., Haines, J.L., Pericak-Vance, M.A., Yan, J., Ticozzi, N., Siddique, T., McKenna-Yasek, D., Sapp, P.C., Horvitz, H.R., Landers, J.E. & Brown, R.H., Jr., (2009). Mutations in the FUS/TLS gene on chromosome 16 cause familial amyotrophic lateral sclerosis. *Science.* Vol. 323, No. 5918, pp. 1205-8.

Lepore, A.C., Dejea, C., Carmen, J., Rauck, B., Kerr, D.A., Sofroniew, M.V. & Maragakis, N.J., (2008a). Selective ablation of proliferating astrocytes does not affect disease outcome in either acute or chronic models of motor neuron degeneration. *Exp Neurol.* Vol. 211, No. 2, pp. 423-32.

Lepore, A.C., Rauck, B., Dejea, C., Pardo, A.C., Rao, M.S., Rothstein, J.D. & Maragakis, N.J., (2008b). Focal transplantation-based astrocyte replacement is neuroprotective in a model of motor neuron disease. *Nat Neurosci*. Vol. 11, No. 11, pp. 1294-301.

Lino, M.M., Schneider, C. & Caroni, P., (2002). Accumulation of SOD1 mutants in postnatal motoneurons does not cause motoneuron pathology or motoneuron disease. *J Neurosci*. Vol. 22, No. 12, pp. 4825-32.

Liu, Y., Jiang, P. & Deng, W., (2011). OLIG gene targeting in human pluripotent stem cells for motor neuron and oligodendrocyte differentiation. *Nat Protoc*. Vol. 6, No. 5, pp. 640-55.

Lobsiger, C.S., Boillee, S., McAlonis-Downes, M., Khan, A.M., Feltri, M.L., Yamanaka, K. & Cleveland, D.W., (2009). Schwann cells expressing dismutase active mutant SOD1 unexpectedly slow disease progression in ALS mice. *Proc Natl Acad Sci U S A*. Vol. 106, No. 11, pp. 4465-70.

Mackenzie, I.R., Bigio, E.H., Ince, P.G., Geser, F., Neumann, M., Cairns, N.J., Kwong, L.K., Forman, M.S., Ravits, J., Stewart, H., Eisen, A., McClusky, L., Kretzschmar, H.A., Monoranu, C.M., Highley, J.R., Kirby, J., Siddique, T., Shaw, P.J., Lee, V.M. & Trojanowski, J.Q., (2007). Pathological TDP-43 distinguishes sporadic amyotrophic lateral sclerosis from amyotrophic lateral sclerosis with SOD1 mutations. *Ann Neurol*. Vol. 61, No. 5, pp. 427-34.

Mackenzie, I.R., Rademakers, R. & Neumann, M., (2010). TDP-43 and FUS in amyotrophic lateral sclerosis and frontotemporal dementia. *Lancet Neurol*. Vol. 9, No. 10, pp. 995-1007.

Magnus, T., Carmen, J., Deleon, J., Xue, H., Pardo, A.C., Lepore, A.C., Mattson, M.P., Rao, M.S. & Maragakis, N.J., (2008). Adult glial precursor proliferation in mutant SOD1G93A mice. *Glia*. Vol. 56, No. 2, pp. 200-8.

Maragakis, N.J. & Rothstein, J.D., (2006). Mechanisms of Disease: astrocytes in neurodegenerative disease. *Nat Clin Pract Neurol*. Vol. 2, No. 12, pp. 679-89.

Marchetto, M.C., Muotri, A.R., Mu, Y., Smith, A.M., Cezar, G.G. & Gage, F.H., (2008). Non-cell-autonomous effect of human SOD1 G37R astrocytes on motor neurons derived from human embryonic stem cells. *Cell Stem Cell*. Vol. 3, No. 6, pp. 649-57.

Miller, R.G., Moore, D.H., 2nd, Gelinas, D.F., Dronsky, V., Mendoza, M., Barohn, R.J., Bryan, W., Ravits, J., Yuen, E., Neville, H., Ringel, S., Bromberg, M., Petajan, J., Amato, A.A., Jackson, C., Johnson, W., Mandler, R., Bosch, P., Smith, B., Graves, M., Ross, M., Sorenson, E.J., Kelkar, P., Parry, G. & Olney, R., (2001). Phase III randomized trial of gabapentin in patients with amyotrophic lateral sclerosis. *Neurology*. Vol. 56, No. 7, pp. 843-8.

Miller, R.G., Mitchell, J.D., Lyon, M. & Moore, D.H., (2007). Riluzole for amyotrophic lateral sclerosis (ALS)/motor neuron disease (MND). *Cochrane Database Syst Rev*. Vol., No. 1, pp. CD001447.

Miller, T.M., Kaspar, B.K., Kops, G.J., Yamanaka, K., Christian, L.J., Gage, F.H. & Cleveland, D.W., (2005). Virus-delivered small RNA silencing sustains strength in amyotrophic lateral sclerosis. *Ann Neurol*. Vol. 57, No. 5, pp. 773-6.

Miller, T.M., Smith, R.A., Kordasiewicz, H. & Kaspar, B.K., (2008). Gene-targeted therapies for the central nervous system. *Arch Neurol*. Vol. 65, No. 4, pp. 447-51.

Nagai, M., Re, D.B., Nagata, T., Chalazonitis, A., Jessell, T.M., Wichterle, H. & Przedborski, S., (2007). Astrocytes expressing ALS-linked mutated SOD1 release factors selectively toxic to motor neurons. *Nat Neurosci*. Vol. 10, No. 5, pp. 615-622.

Neumann, M., Sampathu, D.M., Kwong, L.K., Truax, A.C., Micsenyi, M.C., Chou, T.T., Bruce, J., Schuck, T., Grossman, M., Clark, C.M., McCluskey, L.F., Miller, B.L., Masliah, E., Mackenzie, I.R., Feldman, H., Feiden, W., Kretzschmar, H.A., Trojanowski, J.Q. & Lee,

V.M., (2006). Ubiquitinated TDP-43 in frontotemporal lobar degeneration and amyotrophic lateral sclerosis. *Science*. Vol. 314, No. 5796, pp. 130-3.

Nguyen, M.D., Julien, J.P. & Rivest, S., (2001). Induction of proinflammatory molecules in mice with amyotrophic lateral sclerosis: no requirement for proapoptotic interleukin-1beta in neurodegeneration. *Ann Neurol*. Vol. 50, No. 5, pp. 630-9.

Okita, K., Ichisaka, T. & Yamanaka, S., (2007). Generation of germline-competent induced pluripotent stem cells. *Nature*. Vol. 448, No. 7151, pp. 313-7.

Palmer, T.D., Schwartz, P.H., Taupin, P., Kaspar, B., Stein, S.A. & Gage, F.H., (2001). Cell culture. Progenitor cells from human brain after death. *Nature*. Vol. 411, No. 6833, pp. 42-3.

Park, I.H., Zhao, R., West, J.A., Yabuuchi, A., Huo, H., Ince, T.A., Lerou, P.H., Lensch, M.W. & Daley, G.Q., (2008). Reprogramming of human somatic cells to pluripotency with defined factors. *Nature*. Vol. 451, No. 7175, pp. 141-6.

Perrie, W.T., Lee, G.T., Curtis, E.M., Sparke, J., Buller, J.R. & Rossi, M.L., (1993). Changes in the myelinated axons of femoral nerve in amyotrophic lateral sclerosis. *J Neural Transm Suppl*. Vol. 39, No., pp. 223-33.

Pompl, P.N., Ho, L., Bianchi, M., McManus, T., Qin, W. & Pasinetti, G.M., (2003). A therapeutic role for cyclooxygenase-2 inhibitors in a transgenic mouse model of amyotrophic lateral sclerosis. *FASEB J*. Vol. 17, No. 6, pp. 725-7.

Pramatarova, A., Laganiere, J., Roussel, J., Brisebois, K. & Rouleau, G.A., (2001). Neuron-specific expression of mutant superoxide dismutase 1 in transgenic mice does not lead to motor impairment. *J Neurosci*. Vol. 21, No. 10, pp. 3369-74.

Ralph, G.S., Radcliffe, P.A., Day, D.M., Carthy, J.M., Leroux, M.A., Lee, D.C., Wong, L.F., Bilsland, L.G., Greensmith, L., Kingsman, S.M., Mitrophanous, K.A., Mazarakis, N.D. & Azzouz, M., (2005). Silencing mutant SOD1 using RNAi protects against neurodegeneration and extends survival in an ALS model. *Nat Med*. Vol. 11, No. 4, pp. 429-33.

Raoul, C., Abbas-Terki, T., Bensadoun, J.C., Guillot, S., Haase, G., Szulc, J., Henderson, C.E. & Aebischer, P., (2005). Lentiviral-mediated silencing of SOD1 through RNA interference retards disease onset and progression in a mouse model of ALS. *Nat Med*. Vol. 11, No. 4, pp. 423-8.

Rothstein, J.D., Tsai, G., Kuncl, R.W., Clawson, L., Cornblath, D.R., Drachman, D.B., Pestronk, A., Stauch, B.L. & Coyle, J.T., (1990). Abnormal excitatory amino acid metabolism in amyotrophic lateral sclerosis. *Ann Neurol*. Vol. 28, No. 1, pp. 18-25.

Rothstein, J.D., Van Kammen, M., Levey, A.I., Martin, L.J. & Kuncl, R.W., (1995). Selective loss of glial glutamate transporter GLT-1 in amyotrophic lateral sclerosis. *Ann Neurol*. Vol. 38, No. 1, pp. 73-84.

Rothstein, J.D., Patel, S., Regan, M.R., Haenggeli, C., Huang, Y.H., Bergles, D.E., Jin, L., Dykes Hoberg, M., Vidensky, S., Chung, D.S., Toan, S.V., Bruijn, L.I., Su, Z.Z., Gupta, P. & Fisher, P.B., (2005). Beta-lactam antibiotics offer neuroprotection by increasing glutamate transporter expression. *Nature*. Vol. 433, No. 7021, pp. 73-7.

Ryberg, H., Askmark, H. & Persson, L.I., (2003). A double-blind randomized clinical trial in amyotrophic lateral sclerosis using lamotrigine: effects on CSF glutamate, aspartate, branched-chain amino acid levels and clinical parameters. *Acta Neurol Scand*. Vol. 108, No. 1, pp. 1-8.

Sah, D.W. & Aronin, N., (2011). Oligonucleotide therapeutic approaches for Huntington disease. *J Clin Invest*. Vol. 121, No. 2, pp. 500-7.

Sasaki, S., Shibata, N., Komori, T. & Iwata, M., (2000). iNOS and nitrotyrosine immunoreactivity in amyotrophic lateral sclerosis. *Neurosci Lett*. Vol. 291, No. 1, pp. 44-8.

Shaw, P.J., Forrest, V., Ince, P.G., Richardson, J.P. & Wastell, H.J., (1995). CSF and plasma amino acid levels in motor neuron disease: elevation of CSF glutamate in a subset of patients. *Neurodegeneration*. Vol. 4, No. 2, pp. 209-16.

Smith, R.A., Miller, T.M., Yamanaka, K., Monia, B.P., Condon, T.P., Hung, G., Lobsiger, C.S., Ward, C.M., McAlonis-Downes, M., Wei, H., Wancewicz, E.V., Bennett, C.F. & Cleveland, D.W., (2006). Antisense oligonucleotide therapy for neurodegenerative disease. *J Clin Invest*. Vol. 116, No. 8, pp. 2290-6.

Sreedharan, J., Blair, I.P., Tripathi, V.B., Hu, X., Vance, C., Rogelj, B., Ackerley, S., Durnall, J.C., Williams, K.L., Buratti, E., Baralle, F., de Belleroche, J., Mitchell, J.D., Leigh, P.N., Al-Chalabi, A., Miller, C.C., Nicholson, G. & Shaw, C.E., (2008). TDP-43 mutations in familial and sporadic amyotrophic lateral sclerosis. *Science*. Vol. 319, No. 5870, pp. 1668-72.

Suzuki, M., McHugh, J., Tork, C., Shelley, B., Klein, S.M., Aebischer, P. & Svendsen, C.N., (2007). GDNF secreting human neural progenitor cells protect dying motor neurons, but not their projection to muscle, in a rat model of familial ALS. *PLoS One*. Vol. 2, No. 8, pp. e689.

Takahashi, K. & Yamanaka, S., (2006). Induction of pluripotent stem cells from mouse embryonic and adult fibroblast cultures by defined factors. *Cell*. Vol. 126, No. 4, pp. 663-76.

Takahashi, K., Tanabe, K., Ohnuki, M., Narita, M., Ichisaka, T., Tomoda, K. & Yamanaka, S., (2007). Induction of pluripotent stem cells from adult human fibroblasts by defined factors. *Cell*. Vol. 131, No. 5, pp. 861-72.

Towne, C., Setola, V., Schneider, B.L. & Aebischer, P., (2011). Neuroprotection by gene therapy targeting mutant SOD1 in individual pools of motor neurons does not translate into therapeutic benefit in fALS mice. *Mol Ther*. Vol. 19, No. 2, pp. 274-83.

Turner, B.J., Ackerley, S., Davies, K.E. & Talbot, K., (2010). Dismutase-competent SOD1 mutant accumulation in myelinating Schwann cells is not detrimental to normal or transgenic ALS model mice. *Hum Mol Genet*. Vol. 19, No. 5, pp. 815-24.

Urushitani, M., Sik, A., Sakurai, T., Nukina, N., Takahashi, R. & Julien, J.P., (2006). Chromogranin-mediated secretion of mutant superoxide dismutase proteins linked to amyotrophic lateral sclerosis. *Nat Neurosci*. Vol. 9, No. 1, pp. 108-18.

Van Den Bosch, L., Tilkin, P., Lemmens, G. & Robberecht, W., (2002). Minocycline delays disease onset and mortality in a transgenic model of ALS. *Neuroreport*. Vol. 13, No. 8, pp. 1067-70.

Vance, C., Rogelj, B., Hortobagyi, T., De Vos, K.J., Nishimura, A.L., Sreedharan, J., Hu, X., Smith, B., Ruddy, D., Wright, P., Ganesalingam, J., Williams, K.L., Tripathi, V., Al-Saraj, S., Al-Chalabi, A., Leigh, P.N., Blair, I.P., Nicholson, G., de Belleroche, J., Gallo, J.M., Miller, C.C. & Shaw, C.E., (2009). Mutations in FUS, an RNA processing protein, cause familial amyotrophic lateral sclerosis type 6. *Science*. Vol. 323, No. 5918, pp. 1208-11.

Wang, H., Ghosh, A., Baigude, H., Yang, C.S., Qiu, L., Xia, X., Zhou, H., Rana, T.M. & Xu, Z., (2008). Therapeutic gene silencing delivered by a chemically modified small interfering RNA against mutant SOD1 slows amyotrophic lateral sclerosis progression. *J Biol Chem*. Vol. 283, No. 23, pp. 15845-52.

Wang, L., Sharma, K., Grisotti, G. & Roos, R.P., (2009). The effect of mutant SOD1 dismutase activity on non-cell autonomous degeneration in familial amyotrophic lateral sclerosis. *Neurobiol Dis*. Vol. 35, No. 2, pp. 234-40.

Wang, L., Gutmann, D.H. & Roos, R.P., (2011). Astrocyte loss of mutant SOD1 delays ALS disease onset and progression in G85R transgenic mice. *Hum Mol Genet*. Vol. 20, No. 2, pp. 286-93.

Wernig, M., Meissner, A., Foreman, R., Brambrink, T., Ku, M., Hochedlinger, K., Bernstein, B.E. & Jaenisch, R., (2007). In vitro reprogramming of fibroblasts into a pluripotent ES-cell-like state. *Nature*. Vol. 448, No. 7151, pp. 318-24.

Weydt, P., Yuen, E.C., Ransom, B.R. & Moller, T., (2004). Increased cytotoxic potential of microglia from ALS-transgenic mice. *Glia*. Vol. 48, No. 2, pp. 179-82.

Xiao, Q., Zhao, W., Beers, D.R., Yen, A.A., Xie, W., Henkel, J.S. & Appel, S.H., (2007). Mutant SOD1(G93A) microglia are more neurotoxic relative to wild-type microglia. *J Neurochem*. Vol. 102, No. 6, pp. 2008-19.

Xu, L., Ryugo, D.K., Pongstaporn, T., Johe, K. & Koliatsos, V.E., (2009). Human neural stem cell grafts in the spinal cord of SOD1 transgenic rats: differentiation and structural integration into the segmental motor circuitry. *J Comp Neurol*. Vol. 514, No. 4, pp. 297-309.

Xu, L., Shen, P., Hazel, T., Johe, K. & Koliatsos, V.E., (2011). Dual transplantation of human neural stem cells into cervical and lumbar cord ameliorates motor neuron disease in SOD1 transgenic rats. *Neurosci Lett*. Vol. 494, No. 3, pp. 222-6.

Yamanaka, K., Boillee, S., Roberts, E.A., Garcia, M.L., McAlonis-Downes, M., Mikse, O.R., Cleveland, D.W. & Goldstein, L.S., (2008a). Mutant SOD1 in cell types other than motor neurons and oligodendrocytes accelerates onset of disease in ALS mice. *Proc Natl Acad Sci U S A*. Vol. 105, No. 21, pp. 7594-9.

Yamanaka, K., Chun, S.J., Boillee, S., Fujimori-Tonou, N., Yamashita, H., Gutmann, D.H., Takahashi, R., Misawa, H. & Cleveland, D.W., (2008b). Astrocytes as determinants of disease progression in inherited amyotrophic lateral sclerosis. *Nat Neurosci*. Vol., No., pp.

Yamanaka, S. & Blau, H.M., (2010). Nuclear reprogramming to a pluripotent state by three approaches. *Nature*. Vol. 465, No. 7299, pp. 704-12.

Yu, J., Vodyanik, M.A., Smuga-Otto, K., Antosiewicz-Bourget, J., Frane, J.L., Tian, S., Nie, J., Jonsdottir, G.A., Ruotti, V., Stewart, R., Slukvin, II & Thomson, J.A., (2007). Induced pluripotent stem cell lines derived from human somatic cells. *Science*. Vol. 318, No. 5858, pp. 1917-20.

Zhao, T., Zhang, Z.N., Rong, Z. & Xu, Y., (2011). Immunogenicity of induced pluripotent stem cells. *Nature*. Vol. 474, No. 7350, pp. 212-5.

Zhao, W., Xie, W., Xiao, Q., Beers, D.R. & Appel, S.H., (2006). Protective effects of an anti-inflammatory cytokine, interleukin-4, on motoneuron toxicity induced by activated microglia. *J Neurochem*. Vol. 99, No. 4, pp. 1176-87.

Zhao, W., Beers, D.R., Henkel, J.S., Zhang, W., Urushitani, M., Julien, J.P. & Appel, S.H., (2010). Extracellular mutant SOD1 induces microglial-mediated motoneuron injury. *Glia*. Vol. 58, No. 2, pp. 231-43.

Zhu, S., Stavrovskaya, I.G., Drozda, M., Kim, B.Y., Ona, V., Li, M., Sarang, S., Liu, A.S., Hartley, D.M., Wu, D.C., Gullans, S., Ferrante, R.J., Przedborski, S., Kristal, B.S. & Friedlander, R.M., (2002). Minocycline inhibits cytochrome c release and delays progression of amyotrophic lateral sclerosis in mice. *Nature*. Vol. 417, No. 6884, pp. 74-8.

Zinman, L. & Cudkowicz, M., (2011). Emerging targets and treatments in amyotrophic lateral sclerosis. *Lancet Neurol*. Vol. 10, No. 5, pp. 481-90.

Part 4

Human Genetics in ALS

21

Genetics of Amyotrophic Lateral Sclerosis

Max Koppers[1, 2], Michael van Es[1], Leonard H. van den Berg[1],
Jan H. Veldink[1*] and R. Jeroen Pasterkamp[1, 2*]
[1]*Departments of Neurology, University Medical Center Utrecht,*
[2]*Deparment of Neuroscience and Pharmacology, University Medical Center Utrecht,*
The Netherlands

1. Introduction

Amyotrophic lateral sclerosis (ALS) is a neurodegenerative disease characterized by progressive muscle weakness caused by loss of central and peripheral motor neurons. Symptoms typically have a localized limb or bulbar onset and progress to other muscle groups of the body. Denervation of respiratory muscles and dysphagia leading to respiratory complications are the most common causes of death. There is no cure for this rapidly progressive disease.

Approximately 5% of patients have a family history of ALS (fALS) (Byrne et al., 2011). All other cases are considered to have a sporadic form of the disease (sALS). A twin study of sALS patients has estimated hereditability to be considerable (0.38-0.76), indicating an important genetic component in disease etiology (Al-Chalabi et al., 2010). sALS, therefore, is considered to be a disease of complex etiology with both genetic and environmental factors contributing to disease susceptibility.

This chapter will provide an overview of the current knowledge of the genetics of both fALS and sALS. There will be, however, particular emphasis on two sALS associated regions identified in a large genome wide association study namely, chromosomal region 9p21.2 and 19p13.11. Evidence for the association with these regions as well as the function of the relevant genes in these regions will be discussed.

2. Genetics of familial amyotrophic lateral sclerosis

Familial ALS is a genetically heterogeneous group of diseases for which linkage has been found for over 13 different loci (Table 1). These loci account for approximately 25-30% of all fALS cases. In addition, variants in several other genes have been implicated in fALS but most of these data are still inconclusive. All currently known fALS loci and the genes involved will be briefly discussed in this section.

2.1 ALS1 (SOD1)

Linkage analysis in autosomal-dominant fALS pedigrees associated the copper-zinc superoxide dismutase (*SOD1*) gene on chromosome 21q to ALS. Several point mutations in

*Corresponding authors

Name of Disease	*Locus*	*Gene*	*Protein*	*Inheritance*	*Clinical features*
ALS1	21q22	*SOD1*	Cu/Zn superoxide dismutase	AD/AR	Typical ALS
ALS2	2q33	*ALSin*	ALSin	AR	Juvenile onset, slowly progressive, predominantly upper motor neuron signs
ALS3	18q21	N.K.	-	AD	Typical ALS, disease onset in legs
ALS4	9q34	*SETX*	Senataxin	AD	Childhood/Adolescent onset, slowly progressive, no respiratory and bulbar involvement
ALS5	15q15-21	*SPG11*	Spatacsin	AR	Juvenile onset, slowly progressive
ALS6	16p11.2	*FUS*	Fused in sarcoma	AD/AR	Typical ALS
ALS7	20p13	N.K.	-	AD	Typical ALS
ALS8	20q13	*VAPB*	VAMP-associated protein B	AD	Typical ALS, SMA and atypical ALS
ALS9	14q11	*ANG*	Angiogenin	AD	Typical ALS, frontotemporal dementia, Parkinson's disease
ALS10	1q36	*TARDBP*	TAR-DNA binding protein	AD	Typical ALS
ALS11	6q21	*FIG4*	PI(3,5)P(2)5-phosphatase	AD	Adult onset, prominent corticospinal tract signs
ALS12	10p13	*OPTN*	Optineurin	AD/AR	Adult onset
ALS14	9p13-p12	*VCP*	Valosin-containing protein	AD	Adult onset with or without FTD
ALS-FTD1	9q21-22	N.K.	-	AD	ALS, FTD
ALS-FTD2	9p13.2-21.3	*C9ORF72*	Chromosome 9 open reading frame 72	AD	ALS, FTD
ALS-FTDP	17q21.1	*MAPT*	Microtubule-associated protein tau	AD	Adult onset with FTD
ALS-X	Xcen	N.K.	-	XD	Adult onset

AD = Autosomal dominant, AR = Autosomal recessive, XD = X-linked dominant, FTD = frontotemporal dementia, SMA = spinal muscular atrophy, N.K. = not known, FTDP = frontotemporal dementia with parkinsonism

Table 1. Classification of familial ALS.

SOD1 that co-segregated with the disease were identified in several of these pedigrees (Rosen et al., 1993). To date, over 150 different mutations in *SOD1* have been identified (see http://alsod.iop.kcl.ac.uk). Mutations have been reported in ~20% of fALS patients and in 1-4% of sALS patients (Pasinelli and Brown, 2006; Valdmanis and Rouleau, 2008).
The SOD1 protein is a cytoplasmic enzyme that converts superoxide radicals, a by-product of oxidative phosphorylation, to hydrogen peroxide and molecular oxygen. The exact mechanism by which *SOD1* mutations lead to ALS pathology is unknown although several toxic properties of mutant SOD1 such as aberrant oxidative stress, protein instability, and mitochondrial damage have been proposed to be causative (reviewed in Pasinelli and Brown, 2006). Interestingly, the presence of mutant SOD1 in non-neuronal cells contributes to pathogenesis and is needed for disease progression (Ilieva et al., 2009). *SOD1* mutations most likely result in a toxic gain of function pathology since *SOD1* knockout mice do not develop motor neuron degeneration whereas transgenic mice overexpressing mutant SOD1 show motor neuron degeneration and ALS-like pathology (Gurney et al., 1994; Reaume et al., 1996).

2.2 ALS2 (ALSin)

ALS2 is an autosomal recessive form of juvenile ALS that was first reported in a large consanguineous Tunisian kindred and linkage analysis in this family associated locus 2q33-q35 to ALS (Hentati et al., 1994). This led to the discovery of causal mutations in the gene encoding ALSin (Hadano et al., 2001; Yang et al., 2001). Mutations in *ALSin* have been scarcely reported and do not appear to be a common cause of ALS.
ALSin is a Rab5 and Rac1 guanine exchange factor that acts as a regulator of endosomal/membrane trafficking. The protein is able to promote neurite outgrowth in neuronal cultures through activation of the small GTPase Rac1 (Otomo et al., 2003; Topp et al., 2004). Overexpression of ALSin protects cultured motor neuronal cells from mutant SOD1 toxicity suggesting a neuroprotective role. Mutations in *ALSin* may induce a loss of this neuroprotective function (Kanekura et al., 2004). *ALSin* knockout mice do not develop overt motor neuron disease but degeneration of the corticospinal tract has been reported (Cai et al., 2008; Hadano et al., 2006).

2.3 ALS3 (18q21)

Linkage to chromosome 18q21 was identified in a large European family of which 20 members had autosomal-dominant ALS (Hand et al., 2002). This region contains 50 genes but the causal mutation at this locus remains to be identified.

2.4 ALS4 (SETX)

ALS4 is a rare, childhood- or adolescent-onset, autosomal dominant disease, which is also known as distal hereditary motor neuronopathy with pyramidal features. Linkage to chromosome 9q34 was found in a large family from the USA with 49 affected members (Chance et al., 1998). Sequencing of 19 genes in this locus revealed that missense mutations in the senataxin (*SETX*) gene were the cause of ALS4 in several families (Chen et al., 2004). Since then, mutations have been identified in additional ALS patients from China, Italy and the USA (Avemaria et al., 2011; Hirano et al., 2011; Zhao et al., 2009). Interestingly, mutations in *SETX* leading to a premature termination in the protein product have also been identified in ataxia oculomotor apraxia 2 (Moreira et al., 2004).

Senataxin contains a seven-motif domain characteristic for DNA/RNA helicases. It displays strong homology to several genes involved in RNA processing such as the immunoglobulin mu binding protein 2 gene (*IGHMBP2*), in which mutations are known to cause spinal muscular atrophy with respiratory distress type 1 (Grohmann et al., 2001). SETX was shown to be involved in the termination of RNA transcription (Skourti-Stathaki et al., 2011). It is therefore possible that mutations in *SETX* cause neuronal degeneration due to aberrant RNA processing. Overexpression of wild-type senataxin in primary hippocampal neurons is sufficient to trigger neuronal differentiation by protecting cells from apoptosis and promoting neuritogenesis (Vantaggiato et al., 2011).

2.5 ALS5 (SPG11)

This is the most common form of recessive fALS and is characterized by a juvenile onset. In seven families from Tunisia, Pakistan, and Germany, linkage to chromosome 15q15-21 was found (Hentati et al., 1998). Recently, 12 mutations in the spatacsin (*SPG11*) gene were identified in 10 unrelated pedigrees from Italy, Brazil, Canada, Turkey, and Japan (Orlacchio et al., 2010). Ten out of 12 mutations are frameshift or nonsense mutations. Mutations in *SPG11* are known to cause autosomal recessive hereditary spastic paraplegia with a thin corpus callosum (Stevanin et al., 2007).

Spatacsin contains four putative transmembrane domains, a leucine zipper and a coiled-coil domain. The exact function of spatacsin is unknown although it may play a role in axonal transport (Salinas et al., 2008).

2.6 ALS6 (FUS)

Linkage to a 42-Mb region containing more than 400 genes on chromosome 16 was reported in several families (Sapp et al. 2003). Recently, mutations in the fused in sarcoma/translated in liposarcoma (*FUS/TLS*) gene were shown to cause ALS6 (Kwiatkowski et al., 2009; Vance et al., 2009). Several subsequent studies have identified additional mutations in *FUS* in ALS cohorts from different populations with an overall frequency of ~4% in fALS and ~1% in sALS (Belzil et al., 2009; Corrado et al., 2010; Hewitt et al., 2010; Groen et al., 2010). *FUS* mutations have also been detected in fALS patients with frontemporal dementia (FTD) and patients with juvenile ALS with basophilic inclusions (Bäumer et al., 2010; Huang et al. 2010; Yan et al., 2010).

The *FUS* gene encodes for a DNA/RNA binding protein that is involved in several cellular pathways including the splicing, transport and maturation of RNA (Lagier-Tourenne et al., 2010). FUS positive ubiquitinated cytoplasmic inclusions have been observed in spinal cord tissue of sALS and fALS patients without *SOD1* and *FUS* mutations (Deng et al., 2010). The majority of *FUS* mutations identified reside in its C-terminal nuclear localization signal which results in an abnormal cytoplasmic localization of FUS and localization to stress granules (Bosco et al., 2010; Dormann et al., 2010; Ito et al., 2010). In yeast, overexpression of human FUS leads to toxicity, cytoplasmic inclusions and FUS localization to stress granules as can be seen in ALS patients (Ju et al., 2011; Sun et al., 2011). In addition, transgenic rats overexpressing ALS mutant FUS develop progressive paralysis due to motor axon degeneration as well as neuronal loss in the cortex and hippocampus which are phenotypes seen in ALS and FTD (Huang et al., 2011).

2.7 ALS7 (20p)

Linkage to chromosome 20p was found in a large autosomal dominant fALS pedigree from the USA. A 5-Mb segment was identified that was shared between two affected siblings (Sapp et al., 2003). This region contains 24 genes but no causal mutation has been identified.

2.8 ALS8 (VAPB)

In a large family from Brazil with 28 affected members across 4 generations, linkage was found at chromosome 20q13.3. Sequencing identified a mutation (P56S) in the vesicle associated membrane protein (VAMP)/synaptobrevin-associated membrane protein B (*VAPB*) gene in all affected members of this family (Nishimura et al., 2004). The same mutation was also identified in six additional families with different clinical courses including, ALS8, late-onset spinal muscular atrophy and typical severe ALS with rapid progression. A different mutation (T46I) was detected in a family from the UK (Chen et al., 2010).

The VAPB protein has been implicated in various cellular processes including the formation of the presynaptic terminal in neurons, vesicle trafficking and the unfolded protein response (Chen et al., 2010). Transgenic mice overexpressing ALS mutant VAPB or wild-type VAPB do not develop an overt motor neuron phenotype. However, transgenic mice overexpressing ALS mutant but not wild-type VAPB show TAR DNA-binding protein 43 (TDP-43) positive cytoplasmic inclusions, a pathological hallmark of ALS (Tudor et al., 2010). It has been suggested that mutant VAPB exerts a dominant-negative effect by forming dimeric complexes with wild-type VAPB thereby recruiting it into aggregates (Teuling et al., 2007).

2.9 ALS9 (ANG)

Angiogenin (*ANG*) was identified as a candidate gene for ALS because it is located 237kb downstream of apurinic endonuclease, multifunctional DNA repair enzyme (*APEX*) and because of its functional similarity to vascular endothelial growth factor (VEGF) (Greenway et al., 2004). Both *APEX* and *VEGF* are candidate genes for sALS and will be discussed in the next section. A single nucleotide polymorphism (SNP) in *ANG* was associated with ALS in patients from Ireland and Scotland (Greenway et al., 2004). Missense mutations in *ANG* were found in 4 fALS cases and 11 sALS cases (Greenway et al., 2006). Subsequent sequencing in populations from Europe and the USA identified additional mutations in approximately 2% of fALS cases and 1% of sALS cases (Conforti et al., 2008; Fernández-Santiago et al., 2009; Gellera et al., 2008; Paubel et al., 2008; Wu et al., 2007). However, *ANG* mutations have also been observed in healthy controls suggesting that not all mutations are pathogenic (Corrado et al., 2007). A K17I mutation was identified in a 4-generation family of which one patient presented with ALS, FTD, and Parkinsonism (Van Es et al., 2009a). An obligate carrier did not develop the disease suggesting incomplete penetrance. Two *ANG* mutations (K17I and K54E) were identified in two fALS cases from France who also had a mutation in FUS (Millecamps et al., 2010). An R145C mutation has been observed in a sALS patient with a G93D SOD1 mutation (Luigetti et al., 2011). A recent study showed a significantly higher frequency of *ANG* variants in both ALS and Parkinson's disease (PD) patients which could reflect a genetic susceptibility to widespread neurodegeneration (Van Es et al., 2011).

The ANG protein is a member of the pancreatic ribonuclease superfamily and a potent mediator of new blood vessel formation. In endothelial cells, the protein can promote ribosomal RNA (rRNA) production and cellular proliferation and is able to cleave transfer

RNA which results in inhibition of protein translation (Yamasaki et al., 2009). ANG is also expressed in spinal motor neurons (Sebastià et al., 2009). It is thought that *ANG* mutations cause ALS due to a loss of function and it has been shown that wild-type but not mutant angiogenin is neuroprotective and that mutant angiogenin impairs neurite outgrowth *in vitro* (Sebastià et al., 2009; Subramanian et al., 2008; Wu et al., 2007).

2.10 ALS10 (TARDBP)

TDP-43 was identified as one of the main components of ubiquitinated cytoplasmic inclusions in ALS and FTD (Neumann et al., 2006). Sequencing of the gene encoding this protein (*TARDBP*) identified mutations in ALS patients (Kabashi et al., 2008; Shreedharan et al., 2008). To date over 40 mutations in *TARDBP* have been identified in several different populations with a frequency of ~5% of fALS cases and up to 2% of sALS cases (Corrado et al., 2009; Iida et al., 2010; Millecamps et al., 2010; Ticozzi et al., 2009; Van Deerlin et al., 2008). *TARDBP* mutations have also been observed in ALS-FTD and FTD patients (Benajiba et al., 2009; Gitcho et al., 2009b). Despite the presence of *TARDBP* mutations in only a portion of ALS and FTD patients, TDP-43-positive cytoplasmic inclusions are found in almost all ALS patients but they are also seen in other neurodegenerative diseases such as FTD, Huntington's, Alzheimer's, and Parkinson's disease (Da Cruz and Cleveland, 2011).

TDP-43, like FUS, is a DNA/RNA binding protein that is part of the heterogeneous ribonucleoprotein family. It has a role in gene transcription, regulation of splicing, and mRNA transport and stabilization (Buratti and Baralle, 2010). Except for one truncation mutation, all *TARDBP* mutations identified in ALS patients are missense mutations clustered in the glycine-rich C-terminal region which is involved in protein-protein interactions (Lagier-Tourenne et al., 2010). *TARDBP* mutations lead to an abnormal distribution of the protein to the cytoplasm.

2.11 ALS11 (FIG4)

Mutations in the PI(3,5)P(2)5-phosphatase (*FIG4*) gene on chromosome 6q21 are known to cause a severe form of Charcot-Marie-Tooth (CMT) disease with early onset and loss of sensory and motor neurons, CMT4J (Chow et al., 2007). In a screen for *FIG4* mutations in a large cohort of sALS and fALS patients, several variants were detected that were unique to fALS and sALS patients (Chow et al., 2009). Two mutations were identified in patients diagnosed with primary lateral sclerosis. To date, no other studies have replicated the finding of ALS-associated FIG4 mutations in other cohorts and it is unclear whether *FIG4* mutations are pathogenic in ALS patients.

FIG4 is a phosphoinositide 5-phosphatase that regulates PI(3,5)P2 abundance. PI(3,5)P2 is a signalling lipid that mediates endosomal trafficking to the trans-Golgi network (Rutherford et al., 2006). Pale tremor mice, which are homozygous for null mutations in *FIG4*, show neurodegeneration in sensory and autonomic ganglia, motor cortex, striatum, and cerebellum. Motor neurons in the ventral spinal cord contain vacuoles (Chow et al., 2007). Mutant mice lacking *Vac14*, a gene encoding for a FIG4 interactor, show a similar neurodegeneration (Zhang et al., 2007).

2.12 ALS12 (OPTN)

Using homozygosity mapping in six ALS patients from consanguineous marriages, an overlapping region on chromosome 10 was identified as the candidate region. Screening of

17 genes in this region revealed a homozygous deletion in the gene for optineurin (*OPTN*), a gene known to cause primary open-angle glaucoma, in two siblings and an individual from a different family (Murayama et al., 2010; Rezaie et al., 2002). In addition, a homozygous nonsense (Q398X) mutation was identified in one fALS case (Murayama et al., 2010). Subsequent screening in a larger cohort of fALS and sALS patients identified a heterozygous missense mutation (E478G) in a four individuals with ALS from two families (Murayama et al., 2010). A homozygous E478G mutation was identified in a Japanese fALS case in a different study (Iida et al., 2011). One additional nonsense mutation and one missense mutation in *OPTN* were identified in fALS cases from Italy (Del Bo et al., 2011). Two separate studies identified novel variants in fALS patients but the authors state that these variants may be a genetic predisposition to glaucoma instead of causing ALS (Belzil et al., 2011; Millecamps et al., 2011). One study also detected mutations in sALS patients with a rapid disease progression (van Blitterswijk et al., 2011). Another study could not identify *OPTN* mutations in fALS and sALS patients (Sugihara et al., 2011).

OPTN is a multifunctional protein involved in membrane trafficking, maintainance of the Golgi complex, and exocytosis (Sahlender et al., 2005). OPTN can inhibit the activation of NFκB and it has been proposed that mutations in *OPTN* causing ALS may relieve this inhibition and cause neuronal death (Murayama et al., 2010).

2.13 ALS14 (VCP)

Recently an exome sequencing study detected a mutation in the gene encoding valosin-containing protein (*VCP*) in an Italian family. Subsequent screening in 210 ALS cases from unrelated families identified four mutations in *VCP* in four different families from Italy and the USA (Johnson et al., 2010). Mutations in the gene for *VCP*, located on chromosome 9p13.3, are a known cause for the multi-system degenerative disease inclusion body myopathy with Paget's disease and frontotemporal dementia (IBMPFD) (Watts et al. 2004). IBMPFD, like ALS, is characterized pathologically by TDP-43 inclusions (Weihl et al., 2008).

VCP is an AAA+-ATPase that mediates ubiquitin-dependent extraction of substrates from multiprotein complexes for subsequent recycling or degradation by the proteasome. It plays a role in a variety of cellular functions including Golgi biogenesis, cell cycle regulation, DNA damage repair and protein homeostasis through the ubiquitin-proteasome system (Ju and Weihl, 2010). It is thought that *VCP* mutations result in the impairment of protein degradation trough both the ubiquitin-proteasome system and autophagy leading to the formation of inclusions. *VCP* mutations found in FTD and ALS have been shown to disrupt TDP-43 localization from the nucleus to the cytoplasm which could be caused by the disruption in protein homeostasis (Gitcho et al, 2009a; Ju and Weihl, 2010). In mice, a missense mutation in vacuolar sorting protein 54, the mouse homologue of VCP, causes motor neuron degeneration (Schmitt-John et al., 2005).

2.14 Other fALS associated genes

In addition to the genes listed in the previous sections, several other genes have been implicated in fALS.

Dynactin 1 (*DCTN1*) was discovered as a candidate gene for ALS when a G59S mutation in this gene was identified in a family with a slowly progressive, autosomal dominant form of lower motor neuron disease without sensory symptoms (Puls et al., 2003; Puls et al., 2005). Subsequent sequencing of the *DCNT1* gene in 250 ALS patients revealed the presence of three heterozygous missense mutations in one sALS and three fALS cases with typical ALS (Münch et al., 2004). An additional mutation was detected in a patient with ALS and his brother who had FTD (Münch et al., 2005). The pathogenicity of these variants has however not been established. Screening for *DCTN1* mutations in a cohort of ALS, FTD or ALS-FTD patients did not result in the identification of disease segregating variants (Vilariño-Güell et al., 2009). One of the missense variants identified in a sALS case was also found in controls in the same study (Vilariño-Güell et al., 2009). Interestingly, five mutations in *DCTN1* were found in eight families with Perry syndrome, a disease that is characterized by Parkinsonism and TDP-43- and ubiquitin- positive inclusions (Farrer et al., 2009).

In a 3-generation family with typical ALS, a mutation in the D-amino acid oxidase (*DAO*) gene was identified (Mitchell et al., 2010). However, screening of an additional 322 unrelated fALS cases did not reveal any other causal mutation in this gene (Mitchell et al., 2010). Additional screening will be needed but *DAO* mutations seem to be very rare in ALS.

Because of their structural and functional similarities to FUS, the genes encoding TAF15 RNA polymerase II, TATA box binding protein associated factor (*TAF15*) and Ewing sarcoma breakpoint region 1 (*EWS*) were screened in fALS cases (Ticozzi et al., 2010). Two missense mutations in *TAF15* (A31T and R395Q) were identified in three fALS cases and not in 1159 controls. However, one of the fALS cases with an R395Q mutation also carried a mutation in *TARDBP*. Moreover, the R395Q is in close proximity to two non-pathogenic variants, suggesting it is a benign polymorphism (Ticozzi et al., 2010).

Recently, a mutation in the sigma non-opioid intracellular receptor 1 (*SIGMAR1*) gene was identified in an autosomal recessive family with juvenile ALS (Al-Saif et al., 2011). Interestingly, variants in the 3'UTR of *SIGMAR1* were described in three ALS-FTD families (Luty et al., 2010).

An X-linked dominant ALS locus has been reported but has not been further described (Siddique et al., 1998). Recently, mutations in the gene encoding ubiquitin-like protein ubiquilin 2 (*UBQLN2*) were identified as the cause of dominantly inherited X-linked ALS and ALS/dementia (Deng et al., 2011).

Several family pedigrees contain individuals affected by ALS, FTD or both. The first linkage study performed in 16 of these ALS-FTD families found linkage to chromosome **9q21-q22**, designated as ALS-FTD1 (Hosler et al., 2000). This association has thus far not been replicated in other ALS-FTD families. Linkage to chromosome 9p in ALS-FTD families (ALS-FTD2) has also been reported. A hexanucleotide repeat expansion in the chromosome 9 open reading frame 72 (*C9ORF72*) gene was recently identified as the causal genetic defect of ALS-FTD2 and will be discussed in a next section (Dejesus-Hernandez et al., 2011; Renton et al., 2011). Mutations in the gene encoding microtubule-associated protein tau (*MAPT*) have been reported in patients with ALS or FTD (Hutton et al., 1998).

Finally, mutations in the neurofilament heavy (*NEFH*) gene and the paraoxonase genes (*PON1, 2, 3*) have been identified in fALS cases and these genes will be discussed in more detail in the following section.

3. Genetics of sporadic ALS

Sporadic ALS is considered to be a complex disease, where both genetic and environmental factors contribute to pathogenesis. Several association studies have been performed to identify the genetic contribution in sALS with mixed success, possibly due to the small sample sizes in many of these studies. Although their precise contribution to sALS is often unclear, a few of the risk factors identified to date have been consistently replicated. Furthermore, several of these associated genes have overlapping cellular functions such as in RNA metabolism, vesicle trafficking, and axonal transport. In this section, genes that have been associated with sALS will be discussed (Table 2). In addition to these genes, mutations in several fALS associated genes that were discussed in the previous section have been found in a portion of sALS cases.

Associated Gene	*Protein*	*Positive studies*	*Negative studies*	*Type of association found*	*Additional information*
APEX	Apurinic endonuclease, DNA repair enzyme	2	2	SNP association	Protein has a role in oxidative stress
ATXN2	Ataxin-2	6	0	PolyQ repeats	Intermediate polyQ repeats increase risk for sALS/interaction with TDP-43
CHMP2B	Chromatin modifying protein 2B	2	0	Mutations	Mutations are known to cause FTD. All patients have lower motor neuron signs consistent with PMA.
HFE	Haemo-chromatosis	5	1	SNP association	Mutations cause hereditary haemochromatosis
NEFH	Neurofilament-heavy	5	3	Deletions/ insertions/ mutations	Neurofilament-containing inclusions are a pathological hallmark of ALS
SMN1	Survival motor neuron 1	3	1	Abnormal copy number	*SMN1* deletions cause SMA
SMN2	Survival motor neuron 2	1	5	Deletions	*SMN2* copy number variation affects SMA disease severity
PON1, 2, 3	Paraoxonase	7	3	SNP association/ mutations	Possible gene-environment interaction
PRPH	Peripherin	3	0	Mutations	Peripherin-containing inclusions are a pathological hallmark of ALS. Possible involvement of abnormal splice forms.
VEGF	Vascular-endothelial growth factor	2	6	SNP association	Deletion of HRE in promoter results in an ALS phenotype in mice. Possible gender association.

Table 2. Genes associated with sporadic ALS

3.1 Apurinic endonuclease, multifunctional DNA repair enzyme (APEX1)

A study in 117 Scottish sALS patients showed association of a common SNP resulting in a D148E amino-acid change with ALS (Hayward et al., 1999). This finding was replicated in 169 Irish sALS patients (Greenway et al., 2004). In one study, DNA extracted from CNS tissue from 81 sALS patients was screened but the D184E SNP was not associated with ALS (Tomkins et al., 2000). A different study assessing 134 Italian sALS patients also failed to detect significant association between this SNP and ALS (Coppedè et al., 2010). These inconsistent association results might reflect a population-specific effect of the *APEX1* D184E allele.

APEX1 is involved in DNA repair and maintains and stimulates the DNA binding activity of transcription factors (Fishel and Kelley, 2007). Frontal cortical levels and activity of APEX1 were significantly reduced in 11 ALS patients as compared to six controls (Kisby et al., 1997). However, in a different study, increased expression levels and activity in ALS brain and spinal cord motor neurons were observed (Shaikh and Martin, 2002).

3.2 Ataxin-2 (ATXN2)

In a screen for toxicity modifiers of TDP-43 in yeast, ataxin-2 (ATXN2) was identified (Elden et al., 2010). ATXN2 and TDP-43 form a RNA-dependent complex and are mislocalized in spinal cord motor neurons in ALS patients. *ATXN2* has a polyglutamine (polyQ) region which is normally 22-23 repeats long. Expansion of this region of the protein to 34 repeats causes spinocerebellar ataxia type 2 (SCA2) (Imbert et al., 1996; Pulst et al., 1996; Sanpei et al. 1996). The polyQ repeat length of *ATXN2* was determined in 915 ALS patients and 980 controls and intermediate length polyQ repeats (23-34) were found to be more common in ALS patients and thus may be a risk factor for ALS (Elden et al., 2010). This finding was replicated in several studies with ALS patients from different populations. Interestingly, the exact length of the polyQ repeat region seems to vary between populations (Chen et al., 2011; Daoud et al., 2011; Lee et al., 2011; Ross et al., 2011; Van Damme et al., 2011).

Longer polyQ repeats in ATXN2 possibly stabilize the protein and enhance its interaction with TDP-43. Under stress conditions, increased mislocalization of TDP-43 to the cytoplasm was observed in cells harbouring expanded polyQ repeats in ATXN2 (Elden et al., 2010). ATXN2 was shown to be part of stress granules and interacts with poly-A-binding-protein 1 (PABP), which is involved in poly(A) shortening and translation initiation (Ralser et al., 2005). ATXN2 was also shown to interact with endophilin A1 and A3, which are involved in synaptic vesicle endocytosis (Nonis et al., 2008).

3.3 Chromatin modifying protein 2B (CHMP2B)

A mutation in a splice-site of *CHMP2B* was first identified in a large Danish family with FTD and mutations have since been detected at low frequency in other FTD patients (Skibinski et al., 2005). Screening of the *CHMP2B* gene in ALS patients identified two mutations in two fALS patients. These patients displayed a predominant lower motor neuron phenotype and one of the patients showed signs of FTD (Parkinson et al., 2006). Sequencing of the *CHMP2B* gene in 433 ALS patients identified three missense mutations in one fALS case and three sALS cases (Cox et al., 2010).

The exact function of CHMP2B is unknown but its yeast homologue, vacuolar protein sorting 2 (VPS2), is a component of the ESCRTIII complex (Skibinski et al., 2005). This complex is involved in the trafficking of proteins between plasma membrane, trans-Golgi network, and lysosomes. The *CHMP2B* mutation identified in FTD results in dysmorphic endosomal structures similar to what is seen in ALSin overexpression (Skibinski et al., 2005). In cortical neurons, overexpression of the FTD related CHMP2B splice-site mutant leads to dendritic retraction prior to cell death and the accumulation of autophagosomes (Lee et al., 2007). In hippocampal neurons, the same FTD related CHMP2B mutant causes a decrease in large dendritic spines suggesting that CHMP2B is needed for dendritic spine growth and maturation (Belly et al., 2010).

3.4 Haemochromatosis (HFE)

Mutations in the *HFE* gene are a cause of hereditary haemochromatosis and have been associated with Alzheimer's disease and PD (reviewed by Nandar and Connor, 2011). The first report examining the presence of *HFE* mutations in ALS found no association between two mutations (H63D and C282Y) and ALS patients from the USA (Yen et al., 2004). However, several subsequent studies in a total of 1133 ALS patients and almost 7000 controls individuals from the USA, Ireland, UK, Italy, The Netherlands, and China reported association between the *HFE* H63D polymorphism and an increased risk for ALS (Goodall et al., 2005; He et al, 2011; Restagno et al., 2007; Sutedja et al., 2007; Wang et al., 2004).

The most important function of HFE is the regulation of iron homeostasis by binding to the transferrin receptor and reducing the transport of iron molecules (Feder et al., 1998). When HFE with the H63D mutation binds to the transferrin receptor, iron transport is reduced leading to iron accumulation and increased oxidative stress. In addition, it has been shown that in neuronal cell lines the H63D mutation induces increased oxidative stress, altered glutamate regulation and prolonged ER stress, all cellular processes affected in ALS (Liu et al., 2011; Mitchell et al. 2011).

3.5 Neurofilaments (NEFL, NEFM, NEFH)

One of the pathological hallmarks of ALS is the presence of neurofilament-containing inclusions in the cell body and proximal axon of spinal motor neurons (Delisle and Carpenter, 1984). Neurofilaments are intermediate filaments that constitute the most abundant cytoskeletal element in large myelinated axons. Neurofilaments are formed by the co-polymerization of light (NEFL), medium (NEFM), and heavy (NEFH) subunits, which are each encoded by different genes.

Several lines of evidence suggest a role for neurofilaments in neurodegeneration. Initial evidence came from mouse models overexpressing or deficient for neurofilaments (reviewed in Lariviere and Julien, 2004). Overexpression of NEFL or NEFH resulted in an abnormal accumulation of neurofilaments, as seen in ALS patients, and in axonal atrophy and motor dysfunction but not degeneration. Surprisingly, both overexpression and knockout of neurofilaments in transgenic mutant SOD1 mice increases life span (Couillard-Després et al., 1998; Williamson et al., 1998). This indicates that the role of neurofilaments in ALS is complex and more research is needed to examine the possible contribution of neurofilaments to ALS pathogenesis.

Additional evidence for a role for neurofilaments in ALS comes from genetic studies. Mutations in *NEFL* have been identified in some forms of the sensory and motor neuropathy Charcot-Marie-Tooth disease (Mersiyanova et al., 2000; Shin et al., 2008). The C-terminal tail region of NEFH contains phosphorylation motifs known as KSP repeats. In humans there are two common polymorphic variants of 44 (short) or 45 (long) repeats. Homozygosity for the short repeat allele is associated with Russian sporadic motor neuron disease patients (Skvortsova et al., 2004). Deletions and insertions in the KSP repeats of *NEFH* were detected in ALS patients (Al-Chalabi et al., 1999; Figlewicz et al., 1994; Tomkins et al., 1998). However, another study in 117 unrelated fALS patients could not identify deletions or insertions in the KSP repeats of *NEFH* (Rooke et al., 1996). A missense mutation in the *NEFH* gene was identified in a sALS case and not in controls (Garcia et al., 2006). Moreover, in a recent candidate gene sequencing study, three missense mutations were identified in the *NEFH* gene in two sALS and one fALS case. However, co-segregation of the mutation in the fALS case could not be tested and none of the missense mutations were predicted to be deleterious (Daoud et al., 2011). One study did not identify ALS specific variation in the *NEFH* gene in fALS and sALS samples (Vechio et al., 1996).

3.6 Paraoxonase genes (PON)

The paraoxonase gene cluster consists of 3 genes (*PON1, PON2,* and *PON3*) and is located in an 80-kb block on chromosome 7q21.3-22.1. PON1 and PON3 are primarily expressed in liver where they are associated with high-density lipoproteins, whereas PON2 is ubiquitously expressed (Costa et al., 2005; Draganov et al., 2000; Ng et al., 2002). Both PON1 and PON2 expression has been shown in mouse brain (Giordano et al., 2011). All PON proteins are able to hydrolyze lactones and PON1 is able to detoxify organophosphate pesticides and neurotoxins. Since neurotoxins are not normally present in the body the biological function of PON1 is thought to be protection of low-density lipoproteins from oxidation (Mackness et al., 1991). PON2 and PON3 share this function (Draganov et al., 2000; Ng et al., 2001). A higher incidence of ALS among Gulf war veterans and farmers suggested that chemical exposure may be a risk factor for ALS (Chió et al., 1991; Horner et al., 2003). Because PON proteins reduce oxidation and are able to detoxify neurotoxins these proteins have been investigated for association with ALS.

Polymorphisms in *PON1* and *PON2* as well as a haploblock spanning *PON2* and *PON3* were found to be associated with sALS (Saeed et al., 2006; Slowik et al., 2006). Since then several other studies in different populations have reported association of SNPs in the *PON* genes with sALS (Cronin et al., 2007; Landers et al., 2008; Morahan et al., 2007; Valdmanis et al., 2008). However, a meta-analysis including 4037 cases and 4609 controls from five case-control studies and several genome-wide association studies showed no significant association between *PON* polymorphisms and ALS (Wills et al., 2009). More recently, two other studies failed to detect association between *PON* polymorphisms and ALS (Ricci et al. 2011; Zawislak et al., 2010). In a recent sequencing study, eight mutations in all three *PON* genes were identified in fALS and sALS patients (Ticozzi et al., 2010). Mutations in the *PON* genes might play a role in ALS but additional sequencing is needed to confirm this.

Interestingly, PON1 activity can vary greatly depending on polymorphisms in its coding region (Costa et al., 2005). Thus, mutations in the *PON* genes could affect PON activity and thereby contribute to ALS pathogenesis. Toxicity in neurons caused by oxidative stress was higher in cells from PON2 knockout mice than in wild-type mice, suggesting that PON2 has a protective effect against neurotoxicity caused by oxidative stress (Giordano et al., 2011).

3.7 Peripherin (PRPH)

Peripherin is an intermediate filament similar to neurofilaments and is also associated with axonal spheroids in the proximal axon of spinal cord motor neurons of ALS patients (Corbo and Hays, 1992). It is also present in Lewy body-like inclusions and Bunina bodies that are seen in a portion of ALS patients (He and Hays, 2004; Mizuno et al., 2011). Peripherin is predominantly expressed in the peripheral nervous system and in spinal motor neurons in the central nervous system. After neuronal injury, peripherin expression is upregulated in spinal motor neurons and this upregulation has been linked to axonal regeneration (Troy et al., 1990). However, transgenic mice with wild-type overexpression of peripherin develop a late-onset and selective motor neuron disease characterized by intermediate filament inclusions (Beaulieu et al., 1999). For these reasons, the possibility of *PRPH* mutations in

ALS patients was investigated. Two missense mutations and a frameshift deletion in the PRPH gene have been identified in sALS patients (Corrado et al., 2011; Gros-Louis et al., 2004; Leung et al., 2004). Additional screening of the *PRPH* gene for mutations in larger cohorts of ALS patients and controls is needed to determine the frequency and pathogenecity of *PRPH* mutations.

Expression of abnormal peripherin splice variants has also been suggested to play a role in ALS pathogenesis. A toxic splice variant of peripherin (Per61) was found in motor neurons of mutant SOD1 transgenic mice but not wild-type mice (Robertson et al., 2003). Expression of Per61 has more recently also been observed in mutant TDP-43 transgenic mice but not in wild-type TDP-43 transgenic mice (Swarup et al., 2011). In addition, Per61 specific antibodies stain aggregates in human ALS but not in control spinal cord (Swarup et al., 2011). The presence of abnormal peripherin splice variants (Per28) has also been shown in humans (Xiao et al., 2008). Per28 overexpression results in peripherin aggregation and an upregulation of peripherin expression at the mRNA and protein levels in ALS patients as compared to controls (Xiao et al., 2008). A different study showed expression of Per28 in lumbar spinal cord lysates of ALS patients but not control cases (McLean et al., 2010). Although the functional significance of these abnormal splice forms is unknown they seem to play a role in the development ALS.

3.8 Survival motor neuron (SMN) 1 and 2

Two highly homologous copies of the survival motor neuron gene exist in humans, telomeric *SMN1* and centromeric *SMN2*. *SMN2*, which lacks exon 7 due to a nucleotide difference in a splice enhancer site, produces a less stable SMN protein and has only 20% of the biological function of SMN1 (Lorson et al., 1998). It has been shown that TDP-43 overexpression regulates the inclusion of exon 7 during pre-mRNA splicing of *SMN2* (Bose et al., 2008).

Deletions or mutations in *SMN1* cause the autosomal recessive disorder spinal muscular atrophy (SMA), whereas variation in *SMN2* copy number affects SMA disease severity (Lefebvre et al., 1997). SMA patients with a higher copy number of *SMN2* generally have a milder form of the disease (Gavrilov et al., 1998). SMN1 is widely expressed and functions in the assembly of the spliceosome as part of the SMN complex. SMN1 also interacts with several proteins involved in mRNA editing, transport, splicing, transcriptional regulation, and post-transcriptional processing and modification of rRNA (Eggert et al., 2006). The impaired assembly of the spliceosome could lead to neuronal degeneration.

Thus far, five different studies have failed to detect homozygous *SMN1* deletions in ALS patients (Gamez et al., 2002; Jackson et al., 1996; Moulard et al., 1998; Orrell et al., 1997; Parboosingh et al., 1999). However, an increased frequency of abnormal copy number (one or three copies) of *SMN1* was found in ALS patients compared to controls (Corcia et al., 2002). However, these results were inconsistent with other reports (Corcia et al., 2006; Veldink et al., 2001; Veldink et al., 2005). Recently, a large study was published including new samples of 847 sALS patients and 984 controls, showing that *SMN1* duplications were associated with ALS susceptibility (odds ratio [OR] = 2.07, 95% confidence interval [CI] = 1.34 - 3.20. (Blauw et al, 2011)). A meta-analysis of all previously published data, taking possible heterogeneity between studies into account, confirmed this association with *SMN1* duplications. Other work has shown that homozygous deletions of *SMN2* are associated with sporadic adult-onset lower motor neuron disease (Echaniz-Laguna et al., 2002; Moulard et al., 1998). Homozygous deletions of *SMN2* were also found to be overrepresented in 110 ALS patients (16%) compared to 100 controls (4%) (Veldink et al., 2001). *SMN2* deletions were associated with shorter survival in this study. However, a study by the same group using more ALS and control samples and several other studies did not find a higher frequency of *SMN2* deletions in ALS patients versus controls (Corcia et al., 2006; Gamez et al., 2002; Moulard et al., 1998; Parboosingh et al., 1999; Veldink et al., 2005). The recent meta-analysis showed that there is no increased frequency of homozygous *SMN2* deletions in ALS patients, and that neither *SMN1* nor *SMN2* appear to influence survival or age at onset of disease (Blauw et al. 2011).

Homozygous deletions in *SMN1* or *SMN2* do not play a role in ALS but an abnormal copy number in *SMN1* could increase risk for ALS and it is important to study the consequences on protein level in brain and spinal cord of having three copies of *SMN1* in order to determine the potential damaging effect.

3.9 Vascular endothelial growth factor (VEGF)

VEGF, a protein that stimulates angiogenesis in response to hypoxia, was identified as a candidate gene for ALS based on the finding that a deletion in the hypoxia response element (HRE) in the promoter of this gene in mice, resulting in decreased VEGF expression, led to progressive motor neuron degeneration (Oosthuyse et al., 2001). In addition, *VEGF* gene delivery in muscle and VEGF overexpression prolongs survival in mutant SOD1 transgenic mice. Furthermore, intracerebroventricular VEGF administration prolongs survival in mutant SOD1 transgenic rats (Azzouz et al., 2004; Storkebaum et al., 2005; Wang et al., 2007). Finally, decreased expression of VEGF and its receptor VEGFR2 is observed in spinal cords of ALS patients (Brockington et al., 2006).

Sequencing of the *VEGF* gene and its promotor in ALS patients failed to identify ALS specific mutations (Brockington et al., 2005; Gros-Luois et al., 2003; Lambrechts et al., 2003). However, a large study in 750 ALS patients and over 1200 controls from Sweden, Belgium, and England found association between two haplotypes determined by three SNPs and an increased risk for ALS (Lambrechts et al., 2003). These haplotypes lowered the circulating levels of VEGF and *VEGF* transcription (Lambrechts et al., 2003). This association was replicated in a study with small sample size (Terry et al., 2004). In contrast, subsequent studies could not confirm the association between *VEGF* and ALS in Dutch, British, American, Italian, Polish and Chinese populations (Brockington et al., 2005; Chen et al., 2006; Del Bo et al., 2008a; Golenia et al., 2010; Van Vught et al., 2005; Zhang et al., 2006). Furthermore, a meta-analysis on several of these studies found no association between *VEGF* polymorphisms and ALS (Lambrechts et al., 2009). A study in German ALS patients identified an association of a *VEGF* SNP with sALS in women (Fernández-Santiago et al., 2006). A different SNP was associated with ALS in male patients in a large meta-analysis (Lambrechts et al., 2009). This suggests that the role of *VEGF* in ALS may be gender dependent. An association of *VEGF* SNPs with age of onset in ALS was also reported although no such association was observed in the meta-analysis (Chen et al., 2007; Lambrechts et al., 2009).

In summary, studies in rodent models suggest a role for VEGF in ALS, possibly as a therapeutic target. However, genetic studies do not yet provide conclusive evidence for a genetic role for VEGF in ALS, although gender dependent effects may exist.

3.10 Genome wide association studies in sporadic ALS

Several genome-wide association studies (GWAS) have been performed in sALS patients. These studies have generated association results that have been replicated in the same study but rarely in independent studies. Although several of the associated genes discussed below are plausible to contribute to ALS considering their functional roles, the lack of consistent replication results makes it difficult to firmly establish their role in sALS.

A GWAS in 276 ALS patients and 271 healthy controls identified 34 possible associated SNPs but none of these reached genome-wide significance after Bonferroni correction (Schymick et al., 2007). A SNP near the gene FGGY carbohydrate kinase domain containing (*FGGY*) was reported to be associated in a GWAS in 1152 ALS patients with an odds ratio of 1.35 (Dunckley et al., 2007). However, two replication studies in a total of 2478 sALS patients and 2744 controls did not detect this association (Fernández-Santiago et al., 2011; Van Es et al., 2009b). No mutations in *FGGY* were found by sequencing in 190 ALS patients (Daoud et al., 2010).

A GWAS in 461 ALS patients and 450 controls found a variant in the inositol 1, 4, 5-triphosphate receptor 2 gene (*ITPR2*) to be associated with ALS. This association was replicated in the same study in a cohort of 876 patients and 906 controls and in the combined analysis (Van Es et al., 2007). ITPR2 has a role in glutamate-mediated neurotransmission, regulation of calcium concentration and apoptosis. However, the *ITPR2* association has not been found in a replication study and in subsequent GWAS (Chiò et al., 2009; Cronin et al., 2008; Fernández-Santiago et al., 2011; Laaksovirta et al., 2010; Shatunov et al., 2010; Van Es et al., 2009c).

Variation in the dipeptidyl-peptidase 6 (*DPP6*) gene was found to be significantly associated with sALS in a GWAS performed in a combined GWA data set from the USA and the Netherlands (Van Es et al., 2008). This association was replicated in three additional independent populations from The Netherlands, Sweden, and Belgium (Van Es et al., 2008). The same variant was the top hit in a joint analysis of GWA data sets in an Irish population and the same Dutch and American populations, although it did not reach genome-wide significance (Cronin et al., 2008). Upon addition of a Polish data set the association could not be replicated which could point to a population-specific effect (Cronin et al., 2009). In an Italian cohort of 266 ALS patients association of the same SNP was replicated (Del Bo et al., 2008b). However, subsequent replication studies and GWAS could not find evidence for a role of *DPP6* in ALS (Chiò et al., 2009; Daoud et al., 2010; Fogh et al., 2011; Laaksovirta et al., 2010; Li et al., 2009; Shatunov et al., 2010; Van Es et al., 2009c). Interestingly, in a genome scan for copy number variations, including 4434 ALS patients and over 14000 controls, a suggestive association was found for the *DPP6* locus (Blauw et al., 2010). Not much data is available on the function of DPP6, but it is expressed in brain and able to regulate the activity of neuropeptides and to bind A-type neuronal potassium channels (Nadal et al., 2003).

Another two-stage GWAS in sALS patients was unable to find any associated SNPs that reached genome-wide significance, although suggestive association was found on **chromosome 7p13.3** (Chiò et al., 2009).

Survival analysis in a GWAS using samples from the USA and Europe revealed that a CC genotype of a SNP in the kinesin-associated protein 3 (*KIFAP3*) gene conferred a 14-month survival advantage on ALS patients (Landers et al., 2009). Expression data using RNA from brain tissue and lymphoblasts of patients showed that the favorable genotype significantly decreased KIFAP3 expression (Landers et al., 2009). However, two subsequent studies in two Italian cohorts could not replicate the finding that the CC genotype had a beneficial effect on survival or decreased KIFAP3 expression in ALS patients (Orsetti et al., 2011; Traynor et al., 2010). KIFAP3 is part of the trimeric kinesin 2 motor complex KIF3 which mediates binding between proteins and their cargo. It serves multiple functions including a role in mitosis and intracellular transport of organelles and proteins in various tissues including neurons (Haraguchi et al., 2006; Takeda et al., 2000).

The largest GWAS to date identified two loci, on **chromosome 9p21.2** and **19p13.11**, to be associated with sALS. The genetic variant in 19p13.11 maps to a haplotype within the boundaries of the *UNC13A* gene. Two studies failed to replicate this finding, but were underpowered, and more studies are needed to firmly establish genetic variation in *UNC13A* as being causative to sALS.

The association to chromosome 9p21.2 will be discussed in more detail in the following sections.

4. ALS-FTD2 (9p13.2-21.3)

Several linkage studies associated **chromosome 9p** to ALS-FTD, designated as ALS-FTD2 (Table 3). The first two independent studies found linkage to locus 9p13.2-21.3 in a Dutch and a Scandinavian family (Morita et al., 2006; Vance et al., 2006). Subsequently, eight other linkage studies in families from Canada, France, Belgium, North-America, Australia and Wales showed association to regions on chromosome 9p13.1-q21 (Boxer et al., 2010; Gijselinck et al., 2010; Le Ber et al., 2009; Luty et al., 2009; Momeni et al., 2006; Pearson et al., 2011; Valdmanis et al., 2007; Yan et al., 2006). Individuals in these families were diagnosed with ALS, FTD, and ALS-FTD. However, dementia, psychosis and Parkinsonism were also seen. Besides the co-occurrence of ALS and FTD in families, there is also considerable clinical overlap between ALS and FTD, i.e. mild cognitive abnormalities occur in up to 50% of ALS patients and in approximately 5% of ALS patients FTD is present with marked behavioral changes and language impairment (Elamin et al., 2011; Ringholz et al., 2005). Furthermore, ALS and FTD are both characterized by TDP-43 positive ubiquitinated cytoplasmic inclusions (Neumann et al., 2006). This strongly supports the idea that there is a common genetic contribution to the pathogenesis of both diseases.

A total of 41 genes, four micro RNAs, two pseudogenes, and a non-coding RNA in the associated chromosome 9p region have been screened for mutations but only in one study a premature stop codon in the intraflagellar transport 74 gene (*IFT-74*) was identified in two brothers from one family (Momeni et al., 2006). However, no mutations in *IFT-74* were identified in any of the other ALS-FTD families that were linked to chromosome 9p and it is therefore unlikely that this mutation is the underlying cause in these families.

Interestingly, a recent GWAS in sALS patients found association between ALS and chromosome 9p21.2. 2323 ALS patients and 9013 controls were genotyped and genome-wide significance was found for SNPs on these two loci (van Es et al., 2009c). This finding was replicated in a second, independent cohort of 2532 ALS patients and 5940 controls. The associated SNPs are in a 80-kb linkage disequilibrium (LD) block on chromosome 9 which overlaps with the common region found in the ALS-FTD linkage studies (Figure 1).

Study	*Linkage region*	*Families*	*Country/ Region*	*fALS*	*FTD*	*ALS-FTD*	*Genes screened*	*Mutations*
Yan et al. 2006	9p13.3-p22.1 (D9S1684-D9S1678)	15	N.K.	N.K.	N.K.	N.K.	27	None
Morita et al. 2006	9p13.2-p21.3 (D9S1870-D9S1791)	1	Scandinavia	5	9	-	2	None
Vance et al. 2006	9p13.2-p21.2 (D9S2154-D9S1874)	1	The Netherlands	7	2	3	3	None
Momeni et al. 2006	9p13.2-p22.2 (D9S157-D9S1874)	2	North-America	1	-	9	14	p.Q342X in *IFT-74*
Valdmanis et al. 2007	9p13.3-p22.2 (D9S157-D9S1805)	2	Canada/ France	14	3	4	4	None
Le Ber et al. 2009	9p11.2-p21.2 (AFM218xg11-D9S301)	6	France	9	10	12	29 + 4 miRNAs	None
Luty et al. 2008	9p21.2-q21 (D9S169-D9S167)	1	Australia	2	5	2	11	None
Gijselinck et al. 2010	9p22.3-q21 (D9S235-D9S257)	1	Belgium	1	8	-	17	None
Boxer et al. 2010	9p21.2-p23 (D9S1808-D9S251)	1	USA	2	5	3	10	None
Pearson et al. 2011	9p21.2-p21.2	1	Wales	2	5	1	8	None

Table 3. Overview of linkage studies in ALS-FTD families. N.K. = not known

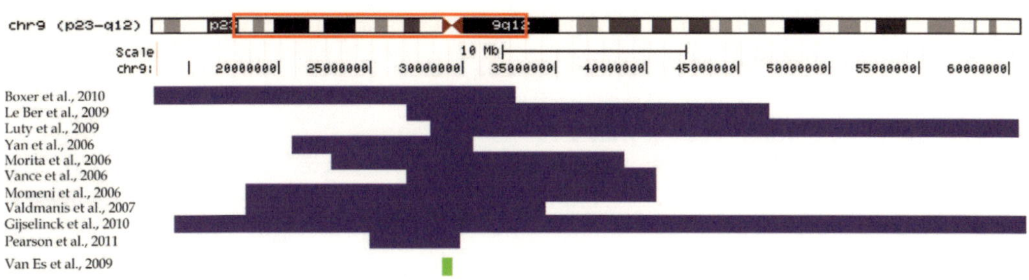

Fig. 1. Schematic overview of the associated regions found by linkage studies and GWAS.

Since this initial report several other GWAS in ALS patients have replicated the association to chromosome 9p21.2. In a GWAS performed on 405 Finnish ALS patients, of whom 93 patients had fALS, and 497 control individuals two association peaks were identified (Laaksovirta et al., 2010). One peak corresponded to the autosomal recessive D90A allele of the SOD1 gene. The other was identified in a 232-kb LD block on chromosome 9p21.2. The association signals in this study were mainly driven by the 93 fALS patients. A 42-SNP risk haplotype across the chromosome 9p21 locus was shared between 41 fALS cases with an odds ratio of 21.0 (Laaksovirta et al., 2010). In another GWAS in an ALS cohort from the UK consisting of 599 ALS patients and 4144 control individuals two SNPs on chromosome 9p21.2 were found to be associated with ALS (Shatunov et al., 2010). A joint analysis including 4132 ALS patients and 8425 controls from this UK cohort and from previously published data from the UK, USA, Netherlands, Ireland, Italy, France, Sweden, and Belgium also showed significant association to the locus on chromosome 9p21.2 (Shatunov et al., 2010). In addition, replication of one of the associated SNPs on chromosome 9p21.2 was found in a GWAS performed in FTD patients when analyzing the ALS-FTD patients only. A different SNP in this locus was significantly associated with FTD (Rollinson et al., 2011). A trend towards significant genome-wide association between chromosome 9p21.2 and FTD was found when analyzing 426 FTD patients with TDP-43 pathology without mutations in the progranulin gene and 2509 control individuals (Van Deerlin et al., 2009). A replication study in Chinese and Japanese sALS patients failed to find association to one of the previously associated SNPs on chromosome 9p21.2 but this might be due to a lack of power (Iida et al., 2011).

In summary, linkage studies in ALS-FTD families and GWAS in sALS, ALS-FTD and FTD patients provide compelling evidence for a role of chromosome 9p21.2 in ALS and/or FTD.

As mentioned, recently two studies identified a GGGGCC hexanucleotide repeat expansion in intron 1 of the *C9ORF72* gene as the cause of chromosome 9p-linked ALS-FTD (Dejesus-Hernandez et al., 2011; Renton et al., 2011).

5. Gene function

A hexanucleotide repeat expansion in the *C9ORF72* gene has recently been identified as the cause of chromosome 9p-linked ALS-FTD. The mechanism as to how this expanded repeat causes ALS is unknown. No causal mutations in *UNC13a* have been identified in ALS patients to date. Close examination of the reported function(s) of the proteins encoded by the *C9ORF72* and *UNC13a* gene may help to design strategies for determining the functional role of these loci in ALS and/or FTD.

In this section the current knowledge of the function of these genes will be discussed in light of a possible contribution to ALS pathogenesis.

5.1 Chromosome 9 open reading frame 72

The *C9ORF72* gene encodes a protein of 481 amino acids. Alternative splicing of this gene is thought to produce five isoforms of which three are protein coding. Isoform 1 contains the entire sequence and consists of 481 amino acids, while isoform 2 and 3 have an asparagine to lysine change at amino acid 222 which results in the truncation of amino acids 223 to 481. Thus far, no C9ORF72 protein has been detected and nothing is known about the function of C9ORF72.

The *C9ORF72* gene has been sequenced in four linkage studies in 39 patients from different families, but no mutations have been identified. No changes in splicing, small deletions or duplications were detected in patients from an ALS-FTD family (Boxer et al., 2010). The gene has been sequenced in 16 sALS patients and 16 controls but no variants specific for sALS were identified (Laaksovirta et al., 2010). Hexanucleotide repeat expansions were recently found to be the most common cause of fALS and familial FTD and were also identified in sALS patients (Dejesus-Hernandez et al., 2011; Renton et al., 2011). The functional consequence of these repeat expansions are however unknown.

Further studies will be needed to characterize the C9ORF72 protein and to establish the consequences of the intronic repeat on ALS pathogenesis.

5.2 UNCoordinated 13 homolog A (UNC13a)

UNC13a is a member of UNC13 family of presynaptic proteins. The protein consists of 1791 amino acids but several isoforms exist. It contains a zinc-finger like C1 domain that is homologous to a diacylglycerol and phorbol ester binding region of protein kinase C (PKC), three C2 domains that are similar to the calcium binding regulatory regions of PKC and synaptotagmin, a calmodulin binding domain and two Munc homology domains (Basu et al., 2005).

In mammals, the Munc13 family comprises four homologous members, Munc13-1, Munc13-2, Munc13-3, and Munc13-4. Deletion mutants of Munc13-1 in mice, the murine homologue of UNC13a, shows that the protein is needed for presynaptic vesicle maturation and fusion competence in glutamergic hippocampal neurons (Augustin et al., 1999). GABA-ergic neurons in the hippocampus show no spontaneous or evoked synaptic transmission in absence of both Munc13-1 and Munc13-2 (Varoqueaux et al., 2002). Neuromuscular junction (NMJ) axon terminals contain Munc13-1 and a splice variant of Munc13-2 (Varoqueaux et al., 2005). Mice deficient in Munc13 due to a double knockout of Munc13-1 and Munc13-2 form specialized neuromuscular endplates. However, the distribution, size and shape of these synapses are altered. Also, muscle morphology is abnormal and a larger number of motor neurons is present in the spinal cord in Munc13-1/2 knockout mice, probably as a result of defective apoptosis. Furthermore, evoked synaptic transmission is impaired in these mutants but spontaneous transmission is unchanged (Varoqueaux et al., 2005). This indicates that vesicle priming in NMJs is partially independent of Munc13-1 or Munc13-2. However, despite the unchanged spontaneous transmission, muscle innervation is aberrant in Munc13-1/2 knockout mice (Varoqueaux et al., 2005).

As exemplified by the defects observed in Munc13-1 and Munc13-1/2 knockout mice, it is plausible that a disruption in UNC13a expression affects motor neurons and muscle innervation. The effect of UNC13a on glutamate exocytosis is also interesting since Riluzole, the only drug with a proven effect on ALS, is a glutamate release inhibitor. Therefore, *UNC13a* is an interesting candidate gene to be investigated further for a role in ALS pathogenesis.

6. Conclusion and future research

The use of linkage analysis, candidate gene studies, and GWAS has led to the identification of several causal loci and genes for fALS and sALS. The overview above clearly shows the extent of heterogeneity in genes that underlie fALS, let alone sALS, illustrating the complex molecular basis of this disease. There is not one dominant biological process that is represented by these genes, although RNA-processing, axonal transport and synaptic dysfunction appear to emerge as being relevant in ALS etiology. Interestingly, several of the genes implicated in these processes are already known to be causal or have been implicated in other neurodegenerative diseases which suggests that there is, at least in part, a common underlying mechanism.

Since these findings explain only about a third of the genetic variability in fALS and a small percentage of the genetic contribution to sALS, there is a clear need for the identification of additional causal loci. This would require the collection of large family pedigrees with many affected individuals, which is difficult in ALS considering the adult onset with rapid disease progression. However, the development of next generation sequencing techniques provides a possible solution to this problem. Using exome and whole-genome sequencing, causal genes can be identified with a small number of affected and unaffected individuals as has been shown in several, mostly autosomal recessive disorders (Choi et al., 2009; Ng et al., 2009). Recently, exome sequencing in two affected individuals from the same family identified *VCP* as a causal gene for fALS, illustrating that this technique is a promising tool for gene identification in ALS as well (Johnson et al., 2010). In addition, the repeat expansion in C9ORF72 was also discovered with the use of whole-genome sequencing (Renton et al., 2011).

The identification of causal genes for ALS has broadened our understanding of this motor neuron degenerative disease. Studying the function of associated genes in neurons and animal models has revealed several possible processes underlying ALS such as RNA processing, axonal transport, glutamate regulation, oxidative stress and synaptic dysfunction. However, the contribution of most genes to ALS pathogenesis has not been resolved. SOD1 and TDP-43 transgenic animal models have provided valuable insights into ALS pathogenesis. Further research using existing animal models of ALS associated genes and the generation of new animal models are needed to further determine their role in the disease. Generation of animal models harbouring repeat expansions in C9ORF72 and ATXN2 could help to reveal the pathogenic mechanisms behind these repeats. The effect of overexpression or knockdown of ALS associated genes and the expression of repeat expansions in motor neurons or motor neuron-like cell lines on protein aggregation and cell survival could also help to unravel the contribution of these genes to ALS. In addition, some associated genes (e.g. *DCTN1*, *PON1/2/3*, *TAF15*, and *VCP*) remain to be sequenced in larger cohorts from different populations in order to determine the actual contribution of these genes to ALS.

Additional new strategies in sALS include a more network oriented approach to gene identification. It is possible to detect networks of genes, proteins and metabolites that are misregulated in ALS, or that determine disease progression. By searching for subtle genetic variation that drives these network perturbations, new genes might be identified that are hard to detect with GWAS. Also, the focus in ALS genetics thus far has been on common variation in exonic DNA. The regulatory part of the genome is challenging to study, but might be relevant as well. This also requires the combined analysis of gene-expression and protein data with data on genetic variation. In addition, recent studies show that tandem repeats in DNA might be also relevant, as exemplified by the ATXN2 and C9ORF72 findings. Typically, this type of variation is hard to detect by current high-throughput methods. Lastly, the type of copy number variation that has not yet been covered very well to date, including variation in microRNAs or inversions, deserves more attention.

In summary, impressive progress in the understanding of the genetics of ALS has been made over the past several years with the identification of several causal genes. However, most of the genetic variability underlying ALS remains to be identified. The use of deep sequencing techniques and functional research will be needed to further broaden our understanding of ALS pathogenesis.

7. Acknowledgements

This work has received funding from the European Community's Health Seventh Framework Programme (FP7/2007-2013) under grant agreement n° 259867, VSB fonds, EURO-MOTOR FP7, The Netherlands ALS Foundation (J.H.V, and L.H.v.d.B.), Neuroscience and Cognition Utrecht (NCU), the Prinses Beatrix Fonds (Kersten Foundation) and the Adessium Foundation (R.J.P., J.H.V. and L.H.v.d.B.). J.H.V. is supported by the Brain Foundation of The Netherlands and J.H.V, R.J.P., and M.K are supported by the Thierry Latran Foundation.

8. References

Al-Chalabi A., et al. (2010). An estimate of amyotrophic lateral sclerosis heritability using twin data. *Journal of Neurology, Neurosurgery, and Psychiatry*, Vol. 81, No. 12, (December 2010), pp. 1342-1346, ISSN 0022-3050

Al-Saif A., Al-Mohanna F. & Bohlega S. (2011). A mutation in Sigma-1 receptor causes juvenile amyotrophic lateral sclerosis. *Annals of Neurology*, 2011, Ahead of print, ISSN 0364-5134

Augustin I., et al. (1999). Munc13-1 is essential for fusion competence of glutamergic synaptic vesicles. *Nature*, Vol. 400, No. 29, (July 2009), pp. 457-461, ISSN 0028-0836

Avemaria F., et al. (2011). Mutation in the senataxin gene found in a patients affected by familial ALS with juvenile onset and slow progression. *Amyotrophic Lateral Sclerosis*, Vol. 12, No. 3, (May 2011), pp. 228-230, ISSN 1748-2968

Azzouz M., et al. (2004). VEGF delivery with retrogradely transported lentivector prolongs survival in a mouse ALS model. *Nature*, Vol. 429, No. 6990, (May 2004), pp. 413-417, ISSN 0028-0836

Badouel C & McNeill H. (2011). Snapshot: The hippo signaling pathway. *Cell*, Vol. 145, No. 3, (April 2011), pp. 484-484.e1, ISSN 1097-4172

Bandyopadhyay S., et al. (2010). A human MAP kinase interactome. *Nature Methods*, Vol. 7, No. 10, (October 2010), pp. 801-805, ISSN 1548-7091

Basu J., et al. (2005). A minimal domain responsible for Munc13 activity. *Nature Structural & Molecular Biology*, Vol. 12, No. 11, (November 2005), pp. 1017-1018, ISSN 1545-9993

Bäumer D., et al. (2010). Juvenile ALS with basophilic inclusions is a FUS proteinopathy with FUS mutations. *Neurology*, Vol. 75, No. 7, (August 2010), pp. 611-618, ISSN 0028-3878

Beaulieu JM, Nguyen MD & Julien JP. (1999). Late onset of motor neurons in mice overexpressing wild-type peripherin. *Journal of Cell Biology*, Vol. 147, No. 3, (November 1999), pp. 531-544, ISSN 0021-9525

Belly A., et al. (2010). CHMP2B mutants linked to frontotemporal dementia impair maturation of dendritic spines. *Journal of Cell Science*, Vol. 123, Pt. 17, (September 2010), pp. 2943-2954, ISSN 0021-9533

Belzil VV., et al. (2009). Mutations in FUS cause FALS and SALS in French and French Canadian populations. *Neurology*, Vol. 73, No. 15, (October 2009), pp. 1176-1179, ISSN 0028-3878

Belzil VV., et al. (2010). Analysis of OPTN as a causative gene for amyotrophic lateral sclerosis. *Neurobiology of Aging*, Vol. 32, No. 3, (March 2011), pp. 555.e13-4, ISSN 1558-1497

Benajiba L., et al. (2009). TARDBP mutations in motoneuron disease with frontotemporal lobar degeneration. *Annals of Neurology*, Vol. 65, No. 4, (April 2009), pp. 470-473, ISSN 0364-5134

Blauw HM., et al. (2010). A large genome scan for rare CNVs in amyotrophic lateral sclerosis. *Human Molecular Genetics*, Vol. 19, No. 20, (October 2010), pp. 4091-4099, ISSN 0964-6906

Blauw HM., et al. *Neurology*, 2011;in press

Bosco DA., et al. (2010). Mutant FUS proteins that cause amyotrophic lateral sclerosis incorporate into stress granules. *Human Molecular Genetics*, Vol. 19, No. 21, (November 2010), pp. 4160-4175, ISSN 0964-6906

Bose JK., et al. (2008). TDP-43 overexpression enhances exon 7 inclusion during the survival of motor neuron pre-mRNA splicing. *Journal of Biological Chemistry*, Vol. 283, No. 43, (October 2008), pp. 28852-28859, ISSN 0021-9258

Boxer AL., et al. (2010). Clinical, neuroimaging and neuropathological features of a new chromosome 9p-linked FTD-ALS family. *Journal of Neurology, Neurosurgery and Psychiatry*, Vol.82, No.2, (February 2011), pp.196-203, ISSN 0022-3050

Brockington A., et al. (2005). Screening of the regulatoy and coding regions of vascular endothelial growth factor in amyotrophic lateral sclerosis. *Neurogenetics*, Vol. 6, No. 2, (May 2005), pp. 101-104, ISSN 1364-6745

Brockington A., et al. (2006). Expression of vascular endothelial growth factor and its receptors in the central nervous system in amyotrophic lateral sclerosis. *Journal of Neuropathology and Experimental Neurology*, Vol. 65, No. 1, (January 2006), pp. 26-36, ISSN 0022-3069

Broeke JHP., et al. (2010). Munc18 and Munc13 regulate early neurite outgrowth. *Biology of the Cell*, Vol. 102, No. 8, (June 2010), pp. 479-488, ISSN 0248-4900

Buratti E & Baralle FE. (2010). The multiple roles of TDP-43 in pre-mRNA processing and gene expression regulation. *RNA Biology*, Vol. 7, No. 4, (July-August 2010), pp. 420-429, ISSN 1547-6286

Byrne S., et al. (2010). Rate of familial amyotrophic lateral sclerosis: a systematic review and meta-analysis. *Journal of Neurology, Neurosurgery, and Psychiatry*, Vol. 82, No. 6, (June 2011), pp. 623-627, ISSN 0022-3050

Cai H., et al. (2008). ALS2/alsin knockout mice and motor neuron diseases. *Neurodegenerative diseases*, Vol. 5, No. 6, (2008), pp. 359-366, ISSN 1660-2854

Calvo A., et al. (2010). Involvement of immune response in the pathogenesis of amyotrophic lateral sclerosis: a therapeutic opportunity? *CNS & Neurological Disorders Drug Targets*, Vol. 9, No. 3, (July 2010), pp. 325-330, ISSN 1871-5273

Chance PF., et al. (1998). Linkage of the gene for an autosomal dominant form of juvenile amyotrophic lateral sclerosis to chromosome 9q34. *American Journal of Human Genetics*, Vol. 62, No. 3, (March 1998), pp. 633-640, ISSN 0002-9297

Chen D., et al. (2007). Association of polymorphisms in vascular endothelial growth factor gene with the age of onset of amyotrophic lateral sclerosis. *Amyotrophic Lateral Sclerosis*, Vol. 8, No. 3, (June 2007), pp. 144-149, ISSN 1748-2968

Chen HJ., et al. (2010). Characterization of the properties of a novel mutation in VAPB in familial amyotrophic lateral sclerosis. *Journal of Biological Chemistry*, Vol. 285, No. 51, (December 2010), pp. 40266-40281, ISSN 0021-9258

Chen W., et al. (2006). Lack of association of VEGF promoter polymorphisms with sporadic ALS. *Neurology*, Vol. 67, No. 3, (August 2006), pp. 508-510, ISSN 0028-3878

Chen Y., et al. (2011). Ataxin-2 intermediate-length polyglutamine: a possible risk factor for Chinese patients with amyotrophic lateral sclerosis. *Neurobiology of Aging*, 2011, Ahead of print, ISSN 0197-4580

Chen YZ., et al. (2004). DNA/RNA helicase gene mutations in a form of juvenile amyotrophic lateral sclerosis (ALS4). *American Journal of Human Genetics*, Vol. 74, No. 6, (June 2004), pp. 1128-1135, ISSN 0002-9297

Chió A., et al. (1991). Risk factors in motor neuron disease: a case-control study. *Neuroepidemiology*, Vol. 10, No. 4, (1991), pp 174-184, ISSN 0251-5350

Chiò A., et al. (2009). A two-stage genome-wide association study of sporadic amyotrophic lateral sclerosis. *Human Molecular Genetics*, Vol. 18, No. 8, (April 2009), pp. 1524-1532, ISSN 0964-6906

Choi M., et al. (2009). Genetic diagnosis by whole exome capture and massively parallel DNA sequencing. *Proceedings of the National Academy of Sciences of the USA*, Vol. 106, No. 45, (November 2009), pp. 19096-19101, ISSN 0027-8424

Chow CY., et al. (2007). Mutation of FIG4 causes neurodegeneration in the pale tremor mouse and patients with CMT4J. *Nature*, Vol. 448, No. 7149, (July 2007), pp. 68-73, ISSN 0028-0836

Chow CY., et al. (2009). Deleterious variants of FIG4, a phosphoinositide phosphatase, in patients with ALS. *American Journal of Human Genetics*, Vol. 84, No. 1, (January 2009), pp. 85-88, ISSN 0002-9297

Conforti FL., et al. (2007). A novel angiogenin gene mutation in a sporadic patient with amyotrophic lateral sclerosis from southern Italy. *Neuromuscular Disorders*, Vol. 18, No. 1, (January 2008), pp. 68-70, ISSN 0960-8966

Coppedè F., et al. (2008). Lack of association between the APEX1 Asp184Glu polymorphism and sporadic amyotrophic lateral sclerosis. *Neurobiology of Aging*, Vol. 31, No. 2, (February 2010), pp. 353-355, ISSN 0197-4580

Corbo M & Hays AP. (1992). Peripherin and neurofilament protein coexist in spinal spheroids of motor neuron disease. *Journal of Neuropathology and Experimental Neurology*, Vol. 51, No. 5, (September 1992), pp. 531-537, ISSN 0022-3069

Corcia P., et al. (2002). Abnormal SMN1 gene copy number is a susceptibility factor for amyotrophic lateral sclerosis. *Annals of Neurology*, Vol. 51, No. 2, (February 2002), pp. 243-246, ISSN 0364-5134

Corcia P., et al. (2006). SMN1 gene, but not SMN2, is a risk factor for sporadic ALS. *Neurology*, Vol. 67, No. 7, (October 2006), pp. 1147-1150, ISSN 0028-3878

Corcia P., et al. (2009). The importance of the SMN genes in the genetics of sporadic ALS. *Amyotrophic Lateral Sclerosis*, Vol. 10, No. 5-6, (October-December 2009), pp. 436-440, ISSN 1748-2968

Corrado L., et al. (2007). Variations in the coding and regulatory sequences of the angiogenin (ANG) gene are not associated to ALS (amyotrophic lateral sclerosis) in the Italian population. *Journal of Neurological Sciences*, Vol. 258, No. 1-2, (July 2007), pp. 123-127, ISSN 0022-510X

Corrado L., et al. (2009). High frequency of TARDBP gene mutations in Italian patients with amyotrophic lateral sclerosis. *Human Mutation*, Vol. 30, No. 4, (April 2009), pp. 688-694, ISSN 1059-7794

Corrado L., et al. (2009). Mutations of FUS gene in sporadic amyotrophic lateral sclerosis. *Journal of Medical Genetics*, Vol. 47, No. 3, (March 2010), pp. 190-194, ISSN 0022-2593

Corrado L., et al. (2010). A novel peripherin gene (PRPH) mutation identified in one sporadic amyotrophic lateral sclerosis patients. *Neurobiology of Aging*, Vol. 32, No. 3, (March 2011), pp. 552.e1-6, ISSN 0197-4580

Costa LG., et al. (2005). Modulation of paraoxonase (PON1) activity. *Biochemical Pharmacology*, Vol. 69, No. 4, (February 2005), pp. 541-550, ISSN 0006-2952

Couillard-Després S., et al. (1998). Protective effect of neurofilament heavy gene overexpression in motor neuron disease induced by mutant superoxide dismutase. *Proceedings of the National Academy of Sciences of the USA*, Vol. 95, No. 16, (August 1998), pp. 9626-9630, ISSN 0027-8424

Cox LE., et al. (2010). Mutations in CHMP2B in lower motor neuron predominant amyotrophic lateral sclerosis (ALS). *PLoS One*, Vol. 5, No. 3, (March 2010), e9872, ISSN 1932-6203

Cronin S., et al. (2007). Paraoxonase promoter and intronic variants modify risk of sporadic amytrophic lateral sclerosis. *Journal of Neurology, Neurosurgery, and Psychiatry*, Vol. 78, No. 9, (September 2007), pp. 984-986, ISSN 0022-3050

Cronin S,. et al. (2007). A genome-wide association study of sporadic ALS in a homogenous Irish population. *Human Molecular Genetics*, Vol. 17, No. 5, (March 2008), pp. 768-774, ISSN 0964-6906

Cronin S., et al. (2008). Screening for replication of genome-wide SNP associations in sporadic ALS. *European Journal of Human Genetics*, Vol. 17, No. 2, (February 2009), pp. 213-218, ISSN 1018-4813

Crow MK. (2010). Type I interferon in organ-targeted autoimmune and inflammatory diseases. *Artrhitis Research and Therapy*, Vol.12, (2010), Suppl.1:S5, ISSN 1478-6354

Da Cruz S & Cleveland DW. (2011). Understanding the role of TDP-43 and FUS/TLS in ALS and beyond. *Current Opinion in Neurobiology*, 2011:Ahead of print

Daoud H., et al. (2010). Analysis of DPP6 and FGGY as candidate genes for amyotrophic lateral sclerosis. *Amyotrophic Lateral Sclerosis*, Vol. 11, No. 4, (August 2011), pp. 389-391, ISSN 1748-2968

Daoud H., et al. (2011). Association of long ATXN2 CAG repeat sizes with increased risk of amyotrophic lateral sclerosis. *Archives of Neurology*, Vol. 68, No. 6, (June 2011), pp. 739-742, ISSN 0003-9942

Dedoni S, Olianas MC & Onali P. (2010). Interferon-β induces apoptosis in human SH-Sy5Y neuroblasto cells through activation of JAK-STAT signaling and down-regulation of PI3K/Akt pathway. *Journal of Neurochemistry*, Vol. 115, No. 6, (December 2010), pp. 1421-1433, ISSN 0022-3042

Dejesus-Hernandez M et al. (2011). Expanded GGGGCC hexanucleotide repeat in noncoding region of C9ORF72 causes chromosome 9p-linked FTD and ALS. *Neuron*, September 2011, Ahead of print.

Del Bo R., et al. (2006). Absence of angiogenic genes modification in Italian ALS patients. *Neurobiology of Aging*, Vol. 29, No. 2, (February 2008), pp. 314-316, ISSN 0197-4580

Del Bo R., et al. (2008). DPP6 gene variability confers increate risk of developing sporadic amyotrophic lateral sclerosis in Italian patients. *Journal of Neurology, Neurosurgery, and Psychiatry*, Vol. 79, No. 9, (September 2008), pp. 1085, ISSN 0022-3050

Del Bo R., et al. (2011). Novel optineurin mutations in patients with familial and sporadic amyotrophic lateral sclerosis. *Journal of Neurology, Neurosurgery, and Psychiatry*, 2001, Ahead of print, ISSN 0022-3050

Delisle MB & Carpenter S. (1984). Neurofibrillary axonal swellings and amyotrophic lateral sclerosis. *Journal of the Neurological Sciences*, Vol. 63, No. 2, (February 1984), pp. 241-250, ISSN 0022-510X

Deng HX., et al. (2010). FUS-immunoreactive inclusions are a common feature in sporadic and non-SOD1 familial amyotrophic lateral sclerosis. *Annals of Neurology*, Vol. 67, No. 6, (June 2010), pp. 739-748, ISSN 0364-5134

Deng HX., et al. (2011). Mutations in UBQLN2 cause dominant X-linked juvenile and adult-onset ALS and ALS/dementia. *Nature*, Vol. 477, No. 7363, (August 2011), pp. 211-215, ISSN 0028-0836

De Weerd NA, Samarajiwa SA & Hertzog PJ. (2007). Type I interferon receptors: biochemistry and biological functions. *Journal of Biological Chemistry*, Vol. 282, No. 28, (July 2007), pp. 20053-20057, ISSN 0021-9258

Dickson SP., et al. (2010). Rare variants create synthetic genome-wide associations. *PLoS Biology*, Vol. 8, No. 1, (January 2010), e1000294, ISSN 1544-9173

Dion PA, Daoud H & Rouleau GA. (2009). Genetics of motor neuron disorders: new insights into pathogenic mechanisms. *Nature Reviews. Genetics*, Vol. 10, No. 11, (November 2009), pp. 769-782, ISSN 1471-0056

Dormann D., et al. (2010). ALS-associated fused in sarcoma (FUS) mutations disrupt Transportin-mediated nuclear import. *EMBO Journal*, Vol. 29, No. 16, (August 2010), pp. 2841-2857, ISSN 0261-4189

Draganov DI., et al. (2000). Rabbit serum paraoxonase 3 (PON3) is a high density lipoprotein-associated lactonase and protects low density lipoprotein against oxidation. *Journal of Biological Chemistry*, Vol. 275, No. 43, (October 2000), pp. 33435-33442, ISSN 0021-9258

Dunckley T., et al. (2007). Whole-genome analysis of sporadic amyotrophic lateral sclerosis. *New England Journal of Medicine*, Vol. 357, No. 8, (August 2007), pp. 775-788, ISSN 0028-4793

Echaniz-Laguna A., et al. (2002). Homozygous exon 7 deletion of the SMN centromeric gene (SMN2): a potential susceptibility factor for adult-onset lower motor neuron disease. *Journal of Neurology*, Vol. 249, No. 3, (March 2002), pp. 290-293, ISSN 0340-5354

Eggert C., et al. (2006). Spinal muscular atrophy: the RNP connection. *Trends in Molecular Medicine*, Vol. 12, No. 3, (March 2006), pp. 113-121, ISSN 1471-4914

Elamin M., et al. (2011). Executive dysfunction is a negative prognostic indicator in patients with ALS without dementia. *Neurology*, Vol. 76, No. 14, (April 2011), pp. 1263-1269, ISSN 0028-3878

Elden AC., et al. (2010). Ataxin-2 intermediate-length polyglutamine expansions are associated with increased risk for ALS. *Nature*, Vol. 466, No.7310, (August 2010), pp.1069-1075, ISSN 0028-0836

Ewing RM., et al. (2007). Large-scale mapping of human protein-protein interactions by mass spectrometry. *Molecular Systems Biology*, Vol. 3, (2007), pp. 89, ISSN 1744-4292

Farrer MJ., et al. (2009). DCTN1 mutations in Perry syndrome. *Nature Genetics*, Vol. 41, No. 2, (February 2009), pp. 163-165, ISSN 1061-4036

Feder JN., et al. (1998). The hemochromatosis gene product complexes with the transferrin receptor and lowers its affinity for ligand binding. *Proceedings of the National Academy of Sciences of the United States of America*, Vol. 95, No. 4, (February 1998), pp.1472-1477, ISSN 0027-8424

Fernández-Santiago R., et al. (2006). Possible gender-dependent association of vascular endothelial growth factor (VEGF) gene and ALS. *Neurology*, Vol. 66, No. 12, (June 2006), pp. 1929-1931, ISSN 0028-3878

Fernández-Santiago R., et al. (2009). Identification of novel Angiogenin (ANG) gene missense variants in German patients with amyotrophic lateral sclerosis. *Journal of Neurology*, Vol. 256, No. 8, (August 2009), pp. 1337-1342, ISSN 1351-5101

Fernández-Santiago R., et al. (2009). No evidence of association of FLJ10986 and ITPR2 with ALS in a large German cohort. *Neurobiology of Aging*, Vol. 32, No. 3, (March 2011), pp. 551.e1-4, ISSN 0197-4580

Figlewicz DA., et al. (1994). Variants of the heavy neurofilament subunit are associated with the development of amyotrophic lateral sclerosis. *Human Molecular Genetics*, Vol. 3, No. 10, (October 1994), pp. 1757-1761, ISSN 0964-6906

Fishel ML & Kelley MR. (2007). The DNA base excision repair protein Ape1/Ref-1 as a therapeutic and chemopreventive target. *Molecular Aspects of Medicine*, Vol. 28, No. 3-4, (June-August 2007), pp. 375-395, ISSN 0098-2997

Fogh I., et al. (2009) No association of DPP6 with amyotrophic lateral sclerosis in an Italian population. *Neurobiology of Aging*, Vol. 32, No. 5, (May 2011), pp. 966-967, ISSN 0197-4580

Gamez J., et al. (2002). Survival and respiratory decline are not related to homozygous SMN2 deletions in ALS patients. *Neurology*, Vol. 59, No. 9, (November 2002), pp. 1456-1460, ISSN 0028-3878

Gavrilov DK., et al. (1998). Differential SMN2 expression associated with SMA severity. *Nature Genetics*, Vol. 20, No. 3, (November 1998), pp. 230-231, ISSN 1061-4036

Gellera C., et al. (2007). Identification of new ANG gene mutations in a large color of Italian patients with amyotrophic lateral sclerosis. *Neurogenetics*, Vol. 9, No. 1, (February 2008), pp. 33-40, ISSN 1364-6745

Gijselinck I., et al. (2010). Identification of 2 loci at chromosome 9 and 14 in a multiplex family with frontotemporal lobar degeneration and amyotrophic lateral sclerosis. *Archives of Neurology*, Vol. 67, No. 5, (May 2010), pp. 606-616, ISSN 0003-9942

Giordano G., et al. (2011). Paraoxonase 2 (PON2) in the mouse central nervous system: A neuroprotective role? *Toxicology and Applied Pharmacology*, (February 2011), Ahead of print, ISSN 0041-008X

Gitcho MA., et al. (2009). VCP mutations causing frontotemporal lobar degeneration disrupt localization of TDP-43 and induce cell death. *Journal of Biological Chemistry*, Vol. 284, No. 18, (May 2009), pp. 12384-12398, ISSN 0021-9258

Gitcho MA., et al. (2009). TARDBP 3´UTR variant in autopsy-confirmed frontotemporal lobar degeneration with TDP-43 proteinopathy. *Acta Neuropathologica*, Vol. 118, No. 5, (November 2009), pp. 633-645, ISSN 0001-6322

Goodall EF., et al. (2005). Association of the H63D polymorphism in the hemochromatosis gene with sporadic ALS. *Neurology*, Vol. 65, No. 6, (September 2005), pp. 934-937, ISSN 0028-3878

Golenia A., et al. (2010). Lack of association between VEGF gene polymorphisms and plasma VEGF levels and sporadic ALS. *Neurology*, Vol. 75, No. 22, (November 2010), pp. 2035-2037, ISSN 0028-3878

Greenway MJ., et al. (2004). A novel candidate region for ALS on chromosome 14q11.2. *Neurology*, Vol. 63, No. 10, (November 2004), pp. 1936-1938, ISSN 0028-3878

Greenway MJ., et al. (2006). ANG mutations segregate with familial and 'sporadic' amyotrophic lateral sclerosis. *Nature Genetics*, Vol. 38, No. 4, (April 2006), pp. 411-413, ISSN 1061-4036

Groen EJ., et al. (2010). FUS mutations in amyotrophic lateral sclerosis in the Netherlands. *Archives of Neurology*, Vol. 67, No. 2, (February 2010), pp. 224-230, ISSN 0003-9942

Grohmann K., et al. (2011). Mutations in the gene encoding immunoglobulin mu-binding protein 2 cause spinal muscular atrophy with respiratory distress type 1. *Nature Genetics*, Vol. 29, No. 1, (September 2001), pp. 75-77, ISSN 1061-4036

Gurney ME., et al. (1994). Motor neuron degeneration in mice that express a human Cu,Zn superoxide dismutase mutation. *Science*, Vol. 264, No. 5166, (June 1994), pp. 1772-1775, ISSN 0036-8075

Hadano S., et al. (2001. A gene encoding a putative GTPase regulator is mutated in familial amyotrophic lateral sclerosis 2. *Nature Genetics*, Vol.29, No.2, (October 2001), pp.166-173, ISSN 1061-4036

Hadano S., et al. (2005). Mice deficient in the Rab5 guanine nucleotide exchange factor ALS2/alsin exhibit age-dependent neurological deficits and altered endosome trafficking. *Human Molecular Genetics*, Vol. 15, No. 2, (January 2006), pp. 233-250, ISSN 0964-6906

Hand CK., et al. (2001). A novel locus for familial amyotrophic lateral sclerosis on chromosome 18q. *The American Journal of Human Genetics*, Vol. 70, No.1, (January 2002), pp.251-256, ISSN 0002-9297

Haraguchi K., et al. (2005). Role of the kinesin-2 family protein, KIF3, during mitosis. *Journal of Biological Chemistry*, Vol. 281, No. 7, (February 2006), pp. 4094-4099, ISSN 0021-9258

Harley IT., et al. (2010). The role of genetic variation near interferon-kappa in systemic lupus erythematosus. *Journal of Biomedicine and Biotechnology*, 2010, ISSN 1110-7243

Hayward C., et al. (1999). Molecular genetic analysis of the APEX nuclease gene in amyotrophic lateral sclerosis. *Neurology*, Vol. 52, No. 9, (June 1999), pp. 1899-1901, ISSN 0028-3878

He X., et al. (2011). H63D polymorphism in the hemochromatosis gene is associated with sporadic amyotrophic lateral sclerosis in China. *European Journal of Neurology*, Vol. 18, No. 2, (February 2011), pp. 359-361, ISSN 1351-5101

He CZ & Hays AP. (2004). Expression of peripherin in ubiquitinated inclusions of amyotrophic lateral sclerosis. *Journal of Neurological Sciences*, Vol. 217, No. 1, (January 2004), pp. 47-54, ISSN 0022-510X

Hentati A., et al. (1994). Linkage of recessive familial amyotrophic lateral sclerosis to chromosome 2q33-q35. *Nature Genetics*, Vol. 7, No. 3, (July 1994), pp. 425-428, ISSN 1061-4036

Hentati A., et al. (1998). Linkage of a commoner form of recessive amyotrophic lateral sclerosis to chromosome 15q15-q22 markers. *Neurogenetics*, Vol. 2, No. 1, (December 1998), pp. 55-60, ISSN 1364-6745

Hergovich A. (2011). MOB control: reviewing a conserved family of kinase regulators. *Cellular Signaling*, Vol. 23, No.9, (September 2011), pp.1433-1440, ISSN 0898-6568

Hervas-Stubss S., et al. (2011). Direct effects of type I interferons on cells of the immune system. *Clinical Cancer Research*, Vol. 17, No. 9, (May 2011), pp. 2619-2627, ISSN 1078-0432

Hewitt C., et al. (2010). Novel FUS/TLS mutations and pathology in familial and sporadic amyotrophic lateral sclerosis. *Archives of Neurology*, Vol. 67, No. 4, (April 2010), pp. 455-461, ISSN 0003-9942

Hirano M., et al. (2010). Senataxin mutations in amyotrophic lateral sclerosis. *Amyotrophic Lateral Sclerosis*, Vol. 12, No. 3, (May 2011), pp. 223-227, ISSN 1748-2968

Horner RD., et al. (2003). Occurrence of amyotrophic lateral sclerosis among Gulf War veterans. *Neurology*, Vol. 61, No. 6, (September 2003), pp. 742-749, ISSN 0028-3878

Hosler BA., et al. (2000). Linkage of familial amyotrophic lateral sclerosis with frontotemporal dementia to chromosome 9q21-q22. *Journal of the American Medical Association*, Vol. 284, No. 13, (October 2000), pp. 1664-1669, ISSN 0098-7484

Huang C., et al. (2011). FUS transgenic rats develop the phenotypes of amyotrophic lateral sclerosis and frontotemporal lobar degeneration. *PLoS Genetics*, Vol. 7, No. 3, (March 2011), pp. e1002011, ISSN 1553-7404

Huang EJ., et al. (2010). Extensive FUS-immunoreactive pathology in juvenile amyotrophic lateral sclerosis with basophilic inclusions. *Brain Pathology*, Vol. 20, No. 6, (November 2010), pp. 1069-1076, ISSN 1015-6305

Hutton M., et al. (1998). Association of missense and 5'-splice-site mutations in tau with the inherited dementia FTDP-17. *Nature*, Vol. 393, No. 6686, (June 1998), pp. 702-705, ISSN 0028-0836

Iida A., et al. (2010). Large-scale screening of TARDBP mutation in amyotrophic lateral sclerosis. *Neurobiology of Aging*, 2010, Ahead of print

Iida A., et al. (2011). Optineurin mutations in Japanese amyotrophic lateral sclerosis. *Journal of Neurology, Neurosurgery and Psychiatry*, (January 2011), ISSN 0022-3050

Iida A., et al. (2011). Replication analysis of SNPs on 9p21.2 and 19p13.11 with amyotrophic lateral sclerosis in East Asians. *Neurobiology of Aging*, Vol. 32, No. 4, (April 2011), pp. 757.e13-4, ISSN 0197-4580

Ilieva H, Polymenidou M & Cleveland DW. (2009). Non-cell autonomous toxicity in neurodegenerative disorders: ALS and beyond. *Journal of Cell Biology*, Vol. 187, No. 6, (December 2009), pp. 761-772, ISSN 0021-9525

Imbert G., et al. (1996). Cloning of the gene for spinocerebellar ataxia 2 reveals a locus with high sensitivity to expanded CAG/glutamine repeats. *Nature Genetics*, Vol. 14, No. 3, (November 1996), pp. 285-291, ISSN 1061-4036

Ito D., et al. (201). Nuclear transport impairment of amyotrophic lateral sclerosis-linked mutations in FUS/TLS. *Annals of Neurology*, 2010, Ahead of print

Jackson M., et al. (1996). Analysis of chromosome 5q13 genes in amyotrophic lateral sclerosis: homozygous NAIP deletion in a sporadic case. *Annals of Neurology*, Vol. 39, No. 6, (June 1996), pp. 796-800, ISSN 0364-5134

Johnson JO., et al. (2010). Exome sequencing reveals VCP mutations as a cause of familial ALS. *Neuron*, Vol. 68, No. 5, (December 2010), pp. 857-864, ISSN 0896-6273

Ju JS & Weihl CC. (2010). Inclusion body myopathy, Paget's disease of the bone and frontotemporal dementia: a disorder of autophagy. *Human Molecular Genetics*, Vol. 19, No. R1, (April 2010), pp. R38-45, ISSN 0964-6906

Ju S., et al. (2011). A yeast model of FUS/TLS-dependent cytotoxicity. *PLoS Biology*, Vol. 9, No. 4, (April 2011), pp. e1001052, ISSN 1545-7885

Kabashi E., et al. (2008). TARDBP mutations in individuals with sporadic and familial amyotrophic lateral sclerosis. *Nature Genetics*, Vol. 40, No. 5, (May 2008), pp. 572-574, ISSN 1061-4036

Kanekura K., et al. (2004). Alsin, the product of ALS2 gene, suppresses SOD1 mutant neurotoxicity through RhoGEF domain by interacting with SOD1 mutants. *Journal of Biological Chemistry*, Vol. 279, No. 18, (April 2004), pp. 19247-19256, ISSN 0021-9258

Kiernan MC., et al. (2011). Amyotrophic lateral sclerosis. *Lancet*, Vol. 377, No. 9769, (March 2011), pp. 942-955, ISSN 0140-6736

Kisby GE, Milne J & Sweatt C. (1997). Evidence of reduced DNA repair in amyotrophic lateral sclerosis brain tissue. *Neuroreport*, Vol. 8, No. 6, (April 1997), pp. 1337-1340, ISSN 0959-4965

Kohler RS., et al. (2010). Differential NDR/LATS interactions with the human MOB family reveal a negative role for human MOB2 in the regulation of human NDR kinases. *Molecular and Cellular Biology*, Vol. 30, No. 18, (September 2010), pp. 4507-4520, ISSN 1098-5549

Kwiatkowski TJ Jr., et al. (2009). Mutations in the FUS/TLS gene on chromosome 16 cause familial amyotrophic lateral sclerosis. *Science*, Vol. 323, No. 5918, (February 2009), pp. 1205-1208, ISSN 1095-9203

Laaksovirta H., et al. (2010). Chromosome 9p21 in amyotrophic lateral sclerosis in Finland: a genome-wide association study. *Lancet Neurology*, Vol. 9, No. 10, (October 2010), pp. 978-985, ISSN 1474-4422

LaFleur DW., et al. (2001). Interferon-κ, a novel type I interferon expressed in human keratinocytes. *Journal of Biological Chemistry*, Vol. 276, No. 43, (October 2001), pp. 39765-39771, ISSN 0021-9258

Lagier-Tourenne C, Polymenidou M & Cleveland DW. (2010). TDP-43 and FUS/TLS: emerging roles in RNA processing and neurodegeneration. *Human Molecular Genetics*, Vol. 19, No. R1, (April 2010), pp. R46-R64, ISSN 0964-6906

Lambrechts D., et al. (2003). VEGF is a modifier of amyotrophic lateral sclerosis in mice and humans and protects motoneuron against ischemic death. *Nature Genetics*, Vol. 34, No. 4, (August 2003), pp. 383-394, ISSN 1061-4036

Lambrechts D., et al. (2009). Meta-analysis of vascular endothelial growth factor variations in amyotrophic lateral sclerosis: increased susceptibility in male carriers of the -2578AA genotype. *Journal of Medical Genetics*, Vol. 46, No. 12, (December 2009), pp. 840-846, ISSN 0022-2593

Landers JE., et al. (2008). A common haplotype within the PON1 promoter region is associated with sporadic ALS. *Amyotrophic Lateral Sclerosis*, Vol. 9, No. 5, (October 2008), pp. 306-314, ISSN 1748-2968

Lariviere RC & Julien JP. (2004). Functions of intermediate filaments in neuronal development and disease. *Journal of Neurobiology*, Vol. 58, No. 1, (January 2004), pp. 131-148, ISSN 0022-3034

Le Ber I., et al. (2009). Chromosome 9p-linked families with frontotemporal dementia associated with motor neuron disease. *Neurology*, Vol. 72, No. 19, (May 2009), pp. 1669-1676, ISSN 0028-3878

Lee JA., et al. (2007). ESCRT-III dysfunction causes autophagosomes accumulation and neurodegeneration. *Current Biology*, Vol. 17, No. 18, (September 2007), pp. 1561-1567, ISSN 0960-9822

Lee T., et al. Ataxin-2 intermediate-length polyglutamine expansions in European ALS patients. *Human Molecular Genetics*, Vol. 20, No. 9, (May 2011), pp. 1697-1700, ISSN 0964-6906

Lefebvre S., et al. (1997). Correlation between severity and SMN protein level in spinal muscular atrophy. *Nature Genetics*, Vol. 16, No. 3, (July 1997), pp. 265-269, ISSN 1061-4036

Li XG., et al. (2009). Association between DPP6 polymorphism and the risk of sporadic amyotrophic lateral sclerosis in Chinese patients. *Chinese Medical Journal*, Vol. 122, No. 24, (December 2009), pp. 2989-2992, ISSN 0366-6999

Lorson CL., et al. (1998). SMN oligomerization defect correlates with spinal muscular atrophy severity. *Nature Genetics*, Vol. 19, No. 1, (May 1998), pp. 63-66, ISSN 1061-4036

Liu Y., et al. (2011). Mutant HFE H63D protein is associated with prolonged endoplasmic reticulum stress and increased neuronal vulnerability. *Journal of Biological Chemistry*, Vol. 286, No. 15, (April 2011), pp. 13161-13170, ISSN 0021-9258

Luty AA., et al. (2008). Pedigree with frontotemporal lobar degeneration – motor neuron disease and Tar DNA binding protein-43 positive neuropathology: genetic linkage to chromosome 9. *BMC Neurology*, Vol. 8, (August 2008), pp. 32, ISSN 1471-2377

Luty AA., et al. (2010). Sigma nonopioid intracellular receptor 1 mutations cause frontotemporal lobar degeneration-motor neuron disease. *Annals of Neurology*, Vol. 68, No. 5, (November 2010), pp. 639-649, ISSN 0364-5134

Mackness MI, Arrol S & Durrington PN. (1991). Paraoxonase prevents accumulation of lipoperoxides in low-density lipoprotein. *FEBS Letters*, Vol. 286, No. 1-2, (July 1991), pp. 151-154, ISSN 0014-5793

McLean J., et al. (2010). Distinct biochemical signatures characterize peripherin isoform expression in both traumatic neuronal injury and motor neuron disease. *Journal of Neurochemistry*, Vol. 114, No. 4, (August 2010), pp. 1177-1192, ISSN 0022-3042

Mersiyanova IV., et al. (2000). A new variant of Charchot-Marie-Tooth disease type 2 is probably the result of a mutation in the neurofilaments-light gene. *American Journal of Human Genetics*, Vol. 67, No. 1, (July 2000), pp. 37-46, ISSN 0002-9297

Millecamps S., et al. (2010). SOD1, ANG, VAPB, TARDBP, and FUS mutations in familial amyotrophic lateral sclerosis: genotype-phenotype correlations. *Journal of Medical Genetics*, Vol. 47, No. 8, (August 2010), pp. 554-560, ISSN 0022-2593

Millecamps S., et al. (2011). Screening of OPTN in French familial amyotrophic lateral sclerosis. *Neurobiology of Aging*, Vol. 32, No. 3, (March 2011), pp. 557.e11-3, ISSN 1558-1497

Mitchell J., et al. (2010). Familial amytrophic lateral sclerosis is associated with a mutation in D-amino acid oxidase. *Proceedings of the National Academy of Sciences of the USA*, Vol. 107, No. 16, (April 2010), pp. 7556-7561, ISSN 0027-8424

Mitchell RM., et al. (2009). HFE polymorphisms affect cellular glutamate regulation. *Neurobiology of Aging*, Vol. 32, No. 6, (June 2011), pp. 1114-1123, ISSN 0197-4580

Mizuno Y., et al. (2011). Peripherin partially localizes in Bunina bodies in amyotrophic lateral sclerosis. *Journal of Neurological Sciences*, Vol. 301, No. 1-2, (March 2011), pp. 14-18, ISSN 0022-510X

Morahan JM., et al. (2006). A gene-environment study of the paraoxonase 1 gene and pesticides in amyotrophic lateral sclerosis. *Neurotoxicology*, Vol. 28, No. 3, (May 2007), pp. 532-540, ISSN 0161-813X

Moreira MC., et al. (2004). Senataxin, the ortholog of a yeast RNA helicase, is mutant in ataxia-ocular apraxia 2. *Nature Genetics*, Vol. 36, No. 3, (March 2004), pp. 225-227, ISSN 1061-4036

Morita M., et al. (2006). A locus on chromosome 9p confers susceptibility to ALS and frontotemporal dementia. *Neurology*, Vol. 66, No. 6, (March 2006), pp. 839-844, ISSN 0028-3878

Moulard B., et al. (1998). Association between centromeric deletions of the SMN gene and sporadic adult-onset lower motor neuron disease. *Annals of Neurology*, Vol. 43, No. 5, (May 1998), pp. 640-644, ISSN 0364-5134

Münch C., et al. (2004). Point mutations of the p150 subunit of dynactin (DCTN1) gene in ALS. *Neurology*, Vol. 63, No. 4, (August 2004), pp. 724-726, ISSN 0028-3878

Münch C., et al. (2005). Heterozygous R1101K mutation of the DCTN1 gene in a family with ALS and FTD. *Annals of Neurology*, Vol. 58, No. 5, (November 2005), pp. 777-780, ISSN 0364-5134

Murayama H., et al. (2010). Mutations of optineurin in amyotrophic lateral sclerosis. *Nature*, Vol. 465, No. 7295, (May 2010), pp. 223-226, ISSN 0028-0836

Nadal MS., et al. (2003). The CD26-related dipeptidyl aminopeptidase-like protein DPPX is a critical component of neuronal A-type K+ channels. *Neuron*, Vol. 37, No. 3, (February 2003), pp. 449-461, ISSN 0896-6273

Nandar W & Connor JR. (2011). HFE gene variants affect iron in the brain. *Journal of Nutrition*, Vol. 141, No. 4, (April 2011), pp. 729S-739S, ISSN 0022-3166

Nardelli B., et al. (2002). Regulatory effect of IFN-κ, a novel type I IFN, on cytokine production by cells of the innate immune system. *Journal of Immunology*, Vol. 169, No. 9, (November 2002), pp. 4822-4830, ISSN 0022-1767

Neumann M., et al. (2006). Ubiquitinated TDP-43 in frontotemporal lobar degeneration and amyotrophic lateral sclerosis. *Science*, Vol. 314, No. 5796, (October 2006), pp. 130-133, ISSN 1095-9203

Nishimura AL., et al. (2004). A mutation in the vesicle-trafficking protein VAPB causes late-onset spinal muscular atrophy and amyotrophic lateral sclerosis. *American Journal of Human Genetics*, Vol. 75, No. 5, (November 2004), pp. 822-831, ISSN 0002-9297

Nonis D., et al. (2008). Ataxin-2 associates with the endocytosis complex and affects EGF receptor trafficking. *Cellular Signalling*, Vol. 20, No. 10, (October 2008), pp. 1725-1739, ISSN

Ng CJ., et al. (2001). Paraoxonase-2 is a ubiquitously expressed protein with antioxidant properties and is capable of preventing cell-mediated oxidative modification of low density lipoprotein. *Journal of Biological Chemistry*, Vol. 276, No. 48, (November 2001), pp. 44444-44449, ISSN 0021-9258

Ng SB., et al. (2009). Targeted capture and massively parallel sequencing of 12 human exomes. *Nature*, Vol. 461, No. 7261, (September 2009), pp. 272-276, ISSN 0028-0836

Oosthuyse B., et al. (2001). Deletion of the hypoxia-response element in the vascular endothelial growth factor promoter causes motor neuron degeneration. *Nature Genetics*, Vol. 28, No. 2, (June 2001), pp. 131-138, ISSN 1061-4036

Orlacchio A., et al. (2010). SPATACSIN mutations cause autosomal recessive juvenile amyotrophic lateral sclerosis. *Brain*, Vol. 133, Pt. 2, (February 2010), pp. 591-598, ISSN 0006-8950

Orozco G, Barrett JC & Zeggini E. (2010). Synthetic associations in the context of genome-wide association scan signals. *Human Molecular Genetics*, Vol. 19, No. R2, (October 2010), pp. R137-R144, ISSN 0964-6906

Orrell RW., et al. (1997). The relationship of spinal muscular atrophy to motor neuron disease: investigation of SMN and NAIP gene deletions in sporadic and familial ALS. *Journal of Neurological Sciences*, Vol. 145, No. 1, (January 1997), pp. 55-61, ISSN 0022-510X

Otomo A., et al. (2003). ALS2, a novel guanine nucleotide exchange factor for the small GTPase Rab5, is implicated in endosomal dynamics. *Human Molecular Genetics*, Vol. 12, No. 14, (July 2003), pp. 1671-1687, ISSN 0964-6906

Parboosingh JS., et al. (1999). Deletions causing spinal muscular atrophy do not predispose to amyotrophic lateral sclerosis. *Archives of Neurology*, Vol. 56, No. 6, (June 1999), pp. 710-712, ISSN 0003-9942

Parkinson N., et al. (2006). ALS phenotypes with mutations in CHMP2B (charged multivesicular body protein 2B). *Neurology*, Vol. 67, No. 6, (September 2006), pp. 1074-1077, ISSN 0028-3878

Pasinelli P & Brown RH. (2006). Molecular biology of amyotrophic lateral sclerosis: insights from genetics. *Nature Reviews Neuroscience*, Vol. 7, No. 9, (September 2006), pp. 710-723, ISSN 1471-003X

Paubel A., et al. (2008). Mutations of the ANG gene in French patients with amyotrophic lateral sclerosis. *Archives of Neurology*, Vol. 65, No. 10, (October 2008), pp. 1333-1336, ISSN 0003-9942

Pearson JP., et al. (2010). Familial frontotemporal dementia with amyotrophic lateral sclerosis and a shared haplotype on chromosome 9p. *Journal of Neurology*, Vol. 258, No. 4, (April 2011), pp. 647-655, ISSN 0340-5354

Pestka S, Krause CD & Walter MR. (2004). Interferons, interferon-like cytokines, and their receptors. *Immunological reviews*, Vol. 202, (December 2004), pp. 8-32, ISSN 0105-2896

Phillips T & Robberecht W. (2010). Neuroinflammation in amyotrophic lateral sclerosis: role of glial activation in motor neuron disease. *Lancet Neurology*, Vol. 10, No. 3, (March 2010), pp. 253-263, ISSN 1474-4422

Puls I., et al. (2003). Mutant dynactin in motor neuron disease. *Nature Genetics*, Vol. 33, No. 4, (April 2003), pp. 455-456, ISSN 1061-4036

Puls I., et al. (2005). Distal spinal and bulbar muscular atrophy caused by dynactin mutation. *Annals of Neurlogy*, Vol. 57, No. 5, (May 2005), pp. 687-694, ISSN 0364-5134

Pulst SM., et al. (1996). Moderate expansion of a normally biallelic trinucleotide repeat in spinocerebellar ataxia type 2. *Nature Genetics*, Vol. 14, No. 3, (November 1996), pp. 269-276, ISSN 1061-4036

Ralser M., et al. (2004). An integrative approach to gain insights into the cellular function of human ataxin-2. *Journal of Molecular Biology*, Vol. 346, No. 1, (February 2005), pp. 203-214, ISSN 0022-2836

Reaume AG., et al. (1996). Motor neurons in Cu/Zn superoxide dismutase-deficient mice develop normally but exhibit enhanced cell death after axonal injury. *Nature Genetics*, Vol. 13, No. 1, (May 1996), pp. 43-47, ISSN 1061-4036

Renton AE et al. (2011). A hexanucleotide repeat expansion in C9ORF72 is the cause of chromosome 9p21-linked ALS-FTD. *Neuron*, September 2011, Ahead of print

Restagno G., et al. (2007). HFE H63D polymorphism is increate in patients with amyotrophic lateral sclerosis of Italian origin. *Journal of Neurology, Neurosurgery and Psychiatry*, Vol. 78, No. 3, (March 2007), pp. 327, ISSN 0022-3050

Rezaie T., et al. (2002). Adult-onset primary open-angle glaucoma caused by mutations in optineurin. *Science*, Vol. 295, No. 5557, (February 2002), pp.1077-1079, ISSN 1095-9203

Ricci C., et al. (2010). Lack of association of PON polymorphisms with sporadic ALS in an Italian population. *Neurobiology of Aging*, Vol. 32, No. 3, (March 2011), pp. 552.e7-13, ISSN 1558-1497

Ringholz GM., et al. (2005). Prevalence and patterns of cognitive impairment in sporadic ALS. *Neurology*, Vol. 65, No. 4, (August 2005), pp. 586-590, ISSN 0028-3878

Robertson J., et al. (2003). A neurotoxic peripherin splice variant in a mouse model of ALS. *Journal of Cell Biology*, Vol. 160, No. 6, (March 2003), pp. 939-949, ISSN 0021-9525

Rollinson S., et al. (2011). Frontotemporal lobar degeneration genome wide association study replication confirms a risk locus shared with amyotrophic lateral sclerosis. *Neurobiology of Aging*, Vol. 32, No. 4, (April 2011), pp. 758.e1-7, ISSN 0197-4580

Rooke K., et al. (1996). Analysis of the KSP repeat of the neurofilament heavy subunit in familial amyotrophic lateral sclerosis. *Neurology*, Vol. 46, No. 3, (March 1996), pp. 789-790, ISSN 0028-3878

Rosen DR., et al. (1993). Mutations in Cu/Zn superoxide dismutase gene are associated with familial amyotrophic lateral sclerosis. *Nature*, Vol. 362, No. 6415, (March 1993), pp. 59-62, ISSN 0028-0836

Ross OA., et al. (2011). Ataxin-2 repeat-length variation and neurodegeneration. *Human Molecular Genetics*, Vol. 20, No. 16, (August 2011), pp. 3207-3212, ISSN 0964-6906

Rual JF., et al. (2005). Towards a proteome-scale map of the human protein-protein interaction network. *Nature*, Vol. 437, No. 7062, (October 2005), pp. 1173-1178, ISSN 0028-0836

Rutherford AC., et al. (2006). The mammalian phosphatidylinositol 3-phosphate 5-kinase (PIKfyve) regulates endosome-to-TGN retrograde transport. *Journal of Cell Science*, Vol. 119, Pt. 19, (October 2006), pp. 3944-3957, ISSN 0021-9533

Saeed M., et al. (2006). Paraoxonase cluster polymorphisms are associated with sporadic ALS. *Neurology*, Vol. 67, No. 5, (September 2006), pp. 771-776, ISSN 0028-3878

Sahlender DA., et al. (2005). Optineurin links myosin VI to the Golgi complex and is involved in Golgi organization and exocytosis. *Journal of Cell Biology*, Vol. 169, No. 2, (April 2005), pp. 285-295, ISSN 0021-9525

Salinas S., et al. (2008). Heriditary spastic paraplegia: clinical features and pathogenic mechanisms. *Lancet Neurology*, Vol. 7, No. 12, (December 2008), pp. 1127-1138, ISSN 1474-4422

Sanpei K., et al. (1996). Identification of the spinocerebellar ataxia type 2 gene using a direct identification of repeat expansion and cloning technique, DIRECT. *Nature Genetics*, Vol. 14, No. 3, (November 1996), pp. 277-284, ISSN 1061-4036

Sapp PC., et al. (2003). Identification of two novel loci for dominantly inherited familial amyotrophic lateral sclerosis. *American Journal of Human Genetics*, Vol. 73, No. 2, (August 2003), pp. 397-403, ISSN 0002-9297

Schmitt-John T., et al. (2005). Mutation of Vps54 causes motor neuron disease and defective spermiogenesis in the wobbler mouse. *Nature Genetics*, Vol. 37, No. 11, (November 2005), pp. 1213-1215, ISSN 1061-4036

Schymick JC., et al. (2007). Genome-wide genotyping in amyotrophic lateral sclerosis and neurologically normal controls: first stage analysis and public release of data. *Lancet Neurology*, Vol. 6, No. 4, (April 2007), pp. 322-328, ISSN 1474-4422

Sebastià J., et al. (2009). Angiogenin protects motoneurons against hypoxic injury. *Cell Death and Differentiation*, Vol. 16, No. 9, (September 2009), pp. 1238-1247, ISSN 1350-9047

Shaikh AY & Martin LJ. (2002). DNA base-excision repair enzyme apurinic/apyrimidinic endonuclease/redox factor-1 is increased and competent in the brain and spinal cord of individuals with amyotrophic lateral sclerosis. *Neuromolecular Medicine*, Vol. 2, No. 1, (2002), pp. 47-60, ISSN 1535-1084

Shatunov A., et al. (2010). Chromosome 9p21 in sporadic amyotrophic lateral sclerosis in the UK and seven other countries: a genome-wide association study. *Lancet Neurology*, Vol. 9, No. 10, (October 2010), pp. 986-994, ISSN 1474-4422

Shin JS., et al. (2008). NEFL Pro22Arg mutation in Charcot-Marie-Tooth disease type 1. *Journal of Human Genetics*, Vol. 53, No. 10, (2008), pp. 936-940, ISSN 1434-5161

Siddique T., et al. (1998). X-linked dominant locus for late-onset familial amyotrophic lateral sclerosis. *American Journal of Human Genetics*, Vol. 63, Suppl. A308.

Skibinski G., et al. (2005). Mutations in the endosomal ESCRTIII-complex subunit CHMP2B in frontotemporal dementia. *Nature Genetics*, Vol. 37, No. 8, (August 2005), pp. 806-808, ISSN 1061-4036

Skourti-Stathaki K, Proudfoot NJ & Gromak N. (2011). Human senataxin resolves RNA/DNA hybrids formed at transcriptional pause sites to promote Xrn2-dependent termination. *Molecular Cell*, Vol. 42, No. 6, (June 2011), pp. 794-805, ISSN 1097-2765

Skvortsova V., et al. (2004). Analysis of heavy neurofilament subunit gene polymorphism in Russian patients with sporadic motor neuron disease (MND). *European Journal of Human Genetics*, Vol. 12, No. 3, (March 2004), pp. 241-244, ISSN 1018-4813

Slowik A., et al. (2006). Paraoxonase gene polymorphisms and sporadic ALS. *Neurology*, Vol. 67, No. 5, (September 2006), pp. 766-770, ISSN 0028-3878

Sreedharan J., et al. (2008). TDP-43 mutations in familial and sporadic amytrophic lateral sclerosis. *Science*, Vol. 319, No. 5870, (March 2008), pp. 1668-1672, ISSN 1095-9203

Stevanin G., et al. (2007). Mutations in SPG11, encoding spatacsin, are a major cause of spastic paraplegia with thin corpus callosum. *Nature Genetics*, Vol. 39, No. 3, (March 2007), pp. 366-372, ISSN 1061-4036

Storkebaum E., et al. (2005). Treatment of motoneuron degeneration by intracerebroventricular delivery of VEGF in a rat model of ALS. *Nature Neuroscience*, Vol. 8, No. 1, (January 2005), pp. 85-92, ISSN 1097-6256

Subramanian V, Crabtree B & Acharya KR. (2007). Human angiogenin is a neuroprotective factor and amyotrophic lateral sclerosis associated angiogenin variants affect neurite extension/pathfinding and survival of motor neurons. *Human Molecular Genetics*, Vol. 17, No. 1, (January 2008), pp. 130-149, ISSN 0964-6906

Sugihara K., et al. (2011). Screening for OPTN mutations in amyotrophic lateral sclerosis in a mainly Caucasian population. *Neurobioloy of Aging*, Vol. 32, No. 10, (October 2011), pp. 1923.e9-1923.e10, ISSN 1558-1497

Sun Z., et al. (2011). Molecular determinants and genetic modifiers of aggregation and toxicity for the ALS disease proten FUS/TLS. *PLoS Biology*, Vol. 9, No. 4, (April 2011), pp. e1000614, ISSN 1545-7885

Sutedja NA., et al. (2007). The association between H63D mutations in HFE and amyotrophic lateral sclerosis in a Dutch population. *Archives of Neurology*, Vol. 64, No. 1, (January 2007), pp. 63-67, ISSN 0003-9942

Swarup V., et al. (2011). Pathological hallmarks of amyotrophic lateral sclerosis/frontotemporal lobar degeneration in transgenic mice produced with TDP-43 genomic fragments. *Brain*, 2011, Ahead of print.

Takeda S., et al. (2000). Kinesin superfamily protein 3 (KIF3) motor transports fodrin-associating vesicles important for neurite building. *Journal of Cell Biology*, Vol. 148, No. 6, (March 2000), pp. 1255-1265, ISSN 0021-9525

Terry PD., et al. (2004). VEGF promoter haplotype and amyotrophic lateral sclerosis (ALS). *Journal of Neurogenetics*, Vol. 18, No. 2, (April-June 2004), pp. 429-434, ISSN 0167-7063

Teuling E., et al. (2007). Motor neuron disease-associated mutant vesicle-associated membrane protein-associated protein (VAP) B recruits wild-type VAPs into endoplasmatic reticulum-derived tubular aggregates. *Journal of Neuroscience*, Vol. 27, No. 36, (September 2007), pp. 9801-9815, ISSN 0270-6474

Ticozzi N., et al. (2009). Mutational analysis of TARDBP in neurodegenerative disease. *Neurobiology of Aging*, 2009, Ahead of print.

Ticozzi N., et al. (2011). Mutational analysis reveals the FUS homolog TAF15 as a candidate gene for familial amyotrophic lateral sclerosis. *American Journal of Medical Genetics B: Neuropsychiatric Genetics*, Vol. 156B, No. 3, (April 2011), pp. 285-290, ISSN 1552-485X

Tomkins J., et al. (2000). Screening of AP endonuclease as a candidate gene for amyotrophic lateral sclerosis (ALS). *Neuroreport*, Vol.11, No. 8 (June 2000), pp. 1695-1697, ISSN 0959-4965

Topp JD., et al. (2004). Alsin is a Rab5 and Rac1 guanine nucleotide exchange factor. *Journal of Biological Chemistry*, Vol. 279, No. 23, (June 2004), pp. 24612-24623, ISSN 0021-9258

Troy CM., et al. (1990). Regulation of peripherin and neurofilaments expression in regenerating rat motor neurons. *Brain Research*, Vol. 529, No. 1-2, (October 1990), pp. 232-238, ISSN 0006-8993

Tudor EL., et al. (2010). Amyotrophic lateral sclerosis mutant vesicle-associated membrane protein-associated protein-B transgenic mice develop TAR-DNA-binding protein-43 pathology. *Neuroscience*, Vol. 167, No. 3, (May 2010), pp. 774-785, ISSN 0306-4522

Valdmanis PN., et al. (2007). Three families with amyotrophic lateral sclerosis and frontotemporal dementia with evidence of linkage to chromosome 9p. *Archives of Neurology*, Vol. 64, No. 2, (February 2007), pp. 240-245, ISSN 0003-9942

Valdmanis PN., et al. (2008). Association of paraoxonase gene cluster polymorphisms with ALS in France, Quebec, and Sweden. *Neurology*, Vol. 71, No. 7, (August 2008), pp. 514-520, ISSN 0028-3878

Valdmanis PN & Rouleau GA. (2008). Genetics of familial amyotrophic lateral sclerosis. *Neurology*, Vol. 70, No. 2, (January 2008), pp. 144-152, ISSN 0028-3878

Van Blitterswijk M., et al. (2011). Novel optineurin mutations in sporadic amyotrophic lateral sclerosis patients. *Neurobiology of Aging*, Ahead of print, ISSN 0197-4580

Vance C., et al. (2006). Familial amyotrophic lateral sclerosis with frontotemporal dementia is linked to a locus on chromosome 9p13.2-21.3. *Brain*, Vol. 129, No. 4, (April 2006), pp. 868-876, ISSN 0006-8950

Vance C., et al. (2009). Mutations in FUS, an RNA processing protein, cause familial amyotrophic lateral sclerosis type 6. *Science*, Vol. 323, No. 5918, (February 2009), pp. 1208-1211, ISSN 1095-9203

Van Damme P., et al. (2011). Expanded ATXN2 CAG repeat size in ALS identifies genetic overlap between ALS and SCA2. *Neurology*, Vol. 76, No. 24, (June 2011), pp. 2066-2072, ISSN 0028-3878

Van Deerlin VM., et al. (2008). TARDBP mutations in amyotrophic lateral sclerosis with TDP-43 neuropathology: a genetic and histopathological analysis. *Lancet Neurology*, Vol. 7, No. 5, (May 2008), pp. 409-416, ISSN 1474-4422

Van Deerlin VM., et al. (2010) Common variants at 7p21 are associated with frontotemporal lobar degeneration with TDP-43 inclusions. *Nature Genetics*, Vol. 42, No. 3, (March 2010), pp. 234-239, ISSN 1061-4036

Van Es MA., et al. (2007). ITPR2 as a susceptibility gene in sporadic amyotrophic lateral sclerosis: a genome-wide association study. *Lancet Neurology*, Vol. 6, No. 10, (October 2007), pp. 869-877, ISSN 1474-4422

Van Es MA., et al. (2008). Genetic variation in DPP6 is associated with susceptibility to amyotrophic lateral sclerosis. *Nature Genetics*, Vol. 40, No. 1, (January 2008), pp. 29-31, ISSN 1061-4036

Van Es MA., et al. (2009). A case of ALS-FTD in a large FALS pedigree with a K17I ANG mutation. *Neurology*, Vol. 72, No. 3, (January 2009), pp. 287-288, ISSN 0028-3878

Van Es MA., et al. (2009). Analysis of FGGY as a risk factor for sporadic amyotrophic lateral sclerosis. *Amyotrophic Lateral Sclerosis*, Vol. 10, No. 5-6, (October-December 2009), pp 441-447, ISSN 1748-2968

Van Es MA., et al. (2009). Genome-wide association study identifies 19p13.11 (UNC13A) and 9p21.2 as susceptibility loci for sporadic amyotrophic lateral sclerosis. *Nature Genetics*, Vol. 41, No. 10 (October 2009), pp. 1083-1087, ISSN 1061-4036

Van Es MA., et al. (2011). Angiogenin variants in Parkinson's disease and amyotrophic lateral sclerosis. *Annals of Neurology*, 2011:Ahead of print

Van Vught PW., et al. (2005). Lack of association between VEGF polymorphisms and ALS in a Dutch population. *Neurology*, Vol. 65, No. 10, (November 2005), pp. 1643-1645, ISSN 0028-3878

Vantaggiato C., et al. (2011). Senataaxin modulates neurite growth through fibroblast growth factor 8 signalling. *Brain*, Vol. 134, Pt. 6, (June 2011), pp. 1808-1828, ISSN 0006-8950

Varoqueaux F., et al. (2002). Total arrest of spontaneous and evoked synaptic transmission but normal synaptogenesis in the absence of Munc13-mediated vesicle priming. *Proceedings of the National Academy of Sciences of the United States of America*, Vol. 99, No. 13, (June 2002), pp. 9037-9042, ISSN 0027-8424

Varoqueaux F., et al. (2005). Aberrant morphology and residual transmitter release at the Munc13-deficient mouse neuromuscular synapse. *Molecular and Cellular Biology*, Vol. 25, No. 14, (July 2005), pp. 5973-5984, ISSN 0270-7306

Veldink JH., et al. (2001). Homozygous deletion of the survival motor neuron 2 gene is a prognostic factor in sporadic ALS. *Neurology*, Vol. 56, No. 6, (March 2001), pp. 749-752, ISSN 0028-3878

Veldink JH., et al. (2005). SMN genotypes producing less SMN protein increase susceptibility to and severity of sporadic ALS. *Neurology*, Vol. 65, No. 6, (September 2005), pp. 820-825, ISSN 0028-3878

Vilariño-Güell C., et al. (2009). Characterization of DCTN1 genetic variability in neurodegeneration. *Neurology*, Vol. 72, No. 23, (June 2009), pp. 2024-2028, ISSN 0028-3878

Wang XS., et al. (2004). Increased incidence of the Hfe mutation in amyotrophic lateral sclerosis and related cellular consequences. *Journal of the Neurological Sciences*, Vol. 227, No. 1 (December 2004), pp. 27-33, ISSN 0022-510X

Wang Y., et al. (2007). Vascular endothelial growth factor overexpression delays neurodegeneration and prolongs survival in amyotrophic lateral sclerosis mice. *Journal of Neuroscience*, Vol. 27, No. 2, (January 2007), pp. 304-307, ISSN 0270-6474

Wang J, Campbell IL & Zhang H. (2007). Systemic interferon-alpha regulates interferon-stimulated genes in the central nervous system. *Molecular Psychiatry*, Vol. 13, No. 3, (March 2008), pp. 293-301, ISSN 1359-4184

Watts GD., et al. (2004). Inclusion body myopathy associated with Paget disease of bone and frontotemporal dementia is caused by mutant valosin-containing protein. *Nature Genetics*, Vol. 36, No. 4, (April 2004), pp. 377-381, ISSN 1061-4036

Weihl CC., et al. (2008). TDP-43 accumulation in inclusion body myopathy muscle suggests a common pathogenic mechanism with frontotemporal dementia. *Journal of Neurology, Neurosurgery and Psychiatry*, Vol. 79, No. 10, (October 2008), pp. 1186-1189, ISSN 0022-3050

Williamson TL., et al. (1998). Absence of neurofilaments reduce the selective vulnerability of motor neurons and slows disease caused by a familial amyotrophic lateral sclerosis-linked superoxide dismutase 1 mutant. *Proceedings of the National Academy of Sciences of the USA*, Vol. 95, No. 16, (August 1998), pp. 9631-9636, ISSN 0027-8424

Wills AM., et al. (2009). A large-scale international meta-analysis of paraoxonase gene polymorphisms in sporadic ALS. *Neurology*, Vol. 73, No. 1, (July 2009), pp. 16-24, ISSN 0028-3878

Wu D., et al. (2007). Angiongenin loss-of-function mutations in amyotrophic lateral sclerosis. *Annals of Neurology*, Vol. 62, No. 6, (December 2007), pp. 609-617, ISSN 0364-5134

Xiao S., et al. (2008). An aggregate-inducing peripherin isoform generated through intron retention is upregulated in amyotrophic lateral sclerosis and associated with disease pathology. *Journal of Neuroscience*, Vol. 28, No. 8, (February 2008), pp. 1833-1840, ISSN 0270-6474

Yamasaki S., et al. (2009). Angiogenin cleaves tRNA and promotes stress-induced translational repression. *Journal of Cell Biology*, Vol. 185, No. 1, (April 2009), pp. 35-42, ISSN 0021-9525

Yan J., et al. (2006). A major novel locus for ALS/FTD on chromosome 9p21 and its pathological correlates. *Neurology*, Vol. 67, No. 1, (July 2006), pp. 186-186b, ISSN 0028-3878

Yan J., et al. (2010). Frameshift and novel mutations in FUS in familial amyotrophic lateral sclerosis and ALS/dementia. *Neurology*, Vol. 75, No. 9, (August 2010), pp. 807-814, ISSN 0028-3878

Yang Y., et al. (2001). The gene encoding alsin, a protein with three guanine-nucleotide exchange factor domains, is mutated in a form of recessive amyotrophic lateral sclerosis. *Nature Genetics*, Vol. 29, No. 2, (October 2001), pp. 160-165, ISSN 1061-4036

Yen AA., et al. (2004). HFE mutations are not strongly associated with sporadic ALS. *Neurology*, Vol. 62, No. 9, (May 2004), pp. 1611-1612, ISSN 0028-3878

Zawiślak D., et al. (2010). The –A162G polymorphism of the PON1 gene and the risk of sporadic amyotrophic lateral sclerosis. *Neurologia I Neurochirurgia Polska*, Vol. 44, No. 3, (May 2010), pp. 246-250, ISSN 0028-3843 (Abstract)

Zhang Y., et al. (2006). VEGF C2578A polymorphism does not contribute to amyotrophic lateral sclerosis susceptibility in sporadic Chinese patients. *Amyotrophic Lateral Sclerosis*, Vol. 7, No. 2, (June 2006), pp. 119-122, ISSN 1748-2968

Zhang Y., et al. (2007). Loss of Vac14, a regulator of the signaling lipid phosphatidylinositol 3,5-biphosphate, results in neurodegeneration in mice. *Proceedings of the National Academy of Sciences of the USA*, Vol. 104, No. 44, (October 2007), pp. 17518-17523, ISSN 0027-8424

Zhao ZH., et al. (2009). A novel mutation in the senataxin gene identified in a Chinese patient with sporadic amyotrophic lateral sclerosis. *Amyotrophic Lateral Sclerosis*, Vol. 10, No. 2, (April 2009), pp. 118-122, ISSN 1748-2968

Genetics of Familial Amyotrophic Lateral Sclerosis

Emily F. Goodall, Joanna J. Bury,
Johnathan Cooper-Knock, Pamela J. Shaw and Janine Kirby
Sheffield Institute for Translational Neuroscience, University of Sheffield, Sheffield, United Kingdom

1. Introduction

Amyotrophic lateral sclerosis (ALS) is a devastating neurodegenerative disorder caused by the selective loss of motor neurones from the cortex, brainstem and spinal cord. For the patient, this results in a progressive loss of muscle function characterised by muscle weakness, atrophy and spasticity that develops into paralysis. Onset is typically in mid-life around ages 50-60 years, however there are juvenile forms with much earlier symptom onset (below 25 years). Disease duration is heterogeneous; however the majority of patients will only survive 2-3 years following initial symptom onset, with death generally resulting from respiratory muscle failure (Worms 2001).

A recent meta-analysis of population based studies revealed that 5% of ALS cases are familial (FALS) and the remaining 95% are sporadic (SALS) with no reported family history (Byrne et al 2011). There is a broad spectrum of inheritance for FALS ranging from fully penetrant, dominantly inherited Mendelian forms to recessive disease with weak penetrance affecting only a few family members (Simpson & Al-Chalabi 2006). The majority of familial cases are clinically and pathologically indistinguishable from sporadic cases, leading to the hypothesis that they share common pathogenic mechanisms. In addition, mutations in several of the FALS genes have also been identified in apparently sporadic disease, suggesting some degree of genetic overlap (Alexander et al 2002; Chio et al 2010; Kabashi et al 2008).

In ALS, cognitive impairment has been reported in up to 51% of cases, with frontotemporal dementia (FTD) present in up to 15% (Gordon et al 2011; Lillo et al 2011; Ringholz et al 2005). In approximately a third of cases, there is a family history of ALS or FTD or both in the family, and genes initially associated with either ALS or FTD are now being found to be associated with both disease phenotypes. This genetic link, in addition to extensive neuropathological evidence (Mackenzie et al 2010) has led to the widely accepted view that ALS and FTD form part of a spectrum of the same neurodegenerative disease process (Geser et al 2010).

2. Overview of genetics of ALS

The inheritance of FALS in many families is atypical with one proband and one or two first/second degree relatives who also have the disease (Valdmanis & Rouleau 2008). The first big breakthrough in the genetics of FALS came in 1993 with the discovery of pathological mutations in the Cu-Zn superoxide dismutase (*SOD1*) gene in ALS patients (Rosen et al 1993). Since then there has been an explosion of research into the mechanism(s) by which *SOD1* mutations cause ALS, however the answer remains elusive. There are now 16 genes associated with Mendelian forms of ALS (Table 1) which have mostly been identified using linkage analysis of rare families with large pedigrees affected by the disease (Lill et al 2011). More recently, studies to identify the proteins found in the ubiquitinated inclusions that are a common neuropathological feature of both ALS and FTD, have identified trans-activation response element (TAR) DNA binding protein of 43kDa (TDP-43) as the major component (Arai et al 2006; Neumann et al 2006). Mutations in the gene encoding TDP-43, *TARDBP*, were subsequently found as a genetic cause of ALS (Sreedharan et al 2008). The genetics of FALS has moved forward rapidly in recent years, providing invaluable insight into disease pathogenesis and allowing the development of animal models to further study the disease and efficacy of therapeutic compounds.

	Type	Locus	Reference
Autosomal Dominant Adult Onset			
Most common genetic causes			
SOD1	ALS1	21q22	(Rosen et al 1993)
TARDBP	ALS10	1p36.22	(Sreedharan et al 2008)
FUS	ALS6	16q12.1-2	(Abalkhail et al 2003)
Less frequent genetic causes			
VAPB	ALS8	20q13.3	(Nishimura et al 2004)
ANG	ALS9	14q11.2	(Greenway et al 2004)
FIG4	ALS11	6q21	(Chow et al 2009)
OPTN	ALS12	10p15-14	(Maruyama et al 2010)
DAO		12q22-23	(Mitchell et al 2010)
VCP		9p13.3	(Johnson et al 2010b)
Autosomal Dominant Juvenile Onset			
SETX	ALS4	9q34	(Chen et al 2004)
Autosomal Recessive			
ALS2	ALS2	2q33-35	(Hentati et al 1994)
ALS+FTD			
SIGMAR1		9p13.3	(Luty et al 2010)
MAPT		17q21	(Sundar et al 2007)
Genetic Loci Linked to Familial ALS			
SPG11	ALS5	15q15-22	(Orlacchio et al 2010)
Unknown	ALS7	20ptel-p13	(Sapp et al 2003)
Unknown	ALS3	18q21	(Hand et al 2002)
UBQLN2	ALSX	Xp11-q12	(Deng et al 2011)
C9ORF72	ALS-FTD1	9p21-q22	(Hosler et al 2000)
Unknown	ALS-FTD2	9p13.2-p21.3	(Vance et al 2006)

Table 1. Summary of the Genetic Causes of Familial ALS

3. Genetic causes of FALS

3.1 Most common genetic causes of autosomal dominant, adult onset ALS

The three most common genetic causes of FALS, together accounting for approximately 30% of cases are mutation of the *SOD1*, *TARDBP* and fused in sarcoma (*FUS*) genes.

3.1.1 ALS1: Cu-Zn superoxide dismutase 1 (*SOD1*)

The first genetic cause of familial ALS was identified by Rosen and colleagues (Rosen et al 1993) when, following analysis of FALS pedigrees demonstrating linkage to chromosome 21, mutations were identified in the *SOD1* gene. Since then, over 150 mutations have been described throughout the 5 exons encoding the gene consisting predominantly of missense mutations, although nonsense mutations, insertions and deletions have also been described (Lill et al 2011). The frequency of *SOD1* mutations is widely reported to be 20% of FALS cases, though this varies across European and North American populations, from 12% in Germany to 23.5% in USA (Andersen 2006). Whilst the majority of mutations are inherited in an autosomal dominant manner, in Scandinavia the p.D90A mutation is polymorphic, (0.5-5% of Scandinavian populations), with the disease manifesting only in individuals who are homozygous (Andersen et al 1995). However, this inheritance pattern is not attributable to the specific amino acid substitution, as p.D90A has been shown to be inherited as an autosomal dominant mutation in other populations. Mutations in *SOD1* have also been identified in sporadic ALS, albeit at lower frequencies, suggesting that some mutations have reduced penetrance. This has been shown in a family where the p.I113T mutation shows age-related penetrance (Lopate et al 2010).

Clinically, *SOD1* mutations are not associated with a distinctive phenotype. Individuals with *SOD1*-related ALS predominantly manifest with limb onset ALS, with symptoms more likely to start in the lower limbs (rather than upper limbs). However, bulbar onset is seen in approximately 7% of *SOD1*-related cases (ALSoD database: http:alsod.iop.kcl.ac.uk). Whilst duration of disease varies widely among *SOD1* mutations, even within members of the same family with the same mutation, the p.A4V mutation has been shown to be associated with a rapid disease progression and only 1-2 years survival (Andersen 2006). In contrast to the indistinguishable clinical phenotype, *SOD1*-related ALS cases appear to have a characteristic pathology distinguished by SOD1 positive, but TDP-43 negative, protein inclusions (Mackenzie et al 2007).

The mature SOD1 protein is a homodimer of 153 amino acid subunits. This free radical scavenging protein converts the superoxide anion to hydrogen peroxide; this in turn is converted to water and oxygen by glutathione peroxidise or catalase. Mutations in *SOD1* cause a toxic gain of function in the resulting mutant protein, though the mechanism(s) by which this brings about selective neurodegeneration of the motor neurones appears to be a complex interplay between multiple interacting pathomechanisms. The main hypotheses involve either an altered redox function or misfolding of the protein leading to aggregation (Rakhit & Chakrabartty 2006). Interestingly, not only have SOD1 positive aggregations been seen in SALS spinal cord, recent work has also shown that a conformation specific antibody raised against mutant SOD1 binds oxidised, but not normal, wild-type SOD1 in a subset of SALS cases thereby linking both *SOD1*-ALS and SALS (Bosco et al 2010).

Identification of *SOD1* led to the generation of many cellular and animal models which mirror aspects of the disease process and enable mechanistic insights and therapeutic approaches to be investigated. Current pathogenic mechanisms associated with mutant

SOD1 include oxidative stress, excitotoxicity, protein aggregation, mitochondrial dysfunction, endoplasmic reticulum stress, inflammatory cascades, involvement of non-neuronal cells and dysregulation of axonal transport. Each of these mechanisms has also been shown to play a role in SALS, demonstrating the relevance of the *SOD1* models to the disease as a whole (Ferraiuolo et al 2011). Therefore, although to date therapeutic agents which have shown promising results in the SOD1 transgenic mouse models have yet to show a beneficial effect in human trials (Benatar 2007), the generation and continued use of these models has greatly extended our knowledge of ALS.

3.1.2 ALS10: Transactive response (TAR) DNA binding protein (*TARDBP*)

The identification of TAR-DNA binding protein (TDP-43) as the major component of ubiquitinated cytoplasmic inclusions in ALS (and FTD) (Neumann et al 2006) led to the gene encoding this protein, *TARDBP*, to be screened in cohorts of FALS. Following the initial report of mutations being identified in exon 6 of the gene (Sreedharan et al 2008), a further 39 nucleotide substitutions have been published; the vast majority of which are in exon 6 and encode non-synonymous changes. The frequency is reported to be 4-5% of FALS cases (Kirby et al 2010; Mackenzie et al 2010), with mutations inherited in an autosomal dominant manner.

Clinically, *TARDBP*-related ALS presents as a classical adult-onset form of ALS; 73% of cases manifest with limb onset and there is a wide range in the age of onset (30-77 years) and disease duration, even in cases carrying the same mutation (e.g. p.M337V), (ALSoD database: http:alsod.iop.kcl.ac.uk). Perhaps the most distinctive feature commented upon, is the absence of dementia in these patients, despite several reports of *TARDBP* mutations in cases of FTD (Borroni et al 2009; Kovacs et al 2009). Neuropathologically, there is no distinction between *TARDBP*-related ALS and SALS cases, with both showing skein and compact ubiquitinated inclusions.

TARDBP encodes several isoforms of a predominantly nuclear protein, of which TDP-43 is the most prevalent. TDP-43 contains 2 RNA recognition motifs (RRM), a nuclear localisation and nuclear export signal, as well as a glycine-rich region in the C-terminus, which is encoded by exon 6. TDP-43 is involved in a variety of roles in the nucleus, including regulation of transcription, RNA splicing, microRNA (miRNA) processing and stabilisation of mRNA. Reports have recently identified RNA molecules which bind to TDP-43 in whole cell extracts using cross linking and immunoprecipitation (CLIP) methodologies (Polymenidou et al 2011; Sephton et al 2011; Tollervey et al 2011; Xiao et al 2011). This has established over 4000 TDP-43 binding targets, including ALS-related genes *FUS* and vasolin containing protein (*VCP*), as well as other RNA processing genes. One target which has been confirmed is the *TARDBP* mRNA. TDP-43 regulates its own transcription by binding to the 3'UTR region of the *TARDBP* mRNA and promoting mRNA instability (Budini & Buratti 2011). In addition, TDP-43 has been shown to interact with mutant, but not wild-type SOD1 mRNA, thereby linking the two distinct genetic pathogenic mechanisms (Higashi et al 2010). In ALS, both in *TARDBP*-related ALS and SALS, TDP-43 is seen to mislocalise to the cytoplasm and form either compact or skein like protein inclusions. It is currently unclear whether a loss of nuclear function or a gain of toxic function (or both) causes motor neuronal cell death. Numerous cellular and animal models for *TARDBP*-related ALS have been generated in multiple species, in order to investigate the mechanisms of TDP-43 associated neurodegeneration (Joyce et al 2011). What is evident from this body of work is that over-expression of not only mutant, but also wild-type *TARDBP* is toxic and that TDP-43 is essential for development, as knockout models show embryonic lethality.

3.1.3 ALS6: Fused in sarcoma (*FUS*)

Mutations in *FUS*, also referred to as translocated in sarcoma (*TLS*), were initially identified both through linkage analysis in a large Cape Verde pedigree manifesting with autosomal recessive ALS and in several autosomal dominant ALS families linked to chr16 (Kwiatkowski et al 2009; Vance et al 2009). Similarly to *TARDBP*, mutations in this second RNA binding protein gene are clustered, rather than spread across the 15 exons encoding FUS; a third occur in exons 5-6 encoding the glycine-rich region and two thirds in exon 13-14 encoding the arginine-glycine-glycine (RGG)-rich domain and the nuclear localisation signal. *FUS* mutations have been shown to account for a further 4-5% of FALS cases (Hewitt et al 2010; Mackenzie et al 2010).

Clinically, *FUS* mutations are associated with limb onset ALS; no bulbar onset cases with *FUS* mutations have been reported to date (ALSoD database: http:alsod.iop.kcl.ac.uk). There is a large range in the age of onset, from 26-80 years and as with *TARDBP* mutations, to date no correlations are evident between specific mutations and clinical characteristics. Pathologically, however, *FUS*-related cases have shown distinctive FUS-positive, TDP-43 negative inclusions. Specifically, those cases with basophilic inclusions and compact neuronal cytoplasmic FUS-positive inclusions had an earlier onset than those ALS cases with skein-like neuronal cytoplasmic inclusions, in whom glial cytoplasmic inclusions were also seen (Baumer et al 2010; Mackenzie et al 2011).

FUS is an RNA/DNA binding protein, which shuttles between the nucleus and cytoplasm. The 526 amino acid protein contains multiple protein domains, including a glutamine-glycine-serine-tyrosine rich domain at the N-terminus, involved in transcriptional activation of oncogenic fusion genes involving *FUS*, a glycine-rich region, a nuclear export signal, an RNA recognition motif and two arginine-glycine-glycine motifs flanking a zinc finger motif. At the C-terminus resides the nuclear localisation signal. Mutations within this region have been shown to disrupt transportin mediated transport of FUS into the nucleus, and cause the formation of FUS containing stress granules in the cytoplasm (Dormann et al 2010; Ito et al 2011a). In contrast, mutations in the glycine-rich region of FUS have yet to demonstrate pathogenicity. The normal function of FUS is poorly understood, though there is evidence for its involvement in alternative splicing, miRNA processing and transportation of mRNA to the dendrites for localised translation. Of the animal and cellular models generated to investigate the mechanisms of mutant FUS, a rat model over-expressing human p.R521C shows progressive paralysis, axonal degeneration and loss of neurones in 1-2 months old rats, whilst rats over-expressing wild-type FUS are pre-symptomatic at 1 year, though they do show learning and memory deficits and loss of cortical neurons (Huang et al 2011). Furthermore, drosophila and yeast models demonstrate FUS toxicity is due to accumulation of mutant protein in the cytoplasm (Kryndushkin et al 2011; Lanson et al 2011).

3.2 Rarer genetic causes of autosomal dominant, adult onset ALS

3.2.1 ALS8: Vesicle associated membrane protein (VAMP) associated protein B (*VAPB*)

ALS8 was first described in a large Brazilian kindred comprised of 28 Caucasian affected male and female family members distributed across four generations. Patients in this family had a characteristic clinical phenotype of a postural tremor, fasciculations and a slowly progressive upper and lower limb weakness with an unusually long duration. Linkage analysis revealed a unique locus at Chr20q13.33 and mutation screening revealed a heterozygous C>T nucleotide substitution, resulting in a p.P56S non-synonymous change within the highly conserved major sperm protein (MSP) domain of VAPB (Nishimura et al 2004).

This exon 2 variant has since been detected in 22 additional individuals from six Brazilian pedigrees in which there is evidence of a founder effect, although it has also been seen in a Japanese and European case (Funke et al 2010; Landers et al 2008; Millecamps et al 2010). The neurodegenerative phenotype associated with this mutation is variable; 3 of the families also had several confirmed cases of autosomal dominant adult onset spinal muscular atrophy (SMA). A second heterozygous point mutation (p.T46I) within the same domain of the VAPB peptide has recently been reported in a single Caucasian from the UK with classical ALS (Chen et al 2010).

VAPB is a type II integral endoplasmic reticulum (ER) membrane protein. It is involved in multiple cellular processes including intracellular trafficking, lipid transport, and the unfolded protein response (Lev et al 2008). Both mutations residing in the MSP domain result in conformational changes which lead to VAPB aggregation and an increase in ER stress (Chen et al 2010; Kim et al 2010; Suzuki et al 2009). Whilst mutations in *VAPB* are only found rarely in FALS patients, *VAPB* shows significantly decreased gene expression in SALS cases compared to age and gender matched neurologically normal controls (Anagnostou et al 2010; Mitne-Neto et al 2011).

3.2.2 ALS9: Angiogenin (*ANG*)

Chr14q11.2 was first proposed as a susceptibility locus for ALS following the strong allelic association in the Irish population with a single nucleotide polymorphism (SNP) (rs11701) residing in the single exon angiogenin (*ANG*) gene (Greenway et al 2004). Mutation screening analysis of a large cohort of Irish, Scottish, English, Swedish and North American ALS cases detected 7 missense mutations in 15 patients, 4 of whom were FALS (Greenway et al 2006). Additional screening of ALS cohorts report *ANG* mutations occurring in both FALS and SALS cases, though at low frequencies (Fernandez-Santiago et al 2009; Gellera et al 2008).

ANG is a member of the pancreatic ribonuclease A (RNaseA) superfamily whose activities are known to be important in protein translation, ribosome biogenesis and cell proliferation (Crabtree et al 2007). The ribonuclease A activity has been shown to be reduced or lost in ANG mutant proteins. ANG is a potent inducer of neovascularization *in vivo* and has been shown to play a key role in neurite outgrowth and pathfinding during early embryonic development (Subramanian et al 2008). Its structure and function are partially homologous to that of vascular endothelial cell growth factor (VEGF); a previously reported genetic susceptibility and disease modifying factor in the development of neurodegeneration (Lambrechts et al 2009), and both VEGF and ANG have been shown to be neuroprotective. A proposed mechanism by which ANG prevents cell death is through inhibiting the translocation of apoptosis inducing factor into the nucleus (Li et al 2011).

3.2.3 ALS11: Factor-induced gene 4 *S.cerevisiae* homolog (*FIG4*)

The Sac1 domain containing protein 3 (SAC3) *FIG4,* located on Chr6q21, was originally identified as the causative gene of Charcot Marie-Tooth disease type 4J (CMT4J); a severe autosomal recessive childhood disorder that is characterised by both sensory and motor deficits (Chow et al 2007). However, in one CMT4J pedigree there was a later onset of disease, with predominantly motor symptoms, similar to ALS (Zhang et al 2008). Screening of a North European cohort of FALS patients revealed 5 heterozygous mutations, resulting in either complete or significant loss of protein (Chow et al 2009). In general, cases of ALS11 are associated with a rapidly progressive disease course of approximately 1-2 years, early bulbar involvement and minimal cognitive dysfunction.

FIG4 encodes the phosphatidylinositol 3,5-bisphosphate 5-phosphatase which controls the cellular abundance of $PI(3,5)P_2$, a signalling lipid that mediates retrograde trafficking of endosomal vesicles to the Golgi apparatus (Michell & Dove 2009). It remains unclear as to whether the deleterious variants of *FIG4* exert an effect by a dominant negative mechanism or through a partial loss of function, as seen in CMT4J patients (Chow et al 2007). Human motor neurones are considered to be particularly susceptible to disruptions in this transport network because of their high membrane component turnover demands from long axonal processes over many decades (Ferguson et al 2010).

3.2.4 ALS12: Optineurin (*OPTN*)

Homozygosity mapping using 4 FALS cases demonstrated linkage to chr10p13 and subsequently mutations in *OPTN*, a gene previously linked to primary open-angle glaucoma (POAG), were identified in these cases (Maruyama et al 2010; Rezaie et al 2002). Mutations were initially found in both homozygous and heterozygous states. However, mutation screening of subsequent cohorts have identified only heterozygous mutations in ALS cases, occurring at a frequency of 3.4% in Japanese populations whilst this was at much lower frequencies in European and North American populations (Belzil et al 2011; Del Bo et al 2011). Interestingly, *OPTN*-related ALS is characterised by a lower limb onset with upper motor neurone involvement and a slow clinical progression.

The gene encodes the ubiquitously expressed optic neuropathy inducing protein which localises to the perinuclear region of the cytoplasm, where it is known to associate with the Golgi apparatus, and plays a key role in a number of biological processes, including vesicular trafficking, signal transduction and gene expression (Chalasani et al 2008). It is anticipated where mutations are inherited in an autosomal recessive manner, that reduced protein levels result in neurotoxicity through a loss of function mechanism. Conversely, the heterozygous missense substitution is predicted to exert a dominant negative effect. Examination of autopsy derived spinal cord tissue revealed extensive OPTN staining of TDP-43 positive intracytoplasmic hyaline inclusion bodies, although this was not replicated in a subsequent study (Hortobagyi et al 2011; Ito et al 2011b).

3.2.5 D-amino acid oxidase (*DAO*)

Following linkage analysis, a rare heterozygous missense mutation in the *DAO* gene, located on chr12q22-23, has been reported to segregate with disease in a single three generational Caucasian pedigree, though there was evidence of incomplete penetrance (Mitchell et al 2010). Those affected showed a rapidly progressive form of classical ALS with a mean disease duration of 21 months. Early bulbar involvement was apparent with limited signs of cognitive impairment. Interestingly, post-mortem immunohistochemical analysis on spinal cord tissue revealed no evidence of TDP-43 positively labelled inclusion bodies within the nuclear or cytoplasmic fractions of residual motor neurones which are normally a distinguishing feature of ALS pathology.

DAO encodes a universally expressed 39.4kDa peroxisomal flavin adenine dinucleotide (FAD)-dependent oxidase that is enriched in the neuronal and glial cell populations of the mammalian brainstem and spinal cord. The mutation results in the formation of an aberrant peptide product proposed to exert a dominant negative effect on the function of the wild type protein; *in vitro* work showed abnormal cellular morphology in cells over expressing the mutant protein, along with reduced cell viability, the presence of large intracellular ubiquitinated aggregates and an increased rate of apoptosis (Mitchell et al 2010).

3.2.6 Valosin containing protein (*VCP*)

Whole exome sequencing of two affected individuals in a large Italian pedigree identified a single heterozygous missense mutation in the *VCP* gene, located on chr9p13.3 (Johnson 2010). Screening of an additional cohort of ALS cases detected further *VCP* mutations at a frequency of 1.74%. There was no distinct phenotype associated with *VCP*-related ALS, with both limb and bulbar onset and an average age of onset of 49 years. Mutations in *VCP* have previously been linked to the autosomal dominant disorder inclusion body myopathy, Paget's disease and FTD (IBMPFD), which is characterised by muscle wasting, associated with osteolytic bone lesions and FTD (Watts et al 2004).

VCP is an evolutionarily conserved AAA+-ATPase that is known to be of importance in multiple biological processes including cell signalling, protein homeostasis, organelle biogenesis and autophagy (Ritson et al 2010), through its role in identifying ubiquitinated proteins in multimeric complexes and mediating their proteasomal degradation. It has been demonstrated both *in vitro* and *in vivo* that aberrant expression of VCP results in the cellular redistribution and mislocalisation of nuclear TDP-43 within the cytoplasm where neurotoxic ubiquitinated and phosphorylated aggregates form (Custer et al 2010; Gitcho et al 2009).

3.3 Genetic causes of autosomal dominant, juvenile onset ALS

3.3.1 ALS4: Senataxin (*SETX*)

The locus responsible for ALS4 was mapped to chr9q34 in an 11 generation pedigree affected by juvenile ALS and later confirmed by analysis of another two families with a similar phenotype (Chance et al 1998; De Jonghe et al 2002; Myrianthopoulos et al 1964). Sequence analysis of this region revealed disease associated mutations in the Senataxin (*SETX*) gene in all three affected families that were inherited in an autosomal dominant pattern (Chen et al 2004). *SETX* mutations are rare, with only four FALS families discovered to date, although mutations in this gene are also associated with ataxia-oculomotor apraxia-2 (AOA2), an autosomal recessive cerebellar ataxia (Anheim et al 2009). ALS4 is characterised by young onset (below the age of 25 years), distal muscle weakness and atrophy, pyramidal signs, an absence of sensory abnormalities while bulbar and respiratory muscles are spared. Disease progression is slow and patients have a normal life span (Chen et al 2004).

The *SETX* gene encodes a ubiquitously expressed DNA/RNA helicase that shares high homology to the yeast Sen1p protein and is suggested to play a role in DNA repair in response to oxidative stress (Suraweera et al 2007). SETX interacts with several RNA processing proteins, including RNA polymerase II, and is proposed to regulate transcription and pre-mRNA processing (Suraweera et al 2009).

3.4 Genetic causes of autosomal recessive ALS

3.4.1 ALS2: Alsin (*ALS2*)

Linkage analysis in a large, inbred Tunisian family mapped the gene responsible for an autosomal recessive form of ALS to chr2p33-q35 (Hentati et al 1994). Subsequent sequencing in this family, and a Saudi pedigree with juvenile primary lateral sclerosis (PLS), revealed mutations in the previously uncharacterised gene now known as *ALS2* (Yang et al 2001). Thus, mutations cause a spectrum of early onset motor neurone disorders including infantile ascending hereditary spastic paraplegia (IAHSP), PLS and ALS (Bertini et al 1993). To date, 19 *ALS2* mutations have been identified in ALS patients, which are characterised by a juvenile onset of limb and facial spasticity with subsequent lower motor neurone signs (Hentati et al 1994; Lill et al 2011). The milder phenotypes of PLS and IAHSP are characterised by isolated upper motor neurone degeneration without lower motor neurone signs (Bertini et al 1993).

The *ALS2* gene is ubiquitously expressed and encodes the Alsin protein which contains three putative guanine-exchange factor (GEF) domains that activate small GTPases (Yang et al 2001). Evidence suggests that loss of Alsin is responsible for motor neurone damage and several groups have now generated *ALS2* knock-out mouse models, but only mild neurological changes have been reported in these animals to date (Cai et al 2008). The pathological mechanism of *ALS2* mutations remains unknown although evidence that Alsin has a role in endosomal transport and glutamate receptor targeting at the synapse offer interesting avenues for further study (Devon et al 2006; Hadano et al 2006; Lai et al 2006).

3.5 Genetic causes of ALS+FTD

3.5.1 Sigma non-opioid intracellular receptor 1 (*SIGMAR1*)

Following linkage analysis of a large multigenerational pedigree to chr9p, mutation screening of 34 genes in the candidate region identified a nucleotide substitution in the 3'UTR of the SIGMAR1 gene which co-segregated with the disease (Luty et al 2010). Two further FALS cases were also identified with 3'UTR substitutions, yet none of the 3 changes were present in controls. Pathological material was available from 2 individuals carrying one of the changes and both TDP-43 and FUS positive inclusions were observed. The SIGMAR1 protein functions as a subunit of the ligand-regulated potassium channel and regulates channel activity (Aydar et al 2002). It was suggested that the 3'UTR alterations alter the stability of the transcript, though how this subsequently causes motor neuronal cell death, is unknown (Luty et al 2010).

3.5.2 Microtubule associated protein tau (*MAPT*)

Pedigrees with clinical features of FTD, ALS and Parkinsonism have been identified with pathogenic mutations in the microtubule associated protein tau (*MAPT*) gene located on chr17 (Hutton et al 1998). Over 40 mutations have been identified to date that either affect the normal function of the tau protein to stabilise microtubules or disrupt alternative splicing leading to changes in the ratio of tau isoforms (Seelaar et al 2011). Affected individuals have a variable age of onset (25-65 years) with disease duration of 3-10 years and usually show symptoms of executive dysfunction, altered personality and behaviour. Many develop a Parkinsonism phenotype and/or other clinical features of 1 or 2 syndromes that may reflect an expansion of affected brain regions over time. Cases affected by an ALS phenotype are rare and so far mutations in *MAPT* have not been described in pure FALS (Boeve & Hutton 2008).

3.6 Genetic loci linked to ALS

3.6.1 ALS5: Spatacsin (*SPG11*)

The study of three consanguineous Tunisian pedigrees originally established linkage of chr15q15-q21 to an autosomal recessive form of ALS (Hentati et al 1998). A more recent study of 25 unrelated FALS families revealed 10 pedigrees with linkage to the same region and disease associated mutations in the spatacsin (*SPG11)* gene (Orlacchio et al 2010). Clinically, FALS patients with linkage to this region experience a juvenile onset, slowly progressive motor neuropathy associated with both upper and lower motor neurone signs. Disease duration is typically over 10-40 years without sensory symptoms and an absence of the feature of thin corpus callosum (Hentati et al 1998; Orlacchio et al 2010).

Mutations in this gene have been previously found to be the most common cause of autosomal recessive hereditary spastic paraplegia with thin corpus callosum (HSP-TCC), a condition characterised by progressive spasticity of lower limbs, mild cognitive impairment and a thin, but otherwise normally structured, corpus callosum (Abdel Aleem et al 2011). All but one of the mutations identified in FALS are also present in HSP-TCC pedigrees and the majority of these are truncating which may suggest a loss of function and a common pathological mechanism between the two conditions (Salinas et al 2008). The *SPG11* gene has 40 exons and encodes the highly conserved Spatacsin protein, which is ubiquitously expressed in the central nervous system (Salinas et al 2008). Although the function of Spatacsin remains unknown, neuropathological studies of HSP-TCC patients with *SPG11* mutations have revealed accumulations of membranous material in non-myelinated axons which are suggestive of axonal transport disturbance (Hehr et al 2007).

3.6.2 ALS7

To date, only one pedigree with ALS7 and linkage to chr20ptel-p13 has been identified (Sapp et al 2003). The family included 15 siblings, two of which were affected by an autosomal dominantly inherited form of ALS with mid-life onset and a rapid disease course of less than 2 years. The authors found probable linkage to a 6.25cM region of chr20 though more individuals from this pedigree are needed to confirm the findings (Sapp et al 2003).

3.6.3 ALS3

One large European kindred affected by an adult onset, autosomal dominant form of ALS has been linked to chr18q21 (Hand et al 2002). Patients in this family present with classical ALS involving progressive weakness in the limbs and bulbar regions with both upper and lower motor neurone signs. A candidate region of 7.5cM was identified on chr18, however, the pathogenic mutation is not yet known (Hand et al 2002).

3.6.4 ALSX

Linkage analysis of a 5-generation pedigree identified an adult onset, dominantly inherited locus on Xp11-q12. The causative gene has very recently been found to be ubiquilin 2 (*UBQLN2*), which encodes a cytosolic ubiquitin-like protein (Deng et al 2011). Mutation screening of additional cohorts of patients found a further 4 missense mutations in unrelated FALS cases, with all mutations affecting proline amino acids in the proline-x-x repeat region near the carboxyl end of the protein. Clinically, age of onset was variable (16-71 years) in the affected individuals, and although males were more likely to have an earlier age of onset, disease duration was similar. Some patients also showed symptoms of dementia. Post-mortem material from two unrelated FALS cases showed the classical skein like inclusions were positive for UBQLN2. The identified missense mutations lead to impairment of the protein degradation pathway in a cell model of *UBQLN2*-related ALS.

3.6.5 ALS-FTD1: 9p21-q22

A locus for FALS that arises in conjunction with FTD has been identified in 5 American families at chr9p21-q22 (Hosler et al 2000). Affected patients had adult onset of either: ALS and FTD, ALS alone or ALS with dementia. Disease duration was typically less than 4 years although one individual had a slow progression and survived for 15 years. No pathogenic mutations have been identified for this region to date (Hosler et al 2000).

3.6.6 ALS-FTD2: 9p13.2-p21.3

Linkage of autosomal dominant FALS and FTD to chr9p13.2-p21.3 has been established in two pedigrees, one large Dutch kindred and a Scandinavian family (Morita et al 2006; Vance et al 2006). Clinically, all members with ALS had definite or probable ALS by the El-Escorial Criteria with mid-life onset and a typical disease course of around 3 years. In the Scandinavian family ALS and FTD occurred separately, in contrast, affected individuals in the Dutch kindred all had features of both conditions. Linkage has been narrowed down to a 12cM (11Mb) region of chr9, however the pathogenic gene mutations have yet to be identified (Morita et al 2006; Vance et al 2006).

4. Conclusion

FALS accounts for 5% of ALS; an underlying mutation has been identified in approximately a third of these cases (Kiernan et al 2011). FALS causing mutations are used as a window into familial and the clinically indistinguishable sporadic disease; generating genetic models of ALS allows investigations into the mechanisms of motor neuronal degeneration, the identification of therapeutic targets and screening for candidate therapeutic agents (Van Damme & Robberecht 2009). However, the discovery of pathogenic mutations in ALS by linkage analysis is difficult because a relatively low prevalence and rapid disease course make large pedigrees difficult to obtain, therefore novel strategies to identify pathogenic mutations are essential (Hand & Rouleau 2002).

With the evolution of next generation sequencing technology, exhaustive sequencing of exonic regions of the genome has been used to identify pathogenic mutations in the *VCP* gene in ALS, and genetic mutations responsible for other diseases have also been identified from relatively few related or unrelated patients (Bowne et al 2011; Hoischen et al 2010; Johnson et al 2010a; Ng et al 2010; Ng et al 2009; Nikopoulos et al 2010; Simpson et al 2011). Exome sequencing, unlike a linkage analysis and positional cloning approach, is not targeted at a candidate region. Therefore it is likely that a large number of potential genetic variations will be discovered; the difficulty then is to determine which, if any, are pathogenic. However, next generation sequencing offers the potential for identifying at least some of the genes responsible for the remaining uncharacterised causes of FALS.

An expanded GGGGCC hexanucleotide repeat in *C9ORF72* has just been published as the cause of 9p-linked ALS-FTD, following next generation sequencing of the disease associated region (Renton et al 2011, DeJesus-Hernandez et al 2011). Expansions have been identified not only in ALS-FTD pedigrees, but also in familial FTD, familial ALS and sporadic ALS. Estimated frequencies vary from 23.5% to 46.4% for familial ALS and 4.1% to 21% for sporadic ALS. The expansion, which is non-coding, is therefore the most common genetic cause of ALS identified to date.

5. Acknowledgments

PJS and JK are funded by the European Community's Health Seventh Framework Programme (FP7/2007-2013) under grant agreement 259867 and by the Motor Neurone Disease Association (MNDA). EFG is also funded by the MNDA.

6. References

Abalkhail H, Mitchell J, Habgood J, Orrell R, de Belleroche J. 2003. A new familial amyotrophic lateral sclerosis locus on chromosome 16q12.1-16q12.2. *Am J Hum Genet* 73:383-9

Abdel Aleem A, Abu-Shahba N, Swistun D, Silhavy J, Bielas SL, et al. 2011. Expanding the clinical spectrum of SPG11 gene mutations in recessive hereditary spastic paraplegia with thin corpus callosum. *European journal of medical genetics* 54:82-5

Alexander MD, Traynor BJ, Miller N, Corr B, Frost E, et al. 2002. "True" sporadic ALS associated with a novel SOD-1 mutation. *Ann Neurol* 52:680-3

Anagnostou G, Akbar MT, Paul P, Angelinetta C, Steiner TJ, de Belleroche J. 2010. Vesicle associated membrane protein B (VAPB) is decreased in ALS spinal cord. *Neurobiol Aging* 31:969-85

Andersen PM. 2006. Amyotrophic lateral sclerosis associated with mutations in the CuZn superoxide dismutase gene. *Curr Neurol Neurosci Rep* 6:37-46

Andersen PM, Nilsson P, Ala-Hurula V, Keranen ML, Tarvainen I, et al. 1995. Amyotrophic lateral sclerosis associated with homozygosity for an Asp90Ala mutation in CuZn-superoxide dismutase. *Nat Genet* 10:61-6

Anheim M, Monga B, Fleury M, Charles P, Barbot C, et al. 2009. Ataxia with oculomotor apraxia type 2: clinical, biological and genotype/phenotype correlation study of a cohort of 90 patients. *Brain : a journal of neurology* 132:2688-98

Arai T, Hasegawa M, Akiyama H, Ikeda K, Nonaka T, et al. 2006. TDP-43 is a component of ubiquitin-positive tau-negative inclusions in frontotemporal lobar degeneration and amyotrophic lateral sclerosis. *Biochem Biophys Res Commun* 351:602-11

Aydar E, Palmer CP, Klyachko VA, Jackson MB. 2002. The sigma receptor as a ligand-regulated auxiliary potassium channel subunit. *Neuron* 34:399-410

Baumer D, Hilton D, Paine SM, Turner MR, Lowe J, et al. 2010. Juvenile ALS with basophilic inclusions is a FUS proteinopathy with FUS mutations. *Neurology* 75:611-8

Belzil VV, Daoud H, Desjarlais A, Bouchard JP, Dupre N, et al. 2011. Analysis of OPTN as a causative gene for amyotrophic lateral sclerosis. *Neurobiology of aging* 32:555 e13-4

Benatar M. 2007. Lost in translation: treatment trials in the SOD1 mouse and in human ALS. *Neurobiol Dis* 26:1-13

Bertini ES, Eymard-Pierre E, Boespflug-Tanguy O, Cleveland DW, Yamanaka K. 1993. In *GeneReviews*, ed. RA Pagon, TD Bird, CR Dolan, K Stephens. Seattle (WA)

Boeve BF, Hutton M. 2008. Refining frontotemporal dementia with parkinsonism linked to chromosome 17: introducing FTDP-17 (MAPT) and FTDP-17 (PGRN). *Arch Neurol* 65:460-4

Borroni B, Bonvicini C, Alberici A, Buratti E, Agosti C, et al. 2009. Mutation within TARDBP leads to frontotemporal dementia without motor neuron disease. *Hum Mutat* 30:E974-83

Bosco DA, Morfini G, Karabacak NM, Song Y, Gros-Louis F, et al. 2010. Wild-type and mutant SOD1 share an aberrant conformation and a common pathogenic pathway in ALS. *Nat Neurosci* 13:1396-403

Bowne SJ, Sullivan LS, Koboldt DC, Ding L, Fulton R, et al. 2011. Identification of Disease-Causing Mutations in Autosomal Dominant Retinitis Pigmentosa (adRP) Using Next-Generation DNA Sequencing. *Investigative Ophthalmology & Visual Science* 52:494-503

Budini M, Buratti E. 2011. TDP-43 Autoregulation: Implications for Disease. *J Mol Neurosci*

Byrne S, Walsh C, Lynch C, Bede P, Elamin M, et al. 2011. Rate of familial amyotrophic lateral sclerosis: a systematic review and meta-analysis. *J Neurol Neurosurg Psychiatry* 82:623-7

Cai H, Shim H, Lai C, Xie C, Lin X, et al. 2008. ALS2/alsin knockout mice and motor neuron diseases. *Neuro-degenerative diseases* 5:359-66

Chalasani ML, Balasubramanian D, Swarup G. 2008. Focus on molecules: optineurin. *Exp Eye Res* 87:1-2

Chance PF, Rabin BA, Ryan SG, Ding Y, Scavina M, et al. 1998. Linkage of the gene for an autosomal dominant form of juvenile amyotrophic lateral sclerosis to chromosome 9q34. *American journal of human genetics* 62:633-40

Chen HJ, Anagnostou G, Chai A, Withers J, Morris A, et al. 2010. Characterization of the properties of a novel mutation in VAPB in familial amyotrophic lateral sclerosis. *J Biol Chem* 285:40266-81

Chen YZ, Bennett CL, Huynh HM, Blair IP, Puls I, et al. 2004. DNA/RNA helicase gene mutations in a form of juvenile amyotrophic lateral sclerosis (ALS4). *American journal of human genetics* 74:1128-35

Chio A, Calvo A, Moglia C, Ossola I, Brunetti M, et al. 2010. A de novo missense mutation of the FUS gene in a "true" sporadic ALS case. *Neurobiology of aging*

Chow CY, Landers JE, Bergren SK, Sapp PC, Grant AE, et al. 2009. Deleterious variants of FIG4, a phosphoinositide phosphatase, in patients with ALS. *Am J Hum Genet* 84:85-8

Chow CY, Zhang Y, Dowling JJ, Jin N, Adamska M, et al. 2007. Mutation of FIG4 causes neurodegeneration in the pale tremor mouse and patients with CMT4J. *Nature* 448:68-72

Crabtree B, Thiyagarajan N, Prior SH, Wilson P, Iyer S, et al. 2007. Characterization of human angiogenin variants implicated in amyotrophic lateral sclerosis. *Biochemistry* 46:11810-8

Custer SK, Neumann M, Lu H, Wright AC, Taylor JP. 2010. Transgenic mice expressing mutant forms VCP/p97 recapitulate the full spectrum of IBMPFD including degeneration in muscle, brain and bone. *Hum Mol Genet* 19:1741-55

De Jonghe P, Auer-Grumbach M, Irobi J, Wagner K, Plecko B, et al. 2002. Autosomal dominant juvenile amyotrophic lateral sclerosis and distal hereditary motor neuronopathy with pyramidal tract signs: synonyms for the same disorder? *Brain : a journal of neurology* 125:1320-5

Del Bo R, Tiloca C, Pensato V, Corrado L, Ratti A, et al. 2011. Novel optineurin mutations in patients with familial and sporadic amyotrophic lateral sclerosis. *J Neurol Neurosurg Psychiatry*

Deng HX, Chen W, Hong ST, Boycott KM, Gorrie GH, et al. 2011. Mutations in UBQLN2 cause dominant X-linked juvenile and adult-onset ALS and ALS/dementia. *Nature*

DeJesus-Hernandez M, Mackenzie IR, Boeve BF, Boxer AL, Baker M, et al. 2011. Expanded GGGGCC Hexanucleotide Repeat in Noncoding Region of C9ORF72 Causes Chromosome 9p-Linked FTD and ALS. *Neuron*

Devon RS, Orban PC, Gerrow K, Barbieri MA, Schwab C, et al. 2006. Als2-deficient mice exhibit disturbances in endosome trafficking associated with motor behavioral abnormalities. *Proceedings of the National Academy of Sciences of the United States of America* 103:9595-600

Dormann D, Rodde R, Edbauer D, Bentmann E, Fischer I, et al. 2010. ALS-associated fused in sarcoma (FUS) mutations disrupt Transportin-mediated nuclear import. *Embo J* 29:2841-57

Ferguson CJ, Lenk GM, Meisler MH. 2010. PtdIns(3,5)P2 and autophagy in mouse models of neurodegeneration. *Autophagy* 6:170-1

Fernandez-Santiago R, Hoenig S, Lichtner P, Sperfeld AD, Sharma M, et al. 2009. Identification of novel Angiogenin (ANG) gene missense variants in German patients with amyotrophic lateral sclerosis. *J Neurol* 256:1337-42

Ferraiuolo L, Kirby J, Grierson AJ, Sendtner M, Shaw PJ. 2011. Molecular and cellular pathways of motor neuron injury in amyotrophic lateral sclerosis. *Nat Rev Neurology* (In Press)

Funke AD, Esser M, Kruttgen A, Weis J, Mitne-Neto M, et al. 2010. The p.P56S mutation in the VAPB gene is not due to a single founder: the first European case. *Clin Genet* 77:302-3

Gellera C, Colombrita C, Ticozzi N, Castellotti B, Bragato C, et al. 2008. Identification of new ANG gene mutations in a large cohort of Italian patients with amyotrophic lateral sclerosis. *Neurogenetics* 9:33-40

Geser F, Lee VM, Trojanowski JQ. 2010. Amyotrophic lateral sclerosis and frontotemporal lobar degeneration: a spectrum of TDP-43 proteinopathies. *Neuropathology* 30:103-12

Gitcho MA, Strider J, Carter D, Taylor-Reinwald L, Forman MS, et al. 2009. VCP mutations causing frontotemporal lobar degeneration disrupt localization of TDP-43 and induce cell death. *J Biol Chem* 284:12384-98

Gordon PH, Delgadillo D, Piquard A, Bruneteau G, Pradat PF, et al. 2011. The range and clinical impact of cognitive impairment in French patients with ALS: A cross-sectional study of neuropsychological test performance. *Amyotroph Lateral Scler*

Greenway MJ, Alexander MD, Ennis S, Traynor BJ, Corr B, et al. 2004. A novel candidate region for ALS on chromosome 14q11.2. *Neurology* 63:1936-8

Greenway MJ, Andersen PM, Russ C, Ennis S, Cashman S, et al. 2006. ANG mutations segregate with familial and 'sporadic' amyotrophic lateral sclerosis. *Nat Genet* 38:411-3

Hadano S, Benn SC, Kakuta S, Otomo A, Sudo K, et al. 2006. Mice deficient in the Rab5 guanine nucleotide exchange factor ALS2/alsin exhibit age-dependent neurological deficits and altered endosome trafficking. *Human molecular genetics* 15:233-50

Hand CK, Khoris J, Salachas F, Gros-Louis F, Lopes AA, et al. 2002. A novel locus for familial amyotrophic lateral sclerosis, on chromosome 18q. *Am J Hum Genet* 70:251-6

Hand CK, Rouleau GA. 2002. Familial amyotrophic lateral sclerosis. *Muscle & Nerve* 25:135-59

Hehr U, Bauer P, Winner B, Schule R, Olmez A, et al. 2007. Long-term course and mutational spectrum of spatacsin-linked spastic paraplegia. *Ann Neurol* 62:656-65

Hentati A, Bejaoui K, Pericak-Vance MA, Hentati F, Speer MC, et al. 1994. Linkage of recessive familial amyotrophic lateral sclerosis to chromosome 2q33-q35. *Nature genetics* 7:425-8

Hentati A, Ouahchi K, Pericak-Vance MA, Nijhawan D, Ahmad A, et al. 1998. Linkage of a commoner form of recessive amyotrophic lateral sclerosis to chromosome 15q15-q22 markers. *Neurogenetics* 2:55-60

Hewitt C, Kirby J, Highley JR, Hartley JA, Hibberd R, et al. 2010. Novel FUS/TLS mutations and pathology in familial and sporadic amyotrophic lateral sclerosis. *Arch Neurol* 67:455-61

Higashi S, Tsuchiya Y, Araki T, Wada K, Kabuta T. 2010. TDP-43 physically interacts with amyotrophic lateral sclerosis-linked mutant CuZn superoxide dismutase. *Neurochem Int* 57:906-13

Hoischen A, van Bon BWM, Gilissen C, Arts P, van Lier B, et al. 2010. De novo mutations of SETBP1 cause Schinzel-Giedion syndrome. *Nat Genet* 42:483-5

Hortobagyi T, Troakes C, Nishimura AL, Vance C, van Swieten JC, et al. 2011. Optineurin inclusions occur in a minority of TDP-43 positive ALS and FTLD-TDP cases and are rarely observed in other neurodegenerative disorders. *Acta Neuropathol* 121:519-27

Hosler BA, Siddique T, Sapp PC, Sailor W, Huang MC, et al. 2000. Linkage of familial amyotrophic lateral sclerosis with frontotemporal dementia to chromosome 9q21-q22. *JAMA : the journal of the American Medical Association* 284:1664-9

Huang C, Zhou H, Tong J, Chen H, Liu YJ, et al. 2011. FUS transgenic rats develop the phenotypes of amyotrophic lateral sclerosis and frontotemporal lobar degeneration. *PLoS genetics* 7:e1002011

Hutton M, Lendon CL, Rizzu P, Baker M, Froelich S, et al. 1998. Association of missense and 5'-splice-site mutations in tau with the inherited dementia FTDP-17. *Nature* 393:702-5

Ito D, Seki M, Tsunoda Y, Uchiyama H, Suzuki N. 2011a. Nuclear transport impairment of amyotrophic lateral sclerosis-linked mutations in FUS/TLS. *Ann Neurol* 69:152-62

Ito H, Nakamura M, Komure O, Ayaki T, Wate R, et al. 2011b. Clinicopathologic study on an ALS family with a heterozygous E478G optineurin mutation. *Acta Neuropathol*

Johnson JO, Mandrioli J, Benatar M, Abramzon Y, Van Deerlin VM, et al. 2010a. Exome Sequencing Reveals VCP Mutations as a Cause of Familial ALS. *Neuron* 68:857-64

Johnson JO, Mandrioli J, Benatar M, Abramzon Y, Van Deerlin VM, et al. 2010b. Exome sequencing reveals VCP mutations as a cause of familial ALS. *Neuron* 68:857-64

Joyce PI, Fratta P, Fisher EM, Acevedo-Arozena A. 2011. SOD1 and TDP-43 animal models of amyotrophic lateral sclerosis: recent advances in understanding disease toward the development of clinical treatments. *Mamm Genome*

Kabashi E, Valdmanis PN, Dion P, Spiegelman D, McConkey BJ, et al. 2008. TARDBP mutations in individuals with sporadic and familial amyotrophic lateral sclerosis. *Nat Genet* 40:572-4

Kiernan MC, Vucic S, Cheah BC, Turner MR, Eisen A, et al. 2011. Amyotrophic lateral sclerosis. *The Lancet* 377:942-55

Kim S, Leal SS, Ben Halevy D, Gomes CM, Lev S. 2010. Structural requirements for VAP-B oligomerization and their implication in amyotrophic lateral sclerosis-associated VAP-B(P56S) neurotoxicity. *J Biol Chem* 285:13839-49

Kirby J, Goodall EF, Smith W, Highley JR, Masanzu R, et al. 2010. Broad clinical phenotypes associated with TAR-DNA binding protein (TARDBP) mutations in amyotrophic lateral sclerosis. *Neurogenetics* 11:217-25

Kovacs GG, Murrell JR, Horvath S, Haraszti L, Majtenyi K, et al. 2009. TARDBP variation associated with frontotemporal dementia, supranuclear gaze palsy, and chorea. *Mov Disord* 24:1843-7

Kryndushkin D, Wickner RB, Shewmaker F. 2011. FUS/TLS forms cytoplasmic aggregates, inhibits cell growth and interacts with TDP-43 in a yeast model of amyotrophic lateral sclerosis. *Protein Cell* 2:223-36

Kwiatkowski TJ, Jr., Bosco DA, Leclerc AL, Tamrazian E, Vanderburg CR, et al. 2009. Mutations in the FUS/TLS gene on chromosome 16 cause familial amyotrophic lateral sclerosis. *Science* 323:1205-8

Lai C, Xie C, McCormack SG, Chiang HC, Michalak MK, et al. 2006. Amyotrophic lateral sclerosis 2-deficiency leads to neuronal degeneration in amyotrophic lateral sclerosis through altered AMPA receptor trafficking. *The Journal of neuroscience : the official journal of the Society for Neuroscience* 26:11798-806

Lambrechts D, Poesen K, Fernandez-Santiago R, Al-Chalabi A, Del Bo R, et al. 2009. Meta-analysis of vascular endothelial growth factor variations in amyotrophic lateral sclerosis: increased susceptibility in male carriers of the -2578AA genotype. *J Med Genet* 46:840-6

Landers JE, Leclerc AL, Shi L, Virkud A, Cho T, et al. 2008. New VAPB deletion variant and exclusion of VAPB mutations in familial ALS. *Neurology* 70:1179-85

Lanson NA, Jr., Maltare A, King H, Smith R, Kim JH, et al. 2011. A Drosophila model of FUS-related neurodegeneration reveals genetic interaction between FUS and TDP-43. *Hum Mol Genet* 20:2510-23

Lev S, Ben Halevy D, Peretti D, Dahan N. 2008. The VAP protein family: from cellular functions to motor neuron disease. *Trends Cell Biol* 18:282-90

Li S, Yu W, Hu GF. 2011. Angiogenin inhibits nuclear translocation of apoptosis inducing factor in a Bcl-2-dependent manner. *J Cell Physiol*

Lill CM, Abel O, Bertram L, Al-Chalabi A. 2011. Keeping up with genetic discoveries in amyotrophic lateral sclerosis: The ALSoD and ALSGene databases. *Amyotrophic lateral sclerosis : official publication of the World Federation of Neurology Research Group on Motor Neuron Diseases* 12:238-49

Lillo P, Mioshi E, Zoing MC, Kiernan MC, Hodges JR. 2011. How common are behavioural changes in amyotrophic lateral sclerosis? *Amyotroph Lateral Scler* 12:45-51

Lopate G, Baloh RH, Al-Lozi MT, Miller TM, Fernandes Filho JA, et al. 2010. Familial ALS with extreme phenotypic variability due to the I113T SOD1 mutation. *Amyotroph Lateral Scler* 11:232-6

Luty AA, Kwok JB, Dobson-Stone C, Loy CT, Coupland KG, et al. 2010. Sigma nonopioid intracellular receptor 1 mutations cause frontotemporal lobar degeneration-motor neuron disease. *Ann Neurol* 68:639-49

Mackenzie IR, Ansorge O, Strong M, Bilbao J, Zinman L, et al. 2011. Pathological heterogeneity in amyotrophic lateral sclerosis with FUS mutations: two distinct patterns correlating with disease severity and mutation. *Acta Neuropathol* 122:87-98

Mackenzie IR, Bigio EH, Ince PG, Geser F, Neumann M, et al. 2007. Pathological TDP-43 distinguishes sporadic amyotrophic lateral sclerosis from amyotrophic lateral sclerosis with SOD1 mutations. *Ann Neurol* 61:427-34

Mackenzie IR, Rademakers R, Neumann M. 2010. TDP-43 and FUS in amyotrophic lateral sclerosis and frontotemporal dementia. *Lancet Neurol* 9:995-1007

Maruyama H, Morino H, Ito H, Izumi Y, Kato H, et al. 2010. Mutations of optineurin in amyotrophic lateral sclerosis. *Nature* 465:223-6

Michell RH, Dove SK. 2009. A protein complex that regulates PtdIns(3,5)P2 levels. *EMBO J* 28:86-7

Millecamps S, Salachas F, Cazeneuve C, Gordon P, Bricka B, et al. 2010. SOD1, ANG, VAPB, TARDBP, and FUS mutations in familial amyotrophic lateral sclerosis: genotype-phenotype correlations. *J Med Genet* 47:554-60

Mitchell J, Paul P, Chen HJ, Morris A, Payling M, et al. 2010. Familial amyotrophic lateral sclerosis is associated with a mutation in D-amino acid oxidase. *Proc Natl Acad Sci U S A* 107:7556-61

Mitne-Neto M, Machado-Costa M, Marchetto MC, Bengtson MH, Joazeiro CA, et al. 2011. Downregulation of VAPB expression in motor neurons derived from induced pluripotent stem cells of ALS8 patients. *Hum Mol Genet*

Morita M, Al-Chalabi A, Andersen PM, Hosler B, Sapp P, et al. 2006. A locus on chromosome 9p confers susceptibility to ALS and frontotemporal dementia. *Neurology* 66:839-44

Myrianthopoulos NC, Lane MH, Silberberg DH, Vincent BL. 1964. Nerve Conduction and Other Studies in Families with Charcot-Marie-Tooth Disease. *Brain : a journal of neurology* 87:589-608

Neumann M, Sampathu DM, Kwong LK, Truax AC, Micsenyi MC, et al. 2006. Ubiquitinated TDP-43 in frontotemporal lobar degeneration and amyotrophic lateral sclerosis. *Science* 314:130-3

Ng SB, Bigham AW, Buckingham KJ, Hannibal MC, McMillin MJ, et al. 2010. Exome sequencing identifies MLL2 mutations as a cause of Kabuki syndrome. *Nat Genet* 42:790-3

Ng SB, Turner EH, Robertson PD, Flygare SD, Bigham AW, et al. 2009. Targeted capture and massively parallel sequencing of 12 human exomes. *Nature* 461:272-6

Nikopoulos K, Gilissen C, Hoischen A, Erik van Nouhuys C, Boonstra FN, et al. 2010. Next-Generation Sequencing of a 40 Mb Linkage Interval Reveals TSPAN12 Mutations in Patients with Familial Exudative Vitreoretinopathy. *The American Journal of Human Genetics* 86:240-7

Nishimura AL, Mitne-Neto M, Silva HC, Richieri-Costa A, Middleton S, et al. 2004. A mutation in the vesicle-trafficking protein VAPB causes late-onset spinal muscular atrophy and amyotrophic lateral sclerosis. *Am J Hum Genet* 75:822-31

Orlacchio A, Babalini C, Borreca A, Patrono C, Massa R, et al. 2010. SPATACSIN mutations cause autosomal recessive juvenile amyotrophic lateral sclerosis. *Brain : a journal of neurology* 133:591-8

Polymenidou M, Lagier-Tourenne C, Hutt KR, Huelga SC, Moran J, et al. 2011. Long pre-mRNA depletion and RNA missplicing contribute to neuronal vulnerability from loss of TDP-43. *Nat Neurosci* 14:459-68

Rakhit R, Chakrabartty A. 2006. Structure, folding, and misfolding of Cu,Zn superoxide dismutase in amyotrophic lateral sclerosis. *Biochim Biophys Acta* 1762:1025-37

Renton AE, Majounie E, Waite A, Simon-Sanchez J, Rollinson S, et al. 2011. A Hexanucleotide Repeat Expansion in C9ORF72 Is the Cause of Chromosome 9p21-Linked ALS-FTD. *Neuron*

Rezaie T, Child A, Hitchings R, Brice G, Miller L, et al. 2002. Adult-onset primary open-angle glaucoma caused by mutations in optineurin. *Science* 295:1077-9

Ringholz GM, Appel SH, Bradshaw M, Cooke NA, Mosnik DM, Schulz PE. 2005. Prevalence and patterns of cognitive impairment in sporadic ALS. *Neurology* 65:586-90

Ritson GP, Custer SK, Freibaum BD, Guinto JB, Geffel D, et al. 2010. TDP-43 mediates degeneration in a novel Drosophila model of disease caused by mutations in VCP/p97. *J Neurosci* 30:7729-39

Rosen DR, Siddique T, Patterson D, Figlewicz DA, Sapp P, et al. 1993. Mutations in Cu/Zn superoxide dismutase gene are associated with familial amyotrophic lateral sclerosis. *Nature* 362:59-62

Salinas S, Proukakis C, Crosby A, Warner TT. 2008. Hereditary spastic paraplegia: clinical features and pathogenetic mechanisms. *Lancet Neurol* 7:1127-38

Sapp PC, Hosler BA, McKenna-Yasek D, Chin W, Gann A, et al. 2003. Identification of two novel loci for dominantly inherited familial amyotrophic lateral sclerosis. *American journal of human genetics* 73:397-403

Seelaar H, Rohrer JD, Pijnenburg YA, Fox NC, van Swieten JC. 2011. Clinical, genetic and pathological heterogeneity of frontotemporal dementia: a review. *J Neurol Neurosurg Psychiatry* 82:476-86

Sephton CF, Cenik C, Kucukural A, Dammer EB, Cenik B, et al. 2011. Identification of neuronal RNA targets of TDP-43-containing ribonucleoprotein complexes. *J Biol Chem* 286:1204-15

Simpson CL, Al-Chalabi A. 2006. Amyotrophic lateral sclerosis as a complex genetic disease. *Biochimica et biophysica acta* 1762:973-85

Simpson MA, Irving MD, Asilmaz E, Gray MJ, Dafou D, et al. 2011. Mutations in NOTCH2 cause Hajdu-Cheney syndrome, a disorder of severe and progressive bone loss. *Nat Genet* 43:303-5

Sreedharan J, Blair IP, Tripathi VB, Hu X, Vance C, et al. 2008. TDP-43 mutations in familial and sporadic amyotrophic lateral sclerosis. *Science* 319:1668-72

Subramanian V, Crabtree B, Acharya KR. 2008. Human angiogenin is a neuroprotective factor and amyotrophic lateral sclerosis associated angiogenin variants affect neurite extension/pathfinding and survival of motor neurons. *Hum Mol Genet* 17:130-49

Sundar PD, Yu CE, Sieh W, Steinbart E, Garruto RM, et al. 2007. Two sites in the MAPT region confer genetic risk for Guam ALS/PDC and dementia. *Hum Mol Genet* 16:295-306

Suraweera A, Becherel OJ, Chen P, Rundle N, Woods R, et al. 2007. Senataxin, defective in ataxia oculomotor apraxia type 2, is involved in the defense against oxidative DNA damage. *The Journal of cell biology* 177:969-79

Suraweera A, Lim Y, Woods R, Birrell GW, Nasim T, et al. 2009. Functional role for senataxin, defective in ataxia oculomotor apraxia type 2, in transcriptional regulation. *Human molecular genetics* 18:3384-96

Suzuki H, Kanekura K, Levine TP, Kohno K, Olkkonen VM, et al. 2009. ALS-linked P56S-VAPB, an aggregated loss-of-function mutant of VAPB, predisposes motor neurons to ER stress-related death by inducing aggregation of co-expressed wild-type VAPB. *J Neurochem* 108:973-85

Tollervey JR, Curk T, Rogelj B, Briese M, Cereda M, et al. 2011. Characterizing the RNA targets and position-dependent splicing regulation by TDP-43. *Nat Neurosci* 14:452-8

Valdmanis PN, Rouleau GA. 2008. Genetics of familial amyotrophic lateral sclerosis. *Neurology* 70:144-52

Van Damme P, Robberecht W. 2009. Recent advances in motor neuron disease. *Current Opinion in Neurology* 22:486-92 10.1097/WCO.0b013e32832ffbe3

Vance C, Al-Chalabi A, Ruddy D, Smith BN, Hu X, et al. 2006. Familial amyotrophic lateral sclerosis with frontotemporal dementia is linked to a locus on chromosome 9p13.2-21.3. *Brain* 129:868-76

Vance C, Rogelj B, Hortobagyi T, De Vos KJ, Nishimura AL, et al. 2009. Mutations in FUS, an RNA processing protein, cause familial amyotrophic lateral sclerosis type 6. *Science* 323:1208-11

Watts GD, Wymer J, Kovach MJ, Mehta SG, Mumm S, et al. 2004. Inclusion body myopathy associated with Paget disease of bone and frontotemporal dementia is caused by mutant valosin-containing protein. *Nat Genet* 36:377-81

Worms PM. 2001. The epidemiology of motor neuron diseases: a review of recent studies. *J Neurol Sci* 191:3-9

Xiao S, Sanelli T, Dib S, Sheps D, Findlater J, et al. 2011. RNA targets of TDP-43 identified by UV-CLIP are deregulated in ALS. *Mol Cell Neurosci* 47:167-80

Yang Y, Hentati A, Deng HX, Dabbagh O, Sasaki T, et al. 2001. The gene encoding alsin, a protein with three guanine-nucleotide exchange factor domains, is mutated in a form of recessive amyotrophic lateral sclerosis. *Nature genetics* 29:160-5

Zhang X, Chow CY, Sahenk Z, Shy ME, Meisler MH, Li J. 2008. Mutation of FIG4 causes a rapidly progressive, asymmetric neuronal degeneration. *Brain* 131:1990-2001

23

A Major Genetic Factor at Chromosome 9p Implicated in Amyotrophic Lateral Sclerosis (ALS) and Frontotemporal Lobar Degeneration (FTLD)

Ilse Gijselinck[1,2], Kristel Sleegers[1,2],
Christine Van Broeckhoven[1,2] and Marc Cruts[1,2]
[1]*Department of Molecular Genetics, VIB, Antwerpen*
[2]*University of Antwerp, Antwerpen*
Belgium

1. Introduction

Amyotrophic lateral sclerosis (ALS) and frontotemporal lobar degeneration (FTLD) are two fatal neurodegenerative diseases for which effective therapies aiming at delaying, halting or preventing the disease are lacking. ALS is the most common motor neuron disorder (Rowland & Shneider, 2001) and FTLD has a prevalence close to that of Alzheimer disease in the population below age 65 years (Rosso et al., 2003). They are considered as both extremes of a spectrum of clinically and pathologically overlapping disorders (Lillo & Hodges, 2009). In addition, there is emerging evidence that FTLD and ALS also share common genetic aetiologies, suggesting that overlapping disease mechanisms are involved in both diseases. Clinically, ALS patients show reduced control of voluntary muscle movement expressed in increased muscle weakness, disturbances of speech, swallowing or breathing, as a result of progressive upper and lower motor neuron degeneration in motor cortex, brainstem and spinal cord, and up to 50% of ALS patients shows mild disturbances in executive functions while a minority also develop overt FTLD (Lomen-Hoerth et al., 2003; Ringholz et al., 2005). FTLD symptoms include behavioural, personality and language disturbances, and also cognitive dysfunctions, due to affected frontal and temporal cortical neurons in the brain. FTLD patients may additionally present with typical clinical signs of ALS in a later stage of the disease (Neary et al., 1998). Pathologically, although in different neuronal cells, TAR DNA-binding protein-43 (TDP-43) is a major constituent of neuronal deposits in both ALS and TDP-43 positive FTLD (FTLD-TDP), the most common pathological FTLD subtype (Arai et al., 2006; Neumann et al., 2006). Five to 10% of ALS patients and up to 50% of FTLD patients has a positive familial history of disease with a Mendelian mode of inheritance indicating a significant contribution of genetic factors in disease aetiology. Although the exact biochemical pathways involved in ALS or FTLD are still unknown, several molecular components were identified in the last twenty years through molecular genetic studies in familial and sporadic patients, which are most likely part of a complex network of cellular mechanisms. Since these genes explain only a minority of patients, further unraveling the genetic heterogeneity is necessary to identify new therapeutic targets. Mutations causing ALS were observed in genes encoding Cu/Zn superoxide dismutase 1 (*SOD1*) (Rosen et al., 1993), TDP-43 (*TARDBP*) (Gitcho et al., 2008; Kabashi et al., 2008; Sreedharan et al., 2008; Van Deerlin et al., 2008; Yokoseki et al., 2008), fused in sarcoma (*FUS*) (Kwiatkowski, Jr. et al., 2009; Vance et al., 2009) and angiogenin (*ANG*) (Greenway et al., 2006), among other genes, while in familial FTLD patients mutations in the genes encoding granulin (*GRN*) (Baker et al., 2006; Cruts et al., 2006), the microtubule-associated protein tau (*MAPT*) (Hutton et al., 1998), the valosin-containing protein (*VCP*) (Watts et al., 2004) and the charged multivesicular body protein 2B (*CHMP2B*) (Skibinski et al., 2005) were found. Recent family-based linkage and population-based association studies identified genetic factors overlapping between ALS and FTLD. For example, mutations in the ALS genes *TARDBP* and *FUS* are occasionally found in FTLD patients (Kovacs et al., 2009; Van Langenhove et al., 2010) and mutations in the FTLD gene *VCP* were also detected in ALS (Johnson et al., 2010). However, most convincing evidence for the genetic overlap comes from the observation that both ALS and FTLD can occur within the same family or within a single patient of a family. More than 15 autosomal dominant families with ALS and FTLD worldwide are causally linked with a major disease locus at chromosome 9p13-p21 (ALSFTD2 locus) (Boxer et al., 2010; Gijselinck et al., 2010; Le Ber et al., 2009; Luty et al., 2008; Momeni et al., 2006; Morita et al., 2006; Pearson et al., 2011; Valdmanis et al., 2007; Vance et al., 2006). The minimally linked region in all these families is about 3.6 Mb in size containing five known protein-coding genes. Moreover, several recent genome-wide association studies (GWAS) in ALS populations from different European origins showed the presence of a major genetic risk factor for ALS at the same chromosome 9p region (Laaksovirta et al., 2010; Shatunov et al., 2010; van Es et al., 2009). The Finnish study narrowed the associated region to a 232 kb linkage disequilibrium (LD) block containing three known genes (*MOBKL2B, IFNK, C9orf72*) and suggested the presence of a major risk gene with high penetrance (Laaksovirta et al., 2010). Likewise, a GWAS in FTLD has implicated the same region (Van Deerlin et al., 2010). This finding was further confirmed in other FTLD and ALS-FTLD cohorts (Rollinson et al., 2011). Together, these data demonstrate that ALS and FTLD share a major common genetic factor on chromosome 9p, most likely showing high mutation frequencies. Despite all attempts of several research groups, the genetic defect(s) underlying both genetic linkage and association to this region have not been identified yet.

In this book chapter we will report and discuss the latest findings in the studies aiming at identifying the chromosome 9 gene defect.

2. Family-based linkage to ALSFTD2 locus on chromosome 9p

Since the original reports of a Dutch and a Scandinavian ALS-FTLD family linked with chromosome 9p21 (Morita et al., 2006; Vance et al., 2006), a growing number of families with inherited ALS and FTLD are reported with significant linkage to the ALSFTD2 locus on chromosome 9p21 (Boxer et al., 2010; Gijselinck et al., 2010; Le Ber et al., 2009; Luty et al., 2008; Valdmanis et al., 2007) (table 1). In all these families patients show similar clinical and pathological characteristics. Clinically, individuals may present with symptoms of both ALS and FTLD, or with ALS or FTLD alone. Pathologically, autopsied patients have TDP-43 positive type 2 (Sampathu et al., 2006) brain inclusions (Boxer et al., 2010; Gijselinck et al., 2010; Le Ber et al., 2009; Luty et al., 2008; Morita et al., 2006; Vance et al., 2006). (table 1)

The minimal candidate region was previously defined by D9S169 (Luty et al., 2008) and D9S1805 (Valdmanis et al., 2007) spanning 7 Mb and was recently reduced to 3.6 Mb between D9S169 (Luty et al., 2008) and D9S251 by Boxer and colleagues (2010) (figure 1). Therefore, several parts of this study were still investigated in the 7 Mb region.

Family	**Origin**	**Max LOD score at 9p21**	**Mean onset age in years (range)**	**Mean disease duration in years (range)**	**TDP-43+**	**# ALS**	**# ALS + FTLD**	**# FTLD**	**References**
Luty	Australian	3.41	53 (43-68)	9 (1-16)	+	2	2	7	(Luty et al., 2008)
DR14	Belgian	3.38	58.1 (51-65)	6.4 (1-17)	+	1	0	10	(Gijselinck et al., 2010)
F2	Dutch	3.02	60.3 (39-72)	3.0 (1-8)	ND	7	3	2	(Vance et al., 2006)
Que23	Canadian	3.01	55.8 (46-58)	2.4 (1.5-3)	ND	5	0	3	(Valdmanis et al., 2007)
VSM20	Irish	3.01	45.7 (35-57)	5.4 (3-10)	+	2	3	5	(Boxer et al., 2010)
F438	Scandinavian	3.00	55.3 (45-64)	4.3 (1-9)	ND	5	0	9	(Morita et al., 2006)
6 families	French	8.0[1]	57.9 (40-84)	3.6 (1-8)	+	9	12	10	(Le Ber et al., 2009)
Que1	French-Canadian	2.51	54.3 (45-63)	4.8 (2-9)	ND	5	3	0	(Valdmanis et al., 2007)
Fr104	Spanish	1.55	ND	ND	ND	4	1	0	(Valdmanis et al., 2007)
F2	North-American	1.5	ND	ND	ND	0	7	0	(Momeni et al., 2006)
Gwent	Brittish	ND	42.2 (31-52)	3.6 (1-13)	+	3	6	0	(Pearson et al., 2011)
F476	North-American	ND	ND	ND	ND	2	3	0	(Momeni et al., 2006)
ALS_A	American	ND	? (35-73)	? (0.5-5)	ND	6	0	0	(Krueger et al., 2009)

Table 1. Genetic, clinical and pathological characteristics of ALS-FTLD families linked or associated with chromosome 9p21 (ND: not determined; [1]summed LODscore in 6 small families, not linked separately)

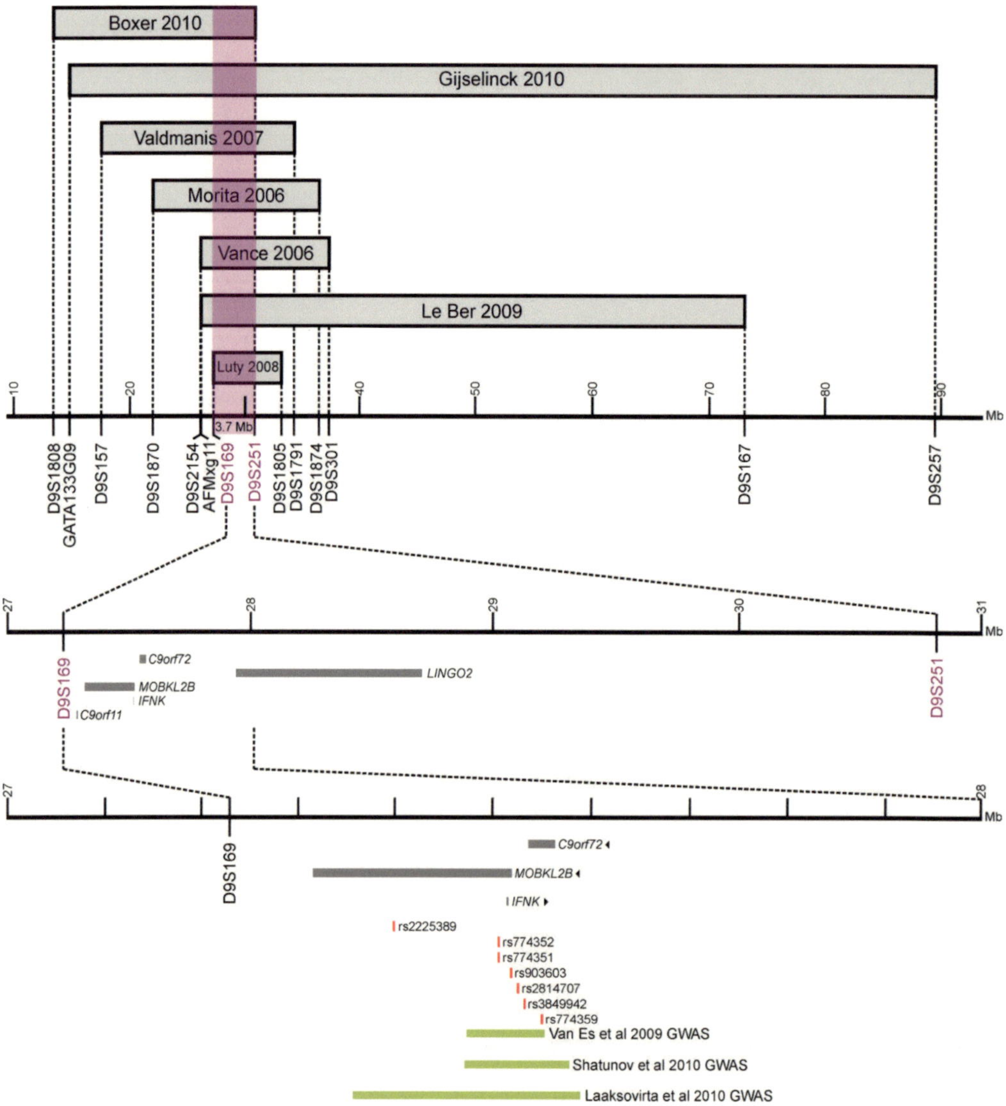

Fig. 1. Schematic representation of the chromosome 9p21 ALS-FTLD locus. Upper panel: grey bars indicate the minimal candidate regions in all reported significantly linked ALS-FTLD families, defining a minimal interval of 3.7 Mb between D9S169 and D9S251 containing five protein coding genes, illustrated with grey lines. Lower panel: associated SNPs in ALS and FTLD GWAS are shown in red and LD blocks or finemapped regions of these GWAS are indicated with green lines. Three genes are located in the associated region.

2.1 Family DR14

We studied a Belgian 4-generation family (family DR14) with autosomal dominant transmission of ALS and FTLD. We collected DNA from 29 family members of whom 3 patients in generation III and 11 at-risk individuals in generation III and IV each (figure 1). Two patients (III.2 and III.12) were diagnosed with FTLD (subtype FTD), while patient III.10 was diagnosed with ALS (figure 2). The mean age at onset was 58.1 ± 4.2 years (N = 9, range 51-65 years) and mean disease duration was 6.4 ± 4.9 years (range 1-17 years). The index patient was clinically diagnosed with familial FTLD (subtype FTD) and pathological TDP-43 positive inclusions were observed in the brain (FTLD-TDP type 2 (Sampathu et al., 2006)). Mutations in the known genes for ALS and dementia were excluded. (Gijselinck et al., 2010)

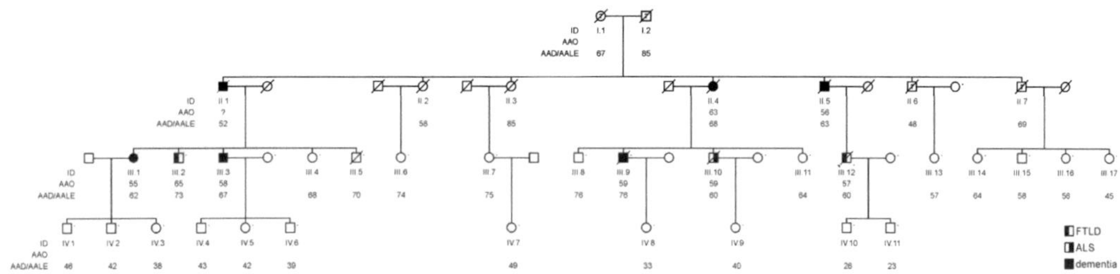

Fig. 2. The pedigree of DR14 consists of four generations. Left-filled and right-filled symbols represent patients with FTLD and ALS respectively. Patients with unspecified dementia are indicated with filled symbols. Open symbols represent unaffected individuals or at-risk individuals with unknown phenotype. Individuals with unclear phenotype are designated with a question mark (?). The arrow indicates index patient III.12. Numbers below the symbols denote age at onset and age at death (AAD) for patients and either age at last examination (AALE) or AAD for unaffected individuals or individuals with unknown phenotype. An asterisk (*) indicates individuals of whom DNA was available.

2.2 Mutation analyses of known genes and conserved regions, and CNV analysis

We performed a genome-wide scan using an in-house developed mapping set of 425 microsatellite markers in 30 multiplex panels with an average distance of 8 cM. Multipoint LOD scores were calculated revealing two loci on chromosome 9 and 14: one at chromosome 9 with a maximal LOD score of 2.71 between D9S1121 and D9S270 and one at chromosome 14 with the highest LOD score of 2.61 between D14S302 and D14S611. Finemapping of the chromosome 9 locus resulted in a significant maximal multipoint LOD score of 3.38 between D9S1833 and D9S1121 at 9p21 and segregation analysis defined a candidate region of 64.6 cM (74.7 Mb) between markers D9S235 and D9S257 on chromosome 9p23-9q21, based on two obligate recombinants (figure 3), harboring 271 protein coding genes (Gijselinck et al., 2010). This region overlaps with the ALSFTD2 locus at chromosome 9p21 but did not reduce the minimally linked region. Therefore, we analyzed the 7 Mb overlap region, including the minimal locus of 3.6 Mb, for mutations. We sequenced all 27 protein-coding genes, either the complete coding sequence of cDNA (N=17) including *MOBKL2B, C9orf72, ACO1, DDX58, TOPORS, NDUFB6, DNAJA1, SMU1, B4GALT1, BAG1, CHMP5, AQP3, NOL6, UBE2R2, UBAP2, WDR40A* and *UBAP1*, or the exons and exon-intron boundaries on gDNA using classical sequencing (N=10). cDNA was prepared from lymphoblasts of two patients and two healthy control individuals of the family not carrying the disease haplotype, treated with or without cycloheximide allowing also the detection of degraded aberrant transcripts.

Mutation analysis on cDNA allows not only detecting simple point mutations and small insertions/deletions but also exon deletions/duplications and alternative transcripts. Similar to other chr9-linked ALS-FTLD families, this mutation analysis did not reveal patient-specific novel variants segregating with disease.

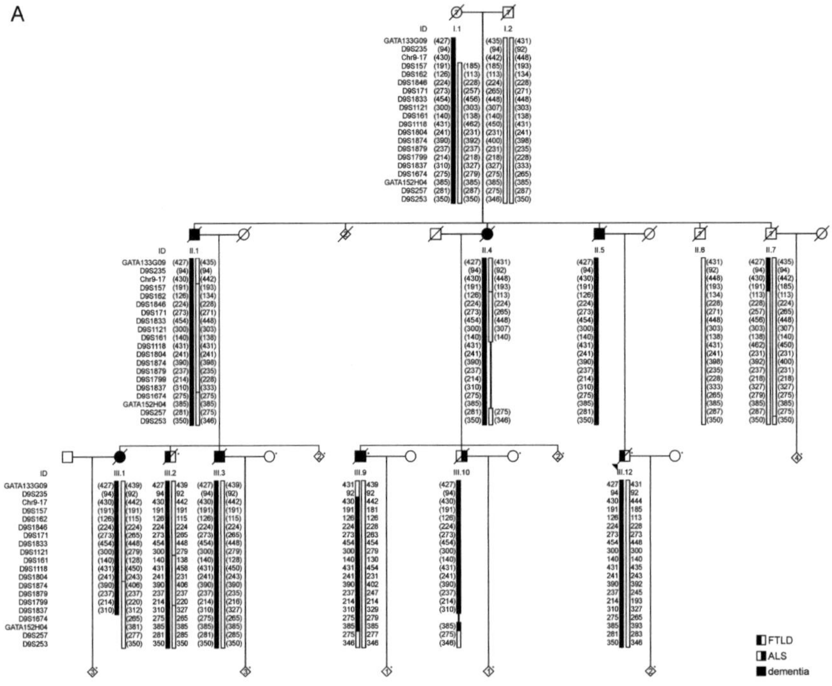

Fig. 3. Segregation of the 9p23-q21 haplotype in family DR14. Haplotypes are based on a selection of 20 informative STR markers at chromosome 9. The black haplotype represents the disease haplotype. Haplotypes for deceased individuals were inferred based on genotype data obtained in their offspring (between brackets). The disease haplotype was arbitrarily set for I.1, and numbers in diamonds indicate the number of genotyped at-risk individuals. An asterisk (*) indicates individuals of whom DNA was available.

Since all coding exons of known genes were excluded for mutations, we selected other evolutionary conserved regions and investigated these sequences for the presence of non-coding variants in evolutionary constrained regulatory elements, e.g. promoters and distant regulatory elements or conserved epigenetic sequence motifs, or coding variants in unknown novel genes (protein coding or non-coding RNA genes). Using the UCSC-PhastCons-mammalian-28way track predicting and scoring the presence of conserved elements in the genome by comparing the sequence between 28 mammalian species, we defined 149 kb of conserved elements throughout the ALSFTD2 locus of 7 Mb. These elements were grouped in 1108 clusters with a total sequence of 465 kb and ranked according to conservation strength. We performed sanger sequencing in two patients and two healthy control individuals of the family not carrying the disease haplotype. In total we sequenced 95 kb of highest conserved elements (total of 260 kb clusters) in the 7 Mb region, not revealing patient-specific novel variants segregating with disease. Of these, 61 kb of conserved regions are located in the minimal candidate region of 3.6 Mb. Using this approach, we excluded mutations in highly conserved regions. However, we did not exclude variants in regions with no or low conservation in mammalian species because it is well known that a substantial number of primate/human-specific exons exist (e.g. Sela et al., 2007) and that the location of regulatory elements is not always highly conserved, even not in mammals e.g. between human and mouse (Ravasi et al., 2010).

In addition, we performed chromosome-specific oligo-based array-comparative genomic hybridization (array-CGH, Nimblegen) at chromosome 9 with a resolution of about 1kb, on the index patient and an independent control individual not carrying the disease haplotype to detect copy number variations (CNVs). The CGH data were analyzed by Signalmap software (Nimblegen) and the scoring program CGHcall, revealing one large CNV (chr9:29082732-29087816) covered by 20 CGH probes. This deletion was confirmed in the index patient by six qPCR fragments demonstrating a deleted region of at least 5273 bp (chr9:29082677-29087949) (data not shown). It did not segregate with disease in DR14 and represented a polymorphism since it was also present in individuals not carrying the disease haplotype and since a frequent CNV had previously been reported at this position (chr9:29082445-29088195) (Cooper et al., 2008). Consequently, these experiments failed to identify a copy number mutation (deletion or insertion) of more than 1 kb (Gijselinck et al., 2010). Cytogenetics excluded large chromosomal rearrangements.

Since all these mutation analyses did not reveal the causal mutation, we hypothesized that the mutation is most likely unusual with respect to location (extragenic or intronic) and/or type (small indel, inversion or other complex rearrangement). Therefore, we performed whole genome sequencing in family DR14 and subsequently analyzed sequences or variants in the linked region.

2.3 Whole genome sequencing

The complete genome sequence of four chromosome 9p disease haplotype carriers of family DR14, including two patients and two asymptomatic individuals was determined using next generation sequencing technology. These family members were selected such that they have a different unaffected haplotype. The sequencing was done with the company Complete Genomics (Mountain View CA, USA, www.completegenomics.com) who provides 35 bp paired-end sequence reads at a high sequence coverage obtained with high-accuracy combinatorial probe anchor ligation (cPAL) sequencing technology (Drmanac et al., 2010; Roach et al., 2010). Also, the paired-end sequencing data enable the identification of copy number variations (CNVs) and other structural variants (SV) including inversions, in addition to single nucleotide polymorphisms (SNPs).

In the 4 genomes, we obtained an average coverage of 62-fold genome sequence and captured both alleles at 95.4% of the genomes. All sequence variants, including SNPs and small indels, were mapped to the human reference genome sequence (NCBI Build 36/hg18). We initially focused on the 3.6 Mb candidate region on chromosome 9p21. We filtered and prioritized variants according to several criteria. First, variants must be present heterozygously in all 4 patients since the disease is segregating in an autosomal dominant manner. As a heterozygous variant might be rarely missed using NGS technology, depending on local sequence coverage and quality, variants detected in three of four patients were also considered. Second, variants were selected that were not catalogued in the dbSNP database (http://www.ncbi.nlm.nih.gov/projects/SNP) and were not found as common polymorphisms (allele frequency ≥ 1%) in the 1000 Genomes

Project (http://www.1000genomes.org). Third, variants in nucleotide stretches were filtered out because they are known to be error-prone in NGS data. This resulted in a total of 189 variants, all located outside coding regions of known genes confirming gene-based mutation analyses. These variants were genotyped in all 29 individuals of the DR14 family using Sanger sequencing and tested for segregation. 120 variants were located on the disease haplotype and were analyzed in a series of 300 neurologically healthy control individuals collected in Flanders, Belgium, i.e. the geographical region of which family DR14 originates, using multiplex Sequenom MassARRAY technology. 37 of these variants were completely absent in 300 control individuals and are all located in untranslated regions or introns of genes, or intergenic. We are currently prioritizing these variants based on evolutionary conservation, regulatory potential, location compatible with cis-acting function on functional candidate genes, etc. Also, we are determining the presence of these variants in a Belgian population of unrelated patients with ALS (N=124), ALS-FTLD (N=21) and FTLD (N=203), aiming to find a possible founder mutation. We already showed evidence for the presence of founder mutations in the Flanders-Belgian FTLD collection, by the *GRN* IVS1+5 G>C founder mutation identified in 19% of familial FTLD (Cruts et al., 2006). We have investigated the patient population for chromosome 9p STR markers and did not find evidence for haplotype sharing with family DR14; however, we cannot exclude the presence of a small, previously undetected founder haplotype.

3. Population-based association for ALS and FTLD to chromosome 9p

In 2009, the first ALS GWAS showing association with a locus at chromosome 9p21 was reported by Van Es and colleagues. They identified genome-wide significance with two SNPs, rs2814707 and rs3849942, almost in complete linkage disequilibrium (LD) with each other and located in an LD block of ~80 kb. Also a third SNP in this LD block (rs774359) showed suggestive association (figure 1). This LD block is situated at the telomeric end of the minimally linked candidate region found in the ALS-FTLD families and contains only three genes: part of *MOBKL2B*, *IFNK* and *C9orf72* (figure 1). Next, data of the first GWAS in FTLD-TDP were suggestive for association of five SNPs (rs774352, rs774351, rs3849942, rs2814707, rs774359) on chromosome 9p21, in the same LD block (Van Deerlin et al., 2010). Subsequently, a Finnish and a British independent ALS GWAS identified genome-wide significance with SNPs rs3849942, rs2814707, rs774359, rs2225389 (Laaksovirta et al., 2010) and with SNPs rs3849942, rs2814707, rs903603 (Shatunov et al., 2010) respectively, all in the same locus at chromosome 9p21. The Finnish study defined a 42-SNP haplotype associated with increased risk of ALS in the Finnish population, located in a 232 kb LD block which overlaps with the previously reported 80 kb LD block (van Es et al., 2009) and the 106.5 kb LD block of the UK study (Shatunov et al., 2010). Because of the unique homogeneous genetic structure of the Finnish isolated population, the extent and structure of LD is different than in other European countries. To date, one study replicated the association of the chr9p21 locus in an ALS-FTLD subpopulation (Rollinson et al., 2011).

To assess the contribution of the chr9p21 risk factor to disease etiology in Belgium, we replicated one of the top SNPs associated in all GWAS reports, rs2814707, in a Belgian population of ALS, ALS-FTLD and FTLD patients. In addition, we performed a meta-analysis of the different published association studies with inclusion of our study.

3.1 Replication study chr9p21 GWAS

We investigated association of the most widely studied GWAS top SNP at chr9p21, rs2814707, in a Flanders-Belgian population of genealogically unrelated patients clinically diagnosed with ALS (N=124), ALS-FTLD (N=21) or FTLD (N=203) according to established consensus criteria (Brooks et al., 2000; Neary et al., 1998), compared to a group of 510 unrelated neurologically healthy control individuals from the same region in Belgium. We genotyped rs2814707 and showed that this SNP is in Hardy-Weinberg Equilibrium. Allelic and genotypic single SNP association was calculated using logistic regression analysis. The SNP showed significant allelic and genotypic association in the total population and highly significant association in the ALS and ALS-FTLD subpopulation reaching a maximal odds ratio of 3.27 in ALS patients homozygous for the minor allele (table 2). In the FTLD subpopulation no association was found, demonstrating that the effect in the total population can entirely be explained by the effect in patients with an ALS phenotype. When we include 21 ALS samples of Bulgarian origin, the relative risk became even higher, compared to Belgians only, indicating that the associated allele is the same between different populations.

SNP ID	Genotype	Controls	ALS, ALS-FTLD and FTLD			ALS and ALS-FTLD		
		N=510	N=348			N=145		
		freq (%)	freq (%)	p-value	OR (95%CI)	freq (%)	p-value	OR (95%CI)
rs2814707	C	77.9	71.3	**0.006**	1.39 (1.10-1.75)	67.0	**0.001**	1.69 (1.25-2.29)
	T	22.1	28.7			33.0		
	CC	59.7	50.4	ref	ref	43.1	ref	ref
	CT	36.5	41.8	0.08	1.31 (0.97-1.77)	47.9	**0.007**	1.76 (1.17-2.64)
	TT	3.8	7.8	**0.008**	2.41 (1.26-4.62)	9.0	**0.005**	3.27 (1.44-7.41)

Table 2. Allelic and genotypic association of a GWAS top SNP in the total population and the ALS/ALS-FTLD subpopulation. P-values are corrected for age at onset or inclusion and gender. (OR: odds ratio; CI: confidence interval)

3.2 Meta analysis on chromosome 9p21

We combined the data from the different GWA studies and our study to determine the relative risk of carrying the risk allele on chromosome 9p21. A meta-analysis of the most widely studied SNP on chromosome 9p21 (rs2814707) underscores the presence of a genetic risk factor for ALS and/or FTLD at this locus. Carriers of the rs2814707 minor allele are at increased risk to develop ALS or FTLD (OR_{meta} 1.29 (95% CI 1.18-1.41), p-value $2.3*10^{-8}$ (Figure 4)). When excluding the GWAS cohorts in which the association was first reported (van Es et al., 2009) to exclude bias because of winner's curse, the strength of the association remains similar (OR_{meta} 1.32 (95%CI 1.17-1.49; p-value $3.5*10^{-6}$). Exclusion of three studies, including our own, which combine FTLD and ALS phenotypes would have resulted in an OR_{meta} 1.24 (95%CI 1.13-1.36); p-value $3.3*10^{-6}$).

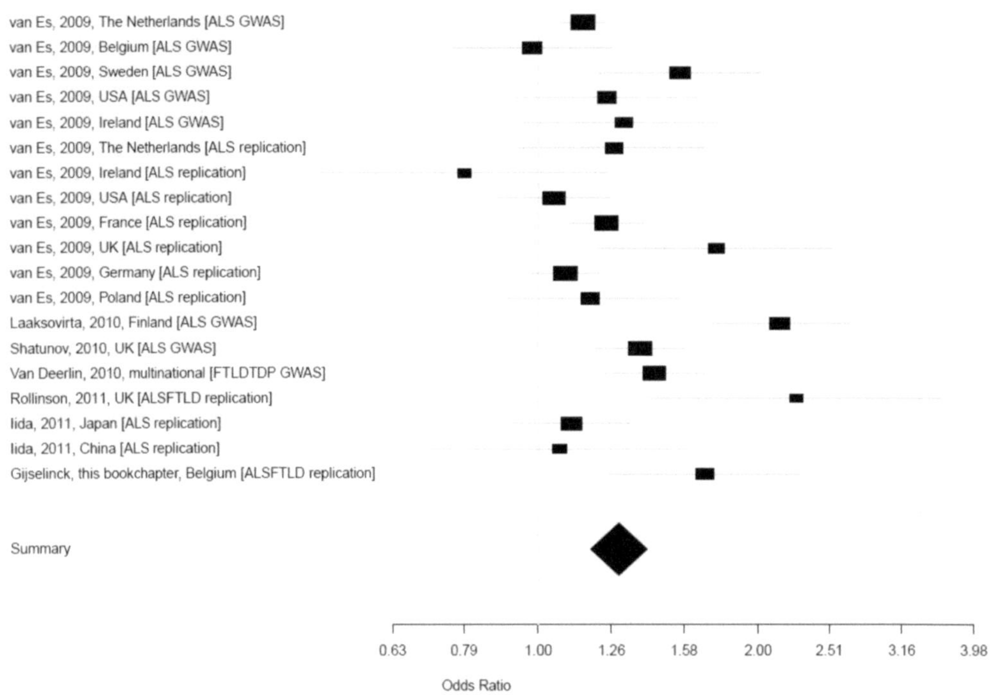

Fig. 4. Forest plot of a random effects meta-analysis of rs2814707. Meta-analysis was conducted in rmeta v2.16, and based on effect estimates and standard errors for the minor allele reported in each individual publication. Odds Ratios and 95% Confidence Intervals are given for each study separately along with a summary Odds Ratio, of the minor allele relative to the major allele. All 9p21 association studies on ALS, ALS-FTLD and FTLD published until July 2011 were included, in addition to our own unpublished data. For the study of Shatunov and colleagues we only included data on the independent UK cohort, to avoid overlap of datasets with previous studies. From Rollinson et al, only data on the Manchester ALS-FTLD cohort are included.

4. Discussion and conclusion

Family-based linkage and population-based association studies in Belgian patients with ALS and/or FTLD provided further evidence for the presence of a major genetic factor on chromosome 9p21 for these diseases.

In the Belgian family DR14 we analyzed the minimally linked region shared in all linked families. We excluded mutations in exons of all known protein-coding genes, in the highest conserved sequences and also copy number mutations of more than 1 kb were excluded. Further we used next generation sequencing technology to sequence the whole genome of four disease haplotype carriers. We are currently analyzing the first selection of variants. If we are left with only a very small number of putative disease-associated variants, we will analyze the complete sequence of the functional unit in which the remaining variants are located in the complete set of ALS, ALS-FTLD and FTLD patients. `Functional unit' in this context means the gene, regulatory element, conserved element or, in the absence of recognizable elements, 1 kb flanking each side of the putative mutation. This might identify additional mutations resulting in the same functional defect as the mutations detected in DR14 and further enhance the likelihood of the variant(s) to be disease-related. Finding such variants will provide strong genetic evidence of a disease causing effect of the variants. Alternatively, in case we do not find a mutation in this first selection of variants, we can use more relaxing filters. Taking into account that dbSNP may include rare clinical variants, rare or non-validated dbSNP SNPs will also be considered (N=91). Also the candidate region can be extended to the next recombinant or to the large DR14 candidate region. Further, regions that are not covered in more than one genome, will be completed using classical sanger sequencing. Finally, structural variants and copy number mutations will be investigated.

More than five years of research in the ALSFTD2 locus in different ALS-FTLD families worldwide did not identify pathogenic mutations yet (table 1), although mutations in two different genes on chromosome 9 outside the minimal candidate region, *IFT74* and *SIGMAR1*, were suggested (Luty et al., 2010; Momeni et al., 2006) but without further confirmation in other families. The fact that the culprit gene is still not found may in part be explained by the fact that families linked with chromosome 9p21 do not all have the same disease haplotype so that different mutations, probably with the same effect on the same gene, are most likely involved. Also, the causal mutations are most likely unusual with respect to position or type. For example, deep intronic mutations or mutations in a distant regulatory element might cause the disease but assessing their effect is rather complicated. Also, identification of small insertions/deletions or inversions is challenging.

In addition, we replicated association in a Belgian cohort of ALS, ALS-FTLD and FTLD patients of two major top SNPs on chromosome 9p21 previously associated in several ALS and FTLD GWA studies. More specifically, we found that the risk haplotype at chromosome 9p21 is most substantially increased in patients with ALS or ALS-FTLD compared to control individuals. The lack of association in the FTLD subpopulation is similar to what was observed in a previous replication study in which association was only found in ALS-FTLD patients (Rollinson et al., 2011). Also, the weakest association signal was found in the FTLD GWAS compared to ALS GWAS. This is the first time that a susceptibility locus for ALS is replicated in different GWA studies and replication studies, underlining the importance of the chromosome 9p21 locus harbouring a risk increasing factor for ALS (and ALS-FTLD) across multiple populations with a high relative risk of disease susceptibility. We are further characterizing this genetic association to reduce the associated region in the Belgian population. We are finemapping the chromosome 9p risk haplotype in great detail in our ALS, FTLD, ALS-FTLD patient cohorts by making a high density SNP map of the complete LD block and using extended association analyses of series of known and newly identified variants in the LD block. These variants were identified in previous publications, hapmap, 1000 Genomes Project and extended genomic sequencing efforts of the linkage disequilibrium block in a selection of ALS and ALS-FTLD patients carrying the associated allele of the GWAS SNPs in a homozygous or heterozygous state. This will finally result in the identification of the functional variant explaining the strong association in the chromosome 9p21 region.

The observation that the chromosome 9p21 region is harboring both disease-causing variants and susceptibility factors with high penetrance, might suggest that different genetic variants with variable degree of biological consequences might be involved. Alternatively, one genetic defect might act as high penetrant susceptibility factor in sporadic patients and as disease-causing factor with reduced penetrance in ALS-FTLD families, carrying also other disease modifying factors. In this respect it is interesting to note that in our studied belgian family DR14 all patients carry in addition to the disease haplotype at chromosome 9p21 also a haplotype in a novel locus at chromosome 14q32, possibly harboring a disease modifying gene (Gijselinck et al., 2010) and of which the sequences are present in the whole genome sequencing data of the family. Combining the family-based and the population-based approach to ultimately find the gene with one or more genetic defects would be of great value. For example, prioritizing the associated LD block in the whole genome sequence analysis of the family could be useful. Further, since in the associated LD block only three genes are located (*IFNK, C9orf72, MOBKL2B*) (figure 1), we could focus on these genes with respect to expression and dosage studies (eg. single exon deletions or duplications) in the family. Also, the region in and around the associated LD block can be saturated with STR markers for sharing studies with the DR14 family to detect a small founder haplotype. Combining all these comprehensive data will bring us closer to the identification of the chromosome 9 gene. As long as the genetic defect underlying linkage and association is not known, the full epidemiological impact of the chromosome 9p gene in familial and non-familial forms of ALS, ALS-FTLD and FTLD cannot be determined. However, the combined evidence emerging from all molecular genetic studies in chromosome 9p21-linked families and in chromosome 9p21 associated ALS/FTLD populations, suggests it is the most important genetic factor contributing to disease in the center of the disease spectrum linking ALS and FTLD (table 1). Moreover, next to the chr9p21 conclusively linked ALS-FTLD families, several other (smaller) families were also reported without conclusive linkage but with several indications pointing towards the presence of a segregating haplotype in the ALSFTD2 locus (Krueger et al., 2009; Le Ber et al., 2009; Momeni et al., 2006; Pearson et al., 2011; Valdmanis et al., 2007; Yan et al., 2008) (table 1). Identification of this major gene will undoubtedly be a steppingstone for subsequent cell biological studies aiming at better understanding of the pathobiology of neurodegenerative processes leading to ALS and FTLD.

5. Acknowledgment

We are grateful to the patients for their cooperation. We further acknowledge the contribution of personnel of the VIB Genetic Service Facility (www.vibgeneticservicefacility.be). This research of the authors was in part funded by the Special Research Fund of the University of Antwerp, the Research Foundation Flanders (FWO-F), the Institute for Science and Technology - Flanders (IWT-F), the Methusalem excellence grant of the Flemish Government, the Interuniversity Attraction Poles program (IUAP) P6/43 of the Belgian Science Policy Office, the Stichting Alzheimer Onderzoek (SAO-FRMA). I.G. is holding a postdoctoral fellowship of FWO-F.

6. References

Arai, T., Hasegawa, M., Akiyama, H., Ikeda, K., Nonaka, T., Mori, H., Mann, D., Tsuchiya, K., Yoshida, M., Hashizume, Y. & Oda, T. (2006). TDP-43 is a component of ubiquitin-positive tau-negative inclusions in frontotemporal lobar degeneration and amyotrophic lateral sclerosis. *Biochem Biophys Res Commun*, 351, 3, 602-611

Baker, M., Mackenzie, I.R., Pickering-Brown, S.M., Gass, J., Rademakers, R., Lindholm, C., Snowden, J., Adamson, J., Sadovnick, A.D., Rollinson, S., Cannon, A., Dwosh, E., Neary, D., Melquist, S., Richardson, A., Dickson, D., Berger, Z., Eriksen, J., Robinson, T., Zehr, C., Dickey, C.A., Crook, R., McGowan, E., Mann, D., Boeve, B., Feldman, H. & Hutton, M. (2006). Mutations in progranulin cause tau-negative frontotemporal dementia linked to chromosome 17. *Nature*, 442, 7105, 916-919

Boxer, A.L., Mackenzie, I.R., Boeve, B.F., Baker, M., Seeley, W.W., Crook, R., Feldman, H., Hsiung, G.Y., Rutherford, N., Laluz, V., Whitwell, J., Foti, D., McDade, E., Molano, J., Karydas, A., Wojtas, A., Goldman, J., Mirsky, J., Sengdy, P., Dearmond, S., Miller, B.L. & Rademakers, R. (2010). Clinical, neuroimaging and neuropathological features of a new chromosome 9p-linked FTD-ALS family. *J Neurol Neurosurg Psychiatry*

Brooks, B.R., Miller, R.G., Swash, M. & Munsat, T.L. (2000). El Escorial revisited: revised criteria for the diagnosis of amyotrophic lateral sclerosis. *Amyotroph Lateral Scler Other Motor Neuron Disord*, 1, 5, 293-299

Cooper, G.M., Zerr, T., Kidd, J.M., Eichler, E.E. & Nickerson, D.A. (2008). Systematic assessment of copy number variant detection via genome-wide SNP genotyping. *Nat Genet*, 40, 10, 1199-1203

Cruts, M., Gijselinck, I., van der Zee, J., Engelborghs, S., Wils, H., Pirici, D., Rademakers, R., Vandenberghe, R., Dermaut, B., Martin, J.J., van Duijn, C., Peeters, K., Sciot, R., Santens, P., de Pooter, T., Mattheijssens, M., Van den Broeck, M., Cuijt, I., Vennekens, K., De Deyn, P.P., Kumar-Singh, S. & Van Broeckhoven, C. (2006). Null mutations in progranulin cause ubiquitin-positive frontotemporal dementia linked to chromosome 17q21. *Nature*, 442, 7105, 920-924

Drmanac, R., Sparks, A.B., Callow, M.J., Halpern, A.L., Burns, N.L., Kermani, B.G., Carnevali, P., Nazarenko, I., Nilsen, G.B., Yeung, G., Dahl, F., Fernandez, A., Staker, B., Pant, K.P., Baccash, J., Borcherding, A.P., Brownley, A., Cedeno, R., Chen, L., Chernikoff, D., Cheung, A., Chirita, R., Curson, B., Ebert, J.C., Hacker, C.R., Hartlage, R., Hauser, B., Huang, S., Jiang, Y., Karpinchyk, V., Koenig, M., Kong, C., Landers, T., Le, C., Liu, J., McBride, C.E., Morenzoni, M., Morey, R.E., Mutch, K., Perazich, H., Perry, K., Peters, B.A., Peterson, J., Pethiyagoda, C.L., Pothuraju, K., Richter, C., Rosenbaum, A.M., Roy, S., Shafto, J., Sharanhovich, U., Shannon, K.W., Sheppy, C.G., Sun, M., Thakuria, J.V., Tran, A., Vu, D., Zaranek, A.W., Wu, X., Drmanac, S., Oliphant, A.R., Banyai, W.C., Martin, B., Ballinger, D.G., Church, G.M. & Reid, C.A. (2010). Human genome sequencing using unchained base reads on self-assembling DNA nanoarrays. *Science*, 327, 5961, 78-81

Gijselinck, I., Engelborghs, S., Maes, G., Cuijt, I., Peeters, K., Mattheijssens, M., Joris, G., Cras, P., Martin, J.J., De Deyn, P.P., Kumar-Singh, S., Van Broeckhoven, C. & Cruts, M. (2010). Identification of 2 Loci at chromosomes 9 and 14 in a multiplex family with frontotemporal lobar degeneration and amyotrophic lateral sclerosis. *Arch Neurol*, 67, 5, 606-616

Gitcho, M.A., Baloh, R.H., Chakraverty, S., Mayo, K., Norton, J.B., Levitch, D., Hatanpaa, K.J., White, C.L., III, Bigio, E.H., Caselli, R., Baker, M., Al Lozi, M.T., Morris, J.C., Pestronk, A., Rademakers, R., Goate, A.M. & Cairns, N.J. (2008). TDP-43 A315T mutation in familial motor neuron disease. *Ann Neurol*, 63, 4, 535-538

Greenway, M.J., Andersen, P.M., Russ, C., Ennis, S., Cashman, S., Donaghy, C., Patterson, V., Swingler, R., Kieran, D., Prehn, J., Morrison, K.E., Green, A., Acharya, K.R., Brown, R.H., Jr. & Hardiman, O. (2006). ANG mutations segregate with familial and 'sporadic' amyotrophic lateral sclerosis. *Nat Genet*, 38, 4, 411-413

Hutton, M., Lendon, C.L., Rizzu, P., Baker, M., Froelich, S., Houlden, H., Pickering-Brown, S., Chakraverty, S., Isaacs, A., Grover, A., Hackett, J., Adamson, J., Lincoln, S., Dickson, D., Davies, P., Petersen, R.C., Stevens, M., de Graaff, E., Wauters, E., van Baren, J., Hillebrand, M., Joosse, M., Kwon, J.M., Nowotny, P., Che, L.K., Norton, J., Morris, J.C., Reed, L.A., Trojanowski, J., Basun, H., Lannfelt, L., Neystat, M., Fahn, S., Dark, F., Tannenberg, T., Dodd, P.R., Hayward, N., Kwok, J.B., Schofield, P.R., Andreadis, A., Snowden, J., Craufurd, D., Neary, D., Owen, F., Oostra, B.A., Hardy, J., Goate, A., van Swieten, J., Mann, D., Lynch, T. & Heutink, P. (1998). Association of missense and 5'-splice-site mutations in tau with the inherited dementia FTDP-17. *Nature*, 393, 6686, 702-705

Johnson, J.O., Mandrioli, J., Benatar, M., Abramzon, Y., Van Deerlin, V.M., Trojanowski, J.Q., Gibbs, J.R., Brunetti, M., Gronka, S., Wuu, J., Ding, J., McCluskey, L., Martinez-Lage, M., Falcone, D., Hernandez, D.G., Arepalli, S., Chong, S., Schymick, J.C., Rothstein, J., Landi, F., Wang, Y.D., Calvo, A., Mora, G., Sabatelli, M., Monsurro, M.R., Battistini, S., Salvi, F., Spataro, R., Sola, P., Borghero, G., Galassi, G., Scholz, S.W., Taylor, J.P., Restagno, G., Chio, A. & Traynor, B.J. (2010). Exome sequencing reveals VCP mutations as a cause of familial ALS. *Neuron*, 68, 5, 857-864

Kabashi, E., Valdmanis, P.N., Dion, P., Spiegelman, D., McConkey, B.J., Vande, V.C., Bouchard, J.P., Lacomblez, L., Pochigaeva, K., Salachas, F., Pradat, P.F., Camu, W., Meininger, V., Dupre, N. & Rouleau, G.A. (2008). TARDBP mutations in individuals with sporadic and familial amyotrophic lateral sclerosis. *Nat Genet*, 40, 5, 572-574

Kovacs, G.G., Murrell, J.R., Horvath, S., Haraszti, L., Majtenyi, K., Molnar, M.J., Budka, H., Ghetti, B. & Spina, S. (2009). TARDBP variation associated with frontotemporal dementia, supranuclear gaze palsy, and chorea. *Mov Disord*, 24, 12, 1843-1847

Krueger, K.A., Tsuji, S., Fukuda, Y., Takahashi, Y., Goto, J., Mitsui, J., Ishiura, H., Dalton, J.C., Miller, M.B., Day, J.W. & Ranum, L.P. (2009). SNP haplotype mapping in a small ALS family. *PLoS One*, 4, 5, e5687

Kwiatkowski, T.J., Jr., Bosco, D.A., Leclerc, A.L., Tamrazian, E., Vanderburg, C.R., Russ, C., Davis, A., Gilchrist, J., Kasarskis, E.J., Munsat, T., Valdmanis, P., Rouleau, G.A., Hosler, B.A., Cortelli, P., de Jong, P.J., Yoshinaga, Y., Haines, J.L., Pericak-Vance, M.A., Yan, J., Ticozzi, N., Siddique, T., McKenna-Yasek, D., Sapp, P.C., Horvitz, H.R., Landers, J.E. & Brown, R.H., Jr. (2009). Mutations in the FUS/TLS gene on chromosome 16 cause familial amyotrophic lateral sclerosis. *Science*, 323, 5918, 1205-1208

Laaksovirta, H., Peuralinna, T., Schymick, J.C., Scholz, S.W., Lai, S.L., Myllykangas, L., Sulkava, R., Jansson, L., Hernandez, D.G., Gibbs, J.R., Nalls, M.A., Heckerman, D., Tienari, P.J. & Traynor, B.J. (2010). Chromosome 9p21 in amyotrophic lateral sclerosis in Finland: a genome-wide association study. *Lancet Neurol*, 9, 10, 978-985

Le Ber, I., Camuzat, A., Berger, E., Hannequin, D., Laquerriere, A., Golfier, V., Seilhean, D., Viennet, G., Couratier, P., Verpillat, P., Heath, S., Camu, W., Martinaud, O., Lacomblez, L., Vercelletto, M., Salachas, F., Sellal, F., Didic, M., Thomas-Anterion,

C., Puel, M., Michel, B.F., Besse, C., Duyckaerts, C., Meininger, V., Campion, D., Dubois, B. & Brice, A. (2009). Chromosome 9p-linked families with frontotemporal dementia associated with motor neuron disease. *Neurology*, 72, 19, 1669-1676

Lillo, P. & Hodges, J.R. (2009). Frontotemporal dementia and motor neurone disease: overlapping clinic-pathological disorders. *J Clin Neurosci*, 16, 9, 1131-1135

Lomen-Hoerth, C., Murphy, J., Langmore, S., Kramer, J.H., Olney, R.K. & Miller, B. (2003). Are amyotrophic lateral sclerosis patients cognitively normal? *Neurology*, 60, 7, 1094-1097

Luty, A.A., Kwok, J.B., Dobson-Stone, C., Loy, C.T., Coupland, K.G., Karlstrom, H., Sobow, T., Tchorzewska, J., Maruszak, A., Barcikowska, M., Panegyres, P.K., Zekanowski, C., Brooks, W.S., Williams, K.L., Blair, I.P., Mather, K.A., Sachdev, P.S., Halliday, G.M. & Schofield, P.R. (2010). Sigma nonopioid intracellular receptor 1 mutations cause frontotemporal lobar degeneration-motor neuron disease. *Ann Neurol*, 68, 5, 639-649

Luty, A.A., Kwok, J.B., Thompson, E.M., Blumbergs, P., Brooks, W.S., Loy, C.T., Dobson-Stone, C., Panegyres, P.K., Hecker, J., Nicholson, G.A., Halliday, G.M. & Schofield, P.R. (2008). Pedigree with frontotemporal lobar degeneration--motor neuron disease and Tar DNA binding protein-43 positive neuropathology: genetic linkage to chromosome 9. *BMC Neurol*, 8, 32

Momeni, P., Schymick, J., Jain, S., Cookson, M.R., Cairns, N.J., Greggio, E., Greenway, M.J., Berger, S., Pickering-Brown, S., Chio, A., Fung, H.C., Holtzman, D.M., Huey, E.D., Wassermann, E.M., Adamson, J., Hutton, M.L., Rogaeva, E., George-Hyslop, P., Rothstein, J.D., Hardiman, O., Grafman, J., Singleton, A., Hardy, J. & Traynor, B.J. (2006). Analysis of IFT74 as a candidate gene for chromosome 9p-linked ALS-FTD. *BMC Neurol*, 6, 44

Morita, M., Al Chalabi, A., Andersen, P.M., Hosler, B., Sapp, P., Englund, E., Mitchell, J.E., Habgood, J.J., de Belleroche, J., Xi, J., Jongjaroenprasert, W., Horvitz, H.R., Gunnarsson, L.G. & Brown, R.H., Jr. (2006). A locus on chromosome 9p confers susceptibility to ALS and frontotemporal dementia. *Neurology*, 66, 6, 839-844

Neary, D., Snowden, J.S., Gustafson, L., Passant, U., Stuss, D., Black, S., Freedman, M., Kertesz, A., Robert, P.H., Albert, M., Boone, K., Miller, B.L., Cummings, J. & Benson, D.F. (1998). Frontotemporal lobar degeneration: a consensus on clinical diagnostic criteria. *Neurology*, 51, 6, 1546-1554

Neumann, M., Sampathu, D.M., Kwong, L.K., Truax, A.C., Micsenyi, M.C., Chou, T.T., Bruce, J., Schuck, T., Grossman, M., Clark, C.M., McCluskey, L.F., Miller, B.L., Masliah, E., Mackenzie, I.R., Feldman, H., Feiden, W., Kretzschmar, H.A., Trojanowski, J.Q. & Lee, V.M. (2006). Ubiquitinated TDP-43 in frontotemporal lobar degeneration and amyotrophic lateral sclerosis. *Science*, 314, 5796, 130-133

Pearson, J.P., Williams, N.M., Majounie, E., Waite, A., Stott, J., Newsway, V., Murray, A., Hernandez, D., Guerreiro, R., Singleton, A.B., Neal, J. & Morris, H.R. (2011). Familial frontotemporal dementia with amyotrophic lateral sclerosis and a shared haplotype on chromosome 9p. *J Neurol*, 258, 4, 647-655

Ravasi, T., Suzuki, H., Cannistraci, C.V., Katayama, S., Bajic, V.B., Tan, K., Akalin, A., Schmeier, S., Kanamori-Katayama, M., Bertin, N., Carninci, P., Daub, C.O., Forrest, A.R., Gough, J., Grimmond, S., Han, J.H., Hashimoto, T., Hide, W., Hofmann, O., Kamburov, A., Kaur, M., Kawaji, H., Kubosaki, A., Lassmann, T., van, N.E.,

MacPherson, C.R., Ogawa, C., Radovanovic, A., Schwartz, A., Teasdale, R.D., Tegner, J., Lenhard, B., Teichmann, S.A., Arakawa, T., Ninomiya, N., Murakami, K., Tagami, M., Fukuda, S., Imamura, K., Kai, C., Ishihara, R., Kitazume, Y., Kawai, J., Hume, D.A., Ideker, T. & Hayashizaki, Y. (2010). An atlas of combinatorial transcriptional regulation in mouse and man. *Cell*, 140, 5, 744-752

Ringholz, G.M., Appel, S.H., Bradshaw, M., Cooke, N.A., Mosnik, D.M. & Schulz, P.E. (2005). Prevalence and patterns of cognitive impairment in sporadic ALS. *Neurology*, 65, 4, 586-590

Roach, J.C., Glusman, G., Smit, A.F., Huff, C.D., Hubley, R., Shannon, P.T., Rowen, L., Pant, K.P., Goodman, N., Bamshad, M., Shendure, J., Drmanac, R., Jorde, L.B., Hood, L. & Galas, D.J. (2010). Analysis of Genetic Inheritance in a Family Quartet by Whole-Genome Sequencing. *Science*

Rollinson, S., Mead, S., Snowden, J., Richardson, A., Rohrer, J., Halliwell, N., Usher, S., Neary, D., Mann, D., Hardy, J. & Pickering-Brown, S. (2011). Frontotemporal lobar degeneration genome wide association study replication confirms a risk locus shared with amyotrophic lateral sclerosis. *Neurobiol Aging*, 32, 4, 758-7

Rosen, D.R., Siddique, T., Patterson, D., Figlewicz, D.A., Sapp, P., Hentati, A., Donaldson, D., Goto, J., O'Regan, J.P., Deng, H.X. & . (1993). Mutations in Cu/Zn superoxide dismutase gene are associated with familial amyotrophic lateral sclerosis. *Nature*, 362, 6415, 59-62

Rosso, S.M., Donker, K.L., Baks, T., Joosse, M., de, K., I, Pijnenburg, Y., de Jong, D., Dooijes, D., Kamphorst, W., Ravid, R., Niermeijer, M.F., Verheij, F., Kremer, H.P., Scheltens, P., van Duijn, C.M., Heutink, P. & van Swieten, J.C. (2003). Frontotemporal dementia in The Netherlands: patient characteristics and prevalence estimates from a population-based study. *Brain*, 126, Pt 9, 2016-2022

Rowland, L.P. & Shneider, N.A. (2001). Amyotrophic lateral sclerosis. *N Engl J Med*, 344, 22, 1688-1700

Sampathu, D.M., Neumann, M., Kwong, L.K., Chou, T.T., Micsenyi, M., Truax, A., Bruce, J., Grossman, M., Trojanowski, J.Q. & Lee, V.M. (2006). Pathological heterogeneity of frontotemporal lobar degeneration with ubiquitin-positive inclusions delineated by ubiquitin immunohistochemistry and novel monoclonal antibodies. *Am J Pathol*, 169, 4, 1343-1352

Sela, N., Mersch, B., Gal-Mark, N., Lev-Maor, G., Hotz-Wagenblatt, A. & Ast, G. (2007). Comparative analysis of transposed element insertion within human and mouse genomes reveals Alu's unique role in shaping the human transcriptome. *Genome Biol*, 8, 6, R127

Shatunov, A., Mok, K., Newhouse, S., Weale, M.E., Smith, B., Vance, C., Johnson, L., Veldink, J.H., van Es, M.A., van den Berg, L.H., Robberecht, W., Van, D.P., Hardiman, O., Farmer, A.E., Lewis, C.M., Butler, A.W., Abel, O., Andersen, P.M., Fogh, I., Silani, V., Chio, A., Traynor, B.J., Melki, J., Meininger, V., Landers, J.E., McGuffin, P., Glass, J.D., Pall, H., Leigh, P.N., Hardy, J., Brown, R.H., Jr., Powell, J.F., Orrell, R.W., Morrison, K.E., Shaw, P.J., Shaw, C.E. & Al-Chalabi, A. (2010). Chromosome 9p21 in sporadic amyotrophic lateral sclerosis in the UK and seven other countries: a genome-wide association study. *Lancet Neurol*, 9, 10, 986-994

Skibinski, G., Parkinson, N.J., Brown, J.M., Chakrabarti, L., Lloyd, S.L., Hummerich, H., Nielsen, J.E., Hodges, J.R., Spillantini, M.G., Thusgaard, T., Brandner, S., Brun, A.,

Rossor, M.N., Gade, A., Johannsen, P., Sorensen, S.A., Gydesen, S., Fisher, E.M. & Collinge, J. (2005). Mutations in the endosomal ESCRTIII-complex subunit CHMP2B in frontotemporal dementia. *Nat Genet*, 37, 8, 806-808

Sreedharan, J., Blair, I.P., Tripathi, V.B., Hu, X., Vance, C., Rogelj, B., Ackerley, S., Durnall, J.C., Williams, K.L., Buratti, E., Baralle, F., de Belleroche, J., Mitchell, J.D., Leigh, P.N., Al Chalabi, A., Miller, C.C., Nicholson, G. & Shaw, C.E. (2008). TDP-43 mutations in familial and sporadic amyotrophic lateral sclerosis. *Science*, 319, 5870, 1668-1672

Valdmanis, P.N., Dupre, N., Bouchard, J.P., Camu, W., Salachas, F., Meininger, V., Strong, M. & Rouleau, G.A. (2007). Three families with amyotrophic lateral sclerosis and frontotemporal dementia with evidence of linkage to chromosome 9p. *Arch Neurol*, 64, 2, 240-245

Van Deerlin, V.M., Leverenz, J.B., Bekris, L.M., Bird, T.D., Yuan, W., Elman, L.B., Clay, D., Wood, E.M., Chen-Plotkin, A.S., Martinez-Lage, M., Steinbart, E., McCluskey, L., Grossman, M., Neumann, M., Wu, I.L., Yang, W.S., Kalb, R., Galasko, D.R., Montine, T.J., Trojanowski, J.Q., Lee, V.M., Schellenberg, G.D. & Yu, C.E. (2008). TARDBP mutations in amyotrophic lateral sclerosis with TDP-43 neuropathology: a genetic and histopathological analysis. *Lancet Neurol*, 7, 5, 409-416

Van Deerlin, V.M., Sleiman, P.M., Martinez-Lage, M., Chen-Plotkin, A., Wang, L.S., Graff-Radford, N.R., Dickson, D.W., Rademakers, R., Boeve, B.F., Grossman, M., Arnold, S.E., Mann, D.M., Pickering-Brown, S.M., Seelaar, H., Heutink, P., van Swieten, J.C., Murrell, J.R., Ghetti, B., Spina, S., Grafman, J., Hodges, J., Spillantini, M.G., Gilman, S., Lieberman, A.P., Kaye, J.A., Woltjer, R.L., Bigio, E.H., Mesulam, M., Al-Sarraj, S., Troakes, C., Rosenberg, R.N., White, C.L., III, Ferrer, I., Llado, A., Neumann, M., Kretzschmar, H.A., Hulette, C.M., Welsh-Bohmer, K.A., Miller, B.L., Alzualde, A., de Munain, A.L., McKee, A.C., Gearing, M., Levey, A.I., Lah, J.J., Hardy, J., Rohrer, J.D., Lashley, T., Mackenzie, I.R., Feldman, H.H., Hamilton, R.L., Dekosky, S.T., van der Zee, J., Kumar-Singh, S., Van, B.C., Mayeux, R., Vonsattel, J.P., Troncoso, J.C., Kril, J.J., Kwok, J.B., Halliday, G.M., Bird, T.D., Ince, P.G., Shaw, P.J., Cairns, N.J., Morris, J.C., McLean, C.A., DeCarli, C., Ellis, W.G., Freeman, S.H., Frosch, M.P., Growdon, J.H., Perl, D.P., Sano, M., Bennett, D.A., Schneider, J.A., Beach, T.G., Reiman, E.M., Woodruff, B.K., Cummings, J., Vinters, H.V., Miller, C.A., Chui, H.C., Alafuzoff, I., Hartikainen, P., Seilhean, D., Galasko, D., Masliah, E., Cotman, C.W., Tunon, M.T., Martinez, M.C., Munoz, D.G., Carroll, S.L., Marson, D., Riederer, P.F., Bogdanovic, N., Schellenberg, G.D., Hakonarson, H., Trojanowski, J.Q. & Lee, V.M. (2010). Common variants at 7p21 are associated with frontotemporal lobar degeneration with TDP-43 inclusions. *Nat Genet*, 42, 3, 234-239

van Es, M.A., Veldink, J.H., Saris, C.G., Blauw, H.M., van Vught, P.W., Birve, A., Lemmens, R., Schelhaas, H.J., Groen, E.J., Huisman, M.H., Van Der Kooi, A.J., De, V.M., Dahlberg, C., Estrada, K., Rivadeneira, F., Hofman, A., Zwarts, M.J., van Doormaal, P.T., Rujescu, D., Strengman, E., Giegling, I., Muglia, P., Tomik, B., Slowik, A., Uitterlinden, A.G., Hendrich, C., Waibel, S., Meyer, T., Ludolph, A.C., Glass, J.D., Purcell, S., Cichon, S., Nothen, M.M., Wichmann, H.E., Schreiber, S., Vermeulen, S.H., Kiemeney, L.A., Wokke, J.H., Cronin, S., McLaughlin, R.L., Hardiman, O., Fumoto, K., Pasterkamp, R.J., Meininger, V., Melki, J., Leigh, P.N., Shaw, C.E., Landers, J.E., Al-Chalabi, A., Brown, R.H., Jr., Robberecht, W., Andersen, P.M.,

Ophoff, R.A. & van den Berg, L.H. (2009). Genome-wide association study identifies 19p13.3 (UNC13A) and 9p21.2 as susceptibility loci for sporadic amyotrophic lateral sclerosis. *Nat Genet*, 41, 10, 1083-1087

Van Langenhove, T., van der Zee, J., Sleegers, K., Engelborghs, S., Vandenberghe, R., Gijselinck, I., Van den Broeck, M., Mattheijssens, M., Peeters, K., De Deyn, P.P., Cruts, M. & Van, B.C. (2010). Genetic contribution of FUS to frontotemporal lobar degeneration. *Neurology*, 74, 5, 366-371

Vance, C., Al Chalabi, A., Ruddy, D., Smith, B.N., Hu, X., Sreedharan, J., Siddique, T., Schelhaas, H.J., Kusters, B., Troost, D., Baas, F., de, J., V & Shaw, C.E. (2006). Familial amyotrophic lateral sclerosis with frontotemporal dementia is linked to a locus on chromosome 9p13.2-21.3. *Brain*, 129, Pt 4, 868-876

Vance, C., Rogelj, B., Hortobagyi, T., De Vos, K.J., Nishimura, A.L., Sreedharan, J., Hu, X., Smith, B., Ruddy, D., Wright, P., Ganesalingam, J., Williams, K.L., Tripathi, V., Al Saraj, S., Al Chalabi, A., Leigh, P.N., Blair, I.P., Nicholson, G., de Belleroche, J., Gallo, J.M., Miller, C.C. & Shaw, C.E. (2009). Mutations in FUS, an RNA processing protein, cause familial amyotrophic lateral sclerosis type 6. *Science*, 323, 5918, 1208-1211

Watts, G.D., Wymer, J., Kovach, M.J., Mehta, S.G., Mumm, S., Darvish, D., Pestronk, A., Whyte, M.P. & Kimonis, V.E. (2004). Inclusion body myopathy associated with Paget disease of bone and frontotemporal dementia is caused by mutant valosin-containing protein. *Nat Genet*, 36, 4, 377-381

Yan J, Slifer S, Siddique N, Chen W, Yong S, Erdong L, Haines JL, Pericak-Vance M, Siddique T. 2008. Fine-Mapping and Candidate Gene Sequencing of the Chromosome 9p Locus of ALS/FTD.

Yokoseki, A., Shiga, A., Tan, C.F., Tagawa, A., Kaneko, H., Koyama, A., Eguchi, H., Tsujino, A., Ikeuchi, T., Kakita, A., Okamoto, K., Nishizawa, M., Takahashi, H. & Onodera, O. (2008). TDP-43 mutation in familial amyotrophic lateral sclerosis. *Ann Neurol*, 63, 4, 538-542

Part 5

Clinical Research in ALS

24

Multidisciplinary Rehabilitation in Amyotrophic Lateral Sclerosis

Louisa Ng and Fary Khan
Royal Melbourne Hospital and University of Melbourne
Australia

1. Introduction

Amyotrophic Lateral Sclerosis (ALS) is the most common chronic neurodegenerative disorder of the motor system in adults. It is a relatively rare disease with a reported population incidence of between 1.5 and 2.5 per 100,000 per year worldwide and a gender ratio of 3:2 men: women. Amyotrophic Lateral Sclerosis is characterized by the loss of motor neurons in the cortex, brain stem, and spinal cord, manifested by upper and lower motor neuron signs and symptoms affecting bulbar, limb, and respiratory muscles. Death usually results from respiratory failure and follows on average two to four years after onset, but some may survive for a decade or more.

Amyotrophic Lateral Sclerosis is a devastating condition with unknown aetiology and no current cure. The symptoms in ALS are diverse and challenging and include weakness, spasticity, limitations in mobility and activities of daily living, communication deficits and dysphagia, and in those with bulbar involvement, respiratory compromise, fatigue and sleep disorders, pain and psychosocial distress. The International Classification of Functioning, Disability and Health (ICF) (World Health Organization, 2001), defines a common language for describing the impact of disease at different levels: impairment (body structure and function), limitation in activity and participation (see Figure 1). Within this framework ALS related impairments (weakness, spasticity), can limit ''activity'' or function (decreased mobility, self-care, pain) and ''participation'' (driving, employment, family, social reintegration). ''Contextual factors'', such as environmental (extrinsic) and personal factors (intrinsic) interact with all the other constructs to shape the impact of ALS on patients and their families. The impact of ALS upon patients, their caregivers (often family members) and on society is substantial, often beginning long before the actual diagnosis is made, and increasing with increasing disability and the need for medical equipment and assisted care (Klein and Forshew, 1996).

Given the broad spectrum of needs, current management spans from diagnosis (acute neurological needs) through to symptomatic and supportive rehabilitation and palliative care. The interface between neurology, rehabilitation and palliative care is of utmost importance to ensure co-ordinated care for persons with ALS rather than duplicating services (Royal College of Physicians National Council for Palliative Care and British Society of Rehabilitation Medicine, 2008). It should be noted however that the focus of this chapter is on the rehabilitation phases, hence discussion of acute neurological and palliative care aspects are limited.

Rehabilitation is defined as "a problem solving educational process aimed at reducing disability and increasing participation experienced by someone as a result of disease or injury" (Wade, 1992). Although it is sometimes effective in reducing impairment, its principal focus is to reduce symptoms and limitations at the level of activity and participation, through holistic interventions, which incorporate personal and environmental factors. The multidisciplinary rehabilitation team (see Figure 2) comprises of a group of clinical professionals with expertise in ALS, directed by a physician, who work as an integrated unit to provide seamless care which is patient-centred, flexible and responsive to the evolving nature of the condition (Hardiman, 2007). The role of multidisciplinary rehabilitation in ALS is supported by a recent Cochrane review (Ng et al., 2009) which suggested some advantage for quality of life without increasing healthcare costs, reduced hospitalisation and improved disability with conflicting evidence for survival.

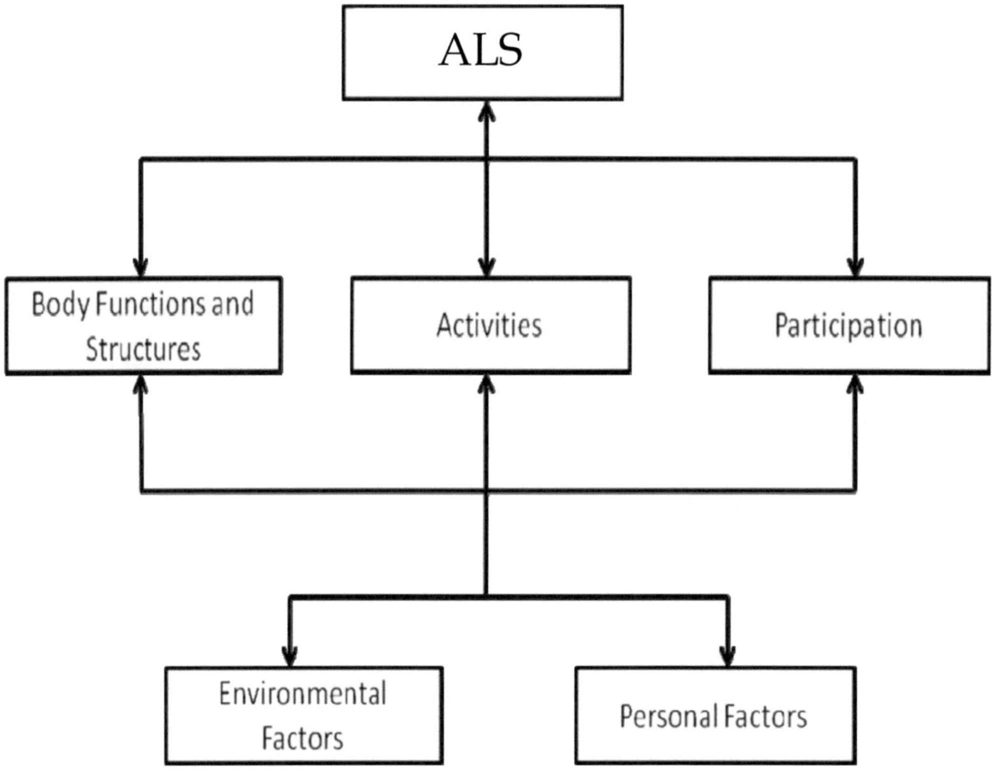

Fig. 1. The interaction between the various domains of the International Classification of Functioning, Disability and Health (adapted from (World Health Organization, 2001))

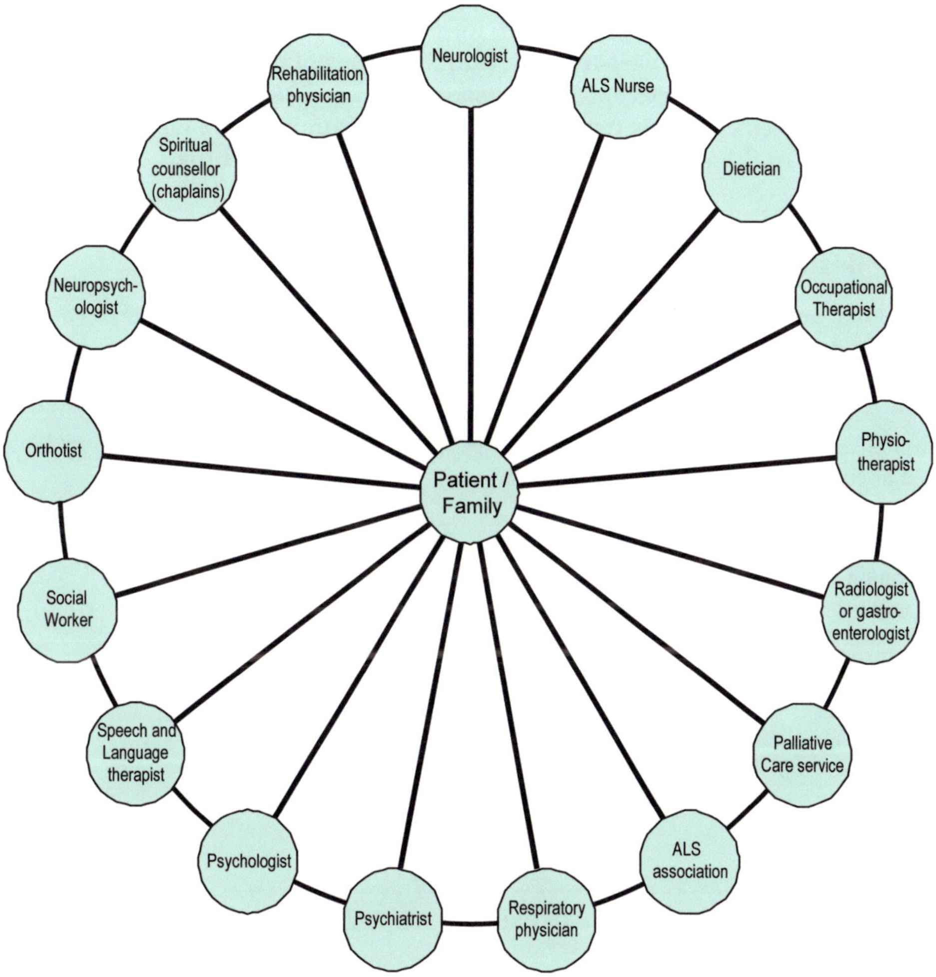

Fig. 2. The multidisciplinary rehabilitation team in ALS (adapted from (Hardiman, 2007))

A proposed model for service interaction in caring for persons with ALS shows involvement of neurologists and palliative care teams in the acute and terminal phases of care, with a relatively smaller role for rehabilitation physicians. However rehabilitation plays a major role in long-term care and support (over years) in the more slowly progressive phase (Royal College of Physicians National Council for Palliative Care and British Society of Rehabilitation Medicine, 2008). Early rehabilitation intervention and treatment has much to contribute to improve health and quality of life prior to accumulation of disability through symptomatic and supportive therapies to enhance functional independence and community integration and reduce barriers (such as lack of knowledge about treatment, economic constraints) (Kemp, 2005). Disability management in ALS should also be planned, with deficits should be anticipated (over time) to avoid "crisis management". As patients deteriorate the rehabilitation and palliative care approaches can overlap, i.e. "neuropalliative rehabilitation". Key skills in neuropalliative rehabilitation include: understanding disease progression, symptom control,

managing expectations, issues relating to communication, addressing end of life issues, legal issues (mental capacity, wills), specialist interventions (ventilation), equipment needs, counselling and support, and welfare advice (Royal College of Physicians National Council for Palliative Care and British Society of Rehabilitation Medicine, 2008).
The literature presented in this review includes all levels of evidence for multidisciplinary rehabilitation of ALS (including randomised and clinical controlled trials, case studies and expert opinion).

2. Rehabilitation issues in ALS

Amyotrophic Lateral Sclerosis is a fatal disease with a challenging progressive course that results in a broad and ever-changing spectrum of care needs. Symptoms are varied (see Table 1) and need to be carefully assessed and managed. The timing of provision of appropriate care is important as whilst information needs to be provided when patients are psychologically in the right frame of mind, the options of certain interventions may be time-limited as the disease continues to progress.

Weakness	94%
Dysphagia	90%
Dyspnoea	85%
Pain	73%
Weight loss	71%
Speech issues	71%
Constipation	54%
Cough	48%
Sleep issues	29%
Emotional lability	27%
Drooling	25%

Table 1. Symptoms experienced by ALS patients (adapted from (Oliver, 1996))

2.1 Respiratory dysfunction

Most deaths in ALS are due to respiratory failure from respiratory muscle weakness, hence the diagnosis and management of respiratory symptoms is important (Figure 3) (Miller et al., 2009a). Counselling may be initiated at the time of diagnosis especially if respiratory symptoms are present and/or forced vital capacity (FVC) is <60% of predicted. Early symptoms may be suggestive of nocturnal hypoventilation (eg. frequent arousals, morning headaches, excessive daytime sleepiness, vivid dreams) rather than overt dyspnoea (Miller et al., 2009a). It is important to discuss the options of respiratory choices, including tracheostomy and ventilatory support well before these are clinically indicated to enable advance planning or directives. It is also important to offer patients information about the terminal stages of ALS and reassure regarding terminal hypercapnoeic coma and resulting peaceful death, as many may fear "choking to death" (Borasio et al., 2001b).
Respiratory function should be evaluated every three months from the time of diagnosis. Whilst FVC is the most commonly used (Melo et al., 1999) and significantly predicts survival (Czaplinski et al., 2006), it can be insensitive to slight changes in muscle strength (Fitting et al., 1999). The maximal sniff nasal inspiratory force (sniff nasal pressure) may be more

appropriate especially in those with bulbar weakness (no mouthpiece) and may be more sensitive to changes in diaphragmatic and respiratory muscle strength (Stefanutti et al., 2000;Lyall et al., 2001). It is also more reliably recorded in the later stages of ALS (Morgan et al., 2005).

Initial management can include chest physiotherapy and postural drainage, especially if the patient has difficulty clearing secretions from the chest (Shaw, 2003). A suction machine may also be helpful. Preventing respiratory infections is a primary goal and pneumococcal and influenza vaccines should be administered. Respiratory muscle exercise can be instituted and may delay the onset of ventilatory failure (Schiffman, 1996).

Non-invasive ventilation (NIV) should be considered in respiratory dysfunction (see Figure 3) especially for nocturnal symptomatic respiratory compromise. A recent Cochrane review concluded that NIV significantly improves quality of life when tolerated and may prolong survival in those with normal to moderately impaired bulbar function especially if used for ≥ 4 hours/day (Radunovic et al., 2009). Successful use of NIV is dependent on respiratory therapists and patients working closely and patiently through the adjustment phase of NIV, especially with selection and tolerance of face masks. A small dose of anxiolytic may assist with the process in select patients. Bulbar involvement and executive dysfunction may also reduce compliance (Miller et al., 2009a).

Invasive ventilation should be offered when longer-term survival is the goal. Counselling is necessary with regards to benefits and burden (expense, intensive physical support with suctioning and nursing care, high caregiver burden) as many may not be able to manage invasive ventilation at home, thus requiring nursing home placement (Kaub-Wittemer et al., 2003;Miller et al., 2009a). There is evidence however that the 10-20% of persons with ALS who undergo invasive ventilation (including those administered at the time of acute respiratory failure without advance discussion) appear to have good acceptance and satisfactory quality of life (Vianello et al., 2010).

2.2 Communication

Dysarthria is common as a result of bulbar involvement and is often a source of significant frustration to the persons with ALS and their families. Early changes include nasality or reduced vocal volume and changes in oral movement rates and speech rates (Yorkston et al., 1993). As weakness and spasticity of the oral and laryngeal muscles increase, imprecise consonant production, hypernasality, harsh vocal quality, slowed rate of speech and breath volumes affect intelligibility (Hillel and Miller, 1989). Speech pathologists can teach the patient to slow speech rate, exaggerate articulation and improve respiratory efficiency through phrasing (Francis et al., 1999). Palatal lift and palatal augmentation prostheses may also be of some use to reduce the hypernasal aspect of dysarthria (Esposito et al., 2000).

As intelligibility in ALS worsens, Augmentative and Alternative Communication (AAC) is required. AACs can improve quality of life by optimising function and assisting with decision making (Brownlee and Palovcak, 2007). AACs range from no or low technology (gestures, communication boards with letters) to high-tech electronic communication devices that allow the user to have voice output (Brownlee and Palovcak, 2007). For example, speech-generating devices such as LightWRITERs are commonly used. These devices can be used as long as there is voluntary motor movement (including eye gaze). The specific access method depends on the abilities of the patient - for example, pointing with a body part or pointer, adapted mice or joysticks or switches and scanning technology can be used. For those who have no voluntary motor control for communication, a recent case study using a brain-computer interface system has been reported and appears promising (Sellers et al., 2010). The emotional aspect of using an alternative form of communication however can result in significant patient resistance and acceptance as the ability to speak and use language is what distinguishes us from all other species (Pinker and Jackendoff, 2005;Brownlee and Palovcak, 2007). Hence, acceptance of an AAC may take weeks to months.

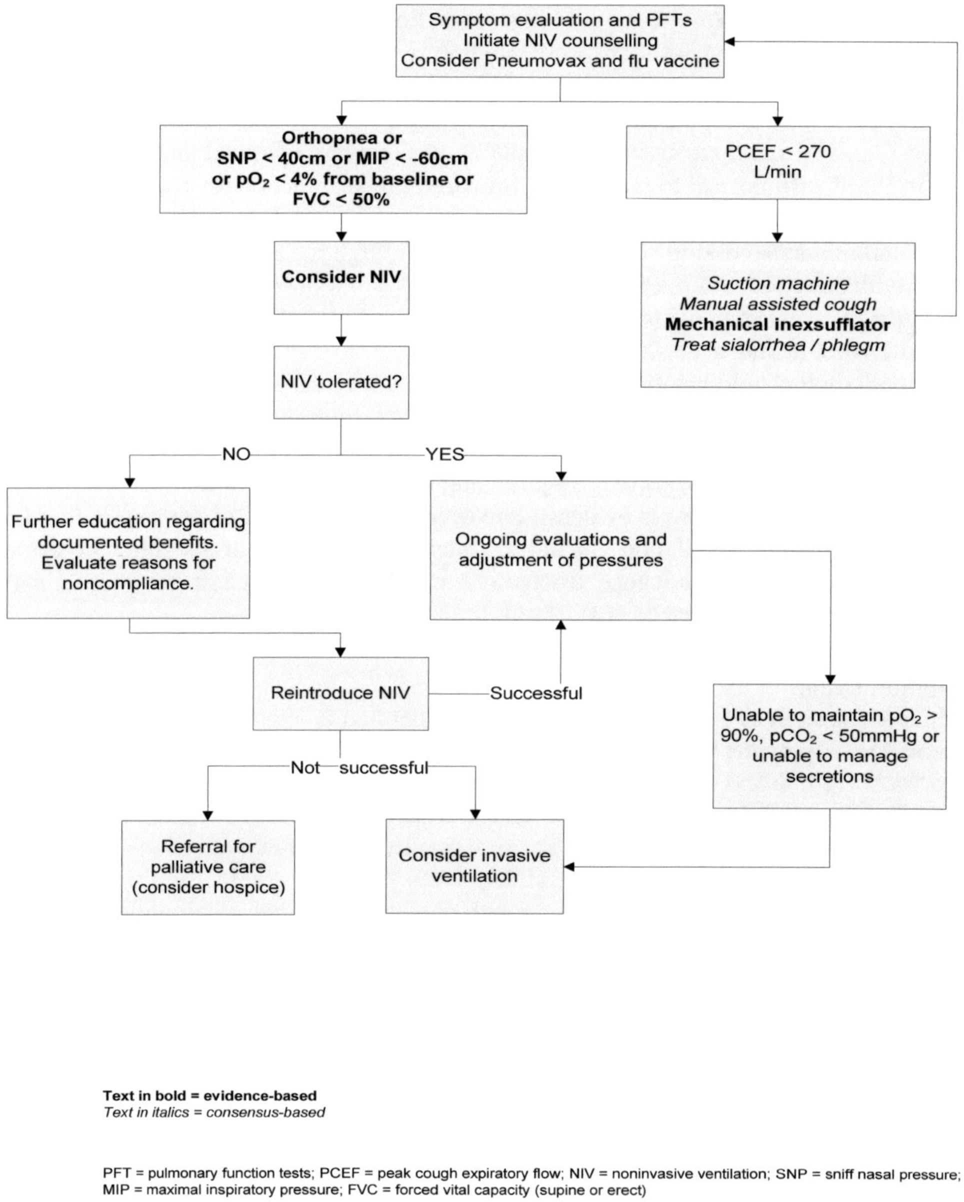

Fig. 3. Respiratory management algorithm in ALS (adapted from (Miller et al., 2009a))

A source of significant frustration for those with speech difficulties is use of the telephone. Technology is available and varies from country to country. In the United States, "Speech to Speech" technology can be used, where trained communication assistants are used by the patient to complete phone calls. They are trained to use superior equipment to hear the caller and place the call, then repeat verbatim what the caller says so the call is completed successfully .

2.3 Swallowing and nutrition

Dysphagia affects a third of persons with ALS at onset and the majority by late disease (Higo et al., 2004). It increases the risk of suboptimal caloric and fluid intake and can worsen weakness and fatigue (Borasio, 2001). Aspiration pneumonia (13%) is a contributor to respiratory complications and is associated with increased mortality with mean survival time post-infection of 2 months (Sorenson et al., 2007).

Difficulties in the oral preparatory stage of swallowing (preparation of food for propulsion to the pharynx) is common (Mayberry and Atkinson, 1986). Symptoms include jaw weakness, fatigue, drooling, choking on food and slow eating. In addition, loss of upper limb function and fear of choking or depression can further impact on self-feeding abilities and oral intake (Slowie et al., 1983). A speech pathologist can evaluate the degree of dysphagia through bed-side assessments and/or further imaging (eg videofluroscopy). Mild dysphagia can be managed with specific interventions such a alteration of food consistency, upright positioning, small bolus size, soft collar for neck extensor weakness and the chin-tuck technique, in which the person flexes their neck to the anterior chest wall as they swallow, narrowing the inlet to the larynx and reducing the chance of food aspiration. Dieticians monitor nutritional status through body weight, percentage weight loss and body mass index. Common advice includes high calorie diets, texture modification and prescription of nutritional supplements (Rio and Cawadias, 2007). Patients may show nutritional compromise even before bulbar symptoms become significant (Slowie et al., 1983) as in addition to muscle wasting, persons with ALS at all stages of disease often do not meet their energy requirements (Kasarskis and Neville, 1996). Dehydration is also a common and important problem contributing to fatigue and thickened secretions (Francis et al., 1999).

As dysphagia progresses, evidence (Level B) suggests a percutaneous endoscopic gastrostomy (PEG) or equivalent (eg. radiologically inserted gastrostomy) is indicated to supplement oral intake (as long as this remains safe) for weight maintenance (Loser et al., 2005). PEGs prolong survival but there is currently little evidence regarding the impact of PEG on quality of life (Langmore et al., 2006). Timing of a PEG can be challenging. Indicators may include weight loss (5-10% of body weight loss implies nutritional risk (Francis et al., 1999)) and reduced FVC. If FVC falls below 50% of predicted (Kasarskis et al., 1999), risks of largyngeal spasm, localised infection, gastric haemorrhage, technical difficulties of PEG placement and respiratory arrest increase (Mazzini et al., 1995;Mathus-Vliegen et al., 1994)).

Sialorrhoea can be a significant issue in ALS and is generally not related to increased saliva production but rather to impaired ability to swallow saliva, combined with facial weakness causing labial incompetence and neck weakness causing the head to tip forward (Francis et al., 1999). Improved positioning, use of a cervical collar and orolingual exercises may be helpful. Medications such as anticholinergics and tricyclics can also be trialled (Schiffman and Belsh, 1996), as can suction machines. In the US, most commonly used medications are amitriptyline, glycopyrrolate, atropine and propantheline (Forshew and Bromberg, 2003). However, medications may further thicken secretions, hence should be used with caution in those with respiratory insufficiency or poor cough. More recently, botulinum toxin injected into the salivary glands (parotid, submandibular) appears to be safe and has been used to treat sialorrhea with beneficial effects lasting approximately 3 months (Verma and Steele, 2006;Contarino et al., 2007). Thick oropharyngeal secretions may be treated with increased fluid intake, humidification of air, cough augmentation, suction machines and guaifenesin (Forshew and Bromberg, 2003).

2.4 Exercise

The effects of exercise and safe therapeutic range in ALS are poorly understood. It is generally thought that weakness and muscle fibre degeneration may be accelerated by overwork or heavy exercise as it is already functioning close to its maximal limits (Johnson and Braddom, 1971). However, inactivity leads to deconditioning and disuse weakness. In addition, muscle and joint spasticity can cause pain, contractures and further loss of function. A recent Cochrane review (Dalbello-Haas et al., 2008) identified two trials (n = 52), which addressed therapeutic exercise in ALS. The trials examined the effects of moderate intensity, endurance type exercise on spasticity, and effects of moderate intensity resistance type exercises in ALS. Although one of the trials reported improvement in function and quality of life, both trials were too small to determine to what extent strengthening exercises were beneficial or harmful in this population (Dalbello-Haas et al., 2008). A more recent pilot study demonstrated that repetitive rhythmic exercise - supported treadmill ambulation training was feasible, tolerated and safe for patients with ALS and appeared to improve work capacity and gait functioning in patients with ALS who were dependent on assistive devices for ambulation (Sanjak et al., 2010). In view of the paucity of evidence to guide exercise prescription, the current recommendations are (Chen et al., 2008):

- Stretching exercise to improve flexibility to maintain muscle length and joint mobility and prevent contractures.
- Strengthening exercise of sub-maximal (low, non-fatiguing) intensity, with degree of resistance tailored to muscle strength.
- Aerobic/endurance exercise may improve cardio-respiratory fitness and is probably safe but adequate oxygenation, aeration and carbohydrate load is important to reduce oxidative stress load. Supported treadmill ambulation training can be considered if available.

2.5 Mobility and activities of daily living

In early stages of disease, rehabilitation aims to prolong independence in mobility and activities of daily living, prevent complications such as falls, contractures, and musculoskeletal pain, maintain strength, range of movement and conditioning through an appropriate exercise program, educate the patient and family about the disease, provide psychological support, evaluate the home for safety and teach energy conservation techniques (Khanna et al., 2007).

As weakness worsens, the physiotherapist can instruct the patient and family in safe transfer techniques (eg. between bed and chair, in and out of cars), optimise gait pattern and provide gait re-training with appropriate gait aids (eg. walking frame, sticks) and orthoses (ankle-foot orthosis to facilitate foot clearance during gait and stabilise knee to prevent falls). Occupational therapists can fabricate with upper limb orthoses to assist with fine motor function. For example, patients with distal weakness can improve hand function with wrists braced in 30° extension which improves efficiency of grip and addition of a universal cuff can assist those with weak grasp in feeding and typing (Francis et al., 1999). Other adaptive equipment is also provided, such as built-up cutlery for eating, Velcro fasteners for dressing, long-handled aids, and bathroom equipment (rails, over-the-toilet frames, bath boards, shower chairs, commodes). Wheelchairs are generally eventually required although introduction of a wheelchair whilst a patient is still ambulant, for intermittent community use, is important to enhance energy conservation. Future needs should be anticipated and considered when prescribing a powered wheelchair (eg. reclining, tilt-in-space, custom seating, and modifiable control system) to optimise independence and social interaction whilst preventing contractures, compression nerve palsies, skin breakdown and aspiration. A motorised scooter may be more appropriate for some patients (Francis et al., 1999). Other equipment such as hospital beds with pressure-relieving mattress and hoists for lifting might also be required. Caregiver training in the use of hoists is important to prevent injury.

A recent study (n=44) (Ng et al., 2011) showed that a small but significant gap exists from the perspective of persons with ALS with regards to advice and assistance relating to continued employment and driving. Healthcare providers may underestimate the importance of maintaining employment as a priority in a fatal condition such as ALS and hence under treat this issue. For these persons, the use of assistive technology may be particularly useful, especially in employment where computer use is crucial. Computer technology is fast advancing and options include different types of keyboards, mouse alternatives, switches, interfaces, mounting systems, integrated communication/computer access packages, software and systems. For those who have some proximal arm control, track balls, type writing sticks and forearm supports may be useful. In persons with ALS who have more severe upper limb weakness, head tracking systems, on-screen keyboards and voice recognition software may be required. Text-entry software such as Dasher (which is free) can be used whenever a full-size keyboard cannot be used such as on a palmtop computer or with a joystick, touchscreen, trackball, headpointer, or eyetracker . There are also many mouse alternatives available -- eyegaze system, foot control mouse, head tracking mouse, joysticks and switch-adapted mouse.

Assistive technology can have a dramatic effect on restoring and maintaining independence, a sense of control and quality of life. Apart from technologies that assist with mobility and communication which have already been discussed, other forms of assistive technology such as environmental control units (ECU) should be considered. Environmental control systems offer sophisticated electronics to enable people with a range of impairments and severe disability to use a wide variety of electrical devices. Aids may include unobtrusive control units (eg. remote control for TV), home security (door intercoms, door release and alarms), adapted telephones (such as hands-free control) and lighting and heating/cooling systems (Wellings and Unsworth, 1997). These environmental control units may be used to facilitate function and decrease reliance on carers, improve family dynamics and improve patients' self-esteem (Wellings and Unsworth, 1997). It is important for patients, families and therapists to work closely together when prescribing and using assistive technology to ensure the correct, safe and optimal use of such aids and equipment; and to anticipate future needs especially with the expense of such technology. Close collaboration with specialised providers of assistive technology that can provide back-up technical support is also crucial.

2.6 Bladder, bowel and sexuality

Although bowel and bladder sphincters are generally spared, bowel, bladder and sexual dysfunction may be much more common (30%) than reported to health professionals by persons with ALS (Ng et al., 2011). These areas are in general poorly studied in ALS. Constipation is common with inactivity and poor nutritional intake, and can be treated with a regular bowel program with intake of fibre/bulking agents and adequate fluids. Suppositories, stool softeners and enemas should be considered. In one of the few studies addressing bladder function in ALS (n=38), 47% had micturition symptoms and urodynamics studies found a range of UMN abnormalities (Hattori et al., 1983). Where urinary urgency is an issue, oxybutinin may be helpful. Contributory factors to incontinence, such as urinary tract infections, drinking large amount of fluids late in the day and dependent oedema causing nocturia when the legs are elevated overnight should be considered and treated. Wasner et al (Wasner et al., 2004) suggested a prevalence of 62% (n=62) in sexual dysfunction with issues including decreased libido and passivity of the patient and partner due to physical weakness and the body image changes. The wide variation in reported prevalence in bowel, bladder and sexual dysfunction suggests that patients may not volunteer this information; hence its inclusion in routine enquiries might help to encourage reporting and thus the facilitation of appropriate treatment, such as sexual counselling and suggestion of specific techniques.

2.7 Pain

Pain is common in ALS (50% in a recent study (Ng et al., 2011)), especially in the later stages. Fatigue and depressive symptoms may also worsen a patient's experience of pain.

Spasticity and muscle spasms are not an uncommon source of pain and with the current paucity of supporting evidence, this is often treated with stretching exercises in combination with a muscle relaxant (baclofen is the drug of choice) (Ashworth et al., 2006). Baclofen should be started at low doses (5mg twice to three times daily) and slowly increased (up to 100mg a day in divided doses). Baclofen however can be associated with muscle weakness. Tizanidine (2mg twice daily up to 24 mg a day) is likely as efficacious but it is associated with dry mouth. Other options include clonidine (25 µg twice a day) which can cause hypotension, drowsiness and bradycardia and benzodiazepines which can cause sedation and habituation and respiratory depression. Dantrolene is not recommended as it can cause excessive muscle weakness in ALS (Krivickas and Carter, 2005). Intrathecal baclofen is rarely required but may be indicated in those with intractable spasticity, needing more than the maximum oral dose (Marquardt and Seifert, 2002). There are few reports of use of botulinum toxin for spasticity in ALS in literature. Caution is advised as persons with ALS may be more prone to developing generalised weakness after being injected with botulinum toxin A to treat spasticity (Mezaki et al., 1996).

Muscle cramps can cause severe pain and discomfort and are a result of spontaneous activity of motor units induced by contraction of shortened muscles (Norris et al., 1957). The list of potentially useful drugs for cramps is extensive, implying efficacy of individual agents is low and variable and the evidence base weak. In the US, quinine (35%), baclofen (19%), phenytoin (10%), and gabapentin (7%) were the preferred agents (Forshew and Bromberg, 2003); in Europe, choices were quinine (58%), benzodiazepines (40%), magnesium (25%) and carbamazepine (23%) (Borasio et al., 2001a). In 2006 however, the US Food and Drug administration restricted the use of quinine sulfate in the US to treatment of

malaria falciparum because of concerns regarding severe adverse events, including cardioarthymias, thrombocytopaenia, severe hypersentivity reactions and serious drug interaction (U.S. Food and Drug Administration, 2006).
In advanced disease, pain often results due to immobility. Musculoskeletal pain from weakness and resulting postural changes can be ameliorated with range of motion exercises, adequate support in sitting and supine positions and proper lifting and transfer techniques to prevent undue traction on weakened joints. Equipment such as motorised beds that slowly rotate from the side to side can be useful for reducing caregiver burden (Francis et al., 1999). Analgesia such as nonsteroidal anti-inflammatory drugs or narcotics (oral or sublingual) may also be required (with careful respiratory status monitoring in the latter). Intramuscular delivery of medications should be avoided due to muscle wasting (Mayadev et al., 2008).

2.8 Fatigue and sleep disorders

Fatigue is a common disability in ALS - 77-83% in recent studies (Ng et al., 2011;Ramirez et al., 2008) but understudied and often overlooked by clinicians (Lou, 2008). It is unrelated to clinical strength as a large component of fatigue in ALS has a central origin (Kent-Braun and Miller, 2000). Fatigue in ALS does not correlate directly with gender, educational level, disease duration, physical function, quality of life, dyspnoea, depression or sleepiness (Ramirez et al., 2008). However, contributory factors may include sepsis (including aspiration), depression and/or anxiety, pain, hypoventilation, positioning, sleep disruption and effortful activity and these should be treated where possible. It may manifest as reduced energy, difficulty in maintaining sustained attention and increased motor weakness, incoordination and gait difficulties. No double-blind, placebo-controlled trials have been performed for treatment of fatigue. Physostigmine is sometimes prescribed but not necessarily effective (Norris et al., 1993). Modafinil appears to be well-tolerated in a recent small open-label study (n=15) and may reduce symptoms of fatigue (Carter et al., 2005). Rehabilitation strategies involve pacing activities (regular rest breaks), energy conservation and fatigue management strategies, addressing sleep disorders, consideration of exercise to improve fitness if appropriate and treating other exacerbating factors.
High incidence of sleep disturbance in ALS has been reported with pain, micturition, and choking listed by patients as the most common causes for awakening (Kinnear et al., 1997 Nov 3-5). Other contributors to poor sleep include abnormal nocturnal movements such as periodic leg movements or fragmentary myoclonus, which was demonstrated on polysomnography in almost all patients with fatigue (Kinnear et al., 1997 Nov 3-5). Such movements may be treated with controlled release carbidopa-levodopa (Sinemet CR) (Sufit, 1997). Antihistamines (eg. diphenhydramine) and other sedatives (eg. Chloral hydrate 250-500mg, benzodiazepines) can also be considered once respiratory causes for sleep disturbance have been ruled out.

2.9 Cognition and behavioural impairment

Cognitive impairment is increasingly recognised in ALS -- 50% are thought to have frontal executive deficits (see Table 2) (Lomen-Hoerth et al., 2003). Visuospatial function, praxis and memory storage are usually spared (Massman et al., 1996;Abrahams et al., 2005;Ringholz et al., 2005). Use of memory aids such as diaries, planners and structured daily routine is encouraged. Other conditions (depression, anxiety, fatigue) and medications (anticholinergics, benzodiazepines) should be monitored as they can worsen cognitive function.

Behavioural changes unrelated to mood or cognition has also been noted although estimates of prevalence vary widely (Woolley and Jonathan, 2008). Marked apathy occurs in an estimated 55% of persons with ALS (Grossman et al., 2007).This correlates with deficits in verbal fluency but not depression, disease duration, FVC or ALSFRS scores and may be related to fatigue, respiratory weakness, impaired sleep, anxiety or medication (Woolley and Jonathan, 2008). It may also be a psychological coping mechanism (Woolley and Jonathan, 2008).

In a subset of persons with ALS (approximately 5%), clear fronto-temporal dementia (also known as fronto-temporal lobar degeneration) is the presenting picture with severe behavioural dysfunction (insidious onset with gradual progression, altered social conduct, impaired regulation of personal conduct, emotional blunting, loss of insight) that begins before motor weakness becomes obvious (Woolley and Jonathan, 2008). In addition, those with fronto-temporal dementia may exhibit disinhibition, restlessness, reduced empathy, lack of foresight, impulsiveness, social withdrawal, verbal stereotypes, verbal or motor perseveration and/or sexual hyperactivity (Neary et al., 1998).

Management of behavioural and cognitive deficits can be challenging and begins with the identification of these issues. An assessment by a neuropsychologist is often helpful in terms of defining the deficits and provision of cognitive and behavioural remediation strategies. Education and counselling of the patient and family is important. No trials have been conducted in efficacy of pharmacological interventions in this area; however the use of antidepressants and antipsychotics may be considered.

Attention and concentration
Working memory
Cognitive flexibility (rigidity)
Response inhibition
"Executive function" - Planning/problem/solving/abstract reasoning
Visual-perceptual skills
Memory
Word generation (fluency)

Table 2 Cognitive deficits in ALS (adapted from (Woolley and Jonathan, 2008))

2.10 Pseudobulbar affect

Pseudobulbar affect describes sudden uncontrollable outbursts of laughter or tearfulness and is a result of bilateral corticobulbar tract degeneration (Rosen and Cummings, 2007). It is common, affecting between 50-70% of persons with ALS (Palmieri et al., 2009) especially those with the bulbar form of ALS. Pseudobulbar affect can have a significant impact on anxiety and emotional frailty (Palmieri et al., 2009), social functioning and relationships in persons with ALS as these sudden, frequent, extreme, uncontrollable emotional outbursts may lead to severe embarrassment and social withdrawal (Moore et al., 1997).

Despite the prevalence of this issue, less than 15% ask for treatment (Meininger, 2005). Education of the persons with ALS and their family and friends assists with understanding and acceptance of these pathological and involuntary outbursts and is an important component of the appropriate treatment of pseudobulbar affect. Crying associated with pseudobulbar affect is easily incorrectly interpreted as depression; laughter may be embarrassing. Pharmacological treatment can include amitryiptiline (10-150mg nocte, starting with 10mg and slowly increasing the dose) which also has the positive benefit on weight loss and loss of appetite (Meininger, 2005) or fluvoxamine (100-200mg daily). A more recent study (n=140) showed that dextromethorphan and quinidine in combination appears to be more effective in reducing the frequency and severity of psudobulbar affect and to improve quality of life) (Brooks et al., 2004). However, side effects are also more common (nausea, dizziness, gastrointestinal complaints) (Brooks et al., 2004).

2.11 Psychosocial issues

ALS is a devastating condition, which takes its toll on the patient and family especially as the disease progresses, and loss of independence occurs. Rates of depression and anxiety are reported to be 0-44% and 0-30% respectively in persons with ALS (Kurt et al., 2007) and depression does not appear to increase in more advanced disease (Rabkin et al., 2005). Quality of life also appears to be more dependent on psychological and existential factors than physical factors (Goldstein et al., 2006b;Simmons et al., 2000). Amongst caregivers, 23% are depressed (Rabkin et al., 2009) and caregiver strain is often significant as a result of increased caregiving time, cognitive impairments in persons with ALS, emotional labour and socio-economic considerations (Chio et al., 2006;Goldstein et al., 2006a;Ray and Street, 2006). Hence, referrals to support groups and counselling and education of patients and their families (often their caregivers) are essential. Frank discussions facilitate understanding of the disease and improve coping skills. Carer support (both physical and emotional) and respite care should be discussed. Referrals to the local ALS associations are also recommended as these provide patients and families with ongoing support, resources and equipment needs. Psychotherapy should also be considered to assist with coping strategies (Matuz et al., 2010). Antidepressants such as amitriptyline and selective serotonin reuptake inhibitors may be used, the former being also useful for other symptoms such as drooling, pseudobulbar affect and insomnia. Anxiety is difficult to measure due to physical confounding symptoms such as shortness of breath, muscle cramps and restlessness. Anxiety can be treated with psychotherapy and training in relaxation and breathing techniques, as well as participation in support groups. It is generally thought that the rates of anxiety increase in the pre-terminal stage (Kurt et al., 2007), hence anxiolytics at this time such as benzodiazepines should be offered. With good support, mental health and quality of life can remain stable despite deteriorating physical health (De Groot et al., 2007).

2.12 End of life issues

It is important to establish an open environment of communication with persons with ALS and their families from the time of diagnosis. Specialist palliative care providers should be involved as early as possible. Discussions should take place early, well before specific decisions need to be made. The actual timing of when to introduce these discussions however can be challenging and will depend on a number of factors including coping skills, depression and anxiety, cultural issues and functional status (Mitsumoto et al., 2005). Some triggers may include the patient or family initiation of discussion, severe psychosocial distress, pain requiring high dosages of analgesia, dysphagia, dyspnoea and functional loss in two body regions (Mitsumoto et al., 2005). Given the progressive nature of the disease, the patient eventually has to choose between life-sustaining therapies (respiratory assistance, feeding tubes) and terminal palliative care whilst considering issues relating to quality of life, burden of therapies, their own wishes and those of their family. It is important that clinicians caring for ALS patients and their families appreciate and communicate the significance of life-threatening symptoms, monitor decision-making capacity, ensure that multiple possible end of life scenarios are anticipated and managed with all options provided (including hospice care), review advance care directives and comprehensively consider and aggressively manage symptoms (McCluskey, 2007).

Medications should be available for all patients who are deteriorating and may be approaching the terminal phase, although the terminal phase may be difficult to recognise as there is usually slow deterioration until a quicker change leads to death within a few days or less (Oliver, 2007). Medications should include morphine to relieve dyspnoea and pain, midazolam to relieve distress and agitation and glycopyrronium bromide or hyoscine hydrobromide to reduce chest secretions, delivered parenterally (Oliver, 2007). Cultural and spiritual issues should also be addressed (Mitsumoto et al., 2005;Albert et al., 2007). Although many persons with ALS fear the terminal stages of ALS, with good palliative care, the later stages can be a time of fulfilment and peace for both persons with ALS and their families (Oliver, 2007).

Bereavement in ALS occurs in both the patient and their family and continues, in families, after the death of the patient. Some families feel relieved of their caregiver burden and the burden of losses for the patient but also have feelings of guilt that they feel these emotions; hence support is vital in this area (Skyes, 2006).

3. Conclusion

ALS is a complex and challenging condition with no cure. Current "gold-standard" management is "multidisciplinary care"which includes neurological, rehabilitative and palliative care. As consistent with the guidelines from the American Academy of Neurology (Miller et al., 2009b) and the World Federation of Neurology (Andersen et al., 2007), multidisciplinary care should be available to all persons with ALS. Where multidisciplinary care is currently available, it should be delivered with a high level of coordination and integration, with evidence-based intervention to ensure holistic and seamless care for persons with ALS and their caregivers. Many areas in ALS are poorly understood, with research often further hindered by the logistical and ethical difficulties. Much more work is needed in the area of evidence-based interventions. At present, much of the evidence has been concentrated in areas such as respiratory and nutritional management. There is paucity of information on effective rehabilitation interventions and very little is understood with regards to the "black box of rehabilitation". For example, evidence to guide exercise prescription (such as strengthening, stretching, aerobic/endurance exercises) is much needed. The use and development of assistive technology is another area that warrants much more attention, as is a better understanding of bowel, bladder and sexuality issues. Further research is also needed into appropriate study designs; outcome measurement; the evaluation of optimal settings, type, intensity or frequency and cost-effectiveness of multidisciplinary care; and the different phases of ALS, covering the spectrum of care required for this patient population. The interface between neurological, rehabilitative and palliative components of care, and caregiver needs should be explored and developed to provide long-term support for this population. Last but not least, national and international guidelines incorporating evidence-based practice in rehabilitation should be further developed to enable optimisation of clinical care and practice.

4. References

The Family Center on Technology and Disability, [Accessed January 2011], Available from: http://www.fctd.info/resources?on=disability&tag=Neurological+Disorders

Abrahams, S.;Leigh P.N. & Goldstein L.H. (2005). Cognitive change in ALS: a prospective study. *Neurology,* Vol. 64, No. 7, pp. 1222-6, 1526-632X (Electronic) 0028-3878 (Linking)

Albert, S.M.;Wasner M.;Tider T.;Drory V.E. & Borasio G.D. (2007). Cross-cultural variation in mental health at end of life in patients with ALS. *Neurology,* Vol. 68, No. 13, pp. 1058-61, 1526-632X (Electronic) 0028-3878 (Linking)

Andersen, P.M.;Borasio G.D.;Dengler R., et al. (2007). Good practice in the management of amyotrophic lateral sclerosis: clinical guidelines. An evidence-based review with good practice points. EALSC Working Group. *Amyotroph Lateral Scler,* Vol. 8, No. 4, pp. 195-213, 1748-2968 (Print) 1471-180X (Linking)

Ashworth, N.L.;Satkunam L.E. & Deforge D. (2006). Treatment for spasticity in amyotrophic lateral sclerosis/motor neuron disease. *Cochrane Database Syst Rev,* Issue 1, pp. CD004156, 1469-493X (Electronic) 1361-6137 (Linking)

Borasio, G.D. (2001). Palliative care in ALS: searching for the evidence base. *Amyotroph Lateral Scler Other Motor Neuron Disord,* Vol. 2 Suppl 1, pp. S31-5, 1466-0822 (Print) 1466-0822 (Linking)

Borasio, G.D.;Shaw P.J.;Hardiman O.;Ludolph A.C.;Sales Luis M.L. & Silani V. (2001a). Standards of palliative care for patients with amyotrophic lateral sclerosis: results of a European survey. *Amyotroph Lateral Scler Other Motor Neuron Disord,* Vol. 2, No. 3, pp. 159-64, 1466-0822 (Print) 1466-0822 (Linking)

Borasio, G.D.;Voltz R. & Miller R.G. (2001b). Palliative care in amyotrophic lateral sclerosis. *Neurol Clin,* Vol. 19, No. 4, pp. 829-47, 0733-8619 (Print) 0733-8619 (Linking)

Brooks, B.R.;Thisted R.A.;Appel S.H., et al. (2004). Treatment of pseudobulbar affect in ALS with dextromethorphan/quinidine: a randomized trial. *Neurology,* Vol. 63, No. 8, pp. 1364-70, 1526-632X (Electronic) 0028-3878 (Linking)

Brownlee, A. & Palovcak M. (2007). The role of augmentative communication devices in the medical management of ALS. *NeuroRehabilitation,* Vol. 22, No. 6, pp. 445-50, 1053-8135 (Print) 1053-8135 (Linking)

Carter, G.T.;Weiss M.D.;Lou J.S., et al. (2005). Modafinil to treat fatigue in amyotrophic lateral sclerosis: an open label pilot study. *Am J Hosp Palliat Care,* Vol. 22, No. 1, pp. 55-9, 1049-9091 (Print) 1049-9091 (Linking)

Chen, A.;Montes J. & Mitsumoto H. (2008). The role of exercise in amyotrophic lateral sclerosis. *Phys Med Rehabil Clin N Am,* Vol. 19, No. 3, pp. 545-57, ix-x, 1047-9651 (Print) 1047-9651 (Linking)

Chio, A.;Gauthier A.;Vignola A., et al. (2006). Caregiver time use in ALS. *Neurology,* Vol. 67, No. 5, pp. 902-4, 1526-632X (Electronic) 0028-3878 (Linking)

Contarino, M.F.;Pompili M.;Tittoto P., et al. (2007). Botulinum toxin B ultrasound-guided injections for sialorrhea in amyotrophic lateral sclerosis and Parkinson's disease. *Parkinsonism Relat Disord,* Vol. 13, No. 5, pp. 299-303, 1353-8020 (Print) 1353-8020 (Linking)

Czaplinski, A.;Yen A.A. & Appel S.H. (2006). Forced vital capacity (FVC) as an indicator of survival and disease progression in an ALS clinic population. *J Neurol Neurosurg Psychiatry,* Vol. 77, No. 3, pp. 390-2, 0022-3050 (Print) 0022-3050 (Linking)

Dalbello-Haas, V.;Florence J.M. & Krivickas L.S. (2008). Therapeutic exercise for people with amyotrophic lateral sclerosis or motor neuron disease. *Cochrane Database Syst Rev,* Issue. 2, pp. CD005229, 1469-493X (Electronic) 1361-6137 (Linking)

De Groot, I.J.;Post M.W.;van Heuveln T.;Van den Berg L.H. & Lindeman E. (2007). Cross-sectional and longitudinal correlations between disease progression and different health-related quality of life domains in persons with amyotrophic lateral sclerosis. *Amyotroph Lateral Scler,* Vol. 8, No. 6, pp. 356-61, 1471-180X (Electronic) 1471-180X (Linking)

Esposito, S.J.;Mitsumoto H. & Shanks M. (2000). Use of palatal lift and palatal augmentation prostheses to improve dysarthria in patients with amyotrophic lateral sclerosis: a case series. *J Prosthet Dent,* Vol. 83, No. 1, pp. 90-8, 0022-3913 (Print) 0022-3913 (Linking)

Fitting, J.W.;Paillex R.;Hirt L.;Aebischer P. & Schluep M. (1999). Sniff nasal pressure: a sensitive respiratory test to assess progression of amyotrophic lateral sclerosis. *Ann Neurol,* Vol. 46, No. 6, pp. 887-93, 0364-5134 (Print) 0364-5134 (Linking)

Forshew, D.A. & Bromberg M.B. (2003). A survey of clinicians' practice in the symptomatic treatment of ALS. *Amyotroph Lateral Scler Other Motor Neuron Disord,* Vol. 4, No. 4, pp. 258-63, 1466-0822 (Print) 1466-0822 (Linking)

Francis, K.;Bach J.R. & DeLisa J.A. (1999). Evaluation and rehabilitation of patients with adult motor neuron disease. *Arch Phys Med Rehabil,* Vol. 80, No. 8, pp. 951-63, 0003-9993 (Print) 0003-9993 (Linking)

Goldstein, L.H.;Atkins L.;Landau S.;Brown R. & Leigh P.N. (2006a). Predictors of psychological distress in carers of people with amyotrophic lateral sclerosis: a longitudinal study. *Psychol Med,* Vol. 36, No. 6, pp. 865-75, 0033-2917 (Print) 0033-2917 (Linking)

Goldstein, L.H.;Atkins L.;Landau S.;Brown R.G. & Leigh P.N. (2006b). Longitudinal predictors of psychological distress and self-esteem in people with ALS. *Neurology,* Vol. 67, No. 9, pp. 1652-8, 1526-632X (Electronic) 0028-3878 (Linking)

Grossman, A.B.;Woolley-Levine S.;Bradley W.G. & Miller R.G. (2007). Detecting neurobehavioral changes in amyotrophic lateral sclerosis. *Amyotroph Lateral Scler,* Vol. 8, No. 1, pp. 56-61, 1748-2968 (Print) 1471-180X (Linking)

Hardiman, O. (2007). Multidisciplinary care in motor neurone disease, In: *The Motor Neurone Disease Handbook,* M. Kiernan, (Ed.), pp. (164), Australasian Medical Publishing Company Limited, Prymont

Hattori, T.;Hirayama K.;Yasuda K. & Shimazaki J. (1983). [Disturbance of micturition in amyotrophic lateral sclerosis]. *Rinsho Shinkeigaku,* Vol. 23, No. 3, pp. 224-7, 0009-918X (Print) 0009-918X (Linking)

Higo, R.;Tayama N. & Nito T. (2004). Longitudinal analysis of progression of dysphagia in amyotrophic lateral sclerosis. *Auris Nasus Larynx,* Vol. 31, No. 3, pp. 247-54, 0385-8146 (Print) 0385-8146 (Linking)

Hillel, A.D. & Miller R. (1989). Bulbar amyotrophic lateral sclerosis: patterns of progression and clinical management. *Head Neck,* Vol. 11, No. 1, pp. 51-9, 1043-3074 (Print) 1043-3074 (Linking)

Johnson, E.W. & Braddom R. (1971). Over-work weakness in facioscapulohuumeral muscular dystrophy. *Arch Phys Med Rehabil,* Vol. 52, No. 7, pp. 333-6, 0003-9993 (Print) 0003-9993 (Linking)

Kasarskis, E.J. & Neville H.E. (1996). Management of ALS: nutritional care. *Neurology,* Vol. 47, No. 4 Suppl 2, pp. S118-20, 0028-3878 (Print) 0028-3878 (Linking)

Kasarskis, E.J.;Scarlata D.;Hill R.;Fuller C.;Stambler N. & Cedarbaum J.M. (1999). A retrospective study of percutaneous endoscopic gastrostomy in ALS patients during the BDNF and CNTF trials. *J Neurol Sci,* Vol. 169, No. 1-2, pp. 118-25, 0022-510X (Print) 0022-510X (Linking)

Kaub-Wittemer, D.;Steinbuchel N.;Wasner M.;Laier-Groeneveld G. & Borasio G.D. (2003). Quality of life and psychosocial issues in ventilated patients with amyotrophic lateral sclerosis and their caregivers. *J Pain Symptom Manage,* Vol. 26, No. 4, pp. 890-6, 0885-3924 (Print) 0885-3924 (Linking)

Kemp, B.J. (2005). What the rehabilitation professional and the consumer need to know. *Phys Med Rehabil Clin N Am,* Vol. 16, No. 1, pp. 1-18, vii, 1047-9651 (Print) 1047-9651 (Linking)

Kent-Braun, J.A. & Miller R.G. (2000). Central fatigue during isometric exercise in amyotrophic lateral sclerosis. *Muscle Nerve,* Vol. 23, No. 6, pp. 909-14, 0148-639X (Print) 0148-639X (Linking)

Khanna, P.;Nations S.P. & Trivedi J.R. (2007). Motor Neuron Diseases, In: *Physical Medicine & Rehabilitation,* R. Braddom, (Ed.), 3rd ed. Saunders Elsevier, Philadelphia

Kinnear, W.;Scriven N.;Orpe V. & Jefferson D. (1997 Nov 3-5). Prevalence of symptoms of sleep disturbance in patients with motor neurone disease [abstract]. *Proceedings of 8th International Symposium on ALS/MND,* Glasgow, Nov 1997

Klein, L.M. & Forshew D.A. (1996). The economic impact of ALS. *Neurology,* Vol. 47, No. 4 Suppl 2, pp. S126-9, 0028-3878 (Print) 0028-3878 (Linking)

Krivickas, L.S. & Carter G.T. (2005). Motor neuron disease, In: *Physical medicine and rehabilitation: principles and practice,* D. J.A., Gans, B.M. & Walsh, N.E., (Eds.), 4th ed. Lippincott Williams & Wilkins, Philadelphia

Kurt, A.;Nijboer F.;Matuz T. & Kubler A. (2007). Depression and anxiety in individuals with amyotrophic lateral sclerosis: epidemiology and management. *CNS Drugs,* Vol. 21, No. 4, pp. 279-91, 1172-7047 (Print) 1172-7047 (Linking)

Langmore, S.E.;Kasarskis E.J.;Manca M.L. & Olney R.K. (2006). Enteral tube feeding for amyotrophic lateral sclerosis/motor neuron disease. *Cochrane Database Syst Rev,* Issue. 4, pp. CD004030, 1469-493X (Electronic) 1361-6137 (Linking)

Lomen-Hoerth, C.;Murphy J.;Langmore S.;Kramer J.H.;Olney R.K. & Miller B. (2003). Are amyotrophic lateral sclerosis patients cognitively normal? *Neurology,* Vol. 60, No. 7, pp. 1094-7, 1526-632X (Electronic) 0028-3878 (Linking)

Loser, C.;Aschl G.;Hebuterne X., et al. (2005). ESPEN guidelines on artificial enteral nutrition--percutaneous endoscopic gastrostomy (PEG). *Clin Nutr,* Vol. 24, No. 5, pp. 848-61, 0261-5614 (Print) 0261-5614 (Linking)

Lou, J.S. (2008). Fatigue in amyotrophic lateral sclerosis. *Phys Med Rehabil Clin N Am,* Vol. 19, No. 3, pp. 533-43, ix, 1047-9651 (Print) 1047-9651 (Linking)

Lyall, R.A.;Donaldson N.;Polkey M.I.;Leigh P.N. & Moxham J. (2001). Respiratory muscle strength and ventilatory failure in amyotrophic lateral sclerosis. *Brain,* Vol. 124, No. Pt 10, pp. 2000-13, 0006-8950 (Print) 0006-8950 (Linking)

Marquardt, G. & Seifert V. (2002). Use of intrathecal baclofen for treatment of spasticity in amyotrophic lateral sclerosis. *J Neurol Neurosurg Psychiatry,* Vol. 72, No. pp. 275-276

Massman, P.J.;Sims J.;Cooke N.;Haverkamp L.J.;Appel V. & Appel S.H. (1996). Prevalence and correlates of neuropsychological deficits in amyotrophic lateral sclerosis. *J Neurol Neurosurg Psychiatry,* Vol. 61, No. 5, pp. 450-5, 0022-3050 (Print) 0022-3050 (Linking)

Mathus-Vliegen, L.M.;Louwerse L.S.;Merkus M.P.;Tytgat G.N. & Vianney de Jong J.M. (1994). Percutaneous endoscopic gastrostomy in patients with amyotrophic lateral sclerosis and impaired pulmonary function. *Gastrointest Endosc,* Vol. 40, No. 4, pp. 463-9, 0016-5107 (Print) 0016-5107 (Linking)

Matuz, T.;Birbaumer N.;Hautzinger M. & Kubler A. (2010). Coping with amyotrophic lateral sclerosis: an integrative view. *J Neurol Neurosurg Psychiatry,* Vol. 81, No. 8, pp. 893-8, 1468-330X (Electronic) 0022-3050 (Linking)

Mayadev, A.S.;Weiss M.D.;Distad B.J.;Krivickas L.S. & Carter G.T. (2008). The amyotrophic lateral sclerosis center: a model of multidisciplinary management. *Phys Med Rehabil Clin N Am,* Vol. 19, No. 3, pp. 619-31, xi, 1047-9651 (Print) 1047-9651 (Linking)

Mayberry, J.F. & Atkinson M. (1986). Swallowing problems in patients with motor neuron disease. *J Clin Gastroenterol,* Vol. 8, No. 3 Pt 1, pp. 233-4, 0192-0790 (Print) 0192-0790 (Linking)

Mazzini, L.;Corra T.;Zaccala M.;Mora G.;Del Piano M. & Galante M. (1995). Percutaneous endoscopic gastrostomy and enteral nutrition in amyotrophic lateral sclerosis. *J Neurol,* Vol. 242, No. 10, pp. 695-8, 0340-5354 (Print) 0340-5354 (Linking)

McCluskey, L. (2007). Amyotrophic Lateral Sclerosis: ethical issues from diagnosis to end of life. *NeuroRehabilitation,* Vol. 22, No. 6, pp. 463-72, 1053-8135 (Print) 1053-8135 (Linking)

Meininger, V. (2005). Treatment of emotional lability in ALS. *Lancet Neurol,* Vol. 4, No. 2, pp. 70, 1474-4422 (Print) 1474-4422 (Linking)

Melo, J.;Homma A.;Iturriaga E., et al. (1999). Pulmonary evaluation and prevalence of non-invasive ventilation in patients with amyotrophic lateral sclerosis: a multicenter survey and proposal of a pulmonary protocol. *J Neurol Sci,* Vol. 169, No. 1-2, pp. 114-7, 0022-510X (Print) 0022-510X (Linking)

Mezaki, T.;Kaji R.;Kohara N. & Kimura J. (1996). Development of general weakness in a patient with amyotrophic lateral sclerosis after focal botulinum toxin injection. *Neurology,* Vol. 46, No. 3, pp. 845-6, 0028-3878 (Print) 0028-3878 (Linking)

Miller, R.G.;Jackson C.E.;Kasarskis E.J., et al. (2009a). Practice parameter update: The care of the patient with amyotrophic lateral sclerosis: drug, nutritional, and respiratory therapies (an evidence-based review): report of the Quality Standards Subcommittee of the American Academy of Neurology. *Neurology,* Vol. 73, No. 15, pp. 1218-26, 1526-632X (Electronic) 0028-3878 (Linking)

Miller, R.G.;Jackson C.E.;Kasarskis E.J., et al. (2009b). Practice parameter update: The care of the patient with amyotrophic lateral sclerosis: multidisciplinary care, symptom management, and cognitive/behavioral impairment (an evidence-based review): report of the Quality Standards Subcommittee of the American Academy of Neurology. *Neurology,* Vol. 73, No. 15, pp. 1227-33, 1526-632X (Electronic) 0028-3878 (Linking)

Mitsumoto, H.;Bromberg M.;Johnston W., et al. (2005). Promoting excellence in end-of-life care in ALS. *Amyotroph Lateral Scler Other Motor Neuron Disord,* Vol. 6, No. 3, pp. 145-54, 1466-0822 (Print) 1466-0822 (Linking)

Moore, S.R.;Gresham L.S.;Bromberg M.B.;Kasarkis E.J. & Smith R.A. (1997). A self report measure of affective lability. *J Neurol Neurosurg Psychiatry,* Vol. 63, No. 1, pp. 89-93, 0022-3050 (Print) 0022-3050 (Linking)

Morgan, R.K.;McNally S.;Alexander M.;Conroy R.;Hardiman O. & Costello R.W. (2005). Use of Sniff nasal-inspiratory force to predict survival in amyotrophic lateral sclerosis. *Am J Respir Crit Care Med,* Vol. 171, No. 3, pp. 269-74, 1073-449X (Print) 1073-449X (Linking)

Neary, D.;Snowden J.S.;Gustafson L., et al. (1998). Frontotemporal lobar degeneration: a consensus on clinical diagnostic criteria. *Neurology,* Vol. 51, No. 6, pp. 1546-54, 0028-3878 (Print) 0028-3878 (Linking)

Ng, L.;Khan F. & Mathers S. (2009). Multidisciplinary care for adults with amyotrophic lateral sclerosis or motor neuron disease. *Cochrane Database Syst Rev,* Issue. 4, pp. CD007425, 1469-493X (Electronic) 1361-6137 (Linking)

Ng, L.; Talman, P. & Khan F. (2011). Motor Neurone Disease: Disability profile and service needs in an Australian cohort. *Int J Rehabil Res,* Vol 34, No. 2, pp.151-9.

Norris, F.H., Jr.;Gasteiger E.L. & Chatfield P.O. (1957). An electromyographic study of induced and spontaneous muscle cramps. *Electroencephalogr Clin Neurophysiol,* Vol. 9, No. 1, pp. 139-47, 0013-4694 (Print) 0013-4694 (Linking)

Norris, F.H.;Tan Y.;Fallat R.J. & Elias L. (1993). Trial of oral physostigmine in amyotrophic lateral sclerosis. *Clin Pharmacol Ther,* Vol. 54, No. 6, pp. 680-2, 0009-9236 (Print) 0009-9236 (Linking)

Oliver, D. (1996). The quality of care and symptom control--the effects on the terminal phase of ALS/MND. *J Neurol Sci,* Vol. 139 Suppl, pp. 134-6, 0022-510X (Print) 0022-510X (Linking)

Oliver, D. (2007). Palliative care, In: *The motor neurone disease handbook,* M. Kiernan, (Ed.), pp. (186-195), Australasian Medical Publishing Company Limited, Prymont

Palmieri, A.;Abrahams S.;Soraru G., et al. (2009). Emotional Lability in MND: Relationship to cognition and psychopathology and impact on caregivers.*J Neurol Sci,* Vol. 278, No. 1-2, pp. 16-20, 0022-510X (Print) 0022-510X (Linking)

Pinker, S. & Jackendoff R. (2005). The faculty of language: what's special about it? *Cognition,* Vol. 95, No. 2, pp. 201-36, 0010-0277 (Print) 0010-0277 (Linking)

Rabkin, J.G.;Albert S.M.;Del Bene M.L., et al. (2005). Prevalence of depressive disorders and change over time in late-stage ALS. *Neurology,* Vol. 65, No. 1, pp. 62-7, 1526-632X (Electronic) 0028-3878 (Linking)

Rabkin, J.G.;Albert S.M.;Rowland L.P. & Mitsumoto H. (2009). How common is depression among ALS caregivers? A longitudinal study. *Amyotroph Lateral Scler,* Vol. 10, No. 5-6, pp. 448-55, 1471-180X (Electronic) 1471-180X (Linking)

Radunovic, A.;Annane D.;Jewitt K. & Mustfa N. (2009). Mechanical ventilation for amyotrophic lateral sclerosis/motor neuron disease. *Cochrane Database Syst Rev,* Issue. 4, pp. CD004427, 1469-493X (Electronic) 1361-6137 (Linking)

Ramirez, C.;Piemonte M.E.;Callegaro D. & Da Silva H.C. (2008). Fatigue in amyotrophic lateral sclerosis: frequency and associated factors. *Amyotroph Lateral Scler,* Vol. 9, No. 2, pp. 75-80, 1471-180X (Electronic) 1471-180X (Linking)

Ray, R.A. & Street A.F. (2006). Caregiver bodywork: family members' experiences of caring for a person with motor neurone disease. *J Adv Nurs,* Vol. 56, No. 1, pp. 35-43, 0309-2402 (Print) 0309-2402 (Linking)

Ringholz, G.M.;Appel S.H.;Bradshaw M.;Cooke N.A.;Mosnik D.M. & Schulz P.E. (2005). Prevalence and patterns of cognitive impairment in sporadic ALS. *Neurology,* Vol. 65, No. 4, pp. 586-90, 1526-632X (Electronic) 0028-3878 (Linking)

Rio, A. & Cawadias E. (2007). Nutritional advice and treatment by dietitians to patients with amyotrophic lateral sclerosis/motor neurone disease: a survey of current practice in England, Wales, Northern Ireland and Canada. *J Hum Nutr Diet,* Vol. 20, No. 1, pp. 3-13, 0952-3871 (Print) 0952-3871 (Linking)

Rosen, H.J. & Cummings J. (2007). A real reason for patients with pseudobulbar affect to smile. *Ann Neurol,* Vol. 61, No. 2, pp. 92-6, 0364-5134 (Print) 0364-5134 (Linking)

Royal College of Physicians National Council for Palliative Care and British Society of Rehabilitation Medicine (2008). Long Term Neurological Conditions: Management at the interface between neurology, rehabilitation and palliative care. *Concise guidance to good practice series,* Royal College of Physicians, London

Sanjak, M.;Bravver E.;Bockenek W.L.;Norton H.J. & Brooks B.R. (2010). Supported treadmill ambulation for amyotrophic lateral sclerosis: a pilot study. *Arch Phys Med Rehabil,* Vol. 91, No. 12, pp. 1920-9, 1532-821X (Electronic) 0003-9993 (Linking)

Schiffman, P.L. (1996). Pulmonary function and respiratory management of the ALS patient, In: *Amyotrophic Lateral Sclerosis: diagnosis and management for the clinician,* J.M. Belsh & Schiffman, P.L., (Eds.), pp. (333-355), Futura Publishing Company, Armonk (NY)

Schiffman, P.L. & Belsh J.M. (1996). Overall management of the ALS patient, In: *Amyotrophic lateral sclerosis: diagnosis and management for the clinician,* J.M. Belsh & Schiffman, P.L., (Eds.), pp. (271-301), Futura Publishing Company, Armonk (NY)

Sellers, E.W.;Vaughan T.M. & Wolpaw J.R. (2010). A brain-computer interface for long-term independent home use. *Amyotroph Lateral Scler,* Vol. 11, No. 5, pp. 449-55, 1471-180X (Electronic) 1471-180X (Linking)

Shaw, P. (2003). Motor neurone disease, In: *Handbook of neurological rehabilitation,* R.J. Greenwood, Barnes, M.P., McMillan, T.M. & al, (Eds.), 2nd ed, pp. (641-661), Psychology Press, New York

Simmons, Z.;Bremer B.A.;Robbins R.A.;Walsh S.M. & Fischer S. (2000). Quality of life in ALS depends on factors other than strength and physical function. *Neurology,* Vol. 55, No. 3, pp. 388-92, 0028-3878 (Print) 0028-3878 (Linking)

Skyes, N.P. (2006). End of life care, In: *Palliative care in amyotrophic lateral sclerosis - from diagnosis to bereavement,* D. Oliver, Borasio, G.D. & Walsh, D. (Eds.), Oxford University Press, Oxford

Slowie, L.A.;Paige M.S. & Antel J.P. (1983). Nutritional considerations in the management of patients with amyotrophic lateral sclerosis (ALS). *J Am Diet Assoc,* Vol. 83, No. 1, pp. 44-7, 0002-8223 (Print) 0002-8223 (Linking)

Sorenson, E.J.;Crum B. & Stevens J.C. (2007). Incidence of aspiration pneumonia in ALS in Olmsted County, MN. *Amyotroph Lateral Scler,* Vol. 8, No. 2, pp. 87-9, 1748-2968 (Print) 1471-180X (Linking)

Stefanutti, D.;Benoist M.R.;Scheinmann P.;Chaussain M. & Fitting J.W. (2000). Usefulness of sniff nasal pressure in patients with neuromuscular or skeletal disorders. *Am J Respir Crit Care Med,* Vol. 162, No. 4 Pt 1, pp. 1507-11, 1073-449X (Print) 1073-449X (Linking)

Sufit, R. (1997). Symptomatic treatment of ALS *Neurology,* Vol. 48, No. pp. 15S-22S

U.S. Food and Drug Administration. (2006). FDA advances effort against marketed unapproved drugs. FDA orders unapproved quinine drugs from the market and cautions consumers about "off-label" use of quinine to treat leg cramps, [Accessed January 2011], Available from: http://www.fda.gov/NewsEvents/Newsroom/PressAnnouncements/2006/ucm108799.htm

Verma, A. & Steele J. (2006). Botulinum toxin improves sialorrhea and quality of living in bulbar amyotrophic lateral sclerosis. *Muscle Nerve,* Vol. 34, No. 2, pp. 235-7, 0148-639X (Print) 0148-639X (Linking)

Vianello, A.;Arcaro G.;Palmieri A., et al. (2010). Survival and quality of life after tracheostomy for acute respiratory failure in patients with amyotrophic lateral sclerosis. *J Crit Care,* Vol., No. pp., 1557-8615 (Electronic) 0883-9441 (Linking)

Wade, D.T. (1992). *Measurement in Neurology Rehabilitation,* Oxford University Press, Oxford

Wasner, M.;Bold U.;Vollmer T.C. & Borasio G.D. (2004). Sexuality in patients with amyotrophic lateral sclerosis and their partners. *J Neurol,* Vol. 251, No. 4, pp. 445-8, 0340-5354 (Print) 0340-5354 (Linking)

Wellings, D.J. & Unsworth J. (1997). Fortnightly review. Environmental control systems for people with a disability: an update. *BMJ,* Vol. 315, No. 7105, pp. 409-12, 0959-8138 (Print) 0959-535X (Linking)

Woolley, S.C. & Jonathan S.K. (2008). Cognitive and behavioral impairment in amyotrophic lateral sclerosis. *Phys Med Rehabil Clin N Am,* Vol. 19, No. 3, pp. 607-17, xi, 1047-9651 (Print) 1047-9651 (Linking)

World Health Organization (2001). International Classification of Functioning, Disability and Health (ICF). Geneva: World Health Organization

Yorkston, K.M.;Strand E.;Miller R.;Hillel A. & Smith K. (1993). Speech deterioration in amyotrophic lateral sclerosis: implications for the timing of intervention. *J Med Speech-Language Pathol,* Vol. 1, pp. 35-46

25

Assessment and Management of Respiratory Dysfunction in Patients with Amyotrophic Lateral Sclerosis

Daniele Lo Coco et al.*

ALS Clinical Research Center, Dipartimento di Biomedicina Sperimentale e Neuroscienze Cliniche (BioNeC), University of Palermo, Palermo, Italy

1. Introduction

Amyotrophic Lateral Sclerosis (ALS) is a relatively rare neurodegenerative disorder that causes progressive dysfunction of voluntary muscle groups secondary to motor neurons death. The relentless involvement of all skeletal muscles of the body, characterized by weakness and atrophy to complete paralysis, invariably involves respiratory muscles (particularly the diaphragm) resulting in a failure to deliver adequate amounts of oxygen to, and remove carbon dioxide from blood. As a result, respiratory failure, frequently complicated by pneumonia related to respiratory muscle weakness and ineffective cough, is the most frequent cause of death in these patients (Lo Coco et al., 2008).

Considering the natural history of ALS, only a few number of patients shows respiratory muscle dysfunction at the onset of the disease (Marti-Fabregas et al., 1995; De Carvalho et al., 1996), and the majority of patients maintains an almost normal pulmonary function for months or years. Patients thus need to be regularly and progressively evaluated to identify early signs of respiratory muscle weakness so that adequate treatment can be implemented. Indeed, in the last few years it has been repeatedly shown that non-invasive positive-pressure ventilation (NIPPV), the treatment of choice for chronic hypoventilation and respiratory failure in ALS, allows a significant improvement in survival and quality of life (Heiman-Patterson & Miller, 2006). Many tests are available to objectively assess the performances of the respiratory system, and there is increasing interest toward those able to sensitively detect mild impairment. Moreover, great attention has to be put on monitoring of cough effectiveness, management of respiratory secretions and prevention of respiratory infections. For all these reasons the management of respiratory dysfunction has become a

---

*Paolo Volanti[2], Domenico De Cicco[2], Antonio Spanevello[3], Gianluca Battaglia[2], Santino Marchese[4], Alfonsa Claudia Taiello[1], Rossella Spataro[1] and Vincenzo La Bella[1]

[1]*ALS Clinical Research Center, Dipartimento di Biomedicina Sperimentale e Neuroscienze Cliniche (BioNeC), University of Palermo, Palermo, Italy*

[2]*Neurorehabilitation Unit, Fondazione Salvatore Maugeri, Mistretta (ME), Italy*

[3]*Università Degli Studi dell'Insubria, Varese, Italy*

[4]*Respiratory Intensive Care Unit, Ospedale Civico ARNAS, Palermo, Italy*

major issue in the multidisciplinary assessment of patients with ALS, and the pulmonologist has gained an increasing role in this process. However, there is still little consensus on pulmonary care worldwide, and clinical practice varies widely from country to country, especially when NIPPV becomes inadequate to support respiratory muscle failure. It is, then, good practice to discuss respiratory issues in advance with the patients and their carers in order to avoid emergency interventions or unwanted treatments, and frequently review these decisions during the course of the disease.

This chapter focuses on the recent advances that have emerged in the management of pulmonary dysfunction in patients with ALS with emphasis on respiratory evaluation and mechanical ventilation.

2. Evaluation of pulmonary function

As already mentioned, when patients with ALS seek medical attention, they do not usually display signs of pulmonary involvement, and do not refer respiratory complaints. However, during the progression of the disease all patients eventually complain of dyspnea with exertion, orthopnea, and poor sleep quality with frequent awakenings, nightmares, early morning headaches or excessive daytime sleepiness (Heffernan et al., 2006; Beneditt & Boitano, 2008). A clinical examination at this point might show respiratory paradox, rapid shallow breathing or accessory muscle contraction. Nevertheless, the observation that many patients may remain asymptomatic even when there is a marked reduction of vital capacity limits the reliability of these signs and symptoms. There are, however, several dyspnea rating scales, such as the Borg dyspnoea score, the baseline dyspnea index and the transition dyspnea index, that have been recently reconsidered and their implementation has been encouraged (Lechtzin et al., 2007a; Just et al., 2010).

In addition to respiratory symptoms and signs, many exams are used in the evaluation of pulmonary function in patients with ALS (Heffernan et al., 2006; Beneditt & Boitano, 2008; Lo Coco et al., 2008; Miller et al., 2009a).

The most widely available measure for detecting respiratory decline is forced vital capacity (FVC) sitting and/or supine. FVC is correlated with survival, and usually presents an almost linear decrease during the course of the disease, but with a marked variability from patient to patient (within 2% to 4% of predicted value per month) (Fallat et al., 1979; Munsat et al., 1988; Schiffman & Belsh, 1993; Stembler et al., 1998; Czaplinski et al., 2006; Lo Coco et al., 2006a).

FVC, however, has some well known limitations, such as low sensitiveness in patients with bulbar involvement, because of reduced buccal strength, or cognitive involvement, and a relative insensitiveness to detect mild or moderate diaphragmatic dysfunction. According to many specialists, supine FVC, although more difficult to perform, has superior sensitivity over seated FVC in predicting survival, is closely correlated with transdiaphragmatic pressure, and then should be always executed in the evaluation of patients with ALS (Varrato et al., 2001; Schmidt et al., 2006; Baumann et al., 2010).

Maximal inspiratory and expiratory pressure (MIP and MEP) are other sensitive measurements, and it has been shown that many patients with an FVC > 70% had abnormal MIP (< -60 cm) (Jackson et al., 2001). However, since many patients are unable to perform the test with the progression of disease, in many centres these two tests are not routinely executed.

Arterial blood gas analysis may also be of help in the evaluation of patients with ALS, especially in those with severe bulbar involvement, since it could reveal resting hypercapnia ($PaCO_2$ > 6.5 kPa) and/or hypoxemia (PaO_2 < 80 mmHg). However, these are usually very late signs of respiratory failure in ALS.
Sniff nasal inspiratory pressure (SNIP) is regarded as a good measure of diaphragmatic strength, and is probably more accurate than FVC, especially at later stages, although even SNIP may underestimate respiratory function in patients with bulbar involvement, because of upper airway collapse. However, a sniff nasal pressure test < 40% of predicted value (or < 60 cmH_2O) is a significant predictor of sleep disordered breathing, nocturnal hypoxemia, hypercapnia and mortality (Fitting et al., 1999; Lyall et al., 2001b; Carrat et al., 2011).
Finally, nocturnal hypoventilation and sleep-disordered breathing are common problems in ALS with the progression of the disease, and can occur even when respiratory muscle function is only mildly affected and in the presence of normal daytime gas exchange (Gay et al., 1991; Ferguson et al., 1996; Arnulf et al., 2000). Nocturnal hypoventilation is particularly severe during rapid eye movements (REM) sleep, when all postural and accessory muscles are physiologically atonic, and only the diaphragm, which may itself be impaired, is left to sustain ventilation and overcome any upper airway resistance (Ferguson et al., 1996). Then, since nocturnal oximetry is easily performed and can be executed domiciliary, it has become frequently used in clinical practice for the evaluation of respiratory involvement in patients with ALS and as a guide to initiate mechanical ventilation. Nocturnal oximetry correlated with survival (mean SaO_2 < 93 mmHg was associated with mean survival of 7 months vs 18 months when mean SaO_2 > 93 mmHg) (Velasco et al., 2002), and nocturnal desaturations < 90% for 1 cumulative minute was a more sensitive indicator of nocturnal hypoventilation than either FVC or MIP (Jackson et al., 2001). Polysomnography is not routinely performed, because is costly and demanding, although it can reveal causes of poor sleep quality different from disordered breathing, such as motor activity during sleep (Lo Coco et al., 2011).

3. Non-invasive mechanical ventilation

Long-term mechanical ventilation in patients with neuromuscular problems was first introduced between 1950 and 1960 in France and Sweden as a consequence of the poliomyelitis epidemics. During the following decades, the concept of home mechanical ventilation expanded rapidly, and long-term non-invasive positive-pressure ventilation (NIPPV) was implemented in many other countries and for many other conditions, including ALS, to treat chronic alveolar hypoventilation.
Chronic alveolar hypoventilation is a state characterized by reduced arterial oxygen tension and increased carbon dioxide tension, which the patient may correct at least partially by voluntary hyperventilation. The underlying mechanisms are not yet fully understood and may involve impairment of lung mechanics or airway function and cough, ventilation-perfusion mismatch, blunted central ventilatory drive, or respiratory muscle fatigue. Abnormalities may occur while awake or during sleep. In most cases, chronic alveolar hypoventilation leads to daytime fatigue, hypersomnia, and changes in psychological function.
The application of ventilatory assistance in ALS, most frequently non-invasively, has led in the last fifteen years to a revolution in respiratory assistance and ventilatory support in these patients, with a significant impact on the natural history of the disorder. Indeed, NIPPV has been shown to alleviate respiratory symptoms, to extend survival considerably,

and to improve quality of life and cognitive functions in most patients (Miller et al., 2009a). At present time, NIV, usually via nasal mask with Bi-level Positive Airway Pressure (BiPAP) machines, is the most effective treatment available for ALS patients (Heiman-Patterson & Miller, 2006).

The first study that investigated the effects of NIPPV in patients with ALS dates back to 1995. In a non-randomized trial of NIPPV, Pinto and colleagues showed that survival was significantly longer in the nine patients that received NIPPV compared to the nine patients that received standard care (Pinto et al., 1995). In the following years, many cohort and retrospective studies, and a single randomized trial confirmed these results in those patients that used the ventilatory device for more than 4 hours/night (defined as tolerant patients) (Aboussouan et al., 1997, 2001; Kleopa et al., 1999; Bourke et al., 2003, 2006; Farrero et al., 2005; Gruis et al., 2005; Lo Coco et al., 2006b). In general, these studies demonstrated a median survival of 10 to 15 months in those who were able to tolerate NIPPV. It was also pointed out that NIPPV treatment could slow the rate of respiratory impairment, while severe bulbar impairment could affect NIPPV tolerance (Pinto et al., 1995; Aboussouan et al., 1997, 2001; Kleopa et al., 1999; Bourke et al., 2003, 2006; Farrero et al., 2005; Gruis et al., 2005; Lo Coco et al., 2006b). Furthermore, many recent studies showed that NIPPV therapy could improve quality of life of patients with ALS (Gelinas et al., 1998; Lyall et al., 2001a; Kaub-Wittemer et al., 2003; Bourke et al., 2003, 2006; Mustfa et al., 2006), although some suggested that the caregivers' burden could become heavier (Gelinas et al., 1998; Kaub-Wittemer et al., 2003). Finally, it has been reported that mechanical ventilation could improve cognitive function after some months of treatment (Newson-Davis et al., 2001).

Notwithstanding the aforementioned effects on respiratory symptoms, quality of life, and survival many studies suggest that the employment of NIPPV in ALS is poor worldwide (Bourke et al., 2002; Lechtzin et al., 2004), with a need for more education of clinicians and patients regarding the benefits of mechanical ventilation earlier in the course of the disease (Bradley et al., 2001). The reasons for such low uptake of NIPPV treatment are multifactorial but are influenced by differences in the experience of physicians, its availability and cost, uncertainty of the benefits and timing for starting ventilation, and concerns that ventilatory support might prolong suffering, render home care less feasible, and lead to dependency or ventilator entrapment (Radunović et al., 2007).

Moreover, there is still debate about the optimal timing to introduce ventilation in these patients and whether early NIPPV initiation could actually lead to increased survival rates. With regard to the first aspect, as previously discussed, there are at present many different guidelines that suggest numerous exams to be performed, including upright and supine spirometry, nocturnal oximetry, blood gas analysis and MIP (Andersen et al., 2005, 2007; Miller et al., 2009a).

Concerning to the effects of early NIPPV introduction in patients with ALS, there are some studies that reported increased compliance, quality of life and survival in those patients that received earlier treatment (mainly defined by the evidence of significant desaturations at nocturnal oximetry) (Velasco et al., 2002; Jackson et al., 2001; Pinto et al., 2003; Lechtzin et al., 2007b; Carratù et al., 2009), encouraging earlier use of NIPPV or the use of more sensitive tests to detect chronic alveolar hypoventilation.

According to recently published guidelines, all patients with ALS could benefit from NIPPV therapy, and a trial with this appliance should never be discouraged, although marked bulbar involvement could be associated with reduced tolerance and maybe survival (Miller et al., 2009a). Indeed, the increased risk of aspiration in patients with bulbar onset and problems because of difficulties in clearing secretions or obstructions, such as those related to abnormal function of the vocal cords, should be considered.

In our experience NIPPV can be well tolerated by both patients and caregivers, even in patients with bulbar involvement, especially if an intensive educational training and adaptation on NIPPV can be performed (Volanti et al., 2011). Special importance, then, should be deserved to adaptation and compliance during the first few weeks of NIPPV use, since this could be a crucial step in determining the efficacy of the treatment.

Factors predicting survival following NIPPV include advanced age, airway mucus accumulation and lower body mass index (Peysson et al., 2008; Lo Coco et al., 2006). Noncompliance with NIPPV has been related to frontotemporal dysfunction and severe bulbar involvement, whereas compliance with the treatment was associated with young age, preserved upper limb function, symptoms of orthopnea and dyspnea, use of percutaneous endoscopic gastrostomy (PEG), speech devices, and riluzole (Bourke et al., 2003, 2006; Gruis et al., 2005; Olney et al., 2005; Jackson et al., 2006). Nocturnal hypercapnea has also been recently indicated as a predictor of good compliance with subsequent NIPPV treatment (Kim et al., 2011). Oxygen supplementation should be avoided unless provided with mechanical ventilation or to treat dyspnea as a palliative, periodically monitoring CO_2 levels. In fact oxygen therapy may reduce respiratory drive particularly during sleep and has been associated with CO_2 retention and a less favourable outcome than ventilation (Bach et al., 1998; Gay & Edmonds, 1995).

At present, worldwide accepted guidelines propose NIPPV initiation in the presence of respiratory symptoms, and/or evidence of respiratory muscles weakness (FVC ≤ 80% of predicted or SNIP ≤ 40 cmH_2O), evidence of significant nocturnal desaturation on overnight oximetry (< 90% for > 5% of the time asleep) or a morning arterial $PaCO_2$ > 6.5 kPa (Radunović et al., 2007; Miller et al., 2009a).

4. Physiotherapy and management of airway secretions

Physiotherapy is a useful palliative adjunction in the treatment on ALS, in particular in the management of respiratory secretions (Lo Coco et al., 2008). Indeed, during the course of the disease progressive inspiratory and expiratory muscle weakness and bulbar innervated muscle dysfunction result in ineffective cough reflex. Coughing, an important part of the airway defence aiding in the removal of secretions, consists of three components: an inspiratory phase, a compressive phase with glottic closure, and an expulsive phase resulting from sudden glottic opening. Patients with ALS may develop impairment of any of these three phases, and as a result, clearance of respiratory secretions may become problematic, leading to further pulmonary complications.

The effectiveness of mucus clearance is largely dependent on the magnitude of peak cough flows (PCFs) (King et al., 1985), which can be measured using a standard peak flow meter adapted to an anesthesia face mask. A PCF of < 2.7 L/s has been suggested to indicate an ineffective cough (Bach & Saporito, 1996; Tzeng & Bach, 2000). However, since PCF decreases during respiratory tract infections, when the pressure generated by expiratory muscles is reduced (Poponick et al., 1997), it has been suggested that once a patient's PCF is < 4.5 L/s, particularly in the presence of bulbar dysfunction, there is a risk for pulmonary complications (Bach et al., 1997; Sancho et al., 2007). That threshold could be an appropriate time to implement assisted cough techniques. Moreover, patients with a mean PCF above

337 L/min had a significantly greater chance of being alive at 18 months (Chaudri et al., 2002).

Methods of treatment include breathing exercises, postural drainage, exercise regimens and the use of assisted cough techniques (Lo Coco et al., 2008).

Medications with mucolytics like guaifenesin or N-acetylcysteine, a β-receptor antagonist (such as metoprolol and propanolol), nebulized saline, or an anticholinergic bronchodilator such as ipratropium are widely used, although no controlled studies exist in ALS (Miller et al., 2009a).

The benefit of breathing exercises is difficult to evaluate but their main aims can be summarized as: to promote a normal breathing pattern; to teach controlled breathing for use during attacks of dyspnoea; in conjunction with forced expiration technique and postural drainage to assist the removal of secretions; and to maintain the mobility of the chest wall. Patients must be carefully instructed by a physiotherapist and should practise these exercises regularly.

Patients who have excess secretions in the bronchial tree or difficulties in secretions removal may benefit from postural drainage. Postural drainage can be defined as the placement of a patient in various positions so that, with the aid of gravity, secretions may drain from the peripheral to the more central areas of the lung and thus become more easily expectorated. The positions to be used and also the length of time spent in each position must be determined for each patient by a skilled physiotherapist. Clearance of bronchial secretions by postural drainage may be further assisted by the use of deep breathing, percussion and chest vibration, which may be combined with compression of the chest wall and also with the use of the forced expiration technique. However, patients with limited mobility and muscle weakness have difficulty with postural drainage and generally do not benefit from chest physical therapy (Kirilloff et al., 1985). Moreover, intensive cycles of physiotherapy may be exhausting for many patients, particularly those with advanced disease, and may cause arterial desaturation.

Interestingly, a recent double-blind, randomized-controlled trial showed that inspiratory muscle training may potentially strengthen the inspiratory muscles and slow the decline in respiratory function in patients with ALS (Cheah et al., 2009).

Among non-invasive expiratory aids, manually assisted coughing techniques, such as anterior chest compression and abdominal trust, have been shown to be effective in facilitating the elimination of airway secretions in patients with neuromuscular diseases (Massery & Frownfelter, 1990; Bach, 1993a). Nevertheless, manually assisted coughing is labour intensive and often difficult for non-professional caregivers, both during outpatient and in-hospital management, and it depends on precise care provider-patient coordination (Vianello et al., 2005).

The mechanical in-exsufflator (MI-E) is a device that assists patients in clearing bronchial secretions. It consists of a two-stage axial compressor that provides positive pressure (that causes a deep insufflation), thereby generating a forced expiration in which high expiratory flow rates and a high expiratory pressure gradient are generated between the mouth and the alveoli. It is usually applied via a facemask. The use of MI-E has been described to be simple and safe enough for application by non-professional caregivers (Bach, 1993a, 1994), and has been proposed as a complement to manually assisted coughing in the prevention of pulmonary morbidity in neuromuscular patients (Tzeng & Bach, 2000; Bach et al., 1993b). MI-E has also been shown to be helpful in the management of patients with ALS (Sancho et al., 2004) and to be effective in prolonging non-invasive respiratory aids delaying the need for tracheostomy (Bach, 2002). However, this device seems to be ineffective in patients with severe bulbar dysfunction (Bach, 2002; Sancho et al., 2004), perhaps because the application of the exsufflation cycle of MI-E for those patients with weakness of the genioglossus activity due to bulbar dysfunction might produce a dynamic, total, or partial collapse of the upper airway (Sancho et al., 2004).

It is useful to remember that for patients whose vital capacities are less than normal, manually assisted coughing is not optimally effective unless preceded by a maximal lung insufflation, and MI-E is not optimal unless an abdominal trust is applied during the exsufflation (Goncalves & Bach, 2005). Then abdominal trusts and MI-E should be combined together for effective prevention of lower respiratory tract infection and respiratory insufficiency. Failure to correctly administer physical medicine aids continues to make respiratory failure inevitable for the great majority of people with neuromuscular diseases (Goncalves & Bach, 2005).

Finally, high-frequency chest-wall oscillation (HFCWO), another airway-clearance technique, has been recently evaluated in a 12-week randomized, controlled trial on 46 patients with ALS (Lange et al., 2006). HFCWO is a technique that, through generation of high flow in the small airways, is thought to mobilize secretions from the distal airways to the larger airways, from where they can be more easily removed. It has been reported that HFCWO is well tolerated, considered to be helpful by a majority of patients, and decreases symptoms of breathlessness, suggesting that the intervention was useful in the clearance of airway secretions in patients with ALS (Lange et al., 2006). Another study, however, failed to show any benefit in loss of lung function or mortality in 9 patients with ALS (Chaisson et al., 2006).

A part from sustaining respiration with mechanical devices, special consideration should be given to prevention of aspiration and development of pneumonia (Radunović et al., 2007; Miller et al, 2009 a,b). In this regard, it is of fundamental importance the reduction of the amount of salivary secretions through the use of several medications (such as amitriptyline and botulinum toxin injections), devoting adequate amount of time in teaching proper swallowing technique, and maintaining hydration. It is also useful to provide a portable mechanical home suction device. In addition, when dysphagia worsens, placement of a PEG tube should be the preferred option, especially when the respiratory function is not too much compromised. Smoking cessation advice should be offered to all patients who are current smokers. Influenza and pneumococcal immunization should be encouraged during the progression of the disease, although ALS has not been included in specific risk-group recommendations available so far. In case of acute pneumonia, adequacy and length of treatment, proper dosages and intervals of administration, and reduction of delay of initial antibiotic treatment are all important issues (American Thoracic Society, 2005; Lim et al., 2009).

Antibiotic prophylaxis strategies are especially useful to prevent ventilator-associated pneumonia, whereas passive humidifiers or heat–moisture exchangers decrease ventilator circuit colonization, but have not consistently reduced the incidence of ventilator-associated pneumonia, and thus they cannot be regarded as a pneumonia prevention tool (American Thoracic Society, 2005).

5. Invasive mechanical ventilation

ALS is a relentless pathology that causes progressive muscle dysfunction. Therefore respiratory capacity eventually fails, despite NIPPV treatment. Indeed, at first, NIPPV is generally used for intermittent nocturnal support to alleviate symptoms of nocturnal hypoventilation, although as respiratory function worsens, patients tend to require increasing daytime support and eventually continuous support. When all the respiratory aids fail to maintain adequate blood oxygen saturation, the only intervention that allows survival of these patients is invasive mechanical ventilation through a tracheostomy tube. Treatment failure seems not to be dependent on lung or respiratory muscle function but on bulbar dysfunction (Bach et al., 2004).

When placed on invasive ventilation patients are supported from a respiratory point of view; however, the loss of motor neurons goes on progressively, leading to complete paralysis and muscular atrophy. Some patients may eventually reach a "locked in" state in which they cannot communicate at all, because there is also total paralysis of the extraocular muscles. When connected to tracheostomy tubes patients may survive for many years, with respiratory tract infections the most frequent cause of death (Bradley et al., 2002; Hayashi & Oppenheimer, 2003; Lo Coco et al., 2007; Marchese et al., 2008; Vianello et al., 2011). Median survival time usually ranges from 2 to 4 years. Interestingly, the amyotrophic lateral sclerosis functional rating scale (ALSFRS), a disease-specific rating scale that assesses functional impairment, has been shown to predict both length of hospital stay as a result of acute respiratory failure and survival after initiation of invasive ventilation in these patients (Lo Coco et al., 2007).

Notwithstanding its effect on survival, only a minority of patients with ALS receive invasive mechanical ventilation, at least in the western Countries (Moss et al., 1993; Miller et al., 2000; Neudert et al., 2001). On the contrary, in Japan the frequency of invasive ventilation is considerably higher. Many patients are treated in emergency without advance planning, because of a respiratory crisis, whereas the number of patients that electively choose this treatment is low (Moss et al., 1993, 1996; Cazzoli & Oppenheimer, 1996; Lo Coco et al., 2007). Socio-economic reasons may be one of the possible explanations for the low prevalence of invasive ventilation in ALS, given the relatively high costs of this treatment. Moreover there is a need for 24-hour-caregiving, which could be perceived by caregivers and relatives as extremely burdensome. A recent study suggested that the choice of invasive ventilation was consistent with a sustained sense that life was worth living in any way possible, at least for some time and within certain boundaries, although it may involve unrealistic expectations of cure by some (Rabkin et al., 2006). Moreover, the attitudes of the treating physician have also a great influence (Moss et al., 1993), and there is concern that tracheostomy will prolong life beyond the point that the patient can communicate or interact with others.

Despite these many doubts and concerns, the majority of patients that underwent invasive ventilation were positive about their choice (Moss et al., 1993), reporting a satisfying quality of life (Cazzoli & Oppenheimer, 1996; Kaub-Wittemer et al., 2003), and indicating that they would repeat the choice again in the same situation. Caregivers were more frequently burdened and distressed by this intervention and they frequently witnessed a marked reduction of social life activities (Cazzoli & Oppenheimer, 1996; Gelinas et al., 1998; Kaub-Wittemer et al., 2003; Rabkin et al., 2006).

It is good practice that patients together with their families discuss end-of-life issues and preferences with the physician, so that advance directives and patient's wishes are well known in advance of a respiratory crisis (Silverstein et al., 1991; Andersen et al., 2005, 2007). Indeed, once intubated, patients can rarely get free from the ventilator. These preferences should also be reviewed periodically during the course of the disease, since patients' desires concerning life-sustaining interventions might change with disease progression. Ideally, emergency intubation and tracheostomy should be avoided (Andersen et al., 2005, 2007), but this is a much debated question, since there is not universal consent from public authorities. As a result, the percentage of patients that had been tracheotomized without informed consent is very high across studies (Moss et al., 1993, 1996; Cazzoli & Oppenheimer, 1996; Lo Coco et al., 2007).

Symptomatic treatment of severe dyspnea includes use of opioids (morphine) alone or in combination with benzodiazepines (such as lorazepam, diazepam or midazolam), if significant anxiety is present (Voltz & Borasio, 1997; Miller et al., 1999; Andersen et al., 2007; Clemens et al., 2008). Relief of dyspnea using opioids was rated as good by 81% of hospice patients with ALS. (O'Brien et al., 1992). Dose titration against clinical symptoms is recommended and rarely results in life-threatening respiratory depression. Anxiety of choking correlated highly significantly with the intensity of dyspnea (Clemens et al., 2008).

Terminal relentlessness and confusion secondary to hypecapnia could be relieved by administration of neuroleptic drugs (Voltz & Borasio, 1997; Miller et al., 1999; Andersen et al., 2007).

There are some case series offering practical advice for withdrawing both invasive and non-invasive ventilation, including frequent and repeated discussions and counseling with the patient and his family, assessment for discomfort, such as dyspnea, agitation, or anxiety, and symptom management during the withdrawal process with morphine and benzodiazepines (such as diazepam) (Borasio &, Voltz, 1998; Ankrom et al., 2001; O'Mahony et al., 2003). However, there are no controlled studies specifically examining withdrawal of ventilation in ALS (Miller et al., 2009b).

6. Conclusion

Recent publications provided important contributions to many aspects of respiratory care for patients with ALS, such as non-invasive ventilation and assisted cough. There is a need for regular assessment and follow up of respiratory function, and investigations should include daytime assessment of respiratory function (including FVC and SNIP) as well as sleep studies in order to ensure early recognition of patients with respiratory muscle impairment (Lo Coco et al., 2008).

At present time the only approved pharmacological treatment for ALS is riluzole, which extends survival by about 2 months (Miller et al., 2007). On the other hand, NIPPV treatment allows survival for longer periods of time, improves quality of life, and may probably alter the disease course. As a consequence, NIPPV should be considered a major treatment option in patients with chronic hypoventilation or in whom respiratory impairment has become evident during sleep despite normal diurnal respiratory function. Every effort, then, should be made to improve NIPPV implementation in the management of patients with ALS worldwide, since it is still underutilized. The degree of hypoventilation that should prompt introduction of NIPPV must be defined further, even if there is a general tendency toward earlier intervention. Nocturnal hypoventilation could be particularly useful for this purpose.

Prevention of aspiration and pneumonia, and adequate management of bronchial secretions are two other important issues. Adequate treatment of sialorrhea and dysphagia are important in the reduction of pneumonia risk. Insufficient cough is a condition that can be diagnosed by measuring peak cough flow and should, whenever present, be treated in patients with ALS. There is some evidence that the MI-E device could be of help in cough assistance, except for patients with severe bulbar dysfunction, but further research is needed, as well as randomized trials that compare the MI-E with other techniques of assisted coughing.

7. References

Aboussouan, LS; Khan, SU; Meeker, DP; Stelmach, K; Mitsumoto, H. (1997). Effect of noninvasive positive pressure ventilation on survival in ALS. *Ann. Intern. Med.*, vol.127:450-453.

Aboussouan, LS; Khan, Su; Banerjee, M; Arroliga, AC; Mitsumoto, H. (2001). Objective measures of the efficacy of non-invasive positive-pressure ventilation in ALS. *Muscle Nerve*, vol.24:403-409.

American Thoracic Society. (2005). Guidelines for the management of adults with hospital-acquired, ventilator-associated, and healthcare-associated pneumonia. *Am. J. Respir. Crit. Care Med.*, vol.171:388-416.

Andersen, PM; Borasio, GD; Dengler, R; Hardiman, O; Kollewe, K; Leigh, PN; Pradat, PF; Silani, V; Tomik, B; EFNS Task Force on Diagnosis and Management of Amyotrophic Lateral Sclerosis. (2005). EFNS Task Force on managment of amyotrophic lateral sclerosis: guidelines for diagnosing and clinical care of patients and relatives. *Eur. J. Neurol.*, vol.12:921-938.

Andersen, PM; Borasio, GD; Dengler, R; Hardiman, O; Kollewe, K; Leigh, PN; Pradat, PF; Silani, V; Tomik, B; EALSC Working Group. (2007). Good practice in the management of amyotrophic lateral sclerosis: clinical guidelines. An evidence-based review with good practice points. EALSC Working Group. *Amyotroph. Lateral Scler.*, vol.8:195-213.

Ankrom, M; Zelesnick, L; Barofsky, I; Georas, S; Finucane, TE; Greenough, WB 3rd. (2001). Elective discontinuation of life-sustaining mechanical ventilation on a chronic ventilator unit. *J. Am. Geriatr. Soc.*, vol.49:1549-1554.

Arnulf, I; Similowski, T; Salachas, F; Garma, L; Mehiri, S; Attali, V; Behin-Bellhesen, V; Meininger, V; Derenne, JP. (2000). Sleep disorders and diaphragmatic function in patients with ALS. *Am. J. Respir. Crit. Care Med.*, vol.161:849-856.

Bach, JR. (1993). Mechanical insufflation-exsufflation: Comparison of peak expiratory flow with manually assisted and unassisted coughing techniques. *Chest*, vol.104:1553-1562.

Bach, JR; Smith, WH; Michaels, J; Saporito, L; Alba, AS; Dayal, R; Pan, J. (1993). Airway secretion clearance by mechanical exsufflation for post-poliomyelitis ventilator assisted individuals. *Arch. Phys. Med. Rehabil.*, vol.74:170-177.

Bach, JR. (1994). Update and perspective on noninvasive respiratory muscle aids: Part 2. The expiratory aids. *Chest*, vol.105:1538-1544.

Bach, JR & Saporito, LR. (1996). Criteria for extubation and tracheostomy tube removal for patients with ventilatory failure: a different approach to weaning. *Chest*, vol.110:1566-1571.

Bach, JR; Ishikama Y; Kim, H. (1997). Prevention of pulmonary morbidity for patients with Duchenne muscular dystrophy. *Chest*, vol.112:1024-1028.

Bach, JR; Rajaraman, R; Ballanger, F; Tzeng, AC; Ishikawa, Y; Kulessa, R; Bansal, T. (1998). Neuromuscular ventilatory insufficiency: effect of home mechanical ventilator use v oxygen therapy on pneumonia and hospitalization rates. *Am. J. Phys. Med. Rehabil.*, vol.77:8-19.

Bach, JR. (2002). Amyotrophic lateral sclerosis: prolongation of life by noninvasive respiratory aids. *Chest,* vol.122:92-98.

Bach, JR; Bianchi, C; Aufiero, E. (2004). Oximetry and indications for tracheostomy for amyotrophic lateral sclerosis. *Chest,* vol.126:1502-1507.

Baumann, F; Henderson, RD; Morrison, SC; Brown, M; Hutchinson, N; Douglas, JA; Robinson, PJ; McCombe, PA. (2010). Use of respiratory function tests to predict survival in amyotrophic lateral sclerosis. *Amyotroph. Lateral Scler.*, vol.11:194-202.

Beneditt, JO & Boitano L. (2008). Respiratory treatment of amyotrophic lateral sclerosis. *Phys. Med. Rehabil. Clin. N. Am.*, vol.19:559-572.

Borasio, GD & Voltz, R. (1998). Discontinuation of mechanical ventilation in patients with amyotrophic lateral sclerosis. *J. Neurol.*, vol.245:717-722.

Bourke, SC; Williams, TL; Bullock, RE; Gibson, GJ; Shaw, PJ. (2002). Non-invasive ventilation in motor neuron disease: current UK practice. *Amyotroph. Lateral Scler.*, vol.3:145-149.

Bourke, SC; Bullock, RE; Williams, TL; Shaw, PJ; and Gibson, GJ. (2003). Noninvasive ventilation in ALS. Indications and effect on quality of life. *Neurology,* vol.61:171-177.

Bourke, SC; Tomlinson, M; Williams, TL; Bullock, RE; Shaw, PJ; Gibson, GJ. (2006). Effects of non-invasive ventilation on survival and quality of life in patients with amyotrophic lateral sclerosis: a randomised controlled trial. *Lancet Neurol.*, vol.5:140-147.

Bradley, WG; Anderson, F; Bromberg, M; Gutmann, L; Harati, Y; Ross, M; Miller, RG; ALS CARE Study Group. (2001). Current management of ALS: comparison of the ALS CARE Database and the AAN Practice Parameter. *Neurology,* vol.57:500-504.

Bradley, MD; Orrell, RW; Clarke, J; Davidson, AC; Williams, AJ; Kullmann, DM; Hirsch, N; Howard, RS. (2002). Outcome of ventilatory support for acute respiratory failure in motor neuron disease. *J. Neurol. Neurosurg. Psychiatry,* vol.72:752-756.

Carrat, P; Cassano, A; Gadaleta, F; Tedone, M; Dongiovanni, S; Fanfulla, F; Resta, O. (July 2011). Association between low sniff nasal-inspiratory pressure (SNIP) and sleep disordered breathing in amyotrophic lateral sclerosis: Preliminary results. *Amyotroph. Lateral Scler.*, [Epub ahead of print].

Carratù, P; Spicuzza, L; Cassano, A; Maniscalco, M; Gadaleta, F; Lacedonia, D; Scoditti, C; Boniello, E; Di Maria, G; Resta, O. (2009). Early treatment with non invasive positive pressure ventilation prolongs survival in Amyotrophic Lateral Sclerosis patients with nocturnal respiratory insufficiency. *Orphanet J. Rare Dis.*, vol.4:10.

Cazzoli, PA & Oppenheimer, EA. (1996). Home mechanical ventilation for ALS: Nasal compared to tracheostomy-intermittent positive pressure ventilation. *J. Neurol. Sci.*, vol.139(suppl):123-128.

Chaisson, KM; Walsh, S; Simmons, Z; Vender, RL. (2006). A clinical pilot study: high frequency chest wall oscillation airway clearance in patients with amyotrophic lateral sclerosis. *Amyotroph. Lateral Scler.*, vol.7:107-11.

Chaudri, MB; Liu, C; Watson, L; Jefferson, D; Kinnear, WJ. (2000). Sniff nasal inspiratory pressure as a marker of respiratory function in motor neuron disease. *Eur. Respir. J.*, vol.15:539-542.

Chaudri, MB; Liu, C; Hubbard, R; Jefferson, D; Kinnear, WJ. (2002). Relationship between supramaximal flow during cough and mortality in motor neuron disease. *Eur. Respir. J.*, vol.19:434-438.

Cheah, BC; Boland, RA; Brodaty, NE; Zoing, MC; Jeffery, SE; McKenzie, DK; Kiernan, MC. (2009). INSPIRATIonAL - INSPIRAtory muscle Training In Amyotrophic Lateral sclerosis. *Amyotroph. Lateral Scler.*, vol.28:1-9.

Clemens, KE & Klaschik, E. (2008). Morphine in the management of dyspnoea in ALS. A pilot study. *Eur. J. Neurol.*, vol.15:445-450.

Czaplinski, A; Yen, AA; Appel, SH. (2006). Forced vital capacity (FVC) as an indicator of survival and disease progression in an ALS clinic population. *J. Neurol. Neurosurg. Psychiatry*, vol.77:390-392.

De Carvalho, M ; Matias, T ; Coelho, F ; Evangelista, T ; Pinto, A ; Luis, ML. (1996). Motor neuron disease presenting with respiratory failure. *J. Neurol. Sci.*, vol.139(Suppl.):117-122.

Fallat, RJ; Jewitt, B, Bass, M; Kamm, B; Norris, F. (1979). Spirometry in amyotrophic lateral sclerosis. *Arch. Neurol.*, vol.36:74-80.

Farrero, E; Prats, E; Povedano, M; Martinez-Matos, JA; Manresa, F; Escabrill, J. (2005). Survival in amyotrophic lateral sclerosis with home mechanical ventilation. The impact of systematic respiratory assessment and bulbar involvement. *Chest*, vol.127:2132-2138.

Ferguson, KA; Strong, MJ; Ahmad, D; George, FP. (1996). Sleep-disordered breathing in amyotrophic lateral sclerosis. *Chest*, vol.110:664-669.

Fitting, JW; Paillex, R; Hirt, L; Aebischer, P; Schluep, M. (1999). Sniff nasal pressure: A sensitive respiratory test to assess progression of amyotrophic lateral sclerosis. *Ann. Neurol.*, vol.46:887-893.

Gay, PC; Westbrook, PR; Daube, JR; Litchy, WJ; Windebank, AJ; Iverson, R. (1991). Effects of alterations in pulmonary function and sleep variables on survival in patients with ALS. *Mayo Clin. Proc.*, vol.66:686-694.

Gay, PC & Edmonds, LC. (1995). Severe hypercapnia after low-flow oxygen therapy in patients with neuromuscular disease and diaphragmatic dysfunction. *Mayo Clin. Proc.*, vol.70:327-330.

Gelinas, DF; O'Connor, P; Miller, RG. (1998). Quality of life for ventilator-dependent ALS patients and their caregivers. *J. Neurol. Sci.*, vol.160(Suppl. 1):S134-S136.

Goncalves, MR & Bach, JR. (2005). Mechanical insullation.exsufflation improves outcomes for neuromuscular disease patients with respiratory tract infections. A step in the right direction (Commentary). *Am. J. Phys. Med. Rehabil.*, vol.84:89-91.

Gruis, KL; Brown, DL; Schoennemann, A; Zebarah, VA; Feldman, EL. (2005). Predictors of noninvasive ventilation tolerance in patients with amyotrophic lateral sclerosis. *Muscle Nerve*, vol.32:808-811.

Hayashi, H & Oppenheimer, EA. (2003). ALS patients on TPPV. Totally locked-in state, neurologic findings and ethical implications. *Neurology,* vol.61:135-137.

Heffernan, C; Jenkinson, C; Holmes, T; Macleod, H; Kinnear, W; Oliver, D; Leigh, N; Ampong, MA. (2006). Management of respiration in MND/ALS patients: an evidence based review. *Amyotroph. Lateral Scler.,* vol.7:5-15.

Heiman-Patterson, TD & Miller, RG. (2006). NIPPV: A treatment for ALS whose time has come. *Neurology,* vol.67:736-737.

Jackson, CE; Rosenfeld, J; Moore, DH; Bryan, WW; Barohn, RJ; Wrench, M; Myers, D; Heberlin, L; King, R; Smith, J; Gelinas, D; Miller, RG. (2001). A preliminary evaluation of a prospective study of pulmonary function studies and symptoms of hypoventilation in ALS/MND patients. *J. Neurol. Sci.,* vol.191:75-78.

Just, N; Bautin, N; Danel-Brunaud, V; Debroucker, V; Matran, R; Perez, T. (2010). The Borg dyspnoea score: a relevant clinical marker of inspiratory muscle weakness in amyotrophic lateral sclerosis. *Eur. Respir. J.,* vol.35:353-360.

Kaub-Wittemer, D; von Steinbüchel, N; Wasner, M; Laier-Groenveld, G; and Borasio, GD. (2003). Quality of life and psychososcial issues in ventilated patients with amyotrophic lateral sclerosis and their caregivers. *J. Pain and Symptom Manage.,* vol.26:890-896.

Kim, SM; Lee, KM; Hong, YH; Park, KS; Yang, JH; Nam, HW; Sung, JJ; Lee, KW. (2007). Relationship between cognitive dysfunction and reduced vital capacity in ALS. *J. Neurol. Neurosurg. Psychiatry,* vol.78:1387-1389.

Kim, SM; Park, KS; Nam, H; Ahn, SW; Kim, S; Sung, JJ; Lee, KW. (March 2011). Capnography for assessing nocturnal hypoventilation and predicting compliance with subsequent noninvasive ventilation in patients with ALS. *PLoS One,* vol.6(3):e17893. [Epub ahead of print].

King, M; Brock, G; Lundell, C. (1985). Clearance of mucus by simulated cough. *J. Appl. Physiol.,* vol.58:1776-1782.

Kirilloff, LH; Owens, GR; Rogers, RM; Mazzocco, MC. (1985). Does chest physical therapy work? *Chest,* vol.88:436-444.

Kleopa, KA; Sherman, M; Bettle, N; Romano, CJ; Heiman-Patterson, T. (1999). BiPap improves survival and rate of pulmonary function decline in patients with ALS. *J. Neurol. Sci.,* vol.164:82-88.

Lange, DJ; Lechtzin, N; Davey, C; David, W; Heiman-Patterson, T; Gelinas, D; Becker, B; Mitsumoto, H; HFCWO Study Group. (2006). High-frequency chest wall oscillation in ALS: an exploratory randomized, controlled trial. *Neurology,* vol.67:991-997.

Lechtzin, N; Wiener, CM; Clawson, L; Davidson, MC; Anderson, F; Gowda, N; Diette, GB; and the ALS CARE Study Group. (2004). Use of noninvasive ventilation in patients with amyotrophic lateral sclerosis. *Amyotroph. Lateral Scler.,* vol.5:9-15.

Lechtzin, N; Lange, DJ; Davey, C; Becker, B; Mitsumoto, H. (2007). Measures of dyspnea in patients with amyotrophic lateral sclerosis. *Muscle Nerve,* vol.35:98-102.

Lechtzin, N; Scott, Y; Busse, AM; Clawson, LL; Kimball, R; Wiener, CM. (2007). Early use of non-invasive ventilation prolongs survival in subjects with ALS. *Amyotroph. Lateral Scler.,* vol.8:185-188.

Lim WS, Baudouin SV, George RC, *et al.* (2009). BTS guidelines for the management of community acquired pneumonia in adults: update 2009. *Thorax,* vol.64(Suppl. 3):iii1-55.

Lo Coco, D; Marchese, S; Corrao, S; Pesco, MC; La Bella, V; Piccoli, F; Lo Coco, A. (2006). Development of chronic hypoventilation in Amyotrophic Lateral Sclerosis patients. *Respir. Med.,* vol.100:1028-1036.

Lo Coco, D; Marchese, S; Pesco, MC; La Bella, V; Piccoli, F; Lo Coco, A. (2006). Noninvasive positive-pressure ventilation in ALS. Predictors of tolerance and survival. *Neurology,* vol.67:761-765.

Lo Coco, D; Marchese, S; La Bella, V; Piccoli, T; Lo Coco, A. (2007). The amyotrophic lateral sclerosis functional rating scale predicts survival time in amyotrophic lateral sclerosis patients on invasive mechanical ventilation. *Chest,* vol.132:64-69.

Lo Coco, D; Marchese, S; Lo Coco, A. (2008). Recent advances in respiratory care for Motor Neuron Disease, In: *Motor Neuron Disease Research Progress*, R.L. Mancini, (Ed.), 253-269, Nova Science Publishers, Inc., ISBN 978-60456-155-5, New York, U.S.A.

Lo Coco, D; Mattaliano, P; Spataro, R; Mattaliano, A; La Bella, V. (2011). Sleep-wake disturbances in patients with amyotrophic lateral sclerosis. *J. Neurol. Neurosurg. Psychiatry,* vol.82:839-842.

Lomen-Hoerth, C. (2005). The effects of executive and behavioral dysfunction on the course of ALS. *Neurology,* vol.65:1774-1777.

Lyall, RA; Donaldson, N; Fleming, T; Wood, C; Newsom-Davis, I; Polkey, MI; Leigh, PN; Moxham, J. (2001). A prospective study of quality of life in ALS patients treated with noninvasive ventilation. *Neurology,* vol.57:153-156.

Lyall, RA; Donaldson, N; Polkey, MI; Leigh, PN; Moxham, J. (2001). Respiratory muscle strength and ventilatory failure in amyotrophic lateral sclerosis. *Brain,* vol.124:2000-2013.

Marchese, S; Lo Coco, D; Lo Coco, A. (2008). Outcome and attitudes toward home tracheostomy ventilation of consecutive patients: a 10-year experience. *Respir. Med.,* vol.102:430-436.

Marti-Fabregas, J; Dourado, M; Sanchis, J; Miralda, R; Pradas, J; Illa, I. (1995). Respiratory function deterioration is not time-linked with upper-limb onset in amyotrophic lateral sclerosis. *Acta Neurol. Scand.,* vol.92:261-264.

Massery, M & Frownfelter, D. (1990). Assisted cough techniques: There's more than one way to cough. *Phys. Ther. Forum.,* vol.9:1-4.

Miller, RG; Rosenberg, JA; Gelinas, DF; Mitsumoto, H; Newman, D; Sufit, R; Borasio, GD; Bradley, WG; Bromberg, MB; Brooks, BR; Kasarskis, EJ; Munsat, TL; Oppenheimer, EA. (1999). Practice parameter. The care of the patient with ALS (an evidence based review). *Neurology,* vol.52:1311-1323.

Miller, RG; Anderson, FA Jr; Bradley, WG; Brooks, BR; Mitsumoto, H; Munsat, TL; Ringel, SP. (2000). The ALS patient care database: goals, design, and early results. ALS C.A.R.E. Study Group. *Neurology,* vol.54:53-57.

Miller, RG; Mitchell, JD; Lyon, M, Moore, DH. (2007). Riluzole for amyotrophic lateral sclerosis (ALS)/motor neuron disease (MND). *Cochrane Database Syst. Rev.,* vol.1:CD001447.

Miller, RG; Jackson, CE; Kasarskis, EJ; England, JD; Forshew, D; Johnston, W; Kalra, S; Katz, JS; Mitsumoto, H; Rosenfeld, J; Shoesmith, C; Strong, MJ; Woolley, SC; Quality Standards Subcommittee of the American Academy of Neurology. (2009). Practice parameter update: The care of the patient with amyotrophic lateral sclerosis: drug, nutritional, and respiratory therapies (an evidence-based review): report of the

Quality Standards Subcommittee of the American Academy of Neurology. *Neurology*, vol.73:1218-1226.

Miller, RG; Jackson, CE; Kasarskis, EJ; England, JD; Forshew, D; Johnston, W; Kalra, S; Katz, JS; Mitsumoto, H; Rosenfeld, J; Shoesmith, C; Strong, MJ; Woolley, SC; Quality Standards Subcommittee of the American Academy of Neurology. (2009). Practice parameter update: The care of the patient with amyotrophic lateral sclerosis: multidisciplinary care, symptom management, and cognitive/behavioral impairment (an evidence-based review): report of the Quality Standards Subcommittee of the American Academy of Neurology. *Neurology*, vol.73:1227-1233.

Morgan, RK; McNally, S; Alexander, M; Conroy, R; Hardiman, O; Costello, RW. (2005). Use of Sniff nasal-inspiratory force to predict survival in amyotrophic lateral sclerosis. *Am. J. Respir. Crit. Care Med.*, vol.171:269-274.

Moss, AH; Casey, P; Stocking, CB; Roos, RP; Brooks, BR; Siegler, M. (1993). Home ventilation for ALS patients: outcomes, costs, and patient, family, and physician attitudes. *Neurology*, vol.43:438-443.

Moss, AH; Oppenheimer, EA; Casey, P; Cazzolli, PA; Roos, RP; Stocking, CB; Siegler, M. (1996). Patients with amyotrophic lateral sclerosis receiving long-term mechanical ventilation: advance care planning and outcomes. *Chest*, vol.110:249-255.

Munsat, TL; Andres, PL; Finison, L; Conlon, T; Thibodeau, L. (1988). The natural history of motorneuron loss in amyotrophic lateral sclerosis. *Neurology*, vol.38:409-413.

Mustfa, N; Walsh, E; Bryant, V; Lyall, RA; Addington-Hall, J; Goldstein, LH; Donaldson, N; Polkey, MI; Moxham, J; Leigh, PN. (2006). The effect of noninvasive ventilation on ALS patients and their caregivers. *Neurology*, vol.66:1211-1217.

Neudert, C; Oliver, D; Wasner, M; Borasio, G. (2001). The course of the terminal phase in patients with amyotrophic lateral sclerosis. *J. Neurol.*, vol.248:612-616.

Newson-Davis, IC; Lyall, RA; Leigh, PN; Morham, J; Goldstein, LH. (2001). The effect of NIPPV on cognitive function in ALS: a prospective study. *J. Neurol. Neurosur. Psychiatry*, vol.71:482-487.

O'Brien, T; Kelly, M; Saunders, C. (1992). Motor neuron disease: a hospice perspective. *BMJ*, vol.304:471-473.

Olney, RK; Murphy, J; Forshew, D; Garwood, E; Miller, BL; Langmore, S; Kohn, MA; Lomen-Hoerth, C. (2005). The effects of executive and behavioral dysfunction on the course of ALS. *Neurology*, vol.65:1774-1777.

O'Mahony, S; McHugh, M; Zallman, L; Selwyn, P. (2003). Ventilator withdrawal: procedures and outcomes. Report of a collaboration between a critical care division and a palliative care service. *J. Pain Symptom Manage.*, vol.26:954-961.

Peysson, S; Vandenberghe, N; Philit, F; Vial, C; Petitjean, T; Bouhour, F; Bayle, JY; Broussolle E. (2008). Factors predicting survival following noninvasive ventilation in amyotrophic lateral sclerosis. *Eur. Neurol.*, vol.59:164-171.

Pinto, A; de Carvalho, M; Evangelista, T; Lopes, A; Sales-Luis, L. (2003). Nocturnal pulse oximetry: a new approach to estabilish the appropriate time for non-invasive ventilation in ALS patients. *Amyotroph. Lateral Scler.*, vol.4:31-35.

Pinto, AC; Evangelista, T; Carvalho, M; Alves, MA; Sales Luis, ML. (1995). Respiratory assistance with a non-invasive ventilator (BiPaP) in motor neuron disease/ALS patients: survival rates in a controlled trial. *J. Neurol. Sci.*, vol.129(Suppl.):19-26.

Poponick, JM; Jacobs, I; Supinski, G; Di Marco AF. (1997). Effect of upper respiratory tract infection in patients with neuromuscular disease. *Am. J. Resp. Crit. Care Med.*, vol.156.659-664.

Rabkin, JG; Albert, SM; Tider, T; Del Bene, ML; O'Sullivan, I; Rowland, LP; Mitsumoto, H. (2006). Predictors and course of elective long-term mechanical ventilation: A prospective study of ALS patients. *Amyotroph. Lateral Scler.*, vol.7:86-95.

Radunović, A; Mitsumoto, H; Leigh, PN. (2007). Clinical care of patients with amyotrophic lateral sclerosis. *Lancet Neurol.*, vol.6:913-25.

Sancho, J; Servera, E; Diaz, J; Marin J. (2004). Efficacy of mechanical insufflation-exsufflation in medically stable patients with amyotrophic lateral sclerosis. *Chest*, vol.125:1400-1405.

Sancho, J; Servera, E; Diaz, J; Marin J. (2007). Predictors of ineffective cough during a chest infection in stable ALS patients. *Am. J. Resp. Crit. Care Med.*, vol.175:1266-1271.

Schiffman, PL & Belsh, JM. (1993). Pulmonary function at diagnosis of ALS. Rate of deterioration. *Chest*, vol.103:508-513.

Schmidt, EP; Drachman, DB; Wiener, CM; Clawson, L; Kimball, R; Lechtzin, N. (2006). Pulmonary predictors of survival in amyotrophic lateral sclerosis: Use in clinical trial design. *Muscle Nerve*, vol.33:127-132.

Silverstein, MD; Stocking, CB; Antel, JP; Beckwith, J; Roos, RP; Siegler, M. (1991). Amyotrophic lateral sclerosis and life-sustaining therapy: patients' desires for information, participation in decision making, and life-sustaining therapy. *Mayo Clin. Proc.*, vol.66:906-913.

Stembler, N; Charatan, M; Cederbaum, JM; and the ALS CNTF Treatment Study Croup. (1998). Prognostic indicators of survival in ALS. *Neurology*, vol.50:66-72.

Tzeng, AC & Bach, JR. (2000). Prevention of pulmonary morbidity for patients with neuromuscular disease. *Chest*, vol.118:1390-1396.

Varrato, J; Siderowf, A; Damiano, P; Gregory, S; Feinberg, D; McCluskey, L. (2001). Postural change of forced vital capacity predicts some respiratory symptoms in ALS. *Neurology*, vol.57:357-359.

Velasco, R; Salachas, F; Munerati, E; Le Forestier, N; Pradat, PF; Lacomblez, L; Orvoen Frija, E; Meininger, V. (2002). Nocturnal oximetry in patients with amyotrophic lateral sclerosis: role in predicting survival. *Rev. Neurol.*, vol.158:575-578.

Vianello, A; Corrado, A; Arcaro, G; Gallan, F; Ori, C; Minuzzo, M; Bevilacqua, M. (2005). Mechanical insullation.exsufflation improves outcomes for neuromuscular disease patients with respiratory tract infections. *Am. J. Phys. Med. Rehabil.*, vol.84:83-88.

Vianello, A; Arcaro, G; Palmieri, A; Ermani, M; Braccioni, F; Gallan, F; Soraràu, G; Pegoraro, E. (2011). Survival and quality of life after tracheostomy for acute respiratory failure in patients with amyotrophic lateral sclerosis. *J. Crit. Care*, vol.26:329.e7-14.

Volanti, P; Cibella, F; Sarvà, M; De Cicco, D; Spanevello, A; Mora, G; La Bella, V. (2011). Predictors of non-invasive ventilation tolerance in amyotrophic lateral sclerosis. *J. Neurol. Sci.*, vol.303:114-118.

Voltz, R & Borasio, GD. (1997). Palliative therapy in the terminal stage of neurological disease. *J. Neurol.*, vol.244(Suppl. 4):S2-10.

26

Nutritional Care in Amyotrophic Lateral Sclerosis: An Alternative for the Maximization of the Nutritional State

Luciano Bruno de Carvalho-Silva
Federal University of Alfenas- MG (UNIFAL-MG); Center for Food Security Studies (NEPA), State University of Campinas (UNICAMP)
Brazil

1. Introduction

Amyotrophic lateral sclerosis (ALS) is characterized by progressive paralysis secondary to the impairment of the motor neurons, upper motor neuron and lower motor neuron. The most common symptoms and signs are atrophy and muscle weakness, fasciculations, cramps, hypertonia and hyperreflexia. In more advanced stages, decreased respiratory muscle strength, progressive loss of body weight and changes in food intake are observed (Nelson et al., 2000).

Several factors are inherent to the food intake in ALS, such as: lack of appetite, dysphagia, weakness, dyspnoea, and depression (Stanich et al., 2004; Nelson et al., 2000; Kasarskis et al., 1996; Welnetz, 1990; Slowie et al., 1983). ALS patients usually have rapid weight loss associated with reduced food intake, increased feeding time, fatigue, dehydration and depression (Wright et al., 2005). The combination of these factors may result in increased energy expenditure and therefore hypercatabolism.

Different studies confirm the correlation between the reduced Body Mass Index (BMI) and the decreased survival in subjects with ALS and the decreased food intake and decrease in tricipital skinfold (TSF) (Kasarskis et al., 1996; Desport et al., 2003; Desport et al., 1999; Desport et al., 2001; Heffernan et al., 2004; Slowie et al. 1983). They also show a high percentage of weight loss, greater than 15% (Mazzini et al. 1995), and prevalence of malnutrition.

Dysphagia, a common symptom with the disease progression, is a factor that makes difficult the maintenance of oral feeding, increasing the respiratory complications, with initiation of invasive ventilation, difficulty to move the patient for the outpatient care and depression (Mazzini et al., 1995).

In this context, taking the nutritiontal impairment experienced by ALS subjects into account, this chapter aims to discuss the key strategies of nutritional care of patients with ALS, with a tool for maximizing the nutritional status.

2. Amyotrophic lateral sclerosis and nutritional status

2.1 Food intake in ALS

Few studies on food intake in patients with ALS are available in the literature. Among these studies, Kasarskis et al. (1996) studies stand out, which found that 70% of the subjects experienced energy intake below the RDA and 84% of the patients experienced protein intake above the RDA. Slowie et al. (1983) found, as well as Kasarskis et al. (1996), 70% of inadequacy for energy, using the 24-hour recall in patients with ALS. Stanich et al. (2004), found values above the RDA for lipids in most ALS patients chosen in their study.

Silva et al. (2007a and 2007b) analyzed the nutritional profile of patients treated in Dysphagia and Neuromuscular Outpatient Clinics of the Hospital das Clínicas of Unicamp – HC/UNICAMP. Interdisciplinary assessments were performed, revealing a low caloric intake of approximately 1600 kcal for men. In women, a low caloric intake (approximately 1700 kcal/day) was also observed.

In another study conducted by Silva et al. (2008a) the food intake was quantitatively and qualitatively assessed in ALS patients regularly followed at the neuromuscular outpatient clinic of the HC-UNICAMP. The foods most consumed daily were oil, rice, beans, French bread and milk. The food was found to be inadequate regarding energy, fiber, calcium and vitamin E. A significant difference was observed between patients with ALS of bulbar and appendicular predominance, whereas, in patients with higher appendicular manifestation, a higher energy intake ($p=0.02$) of saturated fat ($p=0.03$), monounsaturated fat ($p=0.04$) and polyunsaturated fat ($p=0.001$), as well as cholesterol ($p=0.001$) and fibers ($p=0.001$) was observed when compared with the ALS of bulbar predominance. A higher swallowing impairment observed in patients with bulbar predominance may have influenced the qualitative and quantitative intake. While feeding is impacted by the disease features, the per capita income of patients seems to have influenced the low qualitative consumption of food. Based on the results obtained, the authors suggested that guidance regarding the consumption of foods and preparations with a higher content of high-biological proteins, fibers, calcium, and vitamin E is necessary.

In ALS, as in most neuromuscular diseases, changes can also be observed, which increase the muscle catabolism, directly impacting protein synthesis and mineral excretion. In the initial stages of the disease, according to the study conducted in 94 patients with ALS, it was observed no deficiency of vitamins E and C, but upon disease progression, clinical and biochemical manifestations of such deficiency were observed (Ludolph, 2006).

To estimate the dietary intake, some countries in Europe and Canada use as main practices the 24-hour recall, 3-day and 7-day food record. To estimate the energy requirements, professionals have used the equations of Schofield (1985) and Harris and Benedict (1919). To estimate the adequacy of macronutrients, the researchers used the standards of the Recommended Dietary Allowances (NCR, 1989), Department of Health (1991) and the Institute of Medicine (IOM, 2002; IOM, 2001; IOM 2000; IOM 1997).

To estimate the energy requirements, the most used equation was that of Harris and Benedict (1919) modified by Long; Schaffel; Geiger (1979).

According to Harris and Benedict:

$$\text{Men:}\quad BMR^* = 66 + (13.7 \text{ x mass in kg}) + (5 \text{ x height in cm}) - (6.8 \text{ x age in years})$$

$$\text{Women:}\quad BMR^* = 655 + (9.6 \text{ x mass in kg}) + (1.7 \text{ x height in cm}) - (4.7 \text{ x age in years})$$

*BMR = basal metabolic rate

Modified by Long; Schaffel; Geiger (1979):

VET* = BMR x activity factor x injury factor

*TEV = total energy value

The activity factor is considered as 1.2 for patients unable to walk and 1.3 for patients able to walk. The injury factor is considered as 1.1 for chronic diseases (Long; Schaffel; Geiger, 1979). Considering a higher energy expenditure (10-20%) for individuals with ALS (Piquet, 2006), some professionals also employ 35 kcal/kg current body weight.
For water intake, the estimation according to Thomas (2001) should be 30-35mL/kg, taking the age into account.

2.2 Anthropometry and body composition

The nutritional status can be evaluated through objective methods, such as: anthropometry, body composition, biochemical parameters and dietary consumption; or subjective methods, such as: physical examination and subjective global assessment. Anthropometry involves obtaining measures of body size, their proportions and the relationship with standards that reflect the development of adult subjects. The most used measures are weight, height, circumferences and skinfolds (Almeida et al., 2010; Silva et al., 2008b; Silva et al., 2008c; Stanich et al., 2004; Kasarskis et al., 1996; Slowie et al., 1983).

2.2.1 Weight (W)

For patients unable to walk, in the absence of a metabolic scale, the weight is measured using a wheelchair. Prior to patient's weighing, the wheelchairs are weighted and their weight is deducted at the time of calibration of the scale. In patients able to walk, the body weight is measured standing on platform type or digital scales (Silva et al., 2008b; Stanich et al., 2004). The weight can also be measured in chair scales, available in the market.

2.2.2 Height (H)

The height for individuals unable to walk is measured with the subject seated closest to the edge of the chair with his/her left knee bent at 90 degrees. The length between the plantar surface and the knee is measured with the help of a measuring tape. The height is estimated according to the equations proposed by Chumlea; Roche; Steinbaugh (1985), where:

$$\text{Men's height} = \left[64.19 - (0.04 \text{ x age in years})\right] + (2.02 \text{ x knee height in cm})$$

$$\text{Women's height} = [84.88 - (0.24 \text{ x age in years}) + (1.83 \text{ x knee height in cm})$$

2.2.3 Body mass index (BMI)

Usually, body mass-height ratio is used as an indicator of body mass index (BMI = body mass kg/height m^2).
The BMI classification is described below:

- BMI < 16 kg/m^2: severe malnutrition
- 16 - 16.9 kg/m^2: moderate malnutrition
- 17.0 - 18.49 kg/m^2: mild malnutrition
- 18.5 - 24.9 kg/m^2: eutrophic
- 25.0 - 29.9 kg/m^2: overweight
- 30.0 - 34.9 kg/m^2: grade I obesity
- 35.0 - 39.9 kg/m^2: grade II obesity
- >40 kg/m^2: grade III obesity (World Health Organization, 1985)

Kasarskis *et al.* (1996) confirm the correlation between reduced BMI and decreased life expectancy. In studies carried out by Mazzini *et al.* (1995), 53% of ALS patients showed BMI < 20Kg/m^2 and 55% had weight loss > 15% of usual weight.

2.2.4 Arm circumference (AC)

The arm circumference is measured at the non-dominant arm extended along the body, measured at the midpoint between the acromion and the olecranon process, using a flexible, non-elastic, plastic measuring tape (Lohman; Roche; Martorell, 1991). Desport; Maillot (2002) uses the AC to calculate the arm muscle circumference (AMC) and monitor the nutritional status of patients with ALS.

2.2.5 Skinfolds

Tricipital skinfold (TSF) is determined along the longitudinal axis of the arm, on its posterior face, whereas its exact point of repair is the average distance between the superior lateral edge of the acromion and the olecranon.

Bicipital skinfold (BSF) is determined towards the longitudinal axis of the arm, on its anterior face, in the mid-point of the humeral biceps.

Subscapular skinfold (SCSF) is obtained obliquely to the longitudinal axis following the direction of the ribs, and located 2 cm distant from the lower angle of the scapula.

Suprailiac skinfold (SISF) is measured by slightly placing the patient's right arm behind, trying not to influence the attainment of the measure. This fold is obliquely individualized 2 cm above the anterior superior iliac crest, at the anterior axillary line.

To evaluate the AC and skinfolds, the reference standard used is the work of Frisancho (1981).

2.3 Classification of nutritional status

According to the Percentile Distribution Table, the percentage of adequacy for the abovementioned parameters is calculated by considering the 50th percentile (P50) as standard.

$$\% \text{ adequacy} = \text{studied parameter value} / \text{P50 value} \times 100$$

Values in Table 1 are used for the classification of nutritional status.

Parameters	Obesity	Overweig ht	Eutrophy	mild PEM[1]	moderate PEM	severe PEM
AC[2]	≥ 120%	120-110%	110-90%	90-80%	80-70%	≤ 70%
TSF[3]	≥120%	120-110%	110-90%	90-80%	80-70%	≤ 70%

[1]PEM: Protein-energy malnutrition; [2]AC: arm circumference; [3]TSF: Tricipital skinfold.

Table 1. Classification of nutritional status according to the parameters proposed by Blackburn; Harvey (1982) and Blackburn; Thornton (1979).

For the determination of the nutritional status, the anthropometric parameters are analyzed together. The values obtained according to the percentage adequacy are classified by Protein-Energy Malnutrition (PEM) Score. The PEM Score is the sum of all parameters of nutritional assessment in percentage adequacy divided by the number of parameters assessed (Blackburn; Harvey, 1982).

$$\text{PEM Score} = \frac{\%\ \text{adq OW} + \%\ \text{adq TSF} + \%\ \text{adq AC} + \%\ \text{adq AMC} + \%\ \text{adq AMA}}{\text{Numbers of parameters}}$$

% adq OW = % adequacy from the optimal weight
% adq TSF = % adequacy of tricipital skinfold
% adq AC = % adequacy of arm circumference
% adq AMC = % adequacy of arm muscle circumference
% adq AMA = % adequacy of arm muscle area
The value obtained by PEM score allows for the classification of patients as:
Eutrophy: > 100%
Mild PEM: < 100% and > 80%
Moderate PEM: < 80% and > 60%
Severe PEM: < 60%

2.3.1 Percentage of weight loss (% WL)

The percentage change of usual weight or percentage of weight loss (% WL) is determined using the patient's usual and current weights, as per the following equation:

$$\%\ \text{WL} = \frac{\text{Usual Weight} - \text{Current Weight}}{\text{Usual Weight}} \times 100$$

The % WL highly reflects the extent of the disease. Patients with % WL values > 10% are classified as malnourished and above 10% severe malnutrition (Mahan; Escott-Stump, 2005).

2.4 Bioelectrical impedance analysis

Bioelectrical impedance analysis (BIA) is a non-invasive technique that can be used to estimate body composition. The method uses low amperage current (single or multiple frequencies) that passes between two electrodes placed on the skin under the assumption that the current resistance (impedance) ranges on an inversely proportional basis to the fluid contained in the tissues and the content of electrolytes. BIA has a good correlation with body composition made with the isotope dilution, under controlled conditions (O'Brien; Young; Sawka, 2002).

In ALS, due to the limitations and difficulties during nutritional assessment, BIA has been a good tool in nutritional diagnosis. It is an easy, non-invasive technique, where fat-free and fat mass are obtained, in addition to the estimation of the degree of hydration. In 2003, the equation for BIA was validated in patients with ALS through cross-sectional and longitudinal studies, which was optimized at 50 kHz (Desport et al., 2003).

2.5 Dual-emission X-ray absorptiometry (DEXA)

The dual-emission X-ray absorptiometry (DEXA) is an invasive method that has become a popular measure for the assessment of body composition in developed countries (Madsen; Jensen; Sorensen, 1997; Tothill et al., 1996; Snead; Birge; Kohrt, 1993). This method allows the structural assessment of body composition, dividing the body mass by three basic components: mineral- and fat-free soft tissue, bone mineral content and fat (Laskey, 1996).

Some studies show the use of such technique in ALS patients (Tadan et al., 1998; Nau et al., 1995; Kanda et al., 1994), however Desport et al. (2003) emphasizes the equipment is very expensive, and the fact that the patient remains in a horizontal position with his/her arms extended along the body for more than 10 minutes can be a problem for subjects with ALS.

In a study conducted by Rio and Cawadias (2007), it was discussed the main techniques adopted by nutritionists of some centers for the treatment of ALS in Europe and Canada for nutritional assessment of ALS subjects. The researchers found only 22% of nutritionists had more than 4 years of experience in ALS. Amongst the most used nutritional assessment methods were weight, % WL, BMI and arm circumference, used by 100%, 96%, 83%, and 9% of the professionals, respectively. The bioelectrical impedance, validated by Desport et al. in 2003, as well as DEXA, were not reported by the professionals from the centers investigated by Rio and Cawadias.

Analyzing the measures adopted by the relevant literature, in ALS, as well as in other diseases, the use of parameters such as weight, % WL and BMI, as well as skinfolds, BIA, DEXA and indirect calorimetry can also be observed (Rio; Cawadias 2007; Desport et al., 2003; Desport et al., 2001; Silani; Kasarkis, Yanagisawa, 1998).

3. Dysphagia and ALS

With the clinical progression of ALS, manifestations such as dysarthria (speech impairment), dyspnoea (breathing alteration), dysphonia (voice alteration) and dysphagia (swallowing alteration) are common. These manifestations occur as a result of progressive respiratory muscle dysfunction, caused by motor neuron degeneration of corticobulbar tract (Chiappetta; Oda, 2004).

In 17 to 30% of ALS patients, bulbar muscles, especially the muscle groups of the velum and tongue are the first ones affected, resulting in progressive dysphagia, and therefore difficulty in swallowing food and liquids (Calia; Annes, 2003; Mitsumoto; Norris, 1994; Gubbay et al., 1985).

The oro-laryngo-pharyngeal weakness affects the survival of subjects with ALS, especially because of the continuous risk of aspiration pneumonia and sepsis, and the inadequate food intake, which can result in malnutrition (Karsarkis et al., 1996).

Malnutrition due to dysphagia, or other factors associated, such as muscle atrophy and diaphragm weakness, increases the relative risk of death almost eight times in ALS patients (Mitsumoto et al., 2003; Desport et al., 1999).

The involvement of the tongue muscles and lip orbicular muscles, upon ALS progression, triggers a decrease in pressure wave, pharyngeal peristalsis, and elevation and anteriorization of larynx, causing choking, even with saliva (Watts; Vanryckeghem, 2001; Strand et al., 1996).

In ALS, dysphagia for liquids is more common than for solids. The early escape, that is, when the food reaches the vallecula prior to initiation of pharyngeal swallowing, is more frequent with thin liquids and is the leading cause of tracheal aspiration. Pharyngeal residues are more commonly observed throughout the course of the disease. The pasty and solid consistencies may cause laryngeal penetration and tracheal aspiration after swallowing. Swallowing disorders occur due to the influence of oral transit, decreased movement of the tongue base, decreased elevation and anteriorization of the larynx and decreased pharyngeal contraction (Chiappetta; Oda, 2004; Logeman, 1998; Campbel; Enderby, 1984; apud Chiappetta, 2005).

In order to minimize respiratory and nutritional complications in the treatment of dysphagia, interdisciplinary assessment is extremely important, and the modification of the texture of foods is an alternative for the maintenance of the oral route.

3.1 Influence of viscosity

Food viscosity is one of the most important variables of swallowing. Thin liquids make difficult swallowing by patients with reduced laryngeal control, since they are quickly swallowed and do not maintain their shape inside the oral cavity, which can prematurely leak into the pharynx and, thus, penetrate the airways still open. To avoid such effect, the optimal viscosity must be determined so the swallowing may occur safety (Macedo & Furkim, 2000).

Viscosity influences many aspects of the assessment and management of dysphagia. It can be defined as the fluid resistance to the flow and is measured in Centipoise (ctps or cPs) (Silva et al, 2010).

There are different types of viscosity that can be easily achieved using commercial thickeners. These types can be classified in centipoise (cP) values (Table 1) as thin (1-50 cP), nectar (51-350 cP), honey (351-1750 cP) and pudding (> 1750 cP).

Classification	Viscosity (cP)
Thin	1-50
Nectar	51-350
Honey	351-1750
Pudding	> 1750

Source: ADA, 2002.

Table 2. Classification of viscosity, in centipoise (cP) values, according to the ADA (2002), for the nutritional care of subjects with dysphagia.

4. Nutritional therapy

Patients with symptoms of dysphagia limiting their intake of foods and liquids, hospitalized or at home, should be considered those at high risk of experiencing nutritional deficiencies and consequently should be treated.

Appropriate nutrition and hydration in patients with dysphagia are based on a complex balance between preparation, intake and absorption of foods and drinks (Steele & Lieshout, 2004).

When diagnosing the cause and severity of dysphagia, healthcare professionals can determine the texture of foods and the thickness of fluids for a safer swallowing by dysphagic patients, since the consistency of the diet should be individualized according to the type and extent of dysfunction. In case the recipe is not followed, the subject may face serious consequences for health (Silva et al, 2010; Macedo & Furquim, 2000).

Table 1 shows an example of a modified diet with restriction of "thin liquids" (1-50 cP) and solids for subjects with dysphagia and swallowing impairment.

Meal	Food	Ingredients (Servings)	Viscosity (cP)
Breakfast:	Dried milk porridge Mashed banana	Milk: 100 mL Dried Milk: 25 g 1 unit - 90 g	910 2.900
Snack:	Thickened papaya juice	Water: 30 mL Papaya: 170 g	870
Lunch:	Spaghetti and basil soup (liquefied) Thickened orange juice	Spaghetti (125 g), vegetable oil (2 tablespoons), onion (1 unit), mashed garlic cloves (2 units), nut (60 g), chicken bouillon (70 mL), fresh basil leaves (30 g), salt to taste, grated cheese (1 dessert spoon). Orange juice: 200 mL Thickener: 10 g	2.440 320
Snack:	Juice of fruits (papaya, banana and apple)	Cold fluid milk (10°) (200 mL), papaya (100 g), banana (90 g), apple (50 g)	1.090
Dinner:	Vegetable broth Lemon Mousse	Water (2 L), turnips (2 units), carrots (2 units), garlic clove (1 unit), onion (1 unit), arracacha (1 unit), bunch of watercress (1 unit), basil (to taste), salt (to taste), and a drizzle of olive oil, raw large potato (1 unit) 100 g	4.680 8.000
Supper:	Maize porridge	Milk: 100 mL Maize bran: 25 g	840

* Adapted from Peres, Manzano and Silva (2007).

Table 3. Modified diet with restriction of "thin liquids" (1-50 cP) and "solids" for subjects with dysphagia and swallowing impairment. Features: Soft, wet and liquefied foods. Liquid foods are all thickened. The example menu contains approximately 2,000 kilocalories.

Changes in viscosity of foods and fluids can be achieved with the help of commercial thickeners. The choice of thickening agent is critical to achieve a homogeneous and lasting consistency. The thickeners should interfere as little as possible with the sensory properties of liquids (Silva et al, 2010)

Several agents can be used as food thickeners. Such thickeners are mostly composed of polysaccharides (carbohydrates), such as gums and starches, in addition to pectins and cellulose derivatives. Among them, the modified starch is one of the most used, since the starch physically or chemically treated improves the properties of thickening, cohesion, stability, gelatinization, luster and taste of the natural starch. In addition, they can also maximize the nutritional and water intake, facilitating a wide variety of textures (Silva & Ikeda, 2009). Therefore, these modified starch-containing thickeners can be used to prevent dehydration of subjects with dysphagia (Ada, 2002). However, the commercial thickeners are very expensive (approximately R$ 40.00 BRL/200 g), which limits the purchase and adjustment of the correct consistency.

It is known that the intake may be maximized by adjusting the consistency of foods through simple and low-cost techniques, without using commercial thickeners that are very expensive (Silva & Ikeda, 2009; Whelan, 2001). Thickening of foods by using the own foods in several preparations so as to adjust the correct consistency is still unknown by many patients, caregivers and healthcare professionals, limiting the food intake, resulting in high rates of malnutrition, dehydration and pulmonary aspiration, and increasing the risk of death[32]. These techniques are designed for this population, especially regarding the amount of food in household measures necessary to achieve optimal viscosity, according to the ADA standard (Silva et al., 2006a).

In 2006, researches were conducted in order to develop a guide with recent literature survey, standardized preparations for patients with dysphagia, viscosities adjusted according to the ADA, chemical composition and photographic record for healthcare professionals, caregivers and patients with dysphagia, for a safe dietary intake (Silva et al., 2006b). Studies like this are still scarce for this population.

The poor knowledge of the fundamental physical characteristics of the consistency of the preparations is considered a limiting factor to adjust the viscosity, which does not ensure a safe intake. Figure 1 shows a photographic representation of a preparation of heart of palm cream with the consistency of pudding. Its main characteristic is the formation of a heavy cake, in which there is low adherence on the spoon surface, forming no continuous filaments.

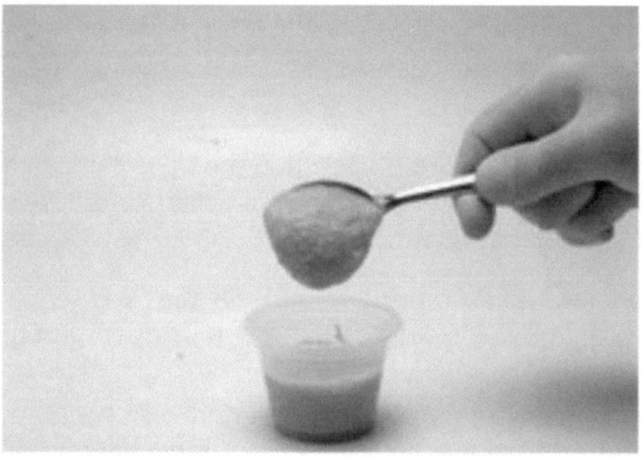

Fig. 1. Photographic representation of a preparation (heart of palm cream) with pudding consistency. pH = 3.73; viscosity = 2000 cP; amount of water for dilution = 0 mL

Figure 2 shows a photographic representation of the same preparation with the consistency of honey, in which there is a formation of continuous filament with the base of the spoon forming a characteristic "V".

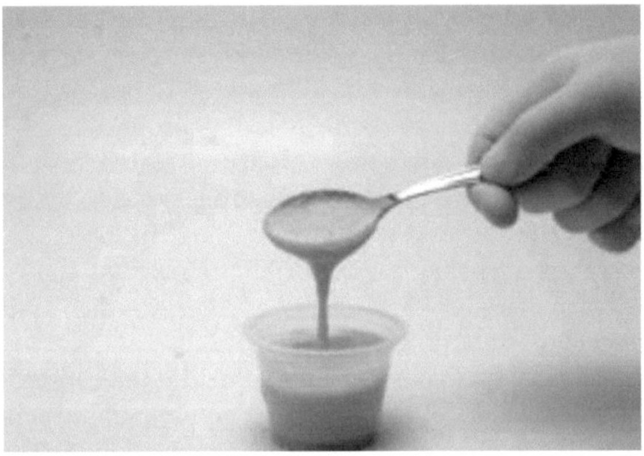

Fig. 2. Photographic representation of a preparation (heart of palm cream) with honey consistency. pH = 3.69; viscosity = 1080 cP; amount of water for dilution in 100 mL of the recipe with pudding viscosity = 14.23 mL

In the photographic representation of the nectar consistency (Figure 3), there is a formation of continuous filament thinner than the previous one, without a characteristic "V" at the base of the spoon.

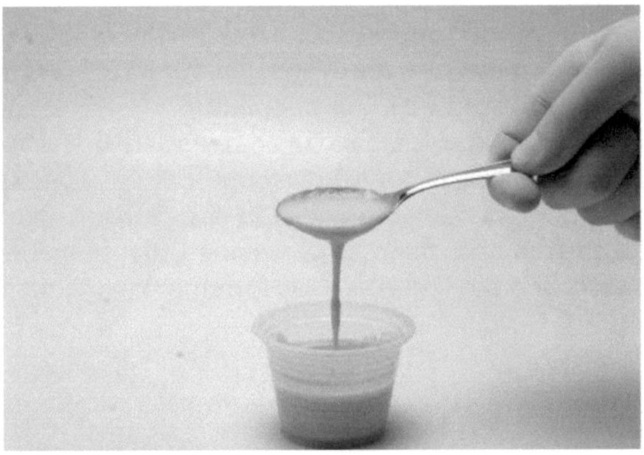

Fig. 3. Photographic representation of a preparation (heart of palm cream) with nectar consistency. pH = 3.71; viscosity = 240 cP; amount of water for dilution in 100 mL of the recipe with pudding viscosity = 42.88 mL

Figure 4 shows a photographic representation of the thin consistency of the same preparation; as the name implies, there is no formation of continuous filament, but only drops that fall from the spoon.
These alternatives are considered simple, low-cost and safe, and are extremely important to ensure a better quality of life for patients without dysphagia, without limiting the need for commercial thickeners, but guidelines concerning how to follow a correct preparation are still necessary. Currently, there are discussions on the improvement of the quality of

life and reduction of potential complications, through education/health promotion programs, including specialized procedures and orientation programs for caregivers (Santoro, 2008)

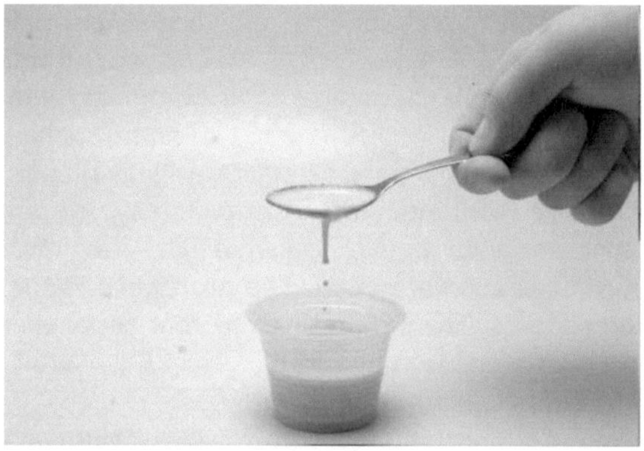

Fig. 4. Photographic representation of a preparation (heart of palm cream) with thin consistency. pH = 5.36; viscosity = 46 cP; amount of water for dilution in 100 mL of the recipe with pudding viscosity = 107.14 mL

Periodic and appropriate reassessments of the swallowing condition are critical aspects for the prevention/recovery from malnutrition. One study assessed the adequacy of the diet of elderlies admitted to nursing homes, where 91% of the patients had diets with a consistency below what they could tolerate safely. Both the nutritional status and the quality of life may be affected when patients are maintained on diets with inappropriate viscosity (Souza et al., 2003)

Patients with dysphagia may experience satiety quickly when they are given an extremely concentrated meal. Instead of providing three meals a day, these patients should receive smaller and more frequent portions (Silva et al., 2003). Of note, for patients with dysphagia, difficulty in performing the swallowing movements worsens when they are most tired. This is especially important for patients with diseases like Parkinson's, for which the medication effect can be reduced during the day, further reducing the patient's ability to swallow (Sachdev, 2005). The correct positioning of the patient may be of great help during meals, but it is important to follow the instructions of a speech therapist & audiologist.

If there is a high risk of aspiration or oral intake is insufficient to maintain the good nutritional status, the possibility of an alternative nutritional support must be considered. A soft and well tolerable tube can be inserted and radiologically guided. Percutaneous endoscopic gastrostomy is performed by inserting a gastrostomy tube into the stomach through a percutaneous abdominal route guided by the endoscopist and, if available, surgical gastrostomy is preferable (Ickenstein, 2003; Nguyen et al., 2006).

Therefore, the guidance on an individualized diet, precautions on the risk of aspiration, and appropriate choice regarding the route of access for feeding, help to prevent malnutrition in patients with dysphagia, where the care of a multidisciplinary team is required for the patient's welfare, as well as for a better quality of life. Nonetheless, the absence of detailed descriptions on the procedures for nutritional therapy makes unfeasible their efficient replication (Nguyen et al., 2006).

4.1 Nutritional support

Nutritional support may delay the weight loss and muscle atrophy. Researchers have shown the weight loss associated with bulbar changes (dysphagia and breathing) require early and specific nutritional support (Kasarskis *et al.*, 1996; Slowie *et al.*, 1983).

Constant muscle atrophy, characteristic of progressive diseases, may mask the increased metabolic demand. The increased baseline energy expenditure of patients with ALS occurs since the energies are focused on the maintenance of pulmonary ventilation (Stanich *et al.*, 2004; Kasarskis *et al.*, 1996; Nau *et al.*, 1995; Shimizu; Hayashi; Tanabe, 1991).

In a study of ALS patients, under the oral nutritional supplementation program, there was a progressive decrease in body mass index (BMI) in patients with progressive bulbar palsy and preservation of such variables in ALS patients. The lean mass/fat mass ratio was maintained during the study for both groups. The nutritional status classification has not changed for 70% of the patients. The results showed that supplementation prevented the worsening of nutritional status, but was unable to correct the overall averages of adequacy (Stanich et al., 2004).

In clinical practice, the use of supplements of vitamins, especially vitamin E, is common. The supplementation of this vitamin, with quantity still not defined, is expected to improve the nutritional profile of subjects with ALS (Borasio; Voltz, 1997). Oral supplementation with creatine monohydrate at 3g/day showed no improvement of nutritional status in ALS. However, the energy and protein supplementation is used by many professionals, and has proven to be efficient in the nutritional status of subjects with ALS (Rio; Cawadias, 2007; Heffernan et al., 2004).

Silva et al., (2010) evaluated the efficacy of oral supplementation with milk whey proteins and modified starch (70%WPI:30%MS), on nutritional and functional parameters of patients with ALS. Sixteen patients were randomized to two groups, treatment (70%WPI:30%MS) and control (maltodextrin). They underwent prospective nutritional, respiratory and functional assessment for 4 months. Patients in the treatment group presented weight gain, increased BMI, increased arm muscle area and circumference, higher albumin, white blood cell and total lymphocyte counts, and reduced creatine-kinase, aspartate aminotransferase and alanine aminotransferase. In the control group, biochemical measures did not change, but weight and BMI declined. The results indicate that the agglomerate 70%WPI:30%MS may be useful in the nutritional therapy of patients with ALS.

4.2 Alternative feeding in ALS

Different authors report the need for alternative routes of nutrition from the following criteria: vital capacity of approximately 50% of the expected value, presence of moderate to severe dysphagia and 10% reduction in body weight over the past three months. (Stanich *et al.*, 2004; Mitsumoto *et al.*, 2003; Albert *et al.*, 2001; Silani; Kasarskis; Yanagisawa, 1998; Lisbeth et al., 1994).

Percutaneous endoscopic gastrostomy (PEG) is an option for the symptomatic treatment of patients with ALS (Miller et al., 1999).

When comparing the use of enteral nutrition via nasogastric tube and percutaneous endoscopic gastrostomy (PEG) in patients with ALS, there is a significant difference in the body mass index (BMI) of patients with PEG compared to those with a nasogastric tube, as well as a better social acceptance and, consequently, quality of life of the patients studied, supporting the use of this technique when oral intake is not safe (Mazzini et al., 1995).

5. Conclusions

This chapter was conducted to support the hypothesis of the thesis and gathers scientific information listing the main practices for assessment, from the nutritional point of view, in patients with ALS. The relevant literature available for consultation is limited. Studies on food intake, specific techniques for assessment of nutritional status, and the use of supplements are scarce. However, the follow-up of nutritional status by monitoring the anthropometric evolution, body composition and clinical signs, such as dysphagia, may improve the quality of life of subjects with ALS.

6. References

ADA. (2002). National Dysphagia Diet Task Force. *National Dysphagia Diet: Standardization for Optimal Care.* The American Dietetics Association. pp 47

Albert, SM., Murphy, PL., Del Bene, M., Rowland, LP., Mitsumoto, H. (2001). Incidence and predictors of GEP placement in ALS/MND. *Journal of Neurological Sciences,* Vol.191, pp 115-119

Barros, PB., Manzano, FM., Silva, LBC. (2006). *Manual de Técnicas e Receitas para Espessamento de Alimentos: utilização de diferentes amidos espessantes,* São Paulo: Cescorf pp 10-68. *(In Portuguese)*

Blackburn, GL., Havey, KB. (1982). Nutritional assessment as a routine in clinical medicine. *Postgraduate Medicine,* Vol. 71, pp 46-63

Blackburn, GL., Thorrnton, PA. (1979). Nutrition assessment of the hospitalized patient. *Medicine Clinical Nutrition of American,* Vol 63, pp. 1103-1115

Borasio, GD., Voltz, R. (1997). Palliative care in amyotrophic lateral sclerosis. *Journal of Neurology,* Vol. 244, pp.S11-S7. Supl. 4.

Calia, LC., Annes, M. (2003). Afecções neurológicas periféricas. In: Levy, JA.; Oliveira, AS. *Reabilitação em doenças neurológicas – guia terapêutico prático.* São Paulo: Atheneu, pp. 31-64. *(In Portuguese)*

Campbell, MJ., Enderby, P. (1984). Management of motor neurone disease. *Journal of theNeurological Sciences,* Vol 64, pp. 65–71

Carvalho-Silva, LBC. (2011). Anthropometric wrist and arm circumference and their derivations: application to amyotrophic lateral sclerosis. In *Handbook of Anthropometry:Physical Measuresof Human Form in Health and Disease.* New York: Springer. DOI 10.1007/978-1-4419-1788-1_39.

Chiappetta, ALML. (2005). *Disfagia Orofaríngea em Pacientes com Doença do Neurônio Motor/Esclerose Lateral Amiotrófica.* São Paulo. 124. Tese (Doutor em Ciências) - Escola Paulista de Medicina, Universidade Federal de São Paulo.

Chiappetta, ALML., Oda, AL. (2004). Doenças neuromusculares. In: Ferreira, L. P., Benefilopes, D. M., Limongi, S. C. Ed. *Tratado de fonoaudiologia.* São Paulo: Roca, pp. 330-342

Chumlea, MAC., Roche, AF., Steinbaugh, ML. (1958). Estimating stature from knee height for persons 60 to 90 years of age. *Journal of American Geriatrics Society,* Vol. 33, pp. 116-120

Department of health. (1991). Report on health and social subjects. *Dietary reference values for food energy and nutrients for the UK*. No. 41

Desport, JC., Preux, PM., Bouteloup-Demange, C., Clavelou, P., Beaufrère, B., Bonnet, C., Couratier, P. P. (2003). Validation of bioelectrical impedance analysis in patients with amyotrophic lateral sclerosis. *American Journal of Clinical Nutrition,* Vol. 77, pp. 1179-1185

Desport, JC., Preux, PM., Magy, L., Boirie, Y., Vallat, JM., Beaufrère, B., Couratier, P. (2001). Factor correllted with hypermetabolism in patients with amyotrophic lateral sclerosis. *American of Journal Clinical Nutrition,* Vol. 74, pp. 328-3

Desport, JC., Preux, PM., Truong, TC., Vallat, JM., Sautereau, D., Couratier, P. (1999). Nutritional status is a prognostics factor for survival in ALS patients. *Neurology,* Vol. 53, pp. 1059-1063

Desport, JC., Maillot, F. Nutrition et Sclérose Latérale Amyotrophique (SLA). (2002). *Nutrition Clinique et Métabolisme,* Vol. 16, pp. 91-96

Frisancho, AR. (1981). New norms of upper limb fat and muscle areas for assessment of nutritional status. *American of Journal Clinical Nutrition,* Vol. 34, pp. 540-545

Gubbay, SS., Kahana, E., Zilber, N., Cooper, G., Pintov, S., Leibowitz, Y. (1985). Amyotrophic lateral sclerosis. A study of its presentation and prognosis. *Journal of Neurology,* Vol. 232, pp. 295-300

Harris, JA., Benedict, FG. (1919). A biometric study of basal metabolism in man. Washington, DC: Carnegie Istitute of Washington.

Heffernan, C., Jenkinson, C., Holmes, T., Feder, G., Kupfer, R., Leigh, R., McGowan, P. N., Rio, A., Sidhu, P. S. Nutritional management in MND/ALS patients: an evidence based review. *Amyotrophic Lateral Sclerosis and Other Motor Neuron Disorders,* Vol. 5, pp.72-83

Ickenstein GW., Kelly PJ., Furie K.L, Ambrosi D., Rallis N., Goldstein R et al. (2003). Predictors of feeding gastrostomy: tube removal in stroke patients with dysphagia. *Journal of Stroke and Cerebrovascular Diseases,* Vol.12(4), pp.169-74

Institute of medicine. (2002). Energy. In: Dietary Reference Intakes for energy, carbohydrate, fiber, fatty acids, cholesterol, protein, and amino acids. Washington, D.C.: The National Academy Press. <http://www.nap.edu> [2011 July 14].

Institute of medicine. (2001). In: Dietary Reference Intakes for vitamin A, vitamin K, arsenic, boron, chromium, copper, iodine, iron, manganese, molybdenum, nickel, silicon, vanadium, and zinc. Washington, D.C.: The National Academy Press, 2001. <http://www.nap.edu> [2011 July 14].

Institute of medicine. (2000). In: Dietary Reference Intakes for vitamin C, vitamin E, selenium, and carotenoids. Washington, D.C.: The National Academy Press. <http://www.nap.edu> [2011 July 14].

Institute of medicine. (1997). In: Dietary Reference Intakes for calcium, phosphorous, magnesium, vitamin D, and fluoride. Washington, D.C.: The National Academy Press. <http://www.nap.edu> [2007 Abril 14].

Kanda, F., Fujii, Y., Takahashi, L., Fujita, T. (1994). Dual-energy X-ray absorptiometry in neuromuscular diseases. *Muscle and Nerve,* Vol. 17, pp. 413-415

Kasarskis, E., Berryman, S., Vanderleest, JG., Schneider, AR., McClain, CJ. (1996). Nutritional status of patients with amyotrophic lateral sclerosis: relation to the proximity of death. *American Journal of Clinical Nutrition*, Vol. 63, pp.130-137

Lisbeth, MH., Mathus, V., Louwerse, LS., Merkus, MP., Tytgat, GNJ., Vianney, JMB. (1994). Percutaneous endoscopic gastrostomy in patients with amyotrophic lateral slerosis and impaired pulmonary function. *Gastrointestinal Endoscopy*, Vol. 40, pp. 463-469

Lohman, TG., Roche, AF., Martorell, R. (1991). *Anthropometric standardization reference manual.* Abrindged edition.

LONG, CL., Schaffel, N., Geiger, JW. (1979). Metabolic response to injury and illness: Estimation of energy and protein needs from indirect calorimetry and nitrogen balance. *Journal of Parenteral and Enteral Nutrition,* Vol. 3, pp. 452-456

Ludolph, AC. (2006). 135th ENMC International Workshop: Nutrition in amyotrophic lateral sclerosis 18-20 of March 2005, Naarden, The Netherlands. *Neuromuscular Disorders,* pp. 1-9

Macedo EDG, Furkim AM. (2000). *Manual de cuidados do paciente com disfagia.* São Paulo: Lovise. (In Portuguese)

Madsen, OR., Jensen, JEB., Sorensen, OH. (1997). Validation of a dual energy x- ray absortiometer: measurement of bone mass and soft tissue composition. European *Journal Applied Physiology*, Vol. 75, pp. 554-558

Mahan, K., Escott-Stump, S. (2005). Krause: alimentos, nutrição e dietoterapia. 11ª ed. São Paulo: Ed. Roca, 407 p. (In Portuguese)

Mazzini, L., Corrá, T., Zaccala, M., Mora, G., Del Piano, M., Galante, M. (1995). Percutaneous endoscopic gastrostomy and enteral nutrition in amyotrophic lateral sclerosis. *Journal of Neurology*, Vol. 242, pp. 695-698

Miller, R. G., Rosenberg, J. A., Gelinas, D. F., Mitsumoto, H., Newman, D., Sufit, R. (1999). Practice parameter: The care of the patient with amyotrophic lateral sclerosis (an evidence-based review). *Neurology*, Vol. 52, pp. 1311- 1323

Mitsumoto, H., Davidson, M., Moore, D., Gad, N., Brands, M., Ringel, S., Rosenfeld, J., Shefner, JM., Strong, MJ., Sufit, R., Anderson, FA. (2003). ALS CARE Study Group Percutaneous endoscopic gastrostomy (GEP) in patients with ALS and bulbar dysfunction. *ALS and other motor disorders*, Vol. 4, pp. 177-185

Mitsumoto, H., Norris, FH. (1994). *Amyotrophic Lateral A Comprehensive Guide to management,* pp. 342

National Research Council (US). (1989). *Recommended dietary allowances.* Washington: National Academic Press

Nau, KL. Individuals with amyotrofic lateral sclerosis are in caloric balance despite losses in mass. *Journal of the Neurological Sciences*, Vol. 192, pp.S47-S49

Nau, KL., Bromberg, MB., Forsshew, DA., Katch, VL. (1995). Individuals with amyotrophic lateral sclerosis are in caloric balance despite losses in mass. *Journal of the Neurological Sciences*, Vol. 129, pp. 47-49

Nelson, LM., Matkin, C., Longstreth, WT, McGuire, V. (2000). Population - based case - control study of amyotrophic lateral sclerosis in Western Washington State. II. Diet. *American Journal of Epidemiology*, Vol. 151, pp. 164-173

Nguyen NP, Moltz CC, Frank C, Vos P, Smith HJ, Nguyen PD, Nguyen LM, Dutta S, Lemanski C, Sallah S. (2006). Impact of swallowing therapy on aspiration rate following treatment for locally advanced head and neck cancer. *Oral Oncol.* Vol 43, pp.352-7

O'Brien, C., Young, AJ., Sawka, MN. (2002). Bioelectrical impedance to estimate changes in hydration status. International Journal of Sports and Medicine,Vol. 23, pp. 361-366

Piquet, MA. Nutritional Approach for patients with amyotrophic lateral sclerosis. *Revue Neurologique,* Vol. 2, pp. S177-4S187. (In French)

Rio, A., Cawadias, E. (2007). Nutritional advice and treatment by dietitians to patients with amyotrophic lateral sclerosis/motor neurone disease: a survey of current practice in England, Wales, Northern Ireland and Canada. *Journal of Human Nutrition and Dietetics,* Vol. 20, pp. 1-13

Sachdev PS. (2005). Neuroleptic-induced moviment disorders: an overview. *Psychiatr. Clin. N.Am,* Vol.28, pp.255-274

Santoro PP. (2008). Disfagia orofaríngea: panorama atual, epidemiologia, opções terapêuticas e perspectivas futuras. *Rev. CEFAC.* 10(2)

Schofield, WN. (1985). Predicting basal metabolic rate, new standards and a review of previous work. *Human Nutrition Clinical Nutrition,* Vol. 39, pp. 5-41

Shimizu, T., Hayashi, H., Tanabe, H. (1991). Energy metabolism of ALS patients Ander mechanical ventilation and tube feeding. *Clinical neurology and neurosurgery,* Vol. 31, pp. 255-259

Silani V., Kasarkis, E. J., Yanagisawa, N. (1998). Nutritional management in amyotrophic lateral sclerosis: a worldwide perspective. *Journal of Neurology,* Vol. 243, pp. S13-S19, 1998. Supl. 2.

Silva, LBC., Mourao, LF., Silva, AA., Lima, NMFV., Almeida, SRM., Franca Júnior, MC., Anamarli, N., Amaya-Farfán, J.. (2010). Effect of nutritional supplementation with milk whey proteins in amyotrophic lateral sclerosis patients. *Arquivos de Neuro-Psiquiatria,* Vol. 68, pp. 1

Silva, LBC., Ikeda, CM.. (2009). Cuidado nutricional na disfagia: uma alternativa para maximização do estado nutricional. *Revista Brasileira de Nutrição Clínica,* Vol. 27, pp. 1 *(in Portuguese)*

Silva, LBC., Mourao, LF., Silva, AA., Lima, NMFV., Franca Junior, M., Nucci, A., Amaya-Farfan, J. (2008a). Avaliação da ingestão alimentar de indivíduos com Esclerose Lateral Amiotrófica. *Revista Brasileira de Nutrição Clínica,* vol. 23, pp. 5-12 *(in Portuguese)*

Silva, LBC., Figueira, M.L., Silva, AA, Lima, NMFV., Almeida, SR., Franca Júnior, MC., Anamarli, N. Amaya-Farfán, J.. (2008b). Amyotrophic lateral sclerosis: combined nutritional, respiratory and functional assessment. *Arquivos de Neuro-Psiquiatria,* Vol. 66, pp. 354

Silva, LBC., Antunes, A., E., Botelho I., Paula A., Silva, A., A., Amaya-Farfan, J. (2008c). Nutrition and dysphagia: body mass index, food consistency and food intake. *Revista Brasileira de Nutrição Clínica.* Vol.6, pp. 23-91

Silva, LBC., Mourão, L., Lima, NMFV., Almeida, SRM., Franca, MJ., Nucci, A., Amaya-Farfan, J. (2007a). *Amyotrophic lateral sclerosis: nutritional status and functional conditions,* Annual Dysphagia Research Society Meeting, Vancouver, Canada, March 8-10

Silva, LBC., Mourão, L., Lima, NMFV., Almeida, SRM., Franca, MJ., Nucci, A., Amaya-Farfan, J. (2007b). *Amyotrophic Lateral Sclerosis (ALS): Nutritional profile and swallowing ability in patients with dysphagia,* Annual Dysphagia Research Society Meeting, Vancouver, Canada, March 8-10

Silva LBC., Mourão L., Lima NMFV., Aldeia SEM., Franca MJ., Nucci A. et al. (2007c). Amyotrophic lateral sclerosis (ALS): nutritional profile and swallowing ability in patients with dysphagia. *Annual Dysphagia Research Society Meeting,* Vancouver; Mar 8-10. Canada: 2007.

Silva LBC., Manzano FM., Moura RMX., Marques IL., Peres SPBA. (2006a). Viscosidade na terapia nutricional da disfagia: como espessar e alcançar a consistência desejada utilizando diferentes espessantes comerciais? 14° Congresso Latinoamericano de Nutrición; Nov 12-16. Florianópolis: 2006. *(In Portuguese)*

Silva LBC., De Paula A., Botelho I., Silva AA. (2006b). Perfil nutricional e de deglutição de pacientes atendidos no ambulatório de disfagia do HC-/Unicamp. 14° Congresso Latinoamericano de Nutrición; 2006 Nov 12-16. Florianópolis: 2006. *(In Portuguese)*

Souza BBA., Martins C., Campos DJ., Balsini ID., Meyer LR. (2003). *Nutrição e disfagia: guia para profissionais,* pp. 9-12.

Slowie, LA., Paige, MS., Antel, JP. (1983). Nutritional considerations in the management of patients with ALS amyotrophic lateral sclerosis. *Journal of the American Dietetic Association,* Vol. 83, pp. 44-47

Stanich, P., Pereira, AML., Chiappeta, ALML., Nunes, M., Oliveira, ASB., Gabbai, AA. (2004). Suplementação nutricional em pacientes com doença do neurônio motor/esclerose lateral amiotrófica.*Revista Brasileira de Nutrição Clínica,* Vol. 19, pp.70-78. *(in Portuguese)*

Steele CM., Van Lieshout PH. (2004). Influence of bolus consistency on lingual behaviors in sequential swallowing. *Dysphagia,* Vol.19, pp. 192-206

Strand, EA., Miller, RM., Yorkston, KM., Hillel, AD. (1996). Management of oral pharyngeal dysphagia symptoms in amyotrophic lateral sclerosis. *Dysphagia,* Vol. 11, pp. 129-139

Tadan, R., Krusinski, PB., Hiser, JR. (1998). *The validity and sensitivity of dual energy X-ray absorptiometry in estimulating lean body mass in amyotrophic lateral sclerosis.* In: Proceedings of the 9th International Symposium on ALS/MND, Munich, 16-18 November 1998. Munich: ALS Association, 1998. 48 p.

Thomas, B. (2001). *Manual of Dietetic Practice.* 3 rd edition. Oxford: Blackwell Science Ltd

Tothill, P., Han, TS., Avenell, A., McNeill, G., Reid, DM. (1996). Comparisons between fat measurements by dual-energy x-ray absorptiometry, underwater weighing and magnetic resonance imaging in healthy women. *European Journal of Clinical Nutrition,* Vol. 50, pp. 747-752

Watts, C. R., Vanryckeghem, M. (2001). Layngeal dysfunction in Amyotropic Lateral Sclerosis: a review and case report. *BMC Ear, Nose and Throat disorders.*

Welnetz, K. (1990). Maintaining adequate nutrition and hydration in the dysphagic ALS patient. *Journal of Continuing Education in Nursing,* Vol. 21, pp. 62-71

Whelan K. (2001). Inadequate fluid intakes in dysphagic acute stroke. *Clinical Nutrition*, Vol. 20, pp. 423-28

Wright, L., Cotter, D., Hickson, M., Frost, G. (2005). Comparison of energy and protein intakes of older people consuming a texture modified diet with a normal hospital diet. *Journal of Human Nutrition and Dietetics*, Vol. 18, pp. 213-219

27

How to Assess Disease's Severity and Monitor Patients with Amyotrophic Lateral Sclerosis: Lessons from Neurophysiology

Ferdinando Sartucci[1,2,3], Tommaso Bocci[1,4], Lucia Briscese[1], Chiara Pecori[1,3], Chiara Rossi[1] and Fabio Giannini[4]
[1]*Department of Neuroscience, Unit of Neurology, Pisa University Medical School,*
[2]*Institute of Neuroscience, CNR, Pisa,*
[3]*Department of Neuroscience, Unit Outpatients Neurological Activity, Pisa University Medical School, Pisa,*
[4]*Department of Neurological Neurosurgical and Behavioural Sciences, Siena University Medical School, Siena,*
Italy

1. Introduction

Amyotrophic Lateral Sclerosis (ALS) is a fatal, neurodegenerative disorder affecting upper and lower motor neurons; it's the commonest of the motor unit diseases in Europe and North America, characterized by a broad spectrum of clinical presentations mimicking vertebral stenosis, motor polyradiculoneuropathies and myopathies (Juergens et al., 1980; Swash, 2001). Striking asymmetry and selective involvement of individual groups of muscles, especially of hand and forearm, are typical early features of the disease. On average, delay from onset of symptoms to diagnosis is about 14 months and expected survival commonly ranges from months to a few years (Andersen et al., 2007).
Clinical neurophysiology in ALS plays a fundamental role both in the diagnosis of suspected disease and in the assessment of its severity and progression, offering a promising perspective to quantify muscle involvement and evaluate response to therapy (Brooks et al., 2000; Olney and Lomen-Hoerth, 2000; Beghi et al., 2002). Neuroimaging using magnetic resonance imaging (MRI), magnetic resonance spectroscopy (1HMRS), positron emission tomography (PET) and functional MRI may prove valuable results (Pohl et al., 2001), although they are complex, expensive and not always available. On the other hand, blood tests are necessary: hypoglycaemia insulinoma-related and autoimmune hyperthyroidism can be mistaken for ALS as they cause generalized muscle weakness, sometimes accompanied by fasciculations without a significant sensory impairment. Spinal fluid analysis could be helpful to rule out rare conditions closely mimicking ALS, such as meningeal infiltration with lymphoma, multifocal motor neuropathy (MMN) or a motor variant of inflammatory demyelinating neuropathy (CIDP). EMG investigation, usually performed with concentric needle electrodes (Daube et al., 2000), plays an essential role in the diagnosis and monitoring of ALS (Bromberg et al., 1993; Eisen, 2001; de Carvalho et al.,

2005b). Amplitude, duration, area, shape, stability on repeated discharges of motor units (MU) and activity at full effort are parameters conventionally used to evaluate disease's stage. EMG may also assess the presence of activity of the denervation-reinnervation process and number of functioning motor units by evaluating recruitment-activation pattern (Brooks et al., 2000; Finsterer and Fuglsang-Frederiksen, 2001). However, these parameters represent only indirect indicators of the number of surviving muscle fibers.

A particular method to evaluate the full MU is the so-called macro-EMG (Stålberg, 1980; Stålberg and Fawcett, 1982; Stålberg, 1983; Dengler et al., 1990). This technique provides information from a larger area of the muscle than traditional needle EMG methods. The signal is recorded by most of the fibers inside the entire MU and is often employed to follow the degree of reinnervation. That represents a quantitative technique and can be applied to follow progression and effects of putative therapies (de Carvalho et al., 2005a; de Carvalho et al., 2005b) by evaluating size of individual MU (Stålberg, 1983; Guiloff et al., 1988).

Among quantitative electrodiagnostic (EDX) techniques, the methodology of Motor Unit Number Estimation (MUNE) has been previously employed in measuring loss of functioning MU in ALS patients (McComas et al., 1971; Daube, 1995; McComas, 1995; Wang and Delwaide, 1998; Gooch and Shefner, 2004; Daube, 2006; Sartucci et al., 2007).

2. Know your enemy. The useful association of MUNE and macro-EMG

MUNE is very sensitive in documenting disease progression in ALS. Some studies combining MUNE and standard electromyography showed a highly significant correlation between motor unit loss, clinical quantitative features and variations in compound motor action potential (CMAP) amplitude over time (Liu et al., 2009). That is not surprising considering their different targets; while MUNE assesses motor unit loss, changes in CMAP amplitude and duration also account for collateral reinnervation. A few longitudinal studies using MUNE in some ALS patients have been reported that MUNE decreases as the disease progresses and that MUNE is a very reliable and reproducible method in patients with ALS (Olney et al., 2000; Kwon and Lee, 2004; Boe et al., 2007; Hong et al., 2007; Sartucci et al., 2007; Sartucci et al., 2011). Its inter-individual and intra-individual reproducibility linearly increases as disease progresses, making this technique particularly useful in the symptomatic stage of the disease (Sartucci et al., 2007; Sartucci et al., 2011). However, results from MUNE might seem contradictory or not always conclusive in view of many studies were made on animals; in comparison with transgenic mice, it's worth remembering that the majority of cases of ALS are sporadic and the SOD-1 GD^{93A} represents only about 20% of patients with hereditary ALS (Shefner et al., 2002; Zhou et al., 2007).

We routinely use the standard incremental technique, known as the McComas technique. Despite some limitations in comparison with statistical MUNE (alternation of motor unit, inability to recognize small motor units, small sample size), it is more reliable and less complex; in addiction, statistical MUNE cannot identify instable MUPs since it is based on the assumption that variability is due solely to the number of motor units responding in an intermittent manner (Shefner et al., 2007).

On the other hand, use of Macro-EMG is limited to muscles from which electrical activity can be elicited without any interference from other muscles (de Koning et al., 1988); moreover, it's difficult to perform it in the hands during the course of the disease due to the strong wasting of the intrinsic hand muscles. Because of these limitations, our twenty-years experience led us to combine the two techniques in order to improve diagnostic accuracy.

3. Methodological and technical considerations

The most used MUNE technique relays on manual incremental stimulation of the motor nerve, known as the McComas technique (McComas, 1995), modified by Ballantyne and Stålberg. The following test settings were used: sweep duration 50 ms, gain 2 mV/Div for M wave, 0.5 mV/Div for each step; filters 20 - 10 KHz (Keypoint Clinical Manual, 1999). The use of specific software for MUNE detects "alternation", eliminates subjectivity and the sampling of artifactually small motor units in ALS patients (McComas, 1995; Hong et al., 2007); ten incremental steps are commonly recorded (Sartucci et al., 2007).
Percutaneous stimuli were delivered over musculocutaneous nerve immediately below axilla, recording from BB muscles, and ulnar nerve at the wrist by recording from the ADM muscle of the same upper limb (Sartucci et al., 2007; Sartucci et al., 2011). Signals are detected with common surface electrodes, Ag/AgCl type, tapered on the cutis over the target muscles with a common muscle-belly tendon montage. In those patients who underwent follow-up after several months, each test was performed exactly on the same side with the same electrode position (spatial coordinates have been annotated in patients schedule).
At least two consecutive MUNE measures are usually performed on each patient to verify the consistency of our results; when required, further estimation was made until the MUNE was clearly stable. The mean of the two or more tests was calculated (Henderson et al., 2007). The results showed an excellent reproducibility with test-retest correlation coefficients ranging from 0.75 to 0.86 (Sartucci *et al.*, 2007).
The standard macro-EMG method is routinely applied in our patients (Stålberg, 1983). We employ a recording electrode, consisting of a modified single fibre EMG (SFEMG) electrode with the cannula Teflon insulated except for the distal 15 mm. The SFEMG recording surface is exposed 7.5 mm from the tip and the recording is made using two channels: the first one in whom the SFEMG activity is displayed (using the cannula as reference) and used to identify the MU and trigger the averaging procedure (band-pass filter for this channel: 500-10 kHz); fiber density (FD) of the triggering single fibre electrode is recorded. The second channel averaged the activity from the cannula until a smooth baseline and a constant macro MUP was obtained (Filter pass-band: 5-10 kHz).
Total area between the curve and the baseline, the maximal peak-to-peak amplitude (macro-MUP) during the total sweep time of 70 ms are measured (Bauermeister and Jabre, 1992). Results are expressed as individual area values from at least 20 recordings. The relative macro amplitude is expressed as the obtained mean value (Stålberg, 1983). Fibre density is expressed as number of time locked spikes obtained on the SFEMG channel (Sanders and Stålberg, 1996).

4. Our experience

Compared with previous studies (Bromberg et al., 1993; de Carvalho et al., 2005b), our idea was taking into consideration simultaneously Macro-EMG and MUNE changes, both in proximal and distal muscles, in the same sample of patients with a one-year follow-up.
Sixty-one ALS patients (34 male: mean age ± SD 60.0 ± 15.5, range 20-82 yrs; 27 female: mean age ± SD 62.0 ± 9.2 yrs, range 30-82 years), were enrolled in the study and examined basally (T0) and every 4 months (T1, T2 and T3). Macro Motor Unit Potentials (macro MUPs) were derived from Biceps Brachialis (BB) muscle; MUNE was performed both in BB and Abductor Digiti Minimi (ADM) muscles of the same side. Thirty-three healthy volunteers (13 women and 20 men, mean age: 57.7 ± 13.8 years, range 28 - 77 years) served as controls.

All patients had probable or definite ALS, according to the criteria of the World Federation of Neurology (Brooks et al., 2000).
The sample group of patients included cases with a disease duration from clinical onset of symptoms to the time of the first examination less than 48 months (mean ± 1SD: 12.2 ± 11.0 months); only few cases had a disease duration behind this limit (11 patients; about 14.3 %). Twenty-two patients presented a bulbar onset and the remaining a spinal one (Brooks et al., 2000). Muscle strength over time was evaluated by MRC score for all muscles (0-5 grading system). Forty patients were in treatment with riluzole (Rilutek® 50 mg), at a mean daily dosage of 100 mg (50 mg BID) throughout the entire period of EDX follow-up.
In twenty-nine patients (subgroup 1, SG1: 19 males and 10 females; mean age ± 1SD: 60,0 ± 11,8 years; range 30-78 years; spinal/bulbar onset: 22/7; mean disease duration 29,7 months) macro EMG was repeated after 4 months (T1). Among the second subgroup, eleven patients (subgroup 2, SG2: 8 males and 3 females; mean age ± SD: 57,0 ± 12,8 years; range 30–72 years; spinal/bulbar onset: 10/1; mean disease duration 31 months) were re-tested after 8 months (T2) and in 8 (Subgroup 3, SGP3; 7 males and 1 female; mean age ± SD: 58,0 ± 13,6 years; range 31-82 years; spinal/bulbar onset: 7/1; mean disease duration 37 months) after 12 months from the first examination.
Both patients and controls gave their written informed consent prior to participation in the study that had been approved by the local ethical Committee and followed the tenets of Helsinki.

5. Results

Macro-EMG in control subjects showed a mean area 1139.9 ± 182.8 μVms, a mean amplitude of 168.0 ± 63.7 μV, and a FD 1.24 ± 0.13 (a summary of results is given in *Figures 1* and 2).

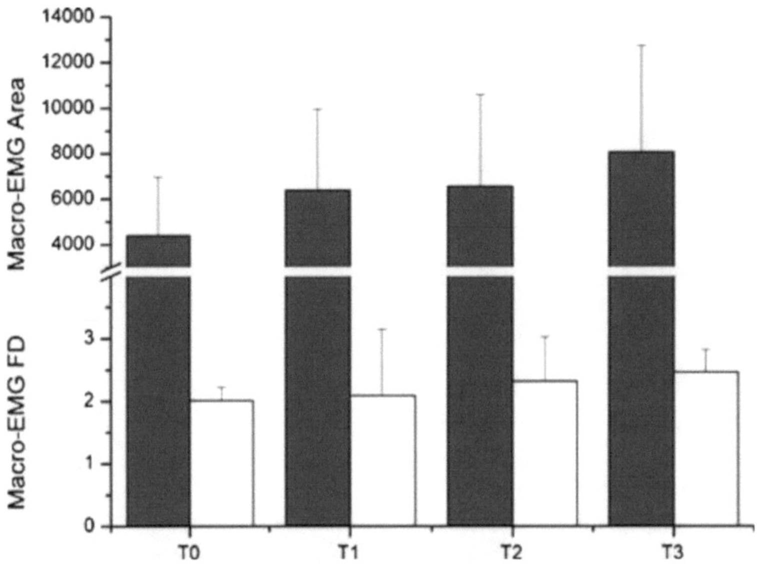

Fig. 1. Time evolution of macro-EMG FD (white columns) and of macro EMG area (gray columns; note the break and the different scale in ordinate) in ALS pt. The macro EMG area increase continuously with the time, paralleled by FD value, up to T2 (modified from Sartucci et al., 2011).

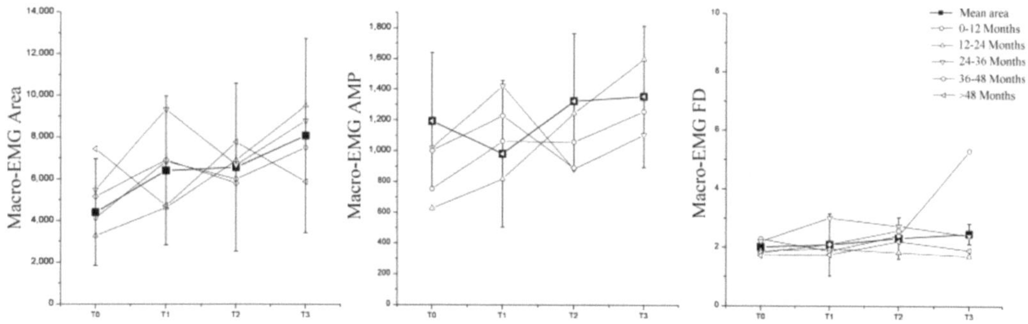

Fig. 2. Time evolution of each macro EMG parameters (area, amplitude and FD) with the time, keeping in the consideration disease duration at the beginning of the observation. Sample with a disease duration of 12-24 months exhibited a more steep slope (modified from Sartucci et al., 2011).

In ALS patients at T0, both Macro-MUP area and FD were above upper normal limits: macro-MUP area was 4397.6 ± 2554.9 µVms (+ 285.8%; $p < 0.001$), mean FD 2.01 ± 0.2 (+62.1%; $p < 0.005$).

The macro EMG MUP area was abnormal in 57 (93.4%). and normal in 4 (6.6%) patients, the FD resulted increased in 55 pt. (90%) and normal in 6 (10%). Macro EMG MUP area and peak-to-peak amplitude exhibited a good correlation (Spearmann coeff. of correlation = 0.888) at every time of testing (Gan and Jabre, 1992).

Macro MUPs area (*Figure* 2) resulted progressively increased at every time, especially at T3 compared with T0: Area: + 45.3% (T1); + 49.0% (T2); + 83.6% (T3); FD showed a trend to increase up to T3: +3.5% (T1); +15.4% (T2); +22.4% (T3) (Fig 2).

FD resulted increased in cases with longer disease duration (*Figure* 2). Anyway, the FD was generally increased when macro EMG amplitude was also increased in the first stage of disease; after less than one year (about 8 months) they showed a large dispersion of value.

MUNE (*Figure* 3) in controls resulted in BB muscle 91.9 ± 18.9, with a mean step area of 2.09 ± 0.7 µV/ms and a Mean Maximal M wave of 131.9 ± 36.0 mV; for the ADM muscle 87.7 ± 14.6, with a mean step area of 1.05 ± 0.4 mV/ms and Mean Maximal M wave of 61.3 ± 21.2 mV. In ALS patients, values were behind normal limits in 56 (91.8%) and within normal limits in 5 (8.2%) in BB muscle; in 60 (98.4%) and in 1 (1.6%) in ADM muscle. Functioning MUs number progressively decreased in both muscles throughout the entire follow-up period. The Pearson's correlation coefficient was 0,61, suggesting the rate and amount of MU decrease was approximately similar in both muscles (Cuturic et al., 2005). In ALS MUNE exhibited a parallel trends in proximal and distal muscles (BB and ADM), independently of disease duration (see *Figures 3 and 4*); mean step area, instead, increased more in BB, especially in patients with longer disease duration. MUP amplitude at T0 did not show any significant difference between females and males, even if a bit higher in males ($p>0.05$, Figure 5).

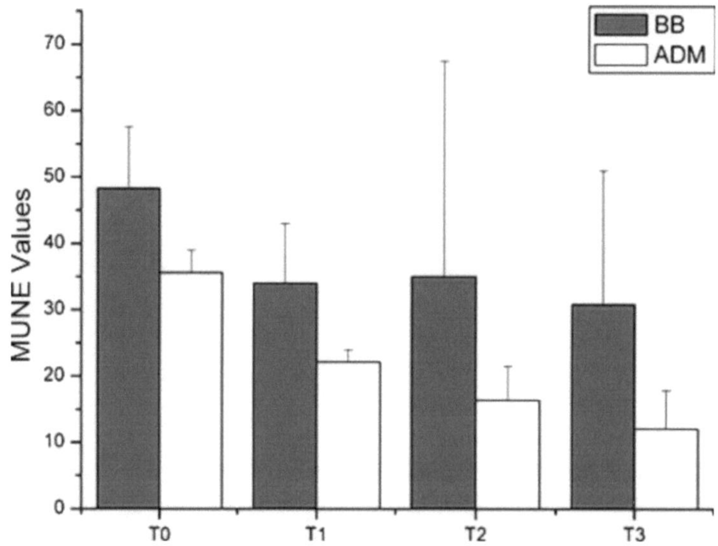

Fig. 3. Histogram showing MUNE values in both BB (gray columns) and ADM (white columns) muscles at every time of measurement. The trends is similar even if more evident in ADM (modified from Sartucci et al., 2011).

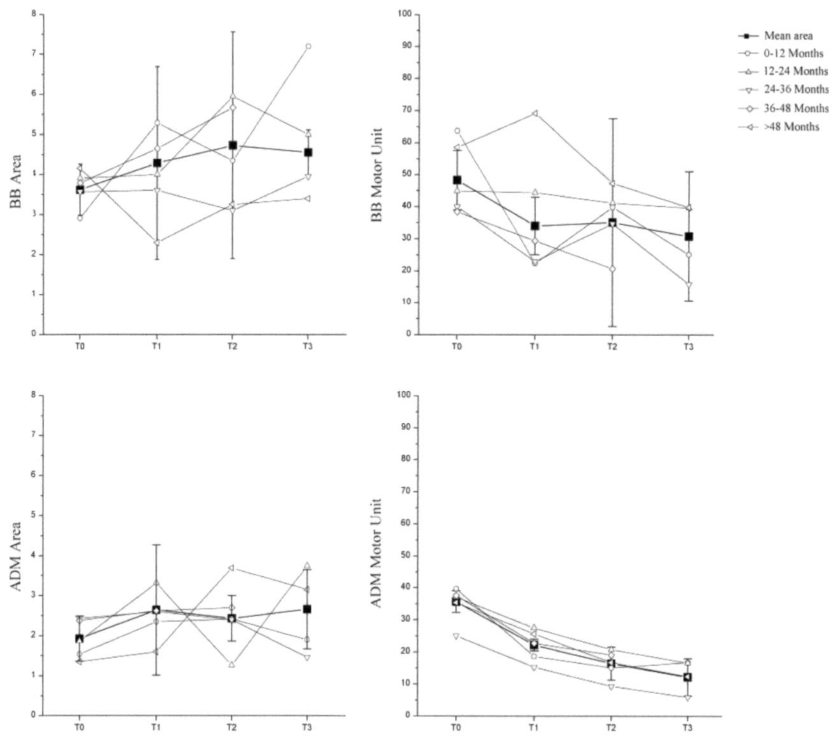

Fig. 4. MUNE values in both BB and ADM muscles at every time of evaluation in pt. with different disease duration and their mean value (filled circles) (modified from Sartucci et al., 2011).

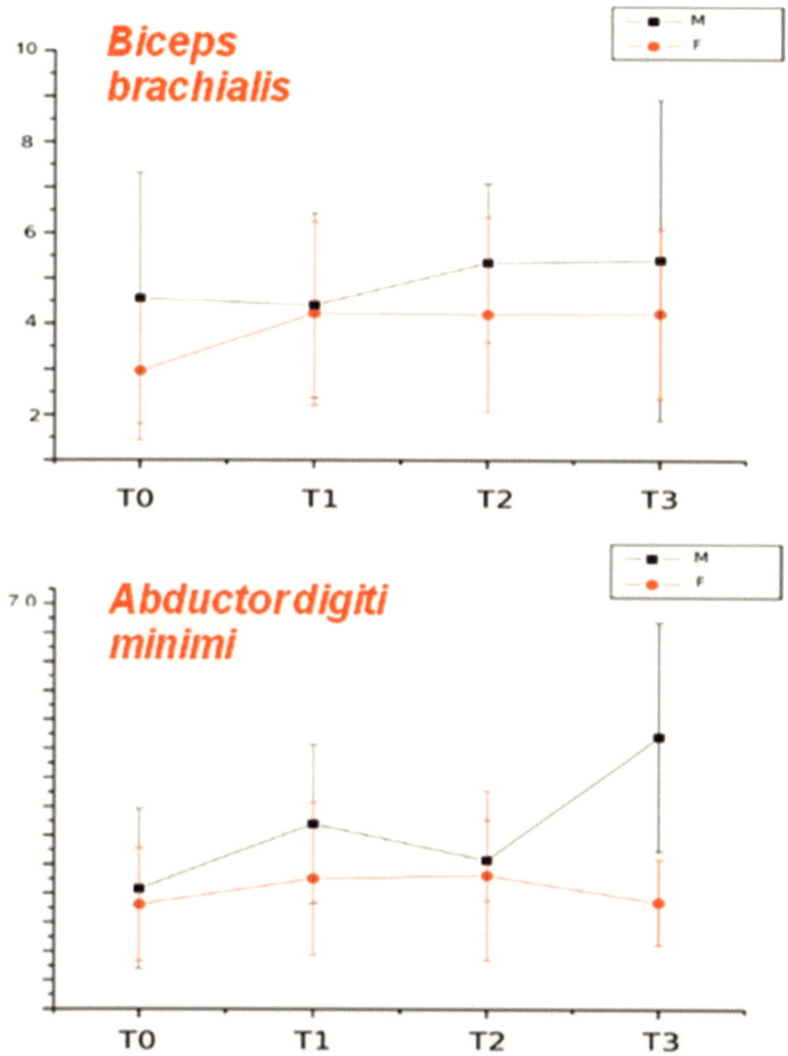

Fig. 5. MUP amplitude at T0 did not show any significant difference between females and males, both in spinal and bulbar form, even if a bit higher in males ($p>0.05$; Sartucci et al., personal data).

5.1 Correlation between macro-MUP and MUNE

All main macro-EMG parameters (area, amplitude and FD), as well as MUNE features (number of MUPs and mean step area either in the BB and ADM), did not disclose any significant difference between patients intaking the drug for both disease type (spinal or bulbar) at any time during the follow-up period (*Figure* 6). As concerns as Macro-EMG area, the difference in the mean values among the different levels of treatment is not great enough to exclude the possibility that the difference is just due to random sampling variability. There is not a statistically significant difference between riluzole vs. control ($p = 0.321$), as confirmed by FD measures over time ($p = 0.588$).

6. Conclusions and unanswered questions

Our study design was a prospective study to evaluate ongoing denervation/reinnervation process. Main aim was to objectively measure the extent of MU loss and the accompanying changes in innervation pattern during the time in ALS patients (Stålberg, 1983; Jabre, 1991), and therefore is often impossible to perform it in a hand muscle in the course of ALS due to the strong wasting of the intrinsic hand muscles; consequently to evaluate distal time disease evolution and its behaviour compared with proximal district we had to use only MUNE.

Area and amplitude of the Macro-MUP reflect number and size of muscle fibers in the motor unit (Schwartz et al., 1976; Stålberg et al., 1976). MUNE instead is the ideal tool for the assessment of disease in which primary defect is MU loss (Strong et al., 1988; Gooch and Shefner, 2004; Daube, 2006; Sartucci et al., 2007).

ALS is featured by repetitive cycles of denervation/reinnervation and the mechanism lead to a variation of fibre density within a given motor unit (Stålberg, 1983; de Carvalho et al., 2005a; de Carvalho et al., 2005b). If this rearrangement is interrupted by new processes of denervation, following further motor neuron loss, this will lead to areas of grouped atrophy and loss of muscle fibers. Reinnervation process are strictly interwoven with lower motor neuron loss; quantization and tracking of MU loss with simultaneously gauging countervailing collateral dynamic innervation may be assessed by combining MUNE and macro-EMG (Gooch and Shefner, 2004; Pouget, 2006). The macro-EMG gives a global view of the MU. First, the physical length of the electrode (15 mm), cover the entire diameter of an average sized MU; the large electrode surface suppresses the contribution of the closest action potentials and favours the relative influence of slow components so including distant fibers (Sanders and Stålberg, 1996).

Macro-EMG parameters in controls were in agreement with data of others authors (Stålberg and Fawcett, 1982; Stålberg, 1983; Jabre, 1991). Both macro-MUP area, amplitude and FD were beyond upper normal limits, as expected, in ALS (Bauermeister and Jabre, 1992; Gan and Jabre, 1992). Macro-EMG parameters progressively increased, at least in the first eight months compared with baseline as proved by coefficient of correlation at each time displaying a progressive increment of correlation up to 8 months, suggesting the process of MU rearrangement begins to fail after 8 months of disease course. Also when macro EMG area and amplitude were increased, FD was parallely increased.

The time elapsed from disease onset plays a fundamental role, since patients included with a diseases duration between 12 and 24 months showed largest changes in Macro EMG features, suggesting a higher efficiency of compensatory mechanisms at least in early stages of disease. Evidence of some MU loss at baseline compared with controls and its trend over time, together with a broader mean step area, yields novel insights into the pathophysiology of MU loss and its relationship to motor function in patients with ALS (Daube et al., 2000; Sartucci et al., 2007). Fluctuation of MU estimates between separate time could suggest reversible motoneurons dysfunction (Gooch and Shefner, 2004). The coefficient of correlation for MUNE - macro EMG mean area regression line was not significant (= - 0.17) in BB muscle, suggesting that both processes go on in some way independently. In more advanced stages, a decline of the strength of the surviving MUs, especially those with higher thresholds, seems to contribute to the progressive muscle weakness, in addition to both corticospinal degeneration and reduction in motoneurons number (Dengler et al., 1990). Our study also showed a significant correlation between MRC scores and EDX measurements throughout the whole course of the disease only for ADM muscle. The absence of a significant correlation between MUNE and MRC values ($p > 0.05$) for BB could confirm the specificity of EDX investigations to track over time changes in muscle MU features and number. Muscle strength seems to decline more linearly than MUNE values: that could be explained, as recently suggested by Liu et al. (2009) with the persistence of a small proportion of lower motor neurons long-term surviving.

6.1 Gender and amyotrophic lateral sclerosis. Lessons from motor unit estimation

Another interesting result is about gender differences (*Figure 5*); in fact, some studies have reported a significant male predominance until the sixth decade of life and an older average age at onset for females, sometimes explained with a possible protective effect of estrogen. In our experience, MUP amplitude at T0 did not show any significant difference between females and males, even if a bit higher in males: MUP amplitudes were 86.9 ± 21.2 μV and 84.1 ± 17.5 μV for the biceps brachii and abductor digiti minimi muscle, respectively, in females, 90.7 ± 17.3 μV and 88.2 ± 16.8 μV in males ($p>0.05$). This is only a trend, as gender don't influence motor unit loss neither corresponding decline in MRC values over time. The lack of significant differences between females and males in both spinal and bulbar form, as emerged from our sample, is consistent with results reported by Hegedus (Hegedus et al., 2009): the antioxidant effects of estrogens and their proved role in preventing glutamate-related toxicity *in vitro* (Kruman et al., 1999; Nakamizo et al., 2000) could not delay both the early retraction of nerve terminals from neuromuscular end-plates and the dying-back of the axons during asymptomatic phase *in vivo*, as well as the denervation/reinnervation process in later stages. However, there is a substantial lack of studies describing the contribution of gender in progression of ALS; that's likely due to the discrepancy between humans patients and animal models, in terms of disease and presymptomatic phase duration, absence of sensitive biological markers and different pathogenesis (sporadic vs. SOD1-related; Zhou et al., 2007).

6.2 MUNE and Macro-EMG in evaluating response to treatment

Our investigation was aimed to evaluate also the EDX effects of one of the most common drug employed in the ALS, riluzole (Leigh et al., 2003), on the fundamentals process of ALS: the primary process of motorneurons loss and denervation, and the secondary process of reinnervation. Riluzole is a benzothiazole derivative with a wide range of effects on glutamate pathways including inhibition of presynaptic glutamate release; it is relatively safe and well tolerated. Prescription of riluzole is restricted to patients with probable or definite ALS. At the moment, there is no convincing evidence that treatment at 100 mg daily is associated with a significant increase in survival (Miller et al., 2007); its effects on quality of life and survival are weak especially in older patients (over 75 years), in those with bulbar onset and at more advanced stages (Miller et al., 2003). We did not detect any significant electrophysiological difference between patient intaking the drug and those who didn't (see *Figure 6*), but considering the high attrition rate it's quite difficult to draw any conclusion about the effect of pharmacological treatments on neurophysiological parameters. Future studies are then required to solve this dilemma.

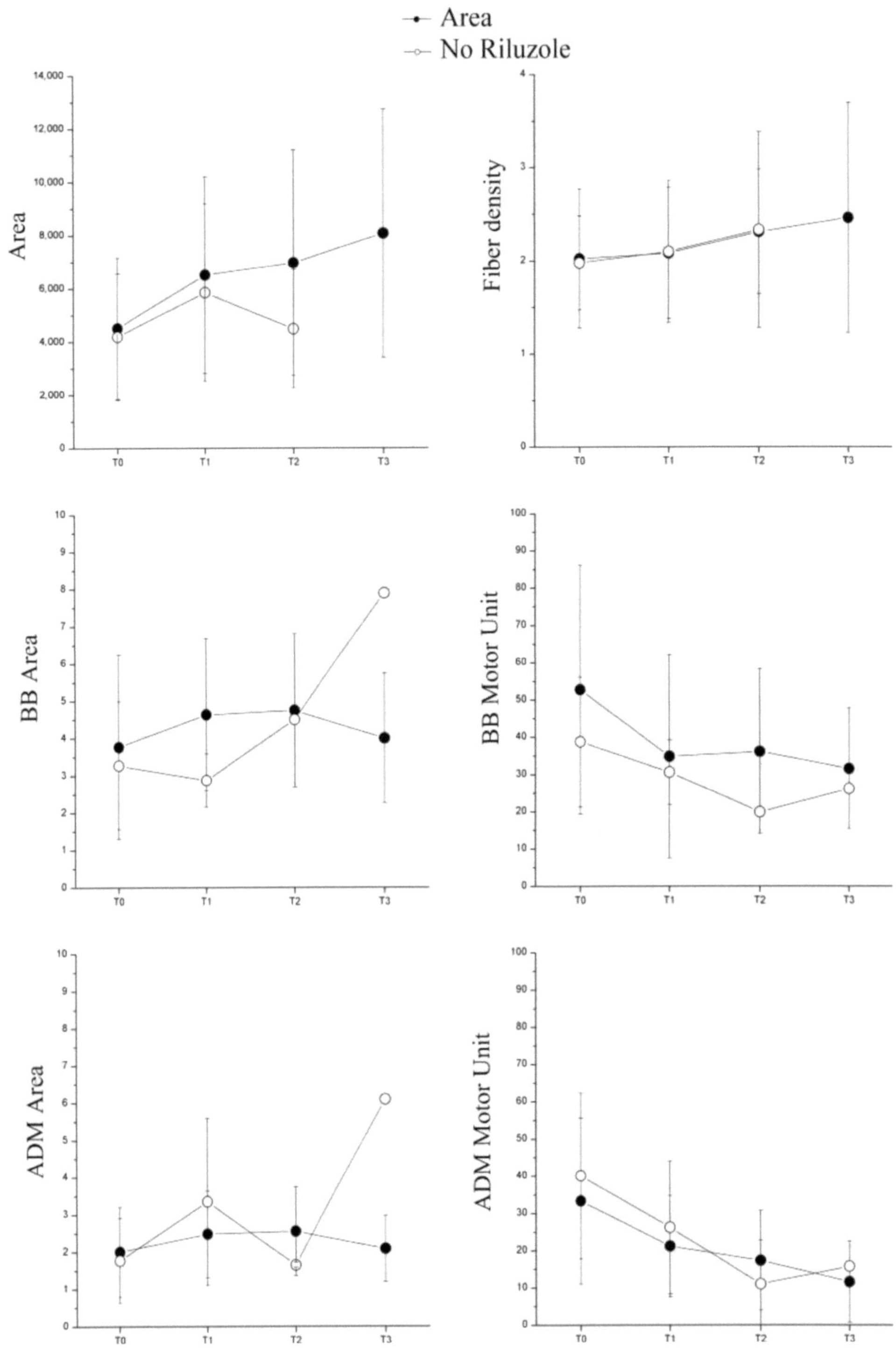

Fig. 6. Effects of Riluzole on the macro EMG and MUNE parameters with the time, in patients intaking (filled circle) or not (empty circle) the drug (modified from Sartucci et al., 2011).

7. References

Andersen PM, Borasio GD, Dengler R, Hardiman O, Kollewe K, Leigh PN, Pradat PF, Silani V, Tomik B (2007), Good practice in the management of amyotrophic lateral sclerosis: clinical guidelines. An evidence-based review with good practice points. EALSC Working Group. Amyotroph Lateral Scler 8:195-213.

Bauermeister W, Jabre JF (1992), The spectrum of concentric macro EMG correlations. Part I. Normal subjects. Muscle Nerve 15:1081-1084.

Beghi E, Balzarini C, Bogliun G, Logroscino G, Manfredi L, Mazzini L, Micheli A, Millul A, Poloni M, Riva R, Salmoiraghi F, Tonini C, Vitelli E (2002), Reliability of the El Escorial diagnostic criteria for amyotrophic lateral sclerosis. Neuroepidemiology 21:265-270.

Boe SG, Stashuk DW, Doherty TJ (2007), Motor unit number estimates and quantitative motor unit analysis in healthy subjects and patients with amyotrophic lateral sclerosis. Muscle Nerve 36:62-70.

Bromberg MB, Forshew DA, Nau KL, Bromberg J, Simmons Z, Fries TJ (1993), Motor unit number estimation, isometric strength, and electromyographic measures in amyotrophic lateral sclerosis. Muscle Nerve 16:1213-1219.

Brooks BR, Miller RG, Swash M, Munsat TL (2000), El Escorial revisited: revised criteria for the diagnosis of amyotrophic lateral sclerosis. Amyotroph Lateral Scler Other Motor Neuron Disord 1:293-299.

Cuturic M, Shamsnia M, Palliyath S (2005), Lateral asymmetry of motor unit number estimate (MUNE). Electromyogr Clin Neurophysiol 45:233-239.

Daube JR (1995), Estimating the number of motor units in a muscle. J Clin Neurophysiol 12:585-594.

Daube JR (2006), Motor unit number estimates--from A to Z. J Neurol Sci 242:23-35.

Daube JR, Gooch C, Shefner J, Olney R, Felice K, Bromberg M (2000), Motor unit number estimation (MUNE) with nerve conduction studies. Suppl Clin Neurophysiol 53:112-115.

de Carvalho M, Chio A, Dengler R, Hecht M, Weber M, Swash M (2005a), Neurophysiological measures in amyotrophic lateral sclerosis: markers of progression in clinical trials. Amyotroph Lateral Scler Other Motor Neuron Disord 6:17-28.

de Carvalho M, Costa J, Swash M (2005b), Clinical trials in ALS: a review of the role of clinical and neurophysiological measurements. Amyotroph Lateral Scler Other Motor Neuron Disord 6:202-212.

de Koning P, Wieneke GH, van der Most van Spijk D, van Huffelen AC, Gispen WH, Jennekens FG (1988), Estimation of the number of motor units based on macro-EMG. J Neurol Neurosurg Psychiatry 51:403-411.

Dengler R, Konstanzer A, Kuther G, Hesse S, Wolf W, Struppler A (1990), Amyotrophic lateral sclerosis: macro-EMG and twitch forces of single motor units. Muscle Nerve 13:545-550.

Eisen A (2001), Clinical electrophysiology of the upper and lower motor neuron in amyotrophic lateral sclerosis. Semin Neurol 21:141-154.

Finsterer J, Fuglsang-Frederiksen A (2001), Concentric-needle versus macro EMG. II. Detection of neuromuscular disorders. Clin Neurophysiol 112:853-860.

Gan R, Jabre JF (1992), The spectrum of concentric macro EMG correlations. Part II. Patients with diseases of muscle and nerve. Muscle Nerve 15:1085-1088.

Gooch CL, Shefner JM (2004), ALS surrogate markers. MUNE. Amyotroph Lateral Scler Other Motor Neuron Disord 5 Suppl 1:104-107.

Guiloff RJ, Modarres-Sadeghi H, Stålberg E, Rogers H (1988), Short-term stability of single motor unit recordings in motor neuron disease: a macro EMG study. J Neurol Neurosurg Psychiatry 51:671-676.

Hegedus J, Putman CT, Gordon T (2009), Progressive motor unit loss in the G93A mouse model of amyotrophic lateral sclerosis is unaffected by gender. Muscle Nerve 39:318-327.

Henderson RD, Ridall PG, Hutchinson NM, Pettitt AN, McCombe PA (2007), Bayesian statistical MUNE method. Muscle Nerve 36:206-213.

Hong YH, Sung JJ, Park KS, Kwon O, Min JH, Lee KW (2007), Statistical MUNE: a comparison of two methods of setting recording windows in healthy subjects and ALS patients. Clin Neurophysiol 118:2605-2611.

Jabre JF (1991), Concentric macro electromyography. Muscle Nerve 14:820-825.

Juergens SM, Kurland LT, Okazaki H, Mulder DW (1980), ALS in Rochester, Minnesota, 1925-1977. Neurology 30:463-470.

Kruman, II, Pedersen WA, Springer JE, Mattson MP (1999), ALS-linked Cu/Zn-SOD mutation increases vulnerability of motor neurons to excitotoxicity by a mechanism involving increased oxidative stress and perturbed calcium homeostasis. Exp Neurol 160:28-39.

Kwon O, Lee KW (2004), Reproducibility of statistical motor unit number estimates in amyotrophic lateral sclerosis: comparisons between size- and number-weighted modifications. Muscle Nerve 29:211-217.

Leigh PN, Abrahams S, Al-Chalabi A, Ampong MA, Goldstein LH, Johnson J, Lyall R, Moxham J, Mustfa N, Rio A, Shaw C, Willey E (2003), The management of motor neurone disease. J Neurol Neurosurg Psychiatry 74 Suppl 4:iv32-iv47.

Liu XX, Zhang J, Zheng JY, Zhang S, Xu YS, Kang DX, Fan DS (2009), Stratifying disease stages with different progression rates determined by electrophysiological tests in patients with amyotrophic lateral sclerosis. Muscle Nerve 39:304-309.

McComas AJ (1995), Motor unit estimation: anxieties and achievements. Muscle Nerve 18:369-379.

McComas AJ, Fawcett PR, Campbell MJ, Sica RE (1971), Electrophysiological estimation of the number of motor units within a human muscle. J Neurol Neurosurg Psychiatry 34:121-131.

Miller RG, Mitchell JD, Lyon M, Moore DH (2003), Riluzole for amyotrophic lateral sclerosis (ALS)/motor neuron disease (MND). Amyotroph Lateral Scler Other Motor Neuron Disord 4:191-206.

Miller RG, Mitchell JD, Lyon M, Moore DH (2007), Riluzole for amyotrophic lateral sclerosis (ALS)/motor neuron disease (MND). Cochrane Database Syst Rev CD001447.

Nakamizo T, Urushitani M, Inoue R, Shinohara A, Sawada H, Honda K, Kihara T, Akaike A, Shimohama S (2000), Protection of cultured spinal motor neurons by estradiol. Neuroreport 11:3493-3497.

Olney RK, Lomen-Hoerth C (2000), Motor unit number estimation (MUNE): how may it contribute to the diagnosis of ALS? Amyotroph Lateral Scler Other Motor Neuron Disord 1 Suppl 2:S41-44.

Olney RK, Yuen EC, Engstrom JW (2000), Statistical motor unit number estimation: reproducibility and sources of error in patients with amyotrophic lateral sclerosis. Muscle Nerve 23:193-197.

Pohl C, Block W, Traber F, Schmidt S, Pels H, Grothe C, Schild HH, Klockgether T (2001), Proton magnetic resonance spectroscopy and transcranial magnetic stimulation for the detection of upper motor neuron degeneration in ALS patients. J Neurol Sci 190:21-27.

Pouget J (2006), [Electroneuromyographic criteria of amyotrophic lateral sclerosis]. Rev Neurol (Paris) 162 Spec No 2:4S34-34S42.

Sanders DB, Stålberg EV (1996), AAEM minimonograph #25: single-fiber electromyography. Muscle Nerve 19:1069-1083.

Sartucci F, Maritato P, Moscato G, Orlandi G, Calabrese R, Domenici GL, Murri L (2007), Motor unit number estimation (mune) as a quantitative measure of disease progression and motor unit reorganization in amyotrophic lateral sclerosis. Int J Neurosci 117:1229-1236.

Sartucci F, Moscato G, Rossi C, Caleo M, Bocci T, Murri L, Giannini F, Rossi A (2011), Macro-EMG and MUNE Changes in Patients with Amyotrophic Lateral Sclerosis: One-Year Follow Up. Int J Neurosci 121(5):257-66.

Schwartz MS, Stålberg E, Schiller HH, Thiele B (1976), The reinnervated motor unit in man. A single fibre EMG multielectrode investigation. J Neurol Sci 27:303-312.

Shefner JM, Cudkowicz ME, Brown RH, Jr. (2002), Comparison of incremental with multipoint MUNE methods in transgenic ALS mice. Muscle Nerve 25:39-42.

Shefner JM, Cudkowicz ME, Zhang H, Schoenfeld D, Jillapalli D (2007), Revised statistical motor unit number estimation in the Celecoxib/ALS trial. Muscle Nerve 35:228-234.

Stålberg E (1983), Macro EMG. Muscle Nerve 6:619-630.

Stålberg E (1980), Macro EMG, a new recording technique. J Neurol Neurosurg Psychiatry 43:475-482.

Stålberg E (1983), Macro EMG. Muscle Nerve 6:619-630.

Stålberg E, Fawcett PR (1982), Macro EMG in healthy subjects of different ages. J Neurol Neurosurg Psychiatry 45:870-878.

Stålberg E, Schwartz MS, Thiele B, Schiller HH (1976), The normal motor unit in man. A single fibre EMG multielectrode investigation. J Neurol Sci 27:291-301.

Strong MJ, Brown WF, Hudson AJ, Snow R (1988), Motor unit estimates in the biceps-brachialis in amyotrophic lateral sclerosis. Muscle Nerve 11:415-422.

Swash M (2001), ALS and motor neuron disorders today and tomorrow. Amyotroph Lateral Scler Other Motor Neuron Disord 2:171-172.

Wang FC, Delwaide PJ (1998), Number and relative size of thenar motor units in ALS patients: application of the adapted multiple point stimulation method. Electroencephalogr Clin Neurophysiol 109:36-43.

Zhou C, Zhao CP, Zhang C, Wu GY, Xiong F, Zhang C (2007), A method comparison in monitoring disease progression of G93A mouse model of ALS. Amyotroph Lateral Scler 8:366-372.

28

Protection of Motor Neurons in Pre-Symptomatic Individuals Carrying SOD 1 Mutations: Results of Motor Unit Number Estimation (MUNE) Electrophysiology

Arun Aggarwal
University of Sydney
Australia

1. Introduction

Amyotrophic lateral sclerosis (ALS) is a progressive degenerative disease of motor neurones. There is a family history in approximately 10% percent of cases. Only 20% of such families have point mutations in the Cu, Zn superoxide dimutase 1 (SOD1) gene. Pre-symptomatic loss of motor neurons has been identified prior to the onset of symptoms in SOD1 mice. This loss was biphasic with initial loss in the pre-symptomatic phase followed by a period of stabilisation and then gradual loss at time of weakness to death. (Kong & Xu, 1998).

In order to determine the time course of motor neurone loss prior to symptomatic onset of disease, a longitudinal study of at-risk asymptomatic individuals (i.e. SOD1 mutation carriers with no neurological symptoms or signs as determined by a neurologist) was performed.

There was no detectable difference in the number of motor units in SOD1 mutation carriers compared to their SOD1 negative family controls. (Aggarwal & Nicholson, 2001). This may indicate that mutation carriers have undetectable loss of motor neurones until rapid and widespread cell death of motor neurones occurs, coinciding with the onset of symptomatic features. This implies that the disease is not the end result of the slow attrition of motor neurones. (Aggarwal, 2009).

The longitudinal study was extended on 20 asymptomatic carriers of the Cu, Zn superoxide dimutase 1 (SOD1) point mutation. In 2 of the 20 mutation carriers, there was a sudden reduction in MUNE, several months prior to the onset of weakness. (Aggarwal & Nicholson 2002), which also occurred in another 3 mutation carriers over the course of the study. (Aggarwal, 2009).

This suggests that gradual pre-clinical loss of motor neurones does not occur in asymptomatic SOD1 mutation carriers and supports the observation that sudden, catastrophic loss of motor neurones occurs immediately prior to the onset of symptoms and the development of the disease, rather than a gradual attrition of motor neurones over time. These results suggest that there may be a biological trigger initiating rapid cell loss, just prior to the onset of symptoms. This observation is an important contribution to the current understanding of the pathogenesis of MND.

Regular follow-up of SOD1 carriers with MUNE may lead to early diagnosis, creating an opportunity for future approaches and therapies aimed at preserving motor neurones rather than replacing lost motor neurones. Detecting the onset of motor neurone loss in asymptomatic individuals will identify those who may benefit from early institution of an active management program to improve their quality of life, until more effective treatment modalities are available for this devastating condition.

2. Background

Amyotrophic lateral sclerosis (ALS) is a group of fatal, neurodegenerative disorders, which is characterised pathologically by progressive degeneration and loss of motor neurones in the anterior horn cells of the spinal cord, motor nuclei of the brainstem and the descending pathways within the corticospinal tracts. The term amyotrophic lateral sclerosis (ALS) is used synonymously with motor neurone disease (MND) in the USA, but in the UK and Australia is used only to refer to patients who have a combination of upper and lower motor neurone dysfunction. (Talbot, 2002).

It is primarily a condition of middle to late life, with onset of symptoms between the ages of 50 and 70 and a mean age of onset of 57.4 years. (Ringel et al., 1993). Occasionally, it arises as early as the 2nd decade or as late as the 9th decade. In a natural history study, the overall median survival is 4.0 years from the onset of symptoms, but only 2.1 years from the time of diagnosis. (Ringel et al., 1993). In a study performed at the Mayo clinic, approximately 50% of patients died within 3 years of referral, but 20% were still alive at 5 years and 10% were still alive at 10 years. (Mulder & Howard, 1976).

Aging, motor neurone diseases and many peripheral neuropathies are all associated with loss of motor neurones or axons. When the disorders are recent or rapidly progressive, the extent of the loss may be indicated by weakness and wasting. In slowly progressive denervating conditions, like MND, loss of more than 50-80% of motor units may occur with little or no clinically apparent weakness.

It has been showed that patients with substantial chronic denervation could maintain normal muscle twitch tension until loss of about 70-80% of motor units occurred. (McComas, 1971). The surviving motor neurones enlarge their territories, through collateral sprouting (reinnervation) to keep pace with cell loss, to maintain the muscle maximum compound muscle action potential (CMAP), until late in the disease. At this point, collateral reinnervation is no longer able to provide full functional compensation. (Campbell et al., 1973).

In MND, needle electromyography often reveals evidence of chronic reinnervation (increased motor unit action potential amplitudes and duration with reduced recruitment), but provides little direct evidence to the extent of motor neurone and axonal loss. The supramaximal CMAP amplitude also provides little direct evidence of the extent of motor neurone loss. Normal CMAP amplitudes might mistakenly suggest that motor neurone loss has not occurred yet. (Shefner, 2001).

Motor unit number estimation (MUNE) is a more reliable method for following changes in neurogenic disorders than the CMAP amplitude. It estimates the number of functioning lower motor neurones innervating a muscle or a group of muscles i.e. the number of motor units, which can be excited by electrical stimulation. It is therefore an indirect measure of motor neurone loss, rather than a measure of primary pathology. It can identify that the number of motor units may be well below normal, in the presence of normal CMAP amplitudes. (Brown, 1976).

Pre-symptomatic loss of motor neurones has been identified in an animal model of the disease (transgenic mice expressing mutant human SOD1-G93A). The initial loss in the pre-symptomatic phase related to severe motor axonal degeneration due to vacuolar changes in motor neurones and a slow decrease in CMAP amplitudes. After a period of stabilisation, there was a gradual loss of motor neurones and a rapid decrease in CMAP amplitude, at the onset of weakness due to myelin alteration. At this point, there was a striking loss of motor units. There was also decrease in evoked motor potentials (an indirect measure of the number of motor units), prior to the onset of symptoms. The onset of disease in transgenic G93A mice involves a sharp decline of muscle strength and a transient explosive increase in vacuoles derived from degenerating mitochondria, but little motor neurone death. These did not die until the terminal stage. (Kong & Xu, 1998). The decline exhibited kinetics consistent with both a constant and exponentially decreasing risk of neuronal death. An escalating risk forced by cumulative damage was not responsible for cell death. (Azzouz et al., 1997).
It is possible that the high metabolic activity in motor neurones, combined with the toxic oxidative properties of the mutant SOD1, causes massive mitochondrial vacuolation in motor neurones, resulting in degeneration, earlier than other neurones, triggering the onset of weakness. The involvement of mitochondrial degeneration in the early stages is consistent with a direct effect of toxicity, mediated by properties gained by the mutant enzyme in catalysing redox reactions. (Beckman et al., 1993).
Until recently, it has not been possible to address this in humans, as pre-symptomatic diagnosis was not possible. Now, with the ability to identify Cu, Zn superoxide dismutase 1, (SOD1) mutation carriers, a group of human pre-symptomatic subjects can be studied to determine whether there was gradual lifelong pre-symptomatic loss of motor neurones or whether sudden catastrophic loss of motor neurones occurs just prior to the onset of clinical symptoms.

3. Familial ALS

The only forms of MND in which a clear cause has been established are the genetic variants. 20% of all familial cases are the dominantly inherited adult onset form of MND, which is clinically indistinguishable from the sporadic form of MND. These are due to a point mutation in the cytosolic Cu, Zn superoxide dismutase 1, (SOD1) gene on long arm of chromosome 21 (21q22.1). (Siddique & Deng, 1996). Mutations in other genes, alsin and the heavy subunit of neurofilament (NEFH) can also result in motor neurone degeneration in humans. Two other genes that have been investigated are the other isoforms of SOD. MnSOD (SOD2) maps to chromosome 6q25 and is primarily located in mitochondria and extracellular SOD (SOD3) maps to chromosome 4p15.2. Neither of these genes have yet to be linked to FALS. (Hand & Rouleau, 2002). There is however genetic heterogeneous and other causal genes remain to be found to explain the vast majority of FALS cases. (Siddique et al., 1989).
The initial study to establish a causal link between the SOD1 gene and familial MND (FALS) identified a total of 11 missense mutations in two exons studied in 13 autosomal dominant MND families. (Rosen et al., 1993). This led to an explosion of SOD1 gene screening in MND pedigrees. To date 112 different mutations in the SOD1 have been found which can lead to changes throughout the protein. There have been 99 substitutions, 5 polymorphisms, 3 insertions, 4 deletions and 1 compound mutation types identified. Mutations have been identified in all five exons of the gene. These include 20 on exon 1, 13 on exon 2, 8 on exon 3,

39 on exon 4 and 29 on exon 5 (Figure 1). There have also been 2 non-exon mutations identified on intron 4 and intron 1 and 14 'apparently' sporadic cases described with 6 different SOD1 mutations. (Shaw et al., 1998).

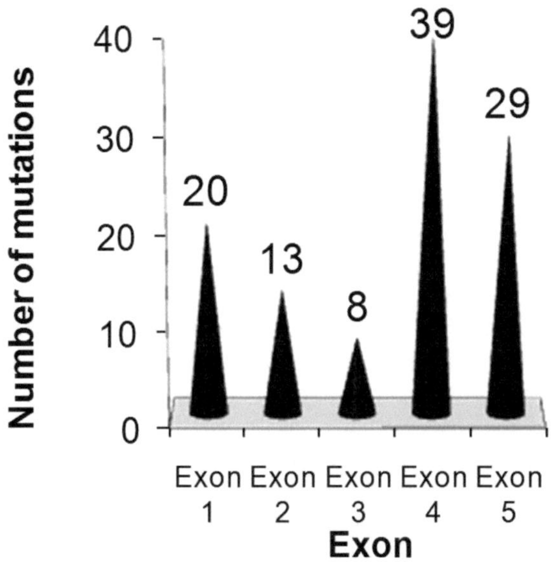

Fig. 1. Number of SOD1 mutations identified for each exon

Most are autosomal dominant in inheritance, but there is one confirmed autosomal recessive mutation, the D90A mutation in exon 4. This is unique in that it exists in dominant families in a heterozygous state, but in a number of pedigrees, specifically those of Scandinavian ancestry, homozygous mutations are required for disease. (Anderson et al., 1997).

Mutations in the heavy polypeptide 200kDa subunit of neurofilaments (NEFH) have been identified in sporadic MND cases, (Figlewicz et al., 1994) and in one FALS case. (Al-Chalabi et al., 1999). Accumulation of neurofilaments in cell bodies and axons of motor neurons is a pathological hallmark of early stages of many neurodegenerative diseases. These mutations lie in the region of the protein involved in cross-linking and thus may disrupt normal aggregation of filaments. Thus far, 1 insertion and 5 deletion mutations have been identified on exon 4. Analysis of the NEFH locus on chromosome 22 however has failed to detect linkage in MND families. (Vechio et al., 1996). Genome search on a large pedigree with autosomal dominant juvenile onset MND found strong evidence for linkage to chromosome 9q34 (ALS4). The average age of onset is 17 years, with slow progression of disease. (Chance et al., 1996). There is also an autosomal recessive, juvenile onset MND, with linkage to a locus on chromosome 15 (ALS5). (Hentati et al., 1998).

The other 90% of all MND patients have the sporadic form. There is no recognisable phenotypic difference between FALS and sporadic MND. The male: female ratio is 1:1 in FALS and 1.7:1 in sporadic MND. (De Belleroche et al., 1995). This decreases with increasing age of onset and approaches 1:1 after the age of 70. (Haverkamp et al., 1995). The site of onset is variable. Survival does not seem to be affected by age or gender, but rather the site of symptom onset. Generally, bulbar onset disease has a worse prognosis, and upper limb onset is more favourable. (Mulder et al., 1986).

It has be postulated that sporadic MND may be the final development of a chain of events that may be set in motion at one or more places in the central nervous system by endogenous and exogenous causes, or both. The aetiology of MND however remains unknown and is probably multifactorial. (Eisen 1995). There is no evidence to support the cause of sporadic MND being due to accumulation of heavy metals in the environment, (Needleman, 1997), deficiencies or excess of essential trace metals, (Mena et al., 1967) or exposure to environmental poisons and industrial solvents. (Leigh, 1997). There is also no evidence to support the cause of sporadic MND being due excessive physical activity or antecedent trauma.

4. Possible patterns of motor neurone loss

In normal healthy individuals, it has been shown that there is little loss of functioning motor neurones before the age of 60. The normal aging process then accounts for loss of approximately 3.9% of the original motor neurone pool per annum after the age of 60. (Brown, 1972). In this situation, the number of motor neurones remain fairly constant up to the age of 60, after which there is a gradual steady decline with age.
MND may be due to a slow attrition of motor neurones over time (Pattern 1 in Figure 2). If this were the case, pre-symptomatic motor neurone loss may be identifiable in SOD1 mutation carriers, as eventually there may be a gradual decline over time (Figure 2).
Another possible course of MND is that normal numbers of motor neurones are maintained until sudden, rapid multi-focal cell death of motor neurones occurs, corresponding with the development of symptoms (Pattern 2 in Figure 2). If this situation, it would be expected that SOD1 mutation carriers have a normal number of motor neurones during the pre-symptomatic phase. In this case, cell death occurs as neurones gradually accumulate damage, secondary to the mutation, which ultimately overwhelms cellular homeostasis. This is the cumulative damage hypothesis. (Clarke et al., 2000).

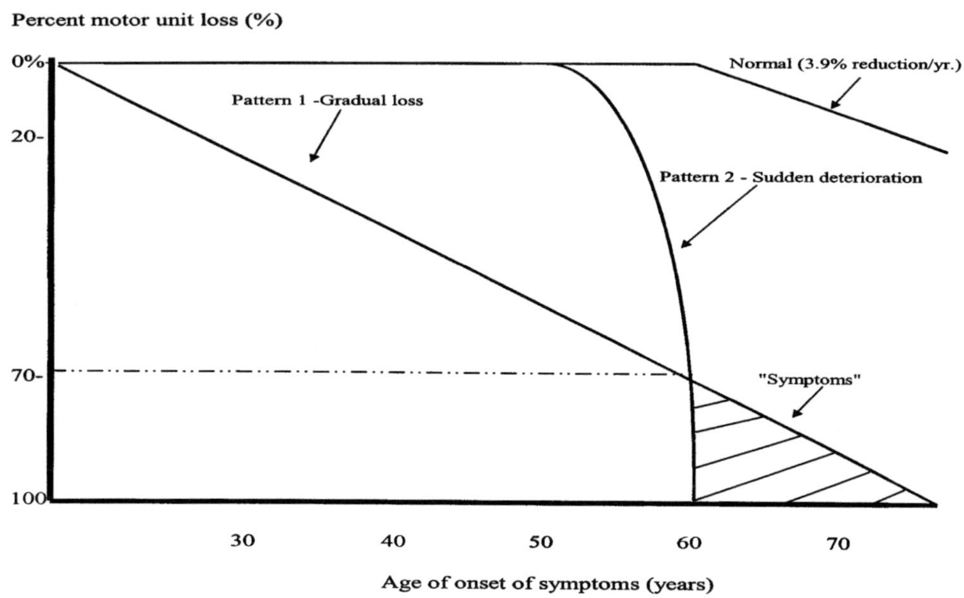

Fig. 2. Diagrammatic representation of possible patterns for motor neurone loss in an individual.

One of the mechanisms most frequently proposed to underlie cumulative damage is oxidative stress, in which an imbalance between the production of reactive oxygen species and cellular antioxidant mechanisms results in chemical modifications of macromolecules, thereby disrupting cellular structure and function. (Robberecht, 2000). A key prediction of the cumulative damage hypothesis is that the probability that any individual neurone will become committed to apoptosis increases as damage accrues within it. A mutant neurone in an older patient will have accumulated a greater amount of damage and is therefore be more likely to die than in a younger patient. Consequently, early in the course of disease, the chance of a cell containing a sufficient amount of damage to initiate apoptosis is small, and the rate of cell loss is correspondingly low. However, as the amount of intracellular damage increases, the chance that a cell will die also increases

It has been shown that the kinetics of neuronal death in a number of inherited neurodegenerative diseases was best explained by models in which the risk of cell death remains constant throughout life of the neurone and that cell death occurred randomly in time and was independent of any other neurone. This implies a "one-hit" biochemical phenomenon in which the mutant imposes an abnormal mutant steady state on the neurone and a single catastrophic event randomly initiates cell death and apoptosis. The principal features of the mutant steady state are that the living mutant neurones function very well for years or even decades and that the predominant feature of the mutant neurones is that they are all at a risk of death. This argues against the multiple environmental factors hypothesis as a cause of MND, as a random process is probably responsible for the initiation of disease. (Clarke et al., 2001).

5. Cu/Zn superoxide dismutase (SOD1) mutations

Linkage studies for familial MND (FALS) on chromosome 21q22.1 led to the identification of point mutations in the gene for Cu/Zn superoxide dismutase (SOD1) as a cause of MND. (Siddique 1991). Superoxide (O2-) is an unstable and highly active molecule, which causes oxidation of cell constituents either directly or through toxic and stable derivatives. The major superoxide dismutase activity in cytoplasm is from SOD1, which consists of 5 small exons that encode 153 highly conserved amino acids with a molecular weight of 16Kda. SOD1 is a homodimer. Within each monomer, there is an active site containing one atom each of copper and zinc. (Radunovic & Leigh, 1996).

The most common SOD1 gene mutation seen in FALS is an alanine to valine shift at codon 4 (Ala4Val). This accounts for 50% of all mutations in the USA. (Rosen, 1993). Of all the clinical variables, only bulbar onset and three specific mutations seem to influence age of onset of MND. Bulbar patients are older when their illness begins, whereas the Gly37Arg and Leu38Val mutations predict an earlier age of onset.). Leu38Val is associated with the earliest onset (mean 35.5 years) and Ile113Thr with the latest onset (mean 58.9 years).

In terms of survival, Ala4Val correlated with the shortest survival of 1.5 years. Whereas, Gly37Arg, Gly41Asp, and Gly93Ala mutation predicted longer survival. The mutations that predict earlier onset are not the same as those that correlate with shortest duration of disease. (Cudkowicz et al., 1997). This suggests that the factors that influence onset of disease differ from those that influence the rate of progression of the disease.

Determining the mechanism by which mutations in the Cu/Zn superoxide dismutase (SOD1) gene triggers the destruction of motor neurones causing MND remains a challenging and complex problem. Five primary hypotheses have been postulated for the pathogenesis of FALS (Figure 3). (Hand & Rouleau, 2002). At present the favoured hypotheses is that the mutation causes disease as a result of a toxic gain of function by the mutant SOD1 provoking selective neurotoxicity, probably disrupting the intracellular homeostasis of copper and/or protein aggregation. (Clevland, 1999).

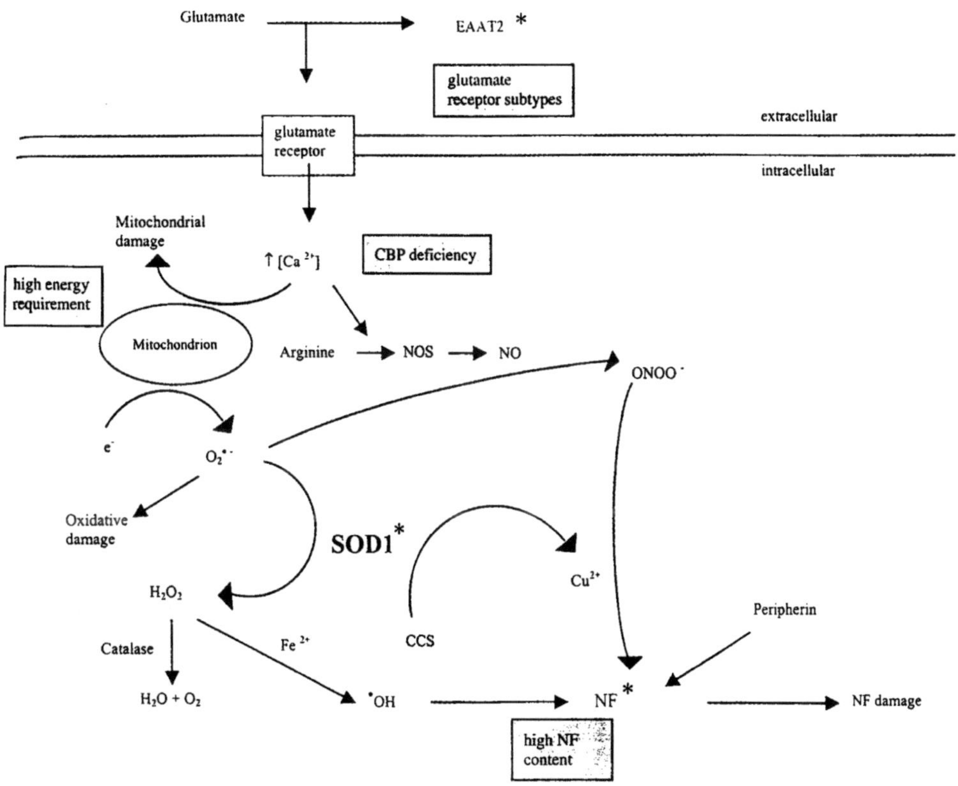

Fig. 3. Pathways that have been implicated in motor neurone cell death in amyotrophic lateral sclerosis (Reproduced from Hand CK. Familial Amyotrophic Lateral Sclerosis. Muscle Nerve 2002; 25:137).

The mutant SOD1 enzyme has altered reactivity with certain substrates, (Noor et al., 2003), in addition to the major superoxide dismutase activity. The SOD1 enzyme catalyses the reduction of hydrogen peroxide (H_2O_2), therefore acting as a peroxidase. This leads to the formation of hydoxyl radicals that can also alter the neurofilament network. Motor neurones have high-energy requirements and thus contain many mitochondria that generate superoxide radials (O_2-) through normal metabolism. SOD1 is an anti-oxidant defence which catalyses conversion of superoxide free radical anion (O2-) to hydrogen peroxide (H_2O_2), which is reduced to H_2O and O_2 by catalse. Mutations at SOD1 binding sites, alter the redox behaviour of the enzyme and destabilise the SOD1 ligand, leading to increased oxidative damage as hydrogen peroxide and its derivatives are toxic to the cell. (Yim et al., 1990).

This supports the hypothesis that the pathogenesis of SOD1 related FALS may be due to increased peroxidase activity of mutant SOD1 resulting in oxidative damage mainly to lipids of the cell membrane.

Mapping of the mutation sites predicted that these mutations destabilise the protein structure, leading to a less active enzyme i.e. "loss of function". This is however not supported by the fact that transgenic mice over expressing SOD1 gene developed disease similar to MND in humans, while those over-expressing normal SOD1 remained unaffected. This suggests that the mutant mice develop the disease independent of the level of SOD1 activity and suggests that the mutant protein itself is selectively toxic to motor neurones and that there is a "gain of toxic function" rather than a "loss of function". (Gurney et al., 1993). Also, although most mutations in SOD1 gene cause decrease in steady state of cytosolic SOD1 activity, Gly37Arg and Asp90Ala, have no significant decrease in SOD1 activity. (Shaw et al., 1998).

As most SOD1 mutations destabilise SOD1 protein (except Asp90Ala), it is possible that the mutant protein, with altered conformation may become unstable and precipitate to form aggregates or inclusions in motor neurons. These aggregates may then disturb normal cell function and lead to cell death. They are easily formed when SOD1 protein stability is decreased because this protein exists in large amounts accounting for 0.5-1% of total cytosolic protein in neurons. Alternations in the length of the coding sequence, folding, solubility or degradation results in the formation of aggregates. (Yim et al., 1990). Structural changes of mutant SOD1 may distort the rim of the electrostatic guidance channel and allow the catalytic site to become exposed and shallow. Molecules that are normally excluded may gain access to the catalytic reactive site. This results in less buffering of copper and zinc, which then become neurotoxic. (Radunovic & Leigh, 1996).

The nitric oxide (NO) produced by nitric oxide synthase (NOS) reacts spontaneously with O_2- to generate peroxynitrite ($ONOO^-$), which nitrosylates proteins leading to damage. Excess NO may also cause an increase in O_2- production by inhibition of mitochondrial electron flow, resulting in further generation of peroxynitrite. This facilitates nitrosylation of tyrosine residues of critical cytosolic proteins thus injuring cells. This reaction is copper dependent. The source of free copper may be mutant SOD1, which cannot accept the ion from the copper chaperone (CCS) protein. Mutant SOD1 possibly exhibit metal mediated cytotoxicities by disrupting the intracellular homeostasis of Cu and Zn, which are potential neurotoxins. (Gurney & Tomasselli, 2000).

The target proteins for nitrosylation include the neurofilament (NF) subunits, which may result in abnormal NF accumulation and subsequent disruption of the NF network and axonal transport, as there is a high neurofilament content in motor neurones. It has also been demonstrated that transgenes encoding mutant NF subunits can directly cause selective degeneration and death of motor neuones. (Cleveland, 1999). Conformational changes have been described in the mutations, Ala4Val, Gly37Arg and His6Arg that may affect the rim of the electrostatic guidance channel coded by exon 3. (Sjalander et al., 1995).

Glutamate is released from the presynaptic terminal activates the glutamate receptor on the postsynaptic cell membrane. It is then cleared from the synaptic cleft by specific glutamate transporters such as EAAT2. (Trotti et al., 1999). Astrocyte (glial cell) dysfunction may result in selective loss of EAAT2, interfering with the normal clearance of glutamate and allowing it to accumulate in the cell membrane and continue to activate the receptor. (Bruijin et al., 1997). Once activated, the glutamate receptor causes a calcium influx and a cascade of toxicity. The neurone does not have the capacity to buffer this efficiently due to a deficiency in calcium binding proteins (CBP's). This results in disturbances in mitochondrial metabolism and as a consequence, motor neurone cell death. (Beal, 1996).

To date, the only effective approved treatment for amyotrophic lateral sclerosis is Riluzole, (Cheah et al., 2010), which has a neuroprotective role, possibly due to pre-synaptic inhibition of glutamate release. (Doble, 1996). Treatment of human ALS patients or transgenic Cu, Zn superoxide dimutase 1 (SOD 1) mice, most commonly produce a modest but significant increase in survival. (Bensimon et al., 1994). It has also been shown to have a small beneficial effect on bulbar function, but not muscle strength. (Miller et al., 2007).

Apoptosis is characterised by a series of cellular changes leading to non-inflammatory cell death. Mitochondrial involvement in the apoptotic pathway also leads to the release of cytochrome c, an activator of the initiator caspase-9, which in turn activates caspase-3, which are executioners in the breakdown of essential cellular proteins. There is evidence that the mutant SOD1 transgene causes motor neurone death in mice through caspase-mediated programmed cell death. (Li et al., 2000). This may then be a target for inhibiting the apoptotic cascade, as it has been shown in a SOD1 transgenic mouse model that a small peptide caspase inhibitor (*zVAD-fmk*), prolonged survival after onset of disease by nearly 70%. (Kosti et al., 1997). It has also been reported that there are elevated levels of *bax* protein in MND spinal motor neurones, which promotes apoptosis. (Mu et al., 1996).

6. Methods

The Department of Molecular Medicine at Concord hospital had a large database of family members with a known family history of MND, who had blood samples collected for DNA, as part of a previous linkage study. From this database, family members were contacted by telephone by the department's genetic counsellor and informed about the study.

The regional committees for Ethics in Medical Research from Central Sydney Area Health Service, Royal North Shore Hospital and Prince Charles Hospital, approved this study.

All individuals participated without knowledge of their mutation status and on the understanding that this would not be revealed to them. Subjects were also aware that the results obtained from the study would not be available to them and that the information would only be used for research purposes. New consents were obtained from all individuals who participated in the study. The neurologist performing the MUNE studies also had no knowledge of their mutation status. The mutation status was only used in the final analysis of results. Subsequently, they were divided into "SOD1 negative family controls" and "asymptomatic SOD1 mutation carriers".

In addition, studies were also carried out on normal individuals, such as department technicians, spouses of SOD1 family members and individuals from the general population who attended MND support meeting and had an interest in helping to advance research into MND. This group was used as "population controls", to test the validity and reproducibility of the MUNE technique used.

Sporadic MND subjects were also initially studied once the MUNE technique had been validated to demonstrate that the MUNE technique used was able to detect a loss of motor neurones, when present. These were used as "positive controls".

6.1 Motor unit number estimation

Motor unit number estimation (MUNE) estimates the number of functioning lower motor neurones innervating a muscle or a group of muscles and is a measure of the primary pathologic process of motor neurone loss. The concept of motor unit number estimation

(MUNE) originated in 1967. At the time there was no satisfactory method of assessing the extent of denervation in muscles during life. Analysis of the density of the electromyographic interference pattern during maximal effort was not quantitative, and required the full co-operation of the patient.

The principle of MUNE is that if one can measure the mean single motor unit amplitude (SMUP), it is possible to obtain an estimate of the total number of motor units in the muscle. The results achieved were comparable with estimates of alpha motor fibres obtained by counting axons in specimens of motor nerves. (McComas, 1971).

MUNE has been performed in a number of different ways, each with their advantages and limitations. (Stein & Yang, 1990). The choice of technique depends on the speed and simplicity of the technique, as well as its accuracy and reproducibility. Some methods sample a very small proportion of the number of motor units innervating a muscle (typically 10-20). The coefficient of variation associated with different methods range from 10-45%. (McComas, 1991). If the variability is too large, then the technique cannot be used to follow motor unit loss reliably over time.

The way the average single motor unit potential (SMUP) size is obtained distinguishes the several techniques available. Most employ electrical stimulation of the motor nerve to determine the sizes of the SMUP, but a few use needle EMG.

Each method measures both the average size of the potentials generated by single motor units - single motor unit potentials (SMUP) and the size of the compound muscle action potential (CMAP) obtained with maximal stimulation of a motor nerve.

The motor unit number estimate is calculated by:

$$\text{MUNE} = \frac{\text{Maximum CMAP amplitude (or area)}}{\text{Average single motor unit potential (SMUP) amplitude or area.}}$$

Whereas the methods of measuring the average SMUP differ, they have common assumptions about the measurement of the supramaximal CMAP and the measurement of the average SMUP.

i. Maximal stimulation of any peripheral motor nerve activates all the muscles innervated by that nerve distal to the point of stimulation. Therefore, measurements of the CMAP are the summation of activity from multiple muscles and the MUNE is more accurately an estimate of the number of motor units in a group of muscles rather than in a single muscle.

For example, the median CMAP recorded at abductor pollicis brevis (APB) is more correctly a "thenar MUNE", as it is a summation of the activity of APB, opponens pollicis, flexor pollicis brevis, and to a lesser extent, the lateral lumbricals.

Extensor digitorum brevis (EDB) on the other hand, is a muscle innervated by the deep peroneal nerve. The only source of interfering muscle action potential is from extensor hallucis longus, which can be reduced by correct position of the stimulating electrodes. The muscle belly is flat in profile, eliminating deeper motor units as a cause of small potentials. The recording electrode is placed transversely across the innervation zone, resulting in a simple biphasic negative-positive M wave.

ii. The motor unit potentials used in the calculation of the average SMUP are representative of those generated by the total population of units. All methods, select a subset of the total population of motor units, measure their sizes and calculate an average SMUP for that subgroup.

iii. Finally, there is a phenomenon caused "alternation". This refers to fluctuations in the CMAP amplitude of the same motor unit with similar stimulation intensities. The thresholds of the first few motor axons excited are not sufficiently separate from one another, so that when graded increases in the stimulus intensity occur, the motor axons excited often overlap and add more than one SMUP to the CMAP being recorded. This can result in an underestimation of the mean SMUP size, as it may appear that there are 7 or 8 motor units when there are only 2 or 3 present, which in turn results in an over-estimation of the MUNE.

6.2 Statistical MUNE method

We used the statistical electrophysiological technique of motor unit number estimation (MUNE), (Daube, 1998), was used to estimate the number of motor units in thenar and extensor digitorum brevis muscles. The statistical method estimates the average size of SMUP's and the number of motor units in a group of muscles innervated by the nerve being stimulated, based on the normal variation of the submaximal CMAP evoked with constant stimuli. No attempt is made to identify individual motor unit potentials. The method relies on the known relation between the variance of multiple measures of step functions and the size of the individual steps when the steps have a Poisson distribution. S.D. Poisson was a French mathematician (1781-1840).

Poisson statistics are useful when the distribution arising for events occur randomly in time or when small particles are distributed randomly in space. They have been used to calculate the number of quanta released from a nerve terminal at the neuromuscular junction when the individual quanta are too small to be distinguished, as in myasthenia gravis. (Lomen-Hoerth & Slawnych, 2003).

In pure Poisson statistics, the size of a series of measurements is multiples of the size of a single component. In a Poisson distribution there is a discrete asymmetrical distribution in which responses are found at some levels and others where there are no responses (Figure 4). (McNeil, 1996).

A pure Poisson distribution has decreasing numbers at higher values. In Poisson distribution, the variance of these 30 measurements is equal to the size of the individual components making up each measurement. The variance can thus provide an estimate of the average size of the SMUP's.

The statistical method looks only at variance of the CMAP and does not require identification of individual components. It can be used when the sizes of SMUP's are too small to be isolated. The statistical method assumes that each motor unit has a similar size and that it is the same size each time it is activated.

Sequences of 30 submaximal stimuli are given. The inherent variability of the threshold of individual axons causes variations in the size of the CMAP. The average change in the submaximal CMAP amplitude caused by alternation (addition and subtraction of motor axons) is derived by Poisson statistics.

The occurrence of alternation with changing units that are activated does not modify the accuracy of the statistical method, because the method is a statistical measurement, a different result is found with each series of 30 stimuli. Therefore, multiple trials are needed to obtain the most accurate measurement. (Olney et al., 2000).

Experimental testing with trials of >300 stimuli has shown that repeated measurement of groups of 30 until the standard deviation of the repeated trials is <10% provides a close estimate of the number obtained with many more stimuli.[86] Estimates of the SMUP size and of the number of motor units are also most reliable if made at multiple different stimulus intensities to test axons with different thresholds.

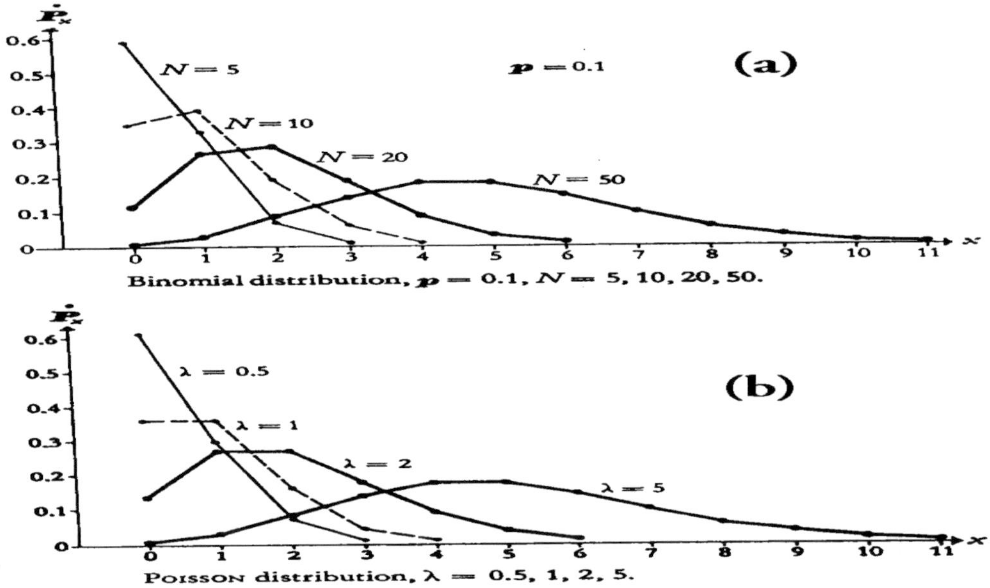

Fig. 4. Graphs illustrating Binomial and Poisson distribution (Reproduced from McNeil D. Statistical Methods. 1996; 184). The top graph (a) illustrates that binomial distribution resembles normal distribution with increasing sample size (n=50). The lower graph (b) illustrates that smaller values (λ=5) result in a normal distribution - Poisson distribution.

MUNE is calculated with the number weighted statistical method, where the mean SMUP amplitude at each level is multiplied by the number of motor units estimated at each level.

The steps in statistical MUNE are as follows:

1. Recording surface electrodes are applied as for standard nerve conduction studies.
2. An initial scan of the CMAP is performed using a series of 30 submaximal stimuli at 1 Hz, increasing in equal increments to identify unusually large steps at which further information is required.
3. On the basis of the scan, three or four 10% stimulus ranges are identified, according to an internal algorithm. Usually, one range includes the smallest step and the other ranges where the steps are >15% (Figure 5).
4. At each intensity, groups of 30 responses are captured at a rate of 3Hz. Estimates are most reliable if 10 groups of 30 responses are recorded. To minimise patient discomfort, however, repetition is repeated until the standard error of the MUNE SMUP size is less than 10%.
5. Statistical MUNE estimates the average size of SMUP's and the number of motor units in a group of muscles innervated by the nerve being stimulated, based on the normal variation of the sub-maximal CMAP evoked with constant stimuli (Figure 6).

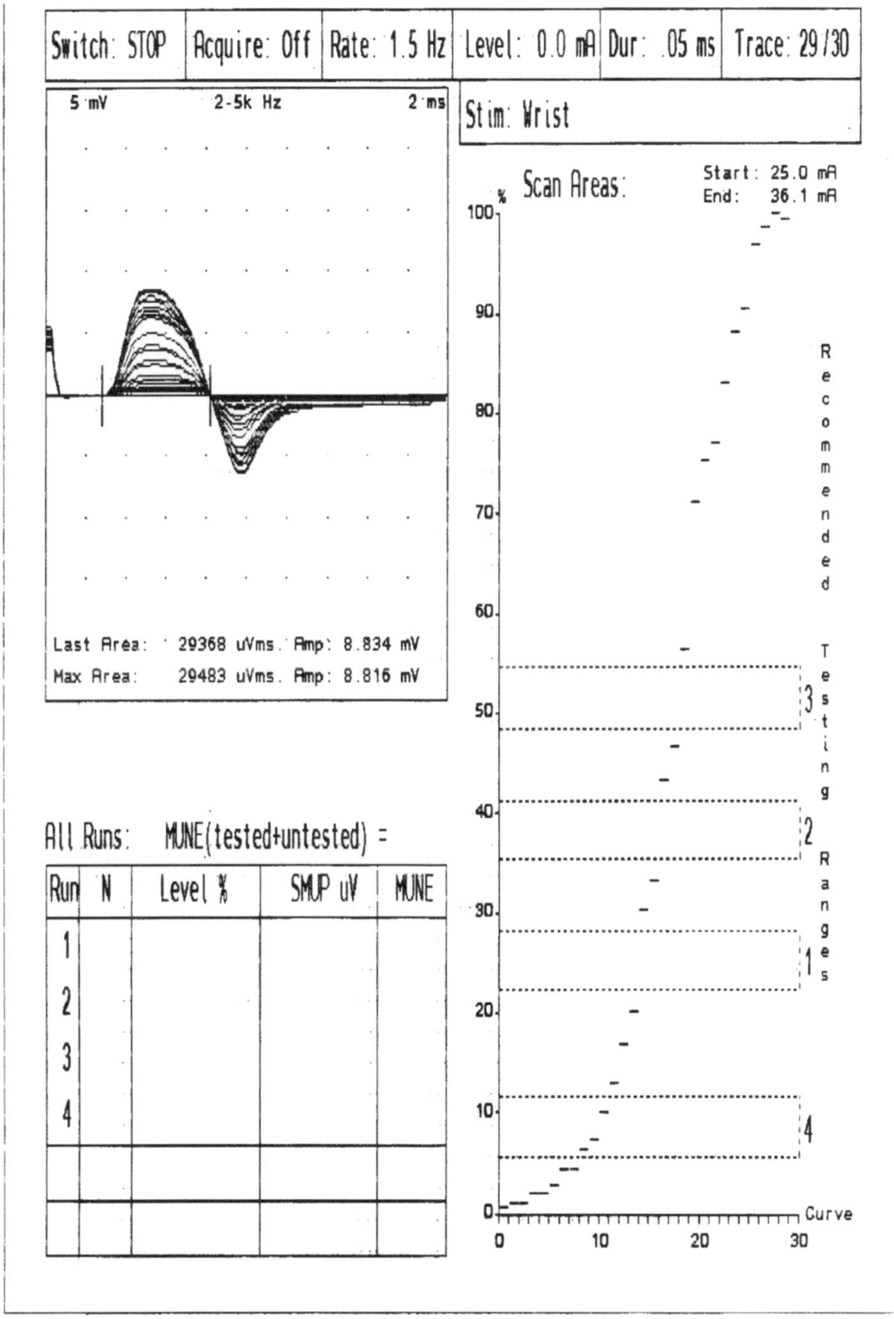

Fig. 5. An initial scan of the CMAP (right) recorded from APB muscles in response to 30 sub-maximal stimuli (x-axis) with equal increments between threshold and maximum stimulation. On the basis of the scan, 10% stimulus ranges are identified, according to an internal algorithm. The CMAP increments are shown at the top left and the eventual table of results in the bottom left corner.

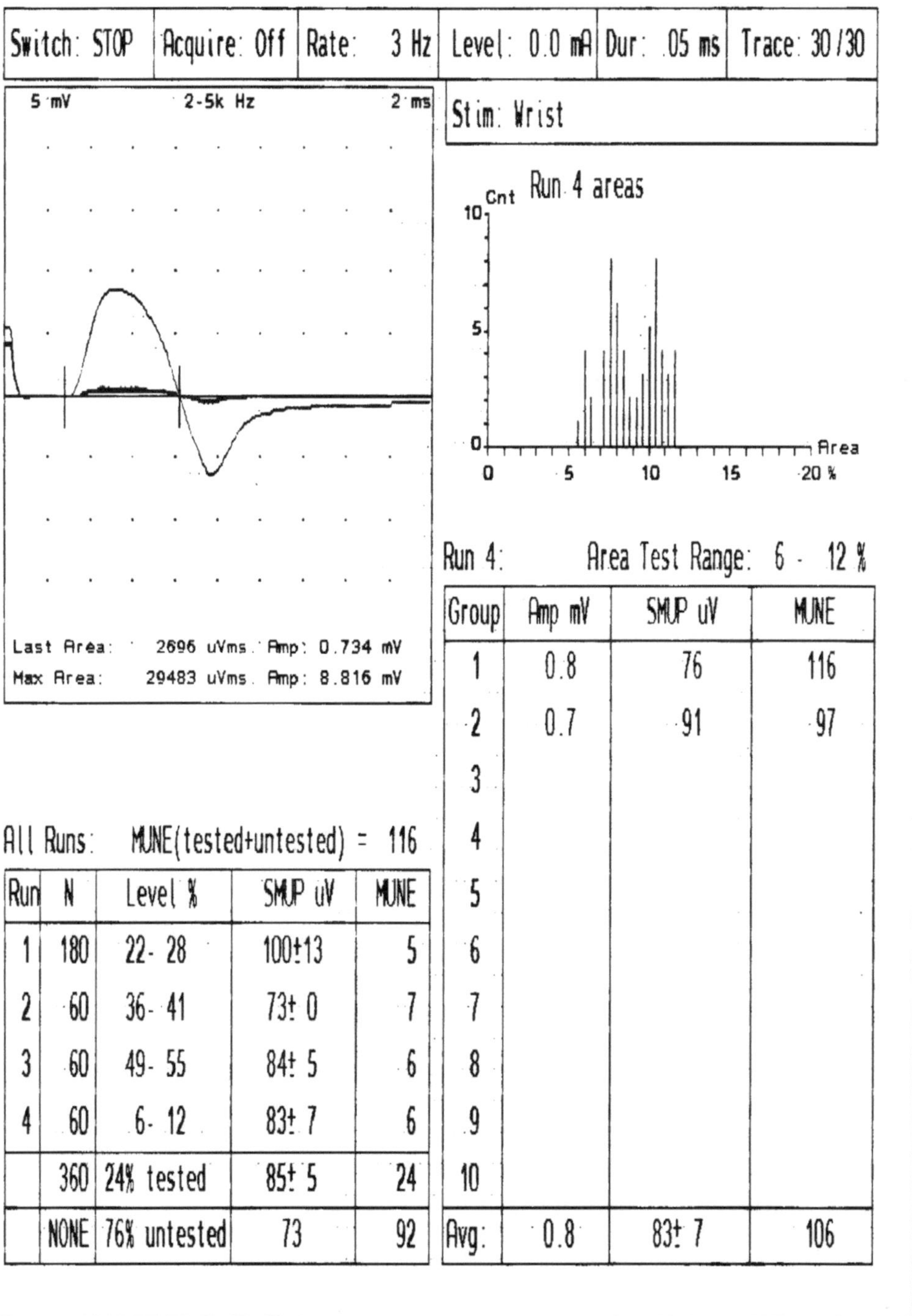

Fig. 6. At each intensity level (runs 1-4), groups of 30 responses are captured at a rate of 3Hz. The CMAP amplitudes are shown at the top left, with the histogram of results at the top right. The thenar MUNE results from repeated trials are shown in the bottom left table.

The statistical technique of estimating the size of the SMUP was performed using proprietary software on a Nicolet Viking IV electromyography machine. This technique uses direct stimulation of the motor nerve. The low frequency filter was set at 2 Hz and the high frequency filter at 5 kHz. The gain for extensor digitorum brevis was set at 2 mV/div and for abductor pollicis brevis studies at 5 mV/div. The sweep speed was 2 ms/div. This method had excellent test-retest reproducibility (+/-2.8%). The method was quick to use and well tolerated.

This technique has been greatly modified since its original description, but numerous studies have shown that MUNE can change systematically in ALS patients when used by experienced technicians, even though evaluator bias needs to be taken into account. (Shefner et al., 2004). The statistical MUNE method has also been shown to be unreliable in the presence of clinical weakness due to motor unit instability. (Shefner, 2009).

Our study however was performed on asymptomatic patients, without clinical weakness.

6.3 MUNE technique

Motor unit numbers were estimated in abductor pollicis brevis (resulting in a thenar MUNE) and the extensor digitorum brevis (EDB) muscle. These muscles were used, as both are easily accessible distal muscles. The electrical activity can be recorded without interference, and in the case of EDB, the muscle belly is flat.

Self-adhesive surface recording electrodes (G1) were placed transversely across the innervation zone of each muscle, resulting in a simple biphasic negative-positive M wave, with G2 placed over a bony prominence. The deep peroneal nerve was stimulated just above the ankle and the median nerve at the wrist with a surface stimulator. This was performed by strapping the stimulating electrode onto the surface of the skin, at the point where the threshold of the nerve to electrical stimulation was at its' lowest. A hand-held stimulator was not used, as reproducibility is enhanced when the stimulating electrodes are fixed to the surface of the skin.

Initially, bilateral thenar and EDB MUNE's were obtained from all subjects. After the reproducibility phase of the study, generally only right-sided studies were performed. Once a reduction in MUNE was identified, bilateral studies were once again performed on selected subjects. The protocol was also modified depending on the subjects' tolerance to the procedure.

Median nerve stimulation at the wrist for thenar MUNE was generally well tolerated by most subjects, as the stimulation intensity required to obtain an adequate response was generally less than 20mA with duration of 0.05-0.1ms.

Peroneal nerve stimulation required for EDB MUNE resulted in slightly more discomfort, as the nerve is located further away from the surface of the skin. The stimulus intensity required, in some cases was up to 50-80mA with duration of between 0.1-0.3ms. Some subjects indicated that they were unwilling to continue to participate in the study due to the discomfort caused by performing EDB MUNE. In these subjects, only thenar MUNE's were performed.

To assess the test-retest reproducibility of the technique, SOD1 family members and population controls were followed over a 1-year period, with thenar and EDB MUNE tests repeated every 3 to 6 months. The difference between MUNE results from the first and second study, and if possible, first and third studies were divided by the MUNE of the first study, and expressed as a percentage change. The results were analysed using Pearson and Spearman correlation coefficients.

All results were entered into a database and analysed using a standard statistical software package (SPSS 9.05 for Windows). For the initial part of the study, the MUNE results from asymptomatic SOD1 mutation carriers were grouped together. Although different mutations in SOD1 have different effects on the progression of the disease once symptoms occur, these different mutations do not influence on the age of onset of symptoms.[67]
Motor unit estimates in carriers were compared to age and sex matched family controls without the SOD1 mutation, and sporadic (non-SOD1) MND patients. To determine whether groups had different numbers of motor units, an unpaired t-test was used. Although there were some outlying results, the distributions were not sufficiently skewed to contradict the use of the t-test. Statistical significance was accepted at a p-value of <0.05.
The group of asymptomatic SOD1 mutation carriers were followed over the next 2 to 5 years, depending on the volunteers' motivation, both clinically and by MUNE. Results were compared to their initial baseline MUNE and the date of the study when this reduction was first detected, was used as the date when motor neurone loss commenced.

6.4 Maximal voluntary isometric contraction testing

It has been suggested that the traditional neurological examination is inadequate for documenting motor performance impairment with reliability. (Hanten et al., 1999). Generally, manual motor testing used in a standard neurological motor examination does not allow objective documentation of change in performance, as it may be influenced by the patient's history and progress. Major changes are apparent, but subtle changes are difficult to determine with accuracy.
There are a number of methods that have been developed to quantify maximal voluntary isometric contraction (MVIC). It has been proposed that this is a clinically useful, reliable, reproducible, time efficient and quantitative measure for monitoring disease progression in MND. (Hoagland et al., 1997). This would be surprising, given that in a slowly progressive denervating process, patients with substantial chronic denervation could maintain normal muscle twitch tension until loss of about 70-80% of motor units occurs. (McComas, 1971).
The methods used to quantify maximal voluntary isometric contraction have included an electronic strain-gauge tensiometer and a hand-held Jamar hydraulic dynamometer. In this study, maximum bilateral isometric grip strength was obtained using the Jamar hydraulic dynamometer to determine whether this correlated with the number of functional motor neurones in the thenar group of muscles, as measured by MUNE. Standardised (middle handle) positioning and instructions were given to all subjects. Handgrip force was measured with subjects in the sitting position and with the arm flexed at 90 degrees. Two trials were performed on each hand, and the best result used for analysis. This method was used as previous studies of grip strength reliability showed that there was no significant difference in reliability between one attempt, the mean score of two or three attempts, or the highest score of three attempts. (Hamilton et al., 1994).
Clinical neurological examination was performed, with power of thumb abduction, finger flexion and finger abduction measured according to the Medical Research Council (MRC) grading system and compared to thenar (APB) MUNE.
Felice showed that in twenty one MND patients, changes in thenar MUNE was the most sensitive outcome measure for following disease progression, when compared to other quantitative tests, such as CMAP, isometric grip strength, forced vital capacity and Medical Research Council manual muscle testing. (Felice, 1997).

7. Results

7.1 Demographics

A total of eighty-eight (88) subjects (45 males and 43 females) gave informed consent. The subjects were divided into four test groups.

1. 24 population controls;
2. 32 SOD1 negative (normal) family controls;
3. 20 asymptomatic (pre-clinical) SOD1 mutation carriers (test group),
   a. 5 subjects with point mutation in exon 4, codon 100, GAA to GGA, Glu to Gly) - glu100gly;
   b. 5 subjects with point mutation in exon 4, codon 113, ATT to ACT, Ile to Thr) - ile113thr;
   c. 5 subjects with point mutation in exon 5; codon 148, GTA to GGA, Val to Gly) - val148gly;
   d. 5 subjects with point mutation in exon 5, codon 148, GTA to GGA, Val to Ile) val148ile.
4. 12 sporadic symptomatic MND patients (positive controls).

There was no statistically significant difference in age distribution between these groups, with a range of 16 to 73 years of age.

7.2 Motor units in asymptomatic FALS (SOD1) carriers

For the initial part of the study, the baseline MUNE results were grouped together and the means of the groups were compared. The initial aim of the study was to determine if MND was due to a slow gradual attrition of motor neurones over time. If this were the case, the group of asymptomatic SOD1 mutation carriers, would be expected to have a reduced number of motor units, indicating the presence of pre-clinical motor neurone loss. Motor unit estimates in the group of asymptomatic SOD1 mutation carriers were compared to age and sex matched family controls without the SOD1 mutation, and sporadic (non-SOD1) MND patients. To determine whether groups had different numbers of motor units, an unpaired t-test was used. Statistical significance was accepted at a p-value of <0.05.

The numbers of motor units in the groups of population controls, SOD1 negative family controls and asymptomatic SOD1 mutation carriers were similar. In population controls the mean thenar MUNE was 148 with a range of 115 - 254, in SOD1 negative family controls was 138 with a range of 106 - 198 and in asymptomatic SOD1 mutation carriers, 144 with a range of 109 - 199. There was no detectable difference in the mean number of thenar motor units in the group of asymptomatic SOD1 mutation carriers compared to the group of SOD1 negative family controls (thenar $p>0.46$), or population controls (thenar $p>0.70$) (Table 1 and Figure 7).

	Thenar (APB) muscle	
	Cases	**MUNE (Range)**
Population Controls	24	148 (115-254)
SOD1 Negative Family Controls	32	138 (106-198)
SOD1 Mutation Carriers	20	144 (109-199)
Sporadic MND patients	12	45 (5-84)

Table 1. Thenar (APB) motor unit number estimates (MUNE number represents mean MUNE).

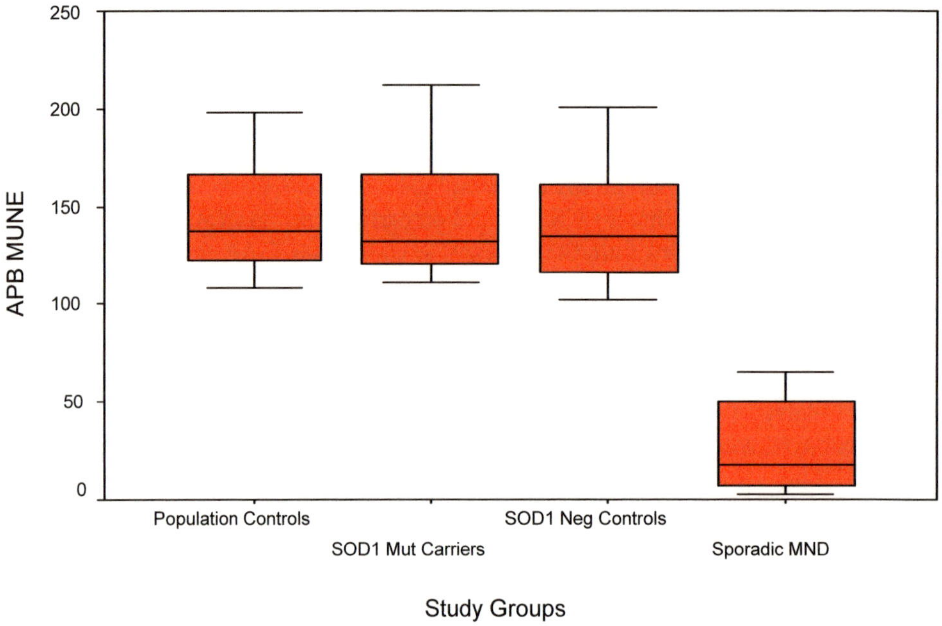

Fig. 7. Baseline thenar (APB) MUNE subdivided into study groups (The lower boundary of the box is the 25th percentile, and the upper border is the 75th percentile of MUNE. The horizontal line inside the box represents the median MUNE. The whispers represent the largest and smallest observed values, i.e. the range). Data is shown in Table 1.

In population controls the mean EDB MUNE was 138 with a range of 119 - 169, in SOD1 negative family controls was 134 with a range of 107 - 180 and in asymptomatic SOD1 mutation carriers, 136 with a range of 111 - 187.

Once again, there was no detectable difference in the mean number of EBD motor units in the group of asymptomatic SOD1 mutation carriers compared to the group of SOD1 negative family controls (EDB p>0.95), or population controls (EDB p>0.50) (Table 2 and Figure 8).

	Extensor Digitorum Brevis	
	Cases	**MUNE (Range)**
Population Controls	13	138 (119-169)
SOD1 Negative Family Controls	30	134 (107-180)
SOD1 Mutation Carriers	14	136 (111-187)
Sporadic MND patients	9	70 (8-82)

Table 2. EDB motor unit number estimates (MUNE number represents mean MUNE).

Symptomatic sporadic MND subjects showed a definite loss of motor units with fewer motor units compared to all other groups (p<0001) with a mean thenar MUNE of 45 with a range of 5 - 84 and a mean EDB MUNE of 70 with a range of 8 - 82 (Tables 1 and 2).

There was no cross over between thenar and EDB MUNE results in symptomatic and asymptomatic subjects.

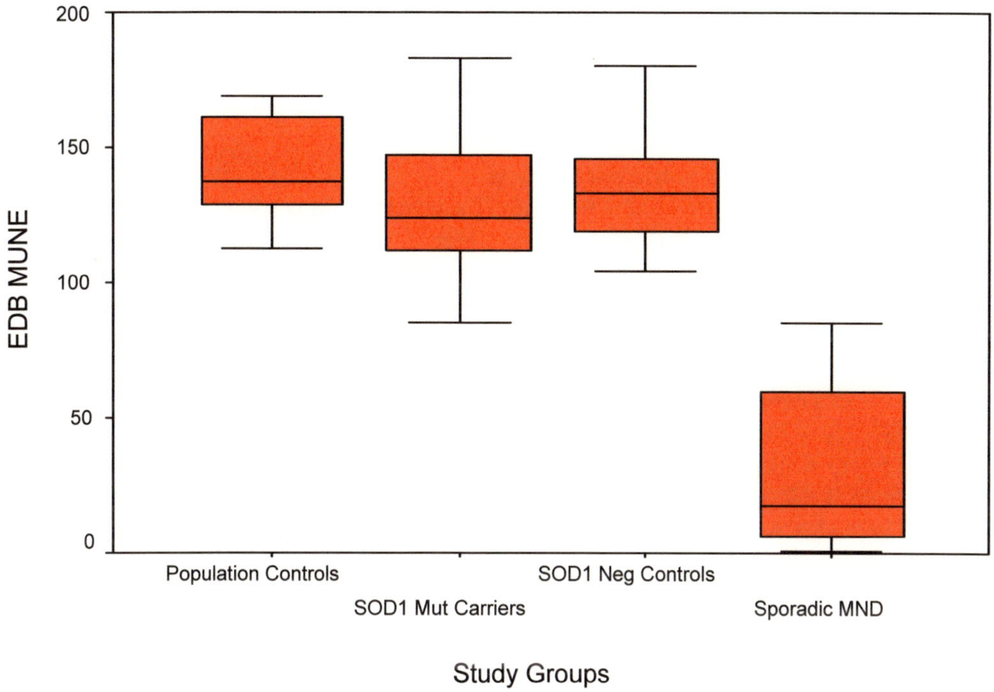

Fig. 8. Baseline EDB MUNE subdivided into study groups (The lower boundary of the box is the 25th percentile, and the upper border is the 75th percentile of MUNE. The horizontal line inside the box represents the median MUNE. The whispers represent the largest and smallest observed values, i.e. the range). Data is shown in Table 2.

7.3 Reproducibility of MUNE technique

To assess the test-retest reproducibility of the technique, 69 of the 88 SOD1 family members and population controls were followed over a 1-year period, with thenar and extensor digitorum brevis (EDB) MUNE tests repeated every 3-6 months, depending on patient availability. The difference between MUNE results from the first and second study, and if possible, first and third studies were divided by the MUNE of the first study, and expressed as a percentage change. The results were analysed using Pearson and Spearman correlation coefficients.

The test-retest correlation of thenar MUNE in asymptomatic subjects was high with a Pearson correlation coefficient of 0.93. The mean difference between MUNE results on separate occasions on the same individual was +/- 3.6%, with a range of 0-11.7% (Table 3).

	Number of Cases	**Mean MUNE**
Thenar 1	88	145.7
Thenar 2	69	140.1
Thenar 3	33	140.0
Thenar Change	**Range (0 - 11.7%)**	**3.6%**

Table 3. Reproducibility of mean thenar (APB) motor unit number estimates in asymptomatic subjects on separate reviews over a one-year period.

For EDB MUNE, the Pearson correlation coefficient was also high, 0.88, with a mean difference between MUNE results on separate occasions on the same individual of +/- 4.6%, with a range of 0-15.7%. The test-retest correlation was high with a Pearson correlation coefficient of 0.91, when groups were broken down into the different study groups.

7.4 Maximal voluntary isometric contraction

Maximal voluntary isometric contraction (MVIC), using the Jamar hand dynamometer was used to measure isometric grip strength to determine whether this correlated with the number of functional motor neurones in the thenar group of muscles as measured by MUNE. Isometric grip strength tests, thenar MUNE and MRC power were performed on 69 asymptomatic subjects twice within a 3-6 month period to assess the test-retest reproducibility of this technique. Pearson correlation coefficients between study 1 and study 2 of right hand grip strength was 0.941, left hand grip strength 0.910 and thenar MUNE results 0.937. These results indicate that the reproducibility of these techniques was high.
Right hand grip strength correlated with left hand grip strength, with Pearson correlation coefficients of 0.959 and Spearman correlation coefficients of 0.956 Two-way analyses of variance showed a no significant difference between the right and left hands (Figure 9). There was no correlation between right grip strength and right thenar motor unit number, with Pearson correlation coefficients of 0.483 and Spearman correlation coefficient of 0.34 (Figure 10).

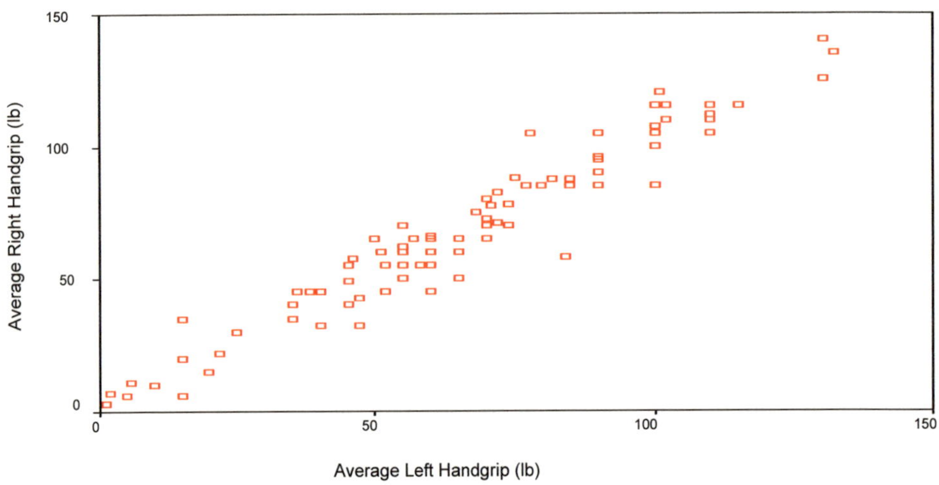

Fig. 9. Graph showing the correlation between right and left handgrip

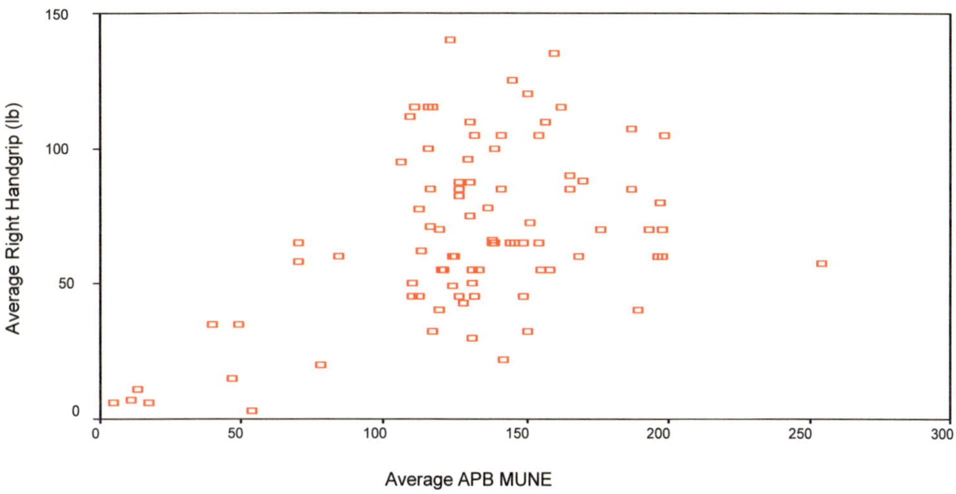

Fig. 10. Scatter graph showing the lack of correlation between right handgrip and right thenar (APB) MUNE

7.5 Detection of pre-symptomatic motor neurone loss in SOD1 mutation carriers

The MUNE results, after validating their reproducibility, were used as a baseline to follow the number of motor units over time in individual pre-symptomatic SOD1 mutation carriers over the next 2-5 years, to determine whether pattern of motor neurone loss is either a slow attrition of motor neurones over time or whether normal numbers of motor neurones are maintained until sudden, rapid multi-focal cell death of motor neurones occurs, corresponding with the development of symptoms.

During the course of the study, 5 of the SOD1 mutation carriers developed leg weakness. A significant fall in motor unit number was detected in these 5 SOD1 mutation carriers, were there was a detectable reduction of motor units, 4-10 months prior to the onset of weakness and the diagnosis of familial ALS being made. There was no detectable loss of motor units in the other 15 SOD1 mutation carriers or in the group of SOD1 mutation negative relatives, during the study period.

In individual cases, there was:

51% loss of motor units, 4 months prior to onset of weakness in Case 1

37% loss of motor units, 10 months prior to onset of weakness in Case 2

28% loss of motor units, 6 months prior to onset of weakness in Case 3

46% loss of motor units, 6 months prior to onset of weakness in Case 4

68% loss of motor units, 8 months prior to onset of weakness in Case 5

There was further motor unit loss as weakness progressed, at which point the diagnosis of MND was confirmed.

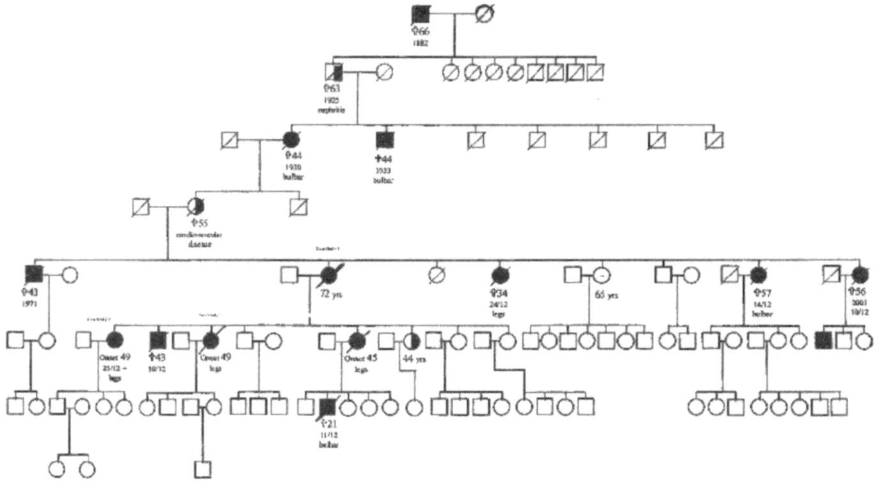

Fig. 11. Pedigree of cases 1, 2 and 3

7.5.1 Case study 1

A 48-year-old lady from a family with a strong history of familial ALS. Pedigree is shown in Figure 11. This family has a point mutation in the SOD1 gene at val148gly. At the time of recruitment, October 1998, the subject was asymptomatic, with a normal neurological examination and no evidence of wasting, weakness or fasciculations. Progress MUNE results are shown in Table 4 and Figure 12.

Months before and after weakness	-26	-24	-21	-13	-7	-4	0	+3	+5	+8	+17
Date of study	Oct-98	Dec-98	Mar-99	Nov-99	Jul-00	Nov-00	Mar-01	Jun-01	Aug-01	Nov-01	Aug-02
R Handgrip	60	65	68	60	60	65	65	62	60	45	Died
R Thenar MUNE	130	131	126	131	115	113	115	110	83	49	
L Handgrip	60	60	60	60	60	60	55	45	37	18	
L Thenar MUNE	122		114	110		122	83	52	40	0	
R EDB power	5/5	5/5	5/5	5/5	5/5	5/5	5/5	3/5	0/5	0/5	
R EDB MUNE	124	120	132	116	116	114	114	72	53	0	
L EDB power	5/5	5/5	5/5	5/5	5/5	5/5	0/5	0/5	0/5	0/5	
L EDB MUNE	130			125		64	0	0	0	0	

Table 4. Case 1 progressive handgrip, dorsiflexion power and thenar and EDB MUNE results

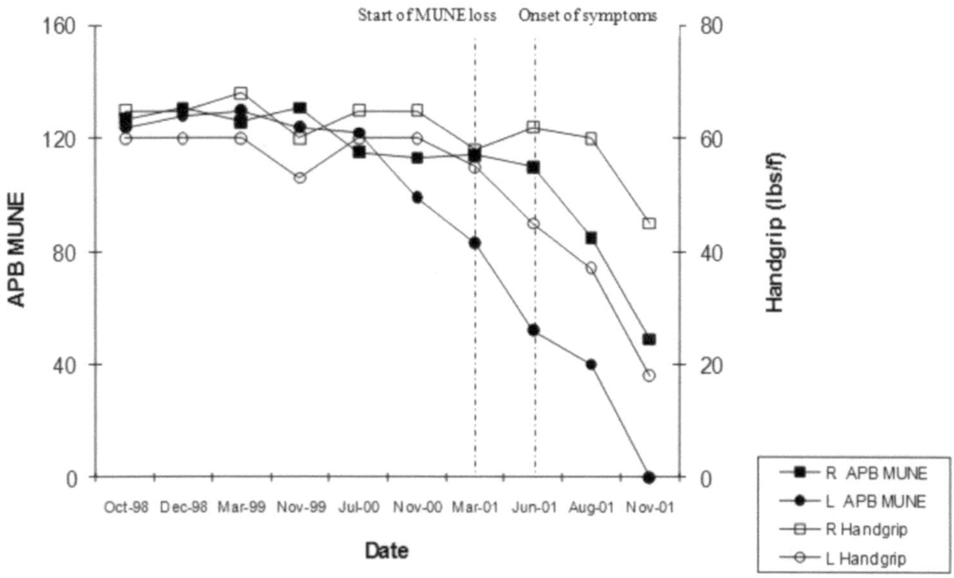

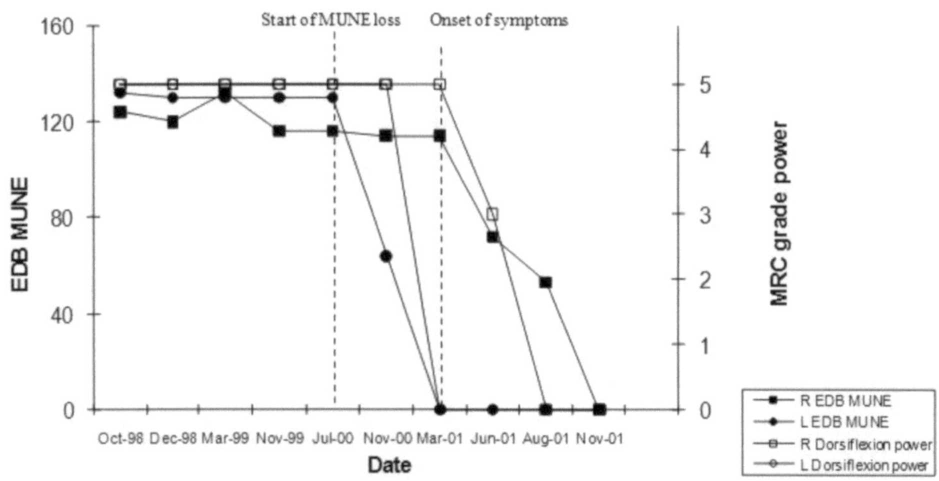

Fig. 12. Progressive results of case 1 showing the change in APB and EDB motor unit estimates over time in relation to handgrip strength and power. There is a reduction of APB and EDB MUNE prior to the onset of weakness.

The MUNE results remained stable over the first 2 years of the study. By November 2000, her left EDB MUNE had dropped to 64 (total reduction of 51%), but she only developed wasting and weakness of the anterior compartment muscles of her left leg, 4 months later, when she had MRC grade 2/5 of dorsiflexion and eversion, 3/5 plantarflexion and inversion 3/5. Proximal muscles, upper limb and right leg muscles were normal. Deep tendon reflexes were brisk in the upper and lower limbs. Over the next 6 months, her right thenar MUNE from 130 to 115 (12%) She had no detectable right arm weakness at the time and her handgrip strength remained at around 65 pounds.

An independent neurologist performed needle EMG, which showed extensive denervation in left leg muscles with fibrillation potentials in the left tibialis posterior, gastrocnemius, vastus medialis and L5/S1 paraspinal muscles. There were no changes in the right vastus medialis, biceps brachialis, triceps, left deltoid and the tongue. It was felt that these changes were not enough to make a diagnosis of ALS. She went on to have a MRI scan of her lumbar spine showed degenerative disc disease of L4/5 and L5/S1, with no evidence of neural compression.

Over the next 6 months, her right EDB MUNE continued to drop from 114 to 72 and subsequently to 53, a 54% reduction. Her left thenar MUNE also dropped from 122 to 83 motor units, a 36% reduction. Her right foot power remained normal until August 2001, 7 months after the reduction was noted. At that time, she developed upper limb weakness, with a reduction of left handgrip strength to 45 pounds.

Repeat needle EMG examination showed severe denervation in the left tibialis anterior and gastrocnemius, but still no changes in proximal right lower limb or upper limb muscles. Once again, this was considered not to be diagnostic for ALS. Her EDB and thenar MUNE however continued to drop and she developed upper and lower limb weakness and became wheelchair bound. She subsequently died with respiratory failure in August 2002.

7.5.2 Case study 2

A 43-year-old sister of case 1. She had the same strong family history of ALS, with a point mutation in SOD1 gene at val148gly. Her pedigree is shown in Figure 11. She was asymptomatic at the time of recruitment with a normal neurological examination, and no evidence of wasting, weakness or fasciculation. Her right and left thenar MUNE's remained stable for the first 2½ years of the study at around 115-120 motor units. Progress MUNE results are shown in Table 5 and Figures 14.

Months pre and post weakness 1st detected	-42	-40	-37	-29	-20	-10	0	+11	+21	+27
Date of study	Oct-98	Dec-98	Mar-99	Nov-99	Jul-00	Jan-01	Nov-01	Oct-02	Aug-03	Feb-04
R Handgrip	60	60	65	65	60	70	65	65	65	65
R Thenar MUNE	111	111	117	119	120	114	96	97	86	85
L Handgrip	60	55	60	65	63	65	65	60	60	60
L Thenar MUNE	117				119	111	89	86	79	81
R EDB power	5/5	5/5	5/5	5/5	5/5	5/5	4+/5	4+/5	4+/5	4+/5
R EDB MUNE	104	111	119	108	104	92	71	75	75	65
L EDB power	5/5	5/5	5/5	5/5	5/5	5/5	5/5	5/5	5/5	5/5
L EDB MUNE	112						89	80	80	81

Table 5. Case 2 progressive handgrip, dorsiflexion power and thenar and EDB MUNE results

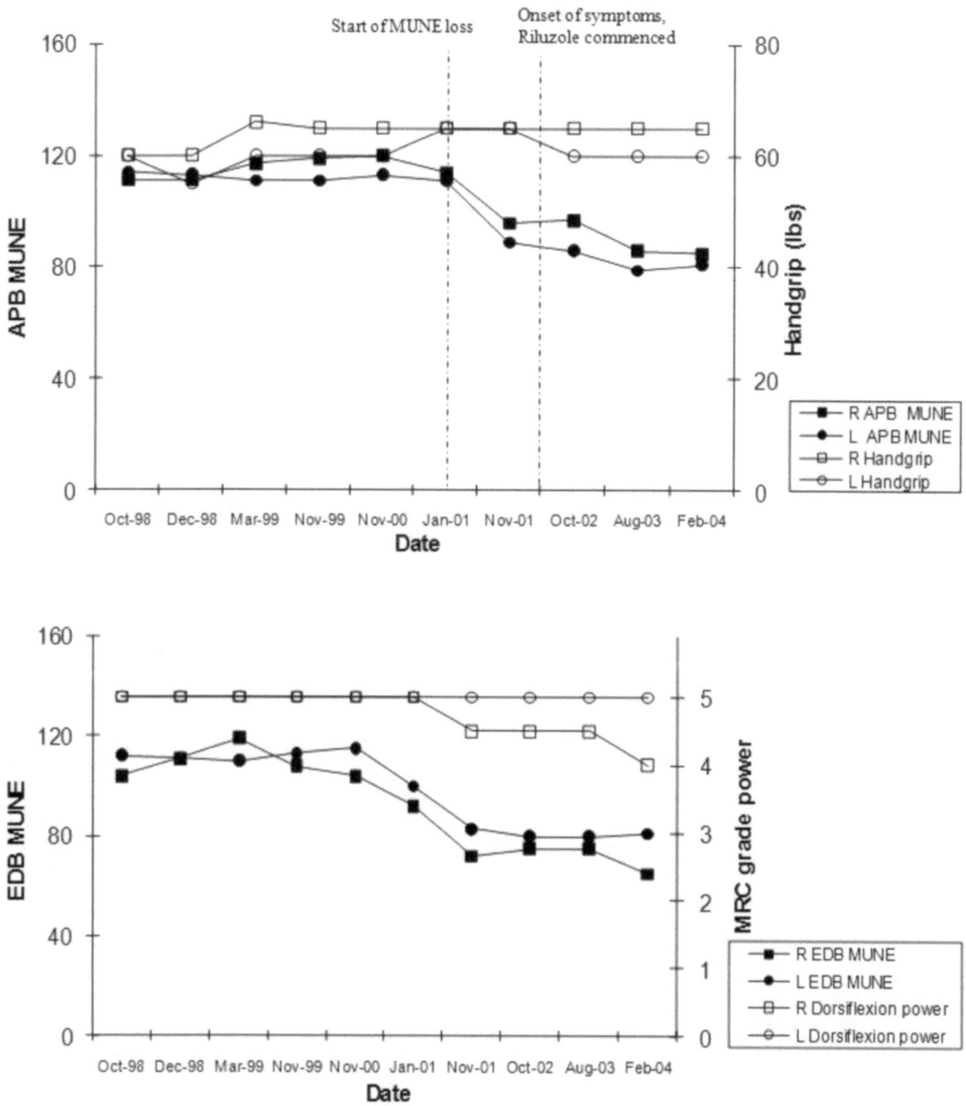

Fig. 14. Progressive results of case 2 showing the change in APB and EDB motor unit estimates over time in relation to handgrip strength and power. There is a reduction of APB and EDB MUNE even though strength has remained stable.

Over the next 6 months, there was a reduction in her right thenar MUNE to 96 (20%) and her left thenar MUNE to 89 (19%), with no detectable weakness. Her right EDB MUNE also dropped from 111 to 92 (17%), but she only had detectable weakness 10 months later of MRC grade 4+/5 in right dorsiflexors, at which time her right EDB MUNE had dropped further to 71 motor units (35%). The left EDB MUNE also dropped from a baseline of 112 (2 years previously) to 89 (20%), but with no detectable weakness.
An independent neurologist performed needle EMG examination, which showed high amplitude motor units with reduced recruitment in vastus medialis, tibialis anterior and

extensor carpi radialis longus, bilaterally but no fibrillation potentials were seen. It was felt that these changes were not enough to make the diagnosis of ALS.
In view of her strong family history, a presumed diagnosis of familial ALS was made and she was commenced on Riluzole in February 2002.
Over the next 3 years, her EDB MUNE results have stabilised. Her weakness has not progressed significantly. In February 2004, she still had MRC grade 4+/5 power of her right dorsiflexors and no symptomatically apparent weakness in her left dorsiflexors or upper limbs.

7.5.3 Case study 3

A 68 year-old mother of case 1 and 2. She had the same family history of ALS, with a point mutation in SOD1 gene at val148gly. Her pedigree is shown in Figure 12. She was also asymptomatic at the time of recruitment. Her right and left thenar MUNE's remained stable at around 130 motor units. Due to her age, she was not followed as regularly as her daughters.
On her review in November 2001, there had been a reduction of her right thenar MUNE to 98 (23%) and her left thenar MUNE to 98 (25%), with no detectable weakness. Her right EDB MUNE also dropped from 147 to 106 (28%), but she did not have any detectable weakness. She subsequently developed voice change 6 months later in May 2002, and died of respiratory failure in August 2002. Progress MUNE and handgrip results are shown in Table 6.

Months pre and post weakness 1st detected	**-43**	**-41**	**-38**	**-6**	**0**	**+3**
Date of study	Oct-98	Dec-98	Mar-99	Nov-01	May-02	Aug-02
R Handgrip	55	55	55	55	Voice	Died
R Thenar MUNE	127	135	130	98	Change	
L Handgrip	60	50	50	45		
L Thenar MUNE	130			125		
R EDB power	5/5	5/5	5/5	5/5		
R EDB MUNE	147	153	150	106		

Table 6. Case 3 progressive handgrip, dorsiflexion power and thenar and EDB MUNE results

7.5.4 Case study 4

A 48-year-old lady with a strong family history of ALS. This family had a point mutation in SOD1 gene at glu100gly. At the time of recruitment, the subject was asymptomatic, with a normal neurological examination and no evidence of wasting, weakness or fasciculations. Progress MUNE results are shown in Table 7.
The MUNE results remained stable over the first 2½ years of the study. Her right EDB MUNE results remained stable at around 120 motor units. It was then noted that her left EDB MUNE had dropped from 118 to 64 (46% reduction) and her right thenar MUNE had also dropped from 153 to 123 (20% reduction). She did not have any detectable weakness of her upper or lower limbs. Needle EMG showed neurogenic changes, but not sufficient to fulfil the criteria for ALS.

She subsequently developed left lower leg weakness with inversion and eversion of MRC grade 3/5 and dorsiflexion and plantarflexion 4/5, 6 months later. Her disease progressed rapidly and died within the 4 months of diagnosis, in March 2002 of respiratory failure.

Months pre and post weakness 1st detected	**-33**	**-30**	**-25**	**-14**	**-6**	**0**	**+4**
Date of study	Apr-98	Jul-98	Dec-98	Nov-99	Apr-01	Oct-01	Mar-02
R Handgrip	60	66	70	80	60	70	Died
R Thenar MUNE	149	144	142	151	153	123	
L Handgrip	50	60	65	60	55	58	
L Thenar MUNE	128						
R EDB power	5/5	5/5	5/5	5/5	5/5	5/5	
R EDB MUNE	126	132	137	119	118	118	
L EDB power	5/5	5/5	5/5	5/5	5/5	3/5	
L EDB MUNE	123			118	64	42	

Table 7. Case 4 progressive handgrip, dorsiflexion power and thenar and EDB MUNE results

7.5.5 Case study 5

A 44-year-old man with a strong family history of ALS and a 2nd cousin once removed of case 4. His family also had a point mutation in SOD1 gene at glu100gly. At the time of recruitment, the subject was asymptomatic, with a normal neurological examination and no wasting, weakness or fasciculations. Progress MUNE results are shown in Table 8.

Months pre and post weakness 1st detected	**-50**	**-48**	**-44**	**-35**	**-22**	**-8**	**0**
Date of study	May-98	Jul-98	Nov-98	Aug-99	Sep-00	Nov-01	Jul-02
R Handgrip	115	110	120	115	110	115	120
R Thenar MUNE	127	117	107	116	138	116	121
L Handgrip	100	100	105	105	105	100	100
L Thenar MUNE	135					122	120
R EDB power	5/5	5/5	5/5	5/5	5/5	0/5	0/5
R EDB MUNE	125	114	129	106	115	0	0
L EDB power	5/5	5/5	5/5	5/5	5/5	5/5	4/5
L EDB MUNE	127				114	36	0

Table 8. Case 5 progressive handgrip, dorsiflexion power and thenar and EDB MUNE results

The MUNE results remained stable over the first 3 years of the study. The right EDB MUNE dropped from 115 down to being not recordable. Thenar MUNE remained stable at about 130 motor units. He had occasional fasciculations in the right quadriceps region, weakness of the right quadriceps and MRC grade 0/5 weakness of right dorsiflexion. He was unsure as to when weakness developed. Needle EMG showed changes of active and chronic denervation limited to the right quadriceps muscle, which was not considered diagnostic for ALS.

Over the next 6 months, there was a reduction of the left EDB MUNE as well from 114 to 36 (68% reduction), but with no detectable weakness. In July 2002, 8 months later, he was reviewed by his neurologist and was found to have only slightly reduced left ankle power with MRC grade 4/5 and weakness of knee flexion bilaterally. He progressed rapidly after that and by October 2002 had bilateral lower limb weakness to a point were he was unable to stand without assistance and became wheelchair bound. He commenced Riluzole, in May 2003, but over the next year there was progression of upper limb weakness. Currently, his forced lung capacity is around 30% and he is using BiPAP ventilation at night and receives PEG feeding.

8. Conclusion

Motor neurone disease (MND) is a group of fatal, progressive neurodegenerative disorders, with an overall median survival is approximately 4.0 years from the onset of symptoms. By the time most patients with MND are aware of clinical weakness and seek review by their primary physician or neurologist, a significant proportion of motor units have already been lost. Early detection of motor neurone loss in clinically apparently unaffected muscles is therefore important to establish an early diagnosis of the condition.

Motor unit number estimates in the group of asymptomatic SOD1 mutation carriers were compared to age and sex matched family controls without the SOD1 mutation, and sporadic (non-SOD1) MND patients. There was no detectable difference in the number of thenar motor units in the group of asymptomatic SOD1 mutation carriers compared to the group of SOD1 negative family controls (thenar $p>0.46$), or population controls (thenar $p>0.70$).. In addition, there was no detectable difference in the number of EBD motor units in the group of asymptomatic SOD1 mutation carriers compared to the group of SOD1 negative family controls (EDB $p>0.95$), or population controls (EDB $p>0.50$). Symptomatic sporadic MND subjects showed a definite loss of motor units with fewer motor units compared to all other groups ($p<0.001$). There was no overlap between MUNE results in symptomatic and asymptomatic subjects.

These results indicate that the group of asymptomatic carriers of the SOD1 mutation have no significant difference in the number of motor neurones, when compared to age and sex matched controls. All carriers had a full complement of motor neurones during the asymptomatic phase, indicating that mutation carriers have normal survival of motor neurones and that symptomatic MND is not the end result of a slow attrition of motor neurones. This implies that gradual pre-symptomatic loss of motor neurones does not occur in asymptomatic SOD1 mutation carriers. This supports the observation that sudden, catastrophic loss of motor neurones occurs immediately prior to the onset of symptoms and the development of the disease, rather than a gradual attrition of motor neurones over time. These results suggest that there may be a biological trigger initiating rapid cell loss, just prior to the onset of symptoms. This observation is an important contribution to the current understanding of the pathogenesis of MND. (Aggarwal & Nicholson, 2001).

The statistical MUNE technique was used for the study. This technique has been greatly modified since its original description, but numerous studies have shown that MUNE can change systematically in ALS patients when used by experienced technicians, even though evaluator bias needs to be taken into account. Shefner demonstrated that the statistical MUNE was unreliable in the presence of clinical weakness due to motor unit instability. The difference is that our study was performed on asymptomatic patients, without clinical weakness.

It also showed that MUNE may be used as a reliable method of pre-symptomatic detection of motor unit loss in SOD1 mutation carriers. Following 69 SOD1 family members and population controls over a 1-year period, with thenar and EDB MUNE tests repeated every 3 to 6 months, assessed the test-retest reproducibility of the technique. The mean difference between thenar MUNE results on separate occasions in asymptomatic subjects was +/- 3.6%, with a range of 0-11.7%, and +/- 4.6%, with a range of 0-15.7% in EDB MUNE. These results indicate that the reproducibility of this technique and the results achieved was high, so that individual results could be used as a baseline for serial MUNE studies. (Aggarwal, 2009).

During the course of the study, however, a significant fall in motor unit number was detected in 5 of the SOD1 mutation carriers, several months before the onset of weakness and the diagnosis of motor neurone disease (MND) being made. There was no detectable loss of motor units in the other 15 SOD1 mutation carriers or in the group of SOD1 mutation negative relatives. From the study, a threshold MUNE of less than 100 was considered to imply that symptoms were imminent.

In individual cases, there was a reduction of 68% 8 months prior, 51% 4 months prior, 46% 6 months prior, 35% 10 months prior and 28% 6 months prior to the onset of weakness. Further motor unit loss occurred as weakness progressed and the diagnosis of MND being made.

Case 1 was a 48-year-old lady from a family with a strong history of familial MND, with a point mutation in the SOD1 gene at val148gly. At the time of recruitment in October 1998, she was asymptomatic. Her MUNE results remained stable over the first 2½ years, after which her left EDB MUNE dropped by 51%, and she only had detectable weakness of her left foot 4 months later with wasting and weakness of the anterior compartment muscles of her left leg of MRC grade 2-3/5. Over the next 6 months, her right EDB MUNE dropped by 56%, but she only developed right foot weakness 3 months later in June2001.

Her 43-year-old sister also showed a reduction in MUNE prior to the onset of symptoms. About 3 years into the study, there was a reduction in her right thenar MUNE to 96 (20%) and her left thenar MUNE to 89 (19%), with no detectable weakness. Her right EDB MUNE also dropped by 17%, but she only had detectable weakness 10 months later of MRC grade 4+/5 in right dorsiflexors, at which time her right EDB MUNE had dropped by a total of 35%. In view of her strong family history, a presumed diagnosis of MND was made and she was commenced on Riluzole in February 2002. Over the last 2 years, her EDB MUNE have not shown any decline. Her weakness has not progressed significantly, as on her last review in February 2004, she still had MRC grade 4/5 power of her right dorsiflexors and no clinically apparent weakness in her left dorsiflexors or upper limbs. It is possible that since "treatment" was commenced prior to the loss of a significant number of motor neurones, this may have slowed down the progression of the disease in this individual case. (Aggarwal & Nicholson, 2002).

Her mother also had a detectable reduction right thenar MUNE of 23% and left thenar MUNE of 25%, with no clinically apparent weakness. Her right EDB MUNE also dropped by 28%, with no detectable weakness. She subsequently developed bulbar symptoms 6 months and died of respiratory failure.

Case 4 was a 48-year-old lady with a strong family history of MND and a point mutation in SOD1 gene at glu100gly. At the time of recruitment, she was asymptomatic and her MUNE results remained stable over the first 3 years of the study. It was then noted that her reduction of her left EDB MUNE of 46% reduction, but with no detectable weakness. She subsequently developed left lower leg weakness of MRC grade 3/5 about 6months later.

Finally, her 2nd cousin, once removed, is a 44-year-old man who also had a point mutation in SOD1 gene at glu100gly. His MUNE results also remained stable over the first 3 years of the study. The right EDB MUNE dropped from 115 down to being not recordable over a 12-month period. At that time, he had occasional fasciculations in the right quadriceps region and MRC grade 0/5 weakness of right dorsiflexion. He was unsure as to when the weakness had developed. Over time, his left EDB MUNE has reduced by 68%, but his left ankle power remained normal until 8 months later, when it reduced slightly to MRC grade 4/5.

This study also shows that there can be substantial loss in MUNE and still have an essentially normal EMG with minimal signs of acute denervation or motor unit potential remodelling, as one would expected that at a minimum, the muscles with transiently reduced MUNE numbers should have reduced recruitment during EMG studies.

Four of the five SOD 1 mutation carriers who had a pre-symptomatic loss of motor neurones had needle EMG studies performed by an independent neurologist, which showed neurogenic changes but not sufficient to fulfil the criteria to make the diagnosis of MND. All had a reduction in MUNE at the time of the EMG study of which the independent neurologist was not aware. This implies that MUNE may be a more reliable and sensitive method for diagnosing MND than needle EMG. MUNE can be used as a non-invasive method of predicting impending decline in motor neurones and estimating the rate of neuronal death in asymptomatic subjects. This indicates that loss of motor neurones is detectable in the pre-symptomatic phase and this loss was detectable before significant needle EMG changes of pathology occur. McComas showed that patients with substantial chronic denervation could maintain normal muscle twitch tension until loss of about 70-80% of motor units, before collateral reinnervation was unable to provide functional compensation, and this is the probable explanation of this finding.

As MUNE is a measure of the primary pathologic process of motor neurone loss and can identify that the number of motor units are reduced, even in the presence of a non-diagnostic needle EMG. Needle electromyography may reveal evidence of chronic reinnervation, but provides little direct evidence to the extent of motor neurone and axonal loss.

This lack of corroboration with needle EMG in the pre-symptomatic stage requires a paradigm shift in the traditional concept that needle EMG is the "gold" standard for the diagnosis of ALS. We are aware that traditional neurologists and neurophysiologists will find this difficult to accept, as it would be expected that at a minimum, the muscles with transiently reduced MUNE numbers should have reduced recruitment during EMG studies. It is hard to understand physiologically how there can be substantial loss in MUNE and still have normal EMG with no signs of acute denervation or motor unit potential remodelling. These cases clearly indicate that loss of motor neurones is detectable in the pre-symptomatic phase and this loss was detectable before significant needle EMG changes of pathology occur. Even though some may argue that a reduction in MUNE cannot be used to support or diagnosis FALS, once changes occur on conventional EMG studies, the window of opportunity to influence the progression of this condition has been missed.

Maximum isometric grip strength using the Jamar hydraulic dynamometer also does not correlate with the number of functional motor neurones in thenar group of muscles as measured using the statistical method of MUNE, indicating that MUNE is a more sensitive test than MVIC for monitoring disease progression in MND. It has also been shown that MUNE is able to identify deterioration in functional motor units before handgrip maximal voluntary isometric contraction (MVIC).

This confirms McComas' observation that patients with substantial chronic denervation could maintain normal muscle twitch tension until loss of about 70-80% of motor units occurs. This suggests that handgrip MVIC is not as sensitive as thenar MUNE for monitoring disease progression, as it is unable to detect early motor neurone loss due to the presence of compensatory mechanisms. The surviving motor neurones enlarge their territories, through collateral sprouting (reinnervation) until late in the disease, when collateral reinnervation is no longer able to provide full functional compensation. Thenar MUNE however does examine all of the motor units that are involved in handgrip MVIC, as forearm flexors and ulnar-innervated muscles are involved in the generation of handgrip MVIC. It also confirms Felice's study which showed that in patients with MND, changes in thenar MUNE was the most sensitive outcome measure for following disease progression, when compared to other quantitative tests, such as CMAP, isometric grip strength, forced vital capacity and Medical Research Council manual muscle testing.

As motor neurone loss once it occurs is rapid and precipitous, any potential treatment will need to be given early to SOD1 mutation carriers. Once the disease progresses, resulting in functional impairment and disability, restorative treatments to replace lost motor neurones becomes less feasible. To date there have been a number of drugs which have undergone clinical trials in MND, for which there is no evidence of benefit. These include creatinine, high dose vitamin E, Gabapentin and nerve growth factors such as brain derived neurotrophic factor and insulin-like growth factor-1. If effective treatment for MND were to be developed to arrest the process of degeneration, therapies aimed at preserving functional motor neurones would be more feasible. This requires the ability to be able to identify individuals at risk of developing the disease, which currently are SOD1 mutation carriers.

Currently, the only effective approved treatment for MND is Riluzole, which has a neuroprotective role, possibly due to pre-synaptic inhibition of glutamate release. Riluzole is an anti-glutamate agent that has been approved for the treatment of patients with amyotrophic lateral sclerosis in most countries. There have been a least three large randomised trials involving hundreds of patients that have been unable to show that Riluzole is a disease altering agent nor does it have any restorative reports.

In one of the cases in the study, Riluzole was commenced once she developed mild weakness. At the time, there was a slight reduction in MUNE, but conventional needle EMG examination did not fulfil the criteria to make the diagnosis of MND. In view of her strong family history and positive genetic testing, a presumed diagnosis of MND was made. Since commencing Riluzole there has been no significant reduction in her EDB MUNE over the last 2 years, and her weakness of right dorsiflexors has only progressed marginally from MRC grade 4+/5 to 4/5 power. It is possible that since "treatment" was commenced prior to the loss of a significant number of motor neurones, this may have slowed down the progression of the disease in this individual case. Early in the course of ALS, the rate of cell death is low as the amount of neuronal damage caused by the mutation is small. As the amount of intracellular damage increases, a critical threshold is reached, which overwhelms cellular homeostasis, resulting in rapid apoptosis and cell death. The increase in MUNE numbers may be either due to reinnervation of the damaged muscle or repair of poorly functioning synapses, at the early stage of the disease, without resulting in a change in CMAP.

We would argue that previous trials have all be performed in the symptomatic phase of the disease when 70-80% of motor units have already been lost, rather than in the pre-symptomatic phase of the disease, when the therapeutic benefit might change, as "treatment" is commenced prior to significant motor neurone loss occurring and therefore, the progression of disease can be slowed down. MUNE numbers are believed to reduce because of remodelling of the motor unit and in our study, the compound muscle action potential amplitudes (CMAP) were retained as early in the course of the disease, the rate of cell death is low. The increase in MUNE numbers may be either due to reinnervation of the damaged muscle or repair of poorly functioning synapses, at the early stage of the disease, without resulting in a change in CMAP.

This longitudinal study showed that it was possible to detect loss of motor neurones in the pre-symptomatic stage of MND in humans. This study provided further evidence that considerable motor neurone loss occurred just before the onset of symptoms or weakness. (Aggarwal, 2009).

This study indicates that SOD1 mutation carriers have normal survival of motor neurones, with as carriers had a full complement of motor neurones during the asymptomatic phase. Significant pre-symptomatic loss of motor neurones did not occur in asymptomatic SOD1 mutation carriers. Sudden and widespread motor neurone death occurs at the time development of the symptomatic symptoms, rather than life-long motor neurone loss. Sudden, catastrophic and multifocal loss of motor neurons occurs immediately prior to the onset of symptoms and the development of MND. This suggests that there may be a biological trigger initiating rapid cell loss, just prior to the onset of symptoms, rather than life-long motor neurone loss. Also, if the trigger initiating motor neurone loss can be identified, it may be possible to prevent motor neurone loss in familial ALS and develop treatments for sporadic MND. The mutant SOD1 protein itself cannot be the trigger, as it is constantly expressed. There may however be a gradual accumulation of a toxic product, possibly SOD1, which has changed into a new toxic conformation or aggregate, resulting in neuronal damage. The possibility of an individual neuron undergoing apoptosis increases as damage accumulates . This cumulative damage may be due to oxidative stress, resulting in disruption of the cellular structure and function.

Neurofilament heavy polypeptide (NF-H) is an abundant stable cytoplasmic protein located in neuronal cells in large axons and may be used as a cell type marker. Abnormal accumulation of NF-H in motor neurones is associated with ALS, but it is unclear to what extent these contribute to human disease. Analysis of blood serum markers looking for increased levels of NF-H was not performed in this study, but would be interesting to be done in the future to the compare levels of NF-H in the carriers.

The results of this study indicate that the risk of cell death probably remains constant throughout life of the neurone and that cell death occurs randomly in time and is independent of that of any other neurone. This suggests a "one-hit" biochemical phenomenon in which the mutation imposes an abnormal mutant steady state on the neurone and a single catastrophic event randomly initiates cell death and apoptosis. Early in the course of MND, the rate of cell death is low as the amount of neuronal damage caused by the mutation is small. The delay in clinical onset was thought to reflect the gradual accumulation of damage within the neurones, as a result of the mutation, which ultimately overwhelms cellular homeostasis leading to cell death. The living mutant neurons function very well for years or decades but the probability that an individual neurone undergoes apoptosis increases as damage accumulates within it. A mutant neurone in an older patient will have accumulated a greater amount of damage and will therefore be more likely to die than in a younger patient. Consequently, early in the course of disease, the chance of a cell containing a sufficient amount of damage to initiate apoptosis is small, and the rate of cell loss is correspondingly low. The mutant neurones appear to function normally for decades, with weakness only occurring once apoptosis and cell death occurs due to a gradual accumulation of damage within the cell. Therapies aimed at preserving motor neurones may be more feasible than trying to replace lost motor neurones. A number of treatment or preventative strategies arise, such as measures to diminish SOD1 aggregation or interactions to specifically reduced apoptosis in motor neurones. As motor neurone loss at this stage is rapid and precipitous, any potential treatment will need to be given much earlier in SOD1 mutation carriers.

Determining the mechanism by which mutations in the Cu/Zn superoxide dismutase (SOD1) gene triggers the destruction of motor neurones causing MND remains unknown. At present, the favoured hypothesis is that the mutation causes disease as a result of a toxic gain of function by the mutant SOD1 provoking selective neurotoxicity, probably disrupting the intracellular homeostasis of copper and/or protein aggregation. However, as the amount of intracellular damage increases, the chance that a cell will die also increases. This cumulative damage may be due to oxidative stress, in which an imbalance between the production of reactive oxygen species and cellular antioxidant mechanisms results in chemical modifications of macromolecules, thereby disrupting cellular structure and function. It is possible that the high metabolic activity in motor neurones, combined with the toxic oxidative properties of the mutant SOD1, causes massive mitochondrial vacuolation in motor neurones, resulting in degeneration, earlier than other neurones, triggering the onset of weakness. Prominent cytoplasmic intracellular inclusions in motor neurones and within astrocytes surrounding them developed by the onset of clinical disease and in some cases represented the first pathological sign of disease. These aggregates increased in number as the disease progressed. This indicates that the mutant SOD1 toxicity is mediated by damage to mitochondria in motor neurones and this damage triggers the functional decline of motor neurones and the clinical onset of symptoms. The absence of motor neurone death in the early stages of the disease indicates that the majority of motor neurones could be rescued after early clinical diagnosis.

Regular follow-up of SOD1 carriers with MUNE may lead to early diagnosis, creating an opportunity for future novel approaches and therapies aimed at preserving motor neurones rather than replacing lost motor neurones. If the trigger initiating motor neurone loss can be identified, it may be possible to prevent motor neurone loss in familial ALS. At this stage, detecting the onset of motor neurone loss in asymptomatic individuals will identify those who may benefit from early institution of an active management program to improve their quality of life, until more effective treatment modalities become available for this devastating condition This observation is an important contribution to the current understanding of the pathogenesis of MND, as it shows that motor neurone disease does not seem to be the end result of slow attrition of motor neurones. MUNE may be able to be used as a method of pre-symptomatic testing of individuals who on genetic testing are SOD1 mutation carriers. Regular follow-up of SOD1 carriers with MUNE may lead to early diagnosis, creating an opportunity for future novel approaches and therapies aimed at preserving motor neurones rather than replacing lost motor neurones.

9. Acknowledgments

Prof. Garth Nicholson who introduced me to research into motor neurone disease and his continuing support. Prof. David Burke and Assoc. Prof. Alastair Corbett for their professional guidance and Prof. Jasper Daube for his technical assistance regarding the technique used in this research. The research was supported by the Motor Neurone Disease Association of NSW (Northern Region), ANZAC Health and Medical Research Foundation, Motor Neurone Disease Research Institute of Australia Inc. and the Nerve Research Foundation.

10. References

Aggarwal, A. (2009). Motor unit number estimation in asymptomatic familial amyotrophic lateral sclerosis. *Supplements to Clinical Neurophysiology.* 60:163-169.

Aggarwal, A. (2009). Detection of pre-clinical motor unit loss in familial amyotrophic lateral sclerosis. *Supplements to Clinical Neurophysiology.* 60:171-179.

Aggarwal, A. & Nicholson, GA. (2001). Normal complement of motor units in asymptomatic familial (SOD1 mutation) amyotrophic lateral sclerosis. J. *Neurology, Neurosurgery and Psychiatry.* 17 (4), 472-48.

Aggarwal, A. & G, Nicholson. (2002). Detection Of pre-clinical motor neurone loss in SOD1 mutation carriers using motor unit number estimation. *J of Neurology, Neurosurgery & Psychiatry.* 73(2):199-201.

Al-Chalabi, A., Andersen, P.M., Nilsson, P., Chioza, B., Andersson, J.L., Russ, C., Shaw, C.E., Powell, J., Leigh, P.N. (1999). Deletions of the heavy neurofilament subunit tail in amyotrophic lateral sclerosis. *Hum Mol Genet.*8: 157-164.

Andersen, P.M., Nilsson, P., Keranen, M.L., Forsgren, L., Hagglund, J., Karlsborg, M., Ronnevi, L.O., Gredal, O., Marklund, S.L. (1997). Phenotypic heterogenicity in motor neurone disease patients with CuZn superoxide dismutase mutations in Scandinavia. *Brain.* 120:1723-1737.

Azzouz, M., Leclerc, N., Gurney, M., Warter, J,M., Poindron, P. & Borg, J. (1997). Progressive motor neuron impairment in an animal model of familial amyotrophic lateral sclerosis. *Muscle Nerve.*20: 45-51.

Beal, M.F. (1996). Mitochondria, free radicals and neurodegeneration. *Curr Opin Neurobiol.* 6: 661-666.

Beckman, J.S., Carson, M., Smith, C.D. & Koppenol, W.H. (1993). ALS, SOD and peroxinitrate. *Nature.*364: 584.

Bensimon, G., Lacomblez, L. & Meiniger, V. (1994). A controlled trial of Riluzole in amyotrophic lateral sclerosis. ALS/Riluzole study group. *N Engl J Med.* 330 (9): 585-591.

Brown, W.F. (1972). A method for estimating the number of motor units in thenar muscles and the changes in motor unit counting with aging. *J Neurol Neurosurg Psychiatry.*35: 845-852.

Bruijn, L.I., Becher, M.W., Lee, M.K., Anderson, K.L., Jenkins, N.A., Copeland, N.G., Sisodia, S.S., Rothstein, J.D., Borchelt, D.R., Price, D.L.& Cleveland, D.W. (1997). ALS-linked SOD1 mutant G85R mediates damage to astrocytes and promotes rapidly progressive disease with SOD1-containing inclusions. *Neuron.* 18: 327-338.

Campbell, M.J., McComas, A.J. & Petito, F. (1973). Physiological changes in ageing muscles. *J Neurol Neurosurg Psychiatry.* 36: 174-182.

Chance, P.F., Rabin, B.A., Ryan, S.G., Ding, Y., Scavina, M., Crain, B., Griffith, J.W., Cornblath, D.R. (1998). Linkage of the gene for an autosomal dominant form of juvenile amyotrophic lateral sclerosis to chromosome 9q34. *Am J Hum Genet.* 62: 633-640.

Cheah, B.C., Vucic, S., Krishnan, A.V., Kiernan, M.C. (2010). Riluzole, neuroprotection and amyotrophic lateral sclerosis. *Curr Med Chem* 17(18): 1942-49.

Clarke, G., Collins, R.A., Leavitt, B.R., Andrews, D.F., Hayden, M.R., Lumsden, C.J. & McInnes, R,R. (2000). A one hit model of cell death in inherited neuronal degenerations. *Nature.* 406: 195-199.

Clarke, G., Lumsden, C.J. & McInnes, R.R. (2001). Inherited neurodegenerative disease: the one hit model of neurodegeneration. *Human Molecular Genetics.* 10: 2269-2275.

Cleveland, D.W. (1999). From Charcot to SOD1: Mechanisms of selective motor neuron death in ALS. *Neuron.* 24: 515-520.

Cudkowicz, M.E., McKenna-Yasek, D., Sapp, P.E., Chin, W., Geller, B., Hayden, D.L., Schoenfeld, D.A., Hosler, B.A., Horvitz, H.R., Brown, R.H. Jr. (1997). Epidemiology of mutations in superoxide dismutase in amyotrophic lateral sclerosis. *Ann Neurol.* 41: 210-221.

Daube, J.R. (1995). Estimating the number of motor units in a muscle. *J Clin Neurophysiol.* 12(6): 585-594.

de Belleroche, J., Orrell, R., King, A. J. (1995). Medical Genetics. Familial amyotrophic lateral sclerosis/motor neurone disease (FALS): a review of current developments. *J Med Genet.* 32: 841-847.

Doble, A. (1996). The pharmacology and mechanism of action of riluzole. *Neurology.* 47: S233-241.

Eisen, A. (1995). Amyotrophic lateral sclerosis is a multifactorial disease. *Muscle Nerve.* 18:741-752.

Felice, K.J. (1997). A longitudinal study comparing thenar motor unit number estimation to other quantitative tests in patients with amyotrophic lateral sclerosis. *Muscle Nerve.* 20: 179-185.

Figlewicz, D.A., Krizus, A., Martinoli, M.G., Meininger, V., Dib, M., Rouleau, G.A., Julein, J.P. (1994). Variants of the heavy neurofilament subunit are associated with the development of amyotrophic lateral sclerosis. *Hum Mol Genet* 3: 1757-1761.

Gurney, M.E., Pu, H., Chiu, A.Y., Dal Canto, M.C., Polchow, C.Y., Alexander, D.D., Caliendo, J., Hentati, A., Kwon, Y.W., Deng, H.X., Chen, W., Zhai, P., Sufit, R.L. & Siddique, T. (1994). Motor neuro degeneration in mice that express a human Cu/Zn superoxide dismutase mutation. *Science.* 264: 1772-1775.

Gurney, M.E., Tomasselli, A.G., Heinrikson, R.L. (1994). Stay the Executioner's hand. *Science* 2000; 288: 283-284.

Hamilton, A., Balnave, R. & Adam, R. Grip strength reliability. *J Hand Therapy.* 7(3): 163-170.

Hand, C.K. & Rouleau, G.A. (2002). Familial Amyotrophic Lateral Sclerosis. *Muscle Nerve.* 25: 135-159.

Hanten, W.P., Chen, W.Y., Austin, A.A., Brooks, R.E., Carter, H.C., Law, C.A., Morgan, M.K., Sanders, D.J., Swan, C.A. & Vanderslice, A.L. (1993). Maximum grip strength in normal subjects from 20 to 64 years of age. *J. Hand Therapy.* 12(3): 193-200.

Haverkamp, L.J., Appel, V., Appel, S.H. (1995). Natural history of amyotrophic lateral sclerosis in a database population. Validation of a scoring system and a model for survival prediction. *Brain.* 118: 707-719.

Hentati, A., Pericak-Vance, M.A., Nijhawan, D., Ahmed, A., Yang, Y., Rimmler, J., Hung, W-Y., Schlotter, B., Ahmed, A., Ben Hamida, M., Hentati, F., Siddique, T. (1998). Linkage of a commoner form of recessive amyotrophic lateral sclerosis to chromosome 15q15-q22 markers. *Neurogenetics.* 2: 55-60.

Hoagland, R.J., Mendoza, M., Armon, C., Barohn, R.J., Byran, W.W., Goodpasture, J.C., Miller, R.G., Parry, G.J., Petjan, J.H., Ross, M.A. & the Syntex / Synergen Neuroscience Joint Venture rhCNTF ALS Study Group. (1997). Reliability of maximal isometric contraction testing in multicenter study of patients with amyotrophic lateral sclerosis. *Muscle Nerve.* 20: 691-695.

Kong, J. & Xu,Z. (1998). Massive mitochondria degeneration in motor neurons triggers the onset of amyotrophic lateral sclerosis in mice expressing a mutant SOD1. *J Neurosci.* 18: 3241-3250.

Kosti, V., Jackson-Lewis, V. & Bilbao, F.D. (1997). Bcl-2: prolonging life in a transgenic mouse model of familial amyotrophic lateral sclerosis. *Science.* 227: 577.

Leigh, P.N. Amyotrophic lateral sclerosis and other motor neurone diseases. (1997). *Current Opinion Neuro Neurosurg.* 3: 567.

Li, M., Ona, V.O., Gueng, C., Chen, M., Jackson-Lewis, V., Andrews, L.J., Olszewski, A.J., Steig, P.E., Przedborski, S. & Friendlander, R.M. (2000). Functional role of caspase-1 and caspase-3 in an ALS transgenic mouse model. *Science.* 288: 335-339.

Lomen-Hoerth, C. & Slawnych, M.P. (2003). Statistical motor unit number estimation: From theory to practice. *Muscle Nerve.* 28: 263-272.

McComas, A.J., Fawcett, P.R.W., Campbell, M.J. & Sica, R.E.P. (1971). Electrophysiological estimation of the number of motor units within a human muscle. *J. Neurology, Neurosurgery and Psychiatry.* 34: 121-131.

McComas, A.J. (1971). Functional compensation in partially denervated muscles. *J Neurol Neurosurg Psychiatry* 34:453-460.

McComas, A.J. (1991). Motor unit estimation: Methods, results and present status. *Muscle Nerve.* 14: 585-597.

McComas, AJ. (1995). Motor unit estimation: The beginning. *J Clin Neurophysiol.* 12(6): 560-564.

McNeil, D. (1996). Statistical Methods.1st Edition. New York. *Wiley & Sons;* 184.

Mena, I., Marin, O., Fuenzalida, S., Cotzias, G.C. (1967). Chronic manganese poisoning. Clinical picture and manganese turnover. *Neurology.* 17: 128-136.

Miller, R.G., Mitchell, J.D., Lyon, M., Moore, D.H. (2007). Riluzole for amyotrophic lateral sclerosis (ALS / motor neuron disease (MND). *Cochrane Database Syst Rev.* 1: CD001447.

Mu, X., He, J, Anderson, M. (1996). Altered expression of bcl-2 and bax mRNA in amyotrophic lateral sclerosis spinal cord motor neurones. *Ann Neurol.* 40: 379.

Mulder, D.W., Howard, F.M. Jr. (1976). Patient resistance and prognosis in amyotrophic lateral sclerosis. *Mayo Clin Proc.*51: 537-541.

Mulder, D.W., Kurland, L.T, Offord, K.P., Beard, C.M. (1986). Familial adult motor neurone disease: amyotrophic lateral sclerosis. *Neurology.* 38: 511-517.

Needleman, H.L. (1997). Exposure to lead: Sources and effects. *N Engl J Med.* 297: 943-945.

Noor, R., Mittal, S., & Iqbal E. (2003). Superoxide dismutase - applications and relevance to human diseases. *Med Sci Monit.* 8(9): 210-215.

Olney, R.K., Yuen, E.C. & Engstrom, J.W. (2000). Statistical motor unit number estimation: Reproducibility and sources of error in patients with amyotrophic lateral sclerosis. *Muscle Nerve.* 23: 193-197.

Radunovic, A., Leigh, P.N. (1996). Cu/Zn superoxide dismutase gene mutations in amyotrophic lateral sclerosis: correlation between genotype and clinical features. *J. Neurology, Neurosurgery and Psychiatry.* 61: 565-572.

Ringel, S.P., Murphy, J.R., Alderson, M.K., Byran, W., England, J.D., Miller, R.G., Petajan, J.H., Smith, S.A., Roelofs, R.I., Ziter, F., Lee, M.Y., Brinkmann, J.R., Almada, A., Gappmaier, E., Graves, J., Herbelin, L., Mendoza, M., Mylar, D., Smith, P. & Yu, P.(1993). The natural history of amyotrophic lateral sclerosis. *Neurology.* 43: 1316-1322.

Robberecht,W. (2000). Oxidative stress in amyotrophic lateral sclerosis. *J. Neuro.* 247 (Suppl. 1): 111-116.

Rosen, D.R., Siddique, T., Patterson, D., Figlewicz, D.A., Sapp, P., Hentati, D., Donaldson, D., Goto, J., O'Regan, J.P., Deng, H.X., Rahmani, Z., Krizus, A., McKenna-Yasek, D., Cayabyab, A., Gaston, S., Berger, M., Tanzi, R.E., Halperin, .J.J, Herzfeldt, B., Van den Bergh, R., Hung, W.Y., Bird, T., Deng, G., Mulder, D.W., Smyth, C., Laing, N.G., Soriano, E., Pericak-Vance, M.A., Haines, J., Rouleau, G.A., Gusella, J.S., Horvitz, H.R. & Brown R.H., Jr. (1993). Mutations in Cu, Zn superoxide dismutase gene are associated with familial amyotrophic lateral sclerosis. *Nature.*362: 59-62.

Shaw, C.E., Enayat, Z.E., Powell, J.F., Anderson, V.E., Radunovic, A., Powell, J.F., Leigh, P.N. (1998). Mutations in all five exons of SOD1 may cause ALS. *Ann Neurol.* 43: 390-394.

Shefner, J.M. (2001). Motor unit number estimation in human neurological diseases and animal models. *Clin Neurophysiolo.* 112: 955-964.

Shefner, JM. (2009). Statistical motor unit number estimation and ALS trials: the effect of motor unit instability. *Suppl Clin Neurophysiol* .60: 135-41

Shefner, J.M., Cudkowicz, M.E., Zhang, H., Schoenfiekd, D. & Jillapalli, D. (2004). Northeast ALS Consortium. The use of statistical MUNE in multicentre clinical trials. *Muscle Nerve.* 30: 463-9.

Sica, R.E.P., McComas, A.J., Upton, A.R.M. & Longmire, D. (1974). Motor unit estimations in small muscles of the hand. *J Neurol Neurosurg Psychiatry.*37: 55-67.

Siddique, T. & Deng, H.X. (1996). Genetics of amyotrophic lateral sclerosis. *Human Mol Gen.* 5: 1465-1470.

Siddique, T., Figlewicz, D.A., Pericak-Vance, M.A., Haines, J.L., Rouleau, G.A., Jeffers, A.J., Sapp, P., Hung, W.Y., Bebout, J., McKenna-Yasek, D., Deng, G., Horvitz, H.R., Gusella, J.S., Brown, R.H., Jr., Roses, A.D. and Collaborators.(1991). Linage of a gene causing familial amyotrophic lateral sclerosis to chromosome 21 and evidence of genetic locus heterogenicity. *N Engl J Med.* 324: 1381-1384.

Siddique, T., Pericak-Vance, M.A. & Brooks, B.R. (1989). Linkage analysis in familial amyotrophic lateral sclerosis. *Neurology*. 39: 919-925.

Sjalander, A., Beckman ,G., Deng, H.Z. (1995). The D90A mutation results in a polymorphism of Cu/Zn superoxide dismutase that is prevalent in northern Sweden and Finland. Hum Mol Genet 1995; 4: 1105-1108.

Stein, R.B. & Yang, J.F. (1990). Methods of estimating the number of motor units in human muscles. *Ann Neurol*. 28: 487-495.

Talbot, K. (2002). Motor neurone disease. *Muscle Nerve*. 25: 513-519.

Trotti, D., Rolfs, A., Danbolt, N.C., Brown, R.H. Jr, Hediger, M.A. (1999). SOD1 mutations linked to amyotrophic lateral sclerosis selectively activates a glial glutamate transporter. *Na Neurosci*. 19: 427-433.

Vechio, J.D., Bruijn, L.I., Xu, Z., Brown, R.H. Jr, (1996). Cleveland ,D.W. Sequence variants in the human neurofilament proteins: absence of linkage to familial amyotrophic lateral sclerosis. Ann Neurol 1996; 40: 603-610.

Yim, M.B., Chock, P.B. & Stadtman, E.R. (1990). Copper, zinc superoxide dismutase catalyses hydroxyl radial production from hydrogen peroxide. *Proc Natl Acad Sci*. 87:5006-5010.

29

Communication Impairment in ALS Patients Assessment and Treatment

Paolo Bongioanni
Neurological Rehabilitation Unit - Neuroscience Department, University of Pisa/NeuroCare onlus Italy

1. Introduction

Amyotrophic lateral sclerosis (**ALS**), also called *Lou Gehrig's disease*, is a rapidly progressive neuromuscular disease that attacks the neurons responsible for controlling voluntary muscles. It belongs to a group of disorders known as *Motor neuron diseases* (*MND*): all these syndromes share a common molecular and cellular pathology comprising degeneration of motor neurons (MNs) in cortex, brainstem and/or spinal cord, and the presence of characteristic ubiquitin and TDP-43-immunoreactive intraneuronal inclusions.

ALS prevalence in Western countries ranges from 2.7 to 7.4 per 100,000 (Worms, 2001). In 90 to 95 percent of all patients with ALS (PALS), the disease occurs sporadically (*sporadic ALS, sALS*); in 5 to 10 percent there is a family history of ALS (*familial ALS, fALS*). Most people developing ALS are between the ages of 40 and 70 years (Haverkamp et al., 1995). The disease is 20% more common in men than in women, although more recent data suggest that the gender ratio may be approaching equality (Logroscino et al., 2008).

The cause of ALS is not known, and it is not clear why ALS strikes some people and not others, but both genetic (Ticozzi et al., 2011) and environmental factors (Callaghan et al., 2011; Calvo et al., 2010; Ferrante et al., 1997) may play a role.

In PALS, both the brain upper MNs (UMNs) and the brainstem or spinal cord lower MNs (LMNs) degenerate or die: unable to function, the muscles gradually weaken, waste away, and twitch, leading to a wide range of disabilities. Patients lose their strength and the ability to move their body, but usually maintain control of eye muscles.

Approximately 70% of PALS have a *spinal form* of the disease: they present with symptoms which may start either distally or proximally in the upper or lower limbs. Some patients see the effects of the disease on a hand or arm, as they experience difficulty with simple tasks requiring manual dexterity, such as buttoning a shirt, writing, or turning a key in a lock; in other cases, symptoms initially affect one of the legs, and patients experience awkwardness when walking or running, or they notice that they are tripping or stumbling more often.

Patients with *bulbar-onset* ALS usually present with dysarthria leading to slow slurred speech or a nasal quality; they may also develop dysphagia for solid or liquids after noticing speech problems; almost all patients with bulbar symptoms complain of sialorrhoea with excessive drooling due to difficulty of swallowing saliva and UMN-type facial weakness, which affects the lower part of the face, causing difficulty with lip seal and blowing cheeks.

The gag reflex is preserved and often brisk, whereas the soft palate may be weak; patients show wasting and fasciculations of the tongue which moves slowly, also due to muscle hypertonia. The other cranial nerves remain intact, although in late stages of the disease patients may very rarely develop a supranuclear gaze palsy or oculomotor palsy (Kobayashi et al., 1999; Okuda et al., 1992).

2. Communication issues in ALS patients

Five functional domains have to be taken into account when communication is concerned: a) motivation to interact; b) cognitive skills (particularly - but not exclusively - those related to language); c) visual and auditory capacities; d) ability to utter sounds and words; and e) writing skills. As a matter of fact, affective disorders, anxiety and emotional discomfort, as well as cognitive impairment or sensory deficits, can compromise communication processes, by interfering directly and/or indirectly with speech and writing performances.

However, ALS does not usually either affect a person's ability to see, smell, taste, hear, or recognize touch; nor impair mind or intelligence - although a small percentage of patients may experience problems with memory or decision-making (Raaphorst et al., 2010; Ringholz et al., 2005), and there is growing evidence that some may even develop a form of dementia (Guedj et al., 2007). On the other hand, since the disease usually does not affect cognitive abilities, PALS are aware of their progressive loss of function and may become anxious and depressed (Patten et al., 2007).

The vast majority of PALS experience a motor speech disorder as the disease progresses: since ALS involves both UMNs and LMNs, it results in *mixed dysarthria* of the *flaccid-spastic* type characterized by effortful, slow productions with short phrases, inappropriate pauses, imprecise consonants, hypernasality, strain-strangled voice, as well as decreased pitch and loudness range (Duffy, 1995; Tomik & Guiloff, 2010).

In the early stages when dysarthria is mild, either spasticity or flaccidity is predominant: initial symptoms typically do not interfere with speech intelligibility and may be limited to a reduction in speaking rate, a change in phonatory quality, or imprecise articulation (Ball et al., 2004_a; Nishio & Niimi, 2000; Yorkston et al., 1993; Yunusova et al., 2010).

Features of *spasmodic dysphonia* (or *focal laryngeal dystonia*) may also occur in PALS, sometimes as the initial clinical symptom (Roth et al., 1996). Typically, laryngeal structure is normal in appearance. When *corticobulbar* involvement prevails (*spastic* forms), there is often a pattern of hyperadduction of the vocal mechanism, and when *bulbar* involvement dominates (*flaccid* forms), there is usually a pattern of hypoadduction.

As disease progresses and dysarthria becomes severe, profound weakness resulting in reduced movement of the speech musculature and severe hypophonia become increasingly common (Yunusova et al., 2010).

Perceptual and acoustic features of dysarthria in ALS have been well studied (Tomik & Guiloff, 2010): the decrease in rate is often associated with increased pause time and enhanced segment durations, particularly for vowel sounds (Green et al., 2004; Tjaden & Turner, 2000; Turner & Weismer, 1993); spectral vowel and consonant properties (e.g., formant frequencies, transition extents and slopes) are also affected, with vowels becoming more centralized and the consonant frequency spectrum less distinct (Kent et al., 1989, 1992; Tjaden & Turner, 1997; Turner et al., 1995; Weismer et al., 1988, 1992, 2001).

Such acoustic findings have been presumed to be due to the disease-related reduction and slowing of articulatory movements (Weismer et al., 1992). Articulatory findings, although limited, support such an interpretation. An early study on articulatory kinematics in two PALS showed slowed articulatory movements, reduced displacement of the tongue and lip, together with exaggerated displacements of the jaw during diadokokinetic tasks (Hirose et al., 1982). A more recent study of articulatory movements in a group of 9 PALS reported an impairment of articulatory speed during vowels (Yunusova et al., 2008): aberrant displacements were found to be word- and vowel-dependent and were more consistently present in movements of the tongue than in those of other articulators, and occasionally in the jaw; the jaw displacements were smaller than normal in words requiring larger articulator movements (e.g., consonant plus low vowel), but were larger than normal in words that only required relatively small jaw movements (e.g., consonant plus high vowel), suggesting difficulty in scaling of the vowel-related movements.

Whereas initially, along a gradual slowing of *speaking rate, speech intelligibility* remains relatively high, it decreases overtime, when dysarthria becomes more and more apparent to PALS themselves and their listeners. Yorkston and co-workers (1993) suggested that speech intelligibility may vary across dysarthric patients depending on the subsystems that are preserved (e.g., relatively less impaired respiratory-phonatory subsystem and the jaw might be associated with better speech intelligibility); the rate of disease progression; and the patient's cognitive status.

Because a person's ability to communicate orally is typically assessed based on speech intelligibility, anticipating the decline in intelligibility in a sensitive way is critical for timely clinical management of bulbar PALS. In this regard, longitudinal studies are, indeed, necessary when the goal of research is to identify early predictors of future changes; additionally, longitudinal studies are advantageous when dealing with heterogeneous populations, as in the case of PALS, since each patient can serve as his own control. Investigations of such a type documented the decline in speech intelligibility and speaking rate (Kent et al., 1992; Mulligan et al, 1994; Nishio & Niimi, 2000; Yorkston et al., 1993); and some studies have also identified several acoustic-based speech markers of disease progression (Mulligan et al., 1994; Ramig et al., 1990).

In their retrospective study of more than a hundred clinical cases, Yorkston and co-workers (1993) reported that speaking rate was a reliable predictor of speech intelligibility decline, by observing a rapid deterioration in speech intelligibility shortly after a decline in speaking rate to 100-120 words per minute. Such a finding was replicated by Ball and co-workers (2002) in a large group of patients with bulbar symptoms of different severity: the authors suggested that speaking rate decline to 100-120 words per minute should serve as a clinical indicator for beginning to support communication by assistive technology.

Moreover, since ALS progresses so rapidly in many subjects, an important goal of clinical management is to anticipate functional changes in patients' performance in order to teach new communication strategies and compensatory skills before the patient's ability to learn these skills is impacted by the severity of their condition. Recently, Yunusova and co-workers (2010) in a longitudinal study on 3 PALS tested the feasibility of using kinematic measures as early predictors of intelligibility decline, trying to understand the relationship between physiologic changes in speech movements and clinical measures of speech performance (such as speaking rate and speech intelligibility). Lip and jaw movements were quantified with respect to their size, speed, and duration.

Results showed that, differently from oral strength measures, changes in lip and jaw movements were related to ALS progression: in two out of 3 PALS, the changes in measures of path distance and speed anticipated the drop in speech intelligibility by approximately 3 months, whereas speaking rate decline was more gradual; and increases in movement duration overtime closely mimicked the pattern of speech intelligibility decline. Overall, the kinematic measures seemed to be sensitive to disease progression: they might therefore be useful clinical markers for initiation of compensatory interventions.

Parallelly to decline in speech intelligibility, *communication effectiveness* is reduced at first in adverse speaking situations, such as noisy crowds, and then in all situations. Ball and co-workers (2004_b) reported that perceptions of communication effectiveness for PALS were quite similar to those of their frequent listeners (spouse or family member) across 10 different social situations: a range of communication effectiveness was reported depending upon the adversity of specific social situations.

Significant dysarthria can lead to frustration on the part of the patient when others are unwilling to spend the time to carefully listen. Friends and healthcare workers may not listen to the patient; there is a temptation to anticipate answers and finish sentences for the patient.

Fatally, at some point in their disease progression, 80 to 95% of PALS are unable to meet their daily communication needs using their natural speech, and finally most become unable to speak at all.

Moreover, upper limb paralysis prevents them from using hands in writing (directly or through computer-linked keyboards or communication devices).

Ultimately, in the so-called "locked-in" cases, a diffuse somatic immobility takes them away any possibility to interact with the world, except by using eye movements - even more unfortunately lost in those PALS classified as having a "super locked-in" syndrome, who may rely only upon their brain electrical waves as a communication tool processed through complex *brain-computer interface* (*BCI*) devices.

3. Functional assessment

Many assessments have been proposed for patient's follow-up in order to analyze the state of motor function and their consequences on activities of everyday life (Couratier et al., 2006). Clinimetric scales must be validated and relatively simple to use, and generate ordinate results allowing statistical analysis: global scales - *Norris Scale* (Norris et al., 1974), *Appel ALS Rating Scale* (Appel et al., 1987), *ALS Severity Scale* (Hillel et al., 1989), and *ALS Functional Rating Scale* (*ALSFRS*) (Cedarbaum & Stambler, 1997) - can be employed to evaluate disability progression.

By using, for instance, ALSFRS - or its revised version, $ALSFRS_R$ (Cedarbaum et al., 1999) - , communication impairment can be assessed through scores on speech function together with those related to handwriting, since people communicate by speaking and/or writing: scores < 2 in both speech and handwriting items correspond to a substantial inability to communicate.

Dysarthric speech can be evaluated through the *Frenchay Dysarthria Assessment* (Enderby & Palmer, 2008) originally developed by Pamela Enderby in 1983, which represents a well-established clinical tool to quantitatively evaluate the organs involved in speech and provides a measurement of intelligibility.

Complete kit includes examiner's manual, 25 rating forms, and intelligibility cards: patient is rated on a number of simple performance tasks related to speech function.

Intelligibility can be measured also through another test developed by Yorkston and co-workers: the *Assessment of Intelligibility of Dysarthric Speech* (Yorkston et al., 1984), a tool for quantifying single-word intelligibility, sentence intelligibility, and speaking rate of adult and adolescent speakers with dysarthria. Standard protocols containing speaker tasks, recording techniques, and listener response formats are employed to obtain a variety of intelligibility and communication efficiency measures.

Yorkston and co-workers (1993) initially suggested that PALS speaking rate reduction precedes decreases in intelligibility; Ball and co-workers (2001, 2002) reported that speaking rate on the *Speech Intelligibility Test - Sentence Subtest* (Yorkston et al., 2007) is a relatively good predictor of PALS intelligibility deterioration. This computerized test supports the efficient measurement of speaking rate in clinical settings; it helps patients and their families monitor changes over time, and reinforces their understanding of speaking rate and intelligibility. Using this test, speaking rate can also be accurately monitored over the telephone if a patient lives at a distance, or is unable to travel (Ball et al., 2005_a): it should be noted, anyway, that speech intelligibility could not be objectively assessed over the telephone, as a clinical measure of understandability.

The *vocal impairment* can be difficult to assess because the voice disorder in dysarthria often occurs along with other impairments affecting articulation, resonance, and respiration: an effective assessment tool is the *Multi-Dimensional Voice Program*, a multi-parameter acoustic analysis (Kent et al., 2003).

4. Treatment

Differently from an acute, self-limited disease with expected recovery, the choice of appropriate therapeutic options for PALS raises more difficult concerns, since one must take into account many personal and ethical considerations. Several decisions by PALS and their families regarding treatment hinge on their concept of the quality of life that will result from such treatments.

At the present time, ALS therapy can be organized under the following multiple modalities: a **pathogenetic treatment** – to counteract MN degeneration; and a **symptomatic treatment** – to reduce impairments in motor abilities including those involved in communication. The appropriate implementation of each one of these types of therapy reflects the difficulties that we now have to face in ALS treatment. Supportive care is best provided by multidisciplinary teams of health care professionals, such as physicians; physical, occupational, and speech therapists; nutritionists; social workers; and home care and hospice nurses (Bede et al., 2011): working with patients and caregivers, these teams can design an individualized plan of medical and physical therapy and provide special equipment aimed at keeping patients as "functional" as possible.

Taking now into account such *a symptomatic approach*, two kinds of therapeutic strategies have to be implemented, those using drugs and those employing assistive/rehabilitative methods and techniques, aids and devices.

4.1 Pharmacological strategies

Physicians can prescribe medications to ameliorate fatigue, ease muscle cramps, control spasticity, and reduce excess saliva and phlegm; drugs also are available to help patients with pain, depression, anxiety, and sleep disturbances (Bede et al., 2011; Gordon, 2011; Guidubaldi et al., 2011; Guy et al., 2011; Miller et al., 1999; $2009_{a,b}$).

It is almost obvious that a patient experiencing less fatigue, pain, anxiety and depression, and controlling better saliva and spasticity, also apart from specific speech and writing motor deficits (which, indeed, are improved by reduced sialorrhoea and muscle hypertonia), will be able to successfully manage his/her language impairment, being more committed to communicate and keep social contacts.

4.2 Non pharmacological strategies

The primary goal of an effective assistive rehabilitation for PALS is the management of disabilities, symptoms and complications arising from the progressive weakness of limb, trunk, and bulbar muscles. Further goals include keeping the patient functioning as independently as possible, and maintaining quality of life even into the terminal stage (Francis et al., 1999).

The rehabilitation program varies depending on whether the patient has a long clinical course or rapid progression of the disease: in the former case, PALS become able to compensate remarkably well for the motor unit loss and are able to continue with their daily activity for several years (Chen et al., 2008). The success of the rehabilitation approach depends on the active participation of the patient who should be a full partner in the therapeutic team even during the advanced stages of the disease. It may be difficult for the physician to discuss such a fatal illness: however, a direct approach allows the patient to deal most effectively with the disease and its physical limitations. This also helps in decisions about the intensity of the therapeutic effort (Bede et al., 2011; Gordon, 2011).

The family and other caregivers should be encouraged to participate in the patient's early rehabilitation program: the family role will then likely increase as weakness progresses, requirements for assistive devices change, and new problems arise in the management of activities of daily living.

4.2.1 Treatment of impaired communication

Loss of effective communication prevents patients from participating in many activities; may lead them to social isolation; and reduces their quality of life: the goal of clinical management of dysarthric PALS is to optimize communication effectiveness for as long as possible. Communication solutions, which may include no-technology, low-technology and high-technology options will be discussed, as well as the importance of psychosocial issues and the factors influencing the use of these systems.

Dysarthric PALS may benefit from working with a *speech therapist*: these health professionals can teach patients adaptive strategies, such as techniques to help them speak louder and more clearly. In early disease stages, patients can be taught to emphasize certain syllables and slow their speech patterns so that others can understand them better: lip and tongue exercises can sometimes help the patient to enunciate words more clearly on a regular basis.

A recent review on ALS communication research (Hanson et al., 2011) concluded that, due to ALS pathophysiology and the intrinsic degenerative nature of disease, speech treatment strategies designed to increase strength or mobility of the oral musculature are not recommended for PALS. Patients or their caregivers, on the contrary, often request oral exercises to improve strength and mobility for speech, as strengthening exercises seem intuitively to them as a way to increase performance: however, such exercise programs should be discouraged, and PALS should be informed that the speaking that they do each day provides a sufficient amount of speech mechanism activity and exercise.

Speech intervention should focus on learning to conserve energy for priority speaking tasks and to rest often to reduce fatigue, instead of increasing effort with speech exercises. PALS speakers should learn to avoid adverse speaking/listening situations by muting the television, inviting people to speak with them in a quiet place rather than in a crowded room, and using voice amplification when speaking in noisy environments to reduce the effort required (Ball et al., 2007; Yorkston et al., 2010).

On the basis of a retrospective study on 25 dysarthric PALS treated with a palatal lift and/or augmentation prosthesis, the use of such devices should be regarded as effective in improving speech: 84% of patients treated with a palatal lift reported reduction of hypernasality (76% benefiting, at least moderately, for 6 months), and 60 % of those treated with a combination of palatal lift and augmentation prosthesis demonstrated improvement in articulation (Esposito et al., 2000).

Writing may be used as a substitute for speech, and devices as simple as paper and pencil, alphabet cards, portable typewriter, and letter boards may be utilized by patients with adequate hand function. Becoming speech more and more difficult to understand, many PALS supplement their speech by identifying the first letter of each word on an alphabet board (*alphabet supplementation*), or by identifying the topic on a communication board (*topic supplementation*).

As ALS progresses, speech therapists can help patients develop ways for responding to yes-or-no questions with their eyes or by other nonverbal means, and can recommend aids such as speech synthesizers and computer-based communication systems: these methods and devices help patients communicate when they can no longer speak or produce vocal sounds.

The technological revolution has expanded communication options for PALS who cannot rely on natural speech and writing. The assistive technologies are categorized as *Augmentative and Alternative Communication* (*AAC*) devices. Four critical features need to be considered within clinical and research domains: language representation, output mode, motor access, and microprocessor units.

Language representation has got remarkable attention for speaking rate enhancement. Whereas most PALS spell and rely on typing as a form of input, they can never approach speech production rates: often the slowness of AAC devices reduces their utility. Nowadays devices are being designed that integrate natural language processing and prediction algorithms for word, utterance and even conversational level units as one tries to approach natural speaking rates.

The **output mode** has seen advances for the storage of digitized voice as well as qualitative improvements to synthetic speech.

Voice banking is often considered as an early treatment option: PALS with intact motor speech skills store their spoken sounds, words, sentences for future use in customized communication devices. The personalized voice and messages can be used along with standard text-to-speech output to retain the PALS' voice signature: engineering efforts to customize synthetic speech to the user's own voice through minimal speech sampling are going on. Scientists and technicians are pursuing the gold standard for a device: bad speech in and good speech out, with attention being paid to recognition of dysarthric speech and production of personalized voices.

Motor access problems are being addressed with visual evoked potentials, detection of alpha and theta waves, and eye gaze recognizers so that head, shoulders, knees and toes are no longer needed: most devices now offer a range of access methods, starting with keyboards, touch screens, a head mouse, and Morse code.

Finally, **microprocessor units** are available in every shape and size to meet user needs, from palmtops to laptops made of magnesium-alloy shells, to software that can be downloaded from the Internet and accessed through any home computer.

AAC has a remarkable importance in dysarthric PALS management. When a person has a severe verbal communication impairment, AAC can meet the overall goals of palliative care: AAC can improve quality of life by optimizing function, assisting with decision making, and providing opportunities for personal growth.

Clinical decision-making related to communication is quite complex as screening, referral, assessment, acquisition of technology, and training must occur in a timely manner, so that when residual speech is no longer effective, AAC strategies are in place to support communication related to personal care, healthcare, social interaction, community involvement. Many reports of use and frequency for the purposes of staying connected and discussing important issues point out that AAC technology can assist the patient-caregiver dyad in maintaining previous relationships. The face-to-face spontaneous conversation mode is used most frequently, despite the slow rate of production, the lack of permanence, and the demands on conversational partners during message generation (Fried-Oken et al., 2006).

PALS, their family members, and, at times, their medical team, usually do not wish to consider an AAC decision until the deteriorating speech intelligibility limits the communication effectiveness: unfortunately, once intelligibility begins to decrease, speech performance often deteriorates so rapidly that there is little time to implement an appropriate AAC intervention. Indeed, appropriate timing of referral for AAC assessment and intervention continues to be a relevant clinical decision-making issue. The speaking rate should be clinically monitored so that the referral for an AAC intervention is initiated in a timely manner: Ball and co-workers (2001, 2002) recommend that patients be referred for AAC assessment when their speaking rates reach 125 words/min (normal value: 190 words/min) on the *Speech Intelligibility Test - Sentence Subtest*) (Yorkston et al., 2007). With sufficient education and preparation, PALS and their caregivers are ready to examine their AAC options timely: nevertheless, speech deterioration can be so rapid anyway that individuals can be left with limited communication options, if they are not really prepared to act in an opportune manner.

Due to the extended AAC use with deteriorating levels of physical control, it is imperative that recommended technology has adjustable access options to meet the range of motor capability as the disease progresses (s. above).

PALS should be fitted with AAC technology that supports multiple access methods, such as allowing them to transition from hand access to scanning and/or head/eye-tracking. Many AAC devices now incorporate a variety of access options so that the technology can continue to meet the needs of the user despite a decline in physical capability: the sensitivity of dynamic touch screens can be adjusted to allow for lighter touch; the improved sensitivity of head-tracking technology has allowed many patients to use this access method with minimal head/neck movement control.

Perhaps the most significant advancement in access technology has occurred with the widespread availability of *eye-tracking systems* to allow cursor control with eye movement to access high-technology AAC devices. As the disease progresses, many PALS require the use of eye-tracking for several reasons. Firstly, compared to other access methods (such as switch-activated scanning), eye-tracking is often reported to be the least fatiguing method

(Gibbons & Beneteau, 2010) and its technology requires relatively little effort (Calvo et al., 2008; Harris & Goren, 2009): eye gaze is natural, and eye muscles generally do not fatigue with use. Secondly, eye gaze may be the only volitional movement that the individual continues to exhibit over time, particularly in cases where invasive ventilation has been chosen (Ball et al., 2010).

BCI technology has generated considerable interest for people who are physically "locked-in", such as PALS in the late stages of the disease. BCI devices translate into computer commands volitional modulation of brain signals which can be recorded from the scalp using electroencephalography (EEG) or magnetoencephalography; from the dura mater or cortical surface using electrocorticography; or from neurons within the cortex.

A common signal for BCI is the P300 event-related potential, a positive deflection in the EEG over parietal cortex, that occurs approximately 300 ms after an "oddball" stimulus: a rare but meaningful stimulus among a series of frequently occurring stimuli. Since the P300 occurs among other ongoing EEG activity, several P300 responses must usually be averaged for the response to be recognized (Polich, 2007). Farwell and Donchin (1988) introduced the first P300-based BCI paradigm: computer presents a 6×6 matrix of letters and commands on-screen and participants attend to the item they wish to select; groups of matrix items are flashed randomly: only flashes of groups containing the attended item should elicit a P300. Items are grouped for flashing as rows and columns: hence, the so-called "*row-column paradigm*" (*RCP*). The computer identifies the attended item as the intersection of the row and column that elicited the largest P300.

The RCP has been tested in various configurations to achieve efficient communication that is practical for in-home use (Krusienski et al., 2006; Lenhardt et al., 2008; Sellers et al., 2006); the paradigm itself has been modified (Guger et al., 2009; Hong et al., 2009; Martens et al., 2009; Salvaris & Sepulveda, 2009; Takano et al., 2009). Unfortunately, none of such alternative paradigms substantially improves P300-based BCI performance. The RCP remains subject to errors that slow communication, cause frustration and diminish attentional resources (Vaughan et al., 2006). Further RCP research could possibly help severely disabled BCI users, who desire speed, accuracy, and ease of use. Moreover, with the RCP, some people are not able to achieve accuracy high enough for practical BCI use (Sellers & Donchin, 2006).

In recognition of these issues, Townsend and co-workers (2010) sought to create an alternative stimulation paradigm that could be faster, more accurate and more reliable than the RCP: they designed the so-called "*checkerboard paradigm*" (*CBP*), using a standard 8×9 matrix of alphanumeric characters and keyboard commands. In the RCP, the 8 columns and 9 rows flash at random: in contrast, in the CBP, the standard matrix is virtually superimposed on a checkerboard which the subjects never actually see. The items in white cells of the standard matrix are segregated into a white 6×6 matrix and the items in the black cells are segregated into a black 6×6 matrix; before each sequence of flashes, the items randomly populate the white or black matrix, respectively. The end result is that the subjects see random groups of 6 items flashing (as opposed to rows and columns), because the virtual rows and columns flash. In other words, the standard matrix never changes: only the pattern of flashing items is changed. After all rows and columns in both matrices have flashed (i.e., 24 flashes, comprising one complete sequence), the program re-randomizes the positions of the items in each virtual matrix and the next sequence of flashes begins (Townsend et al., 2010). The CBP produced a significant increase in BCI performance and user acceptability over the RCP, thus providing a substantially more effective BCI, which is so important for PALS management. Experimental data showed that, whereas average PALS performances were much lower than those of the healthy controls using the RCP, upon switching to the CBP, PALS performed only slightly lower than the healthy controls: patients improved their classification accuracy rates by an average of about 25 % after switching from the RCP to the CBP, whereas accuracy rates of control group improved only of 14 %, thus suggesting that the CBP improvements may be more pronounced for PALS than for healthy controls. In particular, for two patients, the improvement brought them into an accuracy range sufficient for effective BCI control, while previously their accuracy was not consistently enough for effective control.

Non-invasive BCI methods have been utilized more extensively than invasive methods for people with disabilities (Birbaumer & Cohen, 2007; Birbaumer et al., 2008; Gerven et al., 2009): unfortunately, whereas PALS and other patients in "locked-in" conditions have motivated research in this area, very few systems have been successfully used - such as that reported by Townsend and co-workers (2010). It has been postulated that some forms of cognitive impairment and changes in EEG signatures in late ALS stages may contribute to the lack of success using BCI technology (Iversen et al., 2008), as the technology was introduced after the participants had become "locked-in" (Gerven et al., 2009; Münte et al., 1998): really, the most successful application for communication has occurred in people at the beginning stages of ALS (Birbaumer et al., 1999; Birbaumer, 2006; Kubler et al., 2001).

Nowadays, AAC acceptance and use represent two areas of interest for physicians and scientists. Both involve PALS and their caregivers.

In the Ball et al.'s review (2004_b), those who rejected AAC had a co-occurring cognitive deficit or experienced a severe diseases, such as cancer, in addition to ALS.

Fried-Oken and co-workers (2006) reported very positive caregivers' attitudes toward AAC technology: those with greater AAC technology skills got greater rewards associated with caregiving.

In a follow-up study on 15 PALS, Ball and co-workers (2010) examined the acceptance, training, and extended use patterns of eye-tracking technology to support communication.

For 53% of the participants, eye-tracking technology was selected because eye movement was the only viable access option available. More than 90% of the participants reported successful implementation of the technology: the only one patient who was not able to successfully use eye-tracking technology had difficulty with eyelid control. The communicative functions served by eye-tracking devices were extensive: all of the participants used their device to support face-to-face communication, and other functions included group communication, phone, e-mail and internet. More than 40% of the participants also reported using the eye-tracking technology to support other computer-based functions (e.g., word processing, voice-related software programs).

Training and support are an essential component of AAC service delivery for PALS. The significant changes in movement abilities require that service providers not only be proactive in their AAC technology recommendations by fitting up technology options that can meet the changing physical needs over time, but also by supplying adequate training and support to ensure that PALS and their caregivers can successfully implement diachronically these access strategies. Reports of low AAC use often are related to descriptions of minimal training or follow-up (Murphy, 2004).

New advances in AAC technology may need a greater amount of training and intervention than other access options: for instance, implementation of eye-tracking systems often requires for successful technology use trouble-shooting in the form of physical or environmental compensations (Ball et al., 2010). Whereas AAC specialists are professionals who provide the AAC intervention services (such as assessment and initial instruction), AAC facilitators for PALS tend to be family members who typically provide ongoing support (including instruction of new communication partners and caregivers, programming new messages into the AAC device, maintaining the AAC system, and interacting with the technology manufacturer, if necessary) (Beukelman et al., 2008).

In a survey on 68 PALS using AAC technology Ball and co-workers (2005_b) studied the AAC facilitators: almost all of them were family members, the majority with nontechnical backgrounds. They reported to prefer hands-on and detailed step-by-step instruction; and to have received an appropriate training amount (slightly over 2 hours of instruction).

5. Conclusion

Multifunctional impairments of PALS result from a relentlessly progressive muscle weakness, leading ultimately to a widespread body paralysis. In the late disease stages, patients eventually find themselves in a "locked-in" state, totally unable to move neck, trunk and limbs; autonomously breath and feed; and speak, although most of them retain their cognitive skills, thereby assisting impotent at their dreadful somatic decay.

As human beings, and therefore "persons", namely "individuals within a network of relationships", PALS particularly suffer from communication impairment.

Today, much more than in the past, we are able to give interdisciplinary assistance to them, enhancing their possibilities of keeping in touch with their caregivers, friends and other persons, with the aim to maintain their quality of life as high as possible.

Further research is needed to better implement AAC devices and services (trying to optimize communication aids and interfaces, and increase our understanding of acceptance and use of AAC approaches); and to develop new intervention strategies and document their effectiveness.

Anyway, besides scientific and clinical achievements, we look forward to building up in the near future more empathic care strategies for PALS and their families, with respect to them in their dignity of suffering persons.

6. References

Appel, V., Stewart, S., Smith, G. & Appel, S.H. (1987). A rating scale for amyotrophic lateral sclerosis: description and preliminary experience. *Annals of Neurology*, Vol. 22, pp. 328-333

Ball, L.J., Willis, A., Beukelman D.R. & Pattee, G.L. (2001). A protocol for identification of early bulbar signs in amyotrophic lateral sclerosis. *Journal of the Neurological Sciences*, Vol. 191, pp. 43-53

Ball, L.J., Beukelman, D.R. & Pattee, G.L. (2002). Timing of speech deterioration in people with amyotrophic lateral sclerosis. *Journal of Medical Speech-Language Pathology*, Vol. 10, pp. 231-235

Ball, L.J., Beukelman, D.R. & Pattee, G.L. (2004_a). Acceptance of augmentative and alternative communication technology by persons with amyotrophic lateral sclerosis. *Augmentative and Alternative Communication*, Vol. 20, pp. 113-122

Ball, L.J., Beukelman, D.R. & Pattee, G.L. (2004_b). Communication effectiveness of individuals with amyotrophic lateral sclerosis. *Journal of Communication Disorders*, Vol. 37, pp. 197-215

Ball, L.J., Beukelman, D.R., Ullman, C., Maassen, K. & Pattee, G.L. (2005_a). Monitoring speaking rate by telephone for persons with amyotrophic lateral sclerosis. *Journal of Medical Speech-Language Pathology*, Vol. 13, pp. 233-240

Ball, L.J., Schardt, K. & Beukelman, D.R. (2005_b) Primary communication facilitators. *Augmentative Communication News*, Vol. 17, pp. 6-7

Ball, L.J., Beukelman, D.R. & Bardach, L. (2007). AAC intervention for ALS, In: *Augmentative Communication Strategies for Adults with acute or chronic Medical Conditions*, D.R. Beukelman, K. Garrett & K. Yorkston (Eds.), pp. 287-316, Paul H. Brookes, Baltimore, Md, USA

Ball, L.J., Nordness, A., Fager, S.K., Kersch, K., Mohr, B., Pattee, G.L. & Beukelman, D.R. (2010). Eye-gaze access of AAC technology for persons with amyotrophic lateral sclerosis. *Journal of Medical Speech-Language Pathology*, Vol. 18, pp. 11-23

Bede, P., Oliver, D., Stodart, J., van den Berg, L., Simmons, Z., O Brannagáin, D., Borasio. G.D. & Hardiman, O. (2011). Palliative care in amyotrophic lateral sclerosis: a review of current international guidelines and initiatives. *Journal of Neurology, Neurosurgery & Psychiatry*, Vol. 82, pp. 413-418

Beukelman, D.R., Ball, L.J. & Fager, S. (2008). An AAC personnel framework: adults with acquired complex communication needs. *Augmentative and Alternative Communication*, Vol. 24, pp. 255-267

Birbaumer, N., Ghanayim, N., Hinterberger, T., Iversen, I., Kotchoubey, B., Kübler, A. & Perelmouter, J. (1999). A spelling device for the paralysed. *Nature*, Vol. 398, pp. 297-298

Birbaumer, N. (2006). Brain-computer-interface research: coming of age. *Clinical Neurophysiology*, Vol. 117, pp. 479-483

Birbaumer N. & Cohen, L.G. (2007). Brain-computer interfaces: communication and restoration of movement in paralysis. *Journal of Physiology*, Vol. 579, pp. 621-636

Birbaumer, N., Murguialday, A.R. & Cohen, L. (2008). Brain-computer interface in paralysis. *Current Opinion in Neurology*, Vol. 21, pp. 634-638

Callaghan, B., Feldman, D., Gruis, K. & Feldman, E. (2011). The association of exposure to lead, mercury, and selenium and the development of amyotrophic lateral sclerosis and the epigenetic implications. *Neurodegenerative Diseases*, Vol. 8, pp. 1-8

Calvo, A., Chiò, A. & Castellina, E. (2008). Eye tracking impact on quality-of-life of ALS patients, *Proceedings of the Conference on Computers Helping People with Special Needs*, 5101 (*Lecture Notes in Computer Science)*, pp. 70-77

Calvo, A., Moglia, C., Balma, M. & Chiò, A. (2010). Involvement of immune response in the pathogenesis of amyotrophic lateral sclerosis: a therapeutic opportunity? *CNS Neurological Disorders Drug Targets*, Vol. 9, pp. 325-330

Cedarbaum, J.M. & Stambler, N. (1997). Performance of the ALS Functional Rating Scale (ALSFRS) in multicenter clinical trials. *Journal of the Neurological Sciences*, Vol. 152(S), pp. 1-9

Cedarbaum, J.M., Stambler, N., Malta, E., Fuller, C., Hilt, D., Thurmond, B. & Nakanishi, A. (1999). The ALSFRS-R: a revised ALS functional rating scale that incorporates assessments of respiratory function. BDNF ALS Study Group (Phase III). *Journal of the Neurological Sciences*, Vol. 169, pp. 13-21

Chen, A., Montes, J. & Mitsumoto, H. (2008). The role of exercise in amyotrophic lateral sclerosis. *Physical Medicine & Rehabilitation Clinics of North America*, Vol. 19, pp. 545-557

Couratier, P., Torny, F. & Lacoste, M. (2006). [Functional rating scales for amyotrophic lateral sclerosis]. *Revue Neurologie (Paris)*, Vol. 162, pp. 502-507

Duffy, J. (1995). *Motor Speech Disorders: Substrates, Differential Diagnosis, and Management*, Mosby, St. Louis, USA

Enderby, P. & Palmer, R. (2008). *FDA-2. The Frenchay Dysarthria Assessment. Examiner's Manual* (Second edition), Pro-Ed, Austin, Tex, USA

Esposito, S.J., Mitsumoto, H. & Shanks, M. (2000). Use of palatal lift and palatal augmentation prostheses to improve dysarthria in patients with amyotrophic lateral sclerosis: a case series. *Journal of Prosthetic Dentistry*, Vol. 83, pp. 90-98

Farwell, L.A. & Donchin, E. (1988). Talking off the top of your head: toward a mental prosthesis utilizing event-related brain potentials. *Electroencephalography and Clinical Neurophysiology*, Vol. 70, pp. 510-523

Ferrante, R.J., Browne, S.E., Shinobu, L.A., Bowling, A.C., Baik, M.J., MacGarvey, U., Kowall, N.W., Brown, R.H. Jr. & Beal, M.F. (1997). Evidence of increased oxidative damage in both sporadic and familial amyotrophic lateral sclerosis. *Journal of Neurochemistry*, Vol. 69, pp. 2064-2074

Francis, K., Bach, J.R. & DeLisa, J.A. (1999). Evaluation and rehabilitation of patients with adult motor neuron disease. *Archives of Physical Medicine and Rehabilitation*, Vol. 80, pp. 951-963

Fried-Oken, M., Fox, L., Rau, M.T., Tullman, J., Baker, G., Hindal, M., Wile, N. & Lou, J.S. (2006). Purposes of AAC device use for persons with ALS as reported by caregivers. *Augmentative Alternative Communication*, Vol. 20, pp. 209-221

Gerven, M.V., Farquhar, J. & Schaefer, R. (2009). The brain-computer interface cycle. *Journal of Neural Engineering*, Vol. 6, pp. 1-10

Gibbons, C. & Beneteau, E. (2010). Functional performance using eye control and single switch scanning by people with ALS. *Perspectives on Augmentative and Alternative Communication*, Vol. 19, pp. 64-69

Gordon, P.H. (2011). Amyotrophic lateral sclerosis: pathophysiology, diagnosis and management. *CNS Drugs*, Vol. 25, pp. 1-15

Green, J.R., Beukelman, D.R. & Ball, L.J. (2004). Algorithmic estimation of pauses in extended speech samples of dysarthric and typical speech. *Journal of Medical Speech-Language Pathology*, Vol. 12, pp. 149-154

Guedj, E., Ber, I., Lacomblez, L., Dubois, B., Verpillat, P., Didic, M., Salachas, F., Vera, P., Hannequin, D., Lotterie, J.A., Puel, M., Decousus, M., Thomas-Antérion, C., Magne, C., Vercelletto, M., Bernard, A.M., Golfier, V., Pasquier, J., Michel, B.F., Namer, I.,

Sellal, F., Bochet, J., Volteau, M., Brice, A., Meininger, V., French Research Network on FTD/FTD-MND & Habert, M.O. (2007). Brain SPECT perfusion of frontotemporal dementia associated with motor neuron disease. *Neurology*, Vol. 69, pp. 488-490

Guger, C., Daban, S., Sellers, E., Holzner, C., Krausz, G., Carabalona, R., Gramatica, F. & Edlinger, G. (2009). How many people are able to control a P300-based brain-computer interface (BCI)? *Neuroscience Letters*, Vol. 462, pp. 94-98

Guidubaldi, A., Fasano, A., Ialongo, T., Piano, C., Pompili, M., Mascianà, R., Siciliani, L., Sabatelli, M. & Bentivoglio, A.R. (2011). Botulinum toxin A versus B in sialorrhea: a prospective, randomized, double-blind, crossover pilot study in patients with amyotrophic lateral sclerosis or Parkinson's disease. *Movement Disorders*, Vol. 26, pp. 313-319

Guy, N., Bourry, N., Dallel, R., Dualé, C., Verrelle, P., Lapeyre, M. & Clavelou, P. (2011). Comparison of radiotherapy types in the treatment of sialorrhea in amyotrophic lateral sclerosis. *Journal of Palliative Medicine*, Vol. 14, pp. 391-395

Hanson, E., Yorkston, K. & Britton, D. (2011). Dysarthria in amyotrophic lateral sclerosis: a systematic review of characteristics, speech treatment, and AAC options. *Journal of Medical Speech-Language Pathology*. In press.

Harris, D. & Goren, M. (2009). The ERICA eye gaze system versus manual letter board to aid communication in ALS/MND. *British Journal of Neuroscience Nursing*, Vol. 5, pp. 227-230

Haverkamp, L.J., Appel, V. & Appel, S.H. (1995). Natural history of amyotrophic lateral sclerosis in a database population. Validation of a scoring system and a model for survival prediction. *Brain*, Vol. 118, pp. 707-719

Hillel, A.D., Miller, R.M., Yorkston, K., McDonald, E., Norris, F.H. & Konikow, N. (1989). Amyotrophic lateral sclerosis severity scale. *Neuroepidemiology*, Vol. 8, pp. 142-150

Hirose, H., Kiritani, S. & Sawashima, M. (1982). Patterns of dysarthric movement in patients with Amyotrophic Lateral Sclerosis and Pseudobulbar Palsy. *Folia Phoniatrica et Logopaedica*, Vol. 34, pp. 106-112

Hong, B., Guo, F., Liu, T., Gao, X. & Gao, S. (2009). N200-speller using motion-onset visual response. *Clinical Neurophysiology*, Vol. 120, pp. 1658-1666

Iversen, I.H., Ghanayim, N., Kübler, A., Neumann, N., Birbaumer, N. & Kaiser, J. (2008). A brain-computer interface tool to assess cognitive functions in completely paralyzed patients with amyotrophic lateral sclerosis. *Clinical Neurophysiology*, Vol. 119, pp. 2214-2223

Kent, R.D., Kent, J.F., Weismer, G., Martin, R.E., Sufit, R.L. & Rosenbek, J.C. (1989). Relationships between speech intelligibility and the slope of second-formant transitions in dysarthric subjects. *Clinical Linguistics and Phonetics*, Vol. 3, pp. 347-358

Kent, J.F., Kent, R.D., Rosenbek, J.C., Weismer, G., Martin, R. & Sufit, R. (1992). Quantitative description of the dysarthria in women with amyotrophic lateral sclerosis. *Journal of Speech and Hearing Research*, Vol. 35, pp. 723-733

Kent, R.D., Vorperian, H.K., Kent, J.F. & Duffy, J.R. (2003). Voice dysfunction in dysarthria: application of the Multi-Dimensional Voice Program. *Journal of Communication Disorders*, Vol. 36, pp. 281-306

Kobayashi, M., Ikeda, K., Kinoshita, M. & Iwasaki Y. (1999). Amyotrophic lateral sclerosis with supranuclear ophthalmoplegia and rigidity. *Neurological Research*, Vol. 21, pp. 661-664

Krusienski, D.J., Sellers, E.W., Cabestaing, F., Bayoudh, S., McFarland, D.J., Vaughan, T.M. & Wolpaw, J.R. (2006). A comparison of classification techniques for the P300 Speller. *Journal of Neural Engineering*, Vol. 3, pp. 299-305

Kubler, A., Neumann, N., Kaiser, J., Kotchoubey, B., Hinterberger, T. & Birbaumer, N. (2001). Brain-computer communication: self-regulation of slow cortical potentials for verbal communication. *Archives of Physical Medicine and Rehabilitation*, Vol. 82, pp. 1533-1539

Lenhardt, A., Kaper, M. & Ritter, H.J. (2008). An adaptive P300-based online brain-computer interface. *IEEE Transactions on Neural Systems and Rehabilitation Engineering*, Vol. 16, pp. 121-130

Logroscino, G., Traynor, B.J., Hardiman, O., Chiò, A., Couratier, P., Mitchell, J.D., Swingler, R.J. & Beghi, E. for EURALS. (2008). Descriptive epidemiology of amyotrophic lateral sclerosis: new evidence and unsolved issues. *Journal of Neurology, Neurosurgery & Psychiatry*, Vol. 79, pp. 6-11

Martens, S.M., Hill, N.J., Farquhar, J. & Scholkopf, B. (2009). Overlap and refractory effects in a brain-computer interface speller based on the visual P300 event-related potential. *Journal of Neural Engineering*, Vol. 6, pp. 026003

Miller, R.G., Rosenberg, J.A., Gelinas, D.F., Mitsumoto, H., Newman, D., Sufit, R., Borasio, G.D., Bradley, W.G., Bromberg, M.B., Brooks, B.R., Kasarskis, E.J., Munsat, T.L. & Oppenheimer, E.A. (1999). Practice parameter: the care of the patient with amyotrophic lateral sclerosis (an evidence-based review): report of the Quality Standards Subcommittee of the American Academy of Neurology: ALS Practice Parameters Task Force. *Neurology*, Vol. 52, pp. 1311-1323

Miller, R.G., Jackson, C.E., Kasarskis, E.J., England, J.D., Forshew, D., Johnston, W., Kalra, S., Katz, J.S., Mitsumoto, H., Rosenfeld, J., Shoesmith, C., Strong, M.J. & Woolley, S.C., Quality Standards Subcommittee of the American Academy of Neurology. (2009_a). Practice parameter update: The care of the patient with amyotrophic lateral sclerosis: drug, nutritional, and respiratory therapies (an evidence-based review): report of the Quality Standards Subcommittee of the American Academy of Neurology. *Neurology*, Vol. 73, pp. 1218-1226

Miller, R.G., Jackson, C.E., Kasarskis, E.J., England, J.D., Forshew, D., Johnston, W., Kalra, S., Katz, J.S., Mitsumoto, H., Rosenfeld, J., Shoesmith, C., Strong, M.J. & Woolley, S.C., Quality Standards Subcommittee of the American Academy of Neurology. (2009_b). Practice parameter update: The care of the patient with amyotrophic lateral sclerosis: multidisciplinary care, symptom management, and cognitive/behavioral impairment (an evidence-based review): report of the Quality Standards Subcommittee of the American Academy of Neurology. *Neurology*, Vol. 73, pp. 1227-1233

Mulligan, M., Carpenter, J., Riddel, J., Delaney, M.K., Badger, G. & Krusinski, P. (1994). Intelligibility and the acoustic characteristics of speech in amyotrophic lateral sclerosis (ALS). *Journal of Speech and Hearing Research*, Vol. 37, pp. 496-503

Münte, T.F., Tröger, M.C., Nusser, I., Wieringa, B.M., Johannes, S., Matzke, M. & Dengler, R. (1998). Alteration of early components of the visual evoked potential in amyotrophic lateral sclerosis. *Journal of Neurology*, Vol. 245, pp. 206-210

Murphy, J. (2004). "I prefer contact this close": perceptions of AAC by people with motor neurone disease and their communication partners. *Augmentative and Alternative Communication*, Vol. 20, pp. 259-271

Nishio, M. & Niimi, S. (2000). Changes over time in dysarthric patients with amyotrophic lateral sclerosis (ALS): a study of changes in speaking rate and maximum repetition rate (MRR). *Clinical Linguistics and Phonetics*, Vol. 14, pp. 485-497

Norris, F.H., Calanchini, P.R., Fallat, R.J., Pancharis, S. & Jewett, B. (1974). Administration of guanidine in amyotrophic lateral sclerosis. *Neurology*, Vol. 24, pp. 721-728

Okuda, B., Yamamoto, T., Yamasaki, M., Maya, K. & Imai, T. (1992). Motor neuron disease with slow eye movements and vertical gaze palsy. *Acta Neurologica Scandinavica*, Vol. 85, pp. 71-76

Patten, S.B., Svenson, L.W, White, C.M., Khaled, S.M. & Metz, L.M. (2007). Affective disorders in motor neuron disease: a population-based study. *Neuroepidemiology*, Vol. 28, pp. 1-7

Polich, J. (2007). Updating P300: an integrative theory of P3a and P3b. *Clinical Neurophysiology*, Vol. 118, pp. 2128-2148

Raaphorst, J., De Visser, M., Linssen, W.H., De Haan, R.J. & Schmand, B. (2010). The cognitive profile of amyotrophic lateral sclerosis: A meta-analysis. *Amyotrophic Lateral Sclerosis*, Vol. 11, pp. 27-37

Ramig, L.O., Scherer, R.C., Klasner, E.R., Titze, I.R. & Horii, Y. (1990). Acoustic analysis of voice in amyotrophic lateral sclerosis: A longitudinal case study. *Journal of Speech and Hearing Disorders*, Vol. 55, pp. 2-14

Ringholz, G.M., Appel, S.H., Bradshaw, M., Cooke, N.A., Mosnik, D.M. & Schulz, P.E. (2005). Prevalence and patterns of cognitive impairment in sporadic ALS. *Neurology*, Vol. 65, pp. 586-590

Roth, C., Glaze, L., Goding, G. & David, W. (1996). Spasmodic dysphonia symptoms as initial presentation of amyotrophic lateral sclerosis. *Journal of Voice*, Vol. 10, pp. 362-367

Salvaris, M. & Sepulveda, F. (2009). Visual modifications on the P300 speller BCI paradigm. *Journal of Neural Engineering*, Vol. 6, pp. 046011

Sellers, E.W. & Donchin, E. (2006). A P300-based brain-computer interface: initial tests by ALS patients. *Clinical Neurophysiology*, Vol. 117, pp. 538-548

Sellers, E.W., Krusienski, D.J., McFarland, D.J., Vaughan, T.M. & Wolpaw, J.R. (2006). A P300 event-related potential brain-computer interface (BCI): the effects of matrix size and inter stimulus interval on performance. *Biological Psychology*, Vol. 73, pp. 242-252

Takano, K., Komatsu, T., Hata, N., Nakajima, Y. & Kansaku, K. (2009). Visual stimuli for the P300 brain-computer interface: a comparison of white/gray and green/blue flicker matrices. *Clinical Neurophysiology*, Vol. 20, pp. 1562-1566

Ticozzi, N., Tiloca, C., Morelli, C., Colombrita, C., Poletti, B., Doretti, A., Maderna, L., Messina, S., Ratti, A. & Silani, V. (2011). Genetics of familial Amyotrophic Lateral Sclerosis. *Archives Italiennes de Biologie*, Vol. 149, pp. 65-82

Tjaden, K. & Turner, G.S. (1997). Spectral properties of fricative in amyotrophic lateral sclerosis. *Journal of Speech, Language and Hearing Research*, Vol. 40, pp. 1358-1372

Tjaden, K. & Turner, G.S. (2000). Segmental timing in amyotrophic lateral sclerosis. *Journal of Speech, Language and Hearing Research*, Vol. 43, pp. 683-696

Tomik, B. & Guiloff, R.J. (2010). Dysarthria in amyotrophic lateral sclerosis: A review. *Amyotrophic Lateral Sclerosis*, Vol. 11, pp. 4-15

Townsend, G., La Pallo, B.K., Boulay, C.B., Krusienski, D.J., Frye, G.E., Hauser, C.K., Schwartz, N.E., Vaughan, T.M., Wolpaw, J.R. & Sellers, E.W. (2010). A novel P300-based brain-computer interface stimulus presentation paradigm: moving beyond rows and columns. *Clinical Neurophysiology*, Vol. 121, pp. 1109-1120

Turner, G.S., Tjaden, K. & Weismer, G. (1995). The influence of speaking rate on vowel space and speech intelligibility for individuals with ALS. *Journal of Speech and Hearing Research*, Vol. 38, pp. 1001-1013

Turner, G.S. & Weismer, G. (1993). Characteristics of speaking rate in the dysarthria associated with amyotrophic lateral sclerosis. *Journal of Speech and Hearing Research*, Vol. 36, pp. 1134-1144

Vaughan, T.M., McFarland, D.J., Schalk, G., Sarnacki, W.A., Krusienski, D.J., Sellers, E.W. & Wolpaw, J.R. (2006). The Wadsworth BCI Research and Development Program: at home with BCI. *IEEE Transactions on Neural Systems and Rehabilitation Engineering*, Vol. 14, pp. 229-233

Weismer, G., Kent, R.D., Hodge, M. & Martin, R. (1988). The acoustic signatures for intelligibility test words. *Journal of the Acoustical Society of America*, Vol. 84, pp. 1281-1291

Weismer, G., Martin, R., Kent, J.F, & Kent, R.D. (1992). Formant trajectory characteristics of males with amyotrophic lateral sclerosis. *Journal of the Acoustical Society of America*, Vol. 91, pp. 1085-1097

Weismer, G., Jeng, J.Y., Laures, J.S., Kent, R.D. & Kent, J.F. (2001). Acoustic and intelligibility characteristics of sentence production in neurogenic speech disorders. *Folia Phoniatrica et Logopaedica*, Vol. 53, pp. 1-18

Worms, P.M. (2001). The epidemiology of motor neuron diseases: a review of recent studies. *Journal of the Neurological Sciences*, Vol. 191, pp. 3-9

Yorkston, K., Beukelman, D.R. & Traynor, C. (1984). *Assessment of Intelligibility of Dysarthric Speech*, Pro-Ed, Austin, Tex, USA

Yorkston K., Strand, E., Miller, R., Hillel, A. & Smith, K. (1993). Speech deterioration in amyotrophic lateral sclerosis: implications for the timing of intervention. *Journal of Medical Speech-Language Pathology*, Vol. 1, pp. 35-46

Yorkston, K., Beukelman, D.R., Hakel, M. & Dorsey, M. (2007). *Sentence Intelligibility Test, Speech Intelligibility Test*, Madonna Rehabilitation Hospital, Lincoln, Neb, USA

Yorkston, K., Beukelman, D.R., Strand, E. & Hakel, M. (2010). *Management of Motor Speech Disorders in Children and Adults*, Pro-Ed, Austin, Tex, USA

Yunusova, Y., Weismer, G., Westbury, J.R. & Lindstrom, M.J. (2008). Articulatory movements during vowels in speakers with dysarthria and normal controls. *Journal of Speech, Language and Hearing Research*, Vol. 51, pp. 596-611

Yunusova, Y., Green, J.R., Lindstrom, M.J., Ball, L.J., Pattee, G.L. & Zinman, L. (2010). Kinematics of disease progression in bulbar ALS. *Journal of Communication Disorders*, Vol. 43, pp. 6–20.

30

Human Computer Interactions for Amyotrophic Lateral Sclerosis Patients

Ali Bülent Uşaklı
The NCO Academy
Turkey

1. Introduction

In this chapter, alternative communication and device control channels, which are helpful for Amyotrophic lateral sclerosis (ALS) patients, are introduced. In this context, human computer interactions (HCIs) will be discussed in three respects; electrical brain activities, eye movements and hemoglobin level in the blood.

With technological advances, fighting or minimization side effects of the diseases is the main purpose of biomedical research. Under this motto, this chapter focuses on HCIs for individuals suffering from motor neuron diseases. ALS is a progressive neurodegenerative disease caused by the degeneration of motor neurons. ALS or other tetraplegic clinical conditions, otherwise known as the locked-in syndrome, have severe disabilities in controlling muscles and consequently have problems in moving the entire body. Some of these patients can only move their eyes. In severe conditions of the progressive motor neuron diseases, patients cannot move their eyes nor can they speak. Establishing an efficient communication channel without overt speaking and hand motions makes the patient's life a bit easier and increases their quality of life.

ALS occurs in between 4 and 8 out of every 100,000 individuals and only a small percentage of cases arise from a known genetic cause (Parker & Parker, 2007). Concerning other motor neuron diseases or speaking and muscular disabilities, there are more than 100 million potential users in need of alternative channels such as brain computer interface (BCI) for communicating with their environment or for controlling devices (Guger, 2008). Considering life span extension and increasing causes of injuries including traffic accidents and explosions, which may result in spinal cord injuries in serious cases, the need for an efficient communication or control channel has been drastically increasing.

HCIs are a research field which includes interactions such as communication and device/machine control between a user and a computer. The aim of the HCI is to improve performance of the interaction, meaning a minimization of the barrier between the human and the computer. Accurate and fast interpretation of what the user wants to do as well as a correct understanding by the computer of the user's intentions or demand is the aim of this research field.

Man-machine interface (MMI), brain-machine interface (BMI) and BCI can be thought of as applications of HCIs. If communication or control is established directly from the brain, it is called BCI and it is the only method of interaction for the individuals with complete paralysis. Because these research fields are new, there is a need for development in terms of efficiency; meaning accuracy, reliability and quick responses are necessary. Many research groups from all over the world are focusing on HCI applications in order to improve alternative communication channels for the disabled. An efficient alternative channel for communication and control device without overt speaking and muscular movements is important to make life easier for individuals who are suffering from ALS or other illnesses that prevent proper limb and muscular responses. Because of this, the area of study related with HCIs has high expectations and are important for improving quality of life.

In this chapter, ALS related HCI in particular, is discussed. The very common field electroencephalogram (EEG) based BCI and other approaches in this field are presented. With interdisciplinary studies, developing new interfaces and interaction techniques are opening new research fields for investigation. Especially for the paralysis patients, the classical communication or control ways, such as overt speaking or hand motions cannot be used. Using bio-signals such as EEG and its various methodologies (i.e. P300, slow cortical potentials, etc), electrooculogram (EOG), hearth rate (HR) or galvanic skin response (GSR) as well as the hemoglobin level which is related to oxygenation, are the only ways to send messages or control signals to devices regarding user's demands, intentions or expectations. This does not only give the patients the potential ability to give messages on computer screens and control a powered wheelchair or robot arm without muscular movements, but also can be potentially useful for the elderly as well.

The aim of this chapter is to present the state of the art of the technology on HCIs. This chapter also addresses the use of different bio-signals individually or the integrated hybrid/integrated multi-modal system approach for communication and control with high performance. In order to increase performance, processing combined bio-signals and multi-modal integrated systems will be discussed. For this purpose, several bio-signals such as EEG, EOG, and functional near infrared (fNIR) spectroscopy based system research are introduced.

2. Human computer interactions

In general, HCIs are related to the adaptation of a human and a computer. HMIs adapt human demands to the machine. Human computer interface operation requires the effective interaction of two sides; user and system. Here, a system can be an integrated system of computers and a word speller, a robot arm, a powered wheelchair, house appliances such as door locks, TVs or musical instruments, etc. In order to reflect intent/demands, instead of overt speaking or muscular movements, other bio-signals can be used. Effective BCIs may serve as assessment tools and adaptive systems for HCI for able-bodied people and be proven for people with severe motor neuron diseases.

Research in this field is typically focused on several areas of improvement for HCIs in order to increase its usefulness and effectiveness. These areas are:

i. High performance
   a. Accuracy
   b. Reliability
   c. Fast
   d. Robustness
ii. User friendliness (including user training)
iii. Ease of application
iv. Cost effectiveness.

In short, HCI should reflect user demands and expectations accurately and quickly. The next sections of this chapter will introduce the EEG, EOG, NIRS based systems, as they are technologies that show much promise. In addition to these technologies, electrocorticography (ECoG), functional magnetic resonance imaging (fMRI), galvanic skin response (GSR) and heart rate (HR) based systems; and multi-modal integrated design rationale are introduced briefly.

2.1 Brain computer interfaces

From a broad perspective, BMI refers to the interface between a brain and a machine (for review Lebedev & Nicolelis, 2006). In this section, the common term - brain computer interface (BCI) will be presented. BCI can be described as a translation of human intentions into a control signal without using the muscles. The aim of BCI is to provide communication and control for people with severe motor disabilities.

The BCI system translates the signals that are encoded by the user's intentions into messages and control commands. Research in this field has been rapidly growing in neuroscience and bioengineering. Specifically, this technology is promising for users with motor neuron diseases. Table 1 shows the estimated potential users of BCI. According to this table, there are more than 100 million potential users in the world.

Type of the Disease	Number of Patients
Amyotrophic Lateral Sclerosis	400,000/3,000,000
Multiple Sclerosis	2,000,000
Muscular Dystrophy	1,000,000
Brainstem Stroke	10,000,000
Cerebral Palsy	16,000,000
Spinal Cord Injury	5,000,000
Postpolio Syndrome	7,000,000
Guillain-Barre Syndrome	70,000
Other types of Stroke	60,000,000

Table 1. Potential users of BCI in the world (Guger, 2008).

Electrical brain activities (electroencephalography, EEG) related to human intentions can be monitored using electrodes attached to the scalp surface, non-invasively. EEG signals are gross potential of the thousands of neurons, roughly reflecting bodily functions. Because the skull and scalp play the role of a barrier for the electrical signals, EEG signals have low amplitudes (in micro-volts scale) and exist in the 0.5-30 Hz frequency band. Figure 1 shows the ongoing time series EEG signal and its power spectral density. As it is shown from this figure, 8-12 Hz (α band) and 26 Hz (β band) components are dominant.

In order to increase efficiency, brain electrical signals can be recorded by subdural electrodes (electrocorticogram, ECoG), invasively. ECoGs are neuronal activity that is acquired from smaller cortical areas when compared to EEGs. Epidural or subdural recording is less invasive than intra-cortical recording. While their applications are difficult, the resolution of these recordings can be significantly higher than conventional EEG. The BCI usefulness of intra-cortical signals is promising (Wolpaw, 2003).

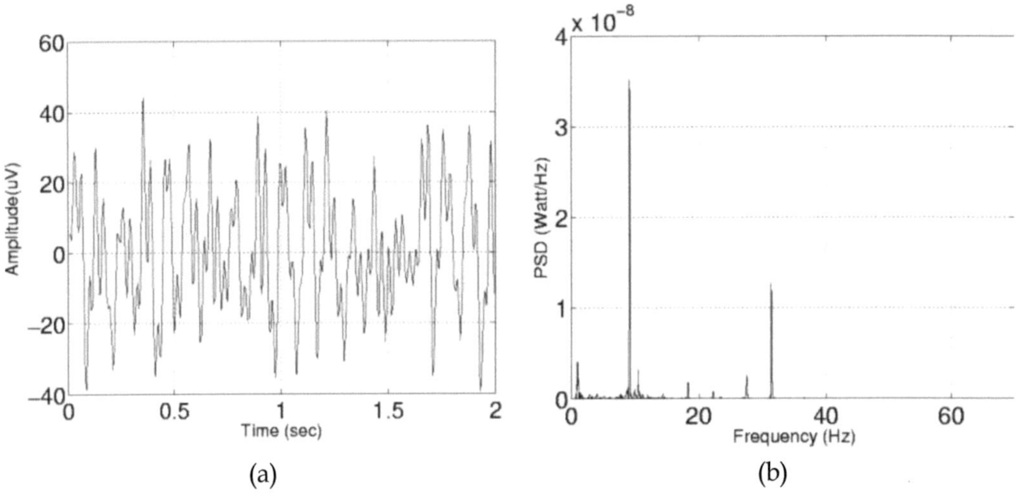

Fig. 1. Ongoing EEG recording from 27-year old male subject's occipital lobe: (a) the time series signal, and (b) power spectral density.

BCI systems can provide a communication and control channel, which bypasses conventional neuromuscular pathways involved in speaking or movement activity made to manipulate objects (Wolpaw et al., 2002). The command for device control can be generated by self-regulated μ rhythms (Wolpaw et al., 2000), motor imagery (Pfurtscheller et al., 2000) or a visual evoked potential (Sutter, 1992).

An EEG based BCI system can use the signals listed below.

- P300 response,
- steady state visual evoked potential (SSVEP),
- event related desynchronisation (ERD),
- slow cortical potential (SCP) and
- sensorimotor rhythm (SMR).

P300 and SSVEP methods require external stimulation that the user has to focus attention on or gaze into flickering lights, which the other methods do not need (self-paced systems). Because of this, the user is not free to decide on performing an action; the user depends on computer software for the synchronization. Each of these methods is advantageous or disadvantageous with respect to performance, information transfer rate and user training time. The BCI systems may not use just one of these approaches, but may use a combination of two or more signals as a hybrid approached system.

As an event related potential (ERP), the common method is using the P300 response (Farwell & Donchin, 1988). The P300 response is elicited between 300 msec and 400 msec after stimulation, as it is shown in figure 2. Because ERPs are so small, for clarity, signal (epoch) averaging is necessary. The latency and amplitude may change from user to user, however the shape of the signal is roughly the same. In addition to using P300 response, SSVEPs (Gao et al, 2003) and SCPs, μ (8-12 Hz) and high β (18-26 Hz) rhythms (sensorimotor applications) are used in BCI applications.

The SSVEP is a brain response evoked mainly in the visual and parietal cortices as a response to flickering visual stimuli. The SSVEP has gained popularity in the BCI research because it provides advantages in terms of speed and robustness. ERD and Event-related synchronization

was quantified by the most reactive frequency bands were chosen then band-pass filtered within those bands. SCPs are slow shifts of the EEG with duration from 300 msec to several seconds. The group of SCPs includes the contingent negative variation, premovement potentials, the Bereitschaftspotential and expectancy waves (Pfurtscheller et al., 2005).
While these approaches are important for the detection of imagery motor activities, the approach of the P300 waveform is very common in BCI applications. As it is shown figure 2, the P300 response is a large, positive potential (conventionally opposite polarization) that has been studied extensively within the context of the oddball paradigm. Donchin and colleagues first reported the use of the P300 for BCI communication (Donchin et al., 2000). International approaches for the detection of P300 speller, a matrix of grey symbols on a dark background (virtual keyboard) are shown in figure 3.

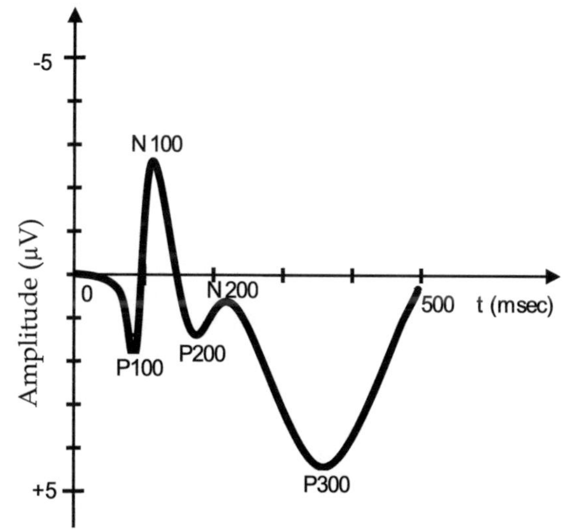

Fig. 2. Typical averaged event related potentials after stimulation. In BCI applications P300 component is extensively used.

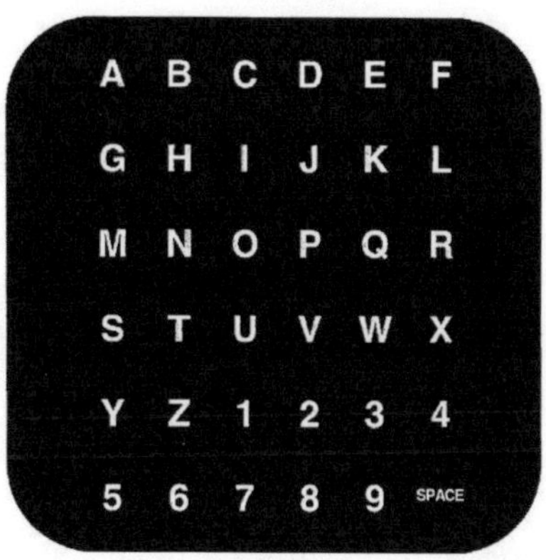

Fig. 3. The matrix for P300 speller. The stimulus matrix monitored by the subject. Typically, one of the rows or columns of the matrix was intensified every 125 ms (The matrix is proposed first by Donchin and colleagues 1988).

The P300 speller paradigm has been common as a promising communication tool. Using the P300, a virtual keyboard without using or requiring any activation of skeletal muscles can be realized (Farwell & Donchin, 1988; Donchin et al., 2000; Sellers & Donchin, 2006). In the virtual keyboard, rows and columns of the matrix were randomly intensified typically every 125 ms. A P300 was produced after attended character is flashed. The attended symbol was selected by averaging responses for rows and columns. Accurate performance is obtained in users with and without motor impairments. Users with ALS are able to use the P300 based, single-stimulus system using either auditory or visual presentations. The Oddball paradigm to implement using the commands: Yes, No, Pass, and End with three presentation modes: auditory, visual, and both auditory and visual were used (Sellers et al., 2006). Detecting P300 signals the mind spelled characters (words, sentences, stories), enable the communication-disabled via internet (van Kokswijk & van Hulle, 2010) were realized.

People can learn to control EEG features consisting of SMR amplitudes and can use this control to move a cursor to a target on a screen. EEG recordings during right and left motor imagery allow users to establish a new communication channel. Such an EEG-based BCI can be used to develop a simple binary response for the control of a device (Guger et al., 2000). To control cursor movement 8-12 Hz (μ) or 18-26 Hz (β) frequency bands over sensorimotor cortex can be used (Fabiani et al., 2004). In the standard one-dimensional application, the cursor moves horizontally from left to right at a fixed rate while vertical cursor movement is continuously controlled by SMR (μ and β rhythms) amplitude over left and/or right sensorimotor cortex (McFarland & Wolpaw, 2005). Intention of movement of left or right index finger, or right foot is recognized in EEG signals (Peters et al., 2001).

The model usually employed in many BCI systems is presented in Figure 4. Here, messages can be word speller output and commands can be for the powered wheelchair, robot hand or domotic (house) appliances control commands.

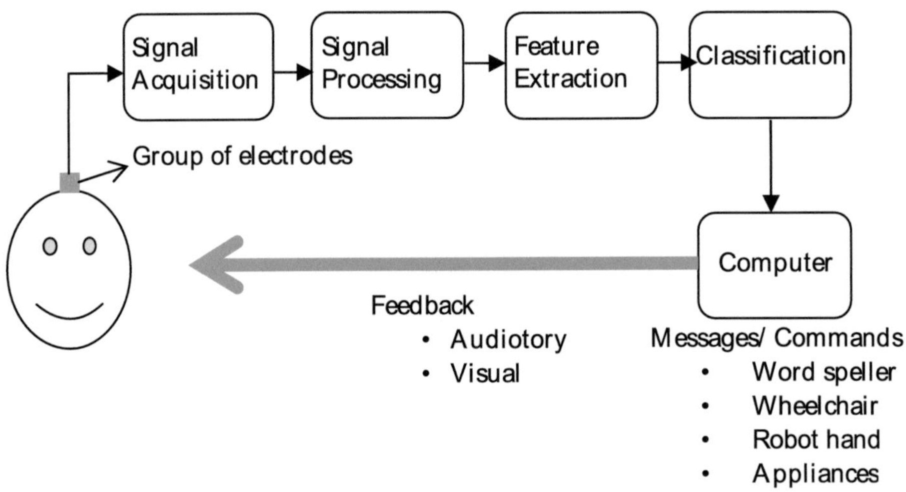

Fig. 4. A Typical BCI system.

To increase usefulness, BCI research groups are focusing several respects. In order to evaluate the usefulness of approaches for user intention, it is important to recognize that intention is normally formatted as a goal (Wolpaw, 2003). This goal may be "Write letter 'A' (On the screen)", "Move forward (powered wheelchair)" "Hit target (cursor)", "Grasp the glass", "Turn on the TV" or "Unlock the door", etc. After real time processing regarding the goal, the next step is goal-directed feedback generation.

The BCI systems may be self-paced. This means that the system allows communication or control whenever the user wishes. These systems' performance determined the true positive rate and the false positive rate. The true positive rate is the percentage of intentional control commands that are correctly detected by the BCI system. False positive rate are false positives generated by the system during the periods for which the user does not intend control.

A synchronous BCI uses external stimulation whereas in asynchronous BCI the subject makes self-paced decisions on when to switch from one mental task to the next. A virtual keyboard and a mobile robot which respond every 0.5 s were developed (Millan & Mourino, 2003). Additionally, an asynchronous BCI analyzes and classifies EEG data continuously (Townsend et al., 2004). These systems are designed to process only one brain state in the ongoing EEG. For this purpose, only one channel may be sufficient. To control a powered wheelchair using a delayed response task a binary classification of left and right movement intentions were classified with a classification rate of over 80% from single trial EEG (Kaneswaran et al., 2010).

In order to improve the BCI system's performance, a rapid transition of various types of parameter estimation and classification algorithms to real-time implementation and testing (Guger, et al., 2001), classification accuracy and communication rate (Turnip et al., 2010) were realized. Identifying errors through the brain's reaction to mistakes is used to improve the robustness, flexibility, and reliability of BCIs (Buttfield et al., 2006). In addition to algorithmic improvement to increase performance, or in other words - high-resolution, multi-channel EEG systems have been developed to enhance the spatial information content of EEG activity. All these factors help to increasing the efficiency of BCI systems.

For standardization of BCI research, there is a documented general-purpose BCI research and development platform known as BCI2000. This platform can incorporate independent or a combination of any brain signals, signal processing methods, output devices and operating protocols (Wolpaw et al., 2003; Schalk, et al., 2004).

As a new approach to drive BCIs, functional magnetic resonance imaging (fMRI), have been used. The temporal resolution of the hemodynamic deoxyhemoglobin changes in the range of 1-2 seconds, while its spatial resolution is generally observable with the current imaging techniques at a few millimeters scale. Local hemodynamic response can be measured by fMRI. Hence, fMRI responses and cortical sources of EEG data are spatially related. It is possible to estimate the cortical activity with a spatial resolution of few millimeters and with a temporal resolution of milliseconds from noninvasive EEG measurements (Astolfi et al., 2010).

Although an fMRI based BCIs noninvasively records activity of the entire brain with a high spatial resolution, they are not suitable for everyday use. They have temporal delays of several seconds. However, they have good spatial resolution and they can sample the activity of deep brain structures (Lebedev & Nicolelis, 2006). An fMRI-based BCI platform which performs data processing and feedback of the hemodynamic brain activity within 1.3 s (Weiskopf et al., 2004), psychophysiological markers (Nijboer et al., 2009), and communication using real-time fMRI (Eklund et al., 2010) were developed. In the later system, the subject in the MR scanner sees a virtual keyboard and steers a cursor to select different letters that can be combined to create words. The cursor is moved to the left by activating the left hand, to the right by activating the right hand, down by activating the left toes and up by activating the right toes (Eklund et al., 2010).

It can be concluded that as an alternative method for communication through speaking and muscular movements, BCIs are allowing communication and control for individuals with motor neuron disease such as ALS. A BCI system consists of recognition by a computation of the patterns of brain electrical activity on the scalp acquired from an array of electrodes. Although this technology is quite useful, it still needs to be developed in terms of efficiency.

2.2 Electrooculography based systems

Paralyzed patients are unable to communicate normally with their environment. For these patients, the only part of their body that is under their control, in terms of muscular movement, is their eyes. Some research in this area has been focused on investigating new efficient communication tools for paralyzed patients to translate their eye movements into appropriate communication messages or control signals.

With eye movements, a potential across the cornea and retina exists. This potential is called the cornea-retinal potential and it is the source of the electrooculogram (EOG). Communicating and controlling with EOG can be used for the disabled. An EOG based HCI device is able to recognize the subject's eye movements by using the electrical activity generated by the eye movements. EOG signals have certain patterns for each kind of eye movement (left, right, up, down, blink or wink). These signal patterns can be acquired and then recognized as signals which can be used for controlling external devices like a virtual keyboard, a powered wheelchair, a robot arm or a movable robot. As a very common application, the EOG-based virtual keyboard provides a means for paralyzed patients to write letters on a screen with eye movements without using a conventional keyboard. An EOG-based system for HCI application is presented in figure 5 and EOG signal samples are shown in figure 6.

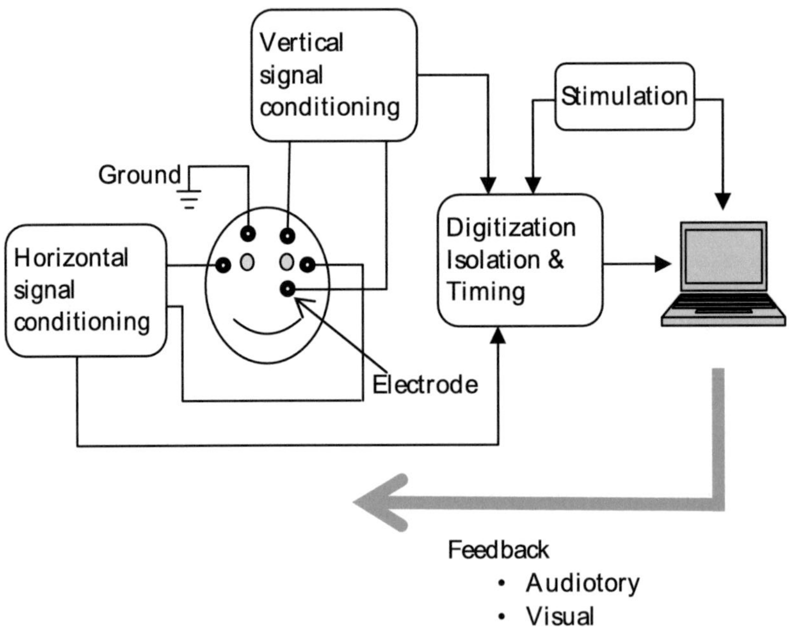

Fig. 5. Typical EOG-based interface.

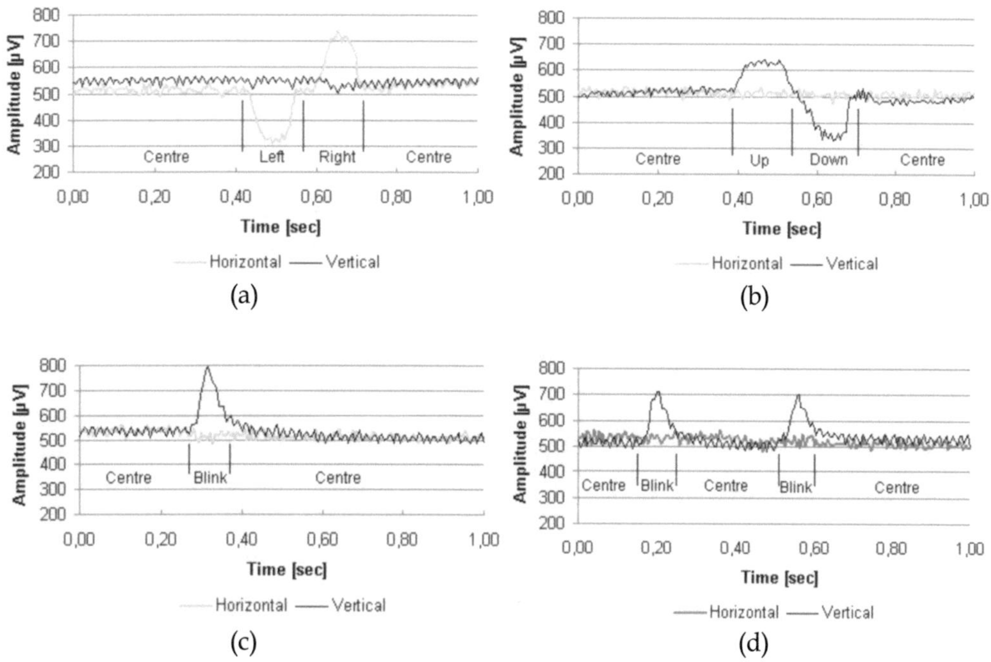

Fig. 6. Voluntary EOG signals: a) Horizontal, b) Vertical, c) Eye blink and d) double blink (Usakli & Gurkan, 2010).

Many studies exist in the literature concerning the application of eye movements to the HCI (Bahill, 1982; Yoshiaki, 1997; Juhola, 1985; Allison et al., 1996; Hutchinson et al., 1989; Norris & Wilson, 1997; Kuno, et al., 1998; Chen et al., 1999; Ihara et al., 2009). The research focused mainly on the word speller. Recognizing eye movements; such as left, right, up and down, and eye blinks to select characters from the virtual keyboard on the screen can use giving a message (Kherlopian et al., 2006; Akan & Argunsah, 2007; Usakli et al, 2009). With the EOG based word speller, it is reported that 5 letter-word such as "Water" can be written in 25 seconds (Usakli & Gurkan, 2010). The menus of this system are shown in figure 7. EOG-controlled cursor interfaces, where the cursor can be controlled by eye movement (Tomita et al., 2006; Tamura et al., 2010) are realized, successfully.

As a communication device, a prototype of a head-mounted display with the eye-gaze detection function was developed which a user can operate by eye movements (Handa & Ebisawa, 2008). With this device, the eye-gaze point was determined from the relative position between the pupil center and the corneal reflection of the light source which were detected by the camera. An eye-gaze controlled navigation and electromyography (EMG) enter (confirm) the selection of letter (Dhillon et al. 2009), and an eye-movement tracking system (Krueger & Stieglitz, 2007; Deng et al., 2009; Septanto et al., 2009) were developed. Another promising EOG based method is a Morse code generator (Wu et al., 2007). Additionally, an EOG-based a powered wheelchair (Barea et al., 2002; Chung-Hsien et al., 2009) and a portable wireless device (Zheng et al., 2009) were realized. The EOG based device allows the patients to generate decisions on a screen by means of simple eye movement signals. These signals can be measured with EMG/EEG electrodes, without the need of complex systems or infra-red cameras. Then, patients are able to select letters on the screen or even communicate basic needs (food drinks, etc.) to the caregiver with a simple movement of their eyes (Usakli et al, 2009). All these studies show that EOG signals can be used as an input for efficient HCI applications. Since the EOG signals are larger, measurement of these signals are easy compared to EEG. This property makes EOG applications much more efficient.

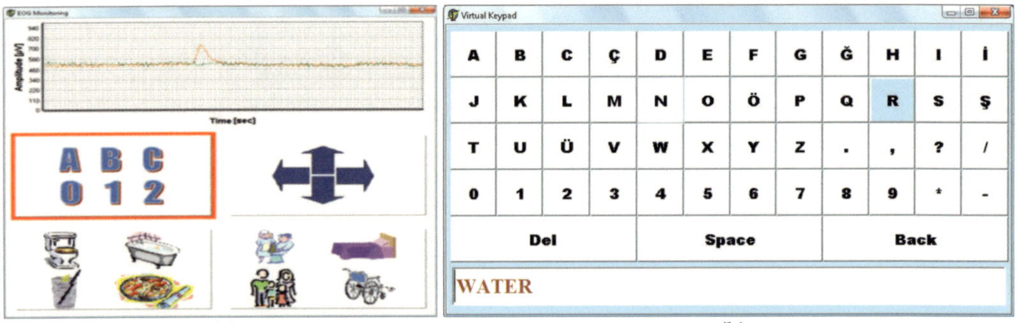

(a) (b)

Fig. 7. The EOG-based user interface (Usakli & Gurkan, 2010): a) Main menu, on the top, vertical and horizontal EOG signals are shown. b) Virtual keyboard: A 5-letter word can be written in 25 seconds.

2.3 Near-infrared spectroscopy based systems

Another approach for noninvasive BCI is based on optical means that measure brain activity by monitoring the hemodynamic response. Near Infrared Spectroscopy (NIRS) optical recording technology measures changes in the brain's oxygen absorption based on the optical properties of hemoglobin. Optical imaging spectroscopy can provide high spatial temporal resolution information about fractional changes in the hemodynamic response to increased neural activity (Mayhev et al, 2000). Human performance and cognitive activities such as attention, working memory, problem solving, etc., can be assessed by fNIR technology (Izzetoglu et al, 2007). NIRS technology usage is growing throughout the world for better understanding cortical activity during cognitive tasks.

NIRS is a spectroscopic method that uses about 800 nm wavelengths in the electromagnetic spectrum. The absorption spectrum in the near-infrared window is presented in figure 8. The level of light absorption related to the amount of oxy-hemoglobin can be measured with detectors. While concentrating, brain uses much more oxygen than normal state. This demand meets with clean blood, then the number of oxy-hemoglobin increases. Therefore, it causes more absorption of the light (Chance et al., 1998). This method gives an idea of oxygenation (changes of (de)oxy-hemoglobin) of blood in cortical capillary vessels.

The primary application of NIRS in the human body is seen through the measurement of the transmission and absorption of NIR light in human body tissues containing information about the changes in hemoglobin concentration. When a specific area of the brain is activated, the localized blood volume in that area changes quickly. Maximum response is observed between the 5th - 9th seconds (Malonek et al. 1997). Optical imaging can measure the location and activity of specific regions of the brain by continuously monitoring blood hemoglobin levels through the determination of optical absorption coefficients.

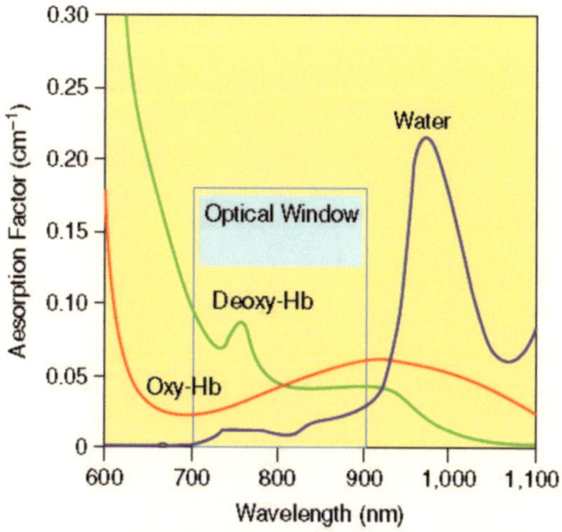

Fig. 8. Absorbtion spectrum in near-infrared window (Izzetoglu et al., 2007).

Figure 9 and 10 show measurement principles of oxygen level in a general NIR system. Photons transmitted with capillary vessels detected by detectors and measured photon intensity related to the oxygen level. fNIR spectroscopy can be used for BCI for the patients with ALS diseases (Bunce et al., 2006); to detect cognitive activity from prefrontal cortex elicited voluntarily (Ayaz et al., 2007).

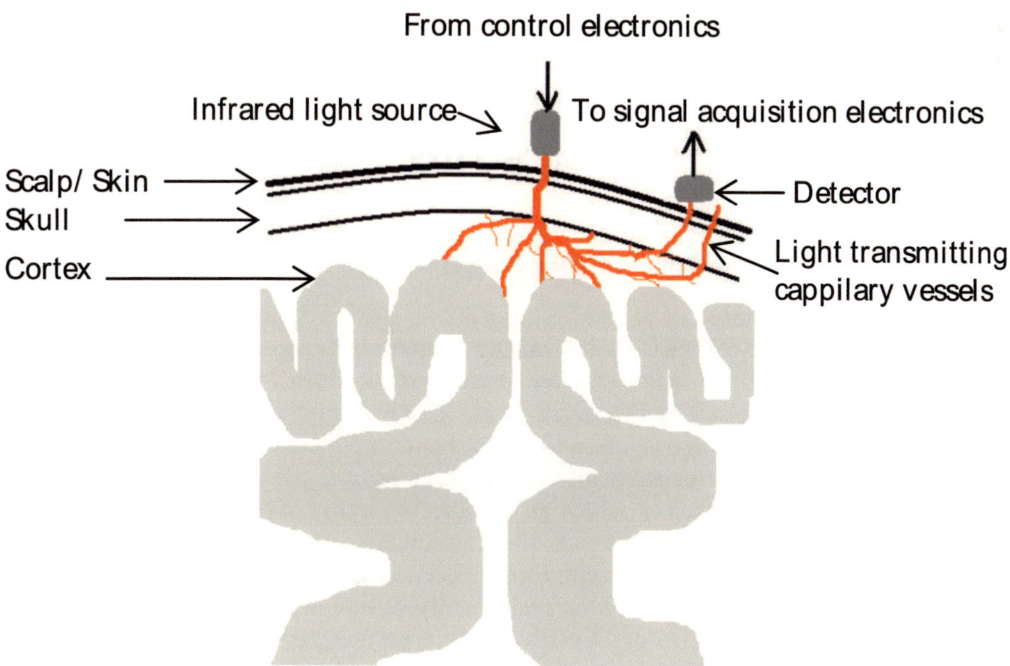

Fig. 9. Measurement of oxygen level in a NIR system. More light absorption means more hemoglobin, and consequently, more oxygenation.

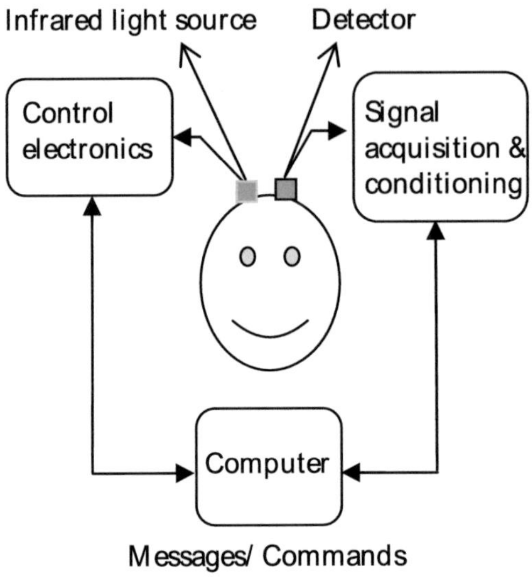

Fig. 10. The block diagram of a NIR system.

2.4 Other approaches

The behavior of active motor units identified via analysis of EMG signals recorded from the first dorsal interosseous muscle using a quadrifilar needle electrode is investigated. According to this study, the motor unit action potential waveforms recorded from patients were more complex than those recorded from control subjects as often observed in motor neuron diseases (Kasi et al., 2009). An eating assistant robot used to assist in eating independence was developed. This assistant robot is useful for people with severe disabilities. A spoon and a camera are attached on the tip of the robotic arm (Takahashi et al., 2001). Additionally, detecting the stress level of the computer user could possibly develop the computers' ability to respond intelligently and help calm negative emotional states of the user during HCI.

3. Feature extraction and classification algorithms

To increase the performance of the HCIs, algorithmic studies related to feature extraction and classification were realized. Motor imagery based BCI, the feature extraction, was performed with an adaptive autoregressive model and the classifier used was an adaptive quadratic discriminant analysis (Vidaurre et al., 2006). A new algorithm for single-trial online classification of imagery left and right hand movements was developed. This algorithm is based on time-frequency information derived from filtering EEG wideband raw data with causal Morlet wavelets, which are adapted to individual EEG spectra (Lemm et al., 2004). For motor imagery EEG, a new EEG recognition algorithm which combined the discrete wavelet transform with the backpropagation neural network was developed (Ming-Ai et al., 2009). According to the results, performance of motor imagery based BCI using a single recording session of EEG or ECoG signals for each subject, is not sufficient. It was relatively easy to obtain classifiable signals quickly from most of the non-paralyzed subjects. However, it was proved that it is impossible to classify the signals obtained from the paralyzed patients by the same methods (Hill, et al., 2006). To detect the ERPs, EEG recordings are transformed into a Haar-wavelet series (Kawakami et al., 1996) and variational Kalman filtering (Sykacek et al., 2004) for adaptive classification in the BCI system was used. The later algorithm translates EEG segments adaptively into probabilities of cognitive states. It allows for nonstationarities in the joint process over cognitive states and generated EEG which may occur during a consecutive number of trials. The wavelet features are used to determine the characteristic of eye movement waveform (Daud & Sudirman, 2010).

A new two-stage approach to extract the μ rhythm component was developed. The first stage uses second-order blind identification with stationary wavelet transform to automatically remove the artifacts. In the second stage, second-order blind identification is applied again to find the μ rhythm component. In this method artifact removal enhances the extraction of the μ rhythm component (Ng & Raveendran, 2009). For classification of motor execution signals, fractal approach provides promising results (Usakli, 2010). An EEG based BCI for users to control a cursor on a computer display is one of the common study area. The developed system uses an adaptive algorithm, based on kernel partial least squares classification, to associate patterns in multichannel EEG frequency spectra with cursor controls (Trejo et al., 2006). For the BCI related classification review can be found in (Lotte et al., 2007).

4. Hybrid approach of human computer interaction

To increase HCI efficiency, hybrid approaches offer good results. Three physiological signals: blood volume pulse, galvanic skin response and pupil diameter, to automatically monitor stress were used, successfully (Zhai et al., 2005). A vision-based multimodal human computer interface system using eye and hand motion tracking was developed. This vision-based virtual interface integrates the function of the motion tracking of eye blinking and hand gestures with the function of their recognition as a virtual interface (Shin & Chun, 2007). EEG error-related signals present a hybrid approach for HCI. This approach uses human gestures to send commands to a computer and exploits brain activity to provide implicit feedback about the recognition of such commands (Chavarriaga et al., 2010).

4.1 Progressing study for hybrid multi-modal human computer interaction

In order to contribute to the HCI field, a novel multi-modal integrated design is completed and establishing an efficient communication and control channel for individuals with motor neuron diseases such as ALS has been continuing. The preliminary results are promising. Using experience in relevant fields such as EEG (Usakli & Gencer, 2007a; Usakli & Gencer, 2007b), EOG (Usakli & Gurkan, 2010; Usakli et al., 2009), BCI prototyping (Erdogan et al, 2009), feature extraction (Usakli, 2010), this novel system attempts to increase usefulness and performance. HR and GSR signals are to be processed with the bio-signals mentioned above, simultaneously. Evaluation of these signals is whether individually or combined, depends on the user. The situation of the severity of the disease also determines the mode of the hybrid multi-mode operation. Through focusing on one of the tasks and sending correct or wrong messages, the bio signals of the subjects will be acquired and processed. Detecting these changes can be used to send data without speaking or control the device.

4.2 Design rationale

The novel system is microcontroller based and battery powered. Data is transferred via optic fiber. To remove the dc level and 50-Hz power line noise, differentiating approach is used. This approach is more successful and practical than the classical methods in the application. After signal conditioning; including filtering and amplification, the analog signal is digitized (at least 12 effective bits) at variable sampling rates and then transferred to the PC via optic fiber. To classify bio-signals, feature extraction with the fractal approach (Usakli, 2010) and wavelet transformed data is applied to artificial neural networks for classification. By using a user-friendly interface, the virtual keyboard and controlling pad allows messages to be given, and some other needs such as cleanup or medical assistance can be selected.

The integrated HCI system provides with high 1) efficiency, 2) usefulness, 3) robustness 4) accurate and reliable output, 5) fast response, 6) user friendly, 7) flexibility, 8) cheap, and 9) designed available components.

5. Conclusions and discussions

ALS is a progressive disease that affects the control of muscle movement by damaging motor neurons. ALS kills the pyramidal neurons of the motor cortex as a corollary muscular functions deteriorate rapidly. For the present, there is no known cure for ALS. Because of these movement and muscular disabilities, these patients need an efficient alternative channel to communicate with their environment or to control devices. In this chapter, HCIs especially BCI technology focused on ALS patients, are presented.

The EEG-based BCI systems represent the only technology for severely paralyzed patients to increase or maintain their communication and control needs. The P300 paradigm for the EEG-based BCI systems is due to the fact that such waveform occurs spontaneously for many of the subjects without need of particular training, which is be useful for increasing the quality of life for the patients. EEG is still the most attractive and popular technology for clinical BCI.

The EOG-based side of the system seems more accurate and fast when compared to the EEG-based systems. It must be noted that the solution for the EOG system is cheaper when compared to the EEG solution and can be used as a first step for the hybrid device for all users. The general idea of a hybrid device is to familiarize the patient with a unique interface, while the user can switch the bioelectric signal for the communication/control of the external devices.

NIRS is a non-invasive optical technique, suitable to assess functional activity by measuring cortical oxygenation (HbO_2) and deoxygenation (Hb). This technology is also a promising and cheap technology for establishing efficient alternative channel, however needs more study on this field to prove ability of efficiency.

In order to increase the usefulness and improve performance, hybrid approaches and multi-modal designs should be investigated. For EEG based BCI systems two or more signal of: P300 response, steady state visual evoked potential, event related desynchronisation, slow cortical potential, sensorimotor rhythms and error-related potentials can be used for an efficient hybrid system. There is no sufficient study in the literature concerning multi-modal system designs. Combination of several bio-signals such as: EEG, EOG, NIRS, HR and GSR, etc offer an improved performance results. The usage of this two or several signals combination may be used depends on the situation of the disability.

6. References

Akan, B. & Argunsah, A.O. (2007). A Human-Computer Interface (HCI) Based on Electrooculogram (EOG) for Handicapped, *Signal Processing and Communications Applications SIU 2007 IEEE 15th,* Eskisehir, Turkey, 11-13 June 2007.

Allison, R.S.; Eizenman, M. & Cheung, B. (1996). Combined Head and Eye Tracking System for Dynamic Testing of the Vestibular System, *IEEE Trans. on Biomedical Engineering,* vol.43, no.11, pp.1073-1082.

Astolfi, L.; Gonzalez Andino, S.; De Vico Fallani, F. & Babiloni, F. (2010). Processing of Brain Signals by Using Hemodynamic and Neuroelectromagnetic Modalities, *Computational Intelligence and Neuroscience,* 2010, ID 934180, pp.1-2.

Ayaz, H.; Izzetoglu, M.; Bunce, S.; Heiman-Patterson & T. Onaral, B. (2007). Detecting Cognitive Activity Related Hemodynamic Signal for Brain Computer Interface Using Functional Near Infrared Spectroscopy, *Neural Engineering, 2007. CNE'07. 3rd International IEEE/EMBS Conference on,* 342, Kohala Coast, HI, USA, 2-5 May 2007.

Bahill, A.T. (1982). Prediction Final Eye Position Halfway Through a Saccade, *IEEE Trans. on Biomedical Engineering,* vol.30, no.12, pp.781-786.

Barea, R.; Boquete, L.; Mazo, M. & Lopez, E. (2002). System for Assisted Mobility Using Eye Movements Based on Electrooculography, *Neural Systems and Rehabilitation Engineering, IEEE Transactions on,* Vol. 10 4, pp. 209 - 218, ISSN: 1534-4320

Bunce, S.; İzzetoglu, M.; İzzetoglu, K.; Onaral, B. & Pourrezaei, K. (2006). Functional Near Infrared Spectroscopy: An Emerging Neuroimaging Modality, *IEEE Engineering in Medicine and Biology Magazine, Special Issue on Clinical Neuroengineering,* 25(4): pp. 54-62.

Buttfield, A.; Ferrez, P.W. & Millan, Jd.R. (2006). Towards a Robust BCI: Error Potentials and Online Learning, *Neural Systems and Rehabilitation Engineering, IEEE Transactions on,* Vol. 14 2, pp. 164 - 168ISSN: 1534-4320

Chance, B.; Anday, E.; Nioka, S.; Zhou, S.; Hong, L.; Worden, .K.; Li, C.; Murray, T.; Ovetsky, Y.; Pidikiti, D. & Thomas, R. (1998). A Novel Method for Fast Imaging of Brain Function, Non-invasively, With Light. *Optics Express,* 2, 10.

Chavarriaga, R.; Biasiucci, A.; Forster, K.; Roggen, D.; Troster, G. & Millan Jdel, R. (2010). Adaptation of Hybrid Human-computer Interaction Systems Using EEG Error-related Potentials, *Conference Proceedings IEEE Eng Med Biol Soc.* pp. 4226-4229, Argentina, Aug. 31-Sept. 4 2010.

Chen, S.; Tsai T. & Luo, C. (1999). Portable Clinical EOG Instrument System, *Proc. of the First Joint BMES/EMBS Conference,* pp.858-859, Atlanta, USA, 13-16 Oct. 1999.

Chung-Hsien, K.; Yi-Chang, C.; Hung-Chyun, C. & Jia-Wun S. (2009). Eyeglasses based electrooculography human-wheelchair interface Systems, *Man and Cybernetics, 2009. SMC 2009. IEEE International Conference on,* San Antonio, TX, USA, pp. 4746 - 4751, ISSN: 1062-922X, 11-14 Oct. 2009.

Daud, W.M.B.W. & Sudirman, R. (2010). A Wavelet Approach on Energy Distribution of Eye Movement Potential Towards Direction, *Industrial Electronics & Applications (ISIEA), 2010 IEEE Symposium on,* Penang, Malaysia, 3-5 Oct. 2010.

Deng, L.Y.; Chun-Liang Hsu Tzu-Ching Lin Jui-Sen Tuan Yung-Hui Chen, (2009). EOG-Based Signal Detection and Verification for HCI, *Machine Learning and Cybernetics, 2009 International Conference on,* 12-15 July 2009, Vol. 6, 3342, Baoding, Hebei, China, ISBN: 978-1-4244-3702-3, 2009

Dhillon, H.S.; Singla, R.; Rekhi, N.S. & Jha, R. (2009). EOG and EMG Based Virtual Keyboard: A Brain-Computer Interface, Computer Science and Information Technology, *ICCSIT 2009. 2nd IEEE International Conference on*, 8-11 Aug. 2009, Beijing, China.

Donchin, E.; Spencer, K.M. & Wijesinghe, R. (2000). The Mental Prosthesis: Assessing the Speed of a P300-Based Brain–Computer Interface, *IEEE Transactions on Rehabilitation Engineering*, Vol. 8, No. 2, pp. 174-178.

Eklund, A.; Andersson, M.; Ohlsson, H.; Ynnerman, A. & Knutsson, H. (2010). A Brain Computer Interface for Communication Using Real-Time fMRI, *Pattern Recognition (ICPR), 2010 20th International Conference on*, Istanbul, Turkey, pp. 3665, ISSN : 1051-4651, 23-26 Aug. 2010.

Erdoğan, B.; Akıncı, B.; Acar, E.; Uşaklı, A. B. & Gençer, N. G. (2009). Prototype Hardware Design for Brain Computer Interface Applications, *14. Biyomedikal Mühendisliği Ulusal Toplantısı*, Izmir, Turkey, 20-22 Mayıs 2009.

Fabiani, G.E.; McFarland, D.J.; Wolpaw, J.R. & Pfurtscheller, G. (2004). Conversion of EEG Activity into Cursor Movement by a Brain-Computer Interface (BCI), *Neural Systems and Rehabilitation Engineering, IEEE Transactions on*, Vol. 12 3, pp. 331 - 338, ISSN: 1534-4320.

Farwell L.A. & Donchin, E. (1988). Talking off the Top of Your Head: A Mental Prosthesis Utilizing Event-Related Brain Potentials, *Electroencephalogr.Clin. Neurophysiol.*, Vol. 70, pp. 510–523.

Gao, X.; Xu, D.; Cheng, M. & Gao, S. (2003). A BCI-Based Environmental Controller for the Motion-Disabled, *Neural Systems and Rehabilitation Engineering, IEEE Transactions on*, Vol. 11, 2, pp. 137 - 140, ISSN: 1534-4320

Gevins, A.; Brickett, P.; Costales, B.; Le, J. & Reutter, B. (1990). Beyond Topographic Mapping: Towards Functional-Anatomical Imaging with 124-Channel EEGs and 3-D MRIs, *Brain Topogr.* 3, pp. 53–64.

Guger C. (2008). Brain Computer Interface, *Lecture notes in The 4th International Summer School on Emerging Technologies in Biomedicine: Advanced Methods for the Estimation of Human Brain Activity and Connectivity, Applications to Rehabilitation Engineering*, Patras, Greece, 29 June - 4 July 2008.

Guger, C. Schlogl, A. Neuper, C. Walterspacher, D. Strein, T. Pfurtscheller, G. (2001). Rapid Prototyping of an EEG-Based Brain-Computer Interface (BCI), *Neural Systems and Rehabilitation Engineerin,g IEEE Transactions on*, Vol. 9 , 1, 49, ISSN : 1534-4320.

Guger, C.; Ramoser, H. & Pfurtscheller, G. (2000). Real-Time EEG Analysis with Subject-Specific Spatial Patterns for a Brain-Computer Interface (BCI), *Rehabilitation Engineering, IEEE Transactions on*, (Dec 2000), Vol. 8 4 , pp. 447 - 456, ISSN: 1063-6528

Handa, S. & Ebisawa, Y. (2008). Development of Head-Mounted Display with Eye-Gaze Detection Function for the Severely Disabled, *Virtual Environments, Human-Computer Interfaces and Measurement Systems, VECIMS 2008 IEEE Conference on*, İstanbul, Turkey, 14-16 July 2008.

Hill, N.J.; Lal, T.N.; Schroder, M.; Hinterberger, T.; Wilhelm, B.; Nijboer, F.; Mochty, U.; Widman, G.; Elger, C.; Scholkopf, B.; Kubler, A. & Birbaumer, N. (2006). Classifying EEG and ECoG Signals Without Subject Training for Fast BCI Implementation: Comparison of Nonparalyzed and Completely Paralyzed Subjects, *Neural Systems and Rehabilitation Engineering, IEEE Transactions on*, Vol. 14, 2 183.

Hutchinson, T.E.; White, K.P.; Martin, W.N.; Reichert K.C. & Frey, L.A. (1989). Human-Computer Interaction Using Eye-Gaze Input, *IEEE Trans. on Systems, Man and Cybernetics*, vol.19, issue 6, pp.1527-1534.

Ihara, T.; Sugi, T.; Eriguchi, M.; Asami, T. & Nakamura, M. (2009). Construction of Simple Communication Method by Use of Neuro-Biological Signals, *ICCAS-SICE, 2009*, pp. 3152, Fukuoka, Japan, 18-21 Aug. 2009.

Izzetoglu, M.; Bunce, S. C.; Izzetoglu, K.; Onaral, B. & Pourrezaei, K. (2007). Functional Brain Imaging, Using Near-Infrared Technology Assessing Cognitive Activity in Real-Life Situations, *IEEE Engineering in Medicine and Biology Magazine*, pp. 38-46.

Juhola, M. (1985). Detection of Saccadic Eye Movements Using a Non-Recursive Adaptive Digital Filter, *Computer Methods and Programs in Biomedicine*, vol.21, pp.81-88.

Kaneswaran, K.; Arshak, K.; Burke, E. & Condron, J. (2010). Towards a Brain Controlled Assistive Technology for Powered Mobility, *Engineering in Medicine and Biology Society (EMBC), 2010 Annual International Conference of the IEEE*, Aug. 31 2010-Sept. 4 2010, Buenos Aires, Argentina, 4176, ISSN : 1557-170X

Kasi, P.K.; Krivickas, L.S.; Meister, M.; Chew, E.; Bonato, P. ; Schmid, M.; Kamen, G. & Pu Liu Clancy, E.A. (2009). Characterization of Motor Unit Behavior in Patients with Amyotrophic Lateral Sclerosis, *Conference on Neural Engineering NER'09 4th International IEEE/EMBS*, Antalya, Turkey, 2009.

Kawakami, T.; Inoue, M.; Kobayashi, Y. & Nakashima, K. (1996). Application of Event Related Brain Potentials to Communication Aids, *Engineering in Medicine and Biology Society, 1996. Bridging Disciplines for Biomedicine, Proceedings of the 18th Annual International Conference of the IEEE*, Vol.: 5, 2229, Amsterdam, Holland, 31 Oct -03 Nov 1996.

Kherlopian, A.R.; Gerrein, J.P.; Yue, M.; Kim, K.E.; Kim, J.W.; Sukumaran, M. & Sajda, P. (2006). Electrooculogram Based System for Computer Control Using a Multiple Feature Classification Model, *Engineering in Medicine and Biology Society, EMBS'06. 28th Annual International Conference of the IEEE*, New York, USA, 2006.

Kuno, Y.; Yagi, T. & Uchikawa, Y. (1998). Development of Eye Pointer with Free Head-Motion, Proc. of the 20th Annual International Conference of the IEEE Engineering in Medicine and Biology Society, Vol. 20, No 4, pp. 1750-1752.

Lebedev, M. A. & Nicolelis, M. A. L. (2006). Brain–machine Interfaces: Past, Present and Future, *Trends in Neurosciences,* Vol. 29 No.9, pp. 536-546.

Lemm, S.; Schafer, C. & Curio, G. (2004). BCI competition 2003-Data Set III: Probabilistic Modeling of Sensorimotor μ Rhythms for Classification of Imaginary Hand Movements, *Biomedical Engineering, IEEE Transactions o,n* Vol. 51 6, pp. 1077 – 1080, ISSN: 0018-9294.

Li, M. A.; Wang, R.; Hao, D. M. & Yang, J.F. (2009). Feature Extraction and Classification of Mental EEG for Motor Imagery, *Natural Computation, 2009 ICNC '09 Fifth International Conference on*, Vol. 2, pp. 139., Tianjin, China, 14-16 Aug. 2009.

Lotte, F.; Congedo, M.; Lécuyer,; A. Lamarche, F. & Arnaldi, B. (2007). A Review of Classification Algorithms for EEG-based Brain-Computer Interfaces, *Journal of Neural Engineering*, Vol.: 4, 2, pp. 1-24, ISSN: 17412560.

Malonek, D.; Dirnagl, U.; Lindauer, U.; Yamada, K.; Kanno, I. & Grinvald, A. (1997). Vascular Imprints of Neuronal Activity: Relationships Between the Dynamics of Cortical Blood Flow, Oxygenation and Volume Changes Following Sensory Stimulation, *Proc. Natl. Acad. Sci.* Vol. 94, pp 14826–14831, USA, December 1997.

Mayhew, J.; Johnston, D.; Berwick, J.; Jones, M.; Coffey, P. & Zheng, Y. (2000). Spectroscopic Analysis of Neural Activity in Brain: Increased Oxygen Consumption Following Activation of Barrel Cortex, *NeuroImage*, 12, pp. 664–675.

McFarland, D.J. & Wolpaw, J.R. (2005). Sensorimotor Rhythm-Based Brain-Computer Interface (BCI): Feature Selection by Regression Improves Performance, *Neural Systems and Rehabilitation Engineering, IEEE Transactions on*, (Sept. 2005), Vol. 13 3, pp. 372 - 379, ISSN: 1534-4320

Millan, J.R.; & Mourino, J. (2003). Asynchronous BCI and Local Neural Classifiers: An Overview of the Adaptive Brain Interface Project, *Neural Systems and Rehabilitation Engineering, IEEE Transactions on*, (June 2003), Vol. 11 2, pp. 159 - 161

Ng, S.C. & Raveendran, P. (2009). Enhanced Rhythm Extraction Using Blind Source Separation and Wavelet Transform, *Biomedical Engineering, IEEE Transactions on*, Vol. 56 , 8, pp. 2024.

Nijboer, F.; Carmien, S.P. ; Leon, E.; Morin, F.O.; Koene, R.A. & Hoffmann, U. (2009). Affective Brain-Computer Interfaces: Psychophysiological Markers of Emotion in Healthy Persons and in Persons with Amyotrophic Lateral Sclerosis, *Affective Computing and Intelligent Interaction and Workshops, ACII 2009. 3rd International Conference on*, Amsterdam, Holland, 10-12 September 2009

Norris, G. & Wilson, E. (1997). The Eye Mouse, an Eye Communication Device, *IEEE Proc. of Bioengineering Conference*, pp.66-67, Durham, N. Carolina , USA, 21-22 May 1997.

Nunez, P. L. (1995). *Neocortical Dynamics and Human EEG Rhythms*, Oxford University Press: New York, 1995, pp. 200-250.

Parker, J.N. & Parker, P.M. (2007). *Amyotrophic Lateral Sclerosis: A Bibliography and Dictionary for Physicians, Patients, and Genome Researchers*, ICON Health Publications, USA, ISBN: 0-497-11327-9, pp. 4.

Peters, B.O.; Pfurtscheller, G. & Flyvbjerg, H. (2001). Automatic Differentiation of Multichannel EEG Signals, (Jan. 2001), Vol. 48 1, pp. 111, ISSN : 0018-9294.

Pfurtscheller, G.; Neuper, C.; Guger, C.; Harkam, W.; Ramoser, H.; Schlögl, A.; Obermaier, B. & Pregenzer, M. (2000). Current Trends in Graz Brain-Computer Interface (BCI) Research, *IEEE Trans. Rehab. Eng.*, vol. 8, pp. 216–219.

Pfurtscheller, G.; Neuper, C. & Birbaumer, N. (2005). Human Brain–Computer Interface, *Motor Cortex In Voluntary Movements, A Distributed System For Distributed Functions*, Alexa Riehle and Eilon Vaadia , (Ed), CRC Press, USA, Chapter 14, pp.1-35.

Schalk, G.; McFarland, D.J.; Hinterberger, T.; Birbaumer, N.; Wolpaw, J.R. (2004). BCI2000: a General-Purpose Brain-Computer Interface (BCI) System, *Biomedical Engineering, IEEE Transactions on* (June 2004), Vol.: 51 6, pp. 1034 - 1043, ISSN: 0018-9294.

Sellers, E. W. & Donchin, E. (2006). A P300-Based Brain-Computer Interface: Initial Tests by ALS Patients, *Clinical Neurophysiology*, 117, pp.538-548.

Sellers, E.W.; Kubler, A. & Donchin, E. (2006). Brain-Computer Interface Research at the University of South Florida Cognitive Psychophysiology Laboratory: The P300 Speller. *Neural Systems and Rehabilitation Engineering, IEEE Transactions on*, Vol.14, No.2, (June 2006) , ISSN : 1534-4320.

Septanto, H.; Prihatmanto, A.S.; Indrayanto, A. (2009). A Computer Cursor Controlled by Eye Movements and Voluntary Eye Winks Using a Single Channel EOG, *Electrical Engineering and Informatics, Selangor, 2009. ICEEI'09. International Conference on*, Issue Date: 5-7 Aug. 2009, pp. 117 - 120.

Shin, G. & Chun J. (2007). Vision-Based Multimodal Human Computer Interface Based on Parallel Tracking of Eye and Hand Motion, *Convergence Information Technology International Conference on*, 21-23 Nov. 2007, pp. 2443, Gyeongju, S. Korea.

Sutter, E. E. (1992). The Brain Response Interface: Communication Through Visually-induced Electrical Brain Response, *J. Microcomput. Appl.*, vol. 15, pp. 31–45.

Sykacek, P.; Roberts, S.J. & Stokes, M. (2004). Adaptive BCI based on Variational Bayesian Kalman Filtering: an Empirical Evaluation, *Biomedical Engineering, IEEE Transactions on*, (May 2004), Vol. 51 5, pp. 719 - 727, ISSN: 0018-9294.

Takahashi, Y.; Hasegawa, N.; Takahashi, K. & Hatakeyama, T. (2001). Human Interface Using PC Display with Head Pointing Device for Eating Assist Robot and Emotional Evaluation by GSR Sensor, *Robotics and Automation, 2001, Proceedings 2001 ICRA IEEE International Conference on*, Vol. 4, pp. 3674, ISSN:1050-4729, Seoul, S. Korea, May 21-26 2001.

Tamura, H.; Miyashita, M.; Tanno, K. & Fuse, Y. (2010). Mouse Cursor Control System Using Electrooculogram Signals, *World Automation Congress WAC 2010*, ISSN : 2154-4824, Kobe, Japan, 19-23 Sept. 2010.

Tomita, Y.; Igarashi, Y.; Honda, S. & Matsuo, N. (1996). Electro-Oculography Mouse for Amyotrophic Lateral Sclerosis Patients, *Bridging Engineering in Medicine and Biology Society Disciplines for Biomedicine Proceedings of the 18th Annual International Conference of the IEEE*, Vol. 5, pp. 1780 - 1781, Amsterdam, Holland, 31 Oct-3 Nov 1996.

Townsend, G.; Graimann, B. & Pfurtscheller, G. (2004). Continuous EEG Classification During Motor Imagery-Simulation of an Asynchronous BCI, *Neural Systems and Rehabilitation Engineering, IEEE Transactions on*, Vol. 12 2, pp. 258 - 265, ISSN: 1534-4320.

Trejo, L.J.; Rosipal, R. & Matthews, B. (2006). Brain-Computer Interfaces for 1-D and 2-D Cursor Control: Designs Using Volitional Control of the EEG Spectrum or Steady-state Visual Evoked Potentials, *Neural Systems and Rehabilitation Engineering, IEEE Transactions on*, Vol. 14 2, pp. 225, ISSN : 1534-4320.

Turnip, A.; Hong, K.S.; Ge, S.S. & Jeong, M. Y. (2010). Neural Networks Training Based on Sequential Extended Kalman Filtering for Single Trial EEG Classification, *Knowledge and Systems Engineering KSE 2010 Second International Conference on*, p. 85, Hanoi, Vietnam, 7-9 October 2010.

Usakli, A. B.; Gurkan, S.; Aloise, F.; Vecchiato, G. & Babiloni, F.(2009). A Hybrid Platform Based on EOG and EEG Signals to Restore Communication for Patients Afflicted with Progressive Motor Neuron Diseases, *31st Annual International Conference of the IEEE EMBS*, pp.543-546, Minneapolis, Minnesota, USA, September 2-6, 2009.

Usakli, A.B. & Gencer N.G., (2007). A USB-Based 256-Channel Electroencephalographic Data-Acquisition System for Electrical Source Imaging of the Human Brain, *Instrumentation Science and Technology*, Vol. 35, pp.255-273.

Usakli, A.B. & Gencer, N.G. (2007). Performance Tests of A Novel Electroencephalographic Data-Acquisition System, *The Fifth International Conference on Biomedical Engineering IASTED BIOMED 2007*, pp. 253-257, Innsbruck, Austria, February 14–16, 2007.

Usakli, A.B. & Gurkan S. (2010). Design of a Novel Efficient Human Computer Interface: An Electrooculagram Based Virtual Keyboard, *IEEE Transaction on Instrumentation and Measurement*, Vol. 59, No.8, pp. 2099-2108.

Usakli, A.B. (2010). Modeling of Movement-Related Potentials Using a Fractal Approach, *Journal of Computational Neuroscience*, Vol.28, No. 3, pp. 595-603.

Van Kokswijk, J. & Van Hulle, M. (2010). Self Adaptive BCI as Service-Oriented Information System for Patients with Communication Disabilities, *New Trends in Information Science and Service Science NISS 2010 4th International Conference on*, pp. 264-269, Gyeongju, S. Korea, 11-13 May 2010.

Vidaurre, C.; Schlogl, A.; Cabeza, R.; Scherer, R. & Pfurtscheller, G. (2006). A Fully On-Line Adaptive BCI, *Biomedical Engineering, IEEE Transactions on*, (June 2006), Vol. 53 6, pp. 1214 - 1219, ISSN: 0018-9294.

Weiskopf, N.; Mathiak, K.; Bock, S.W.; Scharnowski, F.; Veit, R.; Grodd, W.; Goebel, R. & Birbaumer, N. (2004). Principles of a Brain-Computer Interface (BCI) Based on Real-Time Functional Magnetic Resonance Imaging (fMRI), *Biomedical Engineering, IEEE Transactions on*, (June 2004), Vol. 51 6, pp. 966 - 970, ISSN: 0018-9294.

Wolpaw, J. R (2003). Brain-Computer Interfaces: Signals, Methods, and Goals, *Proceedings of the 1st International IEEE EMBS Conference on Neural Engineering*, pp. 584-585, Capri Island, Italy, March 20-22, 2003.

Wolpaw, J.; Birbaumer, N.; McFarland, D.; Pfurtscheller, G. & Vaughan, T. (2002). Brain-Computer Interfaces for Communication and Control, *Electroencephalography and Clinical Neurophysiology*, vol. 113 6, pp. 767-791.

Wolpaw, J.R.; McFarland, D. J. & Vaughan, T. M. (2000). Brain-Computer Interface Research at the Wadsworth center, *IEEE Trans. Rehab. Eng.*, vol. 8, pp. 222–226.

Wolpaw, J.R.; McFarland, D.J.; Vaughan, T.M. & Schalk, G. (2003). The Wadsworth Center Brain-Computer Interface (BCI) Research and Development Program, *Neural Systems and Rehabilitation Engineering, IEEE Transactions on*, (June 2003), Vol.: 11 2 pp. 1 - 4, ISSN: 1534-4320.

Wu, C.M.; Huang, K.G.; Chang, S.H.; Hsu, S.C. & Lin, C.L. (2007). EOG Single Switch Morse Code Translate Input Device for Individuals with the Motor Neuron Disease, *TENCON 2007 - 2007 IEEE Region 10 Conference*, Taipei, Oct. 30-Nov. 2 2007.

Wu, C.M.; Huang, K.G.; Chang, S.H.; Hsu, S.C. & Lin, C.L. (2007). EOG Single Switch Morse Code Translate Input Device for Individuals with the Motor Neuron disease, *ENCON 2007 - 2007 IEEE Region 10 Conference*, Taipei, Taiwan, Oct. 30 2007-Nov. 2 2007.

Yoshiaki, K. (1997). Development of Eye-Gaze Input Interface, *Proc. of 7th International conference on Human Computer Interaction*, pp.44-49.

Zhai, J.; Barreto, A.; Chin, C. & Chao, L. (2005). Realization of Stress Detection Using Psychophysiological Signals for Improvement of Human-computer Interactions, *Southeast Conference Proceedings, IEEE*, pp.415-420, Fort Lauderdale, Florida, USA, 8-10 April 2005.

Zheng, X.; Liu, X. L. J.; Chen, W. & Hao, Y. (2009). A Portable Wireless Eye Movement-Controlled Human-Computer Interface for the Disabled, *Complex Medical Engineering, 2009. CME. ICME International Conference on*, Tempe, Arizona, USA, 9-11 April 2009.

31

Overview of Cognitive Function in ALS, with Special Attention to the Temporal Lobe: Semantic Fluency and Rating the Approachability of Faces

Heike Schmolck[1,3], Paul Schulz[1,2,4] and Michele York[1,2]
[1]*Baylor*
[2]*Veterans Hospital*
[3]*Ruan Neuroscience Center*
[4]*University of Texas*
USA

1. Introduction

Amyotrophic lateral sclerosis (ALS) is a progressive neurodegenerative disorder that affects upper and lower motor neurons and is more recently known to be associated with declines in cognitive and behavioral functions for a subset of patients (Strong, et al., 1996; Strong et al., 2009). The cognitive changes associated with ALS can vary from mild impairments that may or may not affect the individual's daily functioning to more severe cognitive and behavioral changes that meet criteria for a diagnosis of frontotemporal dementia (ALS-FTD). There are at least mild cognitive changes in 40 to 60% of sporadic and familial ALS patients (Massman et al., 1996; Phukan et al., 1996; Ringholz et al., 2005; Wheaton et al., 2007). The cognitive and behavioral changes associated with ALS follow a pattern consistent with involvement of the frontal and temporal lobes (Strong et al., 2009, Hodges et al., 2004), presenting as difficulties with attention, working memory, verbal fluency, and semantic abilities (Abe et al., 1997; Ringholz et al., 2005; Rippon et al., 2006, Schmolck et al., 2007; Strong et al, 1999; Strong et al., 2009). Furthermore, 15% of ALS patients demonstrate more severe cognitive and behavioral changes consistent with ALS-FTD (Lomen-Hoeth et al., 2002; Ringholz et al., 2005; Wheaton et al., 2007), presenting as declines in judgment, problem solving, and reasoning, which are more frontally mediated cognitive functions. In addition to cognitive changes, up to 25% of patients with ALS may also experience significant changes in their behavior, mood, and personality characteristics (Hodges et al., 2004; Kertesz et al., 2005), including a loss of empathy, problems with organization and planning, changes in social behavior and personality, difficulties with impulse control, and apathy.

The temporal lobes are purported to be involved in auditory perception, language comprehension, naming, processing of semantic knowledge and long-term memory storage, high-level visual processing of complex stimuli such as faces and scenes, and episodic memory (Lezak, 1995). In addition, they contain the amygdala and associated limbic areas, which are key structures for processing emotional stimuli and detecting threat from the environment, and are of particular interest for ALS patients. ALS patients show a lack of memory enhancement for highly emotional stimuli (Abrahams et al., 2005). Furthermore, social judgment was found to be decreased in individuals with ALS as compared to healthy controls (Flaherty-Craig et al., 2011). Behavioral dysfunction has been linked to decreased performance on cognitive measures; however it is unclear if these changes present and/or progress independently (Wooley et al., 2009). The relationship between the fontal and temporal cognitive and behavioral changes in ALS is not well understood. Here, we report on two studies examining temporal cognitive changes in ALS.

Indentifying and acknowledging that ALS patients may also be dealing with cognitive and/or behavioral changes in addition to their debilitating motor declines may help their physicians and caregivers to better care for the individual with ALS and anticipate problems that they may experience throughout the disease progression (Hecht et al., 2003). These cognitive changes can affect the everyday social interactions of ALS patients, and they are vital for the execution of more complex tasks such as decision-making, problem solving, and management of occupational demands (e.g., multi-tasking). Patients with these types of impairments have significantly shorter survival than other ALS patients and are twice as likely to be noncompliant with interventions (Woolley et al., 2008). Safety, financial planning, driving, and occupational performance can be of concern in patients who demonstrate impairments in these cognitive domains. Consequently, the predictive value of these cognitive abilities may aid in the clinical management of ALS patients, aiding physicians in making decisions concerning the overall safety of their patients and their patients' ability to work, drive, and manage their medication regimen. Educating the patients and family members to better understand these cognitive and behavioral changes as part of the disease process can help improve the patient's quality of life and reduce the feelings of caregiver burden (Murphy et al., 2009).

2. Rating the approachability of faces in ALS – Too much or not enough fear?

We hypothesize that alterations in emotional cognition indicative of amygdala dysfunction occur in ALS, but are often unrecognized. Changes in the emotional expression of ALS patients are reported by clinicians, and often by patients themselves. Pseudobulbar affect is a common problem. ALS patients also have a lower incidence of depression than patients afflicted with similarly debilitating diseases (Rabkin et al., 2005), and many have a stunning lack of concern regarding their grave illness. They often have a very pleasant personality, which has lead clinicians to call ALS the "nice guy's disease". Emotional lability and mild disinhibition are commonly found.

None of the above observations can be explained satisfactorily by behavioral changes commonly seen with frontal dysfunction alone. Thus, while examining frontal contributions to social and emotional cognitive changes in ALS has been fruitful, other areas that have been implicated in social cognition have not been studied much. In one study, ALS patients have been found to show a lack of memory enhancement for highly emotional stimuli, which is consistent with amygdala dysfunction (Abrahams et al., 2005). We have previously shown in a small group of patients that ALS patients have a tendency to rate faces inappropriately approachable compared to normal controls (Schmolck et al., 2007); this behavior is also consistent with amygdala dysfunction. Lastly, a study by Zimmerman and colleagues (2007) found that over 62% of patients with bulbar ALS had deficits in their ability to properly recognize the emotions of others (emotional perceptual deficits).

Few neuropathologic studies have examined non-frontal areas in ALS brains. In the ALS-Parkinson-dementia complex of Guam, tau and alpha-synuclein aggregates are a common finding in the amygdala (for example, Yamazaki et al., 2000). Case series of sporadic ALS patients with and without dementia have demonstrated ubiquitinated intraneuronal inclusions and spongiform changes in the amygdala and other limbic structures (Kawashima et al., 2001; Kato et al., 1994; also Tsuchiya 2002).

The amygdala is a key structure for processing emotional stimuli and detecting threat from the environment (e.g., Adolphs 2003a; Adolphs 2003b). Patients with bilateral amygdala damage are impaired at recognizing negative basic emotions in facial expressions, most notably fear (e.g., Adolphs et al., 1994; Broks et al., 1998;, Schmolck & Squire 2001) . In a much broader sense, they also have difficulties making social judgments, and interpreting social signals about intentions and internal states (e.g. Adolphs 2003b); for example, patients are differentially impaired at recognizing complex social emotions relative to complex non-social emotions (Adolphs et al., 2002), and assigning emotional states to people (e.g. Fine et al., 2001) and objects (anthropomorphizing; Heberlein & Adolphs, 2004). This is also seen clinically when patients get themselves into unfavorable situations because they are unable to correctly read and act on threatening environmental and social stimuli. Adolphs et al. (1998) replicated this observation most closely in a laboratory experiment, showing that patients indiscriminately rated unfamiliar faces as approachable and trustworthy while controls did not.

We administered the same task to ALS patients hypothesizing that their "nice" personalities and strikingly good morale in facing a debilitating disease might be due, at least in part, to amygdala dysfunction as part of a broader multi-system disorder.

2.1 Participants

91 ALS patients were recruited from the MDA-ALS clinic and the ALSA clinic at Baylor College of Medicine. 78 age and gender matched controls were recruited from 2 groups - family members and friends of ALS patients, as well as patients from the Baylor Cardiology CHF clinic (n = 24). The latter group was chosen to control for the effects of living with a serious life threatening chronic illness. Data from both control groups were combined in the final analysis, as there were no significant differences between groups. Please see Table 1 for demographic characteristics for both groups.

	ALS	CON
Gender		
Male	54.9%	54.3%
Female	45.1%	45.7%
Age		
Mean	50.4	58
Range	22-78	30-84
Disease Type		
Limb onset	61.5%	
Bulbar onset	27.5%	
No information	10.9%	
Disease Duration		
Mean	2.5 years	
Range	0.5 - 14 years	

Table 1. Demographic Characteristics of Participants

2.2 Methods

Participants viewed 60 images of faces (Adolphs et al., 1998) in a pseudo-random order on a computer screen. 40 faces were excluded to reduce testing time. We chose the 20 most approachable, the 20 least approachable, and the 20 intermediate faces. Faces expressed a mix of neutral or emotional expressions. Before viewing, participants were given the following case scenario:

"Imagine you are in a city you do not know well, you are by yourself, it is getting dark and you have lost directions. You see many people on the street. You need to decide who you would like to approach to ask for directions.

We will show you 60 faces. For each face, we would like you to decide how approachable that person is in the particular situation that you are in."

Participants were then instructed to respond with an answer between -3 and 3, and were given examples of what each rating would mean. There was no time limitation. Answers were recorded by the examiner. To minimize gender effects, all faces that had received different ratings ($p < .10$) from male and female controls were eliminated from further analysis; 51 faces remained.

As part of their initial ALS evaluation in the MDA-ALS or ALSA Clinic, several patients (n = 49) were given a comprehensive neuropsychological interview and testing battery and received a cognitive diagnosis: cognitively intact, subtle deficits, mild-to-moderate or severe (FTD) deficits (see Table 2).

2.3 Results

For each participant, three means were calculated - overall mean rating, mean rating for the 10 most approachable faces, and mean rating for the 10 least approachable faces. We then divided participants into Trusters, Suspicious Responders (SR) and Conventional Responders (CR). Participants were labeled Trusters if their average rating for the 10 least approachable faces was above zero; i.e. they regarded even those faces as approachable that controls would not have approached. They were labeled Suspicious Responders if their average rating for the 10 most approachable faces was lower than 1, indicating that they felt faces difficult to approach that controls found very approachable.

While 65.4% of participants in the control group were CR, 62.6% in the ALS group were either Trusters or Suspicious Responders (Figure 1 "minority responders"; Chi square test $p < .001$).

Thirty-one ALS patients were Trusters, 26 were SR, and 34 were CR (34.1%, 28.6% and 37.4%, respectively). In the control group, 16 were Trusters, 11 SR and 51 CR (20.5%, 14.1% and 65.4%, respectively). Both Trusters (34.1% vs. 20.5%) and Suspicious Responders (28.6% vs. 14.1%) were significantly more common in the ALS group (Chi Square tests; both ps < .01) than in the control group.

We previously reported results on 26 patients (Schmolck et al., 2007); only Trusters were identified in that subgroup (n = 14) since that was a common response pattern. In retrospect, the SR pattern was present in 3 patients but not recognized at the time. Our finding in a large group of ALS patients thus not only confirms our earlier results, but also expands them to describe a new common response pattern in the ALS group.

In the subgroup of 49 patients with neuropsychological testing, there was no clear correlation between cognitive diagnosis and performance on the faces task (Table 2). In the small number of patients with FTD (n = 8), half of patients were CR and half of patients were Trusters (Table 2).

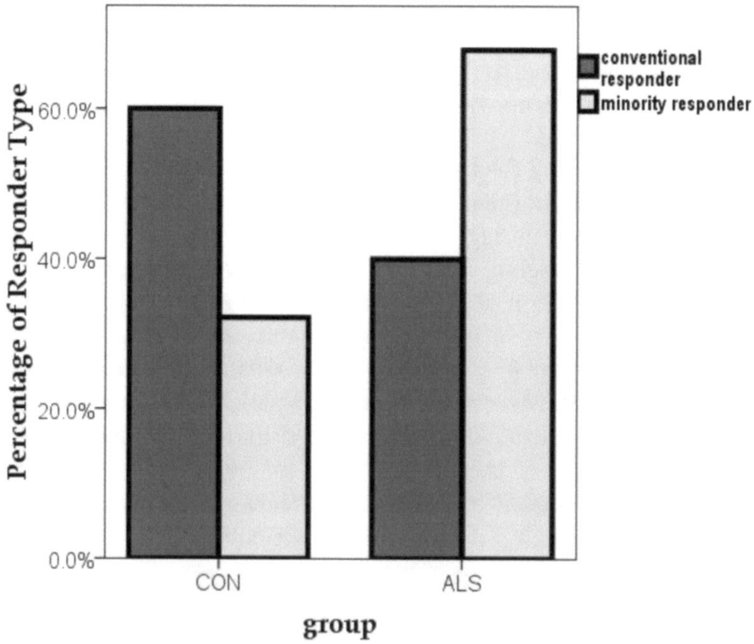

Fig. 1. Significantly more ALS patients were minority responders (Trusters and Suspicious Responders combined)

	Cognitive Diagnosis				
	Intact	Subtle	MiMo	FTD	Total
Conventional Responder	10	3	3	4	20
Truster	10	1	1	4	16
Suspicious Responder	5	2	6	0	13
Total	25	6	10	8	49

Table 2. Cognitive Performance and Responder Type in the subgroup of patients with neuropsychological testing results. MiMo - Mild to moderate impairment

2.4 Discussion

We have shown that more than half of our patients with ALS have an abnormal response pattern. One response pattern (Trusters) shows similar behavioral characteristics to patients with bilateral amygdala damage on a paradigm asking participants to judge the approachability of unfamiliar faces. This difficulty can be generalized as an inability to correctly recognize threat in a given social context. A person with this behavioral pattern would be expected to be trusting, friendly and open to cooperation, and show very little hostility or suspicion. Many clinicians caring for ALS patients have noted this type of personality in ALS patients. The second response pattern is that of overly suspicious behavior (SR). These patients will be overly reluctant to approach unfamiliar faces, also showing poor discrimination between approachable and less approachable faces. These patients show a response pattern that might be seen in autism (e.g. Baron-Cohen et al., 2001), or patients with anxiety disorder or social phobia, which have both been linked to hyperactivity of the amygdala (e.g. Freitas-Ferrari et al., 2010; Blair et al., 2011). Clinically, this patient population might not be easily recognized if not specifically probed by the examiner during history taking.

There are some clues regarding the basic mechanism by which amygdala damage leads to impairments making social judgments from faces. Complex mental states are recognized disproportionately from the eye region of the face, and when making judgments about mental states from the eye region, healthy controls activate the amygdala in functional imaging studies (Baron-Cohen et al., 1999; Baron-Cohen et al., 2001). Bilateral damage to the amygdala has been shown to impair the recognition of negative basic emotions in facial expressions, notably fear (e.g. Adolphs et al., 1994; Calder et al., 1996; Broks et al., 1998; Anderson et al., 2000). Investigating the first patient reported to show this deficit (S.M.), Adolphs and colleagues (2005) demonstrated that her impairment stems from an inability to make normal use of information from the eye region of faces when judging emotions. They traced this deficit to a lack of spontaneous fixations on the eyes during free viewing of faces. Although SM fails to look normally at the eye region in all facial expressions, her selective impairment in recognizing fear is explained by the fact that the eyes are the most important feature for identifying this emotion. It is thus likely that inadequate evaluation of the eye region leads to impairments in the Approachability Task, and perhaps in some real life situations. While this mechanism may explain some of the impairments in social cognition seen in patients with amygdala damage, it would not explain others, such as detection of fear and anger from voices (Scott et al., 1997) impaired anthropomorphizing (Heberlein et al., 2004), or inferring internal mental states (Fine et al., 2001).

Performance on the Approachability Paradigm was not related to frontal dysfunction. While we cannot be certain, this suggests that the response pattern seen in the patients without frontal dysfunction was more likely to be due to amygdala involvement. Healthy volunteers judging the trustworthiness of faces activate the amygdala bilaterally for faces judged untrustworthy in an fMRI paradigm (Winston et al., 2002). Also, even in the presence of overt FTD, only half of the patients had abnormal performance on the Approachability Paradigm.

3. Phonemic and semantic verbal fluency in ALS

Verbal fluency tasks, which require an individual to generate words starting with a specified letter (phonemic fluency) or in a specified category (semantic fluency), have been shown to be sensitive tools for identifying cognitive dysfunction in neurologically impaired populations (Canning, Leach, Struss, Ngo, & Black, 2004; Ho et al., 2002; Fangundo et al., 2008; Libon et al., 2009). Phonemic fluency involves prefrontal and frontal functions because it requires strategic processes for searching the lexicon (Leggio, Silveri, Petrosini, & Molinari,, 2000; Martin, Wiggs, Lalonde, & Mack, 1994), while semantic fluency localizes more to the left anterior temporal lobe, where representations are categorized by meaning (Pihlajamki et al., 2000). Recent functional magnetic resonance imaging (fMRI) studies have verified the neuroanatomical locations involved in phonemic fluency in the left premotor and inferior frontal gyrus and for semantic fluency in the left fusiform and left middle temporal gyrus (Bim et al., 2009; Meinzer et al., 2009). Consequently, by evaluating ALS patient performances on phonemic and semantic fluencies, we were able to investigate frontal and temporal function in ALS patients.

The cognitive substrates underlying verbal fluency have been examined further in neuropsychological studies (Baldo, Schwartz Wilkins & Dronkers, 2006; Troyer, Moscovitch, & Winocur, 1997). Clustering and switching have been shown to be components that underlie verbal fluency performance (Troster et al., 1998; Troyer et al., 1997). Clusters are groups of related words, accessed through memory stores, in which intact performance is purported to rely on temporal lobe functioning. Switching refers to the process of changing from one cluster to another, which has been associated with frontal-lobe-mediated abilities (Troyer et al., 1998). We investigated differences in phonemic and semantic fluency between ALS patients, classified into neurocognitive subgroups, and healthy participants and whether these declines in verbal fluency were due predominantly to changes in clustering, switching, or a combination of the two component processes (Lepow et al., 2010).

3.1 Participants

A total of 49 ALS patients and 25 healthy control participants (HC) were recruited from the Baylor College of Medicine (BCM) ALS Association Clinic. The HC participants were caregivers or family members of the ALS patients who participated in this study. ALS patients' motor functioning was evaluated by the ALS Functional Rating Scale (ALS-FRS), and their site of onset (limb vs. bulbar) was recorded at their initial clinic visit.

A subset of these ALS patients (*N* = 36) underwent a comprehensive neuropsychological assessment, and these data were used to classify participants as cognitively intact (ALS-intact), mildly impaired (ALS-mild), or FTD (ALS-FTD). Patients were coded as ALS-FTD using Strong et al.'s (2009) criteria. Patients were coded as ALS-mild if their neuropsychological evaluation, excluding their performance on phonemic and semantic fluency measures, revealed cognitive deficits (<1.5 *SDs* below the mean for the appropriate normative sample) in one cognitive domain. The ALS cognitive impaired classification (ALSci) described by Strong et al. (2009) is based on impairments in executive functioning only; however, we excluded both phonemic and semantic fluency so as not to classify patients based on the measures under investigation. Hence, additional measures of executive functioning were limited. Consequently, patients were classified based on their entire comprehensive evaluation.

3.2 Methods

3.2.1 Neuropsychological evaluation

The comprehensive neuropsychological assessment examined basic orientation (Mini Mental Status Examination [Folstein Folstein & McHugh, 1975]), attention/ information-processing speed (Wechsler Adult Intelligence Scale-3rd Edition, [WAIS-III; The Psychological Corporation, 1997], Digit Span, Trail Making Test Part A, and Verbal Sustained Attention Test), verbal learning (Rey Auditory Verbal Learning Test [Schmidt, 1996], visual learning (Brief Visual Memory Test-Revised), language (Boston Naming Test [Kaplan, Goodglass, & Weintraub, 1983]), visual-spatial abilities (Rey-Osterrieth Complex Figure Test [Meyers, & Meyers 1995], WAIS-III Block Design), and executive function (Wisconsin Card Sorting Test [Heaton, 1981], Trail Making Test Part B).

3.2.2 Fluency scoring methods

Verbal fluency tests were administered to ALS patients and HC in the following manner: Patients were asked to generate a list of words that began with a specific letter (F, A, & S was used for phonemic fluency) or category (Animals was used for semantic fluency) in a 1-minute period. Prior to administering the test, patients were told that proper nouns and root words with different suffices were not allowed. Words generated (including repetitions and rule breaks) were recorded verbatim. The total number of words generated, excluding repetitions and rule breaks, was the standard measure of analysis and Troyer's (Troyer et al, 1997) scoring methods for clustering and switching were utilized.

3.2.3 Verbal fluency components

Phonemic fluency. Clusters are scored for groups of phonemic words, or words that are similar based on phonemic rules for each letter. Troyer and colleagues (1997) defined parameters for scoring clusters, including: (a) words beginning with the same first two letters, (b) rhyming words, and (c) words that are the same syllabic length and differ only by a vowel sound. For example, *follow, fog, fond, foster, forget* is a cluster of four because the words all begin with the same phoneme, and the cluster size begins with the second word of a cluster. Each word that is not classified in a group of related phonemic words is scored as a cluster of zero. The *number of clusters* is defined as the total sum of individual clusters, including clusters of zero. The *cluster value* is defined as the sum number of consecutive related words excluding the first word of each grouping, or the sum of the values assigned to the clusters. *Switches* are defined as any break between clusters, including clusters of zero.

Semantic fluency. In the semantic fluency task, clusters are composed of words that are semantically related. Troyer's method defines the categories for finding semantic clusters in "Animals" as living environments, zoological categories, and human use, with each supraordinate category containing specific exemplars. The *cluster size* begins with the second word of a cluster. For example the group, *cow, horse, chicken,* and *rooster,* is scored as a cluster of three because they are all farm animals. Number of clusters, cluster value, and switches were calculated as discussed above.

3.3 Results

3.3.1 Participant characteristics

The 49 ALS patients and the 25 HCs did not differ in age or education level (Table 1). There were significantly more female HCs than female ALS patients (p=0.006). Gender correlated significantly with Troyer's average number of switches for phonemic fluency; thus, gender was entered as a covariate in this analysis. There were no significant demographic differences between the three groups of ALS patients coded for degree of cognitive dysfunction (Table 1), including site of onset (p = 0.36) and total ALS-FRS scores (p = 0.34).

Phonemic fluency. ALS patients generated fewer numbers of clusters than did HCs (p = 0.04; Figure 1). ALS patients also generated fewer switches between clusters; however, once gender was entered as a covariate in the analysis, this difference was no longer significant (p =0.14). The number of clusters differed significantly between the ALS groups, with the ALS-intact group scoring higher than the ALS-mild and the ALS-FTD groups (p = 0.004; Table 2). The number of switches also differed between the ALS cognitive groups, with the ALS-intact patients switching more often than both the ALS-mild and the ALS-FTD groups (p =0 .004; Table 2). The cluster value scores did not differ significantly between the ALS groups (p=0 .13).

Table 1	ALS				HC (n=25)	p-value
	Intact (n=13)	Mild (n=17)	FTD (n=7)	Total (n=49)		
Gender (M/F)	8/5	10/7	3/4	28/21	6/19	**0.006**
Age (yrs)	54.2 (8.96)	58.1 (12.1)	61.4 (14.2)	56.1 (11.3)	52.7 (13.0)	0.28
Education (yrs)	14.1 (2.95)	13.3 (1.32)	12.9 (3.44)	13.8 (2.71)	15.2 (2.99)	0.07

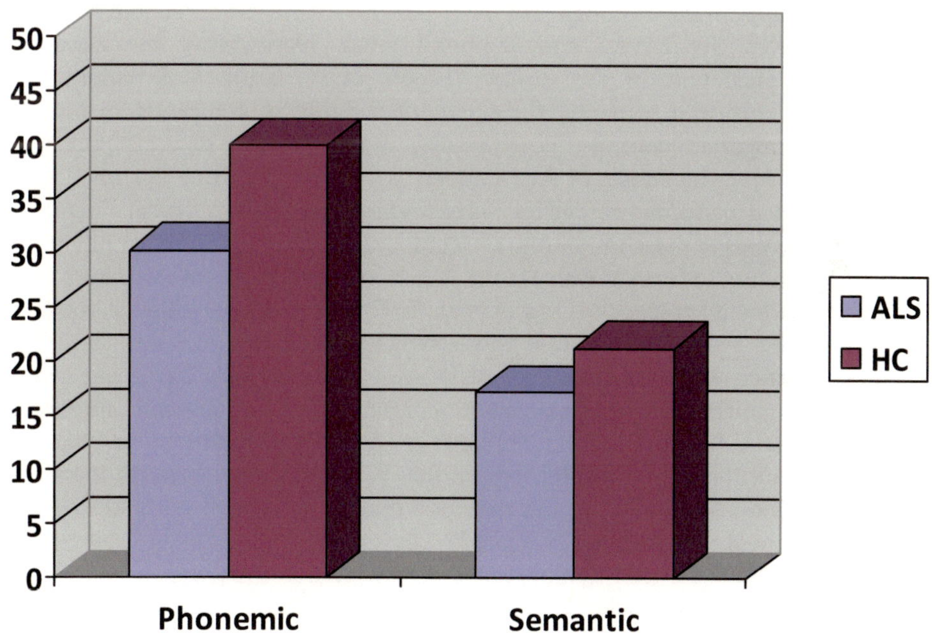

Fig. 1. Total Phonemic and Semantic Fluency Scores for ALS and HC groups

Semantic fluency. The total group of ALS patients generated fewer numbers of clusters (p = 0.01) and made significantly fewer switches between clusters (p =0.03) than did the HCs. The total groups did not differ significantly on the number of words within semantic clusters (cluster value=0.15). The ALS-FTD patients generated a smaller cluster value score than did ALS-intact and ALS-mild groups (p=0.03). The number of clusters and number of switches demonstrated trends toward significant differences between the groups (p=0.07, p= 0.06, respectively; Table 2).

Table 2	ALS intact Mean (SD)	ALS mild Mean (SD)	ALS FTD Mean (SD)	p-value
Total				
Phonemic	37.2 (10.9) [1,2]	30.1 (9.76) [1]	23.3 (6.54) [2]	**0.009**
Semantic	19.0 (5.29) [1,2]	18.3 (5.72) [1]	12.9 (4.05) [2]	**0.02**
Troyer				
Phonemic Fluency				
Number of Clusters	9.84 (2.34)[1,2]	7.15 (2.79)[1]	6.43 (2.17)[2]	**0.004**
Cluster Value	3.20 (1.77)	2.72 (1.62)	1.67 (1.12)	0.13
Switches	8.84 (2.34) [1,2]	6.15 (2.81) [1]	5.43 (2.17) [2]	**0.004**
Semantic Fluency				
Cluster Value	10.94 (3.78)[1]	8.85 (3.83)	6.43 (3.41)[1]	**0.03**
Number of clusters	10.59 (3.73)	8.54 (3.26)	7.29 (1.98)	0.07
Switches	9.59 (3.73)	7.46 (3.20)	6.29 (1.98)	0.06

3.4 Discussion

These results support the findings that ALS patients demonstrate cognitive impairment localizing to both the frontal and temporal lobes, highlighting the frontotemporal neurocognitive phenotype of this disease (Lepow et al., 2010). ALS patients exhibited decreased phonemic and semantic fluency performances as compared to healthy non-neurologically impaired controls. Furthermore, in comparison to ALS patients whose cognition was intact, the subset of ALS patients with mild cognitive dysfunction or ALS-FTD demonstrated performance declines on standard measures of verbal fluency and the component processes of these measures. The component processes of verbal fluency provide a unique opportunity to further evaluate the ALS frontotemporal neurocognitive phenotype from slightly different perspective (Troyer et al., 1997). For phonemic fluency, the intact ALS sample generated fewer clusters and more switches than the ALS-mild and ALS-FTD patients, suggesting temporal involvement in ALS patients, with increasing frontal lobe involvement in patients with greater cognitive dysfunction. For semantic fluency, similar results were obtained with a greater emphasis on declines in clustering or increased temporal lobe dysfunction. These results suggest that verbal fluency measures identify frontal and temporal lobe involvement in the cognitive decline associated with ALS, particularly when the component processes are evaluated.

As a group, the ALS patients demonstrated temporal lobe involvement as compared to individuals without ALS. However, when the ALS patients were stratified based on their level of cognitive dysfunction, the influence of the frontal lobe involvement became more pertinent to their ability to perform this task. In conclusion, the differences in phonemic and semantic fluency scores between ALS patients and HCs suggest temporal lobe involvement in ALS patients with increasing frontal lobe involvement across the neurocognitive spectrum of the disease. A frontotemporal neurocognitive phenotype is revealed in ALS patients who demonstrate cognitive changes.

4. General discussion

Up until the late 1980s, the prevalent view in the neurological literature was that ALS was a pure motor neuron disease only infrequently affecting cognitive function. This view has changed in the last decade with several neuropsychological and functional imaging studies confirming common involvement of cortex outside the motor strip. The concept of primarily frontal lobe dysfunction in motor neuron disease was introduced by Montgomery and Erickson (1987) as well as Iwasaki et al. (1990). Several studies have since confirmed the association between FTLD, executive dysfunction, and ALS (eg. Massman et al., 1996; Strong et al., 2009). The largest study examining cognitive function in ALS to date found that 51% of patients had varying degrees of executive dysfunction (Ringholz et al., 2005; n = 279). These numbers confirmed an earlier study by Lomen-Hoerth and colleagues (2003) who had found evidence for frontal executive deficits in half of their patients, many of whom met criteria for Frontotemporal Lobar Degeneration.

Whereas frontal pathology has become the focus of cognitive investigation in ALS patients, the integrity of temporal structures (apart from the hippocampal formation) in ALS has not received much attention. Temporal pathology is a hallmark of FTLD, and several behavioral observations in ALS patients could suggest temporal pathology.

Several imaging studies and neuropathological investigations suggest that involvement of the temporal cortex, as well as the amygdala and other limbic structures in the disease process is very likely. Kew et al. (1993) showed reduced blood flow (rCBF) in the anterior cingulate cortex, the medial prefrontal cortex (Brodmann area 9 and 10), parahippocampal gyri and the anterior thalamic nuclear complex. Abrahams and colleagues (1995) observed decreased activity across a wide area of the frontal lobes, which also included the insular cortex and thalamic nuclear complex. In a small sample of clinically non-demented patients, there was a decrease in cerebral blood flow of the frontal and temporal lobes, despite normal MR imaging (Kokubo et al., 2003). Recently, a morphometric study of gray matter volume on MR scans revealed significant differences between patients with ALS and normal controls, predominantly in fronto-temporal areas, regardless of cognitive status; that is, the differences in gray matter volume between the ALS group as a whole and the control group were much more extensive than differences between cognitively normal and demented ALS patients (Chang et al., 2005).

There have been a limited number of neuropathological studies looking at frontal and temporal pathology in ALS. Wilson et al. (2001) found changes that where overall more pronounced for cognitively affected patients (ubiquitin positive, alpha-synuclein-negative, and tau-negative neuronal inclusions), most pronounced in the cingulate cortex. Cognitive impairment was uniformly associated with superficial linear spongiosis, a pathologic feature common to several forms of frontotemporal dementia. Wilson and colleagues did not study temporal structures in more detail. In a group of ALS patients with cognitive impairment, and decreased frontal blood flow on SPECT, neuropathologic examination showed spongy degeneration and neuronal loss in the frontal lobe (Abe et al., 1997).

Pathologically, there is also a special tie between semantic dementia, or temporal variant FTD, and ALS. Both FTD-MND (or FTD-ALS) and semantic dementia are characterized by ubiquinated inclusions (FTD-U); the clinical spectrum of patients seen with this histopathological finding varies from ALS, ALS with FTD and semantic dementia without ALS (Davies & Xuereb, 2007). This suggests that patients with ALS caused by this histopathological subtype would be expected to have overt or subtle features of temporal involvement, especially impairments in semantic processing and amygdala function.

Some studies have specifically evaluated the limbic system in sporadic ALS. In the ALS-Parkinson-dementia complex of Guam, tau and alpha-synuclein aggregates are a common finding in the amygdala (e.g., Yamazaki et al., 2000). Case series of sporadic ALS patients with and without dementia have demonstrated ubiquitinated intraneuronal inclusions and spongiform changes in the neostriatum, the amygdala and the parahippocampal gyrus, as well as the temporal pole, anterior cingulate, orbitofrontal cortex and insula (Kawashima et al., 2001; Kato et al., 1994, also Tsuchiya et al., 2002).

We assume that the cognitive findings of decreased semantic fluency and abnormal approachability are the clinical correlate of the changes seen neuroradiologically and neuropathologically and suggest that many ALS patients may, in fact, have both clinically relevant amygdala dysfunction and difficulties with semantic processing.

Performance on the Approachability Paradigm was not related to frontal dysfunction. A similar lack of correlation between amygdala dysfunction and frontal cognitive changes was reported by Zimmerman and colleagues (2007). In their study, among the 8 patients with emotional perceptual impairment, one-half did not have depressive, or memory or cognitive symptoms on screening, whereas the remainder showed dementia symptoms alone or together with depressive symptoms. This finding is important in two ways: First, it suggests the response pattern seen in ALS patients in both studies was in fact due to amygdala involvement as hypothesized and was less likely to be the result of frontal dysfunction

Second, FTLD is known to have several subtypes with variable sites of onset, all of which can be seen in conjunction with ALS. Thus, it is not surprising to find that amygdala dysfunction and frontal dysfunction are not associated. It may be that there are groups of ALS patients that have predominantly temporal dysfunction at onset, while other groups have predominantly frontal onset. This also suggests that more ALS patients have clinical involvement outside the motor strip than the rough estimate of 50% percent from prior studies, which mainly concentrated on frontal cognitive dysfunction.

5. Conclusion

We have shown that more than half of patients with ALS have unusual response patterns on a paradigm asking participants to judge the approachability of unfamiliar faces, suggesting amygdala dysfunction. Performance on this task did not correlate with frontal-executive dysfunction on cognitive testing. Patients also had significantly reduced semantic fluency suggesting involvement of the temporal cortex. Disease involvement outside the motor cortex in ALS is common, and can manifest as frontal, temporal or frontal and temporal dysfunction. Further studies need to be done to clarify the relationship between histopathological subtypes and cognitive patterns.

6. References

Abe K, Fujimura H, Toyooka K, Sakoda S, Yorifuji S & Yanagihara T. (1997) Cognitive function in amyotrophic lateral sclerosis. *J Neurol Sci.* 1997 May 1;148(1):95-100.

Abrahams S, Leigh PN, Kew JJ, Goldstein LH, Lloyd CM & Brooks DJ. (1995) A positron emission tomography study of frontal lobe function (verbal fluency) in amyotrophic lateral sclerosis. *J Neurol Sci.* 1995 May;129 Suppl:44-6.

Abrahams S, Leigh PN, Harvey A, Vythelingum GN, Grise D, Goldstein LH. (2000) Verbal fluency and executive dysfunction in amyotrophic lateral sclerosis (ALS). *Neuropsychologia* 2000;38:734-747.

Adolphs R (2003) Cognitive Neuroscience of Human Social Behavior. *Nature Reviews Neuroscience* 4: 165 – 178

Adolphs R (2003) Is the human amygdala specialized for processing social information? *Ann NY Acad. Sci.* 985: 326 – 340

Adolphs R, Baron-Cohen S & Tranel D (2002) Impaired Recognition of social emotions following amygdala damage. *Journal of Cognitive Neuroscience* 14: 1264 - 1274

Adolphs R, Tranel D & Damasio AR (1998) The human amygdala in social judgment. *Nature.* 1998 Jun 4;393(6684):470-4.

Adolphs R, Gosselin F, Buchanan TW, Tranel D, Schyns P & Damasio AR (2005). A mechanism for impaired fear recognition after amygdala damage. *Nature.* 2005 Jan 6;433(7021):68-72.

Baldo J., Schwartz S., Wilkins D., & Dronkers N. (2006). Role of frontal versus temporal cortex in verbal fluency as revealed by voxel-based lesion symptom mapping. *Journal of the International Neuropsychological Society, 12,* 896-900.

Bim, R. M., Kenworthy, L., Case, L., Caravella, R., Jones, T. B., Bandettini, P. A., et al. (2010). Neural systems supporting phonemic search guided by letter and semantic category cues; A self-paced overt response fMRI study of verbal fluency. *Neurolmage, 49,* 1099-1107. doi:10.1016/j.neuroimage.2009.07.036

Blair KS, Geraci M, Krelitz K, OteroM, Ernst M, Leibenluft E, Blair RJ & Pine DS (2011) The pathology of social phobia is independent of developmental changes in faces processing. *American Journal of Psychiatry* Jun 1 Epub ahead of print

Canning, S. J., Leach, L., Struss, D., Ngo, L., & Black, S. E. (2004). Diagnostic utility of abbreviated fluency measures in Alzheimer disease and vascular dementia. *Neurology, 62,* 556-562.

Chang JL, Lomen-Hoerth C, Murphy J, Henry RG, Kramer JH, Miller BL, Gorno-Tempini ML. (2005) A voxel-based morphometry study of patterns of brain atrophy in ALS and ALS/FTLD. *Neurology* 2005;65:75-8

Davies RR & Xuereb JH (2007) The histopathology of frontotemporal dementia *in* Hodges JR (ed.) *Frontotemporal Dementia Syndromes,* Cambridge University Press, Cambridge pp. 161 - 207

Fagundo, A. B., Lopez, S., Romero, M., Guarch, J., Marcos, T., &. Salamero, M. (2008). Clustering and switching in semantic fluency: Predictors of the development of Alzheimer's disease. *International Journal of Geriatric Psychiatry, 23,* 1007-1013.

Flaherty-Craig, C., Brothers, A., yang, C., Svoboda, R., Simmons, Z. (2011). Decreases in problem solving and anosognosia in amyotrophic lateral sclerosis: Applications of Guilford's structure of intellect theory. *Cogn Behav Neurol;* 24(1): 26-34.

Folstein M. F., Folstein S. E., & McHugh P. R. (1975). Mini-mental state: A practical method for grading the cognitive state of patients for the clinician. *Journal of Psychiatric Research. 12,* 189-198.

Frank B, Haas J, Heinze HJ, Stark E & Munte TF (1997) Relation of neuropsychological and magnetic resonance findings in amyotrophic lateral sclerosis: evidence for subgroups. *Clin Neurol Neurosurg*. 1997 May;99(2):79-86.

Freitas-Ferrari MC, Hallak JE, Trzesniak C, Filho AS. Machado-de-Sousa JP, Chagas MH, Nardi AE, Crippa JA (2010) Neuroimaging in social anxiety disorder: a systematic review of the literature. *Prog Neuropsychopharmacol Biol Psychiatry* 34(4):565-80

Hamann S & Mao H. (2002) Positive and negative emotional verbal stimuli elicit activity in the left amygdala. *Neuroreport*. 2002 Jan 21;13(1):15-9.

Hamann S (2001). Cognitive and neural mechanisms of emotional memory. *Trends Cogn Sci.* 2001 Sep 1;5(9):394-400

Hamann SB, Cahill L, McGaugh JL & Squire LR (1997) Intact enhancement of declarative memory for emotional material in amnesia. *Learn Mem.* 1997 Sep-Oct;4(3):301-9.

Hanagasi HA, Gurvit IH, Ermutlu N, Kaptanoglu G, Karamursel S, Idrisoglu HA, Emre M & Demiralp T (2002) Cognitive impairment in amyotrophic lateral sclerosis: evidence from neuropsychological investigation and event-related potentials. *Brain Res Cogn Brain Res.* 2002 Aug;14(2):234-44.

Iwasaki Y, Kinoshita M, Ikeda K, Takamiya K & Shiojima T. (1990) Neuropsychological dysfunctions in amyotrophic lateral sclerosis: relation to motor disabilities. *Int J Neurosci.* 1990 Oct;54(3-4):191-5.

Heaton, R. K. (1981). *Wisconsin Card Sorting Test manual.* Odessa, FL: Psychological Assessment Resources.

Hecht MJ, Graesel E, Tigges S, et al. (2003) Burden of care in amyotrophic lateral sclerosis. *Palliat Med* 2003;17:327-333.

Ho, A. K., Sahakian, B. J., Robbins, T. W., Barker, R. A., Rosser, A. E., & Hodges, J. R. (2002). Verbal fluency in Huntington's disease: A longitudinal analysis of phonemics and semantic clustering and switching. *Neuropsychologia, 40,*1277-1284.

Hodges JR, Davies RR, Xuereb JH, et al. (2004) Clinicopathological correlates in frontotemporal dementia. *Ann Neurol* 2004;56:399-406.

Kaplan, E., Goodglass, H., &. Weintraub, S. (1983). *The Boston Naming Test.* Philadelphia: Lea & Febiger.

Kato S, Oda M, Hayashi H, Kawata A & Shimizu T. (1994) Participation of the limbic system and its associated areas in the dementia of amyotrophic lateral sclerosis. *J Neurol Sci.* 1994 Oct;126(1):62-9

Kawashima T, Doh-ura K, Kikuchi H & Iwaki T (2001). Cognitive dysfunction in patients with amyotrophic lateral sclerosis is associated with spherical or crescent-shaped ubiquitinated intraneuronal inclusions in the parahippocampal gyrus and amygdala, but not in the neostriatum. *Acta Neuropathol (Berl).* 2001 Nov;102(5):467-72.

Kertesz A, McMonagle P, Blair M, Davidson W, Munoz DG. (2005) The evolution and pathology of frontotemporal dementia. *Brain* 2005;128:1996-2005.

Kew JJ, Goldstein LH, Leigh PN, Abrahams S, Cosgrave N, Passingham RE, Frackowiak RS & Brooks DJ. (1993) The relationship between abnormalities of cognitive function and cerebral activation in amyotrophic lateral sclerosis. A neuropsychological and positron emission tomography study. *Brain.* 1993 Dec;116 (Pt 6):1399-423.

Kilani M, Micallef J, Soubrouillard C, et al. (2004) A longitudinal study of the evolution of cognitive function and affective state in patients with amyotrophic lateral sclerosis. *Amyotroph Lateral Scler Other Motor Neuron Disord* 2004;5:46-54.

Kokubo Y & Kuzuhara S. (2003) Neuroradiological study of patients with amyotrophic lateral sclerosis and parkinsonism-dementia complex on the Kii peninsula of Japan. *Arch Neurol.* 2003 Sep;60(9):1257-61

Leggio, M. G., Silveri, M. C, Petrosini, L., & Molinari, M. (2000). Phonological grouping is specifically affected in cerebellar patients: A verbal fluency study. *Journal of Neurology, Neurosurgery & Psychiatry*, 69, 444-A41.

Lepow, L., Van Sweringen, J., Strutt, A., Jawaid, A., MacAdam, C., Harati, Y., Schulz, P., York, M. (2010). Frontal and temporal lobe involvement on verbal fluency measures in amyotrophic lateral sclerosis. *Jour of Clin and Exp Neuropsych*, 39(9), 913-933.

Lezak M. Neuropsychological Assessment. New York: Oxford University Press, 1995.

Libon, D. J., McMillan, C, Gunawardena, D., Powers, C, Massimo, L., Kahn, A., et al. (2009). Neurocognitive contributions to verbal fluency deficits in frontotemporal lobar degeneration. *Neurology, 73*, 535-542.

Lomen-Hoerth C, Murphy J, Langmore S, Kramer JH, Olney RK & Miller B. (2003) Are amyotrophic lateral sclerosis patients cognitively normal? *Neurology*. 2003 Apr 8;60(7):1094-7.

Loman-Hoerth C, Anderson T, Miller B. (2002) The overlap of amyotrophic lateral sclerosis and frontotemporal dementia. *Neurology* 2002;59:1077-1079.

Martin, A., Wiggs, C. L., Lalonde, F., & Mack, C. (1994). Word retrieval to letter and semantic cues; A double dissociation in normal subjects using interference tasks. *Neuropsychologia, 32*, 1487-1494.

Massman PJ, Sims J, Cooke N, Haverkamp LJ, Appel V & Appel SH. (1996) Prevalence and correlates of neuropsychological deficits in amyotrophic lateral sclerosis. *J Neurol Neurosurg Psychiatry*. 1996 Nov;61(5):450-5

Meinzer, M., Flaisch, T., Wilser, L., Eulitz, C, Karsten, E., Rockstroh, B., et al. (2009). Neural signatures of semantic and phonemic fluency in young and old adults. *Journal of Cognitive Neuroscience, 21*, 2007-2018.

Meyers, J. E., & Meyers, K. R. (1995). *Rey Complex Figure Test and Recognition Trial: Professional Manual*. Odessa, FL: Psychological Assessment Resources.

Montgomery GK & Erickson LM. (1987) Neuropsychological perspectives in amyotrophic lateral sclerosis. *Neurol Clin*. 1987 Feb;5(1):61-81.

Poloni M, Capitani E, Mazzini L & Ceroni M. (1986) Neuropsychological measures in amyotrophic lateral sclerosis and their relationship with CT scan-assessed cerebral atrophy. *Acta Neurol Scand*. 1986 Oct;74(4):257-60.

Murphy, V., Felgoise, S., Walsh, S., Simmons, Z. (2009). Problem solving skills predict quality of life and psychological morbidity in ALS caregivers. *Amyotroph Lateral Scler*; 10(3): 147-153.

Pihlajamki, M., Tanila, H., Hannien, T., Kononen, M., Laakso, M., Partanen, K., et al. (2000). Verbal fluency activates the left medial temporal lobe: A functional magnetic resonance imaging study. *Annals of Neurology, 47*, 470-476.

Phukan J, Pender NP, Hardiman O. Cognitive impairment in amyotrophic lateral sclerosis. (2007) *Lancet Neurol*. 2007 Nov;6(11):994-1003.

Ringholz, G. M., Appel, S. H., Bradshaw, M., Cooke, N. A., Mosnik, D. M., & Schulz, P. E. (2005). Prevalence and patterns of cognitive impairment in sporadic ALS. *Neurology, 65*, 586-590.

Rippon, G. A., Scarmeas, N., Gordon, P., Murphy, P., Albert, S., Mitsumoto, H., Marden, K., Rowland, L., Stern Y. (2006). An observational study of cognitive impairment in amyotrophic lateral sclerosis. Arch Neurol, 63(3); 345-352.

Schmidt M. Rey Auditory and Verbal Learning Test. A handbook. Los Angeles: Western Psychological Services, 1996.

Schmolck, H., Mosnik, D., & Schulz, P. (2007). Rating the approachability of faces in ALS. *Neurology, 69,* 2232-2235.

Schmolck H & Squire LR (2001) Impaired perception of facial emotions following bilateral damage to the anterior temporal lobe. *Neuropsychology.* 2001 Jan;15(1):30-8.

Stark R, Schienle A, Walter B, Kirsch P, Sammer G, Ott U, Blecker C &Vaitl D (2003) Hemodynamic responses to fear and disgust-inducing pictures: an fMRI study. *Int J Psychophysiol.* 2003 Nov;50(3):225-34.

Strong MJ, Grace GM, Orange JB, Leeper HA, Menon RS &Aere C (1999) A prospective study of cognitive impairment in ALS. *Neurology.* 1999 Nov 10;53(8):1665-70.

Strong, M. J., Grace, G. M., Orange, J. B., & Leeper, H. A. (1996). Cognition, language, and speech in amyotrophic lateral sclerosis: A review. *Journal of Clinical and Experimental Neuropsychology 18,* 291-303

Strong MJ, Grace GM, Freedman M, Lomen-Hoerth C, Woolley S, Goldstein LH, et al., (2009) Consensus Criteria for the diagnosis of frontotemporal cognitive and behavioral syndromes in ALS. *Amyotrophic Lateral Sclerosis* 10(3), 131-146

The Psychological Corporation. (1997). *WAIS-III WMS-III technical manual.* San Antonio, TX; The Psychological Corporation.

Troster AI, Fields JA, Testa JA, et al. (1998). Cortical and subcortical influences on clustering and switching in the performance of verbal fluency tasks. *Neuropsychologia.* 36: 295-304.

Troyer, A. K., Moscovitch, M., Winocur, G., Alexander, M. P., & Struss, D. (1998). Clustering and switching on verbal fluency: The effects of focal frontal- and temporal-lobe lesions. *Neuropsychologia, 36,* 499-50.

Troyer, A. K., Moscovitch, M., & Winocur, G. (1997). Clustering and switching as two components of verbal fluency: Evidence from younger and older healthy adults. *Neuropsychology, 11,* 138-146.

Tsuchiya K, Takahashi M, Shiotsu H, Akiyama H, Haga C, Watabiki S, Taki K, Nakano I & Ikeda K. (2002) Sporadic amyotrophic lateral sclerosis with circumscribed temporal atrophy: a report of an autopsy case without dementia and with ubiquitinated intraneuronal inclusions. *Neuropathology.* 2002 Dec;22(4):308-16.

Wheaton, M. W., Salamone, A. R., Mosnik, D. M., McDonald, R. O., Appel, S. H., Schmolck, H. I., et al. (2007). Cognitive impairment in familial ALS. *Neurology, 16,* 1411-1417

Wilson CM, Grace GM, Munoz DG, He BP& Strong MJ (2001) Cognitive impairment in sporadic ALS: a pathologic continuum underlying a multisystem disorder. *Neurology.* 2001 Aug 28;57(4):651-7.

Winston JS, Strange BA, O'Doherty J, Dolan RJ (2002). Automatic and intentional brain responses during evaluation of trustworthiness of faces. *Nature Neuroscience* 5: 277-283

Woolley, S.C. and Katz, J. S. (2008). Cognitive and behavioral impairment in amyotrophic lateral sclerosis. *Phys Med Rehabil Clin N Am,* 19(3); 607-617

Yamazaki M, Arai Y, Baba M, Iwatsubo T, Mori O, Katayama Y & Oyanagi K (2000) Alpha-synuclein inclusions in amygdala in the brains of patients with the parkinsonism-dementia complex of Guam. *J Neuropathol Exp Neurol.* 2000 Jul;59(7):585-91.

Zimmerman EK, Eslinger PJ, Simmons Z, Barrett AM (2007) Emotional perception deficits in amyotrophic lateral sclerosis. *Cognitive and Behavioral Neurology* 20:79-82